S0-BXE-656

Roger A. Côté, MD, FCAP • David J. Rothwell, MD, FCAP
James L. Palotay, DVM • Ronald S. Beckett, MD, FCAP • Louise Brochu

THE SYSTEMATIZED NOMENCLATURE OF HUMAN AND VETERINARY MEDICINE

SNOMED® INTERNATIONAL

Volume II – NUMERIC

Diseases / Diagnoses

Procedures

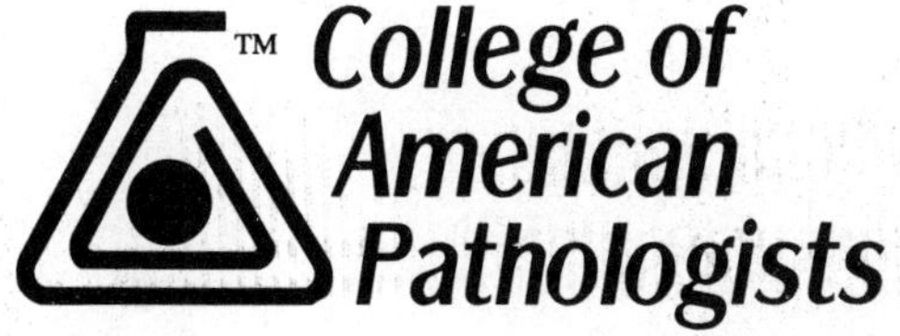

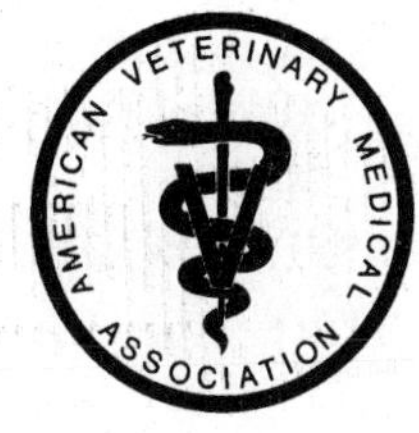

Volume I – Numeric

Topography (**T**)
Morphology (**M**)
Function (**F**)
Living Organisms (**L**)
Chemicals, Drugs, and Biological Products, including Pharmaceutical Manufacturers (**C**)
Physical Agents, Activities, and Forces (**A**)
Occupations (**J**)
Social Context (**S**)
General Linkage-Modifiers (**G**)

Volume II (of IV Volumes) – **Numeric**

Diseases/Diagnoses (**D**)
Procedures (**P**)

Volume III – Alphabetic

Topography (**T**)
Living Organisms (**L**)
Chemicals, Drugs, and Biological Products, including Pharmaceutical Manufacturers (**C**)
Physical Agents, Activities, and Forces (**A**)
Occupations (**J**)
Social Context (**S**)
General Linkage-Modifiers (**G**)

Volume IV – Alphabetic

Diseases/Diagnoses (**D**), including Morphology (**M**) and Function (**F**)
Procedures (**P**)

ISBN 0-930304-48–9
Library of Congress Number 77-154712

Electronic versions (ASCII) are available from:

College of American Pathologists
325 Waukegan Road
Northfield, IL 60093-2750
708/446-8800
708/446-8807 fax

or

American Veterinary Medical Association
1931 N. Meacham Road, Suite 100
Schaumburg, IL 60173-4360
708/925-8070
708/925-1329 fax

Published April 1993

 ***Printed on recycled paper***

Contents

SNOMED
INTERNATIONAL

EDITORS

Roger A.Côté , BA, MD, MS(Path), DSc(Hon), FCAP, FRCP(C), FACMI
Professor of Pathology and Director
Centre de Recherche en Diagnostic Médical Informatisé
Faculty of Medicine
Université de Sherbrooke
Sherbrooke, Quebec

David J. Rothwell, BS, MD, FCAP
Clinical Professor of Pathology
Medical College of Wisconsin
Columbia Hospital
Milwaukee, Wisconsin

Ronald S. Beckett, MD, FCAP
Department of Pathology
Hartford Hospital
Associate Professor of Pathology
University of Connecticut School of Medicine and Dentistry
Hartford, Connecticut

James L. Palotay, DVM, MS, ACVP(dipl)
Scientist (retired)
Oregon Regional Primate Research Center
Beaverton, Oregon

Associate Editor

Louise Brochu
Administrative Assistant
Centre de Recherche en Diagnostic Médical Informatisé
Faculty of Medicine
Université de Sherbrooke
Sherbrooke, Quebec

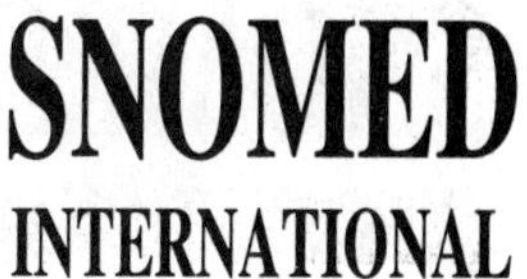

Foreword

Today, around the globe, health care faces terrifying realities. Crises in health care financing and access are compounded worldwide by the AIDS epidemic. Countries are struggling with their own demographic imperatives and new public health challenges like those posed by cigarette smoking in China, cholera in South America, and hepatitis B and C in the United States.

At the same time, there are exhilarating opportunities. Biomedical knowledge continues to grow at an incredible rate, and biotechnology offers new interventions. Computing and communications technologies provide health care professionals with powerful new tools for information handling, making a computer-based patient record 'from womb to tomb' an attainable goal.

Today this goal claims much of the energy and enthusiasm of medical and health informaticians worldwide. They are seizing the opportunities that the new technologies provide, sharing across disciplinary and national boundaries, and moving from theory into practice.

At this time and in this context, the work done by Doctors Roger Côté , David Rothwell, Ronald Beckett, and James Palotay, DVM, in this new 4-volume publication, SNOMED International, has enormous significance. The Systematized Nomenclature of Human and Veterinary Medicine (SNOMED) provides a detailed integrated and structured nomenclature for all aspects of diagnosis and treatment. This new edition represents almost 30 years of cogitation and testing since the original publication of the *Systematized Nomenclature of Pathology* in 1965.

Also available electronically in multiple formats, SNOMED International presents a multidimensional structure that contains the majority of the concepts, both simple and complex, needed to index all of human and veterinary medicine. SNOMED currently contains 130,580 records in 11 modules. For contrast, the Second Edition (1979) of SNOMED contained only 44,587 records. The new edition contains all of the International Classification of Diseases (ICD•9•CM) in the Diseases/Diagnoses module as well as all nursing diagnoses from the North American Nursing Diagnosis Association(NANDA) and a section on nursing procedures.

SNOMED International offers a predefined structured vocabulary, only a few years ago considered an "unobtainable goal". A comprehensive nomenclature, it can serve as the clinical nucleus for a Composite Clinical Data Dictionary (C^2D^2) and provide the infrastructure for computerizing the patient record. A major international effort, SNOMED is currently being translated into multiple languages to allow, for example, a coded patient summary in English to be transferred to Japan and decoded in Japanese.

I commend all of the many contributors to SNOMED International. As we work toward global health through informatics, standards and standard nomenclature will give us the foundation, the infrastructure, upon which our future health care delivery system will rest. The work contained in these volumes will take us well into the 21st century and lead the way to information when, where, and how (W^2H) we need it. I recommend it to you. We owe a debt of gratitude to those who have toiled so long and so hard to produce these pages.

Marion J. Ball, EdD
President
International Medical Informatics Association (IMIA)
January 9, 1993

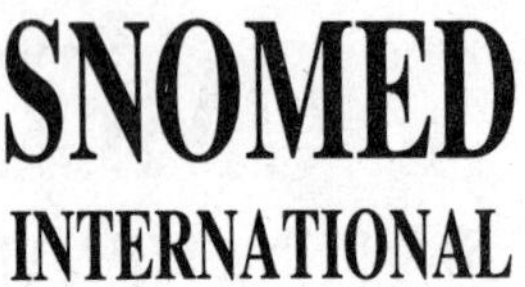

Introduction

SNOMED, the Systematized Nomenclature of Medicine, is a structured nomenclature and classification of the terminology used in human and veterinary medicine. This third edition – SNOMED International – is currently being translated by official representatives in nearly a dozen languages, hence its title. The current printed version is published in four volumes. An electronic version is available in multiple formats.

Terms are assigned to one of eleven independent systematized modules. Over the years numerous terms have been used to describe the different modules of SNOMED. Terms that have been used include axes, fields, dimensions, taxonomies, and thesauri. Each are equivalent terms and can be used interchangeably. For purpose of consistency in this new edition, the term MODULE will be used. Within each module, terms are placed into their natural hierarchies and are assigned a five- or six-digit alphanumeric code.

The code assignment places each term into a related family of medical terms providing context for each term. Codes carry within them a packet of information about the terms they designate. Codes used in this way are not simply a substitute for words – they provide contextual information for each term. This contextual information can be made explicit by any of several notations including frames, conceptual graphs, or other conventions. This feature of SNOMED, each term placed in its natural medical context, makes it particularly suitable for use in expert systems and decision analysis.

Terms may be linked to one another through the use of the G – General Linkage/Modifier module. In this way complex entities or manifestations of disease can be easily represented. These complex linked entities can in turn be decomposed into their elemental parts to whatever level of detail is desired, each represented by a SNOMED termcode. SNOMED International possesses many of the features needed for knowledge representation in medicine. It is, in fact, a data structure that is modular, open-ended and possesses a flexibility suitable for expressing simple and complex concepts and their relations in a highly structured semantically linked data model. It has features that we believe are necessary for a well grounded medical terminology that is capable of "packaging" concepts, i.e., information units into computer processable entities.

SNOMED International is an outgrowth of the second edition of SNOMED, first published in 1979. Its content has been both increased and expanded; eleven modules compared to seven, with the scope of each module expanded or modified. SNOMED International's general structure, however, remains similar in many respects to the second edition of SNOMED, except for the progression from a duodecimal to a hexadecimal system of notation. The hierarchies have been strengthened and often terms are cross-referenced to multiple dimensions establishing hierarchies creating what is, in effect, a series of linked polyhierarchies. Code assignments have changed in this edition; in the electronic version of SNOMED International each term carries a corresponding SNOMED II code so that for those who have established a database in SNOMED II and wish to do so, their database can be automatically transformed to the current version. An additional important feature of SNOMED International is the incorporation of virtually all of the ICD•9•CM terms and codes; most are found in the Diseases/Diagnoses module. It will be possible for users of SNOMED International to use this system as the primary tool for indexing their records and at the same time be provided the necessary ICD•9•CM codes required for reporting.

The relationship between a nomenclature and classification first expressed in the introduction to the second edition of SNOMED remains valid. In the example cited in the second edition, the disease Tuberculosis was given specificity by explicitly capturing the organ, alteration, causative agent, and functional disturbance of a typical patient.

Nomenclature								Classification
T	+	M	+	E	+	F	=	D
Lung	+	Granuloma	+	*M. Tuberculosis*	+	Fever	=	Tuberculous
T-28000	+	M-44060	+	E-2001	+	F-03003	=	D-0188

With these nomenclature and classification categories, any diagnostic level from a presenting problem, sign, or symptom to a complex final, clinical, or pathologic diagnosis can be appropriately and accurately coded for each patient. If a system such as this is used, it is no longer necessary to place patients into predefined categories of a statistical classification.

SNOMED International expands on this model by providing additional modules and categories of even greater specificity. In the new formulation a disease or diagnosis can be given specificity by linking some or all of the other modules and in turn linking these to the procedures that were used to establish that diagnosis.

From this vantage point, any medical encounter can be viewed as:

"a PROCEDURE performed on a SITE makes known a RESULT-FINDING"

To illustrate this model consider the following activities:

Auscultation (PROCEDURE) performed on a **chest** (SITE)
makes known a **murmur** (RESULT-FINDING)

X-ray examination (PROCEDURE) performed on **arm** (SITE)
makes known a **fracture** (RESULT-FINDING)

Electrophoresis (PROCEDURE) performed on **serum** (SITE)
makes known a **monoclonal protein associated with multiple myeloma** (RESULT-FINDING)

Virtually all of the information obtained from a medical encounter can be seen from this perspective. SNOMED International provides a comprehensive tabulation of procedures and anatomic site termcodes each in their separate modules, procedures, and topography. The result-finding terms are distributed across the remaining SNOMED modules, Morphology, Living Organisms, Chemicals-Drugs, Function, Disease, and Physical Agents. Each of these can in turn be linked to one another using the General Linkage/Modifier module. The SNOMED International model becomes:

{ (P) performed at (T) makes known (MLCFD) } G

Module designator	Number of characters in termcode	Number of Characters in term	Records
Topography (**T**)	5	120	12,385
Morphology (**M**)	5	120	4,991
Function (**F**)	5	120	16,352
Living Organisms (**L**)	5	120	24,273
Chemicals, Drugs, and Biological Products (**C**)	5	220	14,138
Physical Agents, Forces, and Activities (**A**)	5	120	1,355
Occupations (**J**)	5	120	1,886
Social Context (**S**)	5	120	433
Diseases/Diagnoses (**D**)	6	200	28,622
Procedures (**P**)	6	220	27,033
General Linkage-Modifiers (**G**)	4	80	1,173
TOTAL	(As of Apri 11, 1993)		132,641

SNOMED International currently contains eleven modules, each an independent taxonomy, representing the semantic categories necessary for describing and indexing virtually all of the events found in the medical record. A brief definition of each of the modules follows:

Topography (12,385 records)
Detailed anatomic terms used in human and veterinary medicine.

Morphology (4,991 records)
Terms used to describe structural changes in the body. It includes an exact replica of the tumor nomenclature found in the morphology section of the International Classification of Diseases for Oncology (ICD–0) 1990.

Function (16,352 records)
Contains terms used to describe both normal and abnormal functions of the body to include physiology and physiopathology with observations and diagnoses made by nursing personnel.

Living Organisms (24,265 records)
Unabridged classification of the animal and plant kingdoms. Included are essentially all of the pathogens and animal vectors of disease.

Chemicals, Drugs, and Biological Products (14,075 records)
A compilation of both generic and proprietary drugs each assigned to their respective class. A full listing of chemicals and plant products are also included.

A Physical Agents, Forces, and Activities (1,355 records)
A listing of those devices and activities commonly associated with disease and trauma.

J Occupations (1,886 records)
The International Labour Office's (ILO) list of occupations.

Social Context (433 records)
A formative listing of social conditions and relationships of importance in medicine.

Diseases / Diagnoses (28,622 records)
A detailed listing of the names of diseases and diagnostic entities encountered in human and veterinary medicine. Essentially all of the diagnostic terms found in the ICD-9-CM are assigned specific and individualized termcodes.

Procedures (27,033 records)
A comprehensive list of the administrative, therapeutic, and diagnostic procedures used by health care personnel. It encompasses all medical specialties.

General Linkage/Modifiers (1,176 records)
A set of linkages, descriptors, and qualifiers used to link or modify terms from each module.

A fuller characterization of structure and content is given in the introduction to each module.

SNOMED International is a detailed, fine grained, semantically typed, comprehensive, and computer-processable terminology used in both human and veterinary medicine. Terms are placed in a data structure in such a way that both simple and complex diagnostic entities and their manifestations can be represented. It will permit the composition of new terms from existing ones giving precise characterization to the new term. SNOMED International is a standardized vocabulary/data dictionary and data structure suitable for use in the computer-based patient record.

College of American Pathologists

325 Waukegan Road Northfield, Illinois 60093-2750 708-446-8800

January 9, 1993

On August 9, 1986, the CAP Board of Governors endorsed the need for a revised edition of the Systematized Nomenclature of Medicine (SNOMED). In order to keep pace with the rapid medical and paramedical changes that have occurred since the last editions of SNOMED and SNOVET appeared in 1979 and 1984, respectively, it was necessary to enhance the scope and capability of SNOMED if it is to remain useful and effective. Seven years later, and with nearly 80,000 added terms, the third edition of SNOMED – *SNOMED International: The Systematized Nomenclature for Human and Veterinary Medicine* – is the most comprehensive system available for managing medical information.

This four volume edition has been updated to reflect current medical knowledge and technology. Many of the changes are subtle, some are substantial. For example, the term Acquired Immune Deficiency Syndrome (AIDS) has been added, while the Etiology field has been expanded into three separate modules – Living Organisms, Chemicals & Drugs, and Physical Agents. A fourth new module – Social Context – has been added and a General Linkage/ Modifier module allows for linking or modifying terms found in each of the other modules.

Perhaps the greatest accomplishment of this monumental task was the cross-referencing of 28,600 terms to corresponding ICD•9•CM codes where applicable. The indexing capabilities are further enhanced by cross-references to the anatomic site, morphologic and functional changes, and etiologic agents.

The need for a unified medical language is a reality. *SNOMED International* is an efficient and effective method for integrating virtually all of the events, observations, and diagnoses found in the medical record into one format. With translations currently underway in ten other countries, *SNOMED International* can serve as our link for communicating and exchanging medical information with colleagues worldwide.

For this outstanding achievement, our appreciation and gratitude to the CAP SNOMED Editorial Board – Roger A. Coté, MD, David J. Rothwell, MD, Ronald S. Beckett, MD – and James Palotay, DVM, who represented the American Veterinary Medical Association and the American College of Veterinary Pathologists – and to the many consultants who contributed to this new edition. We welcome the support and input from all medical specialties as we continue to update and enhance *SNOMED International.*

Donald A. Senhauser, MD, FCAP

President

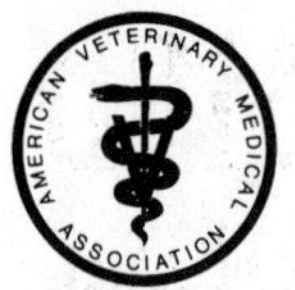

AMERICAN VETERINARY MEDICAL ASSOCIATION
1931 N. MEACHAM ROAD, SUITE 100 • SCHAUMBURG, ILLINOIS 60173-4360
PHONE 708-925-8070 FAX 708-925-1329

January 9, 1993

SNOMED International combines the standard nomenclature of human and veterinary medicine in a single, indexed reference system to enable a unified medical science to serve the health needs of all human and animal life. It reflects the interdependence of life and medicine, and it facilitates the sharing of information and data among the species. That sharing is essential to our learning and understanding more about the processes of health and disease in all species.

The publication of *SNOMED International* culminates a five-year task to assemble and index all of the nomenclature of medicine. This massive undertaking was achieved by the volunteer efforts of physicians and veterinarians who contributed to the work, and to the concentrated effort of four dedicated medical professionals who have devoted almost all of their time to pursue and fulfill their dream to produce a single, comprehensive reference to serve all of medicine. We of the medical professions owe a great deal of gratitude to the editors: Roger A. Côté, MD; David J. Rothwell, MD; James Palotay, DVM; and Ronald S. Beckett, MD for their achievement. We also owe our appreciation to Professor Doctor R .Wingert who, before his untimely death, contributed so much to the indexing theory.

SNOMED International is far more than an update of SNOMED and SNOVET. It uses the science of linguistics to produce a richer, more versatile indexing system for medical language that will provide a more utilitarian knowledge base for automated medical language-data processing.

In addition to its more sophisticated indexing system, *SNOMED International*'s nomenclature now includes terms that were omitted in prior editions of SNOMED and SNOVET as well as new terms that represent new knowledge in human and veterinary medicine since publication of the second edition of SNOMED in 1979 and the publication of SNOVET in 1984. It includes extensive cross-referencing among component axes and with the ICD•9•CM coding system that is widely used in processing medical insurance claims.

We encourage the use of the *SNOMED International* system for the storage of medical record data throughout the veterinary profession. The computer provides the tool to manage massive amounts of information. We can take advantage of that capability only if data is maintained in a common language. SNOMED International provides the ability to record all medical information in a common nomenclature system so it can be correlated and analyzed, regardless of its source.

L. Everett Macomber

L. Everett Macomber, DVM
President

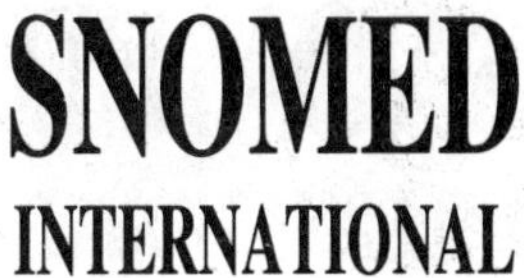

SNOMED
INTERNATIONAL

Consultants and Contributors

James Allen, PhD
Clinical Microbiologist
Columbia Hospital
Milwaukee, Wisconsin

Mr. Michel Boisvert
Informatique Hospitalière, Inc.
St-Bruno, Québec Canada

Thomas J. Bucci, DVM
Director of Pathology Service
National Center for Toxicologic Research
Jefferson, Arkansas

Robert W. Coffin, BA
Director, Data Processing
Oregon Regional Primate Research Center
Beaverton, Oregon

Mark G. Collett, DVM
Department of Pathology
Pretoria University
Faculty of Veterinary Science
Onderstepoort, South Africa

Mr. Jean-Pierre Cordeau, BEng
Department of Biomedical Engineering
Hôpital Sacré-Coeur
Montréal, Québec Canada

Ian R. Dohoo, DVM
Atlantic Veterinary College
University of Prince Edward Island
Charlottetown, Prince Edward Island Canada

Mr. George Dunham
National Institutes of Health
Bethesda, Maryland

Andrew Grant, MD
Department of Clinical Biochemistry
Faculty of Medicine - CHUS
Université de Sherbrooke
Sherbrooke, Québec Canada

Carl Jessen, DVM
College of Veterinary Medicine
University of Minnesota
St. Paul, Minnesota

Pavel Kasal, MD
Department of Medical Informatics
Medical Faculty of Charles University
Prague, Czechoslovakia

Michael Longval, MD
Department of Family Medicine
Faculty of Medicine
Université de Sherbrooke
Sherbrooke, Québec Canada

André Lussier, MD
Department of Rheumatology
Faculty of Medicine
Université de Sherbrooke
Sherbrooke, Québec Canada

James D. McKean, DVM
Ames, Iowa

Arthur McLay, MD
University Department of Pathology
Glasgow Royal Infirmary
Glasgow, Scotland

Frank J. Milne, DVM
Department of Clinical Studies
Ontario Veterinary College
University of Guelph
Guelph, Ontario Canada

Charles A. Montgomery, Jr., DVM
Director, Center for Comparative Medicine
Baylor College of Medicine
Houston, Texas

Roy V. H. Pollock, DVM
Smithkline Beecham Animal Health
Lincoln, Nebraska

Arnold Pratt, MD
Kensington, Maryland

James R. Prine, DVM
Stayton, Oregon

D. L. Proctor, DVM
Lexington, Kentucky

John Saidla, DVM
Cornell University
Ithaca, New York

C. Spencer Streett, DVM
International Research and Development Corporation
Mattawan, Michigan

Frank Stitt, MD
President - Medix Software Systems, Inc.
Key Biscayne, Florida

Richard Talbot, DVM, PhD
Virginia Polytechnic Institute and State University
Blacksburg, Virginia

Sister Gabrielle Tanguay, RN, HRA, MEdHSc
Regional House
Lewiston, Maine

David H. Taylor, DVM
Syracuse, New York

M. A. Thomas, DVM
College Station, Texas

Peter Toner, MD
Department of Pathology
Royal Victoria Hospital
Belfast, Northern Ireland

Walter E. Weirich, DVM
Purdue University
West Lafayette, Indiana

American Veterinary Medical Association
Committee on Standard Nomenclature and Coding

The members of this group constituted a true working committee formed from diverse interest areas within the profession. The Committee showed excellent judgment in electing Doctor Jacob Mosier as its chair. Doctor Arthur Tennyson of the AVMA staff contributed to the success of the committee by a systematic analysis of problems, establishment of priorities, and stimulation of productivity. The AVMA also provided financial and moral support by spearheading a long overdue challenge for uniformity of terminology, which will have a far reaching impact on the veterinary profession specifically and the medical community in general.

It has been through the foresight of the AVMA that funds were provided for the publication of this Systematized Nomenclature of Human and Veterinary Medicine and it will be through the support of the AVMA that progress will continue.

As is evident from the affiliations of the editors, this publication is a joint accomplishment epitomizing comparative medicine.

CHAIR

Jacob E. Mosier, DVM
College of Veterinary Medicine
Kansas State University
Manhattan, Kansas

MEMBERS

Farrel R. Robinson, DVM
Animal Disease Diagnostic Laboratory
Purdue University
West Lafayette, Indiana

Waldo F. Keller, DVM
College of Veterinary Medicine
Michigan State University
East Lansing, Michigan

Edwin I. Pilchard, DVM
USDA - APHIS
Hyattsville, Maryland

James L. Palotay, DVM
Oregon Regional Primate Research Center
Beaverton, Oregon

SNOMED
INTERNATIONAL

American College of Veterinary Pathologists
SNOVET Committee

Early in the development of this Systematized Nomenclature, the Council of the American College of Veterinary Pathologists recognized the value and the impact of a uniform method of information handling. It was through the ACVP's financial and moral support that the first and formative phases of this project were made possible. Through its foresight the need was recognized that this medical information system should not be just a veterinary pathology-based system but would well serve the entire veterinary community. As a consequence, it encouraged adoption of this system by the American Veterinary Medical Association.

CHAIR

James L. Palotay, DVM
Laboratory of Pathology
Oregon Regional Primate Research Center
Beaverton, Oregon

MEMBERS

Thomas J. Bucci, DVM
Director of Pathology Service
National Center for Toxicological Research
Jefferson, Arkansas

Alexander Cameron, DVM
McNeil Pharmaceutical
Spring House, Pennsylvania

B. J. Cooper, DVM
Department of Pathology
New York State College of Veterinary Medicine
Cornell University
Ithaca, New York

D.O. Cordes, DVM
Virginia-Maryland Regional College
of Veterinary Medicine
Virginia Polytechnic and State University
Blacksburg, Virginia

Garret S. Dill, DVM
Battelle Memorial Institute
Columbus Laboratories
Columbus, Ohio

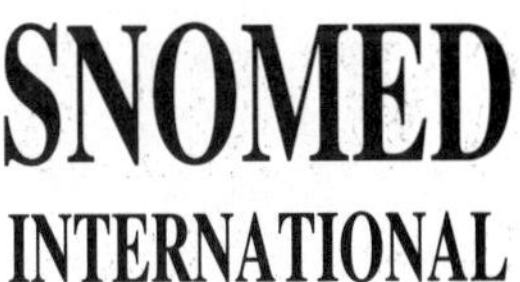

Acknowledgments

The compilation of source documents, the development of an expanded structure, and the editing and publishing of SNOMED International took about five years instead of the original plan of two years. The editors worked on the SNOMED project part time on a voluntary basis as do all of the College of American Pathologists' members. Their dedication to this effort is exemplary. Fortunately, Dr. Jim Palotay, representing the American Veterinary Medical Association and the American College of Veterinary Pathologists, retired from his position at the Oregon Primate Center and was able to devote the last few years to the compilation of the veterinary component of the nomenclature.

Doctor Ronald Beckett, whose involvement with medical nomenclatures dates back to the first SNOP edition, was in a semi-retired position at the Hartford Hospital and was able to compile much practical material for integration into the current SNOMED.

Doctor David Rothwell, although a busy practicing pathologist at Columbia Hospital in Milwaukee, has visited Sherbrooke regularly over the past several years to review material and work on the various aspects of SNOMED. Our FAX machines were humming daily with the exchange of documents. This modern technology was responsible for an open link between the editors and the College office.

Of course, our project would never have materialized without the vision and financial support of the College of American Pathologists. For this liaison we must acknowledge the continuous support of Mr. Gordon Briggs who personally and patiently guided all our requests through the College administration and was responsible for final typesetting and printing as well as the preparation of the electronic formats.

Here at Sherbrooke, thanks to a research project on the computerization of the medical diagnosis, I was relieved of most of my duties as a pathologist for the last three years to work on the completion of SNOMED International. For this enviable situation I must thank sincerely our Medical Faculty Dean, Dr. Michel Bureau.

In the preparation of the alphabetic indices and the alphabetic concordance lists, the Université de Sherbrooke made available to us the services of its computer center. The proximity of this facility saved us much precious time and I must thank Mr. Vaclav Richter and his staff members, Mr. Yves Ponton and Mr. Yves Delorme, who were always available on short notice to perform tasks better done on the larger computers and line printers.

Two other computer specialists, Mr. Michel Boisvert and Mr. Jean-Pierre Cordeau of the Biomedical Engineering Research Center of the Université de Montréal, worked with our team for two years in unravelling computer tapes of information and creating for us specialized look-up and encoding programs. These were most helpful for checking duplicates and for coding the references associated with diagnostic phrases. Their collaboration was indispensable.

Our job would have been impossible without our project administrative assistant, technical editor, computer data base specialist and associate, Ms. Louise Brochu. She had participated in the French translation of SNOMED II, had begun working on SNOMED International part-time, but became full-time about three years ago, supported by our research project. She maintains the data bank of the various thesauri, types in all the original material and follow-up changes, and prepares all the electronic material necessary for typesetting and publication. She has a pivotal role for the entire project. For constantly being available to us and for doing a remarkable job, I want to express our sincere gratitude.

Finally, we want to thank all the contributors, those listed and those forgotten, for sending us over the last three years information for the various thesauri. A special mention goes to Doctors Peter Toner and Arthur McLay for contributing the entire Topography section designed for the electron microscopist. Doctor Michael Longval made a significant contribution in the area of psychiatry and in organizing the drugs and enzymes. Their contributions added significantly to SNOMED International.

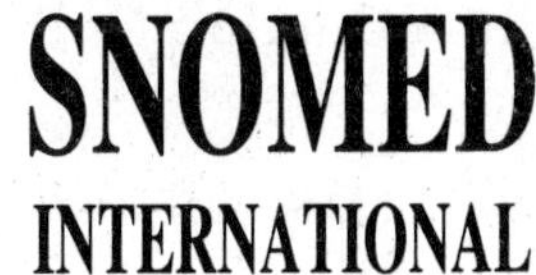

Diseases / Diagnoses

A classification of diseases

The Diseases / Diagnoses module represents a classification of the recognized clinical conditions encountered in human and veterinary medicine. Named diseases, diagnoses, and syndromes are placed within a family of related conditions and assigned to one or multiple categories producing both a monohierarchical and polyhierarchical classification of medical disorders.

Introduction to Diseases / Diagnoses

The Diseases / Diagnoses module is a compilation of disorders that include essentially all of the named diseases, diagnoses, and syndromes used in human and veterinary medicine. These disorders are placed into classes and are arranged either by organ systems or by their underlying etiology.

Ten of sixteen sections found in this module classify disorders in the organ system format that parallels the other SNOMED modules. The remaining six sections categorize disorders as either congenital; metabolic and nutritional; occurring in the pregnancy and perinatal period; injury and poisoning; infectious; or by victim status. Together they form a coherent classification of all the diseases, diagnoses, and syndromes encountered in medicine.

Each term is placed in a hierarchy of related terms, thus all gastrointestinal and all cardiovascular disorders are placed into their respective sections. This, however, does not commit these terms to a single hierarchy of disorders. For example, a gastrointestinal disorder such as Peutz Jaegher syndrome is a congenital disorder as well as a gastrointestinal disorder. This information can be captured using the cross reference feature of SNOMED. Cross references are in effect a mechanism for producing polyhierarchies specifying in detail what additional relationships are known about a disorder and placing terms in more than one hierarchy. Placement of terms into multiple hierarchies is a feature of particular importance for search and retrieval and is a powerful mechanism for knowledge representation.

The Disease/Diagnoses module represents a significant expansion beyond that found in the previous editions of SNOMED. In this edition an attempt has been made to enter all of the diagnostic terminology used in medicine into this one module. For those who wish to do so, this Diseases / Diagnoses module could serve as a single monoaxial index of clinical disease. If this is done however, much of the richness and depth of SNOMED will be lost. Each entry in the Disease/Diagnoses module can be represented by a lesion or change at some site in the body that may have an infectious etiology, be treated with a drug, or exhibit some physiology or biochemical abnormality manifested by a variety of signs and symptoms. All of this information is found in the other SNOMED modules that are complementary to this one. This, in essence, is the distinction between a nomenclature and a classification of disease. The nomens are found in the Topography, Morphology, Living Organisms, Chemicals, Drugs and Biological Products, and Function modules of SNOMED, while disease classes are found in the Disease/Diagnoses module.

This is an additional strength of SNOMED in that it can be used as a statistical classification grouping diseases into classes to fulfill a variety of needs at the institutional and national levels, and, in addition, provide the detailed information about each individual patient or group of patients with a given disorder.

The International Classification of Diseases, ninth edition (ICD–9) and its clinical modification (ICD–9–CM) are statistical classifications of disease used to record the incidence of disease classes. Five-digit codes are used to represent disorders. A single five-digit code may represent a single disorder or, more often, multiple closely related disorders. In this edition of SNOMED, essentially all of the disorders listed in the ICD–9–CM have been isolated, individually listed, and each assigned a specific SNOMED termcode. Most of these are found in the Diseases/Diagnoses module, others are found in the Morphology and Function modules. This provides a 'one-to-one' or 'one-to-many' correspondence between this edition of SNOMED and the ICD–9–CM. It will be possible to index and code using SNOMED, taking advantage of its strengths, while at the same time have available the corresponding ICD–9–CM codes for reporting purposes.

There is an exception, however. Chapter two of ICD–9–CM is devoted to neoplasms; it is not present in SNOMED. In its place, the more specific and highly detailed International Classification of Diseases for Oncology (ICD–O, 1990) is used as the tumor nomenclature. This is found in the SNOMED Morphology module, sections 8 and 9. A translation table between ICD–O Morphology and Chapter Two of ICD–9–CM could be produced if there is an absolute need to do so.

The Diseases/Diagnoses module of SNOMED allows the user to index recognized clinical entities as a coded representation that places that entity into a hierarchy of related entities. The related entities are implicit in the coded representation. By using the cross reference feature of SNOMED, these same entities can be placed in other hierarchies and, in addition, other relationships can be identified and made explicit by this same mechanism.

These same clinical entities can be further defined by using the other SNOMED modules to specify the site, the change, the physiologic alteration, and the signs and symptoms that may be present. SNOMED International offers to the user a single indexing system and a flexible data structure ideally suited for the computerized medical record.

CHAPTER 0 — DISEASES OF THE SKIN AND SUBCUTANEOUS TISSUES

SECTION 0-0 DISEASES OF THE SKIN AND SUBCUTANEOUS TISSUES: GENERAL TERMS, HISTOLOGIC TYPES AND INFECTIONS

0-00 DISEASES OF THE SKIN AND SUBCUTANEOUS TISSUES: GENERAL TERMS AND HISTOLOGIC TYPES

0-000 Diseases of The Skin and Subcutaneous Tissues: General Terms

D0-00000 Disease of skin and subcutaneous tissue, NOS 709.9
(T-01000) (T-03000) (DF-00000)
Dermatosis, NOS 709.9
(T-01000) (T-03000) (DF-00000)

D0-00010 Dermatitis, NOS 692.-
(T-01000) (M-40000)

D0-00012 Acute dermatitis, NOS 692.-
(T-01000) (M-41000)

D0-00014 Subacute dermatitis, NOS 692.-
(T-01000) (M-42000)

D0-00016 Chronic dermatitis, NOS 692.-
(T-01000) (M-43000)

D0-00020 Induration of skin
(T-01000) (M-02712)

D0-00026 Thickening of skin
(T-01000) (M-02610)

D0-00080 Other specified disorder of skin, NEC 709.8
(T-01000) (DF-00000)

0-005 Histologic Types of Inflammatory Skin Disorders

D0-00500 Superficial perivascular dermatitis, NOS
(T-01000)

D0-00501 Interface dermatitis, NOS
(T-01000) (M-40000)

D0-00502 Interface dermatitis, vacuolar type
(T-01000) (M-40000)

D0-00503 Interface dermatitis, lichenoid type
(T-01000) (M-40000)

D0-00505 Spongiotic dermatitis
(T-01000) (M-40000)

D0-00506 Psoriasiform dermatitis
(T-01000) (M-40000)

D0-00507 Spongiotic psoriasiform dermatitis
(T-01000) (M-40000)

D0-00510 Superficial and deep perivascular dermatitis, NOS
(T-01000) (M-40000)

D0-00520 Vasculitis of the skin, NOS
(T-01000) (M-40000)

D0-00522 Neutrophilic vasculitis of skin
(T-01000) (M-40000)

D0-00524 Lymphocytic vasculitis of skin
(T-01000) (M-40000)

D0-00526 Histiocytic vasculitis of skin
(T-01000) (M-40000)
Granulomatous vasculitis of skin
(T-01000) (M-40000)

D0-00528 Small vessel thrombosis of skin
(T-01000) (M-40000)

D0-00530 Nodular and diffuse dermatitis, NOS
(T-01000) (M-40000)

D0-00532 Nodular dermatitis
(T-01000)

D0-00534 Diffuse dermatitis
(T-01000)

D0-00540 Intraepidermal vesicular and pustular dermatitis, NOS
(T-01000)

D0-00541 Spongiotic vesicular dermatitis
(T-01000)

D0-00542 Ballooning vesicular dermatitis
(T-01000)

D0-00543 Acantholytic vesicular dermatitis
(T-01000)

D0-00544 Intragranular vesicular dermatitis
(T-01000)

D0-00545 Intrabasal vesicular dermatitis
(T-01000)

D0-00546 Intraepidermal vesiculopustular dermatitis
(T-01000)

D0-00547 Intraepidermal pustular dermatitis
(T-01000)

D0-00550 Subepidermal vesicular dermatitis
(T-01000)

D0-00560 Folliculitis and perifolliculitis, NOS
(T-01000)

D0-00562 Perifolliculitis
(T-01000)

D0-00564 Folliculitis 704.8
(T-01000)

D0-00570 Fibrosing dermatitis, NOS 709.2
(T-01000) (M-78000)

D0-00572 Fibrosis of the skin 709.2
(T-01000) (M-78000)

D0-00574 Sclerosis of the skin
(T-01000)

D0-00576 Fibrohistiolytic proliferation of the skin
(T-01000)

D0-00580 Panniculitis, NOS 729.30
(T-03000) (M-40000)

D0-00582 Septal panniculitis 729.30
(T-03000) (M-40000)

D0-00584 Lobular panniculitis 729.30
(T-03000) (M-40000)

D0-00590 Panniculitis affecting neck 723.6

D0-00592 Panniculitis affecting back 724.8

D0-00594 Panniculitis affecting sacrum 724.8

0-01 INFECTIONS OF THE SKIN AND SUBCUTANEOUS TISSUES

D0-01000 Infection of skin and subcutaneous tissue, NOS 686.9
(T-01000) (T-03000) (M-40000)

0-011 Carbuncles and Furuncles

D0-01100 Carbuncle of skin and subcutaneous tissue, NOS 680.9
(T-01000) (T-03000) (M-41730)

D0-01101 Carbuncle of face, NOS 680.0
(T-01000) (T-03000) (T-D1200) (M-41730)

D0-01102 Carbuncle of ear 680.0
(T-01000) (T-03000) (T-AB000) (M-41730)

D0-01103 Carbuncle of nose 680.0
(T-01000) (T-03000) (T-21000) (M-41730)

D0-01104 Carbuncle of nasal septum 680.0
(T-01000) (T-03000) (T-21340) (M-41730)

D0-01105 Carbuncle of temple region 680.0
(T-01000) (T-03000) (T-D1150) (M-41730)

D0-01106 Carbuncle of neck 680.1
(T-01000) (T-03000) (T-D1600) (M-41730)

D0-01107 Carbuncle of trunk 680.2
(T-01000) (T-03000) (T-D2000) (M-41730)

D0-01108 Carbuncle of abdominal wall 680.2
(T-01000) (T-03000) (T-D4300) (M-41730)

D0-01109 Carbuncle of back, except buttock 680.2
(T-01000) (T-03000) (T-D2100) (M-41730)

D0-01110 Carbuncle of breast 680.2
(T-01000) (T-03000) (T-04000) (M-41730)

D0-01111 Carbuncle of chest wall 680.2
(T-01000) (T-03000) (T-D3050) (M-41730)

D0-01112 Carbuncle of flank 680.2
(T-01000) (T-03000) (T-D2310) (M-41730)

D0-01113 Carbuncle of pectoral region 680.2
(T-01000) (T-03000) (T-D2235) (M-41730)

D0-01114 Carbuncle of perineum 680.2
(T-01000) (T-03000) (T-D2700) (M-41730)

D0-01115 Carbuncle of umbilicus 680.2
(T-01000) (T-03000) (T-D4220) (M-41730)

D0-01116 Carbuncle of upper arm 680.3
(T-01000) (T-03000) (T-D8200) (M-41730)

D0-01117 Carbuncle of forearm 680.3
(T-01000) (T-03000) (T-D8500) (M-41730)

D0-01118 Carbuncle of axilla 680.3
(T-01000) (T-03000) (T-D8100) (M-41730)

D0-01119 Carbuncle of shoulder 680.3
(T-01000) (T-03000) (T-D2220) (M-41730)

D0-01121 Carbuncle of hand, NOS 680.4
(T-01000) (T-03000) (T-D8700) (M-41730)

D0-01122 Carbuncle of finger, NOS 680.4
(T-01000) (T-03000) (T-D8800) (M-41730)

D0-01123 Carbuncle of thumb 680.4
(T-01000) (T-03000) (T-D8810) (M-41730)

D0-01124 Carbuncle of wrist 680.4
(T-01000) (T-03000) (T-D8600) (M-41730)

D0-01125 Carbuncle of buttock 680.5
(T-01000) (T-03000) (T-D2600) (M-41730)
Carbuncle of gluteal region 680.5
(T-01000) (T-03000) (T-D2600) (M-41730)

D0-01127 Carbuncle of anus 680.5
(T-01000) (T-03000) (T-59900) (M-41730)

D0-01128 Carbuncle of leg, NOS, except foot 680.6
(T-01000) (T-03000) (T-D9400) (M-41730)

D0-01129 Carbuncle of hip 680.6
(T-01000) (T-03000) (T-D2500) (M-41730)

D0-01131 Carbuncle of thigh 680.6
(T-01000) (T-03000) (T-D9100) (M-41730)

D0-01132 Carbuncle of knee 680.6
(T-01000) (T-03000) (T-D9200) (M-41730)

D0-01133 Carbuncle of ankle 680.6
(T-01000) (T-03000) (T-D9500) (M-41730)

D0-01134 Carbuncle of foot 680.7
(T-01000) (T-03000) (T-D9700) (M-41730)

D0-01135 Carbuncle of heel 680.7
(T-01000) (T-03000) (T-D9600) (M-41730)

D0-01136 Carbuncle of toe 680.7
(T-01000) (T-03000) (T-D9800) (M-41730)

D0-01137 Carbuncle of head, except face 680.8
(T-01000) (T-03000) (T-D1100) (M-41730)

D0-01138 Carbuncle of scalp 680.8
(T-01000) (T-03000) (T-D1160)
(M-41730)

D0-01139 Carbuncle of groin 680.2
(T-01000) (T-03000) (T-D7000)
(M-41730)

D0-01140 Carbuncle of other specified site 680.8
(T-01000) (T-03000) (T-.....) (M-41730)

D0-01150 Furuncle of skin and subcutaneous tissue, NOS 680.9
(T-01000) (T-03000) (M-41710)
Boil of skin and subcutaneous tissue, NOS 680.9
(T-01000) (T-03000) (M-41710)

D0-01151 Furuncle of face, NOS 680.0
(T-01000) (T-03000) (T-D1200)
(M-41710)

D0-01152 Furuncle of ear 680.0
(T-01000) (T-03000) (T-AB000)
(M-41710)

D0-01153 Furuncle of nose 680.0
(T-01000) (T-03000) (T-21000)
(M-41710)

D0-01154 Furuncle of nasal septum 680.0
(T-01000) (T-03000) (T-21340)
(M-41710)

D0-01155 Furuncle of temple region 680.0
(T-01000) (T-03000) (T-D1150)
(M-41710)

D0-01156 Furuncle of neck 680.1
(T-01000) (T-03000) (T-D1600)
(M-41710)

D0-01157 Furuncle of trunk 680.2
(T-01000) (T-03000) (T-D2000)
(M-41710)

D0-01158 Furuncle of abdominal wall 680.2
(T-01000) (T-03000) (T-D4300)
(M-41710)

D0-01159 Furuncle of back, except buttock 680.2
(T-01000) (T-03000) (T-D2100)
(M-41710)

D0-0115AV Saddle boil
(T-01000) (T-03000) (T-D2100)
(M-41710)

D0-01160 Furuncle of breast 680.2
(T-01000) (T-03000) (T-04000)
(M-41710)

D0-01161 Furuncle of chest wall 680.2
(T-01000) (T-03000) (T-D3050)
(M-41710)

D0-01162 Furuncle of flank 680.2
(T-01000) (T-03000) (T-D2310)
(M-41710)

D0-01163 Furuncle of groin 680.2
(T-01000) (T-03000) (T-D7000)
(M-41710)

D0-01164 Furuncle of pectoral region 680.2
(T-01000) (T-03000) (T-D2235)
(M-41710)

D0-01165 Furuncle of perineum 680.2
(T-01000) (T-03000) (T-D2700)
(M-41710)

D0-01166 Furuncle of umbilicus 680.2
(T-01000) (T-03000) (T-D4220)
(M-41710)

D0-01167 Furuncle of upper arm 680.3
(T-01000) (T-03000) (T-D8200)
(M-41710)

D0-01168 Furuncle of forearm 680.3
(T-01000) (T-03000) (T-D8500)
(M-41710)

D0-01169 Furuncle of axilla 680.3
(T-01000) (T-03000) (T-D8100)
(M-41710)

D0-01171 Furuncle of shoulder 680.3
(T-01000) (T-03000) (T-D2220)
(M-41710)

D0-01172 Furuncle of hand, NOS 680.4
(T-01000) (T-03000) (T-D8700)
(M-41710)

D0-01173 Furuncle of finger, NOS 680.4
(T-01000) (T-03000) (T-D8800)
(M-41710)

D0-01174 Furuncle of thumb 680.4
(T-01000) (T-03000) (T-D8810)
(M-41710)

D0-01175 Furuncle of wrist 680.4
(T-01000) (T-03000) (T-D8600)
(M-41710)

D0-01176 Furuncle of buttock 680.5
(T-01000) (T-03000) (T-D2600)
(M-41710)
Furuncle of gluteal region 680.5
(T-01000) (T-03000) (T-D2600)
(M-41710)

D0-01178 Furuncle of anus 680.5
(T-01000) (T-03000) (T-59900)
(M-41710)

D0-01179 Furuncle of leg, NOS, except foot 680.6
(T-01000) (T-03000) (T-D9400)
(M-41710)

D0-01181 Furuncle of hip 680.6
(T-01000) (T-03000) (T-D2500)
(M-41710)

D0-01182 Furuncle of thigh 680.6
(T-01000) (T-03000) (T-D9100)
(M-41710)

D0-01183 Furuncle of knee 680.6
(T-01000) (T-03000) (T-D9200)
(M-41710)

D0-01184 Furuncle of ankle 680.6
(T-01000) (T-03000) (T-D9500)
(T-41710)

D0-01185 Furuncle of foot 680.7
(T-01000) (T-03000) (T-D9700)
(M-41710)

0-011 Carbuncles and Furuncles — Continued

D0-01186 Furuncle of heel 680.7
(T-01000) (T-03000) (T-D9600) (M-41710)

D0-01187 Furuncle of toe 680.7
(T-01000) (T-03000) (T-D9800) (M-41710)

D0-01188 Furuncle of head, except face 680.8
(T-01000) (T-03000) (T-D1100) (M-41710)

D0-01189 Furuncle of scalp 680.8
(T-01000) (T-03000) (T-D1160) (M-41710)

D0-01190 Furuncle of other specified site 680.8
(T-01000) (T-03000) (T-.....) (M-41710)

D0-01198 Furunculosis of skin and subcutaneous tissue, NOS 680.9
(T-01000) (T-03000) (M-41718)

0-012 Skin Abscesses

D0-01200 Abscess of skin and subcutaneous tissue, NOS 682.9
(T-03000) (M-41610)

D0-01201 Abscess of digit, NOS 681.9
(T-03000) (T-D2810) (M-41610)

D0-01202 Abscess of finger, NOS 681.00
(T-03000) (T-D8800) (M-41610)

D0-01204 Pulp abscess of finger, NOS 681.01
(T-03000) (T-D8802) (M-41610)
Felon 681.01
(T-03000) (T-D8802) (M-41610)
Whitlow 681.01
(T-03000) (T-D8802) (M-41610)

D0-01210 Abscess of toe, NOS 681.10
(T-03000) (T-D9800) (M-41610)

D0-01220 Abscess of face 682.0
(T-03000) (T-D1200) (M-41610)
Acute abscess of face 682.0
(T-03000) (T-D1200) (M-41610)

D0-01221 Abscess of external cheek 682.0
(T-03000) (T-D1206) (M-41610)

D0-01222 Abscess of chin 682.0
(T-03000) (T-D1210) (M-41610)

D0-01223 Abscess of forehead 682.0
(T-03000) (T-D1110) (M-41610)

D0-01224 Abscess of external nose 682.0
(T-03000) (T-21100) (M-41610)

D0-01225 Abscess of submandibular region 682.0
(T-03000) (T-D1603) (M-41610)

D0-01226 Abscess of temple region 682.0
(T-03000) (T-D1150) (M-41610)

D0-01227 Abscess of neck 682.1
(T-03000) (T-D1600) (M-41610)

D0-01228 Abscess of trunk, NOS 682.2
(T-03000) (T-D2000) (M-41610)

D0-01231 Abscess of abdominal wall 682.2
(T-03000) (T-D4300) (M-41610)

D0-01232 Abscess of back, except buttock 682.2
(T-03000) (T-D2100) (M-41610)

D0-01233 Abscess of chest wall 682.2
(T-03000) (T-D3050) (M-41610)

D0-01234 Abscess of flank 682.2
(T-03000) (T-D2310) (M-41610)

D0-01235 Abscess of groin 682.2
(T-03000) (T-D7000) (M-41610)

D0-01236 Abscess of pectoral region 682.2
(T-03000) (T-D2235) (M-41610)

D0-01237 Abscess of perineum 682.2
(T-03000) (T-D2700) (M-41610)

D0-01238 Abscess of umbilicus 682.2
(T-03000) (T-D4220) (M-41610)

D0-01241 Abscess of upper arm 682.3
(T-03000) (T-D8200) (M-41610)

D0-01242 Abscess of forearm 682.3
(T-03000) (T-D8500) (M-41610)

D0-01243 Abscess of axilla 682.3
(T-03000) (T-D8100) (M-41610)

D0-01244 Abscess of shoulder 682.3
(T-03000) (T-D2220) (M-41610)

D0-01245 Abscess of hand 682.4
(T-03000) (T-D8700) (M-41610)

D0-01246 Abscess of wrist 682.4
(T-03000) (T-D8600) (M-41610)

D0-01251 Abscess of buttock 682.5
(T-03000) (T-D2600) (M-41610)
Abscess of gluteal region 682.5
(T-03000) (T-D2600) (M-41610)

D0-01261 Abscess of leg, NOS, except foot 682.6
(T-03000) (T-D9400) (M-41610)

D0-01262 Abscess of hip 682.6
(T-03000) (T-D2500) (M-41610)

D0-01263 Abscess of thigh 682.6
(T-03000) (T-D9100) (M-41610)

D0-01264 Abscess of knee 682.6
(T-03000) (T-D9200) (M-41610)

D0-01265 Abscess of ankle 682.6
(T-03000) (T-D9500) (M-41610)

D0-01266 Abscess of foot, except toe 682.7
(T-03000) (T-D9700) (M-41610)

D0-01267 Abscess of heel 682.7
(T-03000) (T-D9600) (M-41610)

D0-01271 Abscess of head, except face 682.8
(T-03000) (T-D1100) (M-41610)

D0-01272 Abscess of scalp 682.8
(T-03000) (T-D1160) (M-41610)

D0-01280 Abscess of other specified subcutaneous tissue site 682.8
(T-03000) (T-.....) (M-41610)

D0-01290 Abscess of skin with lymphangitis, NOS
(T-03000) (M-41610) (T-C6010) (M-41000)

D0-01292 Abscess of skin with lymphangitis of digit, NOS 681.9
(T-03000) (M-41610) (T-C6010) (T-D2810) (M-41000)

0-013-014 Cellulitis and Lymphangitis of The Skin

D0-01305 Cellulitis of digit, NOS 681.9
(T-03000) (T-D2810) (M-41650)

D0-01310 Cellulitis of finger, NOS 681.00
(T-03000) (T-D8800) (M-41650)

D0-01311 Onychia of finger 681.02
(T-01607) (T-D8800) (M-41650)
Paronychia of finger 681.02
(T-01607) (T-D8800) (M-41650)
Perionychia of finger 681.02
(T-01607) (T-D8800) (M-41650)
Panaritium of finger 681.02
(T-01607) (T-D8800) (M-41650)

D0-01320 Cellulitis of toe, NOS 681.10
(T-03000) (T-D9800) (M-41650)

D0-01321 Onychia of toe 681.11
(T-01607) (T-D9800) (M-41650)
Paronychia of toe 681.11
(T-01607) (T-D9800) (M-41650)
Perionychia of toe 681.11
(T-01607) (T-D9800) (T-41650)
Panaritium of toe 681.11
(T-01607) (T-D9800) (M-41650)

D0-01322 Cellulitis of face 682.0
(T-03000) (T-D1200) (M-41650)
Diffuse cellulitis of face 682.0
(T-03000) (T-D1200) (M-41650)

D0-01324 Cellulitis of external cheek 682.0
(T-03000) (T-D1206) (M-41650)

D0-01325 Cellulitis of chin 682.0
(T-03000) (T-D1210) (M-41650)

D0-01326 Cellulitis of forehead 682.0
(T-03000) (T-D1110) (M-41650)

D0-01327 Cellulitis of external nose 682.0
(T-03000) (T-21100) (M-41650)

D0-01328 Cellulitis of submandibular region 682.0
(T-03000) (T-D1603) (M-41650)

D0-01329 Cellulitis of temple region 682.0
(T-03000) (T-D1150) (M-41650)

D0-01330 Cellulitis of neck 682.1
(T-03000) (T-D1600) (M-41650)

D0-01332 Cellulitis of trunk, NOS 682.2
(T-03000) (T-D2000) (M-41650)

D0-01334 Cellulitis of abdominal wall 682.2
(T-03000) (T-D4300) (M-41650)

D0-01336 Cellulitis of back, except buttock 682.2
(T-03000) (T-D2100) (M-41650)

D0-01337 Cellulitis of chest wall 682.2
(T-03000) (T-D3050) (M-41650)

D0-01338 Cellulitis of flank 682.2
(T-03000) (T-D2310) (M-41650)

D0-01339 Cellulitis of groin 682.2
(T-03000) (T-D7000) (M-41650)

D0-01341 Cellulitis of pectoral region 682.2
(T-03000) (T-D2235) (M-41650)

D0-01342 Cellulitis of perineum 682.2
(T-03000) (T-D2700) (M-41650)

D0-01343 Cellulitis of umbilicus 682.2
(T-03000) (T-D4220) (M-41650)

D0-01350 Cellulitis of upper arm 682.3
(T-03000) (T-D8200) (M-41650)

D0-01351 Cellulitis of forearm 682.3
(T-03000) (T-D8500) (M-41650)

D0-01352 Cellulitis of axilla 682.3
(T-03000) (T-D8100) (M-41650)

D0-01353 Cellulitis of shoulder 682.3
(T-03000) (T-D2220) (M-41650)

D0-01354 Cellulitis of hand 682.4
(T-03000) (T-D8700) (M-41650)

D0-01355 Cellulitis of wrist 682.4
(T-03000) (T-D8600) (M-41650)

D0-01358 Cellulitis of buttock 682.5
(T-03000) (T-D2600) (M-41650)
Cellulitis of gluteal region 682.5
(T-03000) (T-D2600) (M-41650)

D0-01360 Cellulitis of leg, NOS, except foot 682.6
(T-03000) (T-D9400) (M-41650)

D0-01361 Cellulitis of hip 682.6
(T-03000) (T-D2500) (M-41650)

D0-01362 Cellulitis of thigh 682.6
(T-03000) (T-D9100) (M-41650)

D0-01363 Cellulitis of knee 682.6
(T-03000) (T-D9200) (M-41650)

D0-01364 Cellulitis of ankle 682.6
(T-03000) (T-D9500) (M-41650)

D0-01365 Cellulitis of foot, except toe 682.7
(T-03000) (T-D9700) (M-41650)

D0-01366 Cellulitis of heel 682.7
(T-03000) (T-D9600) (M-41650)

D0-01367 Cellulitis of head, except face 682.8
(T-03000) (T-D1100) (M-41650)

D0-01368 Cellulitis of scalp 682.8
(T-03000) (T-D1160) (M-41650)

D0-01369 Cellulitis of other specified site 682.8
(T-03000) (T-.....) (M-41650)

D0-01370 Cellulitis of skin with lymphangitis, NOS
(T-03000) (M-41650) (T-C6010)
(M-40000)

D0-01372 Cellulitis with lymphangitis of digit, NOS 681.9
(T-03000) (T-C6010) (T-D2810)
(M-41650) (M-41000)

D0-01400 Infectious lymphangitis, NOS
(T-C6010) (M-40000)

D0-01401 Infectious lymphangitis of superficial lymphatics, NOS
(T-C6001) (M-40000)

D0-01402 Infectious lymphangitis of deep lymphatics, NOS
(T-C6002) (M-40000)

D0-01410 Acute lymphangitis, NOS 682.9
(T-C6010) (M-41000)

D0-01411 Acute lymphangitis of face 682.0
(T-C6010) (T-D1200) (M-41000)

0-013-014 Cellulitis and Lymphangitis of The Skin — Continued

D0-01412 Acute lymphangitis of external cheek 682.0
(T-C6010) (T-D1206) (M-41000)
D0-01413 Acute lymphangitis of chin 682.0
(T-C6010) (T-D1210) (T-41000)
D0-01414 Acute lymphangitis of forehead 682.0
(T-C6010) (T-D1110) (M-41000)
D0-01415 Acute lymphangitis of external nose 682.2
(T-C6010) (T-21100) (M-41000)
D0-01416 Acute lymphangitis of submandibular region 682.2
(T-C6010) (T-D1603) (M-41000)
D0-01417 Acute lymphangitis of temple region 682.0
(T-C6010) (T-D1150) (M-41000)
D0-01418 Acute lymphangitis of neck 682.1
(T-C6010) (T-D1600) (M-41000)
D0-01419 Acute lymphangitis of trunk 682.2
(T-C6010) (T-D2000) (M-41000)
D0-01420 Acute lymphangitis of abdominal wall 682.2
(T-C6010) (T-D4300) (M-41000)
D0-01421 Acute lymphangitis of back, except buttock 682.2
(T-C6010) (T-D2100) (M-41000)
D0-01422 Acute lymphangitis of chest wall 682.2
(T-C6010) (T-D3050) (M-41000)
D0-01423 Acute lymphangitis of flank 682.2
(T-C6010) (T-D2310) (M-41000)
D0-01424 Acute lymphangitis of groin 682.2
(T-C6010) (T-D7000) (M-41000)
D0-01425 Acute lymphangitis of pectoral region 682.2
(T-C6010) (T-D2235) (M-41000)
D0-01426 Acute lymphangitis of perineum 682.2
(T-C6010) (T-D2700) (M-41000)
D0-01427 Acute lymphangitis of umbilicus 682.2
(T-C6010) (T-D4220) (M-41000)
D0-01428 Acute lymphangitis of upper arm 682.3
(T-C6010) (T-D8200) (M-41000)
D0-01429 Acute lymphangitis of forearm 682.3
(T-C6010) (T-D8500) (M-41000)
D0-01430 Acute lymphangitis of axilla 682.3
(T-C6010) (T-D8100) (M-41000)
D0-01431 Acute lymphangitis of shoulder 682.3
(T-C6010) (T-D2220) (M-41000)
D0-01432 Acute lymphangitis of hand 682.4
(T-C6010) (T-D8700) (M-41000)
D0-01433 Acute lymphangitis of wrist 682.4
(T-C6010) (T-D8600) (M-41000)
D0-01434 Acute lymphangitis of buttock 682.5
(T-C6010) (T-D2600) (M-41000)
Acute lymphangitis of gluteal region 682.5
(T-C6010) (T-D2600) (M-41000)
D0-01436 Acute lymphangitis of leg, NOS, except foot 682.6
(T-C6010) (T-D9400) (M-41000)
D0-01437 Acute lymphangitis of hip 682.6
(T-C6010) (T-D2500) (M-41000)
D0-01438 Acute lymphangitis of thigh 682.6
(T-C6010) (T-D9100) (M-41000)
D0-01439 Acute lymphangitis of knee 682.6
(T-C6010) (T-D9200) (M-41000)
D0-01440 Acute lymphangitis of ankle 682.6
(T-C6010) (T-D9500) (M-41000)
D0-01441 Acute lymphangitis of foot, except toe 682.7
(T-C6010) (T-D9700) (M-41000)
D0-01442 Acute lymphangitis of heel 682.7
(T-C6010) (T-D9600) (M-41000)
D0-01443 Acute lymphangitis of head, except face 682.8
(T-C6010) (T-D1100) (M-41000)
D0-01444 Acute lymphangitis of scalp 682.8
(T-C6010) (T-D1160) (M-41000)
D0-01445 Acute lymphangitis of other specified site 682.8
(T-C6010) (T-.....) (M-41000)

0-016 Other Infections of The Skin

D0-01600 Pyoderma 686.0
(T-01000) (M-41600)
Pyodermia 686.0
(T-01000) (M-41600)
Purulent dermatitis 686.0
(T-01000) (M-41600)
Suppurative dermatitis 686.0
(T-01000) (M-41600)
Septic dermatitis 686.0
(T-01000) (M-41600)
Pyogenic dermatitis 686.0
(T-01000) (M-41600)
D0-01601 Chancriform pyoderma
(T-01000) (T-D1200) (M-40750)
Pyoderma chancriforme faciei
(T-01000) (T-D1200) (M-40750)
D0-01602 Pyoderma faciale
(T-01000) (T-D1200) (M-41000)
D0-01603 Pyoderma gangrenosum
(T-01000) (M-43000) (G-C008) (M-38000)
D0-01604 Malignant pyoderma
(T-01000) (T-D1100) (T-D1600) (M-40750) (M-40600)
D0-01610V Juvenile pyoderma
(T-01000) (M-41600)
Puppy strangles
(T-01000) (M-41600)
D0-01612V Pyotraumatic dermatitis
Acute moist dermatitis
Hot spots
D0-01614V Infantile pustular dermatosis of puppies
D0-01620 Dermatitis vegetans 686.8
(T-01000) (M-43750) (M-45022)
Pemphigus vegetans, Hallopeau type 686.8
(T-01000) (M-43750) (M-45022)
D0-01640 Bacterid 686.8
(T-01000) (M-01740) (M-01750)
Pustular bacterid of Andrews 686.8
(T-01000) (M-01740) (M-01750)

D0-01642 Pustular bacterid 686.8
(T-01000) (M-01740) (M-01750)

D0-01650 Pyogenic granuloma of skin 686.1
(T-01000) (M-44020)
Septic granuloma of skin 686.1
(T-01000) (M-44020)
Suppurative granuloma of skin 686.1
(T-01000) (M-44020)
Granuloma telangiectaticum of skin 686.1
(T-01000) (M-44020)

D0-01660 Perlèche 686.8
(T-52003) (M-40000) (M-01560)
Angular cheilosis 686.8
(T-52003) (M-40000) (M-01560)
Migrating cheilosis 686.8
(T-52003) (M-40000) (M-01560)
Intertrigo labialis 686.8
(T-52003) (M-40000) (M-01560)
Angular cheilitis 528.5
(T-52003) (M-40000) (M-01560)

D0-01670 Dermatitis infectiosa eczematoides 690.-
(T-01000) (M-01750) (M-01730)
(M-40000)
Infectious eczematoid dermatitis 690.-
(T-01000) (M-01750) (M-01730)
(M-40000)

D0-01680 Fistula of skin, NOS 686.9
(T-01000) (M-39300)

SECTION 0-1 NONINFECTIOUS VESICULAR AND BULLOUS DISEASES

D0-10100 Eczema, NOS 692.-
(T-01000) (M-40000) (F-C3000)
(M-01735) (F-A2300)
Eczematous dermatitis, NOS 692.-
(T-01000) (M-40000) (F-C3000)
(M-01735) (F-A2300)

D0-10101 Acute eczema 692.-
(T-01000) (M-41000) (F-C3000)
(M-01735) (F-A2300)
Erythematous eczema 692.-
(T-01000) (M-41000) (F-C3000)
(M-01735) (F-A2300)

D0-10102 Chronic eczema 692.-
(T-01000) (M-42000) (F-C3000)
(M-01735) (F-A2300)

D0-10106 Occupational eczema 692.-
(T-01000) (M-40000) (F-C3000)
(M-01735) (F-A2300) (G-C001)
(J-00000)
Occupational dermatitis 692.-
(T-01000) (M-40000) (F-C3000)
(M-01735) (F-A2300) (G-C001)
(J-00000)

D0-10120 Nummular eczema
(T-01000) (M-01735) (M-02100)
(F-A2300)
Nummular dermatitis
(T-01000) (M-01735) (M-02100)
(F-A2300)
Nummular eczematous dermatitis
(T-01000) (M-01735) (M-02100)
(F-A2300)
Nummular neurodermatitis
(T-01000) (M-01735) (M-02100)
(F-A2300)
Exudative neurodermatitis
(T-01000) (M-01735) (M-02100)
(F-A2300)

D0-10122 Diffuse neurodermatitis of Brocq 691.8
(T-01000) (M-40000) (M-01735)

D0-10130 Atopic dermatitis, NOS 691.8
(T-01000) (M-43000) (F-C3000)
(M-01735) (F-A2300)
Atopic eczema 691.8
(T-01000) (M-43000) (F-C3000)
(M-01735) (F-A2300)
Allergic eczema 692.-
(T-01000) (M-43000) (F-C3000)
(M-01735) (F-A2300)
Besnier's prurigo 691.8
(T-01000) (M-43000) (F-C3000)
(M-01735) (F-A2300)
Atopic neurodermatitis 691.8
(T-01000) (M-43000) (F-C3000)
(M-01735) (F-A2300)
Allergic dermatitis 692.-
(T-01000) (M-43000) (F-C3000)
(M-01735) (F-A2300)
Prurigo of Besnier 692.-
(T-01000) (M-43000) (F-C3000)
(M-01735) (F-A2300)
Disseminated neurodermatitis 692.-
(T-01000) (M-43000) (F-C3000)
(M-01735) (F-A2300)
Canine atopy
(T-01000) (M-43000) (F-C3000)
(M-01735) (F-A2300)

D0-10132 Flexural eczema 691.8
(T-01000) (M-40000) (M-01735)
(F-A2300)

D0-10134 Infantile eczema 691.8
(T-01000) (M-40000) (M-01735)
(F-A2300)

D0-10135 Acute infantile eczema 691.8
(T-01000) (M-41000)

D0-10136 Chronic infantile eczema 691.8
(T-01000) (M-43000)

D0-10138 Intrinsic allergic eczema 691.8
(T-01000) (F-C3000) (M-01735)
(F-A2300)

D0-10142V Eczema nasi of dogs
Collie nose
Nasal solar dermatitis

D0-10144V Allergic inhalant dermatitis

D0-10150 Diaper rash 691.0
(T-01000) (M-40000) (C-10750)
Napkin rash 691.0
(T-01000) (M-40000) (C-10750)

SECTION 0-1 NONINFECTIOUS VESICULAR AND BULLOUS DISEASES — Continued

D0-10150 (cont.) Diaper dermatitis 691.0
(T-01000) (M-40000) (C-10750)
Diaper erythema 691.0
(T-01000) (M-40000) (C-10750)
Ammonia dermatitis 691.0
(T-01000) (M-40000) (C-10750)
Jacquet's dermatitis 691.0
(T-01000) (M-40000) (C-10750)
Jacquet's erythema 691.0
(T-01000) (M-40000) (C-10750)

D0-10152 Psoriasiform napkin eruption 691.0
(T-01000) (M-40000)

D0-10158V Moist dermatitis of rabbits
Rabbit slobbers

D0-10160 Seborrheic dermatitis 690.-
(T-01000) (M-43000) (F-43003)
Seborrheic eczema 690.-
(T-01000) (M-43000) (F-43003)

D0-10163V Scratches
Greasy heel
Dermatitis verrucosa

D0-10164 Seborrhea sicca 690.-
(T-01000) (T-D1160) (M-43000) (F-41503)
Pityriasis capitis 690.-
(T-01000) (T-D1160) (M-43000) (F-41503)
Dandruff 690.-
(T-01000) (T-D1160) (M-43000) (F-41503)
Pityriasis sicca 690.-
(T-01000) (T-D1160) (M-43000) (F-41503)

D0-10166 Seborrhea adiposa
(T-01000) (F-43003)
Seborrhea oleosa
(T-01000) (F-43003)

D0-10168 Generalized seborrheic dermatitis of infants
(T-01000) (T-D0010) (M-43000) (F-41503)
Leiner's disease
(T-01000) (T-D0010) (M-43000) (F-41503)
Erythroderma desquamativum
(T-01000) (T-D0010) (M-43000) (F-41503)

D0-10170 Generalized exfoliative dermatitis
(T-01000) (M-01780) (M-40000) (F-41503)
Generalized erythroderma
(T-01000) (M-01780) (M-40000) (F-41503)
Pityriasis rubra of Hebra
(T-01000) (M-01780) (M-40000) (F-41503)

D0-10171 Subacute generalized exfoliative dermatitis
(T-01000) (M-01780) (M-42000) (F-41503)

D0-10172 Chronic generalized exfoliative dermatitis
(T-01000) (M-01780) (M-43000) (F-41503)

D0-10180 Id reaction
(T-01000) (M-01700) (F-C3000)

D0-10190 Vesicular eruption of skin, NOS 709.8
(T-01000) (M-01750)

D0-10200 Contact dermatitis, NOS 692.-
(T-01000) (M-40000) (G-4022) (C-50000) (A-00000)
Dermatitis venenata 692.-
(T-01000) (M-40000) (G-4022) (C-50000) (A-00000)

D0-10201 Acute contact dermatitis, NOS
(T-01000) (M-41000)

D0-10202 Subacute contact dermatitis, NOS
(T-01000) (M-42000)

D0-10203 Chronic contact dermatitis, NOS
(T-01000) (M-43000)

D0-10210 Contact dermatitis due to detergents 692.0
(T-01000) (M-40000) (G-C001) (C-22600)

D0-10212 Contact dermatitis due to oils 692.1
(T-01000) (M-40000) (G-C001) (C-20260)

D0-10214 Contact dermatitis due to greases 692.1
(T-01000) (M-40000) (G-C001) (C-20560)

D0-10220 Contact dermatitis due to solvents, NOS 692.2
(T-01000) (M-40000) (G-C001) (C-20530)

D0-10221 Contact dermatitis due to chlorocompound group 692.2
(T-01000) (M-40000) (G-C001) (C-20801)

D0-10222 Contact dermatitis due to cyclohexane group 692.2
(T-01000) (M-40000) (G-C001) (C-20551)

D0-10223 Contact dermatitis due to ester group 692.2
(T-01000) (M-40000) (G-C001) (C-10048)

D0-10224 Contact dermatitis due to glycol group 692.2
(T-01000) (M-40000) (G-C001) (C-21300)

D0-10225 Contact dermatitis due to hydrocarbon group 692.2
(T-01000) (M-40000) (G-C001) (C-20500)

D0-10226 Contact dermatitis due to ketone group 692.2
(T-01000) (M-40000) (G-C001) (C-21500)

DO-10230 Contact dermatitis due to drugs and medicine 692.3
(T-01000) (M-40000) (G-C001) (C-50000)
Dermatitis medicamentosa (drug applied to skin) 692.3
(T-01000) (M-40000) (G-C001) (C-50000)

DO-10231 Contact dermatitis due to arnica 692.3
(T-01000) (M-40000) (G-C001) (L-DA400)
Allergic dermatitis due to arnica 692.3
(T-01000) (M-40000) (G-C001) (L-DA400)

DO-10232 Contact dermatitis due to fungicide 692.3
(T-01000) (M-40000) (G-C001) (C-23700)

DO-10233 Contact dermatitis due to iodine 692.3
(T-01000) (M-40000) (G-C001) (C-11400)

DO-10234 Contact dermatitis due to keratolytic agent 692.3
(T-01000) (M-40000) (G-C001) (C-92200)

DO-10235 Contact dermatitis due to mercurial 692.3
(T-01000) (M-40000) (G-C001) (C-11300)

DO-10236 Contact dermatitis due to neomycin 692.3
(T-01000) (M-40000) (G-C001) (C-52550)

DO-10237 Contact dermatitis due to pediculicide 692.3
(T-01000) (M-40000) (G-C001) (C-91102)

DO-10238 Contact dermatitis due to phenol 692.3
(T-01000) (M-40000) (G-C001) (C-21100)

DO-10239 Contact dermatitis due to scabicide 692.3
(T-01000) (M-40000) (G-C001) (C-91101)

DO-1023AV Flea collar dermatitis
(T-01000) (M-40000) (G-C001) (C-23204)
Contact dermatitis due to dichlorvos
(T-01000) (M-40000) (G-C001) (C-23204)

DO-10240 Contact dermatitis due to other drug, NEC 692.3
(T-01000) (M-40000) (G-C001) (C-50000)

DO-10250 Contact dermatitis due to other chemical product 692.4
(T-01000) (M-40000) (G-C001) (C-10030)
Allergic dermatitis due to other chemical product 692.4
(T-01000) (M-40000) (G-C001) (C-10030)

DO-10251 Contact dermatitis due to acid 692.4
(T-01000) (M-40000) (G-C001) (C-10040)

DO-10252 Contact dermatitis due to adhesive plaster 692.4
(T-01000) (M-40000) (G-C001) (A-13020)

DO-10253 Contact dermatitis due to alkali 692.4
(T-01000) (M-40000) (G-C001) (C-10055)

DO-10254 Contact dermatitis due to caustic agent 692.4
(T-01000) (M-40000) (G-C001) (C-10300)

DO-10255 Contact dermatitis due to dichromate 692.4
(T-01000) (M-40000) (G-C001) (C-12912)

DO-10256 Contact dermatitis due to insecticide 692.4
(T-01000) (M-40000) (G-C001) (C-21300)

DO-10261 Contact dermatitis due to nylon 692.4
(T-01000) (M-40000) (G-C001) (C-20410)

DO-10262 Contact dermatitis due to plastic 692.4
(T-01000) (M-40000) (G-C001) (C-20400)

DO-10263 Contact dermatitis due to rubber 692.4
(T-01000) (M-40000) (G-C001) (C-20030)

DO-10270 Contact dermatitis due to food in contact with skin 692.5
(T-01000) (M-40000) (G-C001) (C-F0000)

DO-10271 Contact dermatitis due to cereal 692.5
(T-01000) (M-40000) (G-C001) (C-F0110)

DO-10272 Contact dermatitis due to fish 692.5
(T-01000) (M-40000) (G-C001) (L-C0000)

DO-10273 Contact dermatitis due to flour 692.5
(T-01000) (M-40000) (G-C001) (C-F0100)

DO-10274 Contact dermatitis due to fruit 692.5
(T-01000) (M-40000) (G-C001) (C-F0200)

DO-10275 Contact dermatitis due to meat 692.5
(T-01000) (M-40000) (G-C001) (C-F0300)

DO-10276 Contact dermatitis due to milk 692.5
(T-01000) (M-40000) (G-C001) (C-F0400)

DO-10280 Contact dermatitis due to plants, except food 692.6
(T-01000) (M-40000) (G-C001) (L-D0000)

DO-10281 Contact dermatitis due to lacquer tree 692.6
(T-01000) (M-40000) (G-C001) (L-D7A25)
Contact dermatitis due to Rhus verniciflua 692.6
(T-01000) (M-40000) (G-C001) (L-D7A35)

SECTION 0-1 NONINFECTIOUS VESICULAR AND BULLOUS DISEASES — Continued

D0-10281 (cont.) Allergic dermatitis due to lacquer tree 692.6
(T-01000) (M-40000) (G-C001) (L-D7A25)
Allergic dermatitis due to Rhus verniciflua 692.6
(T-01000) (M-40000) (G-C001) (L-D7A25)

D0-10282 Contact dermatitis due to poison ivy 692.6
(T-01000) (M-40000) (G-C001) (L-D7A30)
Contact dermatitis due to Rhus toxicodendron 692.6
(T-01000) (M-40000) (G-C001) (L-D7A30)
Allergic dermatitis due to poison ivy 692.6
(T-01000) (M-40000) (G-C001) (L-D7A30)
Allergic dermatitis due to Rhus toxicodendron 692.6
(T-01000) (M-40000) (G-C001) (L-D7A30)

D0-10283 Contact dermatitis due to poison oak 692.6
(T-01000) (M-40000) (G-C001) (L-D7A26)
Contact dermatitis due to Rhus diversiloba 692.6
(T-01000) (M-40000) (G-C001) (L-D7A26)
Allergic dermatitis due to poison oak 692.6
(T-01000) (M-40000) (G-C001) (L-D7A26)
Allergic dermatitis due to Rhus diversiloba 692.6
(T-01000) (M-40000) (G-C001) (L-D7A26)

D0-10284 Contact dermatitis due to poison sumac 692.6
(T-01000) (M-40000) (G-C001) (L-D7A28)
Contact dermatitis due to Rhus venenata 692.6
(T-01000) (M-40000) (G-C001) (L-D7A28)
Allergic dermatitis due to poison sumac 692.6
(T-01000) (M-40000) (G-C001) (L-D7A28)
Allergic dermatitis due to Rhus venenata 692.6
(T-01000) (M-40000) (G-C001) (L-D7A28)

D0-10285 Contact dermatitis due to poison vine 692.6
(T-01000) (M-40000) (G-C001) (L-D7A30)
Contact dermatitis due to Rhus radicans
(T-01000) (M-40000) (G-C001) (L-D7A30)
Allergic dermatitis due to poison vine 692.6
(T-01000) (M-40000) (G-C001) (L-D7A30)
Allergic dermatitis due to Rhus radicans 692.6
(T-01000) (M-40000) (G-C001) (L-D7A30)

D0-10286 Contact dermatitis due to primrose 692.6
(T-01000) (M-40000) (G-C001) (L-D3D11)
Contact dermatitis due to Primula
(T-01000) (M-40000) (G-C001) (L-D3D11)
Allergic dermatitis due to primrose 692.6
(T-01000) (M-40000) (G-C001) (L-D3D11)
Allergic dermatitis due to Primula 692.6
(T-01000) (M-40000) (G-C001) (L-D3D11)

D0-10287 Contact dermatitis due to ragweed 692.6
(T-01000) (M-40000) (G-C001) (L-DA811)
Contact dermatitis due to Senecio jacobae 692.6
(T-01000) (M-40000) (G-C001) (L-DA811)
Allergic dermatitis due to ragweed 692.6
(T-01000) (M-40000) (G-C001) (L-DA811)
Allergic dermatitis due to Senecio jacobae 692.6
(T-01000) (M-40000) (G-C001) (L-DA811)

D0-10288 Contact dermatitis due to other non food plant 692.6
(T-01000) (M-40000) (G-C001) (L-D0000)
Allergic dermatitis due to other non food plant 692.6
(T-01000) (M-40000) (G-C001) (L-D0000)

D0-10310 Contact dermatitis due to solar radiation, NOS 692.70
(T-01000) (M-11100) (G-C001) (A-81074)

D0-10311 Sunburn 692.71
(T-01000) (M-11700) (M-01780) (G-C001) (A-81074)
Solar dermatitis
(T-01000) (M-11700) (M-01780) (G-C001) (A-81074)

D0-10312 Hydroa aestivale 692.79
(T-01000) (M-36760) (G-C001) (A-81074)
Hydroa vacciniforme 692.79
(T-01000) (M-36760) (G-C001) (A-81074)

D0-10312 (cont.) Summer prurigo of Hutchinson 692.99
(T-01000) (M-36760) (G-C001)
(A-81074)

D0-10313 Photodermatitis due to sun 692.79
(T-01000) (M-11700) (F-C3000)
(G-C001) (A-81074)
Photosensitivity due to sun 692.79
(T-01000) (M-11700) (F-C3000)
(G-C001) (A-81074)
Photosentization due to sun 692.79
(T-01000) (M-11700) (F-C3000)
(G-C001) (A-81074)

D0-10318V Trefoil dermatitis
(T-01000) (M-40000) (G-C001)
(F-50440) (L-D6383)
Dermatitis due to ingestion of Medicago polymorpha
(T-01000) (M-40000) (G-C001)
(F-50440) (L-D6383)

D0-10320 Contact dermatitis due to other specified agents 692.8
(T-01000) (M-40000) (G-C001) (C-.....)
(A-.....)

D0-10322 Contact dermatitis due to cosmetics 692.81
(T-01000) (M-40000) (G-C001)
(C-93A00)

D0-10323 Contact dermatitis due to cold weather 692.89
(T-01000) (M-40000) (M-11200)
(G-C001) (A-80212)

D0-10324 Contact dermatitis due to dye 692.89
(T-01000) (M-40000) (G-C001)
(C-22700)

D0-10325 Contact dermatitis due to fur 692.89
(T-01000) (M-40000) (G-C001)
(A-60240)

D0-10326 Contact dermatitis due to hot weather 692.89
(T-01000) (M-40000) (M-11000)
(G-C001) (A-80202)

D0-10327 Contact dermatitis due to infrared rays 692.89
(T-01000) (M-40000) (M-11000)
(G-C001) (A-81090)

D0-10328 Contact dermatitis due to jewelry 692.89
(T-01000) (M-40000) (G-C001)
(A-61000)

D0-10329 Contact dermatitis due to light, except sun 692.89
(T-01000) (M-40000) (G-C001)
(A-81070)

D0-10331 Contact dermatitis due to metal, NOS 692.89
(T-01000) (M-40000) (G-C001)
(C-11800)

D0-10332 Contact dermatitis due to preservative, NOS 692.89
(T-01000) (M-40000) (G-C001)
(C-F1020)

D0-10340 Contact dermatitis due to radiation, NOS 692.89
(T-01000) (M-40000) (M-11600)
(G-C001) (A-81000)

D0-10342 Contact dermatitis due to ultraviolet rays, except sun 692.89
(T-01000) (M-40000) (M-11700)
(G-C001) (A-81060)

D0-10344 Contact dermatitis due to X-rays 692.89
(T-01000) (M-40000) (M-11600)
(G-C001) (A-81050)

D0-10350 Dermatitis due to substances taken internally, NOS 693.9
(T-01000) (M-40000) (G-C001)
(F-50440) (C-00000)

D0-10352 Dermatitis due to drugs and medicines taken internally 693.0
(T-01000) (M-40000) (G-C001)
(F-50440) (C-50000)
Dermatitis medicamentosa due to ingested drugs 693.0
(T-01000) (M-40000) (G-C001)
(F-50440) (C-50000)

D0-10354 Dermatitis due to food taken internally 693.1
(T-01000) (M-40000) (G-C001)
(F-50440) (C-F0000)

D0-10358 Dermatitis due to other specified substance taken internally 693.8
(T-01000) (M-40000)

D0-10400 Bullous dermatosis, NOS 694.9
(T-01000)

D0-10402 Bullous eruption of childhood 694.9
(T-01000)

D0-10410 Dermatitis herpetiformis 694.9
(T-01000)
Dermatosis herpetiformis 694.9
(T-01000)
Duhring's disease 694.9
(T-01000)

D0-10411 Hydroa herpetiformis 694.9
(T-01000)

D0-10412 Juvenile dermatitis herpetiformis 694.2
(T-01000)
Juvenile pemphigoid 694.2
(T-01000)

D0-10414 Impetigo herpetiformis 694.3
(T-01000)

D0-10416 Senile dermatitis herpetiformis 694.5
(T-01000)

D0-10420 Pemphigus, NOS 694.4
(T-01000)

D0-10421 Pemphigus erythematosus 694.4
(T-01000)

D0-10423 Pemphigus foliaceus 694.4
(T-01000)

D0-10425 Malignant pemphigus 694.4
(T-01000)

SECTION 0-1 NONINFECTIOUS VESICULAR AND BULLOUS DISEASES — Continued

D0-10427 Pemphigus vegetans 694.4
(T-01000)

D0-10428 Pemphigus vulgaris 694.4
(T-01000)

D0-10430 Pemphigoid, NOS 694.5
(T-01000)
Benign pemphigus, NOS 694.5
(T-01000)

D0-10431 Bullous pemphigoid 694.5
(T-01000)

D0-10432 Benign mucous membrane pemphigoid 694.6
(T-00400) (M-43000) (G-C009)
(T-AA000) (F-01250)
Cicatricial pemphigoid 694.6
(T-00400) (M-43000) (G-C009)
(T-AA000) (F-01250)
Mucosynechia atrophic bullous dermatitis 694.6
(T-00400) (M-43000) (G-C009)
(T-AA000) (F-01250)
Benign mucous membrane pemphigoid without ocular involvement 694.60
(T-00400) (M-43000) (G-C009)
(T-AA000) (F-01250)

D0-10433 Benign mucous membrane pemphigoid with ocular involvement 694.61
(T-00400) (M-43000) (G-C008)
(T-AA000) (F-01250)

D0-10435 Acquired epidermolysis bullosa
(T-01000)

D0-10438 Other specified bullous dermatosis, NEC 694.8
(T-01000)

D0-10440 Subcorneal pustular dermatosis 694.1
(T-01000)
Sneddon-Wilkinson disease 694.1
(T-01000)
Sneddon-Wilkinson syndrome 694.1
(T-01000)
Pinkus' disease 697.1
(T-01000)

D0-10450 Erythema multiforme, NOS 695.1
(T-01000)

D0-10451 Erythema multiforme, dermal type 695.1
(T-01000)

D0-10452 Erythema multiforme, mixed dermal-epidermal type 695.1
(T-01000)

D0-10453 Erythema multiforme, epidermal type 695.1
(T-01000)

D0-10454 Stevens-Johnson syndrome 695.1
(T-01000)

D0-10455 Lyell's toxic epidermal necrolysis, subepidermal type 695.1

D0-10458 Erythema iris 695.1
(T-01000)

D0-10459 Herpes iris 695.1
(T-01000)

D0-10460 Toxic erythema 695.0
(T-01000)
Erythema venenatum 695.0
(T-01000)

D0-10462 Erythema toxicum neonatorum
(T-01000)

D0-10550 Transient acantholytic dermatosis
(T-01000)

D0-10560 Friction blisters of the skin
(T-01000) (M-14720)

D0-10561 Friction blisters of the soles
(T-02852) (M-14720)

D0-10562 Friction blisters of the palms
(T-02652) (M-14720)

D0-10570 Electrical burn of skin
(T-01000) (M-11100) (G-C001)
(A-81600)

D0-10580 Stasis dermatitis, NOS
(T-01000)

SECTION 0-2 NONINFECTIOUS ERYTHEMATOUS, PAPULAR AND SQUAMOUS DISEASES

D0-20050 Erythematosquamous dermatosis, NOS 690.-
(T-01000) (M-01780)

D0-20102 Allergic urticaria 708.0
(T-01000) (M-36320)

D0-20104 Idiopathic urticaria 708.1
(T-01000) (M-36320)

D0-20106 Urticaria due to cold 708.2
(T-01000) (M-36320)

D0-20108 Urticaria due to heat 708.2
(T-01000) (M-36320)
Thermal urticaria 708.2
(T-01000) (M-36320)

D0-20110 Dermatographic urticaria 708.3
(T-01000) (M-36320)
Dermatographia 708.3
(T-01000) (M-36320)
Factitia urticaria 708.3
(T-01000) (M-36320)

D0-20112 Vibratory urticaria 708.4
(T-01000) (M-36320)

D0-20114 Cholinergic urticaria 708.5
(T-01000) (M-36320)

D0-20120 Chronic urticaria 708.8
(T-01000) (M-36320)
Recurrent periodic urticaria 708.8
(T-01000) (M-36320)

D0-20130 Nettle rash 708.8
(T-01000) (M-36320)

D0-20150 Urticaria pigmentosa, NOS 757.33
(T-01000) (T-C0140) (M-72000)
(M-04013) (M-03130) (F-A2300)
Localized cutaneous mastocytosis, NOS 757.33
(T-01000) (T-C0140) (M-72000)
(M-04013) (M-03130) (F-A2300)

D0-20151 Urticaria pigmentosa, infantile form 757.33
(T-01000) (T-C0140) (M-72000)
(M-04013) (M-03130) (F-A2300)

D0-20152 Urticaria pigmentosa, adult form 757.33
(T-01000) (T-C0140) (M-72000)
(M-04013) (M-03130) (F-A2300)

D0-20153 Urticaria pigmentosa, maculopapular type 757.33
(T-01000) (T-C0140) (M-72000)
(M-01413) (M-03130) (F-A2300)

D0-20154 Urticaria pigmentosa, multiple nodules or plaques 757.33
(T-01000) (T-C0140) (M-72000)
(M-04013) (M-03130) (F-A2300)

D0-20155 Urticaria pigmentosa, solitary cutaneous nodule 757.33
(T-01000) (T-C0140) (M-72000)
(M-04013) (M-03130) (F-A2300)

D0-20156 Urticaria pigmentosa, diffuse erythrodermic type 757.33
(T-01000) (T-C0140) (M-72000)
(M-04013) (M-03130) (F-A2300)

D0-20158 Urticaria pigmentosa, telangiectasia macularis eruptiva perstans 757.33
(T-01000) (T-C0140) (M-72000)
(T-04013) (T-03130) (F-A2300)

D0-20180 Other specified urticaria, NEC 708.8
(T-01000) (M-36320)

D0-20200 Pruritus of skin, NOS 698.9
(T-01000) (F-A2300)
Itch of skin, NOS 698.9
(T-01000) (F-A2300)
Pruritic dermatitis, NOS 698.9
(T-01000) (F-A2300)

D0-20202 Pruritus senilis 698.8
(T-01000) (F-A2300)

D0-20210 Pruritus hiemalis 698.8
(T-01000) (F-A2300)
Winter itch 698.8
(T-01000) (F-A2300)
Xerotic eczema 698.8
(T-01000) (F-A2300)
Asteatotic eczema 698.8
(T-01000) (F-A2300)
Eczema craquelé 698.8
(T-01000) (F-A2300)

D0-20220 Xeroderma, NOS
(T-01000) (M-59020)
Xerodermia, NOS
(T-01000) (M-59020)

D0-20250 Pruritus ani 698.0
(T-02507) (F-A2300)
Anal itch 698.0
(T-02507) (F-A2300)
Perianal itch 698.0
(T-02507) (F-A2300)

D0-20252 Pruritus of genital organs 698.1
(T-80000) (T-90000) (F-A2300)

D0-20300 Prurigo, NOS 698.2
(T-01000)

D0-20310 Prurigo simplex 698.2
(T-01000)
Lichen urticatus 698.2
(T-01000)
Urticaria papulosa of Hebra 698.2
(T-01000)
Prurigo mitis 698.2
(T-01000)
Hebra's prurigo 698.2
(T-01000)
Papular urticaria 698.2
(T-01000)

D0-20314 Prurigo nodularis 698.3
(T-01000)
Hyde's disease 698.3
(T-01000)

D0-22010 Erythematous condition, NOS 695.9
(T-01000) (M-01780)

D0-22012 Menstrual dermatosis 709.8
(T-01000)

D0-22020 Intertrigo 695.89
(T-01000)
Erythema intertrigo 695.89
(T-01000)
Eczema intertrigo 695.89
(T-01000)

D0-22030 Erythema gyratum, NOS
(T-01000)

D0-22032 Erythema gyratum repens
(T-01000)

D0-22034 Erythema annulare centrifugum
(T-01000)

D0-22036 Erythema chronica migrans

D0-22040 Erythema dyschromicum perstans
(T-01000)

D0-22050 Other specified erythematous condition, NEC 695.8
(T-01000)

D0-22100 Psoriasis, NOS 696.1
(T-01000)

D0-22110 Psoriasis vulgaris
(T-01000)
Erythrodermic psoriasis
(T-01000)

D0-22114 Psoriasis with arthropathy 696.0
(T-01000)
Psoriatic arthropathy 696.0
(T-01000)

D0-22120 Generalized pustular psoriasis of von Zumbush
(T-01000)

D0-22122 Generalized pustular psoriasis, exanthematous type
(T-01000)

D0-22124 Acrodermatitis continua of Hallopeau 696.1
(T-01000)
Dermatitis repens 696.1
(T-01000)

SECTION 0-2 NONINFECTIOUS ERYTHEMATOUS, PAPULAR AND SQUAMOUS DISEASES — Continued

D0-22130 Localized pustular psoriasis
(T-01000)
Psoriasis with pustules
D0-22132 Localized acrodermatitis continua of Hallopeau
(T-01000)
D0-22136 Pustular psoriasis of the palms and soles
(T-01000)
D0-22150 Parapsoriasis, NOS 696.2
(T-01000)
D0-22152 Parapsoriasis lichenoides 696.2
(T-01000)
Retiform parapsoriasis 696.2
(T-01000)
Parapsoriasis varigata 696.2
(T-01000)
Poikilodermic parapsoriasis 696.2
(T-01000)
D0-22154 Parapsoriasis en plaques
(T-01000)
D0-22155 Small plaque parapsoriasis
(T-01000)
D0-22156 Large plaque parapsoriasis
(T-01000)
D0-22160 Pityriasis, NOS 696.5
(T-01000)
D0-22161 Pityriasis rosea 696.3
(T-01000)
Pityriasis circinata et maculata 696.3
(T-01000)
D0-22162 Pityriasis rubra pilaris 696.4
(T-01000)
Lichen ruber acuminatus 696.4
(T-01000)
Devergie's disease 696.4
(T-01000)
D0-22163 Pityriasis alba 696.5
(T-01000) (T-D1200) (M-04200) (M-57120)
Pityriasis simplex 696.5
(T-01000) (T-D1200) (M-04200) (M-57120)
Pityriasis streptogenes 696.5
(T-01000) (T-D1200) (M-04200) (M-57120)
D0-22164 Acute lichenoid pityriasis
(T-01000)
Parapsoriasis varioliformis acuta
(T-01000)
D0-22165 Chronic lichenoid pityriasis
(T-01000)
Parapsoriasis varioliformis chronica
(T-01000)
D0-22170 Reiter's disease of the skin
(T-01000)
Keratoderma blennorrhagicum
(T-01000)
Keratosis blennorrhagica
(T-01000)
D0-22180 Gianotti-Crosti syndrome
D0-22200 Lichen, NOS 697.9
(T-01000)
D0-22210 Lichen planus 697.0
(T-01000)
Ruber planus 697.0
(T-01000)
D0-22212 Hypertrophic lichen planus
(T-01000)
D0-22214 Bullous lichen planus
(T-01000)
D0-22220 Lichen planopilaris 697.0
(T-01000)
Lichen planus follicularis
(T-01000)
D0-22230 Lichen nitidus 697.1
(T-01000)
D0-22234 Lichen striatus 697.8
(T-01000)
D0-22240 Lichen ruber moniliformis 697.8
(T-01000)
D0-22250 Lichen simplex chronicus 698.3
(T-01000)
Neurodermatitis circumscripta 698.3
(T-01000)
Local neurodermatitis 698.3
(T-01000)
D0-22256V Acral lick dermatitis
(T-01000)
Feline hyperaesthesia syndrome
(T-01000)
Feline neurodermatitis
(T-01000)
Acral lick granuloma
(T-01000)
Acropruritic granuloma
(T-01000)
D0-22260 Dermatitis factitia 698.4
(T-01000)
Dermatitis artefacta 698.4
(T-01000)
Dermatitis ficta 698.4
(T-01000)
Neurotic excoriation 698.4
(T-01000)
D0-22290 Other specified lichen condition, NEC 697.8
(T-01000)
D0-22300 Parakeratosis of skin, NOS 690.-
(T-01000) (M-74470)
D0-22302 Parakeratosis scutularis
Parakeratosis ostracea
D0-22310 Acquired keratoderma, NOS 701.1
(T-01000) (M-72600)
Hyperkeratosis of skin, NOS 701.1
(T-01000) (M-72600)

D0-22311 Acquired keratoderma palmaris et plantaris 701.1
(T-01000)
Keratoderma climactericum 701.1
(T-01000)
Hyperkeratosis palmoplantaris climacterica 701.1
(T-01000)
D0-22312 Hyperkeratosis follicularis in cutem penetrans 701.1
(T-01000)
D0-22316 Progressive keratoderma tylodes 701.1
(T-01000)
D0-22320 Acquired acanthosis nigricans 701.2
(T-01000)
Keratosis nigricans 701.2
(T-01000)
D0-22330 Confluent and reticulate papillomatosis 701.8
(T-01000)
Gougerot-Carteaud disease 701.8
(T-01000)
Gougerot-Carteaud syndrome 701.8
(T-01000)
D0-22340 Acquired ichthyosis 701.1
(T-01000)
D0-23010 Cutaneous lupus erythematosus, NOS 695.4
(T-01000)
D0-23012 Discoid lupus erythematosus 695.4
(T-01000)
D0-23060V Equine papular dermatitis
(T-01000)
D0-23064V Feline miliary dermatitis
(T-01000)
Scabby cat disease
(T-01000)

SECTION 0-3 VASCULAR DISEASES OF THE SKIN

D0-30000 Vascular disease of the skin, NOS 709.1
(T-01000)
Vascular disorder of skin, NOS 709.1
(T-01000)
D0-30100 Pityriasis lichenoides et varioliformis of Mucha-Habermann
(T-01000)
D0-30112 Pityriasis lichenoides chronica
(T-01000)
D0-30114 Pityriasis lichenoides et varioliformis acuta
(T-01000)
D0-30120 Lymphomatoid papulosis
(T-01000)
D0-30130 Purpura pigmentosa chronica, NOS
(T-01000)
D0-30131 Purpura annularis telangiectodes of Majocchi 709.1
(T-01000)
Purpura annularis telangiectodes 709.1
(T-01000)
Majocchi's purpura 709.1
(T-01000)
D0-30133 Progressive pigmentary dermatosis of Schamberg
(T-01000)
D0-30135 Pigmented purpuric lichenoid dermatitis of Gougerot and Blum
(T-01000)
D0-30137 Eczematid-like purpura of Doucas and Kapetanakis
(T-01000)
D0-30140 Granuloma faciale
(T-01000)
D0-30150 Erythema elevatum diutinum
(T-01000)
D0-30160 Acute febrile neutrophilic dermatosis
(T-01000)
D0-30200 Benign cutaneous periarteritis nodosa
(T-01000)
D0-30230 Malignant atrophic papulosis
(T-01000)
D0-30240 Segmental hyalinizing vasculitis
(T-01000)
Livedo reticularis with ulceration
(T-01000)

SECTION 0-4 DEGENERATIVE DISEASES OF THE SKIN

D0-40000 Degenerative skin disorder, NOS 709.3
(T-01000) (M-50000)
Degeneration of skin, NOS 709.3
(T-01000) (M-50000)
Senile dermatosis, NOS 709.3
(T-01000) (M-50000)
D0-40010 Atrophic condition of skin, NOS 701.9
(T-01000)
Atrophy of skin, NOS 701.9
(T-01000)
Atrophoderma, NOS 701.9
(T-01000)
Atrophica cutis senilis 701.8
(T-01000)
D0-40012 Atrophoderma neuriticum 701.8
(T-01000)
D0-40030 Atrophoderma maculatum 701.3
(T-01000)
Atrophic spots of skin 701.3
(T-01000)
Atrophie blanche of Milian 701.3
(T-01000)
Macular atrophy
(T-01000)
Anetoderma
(T-01000)
D0-40032 Degenerative colloid atrophy 701.3
(T-01000)
D0-40034 Senile degenerative atrophy 701.3
(T-01000)

SECTION 0-4 DEGENERATIVE DISEASES OF THE SKIN — Continued

D0-40036 Circumscribed scleroderma 701.0
(T-01000)
Addison's keloid 701.0
(T-01000)
Localized dermatosclerosis 701.0
(T-01000)
Morphea 701.0
(T-01000)

D0-40040 Cutis laxa, acquired type
(T-01000) (T-1A240) (M-01000)

D0-40041 Cutis laxa senilis 701.8
(T-01000)

D0-40042 Elastosis senilis 701.8
(T-01000)

D0-40100 Solar degeneration
(T-01000)
Actinic degeneration
(T-01000)

D0-40120 Cutis rhomboidalis nuchae
(T-01000)

D0-40130 Nodular elastosis with cysts and comedones of Favre and Racouchot
(T-01000)

D0-40150 Kyrle's disease
(T-01000)

D0-40154 Elastosis perforans serpiginosa 701.1
(T-01000)

D0-40156 Reactive perforating collagenosis
(T-01000)

D0-40160 Hyperkeratosis lenticularis perstans
(T-01000)
Hyperkeratosis lenticularis perstans of Flegel

D0-40170 Acrodermatitis atrophicans chronica 701.8
(T-01000)

D0-40180 Pretibial pigmental patches in diabetes
(T-01000)

D0-40190 Bullosis diabeticorum

D0-40200 Lichen sclerosus et atrophicus, NOS 701.0
(T-01000)

D0-40300 Acroosteolysis, NOS
(T-01000)

D0-40305 Idiopathic acroosteolysis
(T-01000)

D0-40308 Occupational acroosteolysis
(T-01000)

D0-40400 Ulerythema, NOS
(T-01000)

D0-40401 Ulerythema of cheeks
(T-01000) (T-D1206)

D0-40402 Ulerythema of eyebrows
(T-01000) (T-01520)
Folliculitis ulerythematosa reticulata 701.8
(T-01000) (T-01520)
Ulerythema ophryogenes
(T-01000) (T-01520)

D0-40500V Zinc-responsive dermatosis
(T-01000)

D0-40504V Inherited parakeratosis in cattle
(T-01000)
Adema disease
(T-01000)
Imperfect keratogenesis
(T-01000)

D0-40510V Vitamin A-responsive dermatosis
(T-01000)

D0-40520V Neuter-responsive dermatosis
(T-01000)

SECTION 0-5 DISEASES OF THE EPIDERMAL APPENDAGES
0-51 DISEASES OF THE SEBACEOUS GLANDS

D0-51000 Disease of sebaceous glands, NOS 706.9
(T-01310)

D0-51100 Acne, NOS 706.1
(T-01310)

D0-51102 Neonatal acne
(T-01310) (F-88000)
Infantile acne
(T-01310) (F-88000)

D0-51108 Acne atrophica
(T-01310) (G-C008) (M-78060)

D0-51110 Acne vulgaris 706.1
(T-01310)
Common acne 706.1
(T-01310)

D0-51112 Tropical acne
(T-01310)
Acne tropicalis
(T-01310)

D0-51116 Excoriated acne
(T-01310)

D0-51120 Acne necrotica miliaris 706.0
(T-01310) (T-D1160)

D0-51122 Acne varioliformis 706.9
(T-01310) (T-D0110) (T-D1160)
Acne frontalis 706.0
(T-01310) (T-D0110) (T-D1160)

D0-51130 Acne conglobata 706.1
(T-01310)

D0-51135 Pustular acne 706.1
(T-01310)
Acne pustulosa 706.1
(T-01310)

D0-51136 Acne indurata
(T-01310)

D0-51140 Cystic acne 706.1
(T-01310)

D0-51142 Acne fulminans
(T-01310)

D0-51150 Acne rosacea 695.3
(T-01000)
Rosacea 695.3
(T-01000)

D0-51150 (cont.) Acne erythematosa 695.3
(T-01000)

D0-51152 Acne rosacea, erythematous telangiectatic type 695.3
(T-01000)

D0-51153 Acne rosacea, glandular hyperplastic type 695.3
(T-01000)

D0-51154 Acne rosacea, papular type 695.3
(T-01000)

D0-51155 Granulomatous rosacea 695.3
(T-01000)
Perioral dermatitis 695.3
(T-01000)

D0-51156 Rhinophyma 695.3
(T-01000)

D0-51160 Acne of external chemical origin, NOS
(T-01310)

D0-51162 Halogen acne
(T-01310) (G-C001) (C-11000)

D0-51163 Bromide acne
(T-01310) (G-C001) (C-11320)

D0-51164 Chlorine acne
(T-01310) (G-C001) (C-11200)
Chloracne
(T-01310) (G-C001) (C-11200)

D0-51165 Iodide acne
(T-01310) (G-C001) (C-11410)

D0-51170 Acne venenata
(T-01310)
Contact acne
(T-01310)

D0-51171 Acne cosmetica
(T-01310) (G-C001) (C-93A00)

D0-51172 Acne detergicans
(T-01310) (C-22600)

D0-51174 Acne estivalis
(T-01310)

D0-51178 Acne mechanica
(T-01310)

D0-51180V Canine acne
(T-01310)

D0-51182V Feline acne
(T-01310)
Feline fat chin
(T-01310)

D0-51208V Interdigital cyst in dogs

D0-51220 Seborrhea, NOS 706.3
(T-01310) (T-0B120) (F-03473)

D0-51222 Seborrhea capitis 704.8
(T-01400) (T-0B120) (T-B0160) (F-03473)

D0-51230 Asteatosis cutis 706.8
(T-01310) (F-03474)
Xerosis cutis 706.8
(T-01310) (F-03474)

D0-51280 Other specified disease of sebaceous gland, NEC 706.8
(T-01310)

D0-51310V Feline stud tail
(T-01310) (M-72000)

0-52 DISEASES OF THE SWEAT GLANDS

D0-52000 Disorder of sweat glands, NOS 705.9
(T-01380)

D0-52010 Anhidrosis 705.0
(T-01380) (F-03305)

D0-52020 Hypohidrosis 705.0
(T-01380) (F-03304)
Oligohidrosis 705.0
(T-01380) (F-03304)

D0-52040 Miliaria, NOS

D0-52042 Prickly heat 705.1
(T-01381) (M-34000)
Heat rash 705.1
(T-01381) (M-34000)
Miliaria rubra 705.1
(T-01381) (M-34000)
Miliaria tropicalis 705.1
(T-01381) (M-34000)

D0-52044 Miliaria crystallina 705.1
(T-01381) (M-34000)
Sudamina 705.1
(T-01381) (M-34000)

D0-52050 Fox-Fordyce disease 705.82
(T-01320)
Apocrine miliaria 705.82
(T-01320)

D0-52058 Apocrine gland cyst
(T-01320) (M-33400)
Apocrine cyst
(T-01320) (M-33400)
Apocrine cystomatosis
(T-01320) (M-33400)

D0-52060 Dyshidrosis 705.81
Cheiropompholyx 705.81
Pompholyx 705.81
Dyshidria 705.81
Dysidrosis 705.81
Dysidria 705.81
Chiropompholyx 705.81

D0-52070 Granulosis rubra nasi 705.89
(T-01380)

D0-52100 Hidradenitis 705.83
(T-01320) (M-40000)

D0-52110 Hidradenitis suppurativa 705.83
(T-01320) (M-43600)

D0-52210 Bromhidrosis 705.89
(T-01380)
Bromidrosis 705.89
(T-01380)
Osmidrosis 705.89
(T-01380)
Ozochrotia 705.89
(T-01380)

0-52 DISEASES OF THE SWEAT GLANDS — Continued

D0-52220 Chromhidrosis 705.89
(T-01380)
D0-52230 Urhidrosis 705.89
(T-01380)
Uridrosis 705.89
(T-01380)
D0-52250 Sweat gland cyst, NOS
(T-01380) (M-33400)
Sudoriferous cyst, NOS
(T-01380) (M-33400)
D0-52280 Other specified disorder of sweat gland, NEC 705.89
(T-01380)

0-53 DISEASES OF THE HAIR AND HAIR FOLLICLES

D0-53000 Disease of hair and hair follicle, NOS 704.9
(T-01400)
D0-53100 Alopecia, NOS 704.00
(T-01400)
Loss of hair 704.00
(T-01400)
Baldness 704.00
(T-01400)
D0-53102 Male pattern alopecia 704.00
Common baldness 704.00
D0-53106 Female pattern alopecia 704.00
D0-53110 Alopecia areata 704.1
(T-01400)
D0-53112 Ophiasis 704.01
(T-01400)
D0-53120V Atrichia, NOS
(T-01400)
D0-53200 Hypotrichosis, NOS 704.09
(T-01400)
D0-53210 Postinfectional hypotrichosis, NOS 704.09
(T-01400)
D0-53220 Hypertrichosis, NOS 704.1
(T-01400)
Polytrichia, NOS 704.1
(T-01400)
Hypertrichiasis, NOS 704.1
(T-01400)
Polytrichosis, NOS 704.1
(T-01400)
D0-53222 Hypertrichosis lanuginosa 704.1
(T-01400)
D0-53224 Hypertrichosis universalis
D0-53228 Hypertrichosis pinnae auris
Hairy ears
D0-53230 Hirsutism, NOS 704.1
(T-01400)
Hirsuties 704.1
(T-01400)
Pilosis 704.1
(T-01400)
D0-53250 Trichorrhexis, NOS
D0-53251 Trichorrhexis nodosa 704.2
(T-01400)
Clastothrix 704.2
(T-01400)
Trichorrhexis invaginata
Bamboo hair
D0-53260 Trichostasis spinulosa
D0-53270 Atrophic hair 704.2
(T-01400)
D0-53272 Fragilitas crinium 704.2
(T-01400)
Brittle hair
D0-53280 Trichiasis, NOS 704.2
(T-01400)
D0-53288 Cicatricial trichiasis 704.2
(T-01400)
D0-53300 Variation in hair color, NOS 704.3
(T-01400)
D0-53310 Premature canities 704.3
(T-01400)
Premature grayness of hair 704.3
(T-01400)
D0-53320 Heterochromia of hair 704.3
(T-01400)
D0-53330 Poliosis, NOS 704.3
(T-01400)
D0-53332 Acquired poliosis circumscripta 704.3
(T-01400)
D0-53502 Agminate folliculitis
D0-53510 Folliculitis decalvans 704.09
(T-01400)
Pustular folliculitis 704.8
(T-01400) (M-41400)
D0-53513 Alopecia totalis
D0-53514 Alopecia universalis
D0-53515 Alopecia cicatrisata 704.09
(T-01400)
Pseudopelade 704.09
(T-01400)
Pseudopelade of Brocq 704.09
(T-01400)
Cicatricial alopecia 704.09
(T-01400)
Scarring alopecia 704.09
(T-01400)
D0-53516 Alopecia mucinosa
D0-53550 Perifolliculitis capitis abscedens et suffodiens 704.8
(T-01400) (T-B0160) (M-41400) (M-41610) (M-46500)
Folliculitis abscedens et suffodiens 704.8
(T-01400) (T-B0160) (M-41400)
D0-53552 Perifolliculitis of the scalp 704.8
(T-01400) (T-B0160) (M-40000)
D0-53560 Disseminate infundibulo-folliculitis
D0-53570 Sycosis, NOS 704.8
(T-01400) (T-B0200) (M-40000)

D0-53572 Lupoid sycosis 704.8
(T-01400) (T-B0200) (M-41400)
D0-53580 Folliculitis nares perforans
Perforating folliculitis
(T-01000)
D0-53600 Endocrine alopecia
(T-01400)
D0-53610 Psychogenic alopecia
(T-01400)
D0-53620V Collar frictional alopecia
D0-53630V Nutritional alopecia, NOS
D0-53640 Radiation alopecia
D0-53642 Thermal burn alopecia
D0-53644 Frostbite alopecia
D0-53650V Color mutant alopecia
D0-53670V Equine cannon keratosis
Stud crud
D0-53672V Equine linear keratosis
D0-53700 Drug-related alopecia, NOS
Alopecia medicamentosa
D0-53710 Telogen effluvium
D0-53712 Anagen effluvium

0-54 DISEASES OF THE NAILS

D0-54000 Disease of nail, NOS 703.9
(T-01600)
D0-54010 Ingrowing nail 703.0
(T-01600)
Unguis incarnatus 703.0
(T-01600)
D0-54012 Ingrowing nail with infection 703.0
(T-01600)
D0-54100 Dystrophia unguium 703.8
(T-01600)
Onychodystrophy 703.8
(T-01600)
D0-54110 Hypertrophy of nail 703.8
(T-01600)
D0-54120 Koilonychia 703.8
(T-01600)
D0-54130 Leukonychia 703.8
(T-01600)
D0-54132 Leukonychia punctata 703.8
(T-01600)
D0-54134 Leukonychia striata 703.8
(T-01600)
D0-54150 Onychauxis 703.8
(T-01600)
D0-54160 Onychogryposis 703.8
(T-01600)
D0-54170 Onycholysis 703.8
(T-01600)
D0-54200V Equine laminitis
Founder
D0-54202V Metabolic laminitis
D0-54300V Bruised sole
D0-54310V Corns, equine
D0-54320V Canker, equine
D0-54340V Contracted heels
D0-54350V Pyramidal disease
Extensor process disease
Buttress foot
D0-54360V Sandcrack
Toe crack
Quarter crack
D0-54370V Seedy toe
Hollow wall
Dystrophia ungulae
D0-54380V Sheared heels

SECTION 0-6 SKIN ULCERS AND SCARS

D0-60100 Ulcer of skin, NOS 707.9
(T-01000) (M-38000)
D0-60103 Chronic ulcer of skin, NOS 707.9
(T-01000) (M-38020)
D0-60104 Trophic ulcer, NOS 707.9
(T-01000) (M-38120)
Ischemic ulcer, NOS 707.9
(T-01000) (M-38120)
D0-60106 Tropical ulcer, NOS 707.9
(T-01000) (M-38180)
D0-60110 Decubitus ulcer 707.0
(T-01000) (M-10400)
Pressure ulcer 707.0
(T-01000) (M-10400)
Bed sore 707.0
(T-01000) (M-10400)
Decubitus 707.0
(T-01000) (M-10400)
Contact ulcer 707.0
(T-01000) (M-10400)
D0-60116V Saddle sore
Saddle gall
D0-60117V Collar gall
D0-60120 Plaster ulcer 707.0
(T-01000) (M-10400)
D0-60130 Chronic ulcer of lower extremity, NOS 707.1
(T-01000) (T-B9000) (M-38020)
D0-60132 Chronic neurogenic ulcer of lower limb 707.1
(T-01000) (T-B9000) (M-38310)
D0-60134 Chronic trophic ulcer of lower limb 707.1
(T-01000) (T-B9000) (M-38120)
D0-60140 Chronic ulcer of other specified site 707.8
(T-01000) (T-00003) (M-38020)
D0-60142 Chronic neurogenic ulcer of other specified site 707.8
(T-01000) (M-00003) (M-38310)
D0-60144 Chronic trophic ulcer of other specified site 707.8
(T-01000) (T-00003) (M-38120)
D0-60150V Familial acantholysis
D0-61000 Scar of skin, NOS 709.2
(T-01000) (M-78060)
Cicatrix of skin, NOS 709.2
(T-01000) (M-78060)

SECTION 0-6 SKIN ULCERS AND SCARS — Continued

D0-61110 Adherent scar 709.2
(T-01000) (M-78060) (M-78400)

D0-61120 Disfigurement due to scar 709.2
(T-01000) (M-78060)

SECTION 0-7 PIGMENTATION DISORDERS, DRUG ERUPTIONS AND DISORDERS DUE TO PHYSICAL AGENTS

0-70 SKIN PIGMENTATION DISORDERS

D0-70000 Anomalous pigmentation of skin, NOS 709.0
(T-01000)
Dyschromia 709.0
(T-01000)

D0-70010 Café au lait spots 709.0
(T-01000)

D0-70020 Chloasma, NOS 709.0
(T-01000)
Melasma, NOS 709.0
(T-01000)

D0-70022 Idiopathic chloasma 709.0
(T-01000)

D0-70024 Symptomatic chloasma 709.0
(T-01000)

D0-70030 Ephelides 709.0
(T-01000)
Ephelis 709.0
(T-01000)
Freckle 709.0
(T-01000)

D0-70100 Hyperpigmentation of skin, NOS 709.0
(T-01000)

D0-70110 Lentigo, NOS 709.0
(T-01000)
Lentigo simplex 709.0
(T-01000)
Nevus spilus 709.0
(T-01000)

D0-70112 Senile lentigo
Solar lentigo
Liver spot

D0-70120 Melanoderma 709.0
(T-01000)

D0-70122 Parasitic melanoderma
Vagabond's disease
Vagabond's melanosis

D0-70124 Senile melanoderma

D0-70130 Progressive pigmentary dermatosis 709.0
(T-01000)

D0-70140 Pigmented xerodermoid

D0-70150 Tattoo 709.0
(T-01000)

D0-70200 Hypopigmentation of skin, NOS 709.0
(T-01000)

D0-70210 Leukoderma 709.0
(T-01000)

D0-70220 Vitiligo 709.0
(T-01000)

0-71 DRUG ERUPTIONS

D0-71000 Eruption due to drug, NOS
(T-01000) (M-01710) (G-C001)
(C-50000)

D0-71100 Fixed drug eruption, NOS

D0-71102 Fixed drug eruption due to phenolphthalein
(T-01000) (M-01710) (G-C001)
(C-84893)

D0-71110 Bullae and sweat gland necrosis in drug-induced coma

D0-71200 Drug-induced photosensitivity

D0-71210 Photoallergic drug eruption

D0-71220 Phototoxic drug eruption

D0-71224 Chlorpromazine pigmentation

D0-71300 Food-induced photosensitivity

D0-71400 Drug-induced lupus erythematosus, NOS

D0-71410 Drug-induced lupus erythematosus due to procainamide

D0-71420 Drug-induced lupus erythematosus due to hydralazine

D0-71430 Drug-induced lupus erythematosus due to diphenylhydantoin

D0-71510 Bromoderma

D0-71520 Iododerma

D0-71530 Argyria of skin
Pigmentation of skin by silver salts

D0-71540 Mercury pigmentation of skin

D0-71550 Arsenical keratosis of the palms and soles

0-75 SKIN DISORDERS DUE TO PHYSICAL AGENTS AND FOREIGN SUBSTANCES

D0-75100 Polymorphous light eruption, NOS
Allergy to sunlight

D0-75110 Polymorphous light eruption, papular type

D0-75120 Polymorphous light eruption, papulovesicular type

D0-75130 Polymorphous light eruption, eczematous type

D0-75140 Polymorphous light eruption, plaque type

D0-75150 Polymorphous light eruption, diffuse erythematous type

D0-75200 Radiation dermatitis, NOS
Radiodermatitis, NOS

D0-75201 Early radiation dermatitis
Acute radiation dermatitis

D0-75202 Late radiation dermatitis
Chronic radiation dermatitis

D0-75205 Actinic dermatitis
(T-01000)
Actinic dermatosis
(T-01000)

D0-75230 Actinic reticuloid

D0-75310 Calcaneal petechiae
Black heel disease

D0-75500 Foreign body granuloma of skin, NOS 709.4
(T-01000) (M-44140)
Foreign body reaction of the skin, NOS 709.4
(T-01000) (M-44140)

D0-75502 Foreign body granuloma of subcutaneous tissue, NOS 709.4
(T-03000) (M-44140)

D0-75510 Foreign body reaction to oily substance, NOS
(T-01000) (M-44040)

D0-75512 Paraffinoma of skin, NOS
(T-01000) (M-44040)
Lipid granuloma of skin caused by mineral oil
(T-01000) (M-44040)

D0-75520 Silica granuloma of skin
(T-01000) (M-44000)

D0-75530 Starch granuloma of skin
(T-01000) (M-44000)

D0-75540 Interdigital pilonidal sinus
(T-02725) (T-09250)

D0-75550 Zirconium granuloma of skin
(T-01000) (M-44000)

D0-75560 Beryllium granuloma of skin
(T-01000) (M-44000)

D0-75570 Tattoo granuloma
(T-01000) (M-44000)
Foreign body reaction to tattoo dyes
(T-01000) (M-44000)

D0-75600 Skin deposits, NOS 709.3
(T-01000) (M-55000)

D0-75610 Calcinosis cutis 709.3
(T-01000) (M-55500)

D0-75650 Subcutaneous calcification, NOS 709.3
(T-03000) (M-55400)

D0-75655 Calcinosis circumscripta 709.3
(T-03000) (T-13000) (M-55400)

SECTION 0-8 TUMOR-LIKE LESIONS OF THE SKIN

D0-80100 Hypertrophic condition of skin, NOS 701.9
(T-01000) (M-71000)

D0-80110 Corn of toe 700.-
(T-01000) (M-72740)
Clavus 700.-
(T-01000) (M-72740)

D0-80111 Soft corn
Heloma molle

D0-80112 Hard corn
Heloma durum

D0-80120 Keloid scar of skin 701.4
(T-01000) (M-78720)
Cheloid of skin 701.4
(T-01000) (M-78720)
Keloid of skin 701.4
(T-01000) (M-78720)

D0-80122 Hypertrophic scar of skin 701.4
(T-01000) (M-78720)

D0-80130 Abnormal granulation tissue 701.5
(T-01000) (M-45020)
Excessive granulation tissue 701.5
(T-01000) (M-45020)

D0-80132V Exuberant granulation tissue
(T-01000) (M-45020)
Proud flesh
(T-01000) (M-45020)

D0-80160 Leukokeratosis of skin, nOS 702.-
(T-01000) (M-72830)
Leukoplakia of skin, NOS 702.-
(T-01000) (M-72830)

D0-80210 Angioma serpiginosum 709.1
(T-01000)

D0-80212 Angiokeratoma circumscriptum
(T-01000) (M-91410)

D0-80214 Angiokeratoma of Fordyce
(T-98000) (M-91410)
Angiokeratoma of scrotum
(T-98000) (M-91410)

D0-80216 Angiokeratoma of Mibelli
(T-02671) (T-02871) (M-91410)

D0-80250 Epithelial hyperplasia of skin, NOS 709.8
(T-01000) (M-72150)

D0-80300 Pseudolymphoma, NOS
Benign lymphocytoma cutis
Cutaneous lymphoid hyperplasia
Pseudolymphoma of Spiegler-Fendt
Lymphocytoma cutis
Benign cutaneous lymphoid hyperplasia

SECTION 0-9 INFLAMMATORY DISEASES OF THE SUBCUTANEOUS FAT AND NONINFECTIOUS GRANULOMAS

D0-90110 Erythema nodosum, NOS 695.2
(T-03000) (M-40000)

D0-90112 Erythema nodosum, acute form 695.2
(T-03000) (M-41000)

D0-90114 Erythema nodosum, chronic form 695.2
(T-03000) (M-43000)

D0-90120 Erythema induratum 695.2
(T-03000) (M-44000) (M-44700)

D0-90130 Superficial migratory thrombophlebitis
(T-48040) (M-40000) (M-35100)

D0-90150 Relapsing febrile nodular nonsuppurative panniculitis 729.30
(T-03000)
Weber-Christian disease 729.30
(T-03000)

D0-90160 Subcutaneous nodular fat necrosis in pancreatitis
(T-03000)

D0-90170 Cold panniculitis
(T-03000)

SECTION 0-9 INFLAMMATORY DISEASES OF THE SUBCUTANEOUS FAT AND NONINFECTIOUS GRANULOMAS — Continued

D0-90320 Granuloma annulare
D0-90340 Necrobiosis lipoidica, NOS
(T-01000) (T-1A200) (M-50000)
D0-90342 Necrobiosis lipoidica, necrobiotic type
(T-01000) (T-1A200) (M-50000)
D0-90343 Necrobiosis lipoidica, granulomatous type
(T-01000) (T-1A200) (M-50000)
D0-90346 Necrobiosis lipoidica diabeticorum
D0-90350 Subcutaneous rheumatoid nodule
(T-03000)
D0-90400 Subcutaneous emphysema

CHAPTER 1 — DISEASES OF THE MUSCULOSKELETAL SYSTEM AND CONNECTIVE TISSUES

SECTION 1-0 DISEASES OF THE MUSCULOSKELETAL SYSTEM AND CONNECTIVE TISSUES: GENERAL TERMS

D1-00000 Disease of the musculoskeletal system, NOS
Disorder of the musculoskeletal system, NOS
D1-00010 Polymyalgia rheumatica 725.-

SECTION 1-1 DISEASES OF THE CONNECTIVE TISSUES

D1-10000 Collagen disease, NOS 710.9
Diffuse disease of connective tissue, NOS 710.9
D1-10100 Systemic lupus erythematosus 710.0
Disseminated lupus erythematosus 710.0
D1-10200 Systemic sclerosis 710.1
Progressive systemic sclerosis 710.1
Scleroderma 710.1
D1-10220 Acrosclerosis 710.1
D1-10230 CRST syndrome 710.1
Calcinosis cutis, Raynaud's, sclerodactyly and telangiectasia 710.1
D1-10240 CREST syndrome 710.1
Calcinosis cutis, Raynaud's, esophageal dysfunction, sclerodactyly and telangiectasia 710.1
D1-10250 Sicca syndrome 710.2
Sjogren's disease 710.2
D1-10260 Keratoconjunctivitis sicca 710.2
D1-10300 Dermatomyositis 710.3
Polymyositis with skin involvement 710.3
D1-10310 Poikilodermatomyositis 710.3
D1-10320 Polymyositis 710.4
D1-10330 Inclusion body myositis 710.4
D1-10340 Neuromyositis 710.4
D1-10400 Systemic fibrosclerosing syndrome 710.8
D1-10410 Idiopathic multifocal fibrosclerosis, NEC 710.8
D1-10480 Other specified diffuse disease of connective tissue, NEC 710.8

SECTION 1-2 DISEASES OF THE JOINTS

1-20 INFLAMMATORY ARTHROPATHIES

D1-20000 Arthropathy, NOS 716.9
Disorder of joint, NOS 719.9
Joint disease, NOS 716.9
Arthrosis, NOS 716.9
D1-20001 Acute arthropathy 716.9
D1-20002 Subacute arthropathy 716.9
D1-20003 Chronic arthropathy 716.9
D1-20010 Polyarthropathy, NOS 716.5
Multiple joint disease, NOS 716.5
Polyarthrosis, NOS 716.5
D1-20012 Chronic articular rheumatism 716.9
D1-20050 Arthritis, NOS 716.9
D1-20051 Acute arthritis 716.9
D1-20052 Subacute arthritis 716.9
D1-20053 Chronic arthritis 716.9
D1-20060 Polyarthritis, NOS 716.5
D1-20100 Arthropathy associated with infection, NOS 711.-
Infection-associated arthritis, NOS 711.-
D1-20110 Pyogenic arthritis, NOS 711.0
Pyoarthrosis, NOS 711.0
D1-20111 Pyogenic arthritis of shoulder region 711.01
D1-20112 Pyogenic arthritis of upper arm 711.02
D1-20113 Pyogenic arthritis of forearm 711.03
D1-20114 Pyogenic arthritis of hand 711.04
D1-20115 Pyogenic arthritis of pelvic region 711.05
D1-20116 Pyogenic arthritis of thigh 711.05
D1-20117 Pyogenic arthritis of lower leg 711.06
D1-20118 Pyogenic arthritis of ankle 711.07
D1-20119 Pyogenic arthritis of foot 711.07
D1-2011A Pyogenic arthritis of multiple sites 711.09
D1-2011BV Joint-ill
Pyogenic purulent arthritis of newborn
D1-20120 Arthropathy associated with Reiter's disease 711.1
D1-20130 Arthropathy associated with nonspecific urethritis 711.1
D1-20140 Arthropathy in Behcet's syndrome 711.2
D1-20150 Postdysenteric arthropathy 711.3
D1-20160 Arthropathy associated with bacterial disease, NEC 711.4
D1-20170 Arthropathy associated with viral disease, NEC 711.5
D1-20180 Arthropathy associated with a mycosis, NEC 711.6
D1-20190 Arthropathy associated with helminthiasis, NEC 711.7
D1-201A0 Arthropathy associated with other infectious or parasitic disease, NEC 711.8
D1-201B0 Infective arthritis, NOS 711.9
D1-201B1 Infective polyarthritis, NOS 711.9
D1-201C0 Acute infective arthritis, NOS 711.9
D1-201C1 Acute infective polyarthritis, NOS 711.9
D1-201D0 Subacute infective arthritis 711.9
D1-201D1 Subacute infective polyarthritis, NOS 711.9
D1-201E0 Chronic infective arthritis, NOS 711.9
D1-201E1 Chronic infective polyarthritis, NOS 711.9
D1-20210V Quittor
D1-20220V Osselets
D1-20300 Crystal arthropathy, NOS 712.9
Crystal-induced arthritis and synovitis, NOS 712.9
D1-20301 Crystal arthropathy of shoulder region 712.01
D1-20302 Crystal arthropathy of upper arm 712.02

1-20 INFLAMMATORY ARTHROPATHIES — Continued

D1-20303 Crystal arthropathy of forearm 712.03
D1-20304 Crystal arthropathy of hand 712.04
D1-20305 Crystal arthropathy of pelvic region 712.05
D1-20306 Crystal arthropathy of thigh 712.05
D1-20307 Crystal arthropathy of lower leg 712.06
D1-20308 Crystal arthropathy of ankle and foot 712.07
D1-20309 Crystal arthropathy of other site 712.08
D1-2030A Crystal arthropathy of multiple sites 712.09
D1-20400 Arthropathy associated with disorder classified elsewhere 713.-
D1-20402 Polyarthropathy associated with disorder classified elsewhere 713.-
D1-20404 Arthritis associated with disorder classified elsewhere 713.-
D1-20406 Polyarthritis associated with disorder classified elsewhere 713.-
D1-20410 Arthropathy associated with an endocrine or metabolic disorder 713.0
D1-20420 Arthropathy associated with a non-infectious gastrointestinal condition 713.1
D1-20430 Arthropathy associated with a hematological disorder 713.2
D1-20432 Hemophilic arthropathy
D1-20440 Arthropathy associated with a dermatological disorder 713.3
D1-20450 Arthropathy associated with a respiratory disorder 713.4
D1-20460 Arthropathy associated with a neurological disorder 713.5
D1-20461 Charcot's arthropathy 713.5
  Neuropathic arthropathy 713.5
D1-20470 Arthropathy associated with a hypersensitivity reaction 713.6
D1-20480 Arthropathy associated with an other systemic disease 713.7
D1-20490 Arthropathy associated with a condition classifiable elsewhere 713.8
D1-20510V Idiopathic polyarthritis
D1-20520V Progressive feline polyarthritis
D1-20530V Polyarthritis in Greyhounds
D1-20540V Enzootic polyarthritis in goats
D1-20600 Rheumatoid arthritis 714.0
  Atrophic arthritis 714.0
  Chronic rheumatic arthritis 714.0
D1-20610 Felty's syndrome 714.1
  Rheumatoid arthritis, leukopenia and splenadenomegaly 714.1
D1-20618 Rheumatoid arthritis with other visceral or systemic involvement 714.2
D1-20620 Juvenile chronic polyarthritis, NOS 714.3
D1-20622 Polyarticular juvenile rheumatoid arthritis, NOS 714.30
  Juvenile rheumatoid arthritis, NOS 714.30
D1-20623 Chronic polyarticular juvenile rheumatoid arthritis 714.30
D1-20624 Still's disease 714.30
D1-20630 Acute polyarticular juvenile rheumatoid arthritis 714.31
  Acute juvenile rheumatoid arthritis 714.31
D1-20640 Pauciarticular juvenile rheumatoid arthritis 714.32
D1-20644 Monoarticular juvenile rheumatoid arthritis 714.33
D1-20650 Chronic postrheumatic arthropathy 714.4
D1-20652 Chronic rheumatoid nodular fibrosis 714.4
D1-20654 Jaccoud's syndrome 714.4
D1-20660 Extra-articular rheumatoid process, NOS 714.8
D1-20700 Inflammatory polyarthropathy, NOS 714.9
  Inflammatory polyarthritis, NOS 714.9

1-21 DEGENERATIVE JOINT DISEASES AND MISCELLANEOUS ARTHROPATHIES

D1-21000 Degenerative joint disease, NOS 715.9
  Osteoarthrosis, NOS 715.9
  Degenerative arthritis, NOS 715.9
  Degenerative polyarthritis, NOS 715.9
  Hypertrophic arthritis, NOS 715.9
  Hypertrophic polyarthritis, NOS 715.9
  Osteoarthritis, NOS 715.9
D1-21001 Degenerative joint disease of shoulder region 715.-1
D1-21002 Degenerative joint disease of upper arm 715.-2
D1-21003 Degenerative joint disease of forearm 715.-3
D1-21004 Degenerative joint disease of hand 715.-4
D1-21005 Degenerative joint disease of pelvic region 715.-4
D1-21006 Degenerative joint disease of thigh 715.-4
D1-21007 Degenerative joint disease of lower leg 715.-6
D1-21008 Degenerative joint disease of ankle and foot 715.-7
D1-21009 Degenerative joint disease of other site 715.-8
D1-21020 Degenerative joint disease involving multiple joints 715.0
  Generalized osteoarthrosis 715.0
  Primary generalized hypertrophic osteoarthrosis 715.0
D1-21030 Primary localized osteoarthrosis, NOS 715.1
  Idiopathic localized osteoarthropathy, NOS 715.1
D1-21031 Primary localized osteoarthrosis of shoulder region 715.11
D1-21032 Primary localized osteoarthrosis of upper arm 715.12
D1-21033 Primary localized osteoarthrosis of forearm 715.13
D1-21034 Primary localized osteoarthrosis of hand 715.14
D1-21035 Primary localized osteoarthrosis of pelvic region 715.15
D1-21036 Primary localized osteoarthrosis of thigh 715.15

D1-21037 Primary localized osteoarthrosis of lower leg 715.16
D1-21038 Primary localized osteoarthrosis of ankle and foot 715.17
D1-21039 Primary localized osteoarthrosis of other site 715.18
D1-2103A Primary localized osteoarthrosis of multiple sites 715.19
D1-21040 Secondary localized osteoarthrosis, NOS 715.2
D1-21041 Secondary localized osteoarthrosis of shoulder region 715.21
D1-21042 Secondary localized osteoarthrosis of upper arm 715.22
D1-21043 Secondary localized osteoarthrosis of forearm 715.23
D1-21044 Secondary localized osteoarthrosis of hand 715.24
D1-21045 Secondary localized osteoarthrosis of pelvic region 715.25
D1-21046 Secondary localized osteoarthrosis of thigh 715.25
D1-21047 Secondary localized osteoarthrosis of lower leg 715.26
D1-21048 Secondary localized osteoarthrosis of ankle and foot 715.27
D1-21049 Secondary localized osteoarthrosis of other site 715.28
D1-2104A Secondary localized osteoarthrosis of multiple sites 715.29
D1-21050 Coxae malum senilis 715.2
D1-21060 Localized osteoarthrosis uncertain if primary or secondary 715.3
D1-21070 Otto's pelvis 715.3
D1-21080 Osteoarthrosis involving multiple sites but not designated as generalized 715.8
D1-21300 Traumatic arthropathy 716.1
D1-21320 Allergic arthritis 716.2
D1-21330 Climacteric arthritis 716.3
  Menopausal arthritis 716.3
D1-21340 Transient arthropathy 716.4
D1-21360 Unspecified monoarthritis 716.6
D1-21362 Coxitis 716.6
D1-21380 Other specified arthropathy, NEC 716.8

1-22 DERANGEMENTS OF THE JOINTS OTHER THAN VERTEBRAL COLUMN

D1-22010 Derangement of knee, NOS 717.9
  Internal derangement of knee, NOS 717.9
D1-22012 Degeneration of cartilage or meniscus of knee, NOS 717.9
D1-22014 Old rupture of cartilage or meniscus of knee, NOS 717.9
  Old tear of cartilage or meniscus of knee, NOS 717.9
D1-22020 Old bucket handle tear of medial meniscus 717.0
D1-22021 Derangement of anterior horn of medial meniscus 717.1
D1-22022 Derangement of posterior horn of medial meniscus 717.2
D1-22024 Degeneration of internal semilunar cartilage 717.3
D1-22027 Other unspecified derangement of medial meniscus, NEC 717.3
D1-22028 Old bucket handle tear of unspecified cartilage 717.0
D1-22030 Derangement of lateral meniscus, NOS 717.40
D1-22032 Bucket handle tear of lateral meniscus 717.41
D1-22034 Derangement of anterior horn of lateral meniscus 717.42
D1-22035 Derangement of posterior horn of lateral meniscus 717.43
D1-22038 Other derangement of lateral meniscus 717.49
D1-22040 Derangement of meniscus, NEC 717.5
  Derangement of semilunar cartilage, NEC 717.5
D1-22046 Cyst of semilunar cartilage 717.5
D1-22050 Loose body in knee, NOS 717.6
  Joint mice of knee 717.6
D1-22052 Rice bodies of knee joint 717.6
D1-22060 Old disruption of ligament of knee, NOS 717.89
D1-22062 Old disruption of lateral collateral ligament 717.81
D1-22063 Old disruption of medial collateral ligament 717.82
D1-22064 Old disruption of anterior cruciate ligament 717.83
D1-22065 Old disruption of posterior cruciate ligament 717.84
D1-22066 Old disruption of capsular ligament of knee 717.85
D1-22068V Rupture of cruciate ligaments
D1-22069 Old disruption of other ligament of knee 717.85
D1-22100 Chondromalacia of patella 717.7
  Chondromalacia patellae 717.7
  Degeneration of articular cartilage of patella 717.7
D1-22300 Derangement of joint other than knee, NOS 718.9
D1-22310 Articular cartilage disorder, NOS 718.0
D1-22311 Articular cartilage disorder of shoulder region 718.01
D1-22312 Articular cartilage disorder of upper arm 718.02
D1-22313 Articular cartilage disorder of forearm 718.03
D1-22314 Articular cartilage disorder of hand 718.04
D1-22315 Articular cartilage disorder of pelvic region 718.05
D1-22316 Articular cartilage disorder of thigh 718.05

1-22 DERANGEMENTS OF THE JOINTS OTHER THAN VERTEBRAL COLUMN — Continued

D1-22317 Articular cartilage disorder of lower leg 718.06
D1-22318 Articular cartilage disorder of ankle and foot 718.07
D1-22319 Articular cartilage disorder of other site 718.08
D1-2231A Articular cartilage disorder of multiple sites 718.09
D1-22320 Meniscus disorder, other than knee, NOS 718.0
D1-22322 Old rupture of meniscus, other than knee, NOS 718.0
  Old tear of meniscus, other than knee, NOS 718.0
D1-22324 Old rupture of ligaments of joint, other than knee, NOS 718.0
D1-22330 Loose body in joint 718.1
  Joint mice 718.1
  Melon seed bodies in joint 718.1
  Corpora libra in joint
  Free bodies in joint 718.1
D1-22350 Pathological dislocation of joint, NOS 718.20
  Dislocation or displacement of joint, not recurrent or current injury 718.20
  Spontaneous dislocation of joint, NOS 718.20
D1-22351 Pathological dislocation of shoulder region 718.21
D1-22352 Pathological dislocation of upper arm 718.22
D1-22353 Pathological dislocation of forearm 718.23
D1-22354 Pathological dislocation of hand 718.24
D1-22355 Pathological dislocation of pelvic region 718.25
D1-22356 Pathological dislocation of thigh 718.25
D1-22357 Pathological dislocation of lower leg 718.26
D1-22358 Pathological dislocation of ankle and foot 718.27
D1-22359 Pathological dislocation of other site, NEC 718.28
D1-2235A Pathological dislocation of multiple sites 718.29
D1-22360 Recurrent dislocation of joint, NOS 718.30
D1-22361 Recurrent dislocation of shoulder region 718.31
D1-22362 Recurrent dislocation of upper arm 718.32
D1-22363 Recurrent dislocation of forearm 718.33
D1-22364 Recurrent dislocation of hand 718.34
D1-22365 Recurrent dislocation of pelvic region 718.35
D1-22366 Recurrent dislocation of thigh 718.35
D1-22367 Recurrent dislocation of lower leg 718.36
D1-22368 Recurrent dislocation of ankle and foot 718.37
D1-22369 Recurrent dislocation of other site, NEC 718.38
D1-2236A Recurrent dislocation of multiple sites 718.39
D1-22370 Contracture of joint, NOS 718.40
D1-22371 Contracture of joint of shoulder region 718.41
D1-22372 Contracture of joint of upper arm 718.42
D1-22373 Contracture of joint of forearm 718.43
D1-22374 Contracture of joint of hand 718.44
D1-22375 Contracture of joint of pelvic region 718.45
D1-22376 Contracture of joint of thigh 718.45
D1-22377 Contracture of joint of lower leg 718.46
D1-22378 Contracture of joint of ankle and foot 718.47
D1-22379 Contracture of joint of other site, NEC 718.48
D1-2237A Contracture of joint of multiple sites 718.49
D1-22381 Ankylosis of joint of shoulder region 718.51
D1-22382 Ankylosis of joint of upper arm 718.52
D1-22383 Ankylosis of joint of forearm 718.53
D1-22384 Ankylosis of joint of hand 718.54
D1-22385 Ankylosis of joint of pelvic region 718.55
D1-22386 Ankylosis of joint of thigh 718.55
D1-22387 Ankylosis of joint of lower leg 718.56
D1-22388 Ankylosis of joint of ankle and foot 718.57
D1-22389 Ankylosis of joint of other site 718.58
D1-2238A Ankylosis of joint of multiple sites 718.59
D1-22390 Intrapelvic protrusion of acetabulum, NOS 718.6
  Protrusio acetabuli, NOS 718.6
D1-223A0 Other joint derangement, NEC 718.8
D1-223A2 Paralytic flail joint 718.8
D1-223A4 Instability of joint 718.8
  Unstable joint 718.8
D1-22500 Other disorder of joint, NOS 719
D1-22510 Effusion of joint, NOS 719.00
  Hydrarthrosis, NOS 719.00
  Painful swelling of joint
D1-22511 Effusion of joint of shoulder region 719.01
D1-22512 Effusion of joint of upper arm 719.02
D1-22513 Effusion of joint of forearm 719.03
D1-22514 Effusion of joint of hand 719.04
D1-22515 Effusion of joint of pelvic region 719.05
D1-22516 Effusion of joint of thigh 719.05
D1-22517 Effusion of joint of lower leg 719.06
D1-22518 Effusion of joint of ankle and foot 719.07
D1-22519 Effusion of joint of other site, NEC 719.08
D1-2251A Effusion of joint of multiple sites 719.09
D1-22530 Hemarthrosis, NOS 719.10
D1-22531 Hemarthrosis of shoulder region 719.11
D1-22532 Hemarthrosis of upper arm 719.12
D1-22533 Hemarthrosis of forearm 719.13
D1-22534 Hemarthrosis of hand 719.14
D1-22535 Hemarthrosis of pelvic region 719.15
D1-22536 Hemarthrosis of thigh 718.15
D1-22537 Hemarthrosis of lower leg 719.16
D1-22538 Hemarthrosis of ankle and foot 719.17
D1-22539 Hemarthrosis of other site, NEC 719.18
D1-2253A Hemarthrosis of multiple sites 719.19
D1-22540 Villonodular synovitis 719.2
D1-22550 Palindromic rheumatism 719.3
  Hench-Rosenberg syndrome 719.3
  Intermittent hydrarthrosis 719.3

D1-22630 Snapping hip 719.6
Perrin-Ferraton disease 719.6
D1-22660 Other specified disorder of joint, NEC 719.8
D1-22670 Calcification of joint 719.8
D1-22680 Fistula of joint 719.8
D1-22710V Patellar luxation

1-23 DISORDERS OF THE VERTEBRAL COLUMN

D1-23000 Disorder of the vertebral column, NOS 724.9
Dorsopathy, NOS 724.9
Spinal disorder, NOS 724.9
D1-23100 Spondylitis, NOS 720.9
Inflammatory spondylopathy, NOS 720.9
D1-23110 Ankylosing spondylitis, NOS 720.0
Rheumatoid arthritis of spine, NOS 720.0
Marie Strümpell spondylitis 720.0
Rheumatoid spondylitis 720.0
Spondylosis deformans
D1-23140 Spinal enthesopathy, NOS 720.1
D1-23150 Sacroiliitis, NOS 720.2
Inflammation of sacroiliac joint, NOS 720.2
D1-23180 Other inflammatory spondylopathy, NEC 720.89
D1-23190 Inflammatory spondylopathy in disease classified elsewhere 720.81
D1-23300 Spondylosis, NOS 721.9
Spondylarthrosis, NOS 721.9
D1-23310 Spondylosis without mention of myelopathy 721.90
Spinal osteoarthritis 721.90
D1-23312 Spinal arthritis deformans 721.90
Degenerative spinal arthritis 721.90
Hypertrophic spinal arthritis 721.90
D1-23320 Spondylosis with myelopathy, NOS 721.91
Spondylogenic compression of spinal cord, NOS 721.91
D1-23330 Cervical spondylosis without myelopathy 721.0
Cervical osteoarthritis 721.0
D1-23332 Cervical spondyloarthritis 721.0
Cervical arthritis 721.0
D1-23340 Cervical spondylosis with myelopathy 721.1
Spondylogenic compression of cervical spinal cord 721.1
D1-23342 Anterior spinal artery compression syndrome 721.1
D1-23346 Vertebral artery compression syndrome 721.1
D1-23350 Thoracic spondylosis without myelopathy 721.2
Thoracic osteoarthritis 721.2
D1-23352 Thoracic arthritis 721.2
Thoracic spondyloarthritis 721.3
D1-23360 Thoracic spondylosis with myelopathy 721.41
Spondylogenic compression of thoracic spinal cord 721.41
D1-23370 Lumbosacral spondylosis without myelopathy 721.3
Lumbar and sacral osteoarthritis 721.3
D1-23372 Lumbar and sacral arthritis 721.3
Lumbar and sacral spondyloarthritis 721.3
D1-23380 Lumbar spondylosis with myelopathy 721.42
Spondylogenic compression of lumbar spinal cord 721.42
D1-23390 Kissing spine 721.5
Baastrup's syndrome 721.5
Overriding of dorsal spinous processes
D1-23392 Ankylosing vertebral hyperostosis 721.6
D1-23395 Traumatic spondylopathy 721.7
D1-23396 Kümmell's disease 721.7
Kümmell's spondylitis 721.7
D1-23500 Intervertebral disc disorder, NOS 722.90
D1-23510 Displacement of intervertebral disc, site unspecified without myelopathy 722.2
Discogenic syndrome, NOS 722.2
D1-23512 Herniation of nucleus pulposus, NOS 722.2
D1-23514 Intervertebral disc extrusion, NOS 722.2
Intervertebral disc protrusion, NOS 722.2
D1-23515 Intervertebral disc prolapse 722.2
D1-23516 Intervertebral disc rupture 722.2
D1-23517 Neuritis or radiculitis due to displacement of intervertebral disc 722.2
D1-23518 Neuritis or radiculitis due to rupture of intervertebral disc 722.2
D1-23520 Displacement of cervical intervertebral disc without myelopathy 722.0
D1-23522 Brachial neuritis or radiculitis due to displacement of cervical intervertebral disc 722.0
D1-23524 Brachial neuritis or radiculitis due to rupture of cervical intervertebral disc 722.0
D1-23530 Displacement of thoracic intervertebral disc without myelopathy 722.11
D1-23540 Displacement of lumbar intervertebral disc without myelopathy 722.10
D1-23542 Lumbago-sciatica due to displacement of lumbar intervertebral disc 722.10
D1-23544 Neuritis or radiculitis due to displacement of lumbar intervertebral disc 722.10
D1-23546 Neuritis or radiculitis due to rupture of lumbar intervertebral disc 722.10
D1-23550 Schmorl's nodes, NOS 722.30
D1-23552 Schmorl's nodes of thoracic region 722.31
D1-23553 Schmorl's nodes of lumbar region 722.32
D1-23554 Schmorl's nodes of other region, NEC 722.39
D1-23600 Degeneration of intervertebral disc, NOS 722.6
Degenerative disc disease, NOS 722.6
D1-23601 Narrowing of intervertebral disc space, NOS 722.6
D1-23610 Degeneration of cervicothoracic intervertebral disc 722.4
D1-23611 Degeneration of cervical intervertebral disc 722.4
D1-23612 Degeneration of thoracic intervertebral disc 722.51
D1-23614 Degeneration of thoracolumbar intervertebral disc 722.51

1-23 DISORDERS OF THE VERTEBRAL COLUMN — Continued

D1-23616 Degeneration of lumbar intervertebral disc 722.52
D1-23618 Degeneration of lumbosacral intervertebral disc 722.52
D1-23620 Intervertebral disc disorder with myelopathy, NOS 722.70
D1-23622 Intervertebral disc disorder of cervical region with myelopathy 722.71
D1-23624 Intervertebral disc disorder of thoracic region with myelopathy 722.72
D1-23626 Intervertebral disc disorder of lumbar region with myelopathy 722.73
D1-23630 Postlaminectomy syndrome, NOS 722.80
D1-23632 Postlaminectomy syndrome of cervical region 722.81
D1-23634 Postlaminectomy syndrome of thoracic region 722.82
D1-23636 Postlaminectomy syndrome of lumbar region 722.83
D1-23640 Calcification of intervertebral cartilage or disc, NOS 722.90
D1-23642 Calcification of intervertebral cartilage or disc of cervical region 722.91
D1-23644 Calcification of intervertebral cartilage or disc of thoracic region 722.92
D1-23646 Calcification of intervertebral cartilage or disc of lumbar region 722.93
D1-23650 Discitis, NOS 722.90
D1-23652 Discitis of cervical region 722.91
D1-23654 Discitis of thoracic region 722.92
D1-23656 Discitis of lumbar region 722.93
D1-23660 Spinal stenosis in cervical region 723.0
D1-23664 Cervicocranial syndrome 723.2
  Barré-Liéou syndrome 723.2
  Posterior cervical sympathetic syndrome 723.2
D1-23666 Diffuse cervicobrachial syndrome 723.3
D1-23670 Brachial neuritis, NOS 723.4
D1-23671 Brachial radiculitis, NOS 723.4
D1-23672 Cervical radiculitis 723.4
  Radicular syndrome of upper limbs 723.4
D1-23674 Torticollis, NOS 723.5
  Contracture of neck, NOS 723.5
D1-23678 Ossification of posterior longitudinal ligament in cervical region 723.7
D1-23680 Klippel's disease 723.8
D1-23688 Cervical syndrome, NEC 723.8
D1-23690 Unspecified musculoskeletal disorder of the neck 723.9
  Disorder of cervical region, NEC 723.9
D1-23700 Disorder of back, NOS 724.9
D1-23710 Ankylosis of spine, NOS 724.9
D1-23720 Compression of spinal nerve root, NEC 724.9
D1-23730 Spinal stenosis, NOS 724.09
D1-23731 Spinal stenosis other than cervical, NOS 724.00
D1-23732 Spinal stenosis of thoracic region 724.01
D1-23734 Spinal stenosis of lumbar region 724.02
D1-23736 Spinal stenosis of other region, NEC 724.09
D1-23742 Lumbago 724.2
  Low back pain 724.2
  Low back syndrome 724.2
  Lumbalgia 724.2
D1-23746 Sciatica 724.3
  Neuralgia-neuritis of sciatic nerve 724.3
  Sciatic neuralgia 724.3
D1-23750 Thoracic neuritis, NOS 724.4
D1-23752 Thoracic radiculitis, NOS 724.4
D1-23754 Lumbosacral neuritis, NOS 724.4
D1-23756 Lumbosacral radiculitis, NOS 724.4
D1-23758 Radicular syndrome of lower limbs 724.4
D1-23760 Backache, NOS 724.5
  Vertebrogenic pain syndrome, NOS 724.5
D1-23800 Disorder of sacrum, NOS 724.6
D1-23810 Ankylosis of lumbosacral joint 724.6
D1-23812 Ankylosis of sacroiliac joint 724.6
D1-23814 Instability of lumbosacral joint 724.6
D1-23816 Instability of sacroiliac joint 724.6
D1-23830 Disorder of coccyx, NOS 724.70
D1-23832 Hypermobility of coccyx 724.71
D1-23838 Other disorder of coccyx 724.79
D1-23840 Atlantoaxial subluxation
D1-23850 Ossification of posterior longitudinal ligament, NOS 724.8

SECTION 1-3 DISORDERS OF THE SYNOVIA, TENDONS AND BURSAE INCLUDING ENTHESOPATHIES

D1-30000 Enthesopathy of unspecified site, NOS 726.90
D1-30010 Capsulitis, NOS 726.90
D1-30020 Periarthritis, NOS 726.90
D1-30030 Tendinitis, NOS 726.90
  Tendonitis, NOS 726.90
D1-30032V Bowed tendon
D1-30100 Disorder of bursae of shoulder region, NOS 726.10
D1-30110 Disorder of tendon of shoulder region, NOS 726.10
D1-30120 Rotator cuff syndrome, NOS 726.10
D1-30122 Supraspinatus syndrome, NOS 726.10
D1-30140 Adhesive capsulitis of shoulder 726.0
  Frozen shoulder 726.0
D1-30144 Calcifying tendinitis of shoulder 726.11
D1-30146 Bicipital tenosynovitis 726.12
D1-30147 Subcoracoid bursitis 726.19
D1-30148 Subacromial bursitis 726.19
D1-30149 Subdeltoid bursitis 726.19
D1-30150 Periarthritis of shoulder 726.2
D1-30160 Scapulohumeral fibrositis 726.2
D1-30180 Other affections of shoulder region, NEC 726.2
D1-30200 Enthesopathy of elbow region, NOS 726.30
  Enthesopathy of elbow, NOS 726.30

D1-30210 Epicondylitis, NOS 726.32
D1-30220 Medial epicondylitis 726.31
D1-30230 Lateral epicondylitis 726.32
  Golfer's elbow 726.32
  Tennis elbow 726.32
D1-30240 Olecranon bursitis 726.33
  Bursitis of elbow 726.33
D1-30280 Other enthesopathy of elbow, NEC 726.39
D1-30300 Enthesopathy of wrist and carpus, NOS 726.4
D1-30310 Bursitis of wrist 726.4
D1-30312 Bursitis of hand 726.4
D1-30320 Periarthritis of wrist 726.4
D1-30400 Enthesopathy of hip region, NOS 726.5
D1-30410 Bursitis of hip 726.5
D1-30420 Gluteal tendinitis 726.5
D1-30430 Iliac crest spur 726.5
D1-30440 Psoas tendinitis 726.5
D1-30450 Trochanteric tendinitis 726.5
D1-30500 Enthesopathy of knee, NOS 726.60
D1-30510 Bursitis of knee, NOS 726.60
D1-30520 Pes anserinus tendinitis 726.61
D1-30522 Pes anserinus bursitis 726.61
D1-30530 Tibial collateral ligament bursitis 726.62
D1-30532 Pellegrini-Stieda syndrome 726.62
  Calcification of medial collateral ligament of knee 726.62
D1-30540 Fibular collateral ligament bursitis 726.63
D1-30550 Patellar tendonitis 726.64
D1-30552 Prepatellar bursitis 726.65
D1-30554 Infrapatellar bursitis 726.69
D1-30556 Subpatellar bursitis 726.69
D1-30600 Enthesopathy of ankle and tarsus, NOS 726.70
D1-30618 Podagra
D1-30620 Achilles bursitis 726.71
D1-30622 Achilles tendinitis 726.71
D1-30630 Tibialis tendinitis, NOS 726.72
D1-30632 Tibialis anticus tendinitis 726.72
D1-30634 Tibialis posticus tendinitis 726.72
D1-30640 Calcaneal spur 726.73
D1-30650 Peroneal tendinitis 726.79
D1-30680 Other enthesopathy of ankle and tarsus, NEC 726.79
D1-30690 Other peripheral enthesopathy, NEC 726.8
D1-30700V Windgall
  Windpuffs
D1-30710V Curb
D1-30720V Splints
  Interosseous desmitis
D1-30730V Carpitis
  Popped knee
D1-30740V Carpal hygroma
D1-30750V Trochanteric bursitis
  Whirlbone lameness
D1-30760V Capped elbow
  Capped hock
D1-32000 Disorder of synovium, NOS 727.9
D1-32002 Disorder of tendon, NOS 727.9
D1-32004 Disorder of bursa, NOS 727.9
D1-32020 Synovitis, NOS 727.00
D1-32024V Lymphocytic plasmacytic synovitis
D1-32030 Tenosynovitis, NOS 727.00
D1-32040 Synovitis or tenosynovitis in disease classified elsewhere 727.01
D1-32060 Acquired trigger finger 727.03
D1-32070 Radial styloid tenosynovitis 727.04
D1-32080 de Quervain's disease 727.04
D1-32090 Tenosynovitis of hand and wrist, NEC 727.05
D1-32095 Tenosynovitis of foot and ankle, NEC 727.06
D1-32097V Thoroughpin
D1-32098V Bog spavin
  Tarsal hydrarthrosis
D1-32100 Bunion of great toe 727.1
D1-32110 Specific bursitis often of occupational origin 727.2
D1-32112 Beat elbow 727.2
  (T-16000) (T-D8300) (M-40000)
D1-32114 Beat hand 727.2
  (T-16000) (T-D8700) (M-40000)
D1-32116 Beat knee 727.2
  (T-03000) (T-D9200) (M-41650)
D1-32118 Chronic crepitant synovitis of wrist 727.2
D1-32120 Miner's elbow 727.2
D1-32122 Miner's knee 727.2
D1-32130 Bursitis, NOS 727.3
D1-32200 Synovial cyst, NOS 727.40
D1-32210 Ganglion, NOS 727.43
  Benign cystic mucinous tumor, NOS 727.43
D1-32212 Ganglion of joint, NOS 727.41
D1-32214 Ganglion of tendon sheath, NOS 727.42
D1-32215 Ganglion of aponeurosis, NOS 727.42
D1-32216 Cyst of bursa, NOS 727.49
D1-32220 Rupture of synovium, NOS 727.50
D1-32230 Synovial cyst of popliteal space 727.51
  Baker's cyst 727.51
D1-32250 Nontraumatic rupture of tendon, NOS 727.60
D1-32260 Complete rupture of rotator cuff 727.61
D1-32270 Rupture of tendon of biceps, long head 727.62
D1-32280 Rupture of extensor tendons of hand and wrist 727.63
D1-32282 Rupture of flexor tendons of hand and wrist 727.64
D1-32290 Rupture of quadriceps tendon 727.65
D1-32292 Rupture of patellar tendon 727.66
D1-32294 Rupture of Achilles tendon 727.67
D1-322A0 Rupture of other tendons of foot and ankle, NEC 727.68
D1-32300 Other disorder of synovium, tendon or bursa, NEC 727.8
D1-32310 Contracture of tendon sheath 727.81
D1-32312 Acquired short Achilles tendon 727.81
D1-32330 Calcium deposits in tendon and bursa 727.82
  Calcification of tendon, NOS 727.82

SECTION 1-3 DISORDERS OF THE SYNOVIA, TENDONS AND BURSAE INCLUDING ENTHESOPATHIES — Continued

D1-32330 (cont.) Calcific tendinitis, NOS 727.82
D1-32340 Abscess of bursa or tendon 727.89

SECTION 1-5 DISORDERS OF THE MUSCLES, LIGAMENTS, FASCIAE AND OTHER SOFT TISSUES

D1-50010 Disorder of muscle, NOS 728.9
D1-50020 Disorder of ligament, NOS 728.9
D1-50030 Disorder of fascia, NOS 728.9
D1-50040 Disorder of soft tissue, NOS 729.9
D1-50100 Infective myositis, NOS 728.0
D1-50110 Purulent myositis 728.0
    Suppurative myositis 728.0
D1-50200 Muscular calcification, NOS 728.1
D1-50202 Massive calcification in paraplegic 728.10
D1-50210 Muscular ossification, NOS 728.10
D1-50220 Progressive myositis ossificans 728.11
D1-50230 Traumatic myositis ossificans 728.12
D1-50240 Myositis ossificans circumscripta 728.12
D1-50250 Postoperative heterotopic calcification 728.13
D1-50260 Polymyositis ossificans 728.19
D1-50270 Amyotrophia, NOS 728.2
D1-50280 Myofibrosis 782.2
D1-50290 Muscular wasting and disuse atrophy, NEC 728.2
D1-50292V Asymmetrical hindquarter syndrome of pigs
D1-502A0 Arthrogryposis 728.3
D1-502B0 Paraplegic immobility syndrome 728.3
D1-502C0 Other specified muscle disorder, NEC 728.3
D1-50310V Equine rhabdomyolysis
    Azoturia
    Monday morning disease
    Paralytic myoglobinuria
    Tying-up
D1-50320V Exertional rhabdomyolysis
    Capture myopathy
    Overstraining disease
    Idiopathic muscle necrosis
D1-50330V Canine eosinophilic myositis
D1-50332V Bovine eosinophilic myositis
D1-50340V Muscular hypertonicity
    Scottie cramp
D1-50342V Atrophic myositis
D1-50350V Maxillary myositis
D1-50360V Parasitic myositis
D1-50410 Laxity of ligament 728.4
D1-50420 Hypermobility syndrome 728.5
D1-50430 Contracture of palmar fascia 728.6
    Dupuytren's contracture 728.6
D1-50434 Volkmann's contracture 728.6
    Volkmann's syndrome 728.6
D1-50440 Plantar fascial fibromatosis 728.71
D1-50442 Contracture of plantar fascia 728.71
D1-50446 Traumatic plantar fasciitis 728.71
D1-50450 Knuckle pads 728.79
    Garrod's pads 728.79
D1-50460 Nodular fasciitis 728.79
    Pseudosarcomatous fibromatosis 728.79
    Pseudosarcomatous fasciitis 728.79
    Proliferative fasciitis 728.79
D1-50510 Interstitial myositis 728.81
D1-50520 Foreign body granuloma of muscle 728.82
D1-50522 Talc granuloma of muscle 728.82
D1-50530 Nontraumatic rupture of muscle 728.83
D1-50534V Rupture of gastrocnemius muscle or tendon
D1-50540 Diastasis of muscle, NOS 728.84
D1-50542 Diastasis recti 728.84
D1-50600 Rheumatism, NOS 729.0
D1-50610 Fibrositis, NOS 729.0
D1-50611 Primary fibrositis 729.0
D1-50612 Secondary fibrositis 729.0
D1-50630 Myositis, NOS 729.1
D1-50640 Fibromyositis, NOS 729.1
D1-50642 Muscle contracture 728.89
D1-50650 Neuralgia, NOS 729.2
    Paroxysmal nerve pain 729.2
D1-50660 Neuritis, NOS 729.2
D1-50670 Radiculitis, NOS 729.2
D1-50720 Hypertrophy of fat pad of knee 729.31
    Hypertrophy of infrapatellar fat pad 729.31
D1-50730 Fasciitis, NOS 729.4
D1-50740 Pain in limb 729.5
D1-50750 Residual foreign body in soft tissue 729.6
D1-50762 Swelling of limb, NOS 729.81
D1-50780V Muscular steatosis
D1-50790V Stringhalt

SECTION 1-6 DISEASES OF THE BONES

D1-60000 Disease of bone, NOS
D1-60030 Osteodystrophy, NOS
D1-60034 Hepatic osteodystrophy
D1-60036 Disuse osteodystrophy
D1-60060 Osteosclerosis
D1-60080 Disseminated idiopathic skeletal hyperostosis
    DISH
D1-60200 Osteitis, NOS 730.2
    Inflammation of bone, NOS 730.2
D1-60201 Osteitis of shoulder region 730.21
D1-60202 Osteitis of upper arm 730.22
D1-60203 Osteitis of forearm 730.23
D1-60204 Osteitis of hand 730.24
D1-60205 Osteitis of pelvic region 730.25
D1-60206 Osteitis of thigh 730.25
D1-60207 Osteitis of lower leg 730.26
D1-60208 Osteitis of ankle and foot 730.27
D1-60209 Osteitis of other specific site, NEC 730.28
D1-6020A Osteitis of multiple sites 730.29
D1-60210 Osteomyelitis, NOS 730.2
    Pyogenic inflammation of bone, NOS 730.2

D1-60211 Osteomyelitis of shoulder region 730.21
D1-60212 Osteomyelitis of upper arm 730.22
D1-60213 Osteomyelitis of forearm 730.23
D1-60214 Osteomyelitis of hand 730.24
D1-60215 Osteomyelitis of pelvic region 730.25
D1-60216 Osteomyelitis of thigh 730.25
D1-60217 Osteomyelitis of lower leg 730.26
D1-60218 Osteomyelitis of ankle and foot 730.27
D1-60219 Osteomyelitis of other specific site, NEC 730.28
D1-6021A Osteomyelitis of multiple sites 730.29
D1-60220 Acute osteomyelitis, NOS 730.00
  Acute osteomyelitis with or without periostitis 730.00
D1-60221 Acute osteomyelitis of shoulder region 730.01
D1-60222 Acute osteomyelitis of upper arm 730.02
D1-60223 Acute osteomyelitis of forearm 730.03
D1-60224 Acute osteomyelitis of hand 730.04
D1-60225 Acute osteomyelitis of pelvic region 730.05
D1-60226 Acute osteomyelitis of thigh 730.05
D1-60227 Acute osteomyelitis of lower leg 730.06
D1-60228 Acute osteomyelitis of ankle and foot 730.07
D1-60229 Acute osteomyelitis of other specific site, NEC 730.08
D1-6022A Acute osteomyelitis of multiple sites 730.09
D1-60230 Chronic osteomyelitis, NOS 730.10
  Chronic osteomyelitis with or without periostitis 730.10
D1-60231 Chronic osteomyelitis of shoulder region 730.11
D1-60232 Chronic osteomyelitis of upper arm 730.12
D1-60233 Chronic osteomyelitis of forearm 730.13
D1-60234 Chronic osteomyelitis of hand 730.14
D1-60235 Chronic osteomyelitis of pelvic region 730.15
D1-60236 Chronic osteomyelitis of thigh 730.15
D1-60237 Chronic osteomyelitis of lower leg 730.16
D1-60238 Chronic osteomyelitis of ankle and foot 730.17
D1-60239 Chronic osteomyelitis of other specific site, NEC 730.18
D1-6023A Chronic osteomyelitis of multiple sites 730.19
D1-60240 Subacute osteomyelitis with or without periostitis 730.0
D1-60250 Brodie's abscess 730.1
D1-60254 Acute necrosis of bone 730.1
D1-60258 Sclerosing osteomyelitis of Garré 730.1
D1-60260 Periostitis, NOS 730.3
  Periostitis without osteomyelitis 730.3
D1-60261 Periostitis of shoulder region 730.31
D1-60262 Periostitis of upper arm 730.32
D1-60263 Periostitis of forearm 730.33
D1-60264 Periostitis of hand 730.34
D1-60265 Periostitis of pelvic region 730.35
D1-60266 Periostitis of thigh 730.35
D1-60267 Periostitis of lower leg 730.36
D1-60268 Periostitis of ankle and foot 730.37
D1-60269 Periostitis of other specified site, NEC 730.38
D1-6026A Periostitis of multiple sites 730.39
D1-60270 Abscess of periosteum without osteomyelitis 730.3
D1-60274 Abscess of bone, except accessory sinus, jaw or mastoid 730.0
D1-60280 Periostosis without osteomyelitis 730.3
D1-60290 Osteopathy resulting from poliomyelitis 730.7
D1-602A0 Other infections of bone in diseases classified elsewhere 730.8
D1-602B0 Infection of bone, NEC 730.9
D1-60310V Navicular disease
    (T-12450) (M-40000)
  Podotrochlosis
    (T-12450) (M-40000)
  Podotrochilitis
    (T-12450) (M-40000)
D1-60320V Pedal osteitis
D1-60340V Sidebone
D1-60342V Ringbone
D1-60350V Sesamoiditis
D1-60354V Bucked shins
  Sore shins
  Saucer fractures
D1-60356V Bone spavin
D1-60360V Eosinophilic panostitis
D1-60500 Metabolic bone disease, NOS
D1-60510V Feline osteogenesis imperfecta
  Juvenile osteoporosis
D1-61100 Osteitis deformans 731.0
  Osteitis deformans without mention of bone tumor 731.0
  Paget's disease of bone 731.0
D1-61110 Osteitis deformans in disease classified elsewhere 731.1
D1-61120 Hypertrophic pulmonary osteoarthropathy 731.2
  Bamberger-Marie disease 731.2
  Acropachy 731.2
D1-61130V Craniomandibular osteopathy
  Lion jaw
  Craniomandibular hyperostosis
D1-61200 Osteochondropathy, NOS 732.9
  Disease of bone and cartilage, NOS 733.90
D1-61210 Juvenile osteochondrosis of spine, NOS 732.0
  Juvenile osteochondrosis of vertebral epiphyses 732.0
  Scheuermann's disease 732.0
  Vertebral epiphysitis 732.0
  Scheuermann's kyphosis 732.0
  Kyphosis dorsalis juvenilis 732.0
D1-61220 Juvenile osteochondrosis of hip and pelvis 732.1
  Coxa plana 732.1
  Juvenile osteochondrosis of head of femur 732.1

SECTION 1-6 DISEASES OF THE BONES — Continued

D1-61220 (cont.) Pseudocoxalgia 732.1
  Juvenile osteochondrosis of hip 732.1
  Legg-Calvé-Perthes disease 732.1
D1-61226 Juvenile osteochondrosis of pelvis 732.1
D1-61227 Ischiopubic synchondrosis of van Neck 732.1
D1-61228 Juvenile osteochondrosis of iliac crest 732.1
  Juvenile osteochondrosis of Buchanan 732.1
D1-61229 Juvenile osteochondrosis of acetabulum 732.1
D1-6122A Juvenile osteochondrosis of symphysis pubis 732.1
  Juvenile osteochondrosis of Pierson 732.1
D1-61230 Slipped upper femoral epiphysis, NOS 732.2
  Nontraumatic slipped upper femoral epiphysis, NOS 732.2
D1-61240 Juvenile osteochondrosis of upper extremity, NOS 732.3
D1-61241 Juvenile osteochondrosis of capitellum of humerus 732.3
  Juvenile osteochondrosis of head of humerus 732.3
  Panner's disease 732.3
  Haas' disease 732.3
D1-61243 Juvenile osteochondrosis of carpal lunate 732.3
  Kienbock's disease 732.3
D1-61245 Juvenile osteochondrosis of hand, NOS 732.3
D1-61246 Juvenile osteochondrosis of head of metacarpals 732.3
  Mauclaire's disease 732.3
D1-61247 Juvenile osteochondrosis of lower ulna 732.3
  Burns' disease 732.3
D1-61248 Juvenile osteochondrosis of radial head 732.3
  Brailsford's disease 732.3
D1-61250 Juvenile osteochondrosis of lower extremity, NOS 732.4
  Juvenile osteochondrosis of lower extremity, excluding foot, NOS 732.4
D1-61251 Tibia vara 732.4
  Juvenile osteochondrosis of proximal tibia 732.4
  Blount's disease 732.4
D1-61252 Juvenile osteochondrosis of primary patellar center 732.4
D1-61255 Juvenile osteochondrosis of secondary patellar center 732.4
D1-61257 Juvenile osteochondrosis of tibial tubercle 732.4
  Osgood-Schlatter's disease 732.4
D1-61260 Juvenile osteochondrosis of foot, NOS 732.5
D1-61262 Calcaneal apophysitis 732.5
  Epiphysitis of os calcis 732.5
  Juvenile osteochondrosis of calcaneum 732.5
D1-61263 Juvenile osteochondrosis of astragalus 732.5
D1-61266 Juvenile osteochondrosis of second metatarsal 732.5
  Freiberg's infraction 732.5
D1-61267 Juvenile osteochondrosis of fifth metatarsal 732.5
D1-61268 Juvenile osteochondrosis of os tibiale 732.5
D1-61269 Juvenile osteochondrosis of tarsal navicular 732.5
  Kohler's tarsal scaphoiditis 732.5
D1-61300 Juvenile apophysitis, NOS 732.6
D1-61302 Juvenile epiphysitis, NOS 732.6
D1-61304 Juvenile osteochondritis, NOS 732.6
D1-61306 Juvenile osteochondrosis, NOS 732.6
D1-61310 Osteochondritis dissecans 732.7
  Osteochondrosis dessicans
  Idiopathic avascular necrosis
  OCC
D1-61320 Adult osteochondritis of spine 732.8
D1-61330 Other specified form of osteochondropathy, NEC 732.8
D1-61410 Apophysitis, NOS 732.9
D1-61420 Epiphysitis, NOS 732.9
  Physitis
  Physeal dysplasia
  Dysplasia of growth plate
D1-61422 Epiphyseal necrosis, NOS
D1-61430 Osteochondritis, NOS 732.9
D1-61440 Osteochondrosis, NOS 732.9
D1-61500 Osteoporosis, NOS 733.00
D1-61502 Wedging of vertebra, NOS 733.00
D1-61510 Senile osteoporosis 733.01
D1-61514 Menopausal osteoporosis
D1-61514 Postmenopausal osteoporosis 733.01
D1-61520 Idiopathic osteoporosis 733.02
D1-61530 Disuse osteoporosis 733.03
D1-61532 Posttraumatic osteoporosis 733.7
  Sudeck's atrophy 733.7
D1-61540 Drug-induced osteoporosis 733.09
D1-61580 Other disorder of bone and cartilage, NEC 733.-
D1-61604 Collapse of vertebra, NOS 733.1
D1-61622 Local cyst of bone, NOS 733.20
D1-61628 Monostotic fibrous dysplasia 733.29
D1-61640 Hyperostosis of skull 733.3
D1-61642 Hyperostosis interna frontalis 733.3
D1-61644 Leontiasis ossium 733.3
  Leontiasis ossea 733.3
  Leonine bones 733.3
D1-61648V Canine cortical hyperostosis
  Caffey's disease
D1-61650 Aseptic necrosis of bone of unspecified site 733.40
D1-61652 Aseptic necrosis of head of humerus 733.41
D1-61654 Aseptic necrosis of head and neck of femur 733.42
D1-61655 Aseptic necrosis of medial femoral condyle 733.43

D1-61657 Aseptic necrosis of talus 733.44
D1-61659 Aseptic necrosis of other specified site, NEC 733.49
D1-61660 Osteitis condensans 733.5
D1-61662 Piriform sclerosis of ilium 733.5
D1-61670 Tietze's disease 733.6
Costochondral junction syndrome 733.6
D1-61680 Algoneurodystrophy 733.7
D1-61682 Disuse atrophy 733.7
D1-61760 Arrest of bone development or growth 733.91
D1-61770 Epiphyseal arrest 733.91
D1-61800 Chondromalacia, NOS 733.92
D1-61810 Localized chondromalacia 733.92
D1-61820 Systemic chondromalacia 733.92
D1-61830 Tibial plateau chondromalacia 733.92
D1-61840 Diaphysitis 733.99
D1-61880 Relapsing polychondritis 733.99
D1-61910V Cage layer fatigue

SECTION 1-8 ACQUIRED MUSCULOSKELETAL DEFORMITIES

D1-80000 Acquired musculoskeletal deformity, NOS 738.9
D1-80100 Acquired flat foot 734.-
Acquired pes planus 734.-
Acquired talipes planus 734.-
D1-80200 Acquired deformity of toe, NOS 735.9
D1-80210 Acquired hallux valgus 735.0
D1-80220 Acquired hallux varus 735.1
D1-80230 Acquired hallux rigidus 735.2
D1-80240 Acquired hallux malleus 735.3
D1-80250 Acquired hammer toe, other than great toe 735.4
D1-80260 Acquired claw toe 735.5
D1-80280 Other acquired deformity of toe, NEC 735.8
D1-80300 Acquired deformity of forearm, excluding fingers, NOS 736.00
D1-80310 Acquired deformity of elbow, NOS 736.00
D1-80320 Acquired deformity of forearm, NOS 736.00
D1-80330 Acquired deformity of wrist, NOS 736.00
D1-80340 Acquired deformity of hand, NOS 736.00
D1-80350 Acquired cubitus valgus 736.01
D1-80354 Acquired cubitus varus 736.02
D1-80360 Acquired valgus deformity of wrist 736.03
D1-80364 Acquired varus deformity of wrist 736.04
D1-80366 Acquired wrist drop 736.05
D1-80370 Acquired claw hand 736.06
D1-80374 Acquired clubhand 736.07
D1-80400 Acquired deformity of finger, NOS 736.20
D1-80410 Mallet finger 736.1
D1-80420 Boutonnière deformity 736.21
D1-80430 Swan-neck deformity 736.22
D1-80440 Clubbing of fingers 781.5
D1-80480 Other acquired deformity of finger, NEC 736.29
D1-80500 Acquired deformity of hip, NOS 736.30
D1-80510 Acquired coxa valga 736.31
D1-80520 Acquired coxa vara 736.32
D1-80580 Other acquired deformity of hip, NEC 736.39
D1-80600 Acquired deformity of knee, NOS 736.6
D1-80610 Acquired genu valgum 736.41
D1-80620 Acquired genu varum 736.42
D1-80630 Acquired genu recurvatum 736.5
D1-80680 Other acquired deformity of knee, NEC 736.6
D1-80700 Acquired deformity of ankle and foot, NOS 736.70
D1-80710 Acquired equinovarus deformity 736.71
Acquired clubfoot 736.71
D1-80730 Acquired equinus deformity of foot 736.72
D1-80740 Acquired cavus deformity of foot 736.73
D1-80742 Acquired claw foot 736.74
D1-80746 Acquired cavovarus deformity of foot 736.75
D1-80780 Other acquired calcaneus deformity, NEC 736.76
D1-80790 Acquired pes, NEC 936.79
Acquired talipes, NEC 936.79
D1-80800 Acquired deformity of limb, site unspecified 736.9
D1-80810 Acquired unequal leg length 736.81
D1-80820 Acquired deformity of arm, NEC 736.89
D1-80830 Acquired deformity of leg, NEC 736.89
D1-80840 Acquired deformity of shoulder, NEC 736.89
D1-81100 Acquired curvature of spine, NOS 737.9
D1-81102 Acquired hunchback 737.9
D1-81110 Adolescent postural kyphosis 737.0
D1-81120 Acquired kyphosis 737.1
D1-81130 Acquired postural kyphosis 737.10
D1-81140 Kyphosis due to radiation 737.11
D1-81150 Postlaminectomy kyphosis 737.12
D1-81180 Other acquired kyphosis, NEC 737.19
D1-81200 Acquired lordosis 737.2
D1-81210 Acquired postural lordosis 737.20
D1-81250 Postlaminectomy lordosis 737.21
D1-81260 Other postsurgical lordosis 737.22
D1-81280 Other acquired lordosis, NEC 737.29
D1-81300 Idiopathic scoliosis and kyphoscoliosis 737.30
D1-81310 Resolving infantile idiopathic scoliosis 737.31
D1-81320 Progressive infantile idiopathic sclerosis 737.32
D1-81340 Scoliosis due to radiation 737.33
D1-81350 Thoracogenic scoliosis 737.34
D1-81380 Other acquired scoliosis, NEC 737.39
D1-81400 Curvature of spine, NOS 737.40
D1-81410 Kyphosis, NOS 737.41
D1-81420 Lordosis, NOS 737.42
D1-81430 Scoliosis, NOS 737.43
D1-81500 Other curvature of spine, NEC 737.8
D1-81600 Acquired deformity of nose 738.0
D1-81610 Overdevelopment of nasal bones 738.0
D1-81620 Other acquired deformity of head, NEC 738.1
D1-81630 Acquired deformity of neck 738.2
D1-81642 Acquired deformity of chest 738.3
D1-81644 Acquired pectus carinatum 738.3
D1-81646 Acquired pectus excavatum 738.3
D1-81648 Acquired deformity of rib 738.3

SECTION 1-8 ACQUIRED MUSCULOSKELETAL DEFORMITIES — Continued

D1-81700 Acquired deformity of spine, NOS 738.5
D1-81710 Spondylolisthesis, NOS 738.4
Acquired spondylolisthesis, NOS 738.4
Acquired spondylolysis, NOS 738.4
D1-81711 Spondylolisthesis, grade 1 738.4
D1-81712 Spondylolisthesis, grade 2 738.4
D1-81713 Spondylolisthesis, grade 3 738.4
D1-81714 Spondylolisthesis, grade 4 738.4
D1-81720 Degenerative spondylolisthesis 738.4
D1-81800 Acquired deformity of pelvis 738.6
D1-81810 Pelvic obliquity 738.6
D1-81910 Cauliflower ear 738.7
D1-81920 Acquired deformity of clavicle 738.8

SECTION 1-9 NONALLOPATHIC LESIONS, NEC

D1-90000 Nonallopathic lesion, NEC 739.-
D1-90010 Segmental dysfunction 739.-
D1-90020 Somatic dysfunction 739.-
D1-90100 Nonallopathic lesion of head region 739.0
D1-90110 Nonallopathic lesion of occipitocervical region 739.0
D1-90120 Nonallopathic lesion of cervical region 739.1
D1-90130 Nonallopathic lesion of cervicothoracic region 739.1
D1-90140 Nonallopathic lesion of thoracic region 739.2
D1-90150 Nonallopathic lesion of thoracolumbar region 739.2
D1-90160 Nonallopathic lesion of lumbar region 739.3
D1-90170 Nonallopathic lesion of lumbosacral region 739.3
D1-90180 Nonallopathic lesion of sacral region 739.4
D1-90190 Nonallopathic lesion of sacrococcygeal region 739.4
D1-901A0 Nonallopathic lesion of sacroiliac region 739.4
D1-90200 Nonallopathic lesion of pelvic region 739.5
D1-90210 Nonallopathic lesion of hip region 739.5
D1-90220 Nonallopathic lesion of pubic region 739.5
D1-90300 Nonallopathic lesion of lower extremities 739.6
D1-90350 Nonallopathic lesion of upper extremities 739.7
D1-90360 Nonallopathic lesion of acromioclavicular region 739.7
D1-90370 Nonallopathic lesion of sternoclavicular region 739.7
D1-90400 Nonallopathic lesion of rib cage 739.8
D1-90410 Nonallopathic lesion of costochondral region 739.8
D1-90420 Nonallopathic lesion of costovertebral region 739.8
D1-90430 Nonallopathic lesion of sternochondral region 739.8
D1-90500 Nonallopathic lesion of abdomen 739.9

CHAPTER 2 — DISEASES OF THE RESPIRATORY SYSTEM

SECTION 2-0 DISEASES OF THE SINUSES, NOSE, PHARYNX AND LARYNX

2-00 RESPIRATORY DISEASES: GENERAL TERMS

D2-00000 Disease of respiratory system, NOS 519.9
(T-20000) (DF-00000)

D2-00001 Acute respiratory disease, NOS 519.9
(T-20000) (M-41000) (DF-00001)

D2-00003 Chronic respiratory disease, NOS 519.9
(T-20000) (DF-00003)

D2-00010 Disease of upper respiratory system, NOS 478.9
(T-20100) (DF-00000)
Disease of upper respiratory tract, NOS 478.9
(T-20100) (DF-00000)
Upper respiratory disease, NOS 478.9
(T-20100) (DF-00000)

D2-00020 Upper respiratory infection, NOS 465.9
(T-20100) (M-40000) (DE-00000)

D2-00021 Acute upper respiratory infection 465.9
(T-20100) (M-41000) (DE-00000)
Acute URI 465.9
(T-20100) (M-41000) (DE-00000)

D2-00022 Acute upper respiratory infection of multiple sites 465.8
(T-20100) (T-.....) (M-41000) (DE-00000)
Acute URI of multiple sites 465.8
(T-20100) (T-.....) (M-41000) (DE-00000)

D2-00030 Upper respiratory tract hypersensitivity reaction, NOS 478.8
(T-20100) (F-C3000)

D2-00050V Brachycephalic airway obstruction syndrome
(T-20100) (G-C008) (M-34000)

2-01 DISEASES OF THE NASAL SINUSES

2-010-011 Diseases of The Nasal Sinuses: General Terms

D2-01000 Disease of nasal sinus, NOS
(T-22000) (DF-00000)
Disease of accessory sinus, NOS
(T-22000) (DF-00000)

D2-01010 Acute pansinusitis 461.8
(T-22000) (M-41000)

D2-01020 Chronic pansinusitis 473.8
(T-22000) (M-43000)

D2-01070 Polypoid sinus degeneration 471.1
(T-22010) (M-76820) (M-50000)
Woakes' syndrome 471.1
(T-22010) (M-76820) (M-50000)
Woakes' ethmoiditis 471.1
(T-22010) (M-76820) (M-50000)

D2-01100 Sinusitis, NOS
(T-22000) (M-40000)

D2-01110 Acute sinusitis, NOS 461.9
(T-22000) (M-41000)
Acute infection of nasal sinus, NOS 461.9
(T-22000) (M-41000)
Acute inflammation of nasal sinus, NOS 461.9
(T-22000) (M-41000)

D2-01120 Acute abscess of nasal sinus 461.9
(T-22000) (M-41610)

D2-01130 Acute empyema of nasal sinus 461.9
(T-22000) (M-41620)

D2-01140 Acute suppuration of nasal sinus 461.9
(T-22000) (M-41600)
Acute suppurative inflammation of nasal sinus 461.9
(T-22000) (M-41600)

D2-01150 Chronic sinusitis, NOS 473.9
(T-22000) (M-43000)
Chronic infection of sinus, NOS 473.9
(T-22000) (M-43000)

D2-01170 Polyp of nasal sinus, NOS 471.8
(T-22000) (M-76820)
Polyp of accessory sinus, NOS 471.8
(T-22000) (M-76820)

D2-01180 Cyst of nasal sinus 478.1
(T-22000) (M-33440)
Mucocele of nasal sinus 478.1
(T-22000) (M-33440)
Mucous cyst of nasal sinus 478.1
(T-22000) (M-33440)

2-012 Diseases of The Maxillary Sinuses

D2-01200 Maxillary sinusitis, NOS
(T-22100) (M-40000)

D2-01210 Acute maxillary sinusitis 461.0
(T-22100) (M-41000)

D2-01220 Acute abscess of maxillary sinus 461.0
(T-22100) (M-41610)

D2-01230 Acute empyema of maxillary sinus 461.0
(T-22100) (M-41620)

D2-01240 Acute suppuration of maxillary sinus 461.0
(T-22100) (M-41600)
Acute suppurative inflammation of maxillary sinus 461.0
(T-22100) (M-41600)

D2-01250 Chronic maxillary sinusitis 473.0
(T-22100) (M-43000)

D2-01270 Polyp of maxillary sinus 471.8
(T-22100) (M-76820)

2-013 Diseases of The Frontal Sinuses

D2-01300 Frontal sinusitis, NOS
(T-22200) (M-40000)

D2-01310 Acute frontal sinusitis 461.1
(T-22200) (M-41000)

D2-01320 Acute abscess of frontal sinus 461.1
(T-22200) (M-41610)

D2-01330 Acute empyema of frontal sinus 461.1
(T-22200) (M-41620)

D2-01340 Acute suppuration of frontal sinus 461.1
(T-22200) (M-41600)
Acute suppurative inflammation of frontal sinus 461.1
(T-22200) (M-41600)

D2-01350 Chronic frontal sinusitis 473.1
(T-22200) (M-43000)

2-014 Diseases of The Ethmoidal Sinuses

D2-01400 Ethmoidal sinusitis, NOS
(T-22300) (M-40000)

D2-01410 Acute ethmoidal sinusitis 461.2
(T-22300) (M-41000)

D2-01420 Acute abscess of ethmoidal sinus 461.2
(T-22300) (M-41610)

D2-01430 Acute empyema of ethmoidal sinus 461.2
(T-22300) (M-41620)

D2-01440 Acute suppuration of ethmoidal sinus 461.2
(T-22300) (M-41600)
Acute suppurative inflammation of ethmoidal sinus 461.2
(T-22300) (M-41600)

D2-01450 Chronic ethmoidal sinusitis 473.2
(T-22300) (M-43000)

D2-01470 Polyp of ethmoidal sinus 471.8
(T-22300) (M-76820)

D2-01480 Acute antritis 461.0
(T-22360) (M-41000)

D2-01490 Chronic antritis 473.0
(T-22360) (M-43000)

2-015 Diseases of The Sphenoidal Sinuses

D2-01500 Sphenoidal sinusitis, NOS
(T-22400) (M-40000)

D2-01510 Acute sphenoidal sinusitis 461.3
(T-22400) (M-41000)

D2-01520 Acute abscess of sphenoidal sinus 461.3
(T-22400) (M-41610)

D2-01530 Acute empyema of sphenoidal sinus 461.3
(T-22400) (M-41620)

D2-01540 Acute suppuration of sphenoidal sinus 461.3
(T-22400) (M-41600)
Acute suppurative inflammation of sphenoidal sinus 461.3
(T-22400) (M-41600)

D2-01550 Chronic sphenoidal sinusitis 473.3
(T-22400) (M-43000)

D2-01570 Polyp of sphenoidal sinus 471.8
(T-22400) (M-76820)

2-02 DISEASES OF THE NOSE AND NASOPHARYNX

D2-02000 Disease of the nose, NOS
(T-21000) (DF-00000)

D2-02100 Allergic rhinitis, NOS
(T-21000) (M-40000) (F-C3000)

D2-02110 Seasonal allergic rhinitis 477.9
(T-21000) (M-40000) (G-C001) (F-C3000) (F-C1120)
Hay fever 477.9
(T-21000) (M-40000) (G-C001) (F-C3000) (F-C1120)
Spasmodic rhinorrhea 477.9
(T-21000) (M-40000) (G-C001) (F-C3000) (F-C1120)
Allergic rhinitis due to allergen 477.8
(T-21000) (M-40000) (G-C001) (F-C3000) (F-C1120)

D2-02111 Allergic rhinitis due to pollen 477.0
(T-21000) (M-40000) (G-C001) (F-C3000) (L-D0003)
Pollinosis 477.0
(T-21000) (M-40000) (G-C001) (F-C3000) (L-D0003)

D2-02120 Atopic rhinitis
(T-21000) (M-40000) (F-C3000)
Non-seasonal allergic rhinitis
(T-21000) (M-40000) (F-C3000)

D2-02130 Vasomotor rhinitis, NOS
(T-21000) (M-40000)

D2-02190 Atrophy of nasal turbinates
(T-21360) (M-58000)

D2-02200 Hypertrophy of nasal turbinates 478.0
(T-21360) (M-71000)

D2-02210 Rhinolith 478.1
(T-21300) (M-30000)

D2-02230 Acquired deviated nasal septum 470.-
(T-21340) (M-31070)
Acquired deflected nasal septum 470.-
(T-21340) (M-31070)

D2-02300 Abscess of nose 478.1
(T-21000) (M-41610)

D2-02310 Abscess of nasal septum 478.1
(T-21340) (M-41610)

D2-02320 Necrosis of nose 478.1
(T-21000) (M-54000)

D2-02330 Necrosis of nasal septum 478.1
(T-21340) (M-54000)

D2-02340 Ulcer of nose 478.1
(T-21000) (M-38000)

D2-02350 Ulcer of nasal septum 478.1
(T-21340) (M-38000)

D2-02400 Nasal polyp, NOS 471.9
(T-21300) (M-76820)
Polyp of nasal cavity, NOS 471.9
(T-21300) (M-76820)

D2-02500 Rhinitis, NOS 472.0
(T-22010) (M-40000)

D2-02510 Chronic rhinitis 472.0
(T-22010) (M-43000)

D2-02530 Atrophic rhinitis 472.0
(T-22010) (M-45100)

D2-02540 Granulomatous rhinitis 472.0
(T-22010) (M-44000)

D2-02550 Hypertrophic rhinitis 472.0
(T-22010) (M-45200)

D2-02560 Obstructive rhinitis 472.0
(T-22010) (M-45100) (M-34000)

D2-02570 Purulent rhinitis 472.0
(T-22010) (M-40600)

D2-02580 Ulcerative rhinitis 472.0
(T-22010) (M-40750)

D2-02600 Nasal discharge
(T-21300) (M-36850)

D2-02602 Catarrhal nasal discharge
(T-21300) (M-36870)

D2-02604 Purulent nasal discharge
(T-21300) (M-36880)

D2-02606 Hemorrhagic nasal discharge
(T-21300) (M-36850)

D2-02620 Epistaxis 784.7
(T-21000) (M-37000)
Nose bleed 784.7
(T-21000) (M-37000)

D2-02700 Chronic nasopharyngitis 472.2
(T-23000) (M-43000)

D2-02710 Cellulitis of nasopharynx 478.21
(T-23000) (M-41650)

D2-02720 Abscess of nasopharynx 478.29
(T-23000) (M-41610)

D2-02730 Cyst of nasopharynx 478.26
(T-23000) (M-33440)

D2-02740 Edema of nasopharynx 478.25
(T-23000) (M-36300)

D2-02750 Choanal polyp 471.0
(T-23000) (M-76820)
Nasopharyngeal polyp 471.0
(T-23000) (M-76820)

2-03 DISEASES OF THE PHARYNX

D2-03000 Disease of pharynx, NOS 478.20
(T-55000) (DF-00000)

D2-03005 Pharyngitis, NOS 462.-
(T-55000) (M-40000)

D2-03010 Acute pharyngitis, NOS 462.-
(T-55000) (M-41000)
Acute sore throat, NOS 462.-
(T-55000) (M-41000)
Infective pharyngitis, NOS 462.-
(T-55000) (M-41000)

D2-03020 Gangrenous pharyngitis 462.-
(T-55000) (M-40700)

D2-03030 Phlegmonous pharyngitis 462.-
(T-55000) (M-41650)

D2-03040 Suppurative pharyngitis 462.-
(T-55000) (M-40600)

D2-03050 Ulcerative pharyngitis 462.-
(T-55000) (M-40750)

D2-03100 Chronic pharyngitis 472.1
(T-55000) (M-43000)
Chronic sore throat 472.1
(T-55000) (M-43000)

D2-03110 Atrophic pharyngitis 472.1
(T-55000) (M-45100)

D2-03120 Chronic granular pharyngitis 472.1
(T-55000) (M-43000)

D2-03130 Hypertrophic pharyngitis 472.1
(T-55000) (M-45200)

D2-03200 Cellulitis of pharynx 478.21
(T-55000) (M-41650)

D2-03210 Parapharyngeal abscess 478.22
(T-55140) (M-41610)

D2-03220 Retropharyngeal abscess 478.24
(T-55141) (M-41610)

D2-03230 Edema of pharynx 478.25
(T-55000) (M-36300)

D2-03240 Cyst of pharynx 478.26
(T-55000) (M-33440)

D2-03250 Abscess of pharynx 478.29
(T-55000) (M-41610)

D2-03260 Hemorrhage from pharynx 784.8
(T-55000) (M-37000)
Hemorrhage from throat 784.8
(T-55000) (M-37000)

D2-03420 Pharyngeal paralysis
(T-55000) (F-A0840)

D2-03430V Pharyngeal diverticulitis
(T-55060) (M-40000)

2-04 DISEASES OF THE LARYNX

D2-04000 Disease of the larynx, NOS 478.70
(T-24100) (DF-00000)

D2-04100 Laryngitis, NOS 464.0
(T-24100) (M-40000)

D2-04110 Acute laryngitis 464.0
(T-24100) (M-41000)

D2-04120 Edematous laryngitis 464.0
(T-24100) (M-41000) (M-36300)
Laryngeal edema 464.0
(T-24100) (M-41000) (M-36300)

D2-04130 Suppurative laryngitis 464.0
(T-24100) (M-40600)

D2-04150 Ulcerative laryngitis 464.0
(T-24100) (M-40750)

D2-04160 Croup 464.4
(T-24100) (M-34000) (F-11310)
Croup syndrome 464.4
(T-24100) (M-34000) (F-11310)

2-04 DISEASES OF THE LARYNX — Continued

D2-04170 Ozena laryngis 476.0
(T-24110) (M-45100)

D2-04200 Chronic laryngitis, NOS 476.0
(T-24100) (M-43000)

D2-04210 Catarrhal laryngitis 476.0
(T-24100) (M-40500)

D2-04220 Hypertrophic laryngitis 476.0
(T-24100) (M-45200)

D2-04230 Laryngitis sicca 476.0
(T-24100) (M-43000) (M-58000)

D2-04300 Acute laryngopharyngitis 465.0
(T-24100) (T-55000) (M-41000)

D2-04310 Chronic laryngotracheitis 476.1
(T-24100) (T-25000) (M-43000)

D2-04320 Abscess of larynx 478.79
(T-24100) (M-41610)

D2-04330 Necrosis of larynx 478.79
(T-24100) (M-54000)

D2-04350 Acute laryngotracheitis 464.2
(T-24100) (T-25000) (M-41000)

D2-04351 Acute laryngotracheitis without mention of obstruction 464.20
(T-24100) (T-25000) (M-41000)
(G-C009) (M-34000)

D2-04352 Acute laryngotracheitis with obstruction 464.21
(T-24100) (T-25000) (M-41000)
(G-C008) (M-34000)

D2-04360 Perichondritis of larynx 478.71
(T-24150) (M-40000)

D2-04370 Cellulitis of larynx 478.71
(T-24100) (M-41650)

D2-04400 Paralysis of larynx, NOS 478.30
(T-24100) (F-A0840)
Laryngoplegia, NOS 478.30
(T-24100) (F-A0840)

D2-04406 Laryngeal hemiplegia 478.30
(T-24100) (F-A0841)

D2-04410 Stenosis of larynx 478.74
(T-24100) (M-34200)

D2-04412 Obstruction of larynx 478.79
(T-24100) (M-34000)

D2-04420 Laryngeal spasm 478.75
(T-24100) (F-11310)

D2-04440 Pachyderma of larynx 478.79
(T-24100) (M-02610)

D2-04450 Ulcer of larynx 478.79
(T-24100) (M-38000)

D2-04460 Edema of larynx 478.6
(T-24100) (M-36300)

D2-04470 Polyp of larynx 478.4
(T-24100) (M-76800)

D2-04480 Laryngeal granuloma 478.4
(T-24100) (M-44000)

D2-04600 Disease of vocal cords, NOS
(T-24400) (DF-00000)

D2-04610 Paralysis of glottis 478.30
(T-24400) (F-A0840)
Paralysis of vocal cords 478.30
(T-24400) (F-A0840)

D2-04620 Partial unilateral paralysis of vocal cords 478.31
(T-24400) (F-A0841)

D2-04630 Complete unilateral paralysis of vocal cords 478.32
(T-24400) (F-A0842)

D2-04640 Partial bilateral paralysis of vocal cords 478.33
(T-24400) (F-A0843)

D2-04650 Complete bilateral paralysis of vocal cords 478.34
(T-24400) (F-A0844)

D2-04700 Polyp of vocal cord 478.4
(T-24400) (M-76800)

D2-04710 Singers' nodes 478.5
(T-24400) (M-76800) (J-17145)

D2-04720 Abscess of vocal cords 478.5
(T-24400) (M-41610)

D2-04730 Cellulitis of vocal cords 478.5
(T-24400) (M-41650)

D2-04740 Granuloma of vocal cords 478.5
(T-24400) (M-44000)

D2-04750 Leukoplakia of vocal cords 478.5
(T-24400) (M-76830)

D2-04760 Chorditis 478.5
(T-24400) (M-40000)

D2-04810 Edema of glottis 478.6
(T-24440) (M-36300)

D2-04820 Subglottic edema 478.6
(T-24450) (M-36300)

D2-04830 Supraglottic edema 478.6
(T-24455) (M-36300)

D2-04910 Acute epiglottitis 464.3
(T-24000) (M-41000)

D2-04911 Acute epiglottitis without mention of obstruction 464.30
(T-24000) (M-41000) (G-C009)
(M-34000)

D2-04912 Acute epiglottitis with obstruction 464.31
(T-24000) (M-41000) (G-C008)
(M-34000)

SECTION 2-1 DISEASES OF THE TRACHEA

D2-10000 Disease of trachea, NOS
(T-25000) (DF-00000)

D2-10100 Tracheitis, NOS 464.1
(T-25000) (M-40000)

D2-10110 Acute tracheitis 464.1
(T-25000) (M-41000)

D2-10120 Catarrhal tracheitis 464.1
(T-25000) (M-40500)

D2-10140 Acute tracheitis without mention of obstruction 464.10
(T-25000) (M-41000) (G-C009)
(M-34000)

D2-10141 Acute tracheitis with obstruction 464.11
(T-25000) (M-41000) (G-C008)
(M-34000)
D2-10150 Abscess of trachea 478.9
(T-25000) (M-41610)
D2-10160 Cicatrix of trachea 478.9
(T-25000) (M-78060)
D2-10200 Tracheobronchitis, NOS 490.-
(T-25000) (T-26000) (M-40000)
D2-10210 Acute tracheobronchitis 466.0
(T-25000) (T-26000) (M-41000)
D2-10220 Chronic tracheitis 491.8
(T-25000) (M-43000)
D2-10240 Chronic tracheobronchitis 491.8
(T-25000) (T-26000) (M-43000)
D2-10310 Calcification of trachea 519.1
(T-25000) (M-55400)
D2-10320 Stenosis of trachea 519.1
(T-25000) (M-34200)
D2-10330 Ulcer of trachea 519.1
(T-25000) (M-38000)
D2-10500 Tracheostomy complication, NOS 519.0
(T-25000) (M-18800) (G-C008)
(F-01450)
D2-10510 Tracheostomy hemorrhage 519.0
(T-25000) (M-18800) (G-C008)
(M-37000)
D2-10520 Tracheostomy sepsis 519.0
(T-25000) (M-18800) (G-C008)
(DE-00020)
D2-10530 Tracheostomy obstruction 519.0
(T-25000) (M-18800) (G-C008)
(M-34000)
D2-10540 Tracheal stenosis following tracheostomy 519.0
(T-25000) (M-18800) (G-C008)
(M-34200)
D2-10550 Tracheoesophageal fistula following tracheostomy 519.0
(T-25000) (M-18800) (G-C008)
(T-25000) (T-56000) (M-39300)
D2-10600 Acquired tracheal collapse
(T-25000) (M-02580)
D2-10620V Tracheal edema syndrome
(T-25000) (M-36300) (G-C008)
(M-34000) (F-20040)
Honker syndrome of feeder cattle
(T-25000) (M-36300) (G-C008)
(M-34000) (F-20040)
D2-10630V Obstructive tracheal disease
(T-25000) (M-34000)
D2-10640V Segmental tracheal stenosis
(T-25000) (G-A137) (M-34200)

SECTION 2-3 DISEASES OF THE BRONCHI

D2-30000 Disease of bronchus, NOS
(T-26000) (DF-00000)
D2-30100 Bronchitis, NOS 490.-
(T-26000) (M-40000)
D2-30110 Catarrhal bronchitis 490.-
(T-26000) (M-40500)
D2-30200 Acute bronchitis, NOS 466.0
(T-26000) (M-41000)
D2-30201 Acute bronchitis with bronchospasm 466.0
(T-26000) (M-41000) (G-C008)
(F-11310)
D2-30202 Acute bronchitis with obstruction 466.0
(T-26000) (M-41000) (G-C008)
(M-34000)
D2-30220 Subacute bronchitis 466.0
(T-26000) (M-42000)
D2-30230 Croupous bronchitis 466.0
(T-26000) (M-40100) (G-C008)
(F-11310) (F-20040)
Fibrinous bronchitis 466.0
(T-26000) (M-40100) (G-C008)
(F-11310) (F-20040)
Membranous bronchitis 466.0
(T-26000) (M-40100) (G-C008)
(F-11310) (F-20040)
D2-30240 Purulent bronchitis 466.0
(T-26000) (M-40600)
D2-30250 Septic bronchitis 466.0
(T-26000) (M-41000) (G-C008)
(M-54380)
D2-30400 Chronic bronchitis, NOS 491.9
(T-26000) (M-43000)
D2-30410 Simple chronic bronchitis 491.0
(T-26000) (M-43000)
D2-30411 Smokers' cough 491.0
(T-28000) (F-0A000) (F-24120)
D2-30420 Mucopurulent chronic bronchitis 491.1
(T-26000) (M-43500)
Chronic catarrhal bronchitis 491.0
(T-26000) (M-43500)
D2-30430 Purulent chronic bronchitis 491.1
(T-26000) (M-43600)
D2-30440 Fetid chronic bronchitis 491.1
(T-26000) (M-43000)
D2-30500 Chronic obstructive bronchitis 491.2
(T-26000) (M-43000) (G-C008)
(M-34000) (M-33900)
Obstructive chronic bronchitis 491.2
(T-26000) (M-43000) (G-C008)
(M-34000) (M-33900)
Chronic asthmatic bronchitis 491.2
(T-26000) (M-43000) (G-C008)
(M-34000) (M-33900)
Emphysematous bronchitis 491.2
(T-26000) (M-43000) (G-C008)
(M-34000) (M-33900)
Bronchitis with airway obstruction 491.2
(T-26000) (M-43000) (G-C008)
(M-34000) (M-33900)

SECTION 2-3 DISEASES OF THE BRONCHI — Continued

D2-30500 (cont.) Chronic bronchitis with emphysema 491.2
(T-26000) (M-43000) (G-C008)
(M-34000) (M-33900)

D2-30610 Calcification of bronchus 519.1
(T-26000) (M-55400)
Bronchial mineralization
(T-26000) (M-55400)

D2-30620 Stenosis of bronchus 519.1
(T-26000) (M-34200)

D2-30622 Bronchial compression
(T-26000) (M-01460)

D2-30630 Ulcer of bronchus 519.1
(T-26000) (M-38000)

D2-30670 Broncholithiasis 518.89
(T-26000) (M-30010)

D2-30690 Acquired bronchoesophageal fistula
(T-26000) (T-56000) (M-39300)

D2-30700 Bronchiectasis, NOS 494.-
(T-26000) (M-32000)

D2-30710 Childhood bronchiectasis 494.-
(T-26000) (M-32000)

D2-30720 Adult bronchiectasis 494.-
(T-26000) (M-32000)

D2-30730 Cylindrical bronchiectasis 494.-
(T-26000) (M-32002)

D2-30732 Fusiform bronchiectasis 494.-
(T-26000) (M-32003)

D2-30734 Saccular bronchiectasis 494.-
(T-26000) (M-32001)

D2-30740 Traction bronchiectasis 494.-
(T-26000) (M-32000) (G-C001)
(M-78000)

SECTION 2-4 BRONCHIOLAR DISEASES

D2-40000 Bronchiolar disease, NOS
(T-27000) (DF-00000)

D2-40010 Bronchiolitis, NOS
(T-27000) (M-40000)

D2-40020 Acute bronchiolitis, NOS 466.1
(T-27000) (M-41000)
Capillary pneumonia 466.1
(T-27000) (M-41000)

D2-40022 Acute bronchiolitis with bronchospasm 466.1
(T-27000) (M-41000) (G-C008)
(T-26000) (F-11310)

D2-40024 Acute bronchiolitis with obstruction 466.1
(T-27000) (M-41000) (G-C008)
(M-34000)

D2-40100 Obliterative bronchiolitis, NOS
(T-27000) (M-45100)

D2-40110 Acute obliterating bronchiolitis
(T-28000) (M-41000) (M-78000)
(G-C001) (M-02712) (T-27000)

D2-40120 Bronchiolitis exudativa
(T-27000) (M-40000) (M-33200)

D2-40130 Subacute obliterative bronchiolitis
(T-27000) (M-42000) (M-01520)

D2-40140 Chronic obliterative bronchiolitis
(T-27000) (M-43000) (M-01520)

D2-40144 Bronchiolitis fibrosa obliterans
(T-27000) (M-40000) (G-C001)
(M-78000) (M-01520) (T-27040)

D2-40160 Bronchiolectasis 494.-
(T-27000) (M-32000)

D2-40200 Constriction of bronchioles
(T-27000) (M-34260)

D2-40210 Ulceration of bronchioles
(T-27000) (M-38000)

SECTIONS 2-5-6 DISEASES OF THE LUNG

2-500 Diseases of The Lung: General Terms

D2-50000 Disease of lung, NOS 518.89
(T-28000) (DF-00000)

2-501 Non-Infectious Pneumonias

D2-50100 Bronchopneumonia, NOS 485.-
(T-26000) (T-28000) (M-40000)
Lobular pneumonia 485.-
(T-28040) (M-40000)
Segmental pneumonia 485.-
(T-280D0) (M-40000)
Bronchial pneumonia
(T-280D0) (M-40000)

D2-50104V Peribronchial pneumonia
(T-26090) (T-28000) (M-40000)

D2-50110 Hemorrhagic bronchopneumonia 485.-
(T-26000) (T-28000) (M-40790)

D2-50120 Terminal bronchopneumonia 485.-
(T-26000) (T-28000) (M-40000)
(G-A023)

D2-50130 Pleurobronchopneumonia 485.-
(T-26000) (T-28000) (T-29000)
(M-40000)
Pleuropneumonia
(T-26000) (T-29000) (T-29000)
(M-40000)

D2-50140 Pneumonia, NOS 486.-
(T-28000) (M-40000)
Pneumonitis, NOS
(T-28000) (M-40000)

D2-50142V Catarrhal pneumonia
(T-28000) (M-40000) (G-C008)
(T-1A325)

D2-50150 Unresolved pneumonia
(T-28000) (M-40000)

D2-50152 Unresolved lobar pneumonia
(T-28770) (M-40000)

D2-50160V Granulomatous pneumonia, NOS
(T-28000) (M-44000)

D2-50170V Airsacculitis, NOS
(T-28850) (M-40000)

2-503-504 Aspiration Pneumonias

D2-50300 Aspiration pneumonia, NOS 507.0
(T-28000) (M-40000) (G-C001) (F-29200)
Inhalation pneumonia 507.0
(T-28000) (M-40000) (G-C001) (F-29200)

D2-50304 Foreign body pneumonia 507.0
(T-28000) (M-40000) (G-C001) (F-29200) (M-30400)

D2-50310 Aspiration pneumonia due to regurgitated food 507.0
(T-28000) (M-40000) (G-C001) (F-52890) (C-F0000)

D2-50320 Aspiration pneumonia due to regurgitated gastric secretions 507.0
(T-28000) (M-40000) (G-C001) (F-52890) (F-52000)

D2-50330 Aspiration pneumonia due to inhalation of milk 507.0
(T-28000) (M-40000) (G-C001) (F-29200) (C-F0400)

D2-50340 Aspiration pneumonia due to inhalation of vomitus 507.0
(T-28000) (M-40000) (G-C001) (F-29200) (T-50270)

D2-50350 Aspiration pneumonia due to near drowning
(T-28000) (M-40000) (G-C001) (A-A1070)

D2-50400 Pneumonitis due to inhalation of oils 507.1
(T-28000) (M-40000) (G-C001) (F-29200) (C-20260)
Exogenous lipoid pneumonia 507.1
(T-28000) (M-40000) (G-C001) (F-29200) (C-20260)
Lipid pneumonia 507.1
(T-28000) (M-40000) (G-C001) (F-29200) (C-20260)
Lipoid pneumonia 507.1
(T-28000) (M-40000) (G-C001) (F-29200) (C-20260)
Oil aspiration pneumonia 507.1
(T-28000) (M-40000) (G-C001) (F-29200) (C-20260)
Oil pneumonitis 507.1
(T-28000) (M-40000) (G-C001) (F-29200) (C-20260)
Lipid pneumonitis 507.1
(T-28000) (M-40000) (G-C001) (F-29200) (C-20260)

D2-50410 Pneumonitis due to inhalation of essences 507.1
(T-28000) (M-40000) (G-C001) (F-29200) (C-31100)

2-505-506 Pulmonary Emphysemas

D2-50500 Pulmonary emphysema, NOS 492.8
(T-28000) (M-33900)
Emphysema of lung, NOS 492.8
(T-28000) (M-33900)

D2-50510 Obstructive emphysema 492.8
(T-28000) (M-33900) (G-C008) (M-34000)

D2-50520 Centriacinar emphysema 492.8
(T-28000) (T-27040) (M-33900)
Centrilobular emphysema 492.8
(T-28000) (T-27040) (M-33900)

D2-50524 Panacinar emphysema 492.8
(T-28000) (M-33900) (G-C008) (M-32000) (M-34000)
Panlobular emphysema 492.8
(T-28000) (M-33900) (G-C008) (M-32000) (M-34000)
Vesicular emphysema 492.8
(T-28000) (M-33900) (G-C008) (M-32000) (M-34000)
Alveolar emphysema of lung
(T-28000) (M-33900) (G-C008) (M-32000) (M-34000)

D2-50526 Paraseptal emphysema 492.8
(T-28001) (T-28007) (M-33900)
Peripheral lobular emphysema 492.8
(T-28001) (T-28007) (M-33900)
Subpleural emphysema 492.8
(T-28001) (T-28007) (M-33900)

D2-50540 Unilateral emphysema 492.8
(T-28000) (M-33900)
Swyer-James syndrome 492.8
(T-28000) (M-33900)
Unilateral hyperlucent lung 492.8
(T-28000) (M-33900)
MacLeod's syndrome 492.8
(T-28000) (M-33900)

D2-50560 Emphysematous bleb of lung 492.0
(T-28000) (M-33910) (M-33960)
Tension pneumatocele of lung 492.0
(T-28000) (M-33910) (M-33960)

D2-50570 Ruptured emphysematous bleb of lung 492.0
(T-28000) (M-33910) (M-33960) (G-C008) (M-14400)

D2-50580 Giant bullous emphysema 492.0
(T-28000) (M-33900) (M-33960)

D2-50590 Vanishing lung 492.0
(T-28000) (M-33900) (M-33960) (G-A003)

D2-50610 Interstitial emphysema of lung 518.1
(T-28000) (T-28780) (M-33900)

D2-50620 Compensatory emphysema 518.2
(T-28000) (M-33900)

D2-50630V Acute bovine pulmonary emphysema and edema
(T-28000) (M-33900) (M-36300) (DF-00001)
ABPE
(T-28000) (M-33900) (M-36300) (DF-00001)

2-505-506 Pulmonary Emphysemas — Continued

D2-50630V (cont.) Fog fever
(T-28000) (M-33900) (M-36300) (DF-00001)
Atypical interstitial pneumonia
(T-28000) (M-33900) (M-36300) (DF-00001)

D2-50650V Cystic-bullous disease of the lung, NOS
(T-28000) (M-33900) (M-33400)

D2-50660V Gas bubble disease

2-51 ASTHMA

D2-51000 Asthma, NOS 493.9
(T-26000) (F-11310) (F-23310) (F-20060)
Bronchial asthma, NOS 493.9
(T-26000) (F-11310) (F-23310) (F-20060)
Allergic bronchitis, NOS 493.9
(T-26000) (F-11310) (F-23310) (F-20060)
Asthmatic bronchitis, NOS 493.9
(T-26000) (F-11310) (F-23310) (F-20060)

D2-51003V Chronic allergic bronchitis
(T-26000) (F-11310) (F-23310) (F-20060)

D2-51080 Asthma without status asthmaticus 493.90
(T-26000) (F-11310) (F-23310) (F-20060) (G-C009) (D2-51250)

D2-51090 Asthma with status asthmaticus 493.91
(T-26000) (F-11310) (F-23310) (F-20060) (G-C008) (D2-51250)

D2-51100 Extrinsic asthma 493.0
(T-26000) (F-11310) (F-23310) (F-20060) (G-C001) (F-C1120)
Atopic asthma 493.0
(T-26000) (F-11310) (F-23310) (F-20060) (G-C001) (F-C1120)
Childhood asthma 493.0
(T-26000) (F-11310) (F-22310) (F-20060) (G-C001) (F-C1120)
Allergic asthma 493.0
(T-26000) (F-11310) (F-23310) (F-20060) (G-C001) (F-C1120)

D2-51110 Allergic asthma with stated cause 493.0
(T-26000) (F-11310) (F-22310) (F-20060) (G-C008) (C-.....)

D2-51120 Hay asthma 493.0
(T-26000) (F-11310) (F-22310) (F-20060) (G-C008) (D2-02100)
Hay fever with asthma 493.0
(T-26000) (F-11310) (F-22310) (F-20060) (G-C008) (D2-02100)

D2-51180 Extrinsic asthma without status asthmaticus 493.00
(T-26000) (F-11310) (F-22310) (F-20060) (G-C009) (D2-51250)

D2-51190 Extrinsic asthma with status asthmaticus 493.01
(T-26000) (F-11310) (F-22310) (F-20060) (G-C008) (D2-51250)

D2-51200 Intrinsic asthma 493.1
(T-26000) (F-11310) (F-22310) (F-20060)
Late-onset asthma 493.1
(T-26000) (F-11310) (F-22310) (F-20060)
Asthma due to internal immunological process 493.1
(T-26000) (F-11310) (F-22310) (F-20060)

D2-51210 Intrinsic asthma without status asthmaticus 493.10
(T-26000) (F-11310) (F-22310) (F-20060) (G-C009) (D2-51250)

D2-51220 Intrinsic asthma with status asthmaticus 493.11
(T-26000) (F-11310) (F-22310) (F-20060) (G-C008) (D2-51250)

D2-51250 Status asthmaticus 493.9
(T-26000) (F-11310) (F-22310) (F-20060)

D2-51260V Feline allergic bronchitis
(T-26000) (F-11310) (F-23310) (F-20060)
Feline asthma
(T-26000) (F-11310) (F-23310) (F-20060)

D2-51264V Canine allergic bronchitis

2-52-54 ENVIRONMENTAL AND OCCUPATIONAL LUNG DISEASES

2-52 ENVIRONMENTAL AND OCCUPATIONAL LUNG DISEASES: GENERAL DISORDERS

D2-52000 Environmental lung disease, NOS
(T-28000) (DF-00000) (G-C001) (J-00000)

D2-52100 Occupational lung disease, NOS
(T-28000) (DF-00000) (G-C001) (J-00000)
Occupational lung disorder, NOS
(T-28000) (DF-00000) (G-C001) (J-00000)
Occupational respiratory disease, NOS
(T-28000) (DF-00000) (G-C001) (J-00000)
Occupational pulmonary disease, NOS
(T-28000) (DF-00000) (G-C001) (J-00000)
Occupational inhalation disease, NOS
(T-28000) (DF-00000) (G-C001) (J-00000)

D2-52110 Occupational bronchitis, NOS
(T-26000) (M-40000) (J-00000)
Industrial bronchitis, NOS
(T-26000) (M-40000) (J-00000)

D2-52120 Occupational asthma
(T-26000) (F-11310) (F-22310)
(F-20060) (G-C001) (J-00000)
Industrial asthma
(T-26000) (F-11310) (F-22310)
(F-20060) (G-C001) (J-00000)

2-53 PNEUMOCONIOSES

D2-53000 Pneumoconiosis, NOS 505.-
(T-28000) (M-55700)

D2-53020 Coal workers' pneumoconiosis 500.-
(T-28000) (M-55700) (C-20201)
Anthracosis 500.-
(T-28000) (M-55700) (C-20201)
Black lung disease 500.-
(T-28000) (M-55700) (C-20201)
Coal workers' lung 500.-
(T-28000) (M-55700) (C-20201)
Miners' asthma 500.-
(T-28000) (M-55700) (C-20201)
Lung melanosis 500.-
(T-28000) (M-55700) (C-20201)
Pneumomelanosis 500.-
(T-28000) (M-55700) (C-20201)
Coal miners' lung 500.-
(T-28000) (M-55700) (C-20201)
Coal miners' pneumoconiosis 500.-
(T-28000) (M-55700) (C-20201)
Coal pneumoconiosis 500.-
(T-28000) (M-55700) (C-20201)
Colliers' lung 500.-
(T-28000) (M-55700) (C-20201)
Colliers' anthracosis 500.-
(T-28000) (M-55700) (C-20201)
Miners' lung 500.-
(T-28000) (M-55700) (C-20201)
Melanedema 500.-
(T-28000) (M-55700) (C-20201)

D2-53022 Anthracosilicosis 500.-
(T-28000) (M-55700) (C-20201)
(C-10955)

D2-53100 Pneumoconiosis due to silica, NOS 502.-
(T-28000) (M-55700) (G-C001)
(C-10955)

D2-53101 Simple silicosis 502.-
(T-28000) (M-55700) (G-C001)
(C-10955)

D2-53104 Complicated silicosis 502.-
(T-28000) (M-55700) (C-10955)
(F-01450)

D2-53105 Massive silicotic fibrosis of lung 502.-
(T-28000) (M-55700) (C-10955)
(G-C008) (M-78260)

D2-53110 Pneumoconiosis due to silicates, NOS 502.-
(T-28000) (M-55700) (C-10960)
Silicatosis 502.-
(T-28000) (M-55700) (C-10960)

D2-53112 Pneumoconiosis due to talc 502.-
(T-28000) (M-55700) (C-14821)
Talcosis 502.-
(T-28000) (M-55700) (C-14821)
Pulmonary talcosis 502.-
(T-28000) (M-55700) (C-14821)
Talc lung disease 502.-
(T-28000) (M-55700) (C-14821)
Talc pneumoconiosis 502.-
(T-28000) (M-55700) (C-14821)
Talc workers' pneumoconiosis 502.-
(T-28000) (M-55700) (C-14821)

D2-53130 Platinosis
(T-26000) (F-11310) (F-22310)
(F-20060) (G-C001) (C-15311)
Platinum asthma 493.0
(T-26000) (F-11310) (F-22310)
(F-20060) (G-C001) (C-15311)

D2-53140 Asbestosis 501.-
(T-28000) (M-55700) (C-20110)
Amianthosis 501.-
(T-28000) (M-55700) (C-20110)
Asbestos pneumoconiosis 501.-
(T-28000) (M-55700) (C-20110)

D2-53160 Rheumatoid pneumoconiosis 714.81
(T-28000) (M-55700) (C-10955)
(G-C002) (D1-20600)
Caplan's syndrome 714.81
(T-28000) (M-55700) (C-10955)
(G-C002) (D1-20600)
Rheumatoid lung 714.81
(T-28000) (M-55700) (C-10955)
(G-C002) (D1-20600)

D2-53170 Diatomaceous earth disease
(T-28000) (M-55700) (C-10957)
Diatomite disease
(T-28000) (M-55700) (C-10957)

D2-53172 Fullers' earth disease
(T-28000) (M-55700) (C-12012)

D2-53176 Chalicosis
(T-28000) (C-20103) (C-20140)

D2-53180 Liparitosis
(T-28000) (M-55700) (C-10965)

D2-53190 Siderosilicosis
(T-28000) (M-55700) (C-10955)
(C-13031)
Haematite foundry workers' lung
(T-28000) (M-55700) (C-10955)
(C-13031)
Haematite lung
(T-28000) (M-55700) (C-10955)
(C-13031)
Haematite miners' lung
(T-28000) (M-55700) (C-10955)
(C-13031)

2-53 PNEUMOCONIOSES — Continued

D2-53190 (cont.) Haematite pneumoconiosis
(T-28000) (M-55700) (C-10955) (C-13031)
Hematite pneumoconiosis
(T-28000) (M-55700) (C-10955) (C-13031)
Silicosiderosis
(T-28000) (M-55700) (C-10955) (C-13031)
Hematite miners' lung disease
(T-28000) (M-55700) (C-10955) (C-13031)

D2-53200 Pneumoconiosis due to inorganic dust, NOS 503.-
(T-28000) (M-55700) (C-20062)

D2-53201 Benign pneumoconiosis, NOS
(T-28000) (M-55700)
Non-collagenous pneumoconiosis, NOS
(T-28000) (M-55700)

D2-53202 Collagenous pneumoconiosis, NOS
(T-28000) (M-55700) (G-C008) (T-1A050)

D2-53203 Hard metal pneumoconiosis, NOS
(T-28000) (M-55700) (C-11840)

D2-53205 Kaolinosis
(T-28000) (M-55700) (C-12011)
Kaolin pneumoconiosis
(T-28000) (M-55700) (C-12011)

D2-53206 Mixed dust pneumoconiosis
(T-28000) (M-55700) (C-20061)

D2-53210 Aluminosis of lung 503.-
(T-28000) (M-55700) (C-12000)
Aluminosis 503.-
(T-28000) (M-55700) (C-12000)
Aluminosis pulmonum 503.-
(T-28000) (M-55700) (C-12000)
Aluminum pneumoconiosis 503.-
(T-28000) (M-55700) (C-12000)

D2-53215 Bauxite fibrosis of lung 503.-
(T-28000) (M-55700) (C-12014) (G-C008) (M-78000)
Bauxite fume pneumoconiosis 503.-
(T-28000) (M-55700) (C-12014) (G-C008) (M-78000)
Bauxite pneumoconiosis 503.-
(T-28000) (M-55700) (C-12014) (G-C008) (M-78000)
Bauxite workers' disease 503.-
(T-28000) (M-55700) (C-12014) (G-C008) (M-78000)
Corundum smelters' lung 503.-
(T-28000) (M-55700) (C-12014) (G-C008) (M-78000)
Bauxite lung 503.-
(T-28000) (M-55700) (C-12014) (G-C008) (M-78000)
Bauxite pulmonary fibrosis 503.-
(T-28000) (M-55700) (C-12014) (G-C008) (M-78000)
Bauxite fibrosis 503.-
(T-28000) (M-55700) (C-12014) (G-C008) (M-78000)
Shavers' disease 503.-
(T-28000) (M-55700) (C-12014) (G-C008) (M-78000)

D2-53220 Baritosis
(T-28000) (M-55700) (C-12203)
Barium lung
(T-28000) (M-55700) (C-12203)
Baryta miners' disease
(T-28000) (M-55700) (C-12203)
Barium lung disease
(T-28000) (M-55700) (C-12203)

D2-53230 Berylliosis 503.-
(T-28000) (DF-00000) (G-C001) (C-12300)
Beryllium disease 503.-
(T-28000) (DF-00000) (G-C001) (C-12300)
Beryllium poisoning 503.-
(T-28000) (DF-00000) (G-C001) (C-12300)

D2-53231 Acute berylliosis 503.-
(T-28000) (F-C3000) (G-C001) (C-12312)
Acute beryllium disease 503.-
(T-28000) (F-C3000) (G-C001) (C-12312)

D2-53232 Chronic berylliosis 503.-
(T-28000) (M-55700) (C-12300) (G-C008) (M-44000)
Beryllium granuloma 503.-
(T-28000) (M-55700) (C-12300) (G-C008) (M-44000)
Chronic beryllium disease 503.-
(T-28000) (M-55700) (C-12300) (G-C008) (M-44000)
Chronic beryllium lung 503.-
(T-28000) (M-55700) (C-12300) (G-C008) (M-44000)
Chronic beryllium lung disease 503.-
(T-28000) (M-55700) (C-12300) (G-C008) (M-44000)
Chronic beryllium poisoning 503.-
(T-28000) (M-55700) (C-12300) (G-C008) (M-44000)

D2-53240 Cadmium pneumonitis
(T-28000) (M-55700) (C-12602)
Cadmiosis
(T-28000) (M-55700) (C-12602)

D2-53250 Graphite fibrosis of lung 503.-
(T-28000) (M-55700) (C-10506) (G-C008) (M-78000)
Graphitosis 503.-
(T-28000) (M-55700) (C-10506) (G-C008) (M-78000)

D2-53250 (cont.) Graphite pneumoconiosis 503.-
(T-28000) (M-55700) (C-10506)
(G-C008) (M-78000)
Graphite lung disease 503.-
(T-28000) (M-55700) (C-10506)
(G-C008) (M-78000)
Graphite fibrosis 503.-
(T-28000) (M-55700) (C-10506)
(G-C008) (M-78000)

D2-53260 Antimony pneumoconiosis
(T-28000) (M-55700) (C-12100)

D2-53270 Pulmonary siderosis 503.-
(T-28000) (M-55700) (C-13005)
Arc-welders' disease 503.-
(T-28000) (M-55700) (C-13005)
Arc-welders' lung 503.-
(T-28000) (M-55700) (C-13005)
Arc-welders' nodulation 503.-
(T-28000) (M-55700) (C-13005)
Arc-welders' pneumoconiosis 503.-
(T-28000) (M-55700) (C-13005)
Iron oxide lung 503.-
(T-28000) (M-55700) (C-13005)
Pneumoconiosis siderotico 503.-
(T-28000) (M-55700) (C-13005)
Siderotic lung disease 503.-
(T-28000) (M-55700) (C-13005)
Steel grinders' disease 503.-
(T-28000) (M-55700) (C-13005)
Welders' lung 503.-
(T-28000) (M-55700) (C-13005)
Welders' siderosis 503.-
(T-28000) (M-55700) (C-13005)

D2-53272 Silver polishers' lung disease
(T-28000) (M-55700) (C-13700)

D2-53280 Arsine poisoning
(T-28000) (F-20010) (C-27222)

D2-53290 Stannosis 503.-
(T-28000) (M-55700) (C-13921)
Tin miners' lung 503.-
(T-28000) (M-55700) (C-13921)
Tin oxide pneumoconiosis 503.-
(T-28000) (M-55700) (C-13921)
Tin pneumoconiosis 503.-
(T-28000) (M-55700) (C-13921)

D2-532A0 Carbon electrode makers' pneumoconiosis
(T-28000) (M-55700) (C-10500)

D2-532B0 Cobaltosis
(T-28000) (F-20010) (C-14403)
(G-C008) (F-24100) (F-20040)

D2-532C0 Manganese pneumonitis
(T-28000) (M-55700) (C-14900)
Manganese poisoning
(T-28000) (M-55700) (C-14900)
Manganic pneumonia
(T-28000) (M-55700) (C-14900)
Manganic pneumonitis
(T-28000) (M-55700) (C-14900)
Manganism
(T-28000) (M-55700) (C-14900)

D2-532E0 Organophosphate poisoning
(T-28000) (F-20010) (C-23150)
(C-22100)
Organophosphate insecticide poisoning
(T-28000) (F-20010) (C-23150)
(C-22100)

D2-53300 Bituminosis
(T-28000) (M-55700) (C-20204)

D2-53310 Schistosis
(T-28000) (M-55700) (C-20130)
(C-20103)
Slate-workers' lung
(T-28000) (M-55700) (C-20130)
(C-20103)

D2-53400 Pneumonopathy due to inhalation of dust, NOS 504.-
(T-28000) (DF-00000) (G-C001)
(F-20010) (C-20060)

D2-53420 Byssinosis 504.-
(T-28000) (M-55700) (C-30652)
(L-D4D00)
Cotton workers' lung disease 504.-
(T-28000) (M-55700) (C-30652)
(L-D4D00)
Cotton-dust asthma 504.-
(T-28000) (M-55700) (C-30652)
(L-D4D00)

D2-53430 Sisal workers' disease 504.-
(T-28000) (M-55700) (C-30653)
(L-DC100)

D2-53440 Cannabinosis 504.-
(T-28000) (M-55700) (C-30651)
(L-D5101)
Cannabosis 504.-
(T-28000) (M-55700) (C-30651)
(L-D5101)
Hemp-workers' disease 504.-
(T-28000) (M-55700) (C-30651)
(L-D5101)

D2-53450 Weavers' cough 504.-
(T-26000) (M-40000) (M-34000)
(G-C001) (C-30650) (L-44130)
(L-44310) (L-40150)

D2-53460 Flax-dressers' disease 504.-
(T-26000) (M-40000) (M-34000)
(G-C001) (C-30654) (L-D7001)
Strippers' disease 504.-
(T-26000) (M-40000) (M-34000)
(G-C001) (C-30654) (L-D7001)

D2-53500 Respiratory condition due to chemical fumes and vapors, NOS 506.-
(T-20000) (DF-00000) (G-C001)
(C-20070)

D2-53502 Upper respiratory inflammation due to fumes and vapors 506.2
(T-20100) (DF-00000) (G-C001)
(C-20070)

2-53 PNEUMOCONIOSES — Continued

D2-53503 Metal fever, NOS 506.2
(T-20000) (DF-00000) (F-03003)
(G-C001) (C-14118)
Metal-fume fever, NOS 506.2
(T-20000) (DF-00000) (F-03003)
(G-C001) (C-14118)
Monday morning fever 506.2
(T-20000) (DF-00000) (F-03003)
(G-C001) (C-14118)
Monday fever 506.2
(T-20000) (DF-00000) (F-03003)
(G-C001) (C-14118)

D2-53504 Brass-founders' fever 506.2
(T-20000) (DF-00000) (F-03003)
(G-C001) (C-14118)
Foundrymen's fever 506.2
(T-20000) (DF-00000) (F-03003)
(G-C001) (C-14118)
Brass fever 506.2
(T-20000) (DF-00000) (F-03003)
(G-C001) (C-14118)
Brass-founders' disease 506.2
(T-20000) (DF-00000) (F-03003)
(G-C001) (C-14118)
Braziers' disease 506.2
(T-20000) (DF-00000) (F-03003)
(G-C001) (C-14118)
Brass poisoning 506.2
(T-20000) (DF-00000) (F-03003)
(G-C001) (C-14118)
Foundry syndrome 506.2
(T-20000) (DF-00000) (F-03003)
(G-C001) (C-14118)

D2-53505 Spelters' fever 506.2
(T-20000) (DF-00000) (F-03003)
(G-C001) (C-14118)
Zinc-fume fever 506.2
(T-20000) (DF-00000) (F-03003)
(G-C001) (C-14118)
Galvanizers' poisoning 506.2
(T-20000) (DF-00000) (F-03003)
(G-C001) (C-14118)
Zinc-poisoning tremor 506.2
(T-20000) (DF-00000) (F-03003)
(G-C001) (C-14118)

D2-53506 Polymer fume fever
(T-20000) (DF-00000) (G-C001)
(F-24100) (C-2A560)
Teflon shakes
(T-20000) (DF-00000) (G-C001)
(F-24100) (C-2A560)

D2-53510 Bronchitis due to fumes and vapors 506.0
(T-26000) (M-41000) (F-24100)
(G-C001) (C-20070)
Acute chemical bronchitis 506.0
(T-26000) (M-41000) (F-24100)
(G-C001) (C-20070)

D2-53511 Copper fever 506.0
(T-20000) (DF-00000) (G-C008)
(F-24100) (G-C001) (F-20010)
(C-12702)

D2-53520 Smoke inhalation
(T-28000) (F-20010) (A-80320)

D2-53540 Pneumonitis due to fumes and vapors 506.0
(T-28000) (M-40000) (G-C001)
(F-20010) (C-20070)
Chemical pneumonia 506.0
(T-28000) (M-40000) (G-C001)
(F-20010) (C-20070)
Chemical pneumonitis 506.0
(T-28000) (M-40000) (G-C001)
(F-20010) (C-20070)
Chemical workers' lung 506.0
(T-28000) (M-40000) (G-C001)
(F-20010) (C-20070)

D2-53550 Acute pulmonary edema due to fumes and vapors 506.1
(T-28000) (M-36301) (G-C001)
(C-20070)
Acute chemical pulmonary edema 506.1
(T-28000) (M-36301) (G-C001)
(C-20070)

D2-53600 Chronic respiratory condition due to fumes and vapors, NOS 506.4
(T-28000) (DF-00003) (G-C001)
(F-20010) (C-20070)

D2-53610 Chronic diffuse emphysema due to inhalation of chemical fumes and vapors 506.4
(T-28000) (M-33900) (G-C001)
(F-20010) (C-20070)

D2-53620 Chronic obliterative bronchiolitis due to inhalation of chemical fumes and vapors 506.4
(T-27000) (D2-50840) (G-C001)
(F-20010) (C-20070)

D2-53630 Subacute obliterative bronchiolitis due to inhalation of chemical fumes and vapors 506.4
(T-27000) (D2-50835) (G-C001)
(F-20010) (C-20070)

D2-53640 Chronic pulmonary fibrosis due to inhalation of chemical fumes and vapors 506.4
(T-28000) (M-78003) (G-C001)
(F-20010) (C-20070)

D2-53650 Silo-fillers' disease 506.9
(T-28000) (M-36300) (G-C001)
(C-10713)
Silo-fillers' lung 506.9
(T-28000) (M-36300) (G-C001)
(C-10713)
Silo-workers' asthma 506.9
(T-28000) (M-36300) (G-C001)
(C-10713)

D2-53670 Pneumonitis due to solids, NOS 507.-
(T-28000) (M-40000) (G-C001)
(F-29230)

D2-53680 Pneumonitis due to liquids, NOS 507.-
(T-28000) (M-40000) (G-C001)
(F-29280)

D2-53900 Radiation pneumonitis 508.0
(T-28000) (M-40000) (G-C001)
(A-81000)

D2-53910 Fibrosis of lung following radiation 508.1
(T-28000) (M-78000) (G-C001)
(A-81000)

2-54 EXTRINSIC ALLERGIC RESPIRATORY DISEASES

D2-54000 Extrinsic allergic alveolitis, NOS 495.9
(T-28010) (F-C3000)
Hypersensitivity pneumonitis, NOS 495.9
(T-28010) (F-C3000)
Extrinsic allergic bronchiolo-alveolitis, NOS 495.9
(T-28010) (F-C3000)
Hypersensitivity pneumonia, NOS 495.9
(T-28010) (F-C3000)
Allergic alveolitis, NOS 495.9
(T-28010) (F-C3000)
Allergic pneumonitis, NOS 495.9
(T-28010) (F-C3000)
Allergic interstitial pneumonitis, NOS 495.9
(T-28010) (F-C3000)

D2-54010 Detergent asthma 507.8
(D2-54000) (G-C001) (F-66000)
(L-12201)
Detergent workers' lung 507.8
(D2-54000) (G-C001) (F-66000)
(L-12201)
Enzyme detergent lung 507.8
(D2-54000) (G-C001) (F-66000)
(L-12201)
Enzyme detergent respiratory disease 507.8
(D2-54000) (G-C001) (F-66000)
(L-12201)
Enzyme lung 507.8
(D2-54000) (G-C001) (F-66000)
(L-12201)
Enzyme lung disease 507.8
(D2-54000) (G-C001) (F-66000)
(L-12201)

D2-54020 Farmers' lung 495.0
(D2-54000) (G-C001) (L-21301)
Farmers' lung disease 495.0
(D2-54000) (G-C001) (L-21301)
Moldy-hay disease 495.0
(D2-54000) (G-C001) (L-21301)

D2-54040 Bagassosis 495.1
(D2-54000) (G-C001) (L-25704)
(L-25705) (C-30641)
Bagasse disease 495.1
(D2-54000) (G-C001) (L-25704)
(L-25705) (C-30641)
Bagasse workers' disease 495.1
(D2-54000) (G-C001) (L-25704)
(L-25705) (C-30641)
Bagasse workers' lung 495.1
(D2-54000) (G-C001) (L-25704)
(L-25705) (C-30641)
Sugar cane workers' hypersensitivity pneumonitis 495.1
(D2-54000) (G-C001) (L-25704)
(L-25705) (C-30641)

D2-54060 Bird-fanciers' lung, NOS 495.2
(D2-54000) (G-C001) (F-C1000)
(L-82000)
Bird breeders' lung 495.2
(D2-54000) (G-C001) (F-C1000)
(L-82000)
Bird fanciers' disease 495.2
(D2-54000) (G-C001) (F-C1000)
(L-82000)
Avian protein hypersensitivity 495.2
(D2-54000) (G-C001) (F-C1000)
(L-82000)
Bird breeders' disease 495.9
(D2-54000) (G-C001) (F-C1000)
(L-82000)

D2-54061 Budgerigar-fanciers' disease 495.2
(D2-54000) (G-C001) (F-C1000)
(L-96249)
Budgerigar-fanciers' lung 495.2
(D2-54000) (G-C001) (F-C1000)
(L-96249)
Budgerigar-breeders' lung 495.2
(D2-54000) (G-C001) (F-C1000)
(L-96249)

D2-54062 Pigeon-fanciers' disease 495.2
(D2-54000) (G-C001) (F-C1000)
(L-96100)
Pigeon-fanciers' lung 495.2
(D2-54000) (G-C001) (F-C1000)
(L-96100)
Pigeon-breeders' lung 495.2
(D2-54000) (G-C001) (F-C1000)
(L-96100)
Pigeon-breeders' disease 495.2
(D2-54000) (G-C001) (F-C1000)
(L-96100)

D2-54080 Suberosis 495.3
(D2-54000) (G-C001) (F-C1000)
(L-44310) (C-30646)
Cork-handlers' disease 495.3
(D2-54000) (G-C001) (F-C1000)
(L-44310) (C-30646)
Cork-handlers' lung 495.3
(D2-54000) (G-C001) (F-C1000)
(L-44310) (C-30646)

D2-54090 Malt-workers' lung 495.4
(D2-54000) (G-C001) (F-C1000)
(L-44133) (L-44136)
Alveolitis due to Aspergillus clavatus and fumigatus 495.4
(D2-54000) (G-C001) (F-C1000)
(L-44133) (L-44136)

2-54 EXTRINSIC ALLERGIC RESPIRATORY DISEASES — Continued

D2-54090 (cont.) Malt-workers' alveolitis 495.4
(D2-54000) (G-C001) (F-C1000)
(L-44133) (L-44136)
Malt-workers' lung disease 495.4
(D2-54000) (G-C001) (F-C1000)
(L-44133) (L-44136)
Malt fever 495.4
(D2-54000) (G-C001) (F-C1000)
(L-44133) (L-44136)
Malt house workers' cough 495.4
(D2-54000) (G-C001) (F-C1000)
(L-44133) (L-44136)

D2-54100 Mushroom workers' lung 495.5
(D2-54000) (G-C001) (F-C1000)
(L-25700)
Mushroom-workers' disease 495.5
(D2-54000) (G-C001) (F-C1000)
(L-25700)
Mushroom pickers' disease 495.5
(D2-54000) (G-C001) (F-C1000)
(L-25700)

D2-54110 Maple-bark strippers' lung 495.6
(D2-54000) (G-C001) (F-C1000)
(L-49011)
Alveolitis due to Cryptostroma corticale 495.6
(D2-54000) (G-C001) (F-C1000)
(L-49011)
Maple-bark disease 495.6
(D2-54000) (G-C001) (F-C1000)
(L-49011)
Maple-bark strippers' disease 495.6
(D2-54000) (G-C001) (F-C1000)
(L-49011)

D2-54120 Humidifier lung 495.7
(D2-54000) (G-C001) (C-20060)
Air conditioner lung 495.7
(D2-54000) (G-C001) (C-20060)
Humidifier and air conditioning pneumonitis 495.7
(D2-54000) (G-C001) (C-20060)
Ventilation pneumonitis 495.7
(D2-54000) (G-C001) (C-20060)

D2-54140 Cheese-washers' lung 495.8
(D2-54000) (G-C001) (F-C1000)
(L-44311) (L-44325) (L-67001)
Cheese-makers' asthma 495.8
(D2-54000) (G-C001) (F-C1000)
(L-44311) (L-44325) (L-67001)
Cheese-workers' lung 495.8
(D2-54000) (G-C001) (F-C1000)
(L-44311) (L-44325) (L-67001)
Cheese-washers' disease 495.8
(D2-54000) (G-C001) (F-C1000)
(L-44311) (L-44325) (L-67001)

D2-54150 Laboratory animal dander allergy
(D2-54000) (G-C001) (F-C1000)
(T-01796)
Animal dander allergy
(D2-54000) (G-C001) (F-C1000)
(T-01796)
Animal handlers' lung
(D2-54000) (G-C001) (F-C1000)
(T-01796)
Laboratory animal allergy
(D2-54000) (G-C001) (F-C1000)
(T-01796)
Laboratory technician lung
(D2-54000) (G-C001) (F-C1000)
(T-01796)

D2-54160 Coffee-workers' lung 495.8
(D2-54000) (G-C001) (F-C1000)
(L-43131)
Coffee-workers' disease 495.8
(D2-54000) (G-C001) (F-C1000)
(L-43131)

D2-54170 Meat-wrappers' asthma
(D2-54000) (G-C001) (C-.....) (C-.....)

D2-54180 Fish-meal workers' lung 495.8
(D2-54000) (G-C001) (F-62000)
(L-C0000) (L-10000)

D2-54190 Millers' asthma
(D2-54000) (G-C001) (C-20060)
(C-F0110)
Mill-workers' asthma
(D2-54000) (G-C001) (C-20060)
(C-F0110)
Millers' cough
(D2-54000) (G-C001) (C-20060)
(C-F0110)

D2-541A0 Grain fever
(D2-54000) (G-C001) (C-20060)
(L-60001)

D2-541B0 Printers' asthma
(D2-54000) (G-C001) (C-30634)
(L-D6219) (L-D621A)

D2-541C0 Storage disease of the lung
(D2-54000) (G-C001) (C-20074)
Accumulation disease of the lung
(D2-54000) (G-C001) (C-20074)
Hairspray lung
(D2-54000) (G-C001) (C-20074)
Hairspray thesaurosis
(D2-54000) (G-C001) (C-20074)
Hairspray disease
(D2-54000) (G-C001) (C-20074)
Aerosol disease
(D2-54000) (G-C001) (C-20074)

D2-541D0 Tea-tasters' disease
(D2-54000) (G-C001) (C-20060)
(L-40000)
Tea-factory cough
(D2-54000) (G-C001) (C-20060)
(L-40000)

D2-541D0 (cont.) Tea-makers' asthma
(D2-54000) (G-C001) (C-20060) (L-40000)
Tea-tasters' cough
(D2-54000) (G-C001) (C-20060) (L-40000)

D2-541E0 Vinyard sprayers' lung
(D2-54000) (G-C001) (C-20070) (C-12731)

D2-541F0 Wheat weevil disease
(D2-54000) (G-C001) (F-C1000) (L-60951)
Insect-antigen lung
(D2-54000) (G-C001) (F-C1000) (L-60951)

D2-54210 Furriers' lung 495.8
(D2-54000) (G-C001) (F-C1000) (T-01785)

D2-54220 Grain-handlers' disease 495.8
(D2-54000) (G-C001) (C-30645)
Grain-handlers' lung 495.8
(D2-54000) (G-C001) (C-30645)
Cereal-workers' disease 495.8
(D2-54000) (G-C001) (C-30645)
Grain-workers' disease 495.8
(D2-54000) (G-C001) (C-30645)

D2-54260 Sequoiosis 495.8
(D2-54000) (G-C001) (F-C1000) (L-45260)
Red-cedar asthma 495.8
(D2-54000) (G-C001) (F-C1000) (L-45260)
Sequoiasis 495.8
(D2-54000) (G-C001) (F-C1000) (L-45260)

D2-54262 Wood asthma 495.8
(D2-54000) (G-C001) (C-30625)
Wood-workers' asthma 495.8
(D2-54000) (G-C001) (C-30625)
Wood-workers' lung 495.8
(D2-54000) (G-C001) (C-30625)
Wood dust asthma 495.8
(D2-54000) (G-C001) (C-30625)
Saw dust asthma 495.8
(D2-54000) (G-C001) (C-30625)
Wood dust pneumonitis 495.8
(D2-54000) (G-C001) (C-30625)

D2-54280 Bakers' asthma
(D2-54000) (G-C001) (F-C1000) (L-67000) (L-40000) (C-F0100)
Flour asthma
(D2-54000) (G-C001) (F-C1000) (L-67000) (L-40000) (C-F0100)

D2-54290 Feather-pickers' disease
(D2-54000) (G-C001) (C-20060) (T-01790)
Feather asthma
(D2-54000) (G-C001) (C-20060) (T-01790)

D2-54300V Hypersensitivity alveolitis in lungworm infection
(T-28000) (F-C3000) (L-55A72)
Hypersensitivity alveolitis in Dictyocaulus viviparus infection
(T-28000) (F-C3000) (L-55A72)

D2-54310V Bovine allergic alveolitis
(T-28000) (F-C3000) (G-C001) (F-20010) (L-2A000)
Bovine farmers' lung
(T-28000) (F-C3000) (G-C001) (F-20010) (L-2A000)
Bovine hypersensitivity pneumonitis
(T-28000) (F-C3000) (G-C001) (F-20010) (L-2A000)
Hypersensitivity pneumonitis due to inhalation of Micropolyspora faeni spores
(T-28000) (F-C3000) (G-C001) (F-20010) (L-2A000)

D2-54320V Equine allergic pneumonitis
(T-28000) (F-C3000)

SECTION 2-6 OTHER LUNG DISEASES AND CONDITIONS

D2-60000 Chronic obstructive lung disease, NOS 496.-
(T-28000) (DF-00003) (G-C008) (M-34000)
Chronic obstructive lung disease, NEC 496.-
(T-28000) (DF-00003) (G-C008) (M-34000)
COLD 496.-
(T-28000) (DF-00003) (G-C008) (T-01790)
COPD 496.-
(T-28000) (DF-00003) (G-C008) (M-34000)

D2-60010 Chronic nonspecific lung disease, NOS 496.-
(T-28000) (DF-00003)

D2-60020V Heaves
(T-28000) (DF-00003) (G-C008) (M-34000)
Broken wind
(T-28000) (DF-00003) (G-C008) (M-34000)
Chronic alveolar emphysema of horses
(T-28000) (DF-00003) (G-C008) (M-34000)
Chronic obstructive pulmonary disease of horses
(T-28000) (DF-00003) (G-C008) (M-34000)

D2-60100 Adult respiratory distress syndrome, NOS 518.5
(T-28000) (F-00161) (G-C001) (D3-80610)
Shock lung 518.5
(T-28000) (F-00161) (G-C001) (D3-80610)

SECTION 2-6 OTHER LUNG DISEASES AND CONDITIONS — Continued

D2-60100 (cont.) ARDS 518.5
(T-28000) (F-00161) (G-C001) (D3-80610)
Pulmonary insufficiency following shock 518.5
(T-28000) (F-00161) (G-C001) (D3-80610)
Pulmonary insufficiency following surgery 518.5
(T-28000) (F-00161) (G-C001) (D3-80610)
Pulmonary insufficiency following trauma 518.5
(T-28000) (F-00161) (G-C001) (D3-80610)
Post-traumatic pulmonary insufficiency 518.5
(T-28000) (F-00161) (G-C001) (D3-80610)
Traumatic wet lung 518.5
(T-28000) (F-00161) (G-C001) (D3-80610)
Congestive atelectasis 518.5
(T-28000) (F-00161) (G-C001) (D3-80610)
DaNang lung 518.5
(T-28000) (F-00161) (G-C001) (D3-80610)
Vietnam lung 518.5
(T-28000) (F-00161) (G-C001) (D3-80610)

D2-60110 Idiopathic respiratory distress syndrome, NOS 769.9

D2-60200 Respiratory failure, NOS 518.81 —799.1
(T-28000) (F-00150)
Respiratory insufficiency, NOS 786.09
(T-28000) (F-00150)

D2-60210 Acute respiratory failure 518.81
(T-28000) (F-00151)

D2-60220 Acute-on-chronic respiratory failure 518.81
(T-28000) (F-00152)

D2-60230 Chronic respiratory failure 518.81
(T-28000) (F-00153)

D2-60250 Acute respiratory distress, NEC 518.82
(T-28000) (F-00161)
Acute respiratory insufficiency, NEC 518.82
(T-28000) (F-00161)

D2-60260 Respiratory arrest 799.1

D2-60300 Atelectasis, NOS 518.0
(T-28000)
Pulmonary collapse 518.0
(T-28000)
Collapse of lung 518.0
(T-28000)

D2-60302 Discoid atelectasis
(T-28000)
Plate atelectasis
(T-28000)
Plate-like atelectasis
(T-28000)

D2-60303 Linear atelectasis
(T-28000)

D2-60304 Focal atelectasis
(T-28000)
PAtchy atelectasis
(T-28000)
Lobular atelectasis
(T-28000)

D2-60306 Complete atelectasis
(T-28000)

D2-60307 Obstructive atelectasis
(T-28000) (M-34000)

D2-60308 Compression atelectasis
(T-28000) (M-01460)

D2-60320 Middle lobe syndrome 518.0
(T-28300) (M-43000)
Brock syndrome 518.0
(T-28300) (M-43000)

D2-60400 Pulmonary eosinophilia 518.3
(T-28000) (M-43040)
Eosinophilic asthma 518.3
(T-28000) (M-43040)
Eosinophilic pneumonia 518.3
(T-28000) (M-43040)

D2-60420 Allergic pneumonia 518.3
(T-28000) (F-C3000)

D2-60430 Loffler's syndrome 518.3
(T-28000) (F-24100) (F-03003) (M-69010)

D2-60440V PIE syndrome

D2-60500 Acute pulmonary edema, NOS 518.4
(T-28000) (M-36301)
Acute edema of lung, NOS 518.4
(T-28000) (M-36301)

D2-60510 Postoperative pulmonary edema 518.4
(T-28000) (M-36300) (F-06030)

D2-60600 Alveolar pneumopathy, NOS 516.9
(T-28010) (DF-00000)

D2-60610 Parietoalveolar pneumopathy, NOS 516.9
(T-28010) (DF-00000)

D2-60620 Pulmonary alveolar proteinosis 516.0
(T-28010) (M-55000) (F-62000)

D2-60640 Pulmonary alveolar microlithiasis 516.2
(T-28010) (M-30180)

D2-60650 Idiopathic fibrosing alveolitis 516.3
(T-28000) (DF-00001) (M-78000)
Hamman-Rich syndrome 516.3
(T-28000) (DF-00001) (M-78000)
Diffuse idiopathic pulmonary fibrosis 516.3
(T-28000) (DF-00001) (M-78000)
Diffuse interstitial pulmonary fibrosis 516.3
(T-28000) (DF-00001) (M-78000)

D2-60650 (cont.) Hamman-Rich disease 516.3
(T-28000) (DF-00001) (M-78000)
Idiopathic fibrosing alveolitis, acute fatal form 516.3
(T-28000) (DF-00001) (M-78000)

D2-60652 Idiopathic fibrosing alveolitis, subacute form 516.3
(T-28000) (M-78000) (DF-00002)
Scadding syndrome 516.3
(T-28000) (M-78000) (DF-00002)

D2-60654 Idiopathic fibrosing alveolitis, chronic form 516.3
(T-28000) (M-78000) (DF-00003)

D2-60656 Simple pulmonary alveolitis
(T-28010) (M-40000)

D2-60657 Prolonged pulmonary alveolitis
(T-28010) (M-40000)

D2-60658 Asthmatic pulmonary alveolitis
(T-28010) (M-40000)

D2-60659 Tropical pulmonary alveolitis
(T-28000) (M-40000)

D2-60670 Endogenous lipoid pneumonia 516.8
(T-28000) (M-55700) (F-63600)

D2-60680 Interstitial pneumonia 516.8
(T-28780) (M-43000) (M-78000)
Interstitial lung disease 516.8
(T-28780) (M-43000) (M-78000)
Interstitial pneumonitis 516.8
(T-28780) (M-43000) (M-78000)

D2-60682 Desquamative interstitial pneumonia 516.8
(T-28780) (M-43000) (G-C008)
(T-28050) (F-41500)
Desquamative interstitial pneumonitis 516.8
(T-28780) (M-43000) (G-C008)
(T-28050) (F-41500)

D2-60684 Lymphoid interstitial pneumonia 516.8
(T-28780) (M-43010)
Lymphocytic interstitial pneumonia 516.8
(T-28780) (M-43010)

D2-60690 Rheumatic pneumonia 517.1
(T-28000) (M-40000) (G-C002)
(D3-17100)

D2-606A0 Rheumatoid fibrosing alveolitis 714.81

D2-606A2 Diffuse interstitial rheumatoid disease of lung 714.81

D2-61010 Abscess of lung 513.0
(T-28000) (M-41610)

D2-61020 Gangrenous pneumonia 513.0
(T-28000) (M-40700)
Necrotic pneumonia 513.0
(T-28000) (M-40700)
Necrotizing pneumonia 513.0
(T-28000) (M-40700)

D2-61030 Pulmonary gangrene 513.0
(T-28000) (M-54600)

D2-61032 Pulmonary necrosis 513.0
(T-28000) (M-54000)

D2-61100 Pulmonary edema, NOS 514.-
(T-28000) (M-36300)

D2-61110 Chronic pulmonary edema 514.-
(T-28000) (M-36302)

D2-61120 Pulmonary congestion, NOS 514.-
(T-28000) (M-36100)

D2-61130 Chronic pulmonary congestion 514.-
(T-28000) (M-36142)

D2-61140 Pulmonary hemorrhage
(T-28000) (M-37000)
Intra-alveolar hemorrhage
(T-28000) (M-37000)

D2-61150V Exercise-induced pulmonary hemorrhage
(T-28000) (M-37000) (G-C001)
(A-70500)
EIPH
(T-28000) (M-37000) (G-C001)
(A-70500)
Bleeder syndrome
(T-28000) (M-37000) (G-C001)
(A-70500)
Epistaxis in the horse
(T-28000) (M-37000) (G-C001)
(A-70500)

D2-61160 Hypostatic bronchopneumonia 514.-
(T-26000) (T-28000) (M-40000)
(F-10340)

D2-61170 Hypostatic pneumonia 514.-
(T-28000) (M-40000) (F-10340)
Passive pneumonia 514.-
(T-28000) (M-40000) (F-10340)

D2-61210 Pulmonary ossification
(T-28000) (F-12100)

D2-61212 Calcification of lung 518.89
(T-28000) (M-55400)
Pulmonary mineralization 518.89
(T-28000) (M-55400)

D2-61220 Pulmolithiasis 518.89
(T-28000) (M-30000)

D2-61300 Postinflammatory pulmonary fibrosis 515.-
(T-28000) (M-78000) (F-06090)
(M-40000)

D2-61310 Fibrosis of lung, NOS 515.-
(T-28000) (M-78000)
Cirrhosis of lung, NOS 515.-
(T-28000) (M-78000)
Pulmonary fibrosis 515.-
(T-28000) (M-78000)

D2-61320 Chronic fibrosis of lung 515.-
(T-28000) (M-78003)

D2-61330 Atrophic fibrosis of lung 515.-
(T-28000) (M-78000) (M-58000)

D2-61340 Confluent fibrosis of lung 515.-
(T-28000) (M-78000)

D2-61350 Massive fibrosis of lung 515.-
(T-28000) (M-78260)

D2-61360 Perialveolar fibrosis of lung 515.-
(T-28010) (M-78000)

SECTION 2-6 OTHER LUNG DISEASES AND CONDITIONS — Continued

D2-61370 Peribronchial fibrosis of lung 515.-
(T-26000) (M-78000)

D2-61380 Induration of lung, NOS 515.-
(T-28000) (M-02712)

D2-61382 Chronic induration of lung 515.-
(T-28000) (M-02712)

D2-61420 Pseudolymphoma of lung in Sjogren's disease

D2-61430 Pulmonary eosinophilic granuloma

SECTION 2-8 DISEASES OF THE PLEURA, MEDIASTINUM AND DIAPHRAGM

2-80 DISEASES OF THE PLEURA

D2-80000 Disease of pleura, NOS
(T-29000) (DF-00000)

D2-80010 Pleurisy, NOS 511.0
(T-29000) (M-40000)
Pleurisy without effusion 511.0
(T-29000) (M-40000)
Pleuritis, NOS 511.0
(T-29000) (M-40000)

D2-80020 Fibrinous pleurisy 511.0
(T-29000) (M-40300)

D2-80030 Diaphragmatic pleurisy 511.0
(T-29330) (M-40000)

D2-80040 Interlobar pleurisy 511.0
(T-29030) (M-40000)

D2-80050 Calcification of pleura 511.0
(T-29000) (M-55400)

D2-80060 Adhesion of pleura 511.0
(T-29000) (M-78400)
Adhesive pleuritis 511.0
(T-29000) (M-78400)

D2-80070 Adhesion of lung 511.0
(T-29030) (M-78400)

D2-80080 Thickening of pleura 511.0
(T-29000) (M-50060)

D2-80100 Pleural effusion, NOS 511.9
(T-29050) (M-36700)

D2-80110 Hemopneumothorax 511.8
(T-29050) (M-37000) (M-36670)

D2-80120 Hemothorax 511.8
(T-29050) (M-37000)

D2-80130 Hydropneumothorax 511.8
(T-29050) (M-36700) (M-36670)

D2-80140 Hydrothorax 511.8
(T-29050) (M-36710)
Pleural effusion with transudate 511.8
(T-29050) (M-36710)

D2-80150 Pleural effusion due to congestive heart failure
(T-29050) (M-36700) (G-C001)
(D3-16010)

D2-80154 Pleural effusion associated with hepatic disorder
(T-29050) (M-36700) (G-C002)
(T-62000) (DF-00000)

D2-80160 Pleural effusion associated with pancreatitis
(T-29050) (M-36700) (G-C002)
(T-65000) (M-40000)

D2-80170 Neoplastic pleural effusion
(T-29050) (M-36700) (G-C002)
(DF-00400)

D2-80180 Pleural effusion associated with pulmonary infection
(T-29050) (M-36700) (G-C008)
(T-28000) (DE-00000)
Parapneumonic effusion
(T-29050) (M-36700) (G-C008)
(T-28000) (DE-00000)

D2-80200 Pleurisy with effusion, NOS 511.9
(T-29050) (M-40000) (M-36700)
Exudative pleurisy 511.9
(T-29050) (M-40000) (M-36700)

D2-80230 Serofibrinous pleurisy 511.9
(T-29050) (M-40300)
Serous pleurisy 511.9
(T-29050) (M-40300)

D2-80250 Encysted pleurisy 511.8
(T-29000) (M-40000) (M-33400)
(M-78400)

D2-80300 Pneumothorax, NOS 512.8
(T-29050) (M-36670)

D2-80302 Closed pneumothorax 512.8
(T-29050) (M-36670)

D2-80304 Open pneumothorax 512.8
(T-29050) (M-36670)

D2-80310 Acute pneumothorax 512.8
(T-29050) (M-36670) (G-A231)

D2-80320 Chronic pneumothorax 512.8
(T-29050) (M-36670) (G-A270)

D2-80350 Spontaneous pneumothorax 512.8
(T-29050) (M-36670) (G-A549)

D2-80360 Spontaneous tension pneumothorax 512.0
(T-29050) (M-36670) (G-A549)
Tension pneumothorax 512.0
(T-29050) (M-36670) (G-A549)

D2-80370 Chylothorax
(T-29050) (M-36740)

D2-80380 Pseudochylothorax
(T-29050) (M-36700)

D2-80500 Empyema of pleura, NOS 510.9
(T-29050) (M-40620)

D2-80502 Empyema of pleura without fistula 510.9
(T-29050) (M-40620) (G-C009)
(M-39300)

D2-80504 Abscess of thorax 510.9
(T-29050) (M-41610)
Abscess of pleural cavity 510.9
(T-29050) (M-41610)
Pyothorax 510.9
(T-29050) (M-41610)

D2-80510 Pyopneumothorax 510.9
(T-29050) (M-41610) (M-36670)

D2-80530 Purulent pleurisy 510.9
(T-29000) (M-40600)
Suppurative pleurisy 510.9
(T-29000) (M-40600)

D2-80540 Septic pleurisy 510.9
(T-29000) (M-41000) (M-54380)

D2-80550 Seropurulent pleurisy 510.9
(T-29000) (M-40200) (G-C008)
(M-41602)

D2-80560 Fibrinopurulent pleurisy 510.9
(T-29000) (M-41300)

D2-80600 Empyema with fistula, NOS 510.0
(T-29050) (M-40620) (G-C008)
(M-39300)

D2-80610 Empyema with pleural fistula 510.0
(T-29050) (M-40620) (G-C008)
(M-29000) (M-39300)
Empyema with thoracic fistula 510.0
(T-29050) (M-40620) (G-C008)
(T-D3000) (M-39300)

D2-80620 Empyema with bronchopleural fistula 510.0
(T-29050) (M-40620) (G-C008)
(T-26000) (T-29000) (M-39300)

D2-80630 Empyema with hepatopleural fistula 510.0
(T-29050) (M-40620) (G-C008)
(T-62000) (T-29000) (M-39300)

D2-80640 Empyema with mediastinal fistula 510.0
(T-29050) (M-40620) (G-C008)
(T-D3300) (M-39300)

D2-80650 Empyema with bronchocutaneous fistula 510.0
(T-29050) (M-40620) (G-C008)
(T-26000) (T-01000) (M-39300)

2-81 DISEASES OF THE MEDIASTINUM

D2-81000 Disease of mediastinum, NOS
(T-D3300) (DF-00000)

D2-81010 Mediastinitis 519.2
(T-D3300) (M-40000)

D2-81020 Abscess of mediastinum 513.1
(T-D3300) (M-41610)

D2-81100 Fibrosis of mediastinum 519.3
(T-D3300) (M-78000)

D2-81120 Retraction of mediastinum 519.3
(T-D3300) (M-02595)

D2-81150 Hernia of mediastinum 519.3
(T-D3300) (M-31500)

D2-81180 Mediastinal emphysema 518.1
(T-D3300) (M-33900)

D2-81200 Mass in chest, NOS 786.6
Swelling in chest, NOS 786.6
Lump in chest, NOS 786.6

2-82 DISEASES OF THE DIAPHRAGM

D2-82000 Disease of diaphragm, NOS
(T-D3400) (DF-00000)

D2-82010 Diaphragmitis 519.4
(T-D3400) (M-40000)

D2-82020 Rupture of diaphragm
(T-D3400) (M-14400)

D2-82030 Perforation of diaphragm
(T-D3400) (M-39210)

D2-82050 Paralysis of diaphragm 519.4
(T-D3400) (M-A0840)

D2-82060 Diaphragmatic eventration
(T-D3400) (M-31060)

D2-82064 Unilateral caudal displacement of diaphragm
(T-D3400) (M-31050)

D2-82080 Relaxation of diaphragm 519.4
(T-D3400) (M-11160)

D2-82090 Elevated diaphragm
(T-D3400) (M-31060)

D2-82100 Diaphragmatic cyst, NOS
(T-D3400) (M-33400)

D2-82110 Adhesion of diaphragm 568.0
(T-D3400) (M-78400)

D2-82120 Intradiaphragmatic abscess
(T-D3400) (M-41610)

SECTION 2-9 VOICE DISORDERS

2-900 Voice Disorders: General Terms

D2-90000 Voice disorder, NOS
(T-24400) (F-F7000) (DF-00000)
Dysphonia, NOS
(T-24400) (F-F7000) (DF-00000)
Voice disturbance, NOS
(T-24400) (F-F7000) (DF-00000)
Voice impairment, NOS
(T-24400) (F-F7000) (DF-00000)

2-901 Spastic Dysphonias

D2-90100 Spastic dysphonia, NOS 784.49
Spasmodic dysphonia 784.49

D2-90110 Adductor spastic dysphonia, NOS

D2-90120 Psychogenic adductor spastic dysphonia

D2-90121 Adductor spastic dysphonia of conversion reaction

D2-90122 Adductor spastic dysphonia of musculoskeletal tension reaction

D2-90130 Neurologic adductor spastic dysphonia

D2-90131 Adductor spastic dysphonia of organic voice tremor
Adductor spastic dysphonia of essential voice tremor

D2-90132 Adductor spastic dysphonia of dystonia

D2-90140 Idiopathic adductor spastic dysphonia

D2-90160 Abductor spastic dysphonia

D2-90180 Spastic aphonia

D2-90182 Aphonia paralytica

2-902 Neurologic Voice Disorders

D2-90200 Neurologic voice disorder, NOS
  Neurologic dysphonia, NOS
D2-90210 Flaccid dysphonia
D2-90212 Spastic pseudobulbar dysphonia
D2-90214 Mixed flaccid-spastic pseudobulbar dysphonia
D2-90216 Hypokinetic parkinsonian dysphonia
D2-90220 Ataxic dysphonia
D2-90224 Choreic dysphonia
D2-90228 Dystonic dysphonia
D2-90232 Dysphonia of palatopharyngolaryngeal myoclonus
D2-90234 Dysphonia of organic tremor
  Dysphonia of essential tremor
D2-90238 Dysphonia of Gilles de la Tourette's syndrome
D2-90242 Apraxia of phonation
  Apraxic aphonia
D2-90246 Akinetic mutism
D2-90248 Dysprosody of "pseudoforeign dialect"

2-903 Nasal Resonatory Disorders

D2-90300 Nasal resonatory disorder, NOS
D2-90310 Hypernasality syndrome 784.49
  Hypernasality 784.49
  Rhinolalia aperta
  Hyper-rhinolalia
  Open nasality
D2-90320 Hypernasality syndrome due to neurologic disease, NOS
D2-90322 Hypernasality syndrome due to velopharyngeal weakness
D2-90324 Hypernasality syndrome due to velopharyngeal incoordination
D2-90350 Hyponasality syndrome 784.49
  Hyponasality 784.49
  Denasality
  Closed nasality
  Rhinolalia clausa
D2-90352 Posterior rhinolalia clausa
D2-90354 Anterior rhinolalia clausa
  Cul-de-sac resonation
D2-90360 Mixed nasality
  Rhinolalia mixta

2-905 Psychogenic Voice Disorders

D2-90500 Psychogenic voice disorder, NOS
  Functional voice disorder, NOS
D2-90502 Vocal abuse in children
D2-90504 Vocal nodules in children
D2-90506 Vocal nodules in adults
D2-90508 Contact ulcer of vocal folds
D2-90510 Ventricular dysphonia
  Dysphonia plicae ventricularis
D2-90520 Conversion muteness
  Conversion mutism
D2-90522 Conversion aphonia
D2-90524 Conversion dysphonia
D2-90550 Voice disorder due to psychosexual conflict, NOS
D2-90552 Mutational falsetto
  Puberphonia
D2-90556 Voice disorder due to transsexualism
D2-90580 Voice disorder due to iatrogenic factor, NOS

CHAPTER 3 — DISEASES OF THE CARDIOVASCULAR SYSTEM

SECTION 3-0 DISEASES AFFECTING THE ENTIRE CARDIOVASCULAR SYSTEM

3-00 CARDIOVASCULAR DISORDERS: GENERAL TERMS

D3-00000 Disease of cardiovascular system, NOS 459.9 (T-30000)
  Disorder of circulatory system, NOS 459.9 (T-30000)
  Cardiovascular disease, NOS 429.2
  CVD, NOS 429.2
D3-00100 Arteriosclerotic cardiovascular disease, NOS 429.2
  ASCVD 429.2
  Cardiovascular arteriosclerosis 429.2
  Cardiovascular degeneration with arteriosclerosis 429.2
  Cardiovascular disease with arteriosclerosis 429.2
  Cardiovascular sclerosis with arteriosclerosis 429.2
D3-00200 Cardiogenic shock 785.51

3-02 HYPERTENSIVE DISEASES

D3-02000 Hypertensive disease, NOS 401.9 (T-30000)
  High blood pressure 401.- (T-30000)
  Hyperpiesia 401.- (T-30000)
  Hypertensive vascular degeneration 401.- (T-30000)
  Hypertensive vascular disease 401.- (T-30000)
  Hypertension, NOS 401.9 (T-30000)
  Hyperpiesis 401.- (T-30000)
D3-02010 Benign hypertension 401.1 (T-30000)
D3-02020 Malignant hypertension 401.0 (T-30000)
D3-02100 Essential hypertension, NOS
  Systemic primary arterial hypertension 401.- (T-30000)
  Idiopathic hypertension
  Primary hypertension, NOS
D3-02110 Renal hypertension
D3-02112 Low-renin essential hypertension
D3-02114 High-renin essential hypertension
D3-02120 Benign essential hypertension
D3-02130 Malignant essential hypertension
D3-02140 Accelerated essential hypertension
D3-02200 Secondary hypertension, NOS 405.9
D3-02202 Endocrine hypertension
  Adrenal hypertension
D3-02210 Benign secondary hypertension 405.1
D3-02211 Benign secondary renovascular hypertension 405.11
D3-02220 Malignant secondary hypertension 405.0
D3-02221 Malignant secondary renovascular hypertension 405.01
D3-02230 Accelerated secondary hypertension
D3-02500 Hypertensive heart disease, NOS 402.9 (T-32000)
  Hypertensive cardiopathy 402.9 (T-32000)
  Hypertensive cardiomegaly 402.9 (T-32000)
  Hypertensive cardiovascular disease 402.9 (T-30000)
D3-02501 Hypertensive heart disease with congestive heart failure 402.91 (T-32000)
D3-02504 Hypertensive heart disease without congestive heart failure 402.90 (T-32000)
D3-02505 Hypertensive heart and renal disease, NOS 404.9
  Cardiorenal disease, NOS 404.9
D3-02508 Hypertensive heart failure, NOS 402.9 (T-32000)
D3-02510 Benign hypertensive heart disease 402.1 (T-32000)
D3-02511 Benign hypertensive heart disease with congestive heart failure 402.11 (T-32000)
D3-02514 Benign hypertensive heart disease without congestive heart failure 402.10 (T-32000)
D3-02515 Benign hypertensive heart and renal disease 404.1
D3-02520 Malignant hypertensive heart disease 402.0 (T-32000)
D3-02521 Malignant hypertensive heart disease with congestive heart failure 402.01 (T-32000)
D3-02524 Malignant hypertensive heart disease without congestive heart failure 402.00 (T-32000)
D3-02525 Malignant hypertensive heart and renal disease 404.0
D3-02700 Hypertensive renal disease, NOS 403.9 (T-71000)
  Hypertensive nephropathy, NOS 403.9 (T-71000)
D3-02701 Hypertensive renal failure 403.- (T-71000)
D3-02702 Chronic hypertensive uremia 403.-
D3-02703 Nephrosclerosis 403.-
  Chronic arteriosclerotic nephritis 403.-

3-02 HYPERTENSIVE DISEASES — Continued

D3-02703 (cont.) Interstitial arteriosclerotic nephritis 403.-
Arteriosclerosis of kidney 403.-

D3-02704 Arteriolar nephritis 403.-
Arteriosclerosis of renal arterioles 403.-
Arteriolar sclerosis of renal arterioles 403.-

D3-02707 Cardiovascular renal disease 404.-

D3-02710 Renal sclerosis with hypertension 403.-

D3-02720 Benign hypertensive renal disease 403.1

D3-02730 Malignant hypertensive renal disease 403.0

3-04 HYPOTENSIVE DISEASES

D3-04000 Hypotension, NOS 458.9
Hypopiesis 458.9
Arterial hypotension, NOS 458.9

D3-04003 Chronic hypotension 458.1
Permanent idiopathic hypotension 458.1

D3-04100 Orthostatic hypotension 458.0
Postural hypotension 458.0

D3-04103 Chronic orthostatic hypotension 458.0

SECTION 3-1 HEART DISEASES

3-10 HEART DISEASES: GENERAL TERMS

D3-10000 Heart disease, NOS 429.9
(T-32000)
Morbus cordis, NOS 429.9
(T-32000)

D3-10010 Rupture of heart 410.9
(T-32000) (M-14400)

D3-10500 Aneurysm of heart, NOS 414.1
(T-32000) (M-32200)
Aneurysm of heart wall 414.10
(T-32000) (M-32200)
Mural aneurysm of heart 414.10
(T-32000) (M-32200)

D3-10510 Ventricular aneurysm 414.10
(T-32400) (M-32200)

D3-10520 Atrial aneurysm

D3-10530 Acquired arteriovenous fistula of heart 414.19
(T-32000) (M-39370)

D3-10600 Hyperkinetic heart disease 429.82
(T-32000)

D3-10700 Myocardial disease, NOS 429.1

D3-10710 Myocardial degeneration 429.1
Degeneration of heart 429.1
Mural degeneration of heart 429.1
Muscular degeneration of heart 429.1

D3-10720 Fatty degeneration of heart 429.1

3-11 PAPILLARY MUSCLE DISORDERS

D3-11000 Papillary muscle disorder, NOS

D3-11100 Rupture of chordae tendinae 429.5
(T-35160) (T-35330) (M-14400)

D3-11110 Rupture of papillary muscle 429.6
(T-32421) (M-14400)

D3-11120 Atrophy of papillary muscle 429.81
(T-32421) (M-58000)

D3-11122 Degeneration of papillary muscle 429.81
(T-32421) (M-50000)

D3-11124 Scarring of papillary muscle 429.81
(T-32421) (M-78060)

D3-11130 Dysfunction of papillary muscle 429.81
(T-32421) (F-01100)

D3-11132 Incompetence of papillary muscle 429.81
(T-32421) (F-00210)

D3-11134 Incoordination of papillary muscle 429.81
(T-32421) (F-A4202)

D3-11140 Acute infarction of papillary muscle 410.8
(T-32421) (M-54720)

3-12 ANGINAL SYNDROMES

D3-12000 Angina pectoris, NOS 413.9
(T-32000)
Angina, NOS 413.9
(T-32000)
Cardiac angina 413.9
(T-32000)
Angina of effort 413.9
(T-32000)
Anginal syndrome 413.9
(T-32000)
Stenocardia 413.9
(T-32000)

D3-12001 Angina, class I 413.9

D3-12002 Angina, class II 413.9

D3-12003 Angina, class III 413.9

D3-12004 Angina, class IV 413.9

D3-12200 Angina decubitus 413.0
(T-32000)
Anginal chest pain at rest 413.0
(T-32000)

D3-12300 Nocturnal angina 413.0
(T-32000)

D3-12400 Prinzmental angina 413.1
(T-32000)
Variant angina pectoris 413.1
(T-32000)

D3-12500 Status anginosus 413.9
(T-32000)

D3-12600 Syncope anginosa 413.9
(T-32000)

D3-12700 Preinfarction syndrome 411.1
(T-32000) (F-37000)
Intermediate coronary syndrome 411.1
(T-32000) (F-37000)
Unstable angina 411.1
(T-32000) (F-37000)
Crescendo angina 411.1
(T-32000) (F-37000)

D3-12710 Impending infarction 411.1
(T-32000) (F-37000)

D3-12720 Preinfarction angina 411.1
(T-32000) (F-37000)

3-13 CORONARY ARTERY DISEASES

D3-13000 Coronary artery disease, NOS
D3-13010 Coronary atherosclerosis 414.0
(T-43000) (M-52110)
Arteriosclerotic heart disease 414.0
(T-43000) (M-52110)
ASHD 414.0
(T-43000) (M-52110)
Coronary sclerosis 414.0
(T-43000) (M-52000)
D3-13040 Coronary arteriosclerosis 414.0
(T-43000) (M-52000)
Atherosclerotic heart disease 414.0
(T-43000) (M-52110)
D3-13050 Coronary artery atheroma 414.0
(T-43000) (M-52100)
D3-13100 Coronary arteritis 414.0
(T-43000) (M-40000)
Coronary endarteritis 414.0
(T-43000) (M-40000)
D3-13200 Coronary occlusion, NOS 410.9
(T-43000) (M-34000)
Coronary artery occlusion 410.9
(T-43000) (M-34000)
D3-13210 Coronary artery thrombosis 410.9
(T-43000) (M-35110)
D3-13220 Coronary artery embolism 410.9
(T-43000) (M-35300)
D3-13230 Coronary stricture 414.0
(T-43000) (M-34260)
D3-13240 Coronary artery rupture 410.9
(T-43000) (M-14400)
D3-13250 Aneurysm of coronary vessels 414.11
(T-43000) (M-32200)
D3-13312 Left main coronary artery thrombosis 410.9
D3-13314 Left anterior descending coronary artery thrombosis 410.9
D3-13316 Right main coronary artery thrombosis 410.9

3-14-15 ISCHEMIC HEART DISEASES

D3-14000 Ischemic heart disease, NOS 414.9
(T-32000) (F-39340)
D3-14010 Acute ischemic heart disease 411.8
(T-43000) (F-39310)
Acute coronary insufficiency 411.8
(T-43000) (F-39310)
D3-14020 Chronic ischemic heart disease 414.9
(T-32000) (F-39320)
Chronic coronary insufficiency 414.8
(T-43000) (F-39320)
Chronic myocardial ischemia 414.8
(T-32020) (F-39320)
D3-14050 Subendocardial ischemia 411.8
(T-32024) (F-39340)
D3-15000 Myocardial infarction, NOS 410.9
(T-32020) (M-54720)
Cardiac infarction, NOS 410.9
(T-32020) (M-54720)
Infarction of heart, NOS 410.9
(T-32020) (M-54720)
Heart attack, NOS 410.9
(T-32020) (M-54720)
D3-15010 Microinfarct of heart 411.8
(T-32000) (M-54701)
D3-15100 Acute myocardial infarction, NOS 410.9
(T-32020) (M-54720)
D3-15110 Acute myocardial infarction of anterior wall, NOS 410.1
(T-32021) (M-54720)
D3-15111 Acute myocardial infarction of anterolateral wall 410.0
(T-32634) (M-54720)
D3-15112 Acute anteroapical myocardial infarction 410.1
(T-32636) (M-54720)
D3-15113 Acute anteroseptal myocardial infarction 410.1
(T-32631) (M-54720)
D3-15120 Acute myocardial infarction of inferior wall, NOS 410.4
(T-32632) (M-54720)
Acute myocardial infarction of diaphragmatic wall 410.4
(T-32632) (M-54720)
D3-15121 Acute myocardial infarction of inferolateral wall 410.2
(T-32637) (M-54720)
D3-15122 Acute myocardial infarction of inferoposterior wall 410.3
(T-.....) (M-54720)
D3-15130 Acute myocardial infarction of lateral wall 410.5
(T-32023) (M-54720)
D3-15131 Acute myocardial infarction of apical-lateral wall 410.5
(T-.....) (M-54720)
D3-15132 Acute myocardial infarction of basal-lateral wall 410.5
(T-.....) (M-54720)
D3-15133 Acute myocardial infarction of high lateral wall 410.5
(T-.....) (M-54720)
D3-15134 Acute myocardial infarction of posterolateral wall 410.5
(T-32633) (M-54720)
D3-15140 True posterior wall infarction 410.6
(T-32022) (M-54700)
D3-15141 Acute myocardial infarction of posterobasal wall 410.6
(T-.....) (M-54720)

3-14-15 ISCHEMIC HEART DISEASES — Continued

D3-15150 Acute myocardial infarction of atrium 410.8
(T-32100) (M-54720)

D3-15170 Acute myocardial infarction of septum 410.8
(T-32410) (M-54720)
Acute myocardial infarction of septum alone 410.8
(T-32410) (M-54720)

D3-15180 Acute subendocardial infarction 410.7
(T-32024) (M-54720)
Acute nontransmural infarction 410.7
(T-32024) (M-54720)

D3-15200 Old myocardial infarction 412.-
(T-32020) (M-54750)
Healed myocardial infarction 412.-
(T-32020) (M-54750)

D3-15210 Past myocardial infarction diagnosed on ECG or other special investigation, but currently presenting no symptoms 412.-
(T-32020) (M-54750)

D3-15300 Postmyocardial infarction syndrome 411.0
(T-32020) (M-54700) (F-06090) (F-03003) (F-37080)
Dressler's syndrome 411.0
(T-32020) (M-34700) (F-06090) (F-03003) (F-37080)
Postmyocardial infarction pericarditis 411.0

3-16 HEART FAILURE AND OTHER FUNCTIONAL DISORDERS

D3-16000 Heart failure, NOS 428.9
Cardiac failure, NOS 428.9
Myocardial failure, NOS 428.9
Weak heart, NOS 428.9

D3-16010 Congestive heart failure 428.0
Congestive heart disease 428.0

D3-16015 Right heart failure secondary to left heart failure 428.0

D3-16017 Left heart failure 428.1
Acute edema of lung with heart disease 428.1
Acute pulmonary edema with heart disease 428.1
Left ventricular failure 428.1

D3-16110 Cardiac asthma 428.1

D3-16130 Cardiac insufficiency following cardiac surgery 429.4
Heart failure following cardiac surgery 429.4

D3-16140 Cardiac insufficiency due to prosthesis 429.4
Heart failure due to prosthesis 429.4

D3-16150 Postcardiotomy syndrome 429.4

D3-16160 Postvalvulotomy syndrome 429.4

D3-16170 Cardiomegaly 429.3
Cardiac hypertrophy 429.3

D3-16180 Cardiac dilatation 429.3

D3-16184 Ventricular dilatation 429.3

D3-16186 Atrial dilatation

D3-16188 Auricular dilatation

D3-16200V Round heart disease
Spontaneous cardiomyopathy

3-17 RHEUMATIC FEVER AND RHEUMATIC HEART DISEASES

D3-17100 Rheumatic fever, NOS
(T-15000)

D3-17110 Rheumatic fever without heart involvement 390.-
(T-15000) (M-41000)

D3-17112 Active rheumatic fever 390.-
(T-15000) (M-41000)
Acute rheumatic fever 390.-
(T-15000) (M-41000)
Acute rheumatic attack 390.-
(T-15000) (M-41000)

D3-17113 Subacute rheumatic arthritis 390.-
(T-15000) (M-42000)
Subacute articular rheumatism 390.-
(T-15000) (M-42000)

D3-17114 Acute rheumatic arthritis 390.-
(T-15000) (M-41000)
Acute articular rheumatism 390.-
(T-15000) (M-41000)

D3-17116 Rheumatic chorea 392.-
(F-A4510)
Sydenham's chorea 392.-
(F-A4510)
Rheumatic chorea without heart involvement 392.9
(F-A4510)

D3-17117 Rheumatic chorea with heart involvement 392.0
(T-32000) (F-A4510)

D3-17400 Rheumatic heart disease, NOS 398.90
(T-32000)
Rheumatic carditis, NOS 398.90
(T-32000)

D3-17402 Rheumatic pericarditis, NOS
(T-39000) (M-40000)

D3-17410 Acute rheumatic heart disease, NOS 391.9
(T-32000) (M-41000)
Rheumatic fever with heart involvement 391.-
(T-32000) (M-41000)
Acute rheumatic carditis 391.9
(T-32000) (M-41000)
Active rheumatic fever with unspecified type of heart involvement 391.9
(T-32000) (M-41000)
Acute rheumatic fever with unspecified type of heart involvement 391.9
(T-32000) (M-41000)

D3-17420 Acute rheumatic myocarditis 391.2
(T-32020) (M-41000)
Active rheumatic fever with myocarditis 391.2
(T-32020) (M-41000)

D3-17420 (cont.) Acute rheumatic fever with myocarditis 391.2
(T-32020) (M-41000)
Rheumatic myocarditis 398.0
(T-32020) (M-40000) (M-50000)
Rheumatic degeneration of myocardium 398.0
(T-32020) (M-40000) (M-50000)

D3-17430 Acute rheumatic endocarditis 391.1
(T-32060) (M-41000)
Acute rheumatic fever with endocarditis 391.1
(T-32060) (M-41000)
Active rheumatic fever with endocarditis 391.1
(T-32060) (M-31000)

D3-17440 Acute rheumatic pericarditis 391.0
(T-39000) (M-41000)
Active rheumatic fever with pericarditis 391.0
(T-39000) (M-41000)
Acute rheumatic fever with pericarditis 391.0
(T-39000) (M-41000)

D3-17450 Acute rheumatic pancarditis 391.8
(T-32000) (M-41000)

D3-17460 Other acute rheumatic heart disease, NEC 391.8
(T-32000) (M-41000)
Acute rheumatic fever with multiple types of heart involvement, NEC 391.8
(T-32000) (M-41000)

D3-17500 Chronic rheumatic heart disease 398.90
(T-32000) (M-43000)
Chronic rheumatic carditis 398.90
(T-32000) (M-43000)

D3-17510 Chronic rheumatic heart disease with myocarditis 398.0
(T-32020) (M-43000)
Chronic rheumatic myocarditis 398.0
(T-32020) (M-43000)

D3-17520 Chronic rheumatic endocarditis 397.9
(T-32060) (M-43000)
Chronic rheumatic heart disease with endocarditis 397.9
(T-32060) (M-43000)

D3-17530 Chronic rheumatic pericarditis 393.-
(T-39000) (M-43000)

D3-17531 Rheumatic adherent pericaridum 393.-
(T-39000) (M-45000)

D3-17532 Chronic rheumatic mediastinopericarditis 393.-
(T-D3320) (T-39000) (M-43000)

D3-17533 Chronic rheumatic myopericarditis 393.-
(T-32020) (T-39000) (M-43000)

D3-17600 Rheumatic disease of heart valve, NOS

D3-17601 Acute rheumatic fever with valvulitis 391.1
(T-35000) (M-41000)
Active rheumatic fever with valvulitis 391.1
(T-35000) (M-41000)

D3-17602 Rheumatic heart valve stenosis

D3-17603 Rheumatic heart valve regurgitation
Rheumatic heart valve insufficiency
Rheumatic heart valve incompetence

D3-17604 Rheumatic heart valve stenosis with insufficiency
Rheumatic heart valve stenosis with incompetence

D3-17606 Rheumatic heart valve failure

D3-17608 Chronic rheumatic valvulitis 397.9
(T-35000) (M-43000)
Chronic rheumatic heart disease with valvulitis 397.9
(T-35000) (M-43000)

D3-17610 Rheumatic endocarditis 397.9
(T-32060) (M-40000)
Rheumatic disease of endocardium 397.9
(T-32060) (M-40000)
Rheumatic disease of endocardium, valve unspecified 397.9
(T-32060) (T-35000)

D3-17630 Rheumatic disease of mitral valve, NOS 394.9
(T-35300)

D3-17631 Rheumatic mitral stenosis, NOS 394.0
(T-35300) (M-34200)
Rheumatic mitral valve obstruction 394.0
(T-35300) (M-34200)

D3-17632 Rheumatic mitral regurgitation 394.1
(T-35300) (F-32400)
Rheumatic mitral insufficiency 394.1
(T-35300) (F-32400)
Rheumatic mitral incompetence 394.1
(T-35300) (F-32400)

D3-17633 Rheumatic mitral stenosis with regurgitation 394.2
(T-35300) (M-34200) (F-32400)
Rheumatic mitral stenosis with insufficiency 394.2
(T-35300) (M-34200) (F-32400)
Rheumatic mitral stenosis with incompetence 394.2
(T-35300) (M-34200) (F-32400)

D3-17634 Rheumatic mitral valve failure 394.9
(T-35300) (F-00150)

D3-17640 Rheumatic disease of aortic valve, NOS 395.9
(T-35400)
Rheumatic aortic valve disease, NOS 395.9
(T-35400)

D3-17641 Rheumatic aortic stenosis 395.0
(T-35400) (M-34200)
Rheumatic aortic valve obstruction 395.0
(T-35400) (M-34200)

D3-17642 Rheumatic aortic regurgitation 395.1
(T-35400) (F-32400)
Rheumatic aortic insufficiency 395.1
(T-35400) (F-32400)

3-17 RHEUMATIC FEVER AND RHEUMATIC HEART DISEASES — Continued

D3-17642 (cont.) Rheumatic aortic incompetence 395.1
(T-35400) (F-32400)

D3-17643 Rheumatic aortic stenosis with regurgitation 395.2
(T-35400) (T-34200) (F-32400)
Rheumatic aortic stenosis with insufficiency 395.2
(T-35400) (M-34200) (F-32400)
Rheumatic aortic stenosis with incompetence 395.2
(T-35400) (M-34200) (F-32400)

D3-17650 Rheumatic disease of mitral and aortic valves, NOS 396.9
(T-35300) (T-35400)

D3-17651 Rheumatic mitral valve and aortic valve stenosis 396.0
(T-35300) (T-35400) (M-34200)
Rheumatic mitral and aortic valve obstruction 396.0
(T-35300) (T-35400) (M-34200)

D3-17652 Rheumatic mitral valve stenosis and aortic valve insufficiency 396.1
(T-35300) (M-34200) (T-35400) (F-32400)

D3-17653 Rheumatic mitral valve insufficiency and aortic valve stenosis 396.2
(T-35300) (F-32400) (T-35400) (M-34200)

D3-17655 Rheumatic mitral and aortic valve regurgitation 394.3
(T-35300) (T-35400) (F-32400)
Rheumatic mitral and aortic valve insufficiency 396.3
(T-35300) (T-35400) (F-32400)
Rheumatic mitral and aortic valve incompetence 396.3
(T-35300) (T-35400) (F-32400)

D3-17656 Rheumatic involvement of mitral and aortic valves, NEC 396.8
(T-35300) (T-35400)

D3-17660 Rheumatic disease of tricuspid valve, NOS 397.0
(T-35100)
Rheumatic tricuspid valve disease, NOS 397.0
(T-35100)

D3-17661 Rheumatic tricuspid valve stenosis 397.0
(T-35100) (M-34200)
Rheumatic tricuspid valve obstruction 397.0
(T-35100) (M-34200)

D3-17662 Rheumatic tricuspid valve regurgitation 397.0
(T-35100) (F-32400)
Rheumatic tricuspid valve insufficiency 397.0
(T-35100) (F-32400)
Rheumatic tricuspid valve incompetence
(T-35100) (F-32400)

D3-17663 Rheumatic tricuspid valve stenosis with regurgitation 397.0

D3-17664 Rheumatic tricuspid valve failure 397.0

D3-17670 Rheumatic disease of pulmonary valve, NOS 397.1
(T-35200)
Rheumatic pulmonary valve disease, NOS 397.1

D3-17671 Rheumatic pulmonary valve stenosis 397.1
Rheumatic pulmonary valve obstruction 397.1

D3-17672 Rheumatic pulmonary valve insufficiency 397.1
Rheumatic pulmonary valve regurgitation 397.1
Rheumatic pulmonary valve incompetence 397.1

D3-17673 Rheumatic pulmonary valve stenosis with insufficiency 397.1
Rheumatic pulmonary valve stenosis with regurgitation 397.1
Rheumatic pulmonary valve stenosis with incompetence 397.1

D3-17676 Rheumatic pulmonary valve failure 397.1

D3-17700 Congestive rheumatic heart failure 398.91
(T-32000) (F-00150)

D3-17702 Rheumatic left ventricular failure 398.91
(T-32600) (F-00150)

SECTION 3-2 CARDIOMYOPATHIES AND NONRHEUMATIC CARDIAC INFLAMMATORY DISEASES

3-20-23 CARDIOMYOPATHIES

D3-20000 Cardiomyopathy, NOS 425.4
(T-32020)
Myocardiopathy, NOS 425.4
(T-32020)

D3-20010 Obscure cardiomyopathy of Africa 425.2
Becker's disease 425.2
Idiopathic mural endomyocardial disease 424.2

D3-20020 Endomyocardial fibrosis 425.0
(T-32060) (T-32020) (M-78000)

D3-20030 Endocardial fibroelastosis 425.3
(T-32060) (M-78100)
Elastomyofibrosis 425.3
(T-32060) (M-78100)

D3-20040 Nonobstructive cardiomyopathy 425.4
(T-32000)

D3-20100 Primary cardiomyopathy 425.4

D3-20110 Idiopathic cardiomyopathy 425.4
(T-32000)
Primary idiopathic cardiomyopathy 425.4

D3-20120 Familial cardiomyopathy 425.4
(T-32000)
Primary familial cardiomyopathy 425.4

D3-20130 Primary eosinophilic endomyocardial cardiomyopathy 425.4
D3-20140 Primary endomyocardial fibrosis cardiomyopathy 425.0
D3-20200 Secondary cardiomyopathy, NOS 425.9
(T-32000)
D3-21100 Congestive cardiomyopathy 425.4
(T-32000)
Primary dilated cardiomyopathy 425.4
D3-21110 Primary idiopathic dilated cardiomyopathy 425.4
D3-21120 Primary familial dilated cardiomyopathy 425.4
D3-21200 Secondary dilated cardiomyopathy 425.9
D3-21210 Dilated cardiomyopathy secondary to infection, NOS
D3-21211 Dilated cardiomyopathy secondary to viral myocarditis
D3-21212 Dilated cardiomyopathy secondary to bacterial myocarditis
D3-21213 Dilated cardiomyopathy secondary to fungal myocarditis
D3-21214 Dilated cardiomyopathy secondary to protozoal myocarditis
D3-21215 Dilated cardiomyopathy secondary to metazoal myocarditis
D3-21220 Dilated cardiomyopathy secondary to metabolic disorder 425.7
Metabolic cardiomyopathy, NOS 425.7
(T-32000)
D3-21230 Dilated cardiomyopathy secondary to familial storage disease 425.7
D3-21231 Dilated cardiomyopathy secondary to glycogen storage disease 425.7
D3-21232 Dilated cardiomyopathy secondary to mucopolysaccharidosis 425.7
D3-21240 Dilated cardiomyopathy secondary to deficiency, NOS 425.7
D3-21241 Dilated cardiomyopathy secondary to nutritive deficiency 425.7
Nutritional cardiomyopathy, NOS 425.7
(T-32000)
D3-21242 Dilated cardiomyopathy secondary to electrolyte deficiency 425.7
D3-21250 Dilated cardiomyopathy secondary to connective tissue disorder, NOS 425.4
(T-32000)
Cardiovascular collagenosis 425.4
(T-30000)
D3-21251 Dilated cardiomyopathy secondary to systemic lupus erythematosus 425.8
D3-21252 Dilated cardiomyopathy secondary to polyarteritis nodosa 425.8
D3-21253 Dilated cardiomyopathy secondary to rheumatoid arthritis 425.8
D3-21254 Dilated cardiomyopathy secondary to scleroderma 425.8
D3-21255 Dilated cardiomyopathy secondary to dermatomyositis 425.8
D3-21260 Dilated cardiomyopathy secondary to infiltrations 425.8
D3-21261 Dilated cardiomyopathy secondary to amyloidosis 425.7
D3-21262 Dilated cardiomyopathy secondary to sarcoidosis 425.8
D3-21263 Dilated cardiomyopathy secondary to malignancy 425.8
D3-21264 Dilated cardiomyopathy secondary to hemochromatosis 425.8
D3-21265 Dilated cardiomyopathy secondary to granulomas 425.8
D3-21270 Dilated cardiomyopathy secondary to neuromuscular disorders 425.8
D3-21271 Dilated cardiomyopathy secondary to muscular dystrophy 425.8
D3-21272 Dilated cardiomyopathy secondary to myotonic dystrophy 425.8
D3-21273 Dilated cardiomyopathy secondary to Friedreich's ataxia 425.8
D3-21274 Dilated cardiomyopathy secondary to Refsum's disease 425.8
D3-21280 Dilated cardiomyopathy secondary to sensitivity
D3-21281 Dilated cardiomyopathy secondary to alcohol 425.5
Alcoholic cardiomyopathy 425.5
(T-32000)
D3-21282 Dilated cardiomyopathy secondary to radiation
D3-21283 Dilated cardiomyopathy secondary to drug, NOS
D3-21284 Dilated cardiomyopathy secondary to toxic reaction
D3-21290 Dilated cardiomyopathy secondary to peripartum heart disease
D3-22100 Primary restrictive cardiomyopathy 425.4
Restrictive cardiomyopathy 425.4
(T-32000)
Constrictive cardiomyopathy 425.4
(T-32000)
D3-22110 Primary idiopathic restrictive cardiomyopathy 425.4
D3-22130 Primary eosinophilic endomyocardial restrictive cardiomyopathy 425.4
D3-22140 Primary endomyocardial fibrosis restrictive cardiomyopathy 425.4
D3-22230 Restrictive cardiomyopathy secondary to familial storage disease 425.7
D3-22231 Restrictive cardiomyopathy secondary to glycogen storage disease 425.7
D3-22232 Restrictive cardiomyopathy secondary to mucopolysaccharidosis 425.7
D3-22260 Restrictive cardiomyopathy secondary to infiltrations
D3-22261 Restrictive cardiomyopathy secondary to amyloidosis 425.7
D3-22262 Restrictive cardiomyopathy secondary to sarcoidosis 425.8

3-20-23 CARDIOMYOPATHIES — Continued

D3-22263 Restrictive cardiomyopathy secondary to malignancy 425.8
D3-22264 Restrictive cardiomyopathy secondary to hemochromatosis 425.7
D3-22265 Restrictive cardiomyopathy secondary to granulomas
D3-222A0 Restrictive cardiomyopathy secondary to endocardial fibroelastosis 425.9
D3-23000 Hypertrophic obstructive cardiomyopathy 425.1
D3-23100 Primary hypertrophic cardiomyopathy 425.4
  Obstructive cardiomyopathy 425.4
    (T-32000)
  Hypertrophic cardiomyopathy 425.4
    (T-32000)
D3-23110 Primary idiopathic hypertrophic cardiomyopathy 425.4
D3-23120 Primary familial hypertrophic cardiomyopathy 425.4
D3-23210 Hypertrophic cardiomyopathy secondary to neuromuscular disorder, NOS 425.8
D3-23273 Hypertrophic cardiomyopathy secondary to Friedreich's ataxia 425.8

3-26-27 MYOCARDITIDES

D3-26000 Myocarditis, NOS 429.0
D3-26001 Acute myocarditis, NOS 422.90
    (T-32020) (M-41000)
D3-26002 Subacute interstitial myocarditis 422.90
    (T-32020) (M-42000)
D3-26003 Chronic interstitial myocarditis 429.0
D3-26004 Fibroid myocarditis 429.0
D3-26005 Idiopathic myocarditis 422.91
    (T-32020) (M-40000)
  Fiedler's myocarditis 422.91
    (T-32020) (M-40000)
D3-26006 Senile myocarditis 429.0
D3-26007 Isolated diffuse granulomatous myocarditis 422.91
    (T-32020) (M-44000)
  Nonspecific granulomatous myocarditis 422.91
    (T-32020) (M-44000)
D3-26010 Giant cell myocarditis 422.91
    (T-32020) (M-44000)
D3-26020 Rheumatoid carditis 714.2
D3-26100 Myocarditis due to hypersensitivity state, NOS
D3-26200 Myocarditis due to radiation
D3-26300 Toxic myocarditis 422.93
    (T-32020) (M-40000) (C-00220)
D3-26310 Myocarditis due to chemical agent, NOS
D3-26400 Myocarditis due to drug, NOS
D3-26500 Myocarditis due to physical agent, NOS
D3-26700 Myocarditis due to infectious agent, NOS

3-28 ENDOCARDITIDES

D3-28001 Acute endocarditis, NOS 421.9
    (T-32060) (M-41000)
D3-28002 Subacute endocarditis, NOS 421.9
    (T-32060) (M-42000)
D3-28003 Chronic endocarditis, NOS 424.9
    (T-32060) (M-43000)
D3-28005 Valvular endocarditis, NOS 424.9
    (T-32060) (T-35000) (M-43000)
D3-28100 Bacterial endocarditis, NOS 421.0
    (T-32060) (M-40000) (L-10000)
  Infective endocarditis 421.0
    (T-32060) (M-40000) (L-10000)
  Endocarditis lenta 421.0
    (T-32060) (M-40000) (L-10000)
D3-28101 Acute bacterial endocarditis 421.0
    (T-32060) (M-41000) (L-10000)
D3-28102 Subacute bacterial endocarditis 421.0
    (T-32060) (M-42000) (L-10000)
  SBE 421.0
    (T-32060) (M-42000) (L-10000)
D3-28103 Chronic bacterial endocarditis 421.0
    (T-32060) (M-43000) (L-10000)
D3-28110 Purulent endocarditis 421.0
    (T-32060) (M-40600)
D3-28120 Vegetative endocarditis 421.0
    (T-32060) (M-40000) (L-40000)
D3-28130 Malignant endocarditis 421.0
    (T-32060) (M-41750)
  Septic endocarditis 421.0
    (T-32060) (M-41750)
  Ulcerative endocarditis 421.0
    (T-32060) (M-41750)
D3-28140 Endocarditis with infective aneurysm 421.0
    (T-32060) (M-40000) (M-32200)
D3-28150 Acute myoendocarditis 421.9
    (T-32060) (T-32020) (M-41000)
D3-28160 Subacute myoendocarditis 421.9
    (T-32060) (T-32020) (M-42000)
D3-28170 Acute periendocarditis 421.9
    (T-32060) (T-32024) (M-41000)
D3-28180 Subacute periendocarditis 421.9
    (T-32060) (T-32024) (M-42000)

3-29 NONRHEUMATIC HEART VALVE DISORDERS

D3-29000 Nonrheumatic heart valve disorder, NOS
D3-29001 Heart valve stenosis, NOS 424.90
    (T-35000) (M-34200)
D3-29002 Heart valve regurgitation, NOS 424.90
    (T-35000) (F-32400)
  Heart valve insufficiency, NOS 424.90
    (T-35000) (F-32400)
  Heart valve incompetence, NOS 424.90
    (T-35000) (F-32400)
D3-29007 Chronic valvulitis, NOS 424.9
    (T-32060) (T-35000) (M-43000)

D3-29010 Mitral valve disorder, NOS 424.0
(T-35300)
D3-29011 Mitral valve stenosis, NOS 424.0
(T-35300) (M-34200)
D3-29012 Mitral valve regurgitation, NOS 424.0
(T-35300) (F-32400)
Mitral valve insufficiency, NOS 424.0
(T-35300) (F-32400)
Mitral valve incompetence, NOS 424.0
(T-35300) (F-32400)
D3-29020 Aortic valve disorder, NOS 424.1
(T-35400)
D3-29021 Aortic valve stenosis, NOS 424.1
(T-35400) (M-34200)
D3-29022 Aortic valve regurgitation, NOS 424.1
(T-35400) (F-32400)
Aortic valve insufficiency, NOS 424.1
(T-35400) (F-32400)
Aortic valve incompetence, NOS 424.1
(T-35400) (F-32400)
D3-29040 Tricuspid valve disorder, NOS 424.2
(T-35100)
D3-29041 Tricuspid valve stenosis, NOS 424.2
(T-35100) (M-34200)
D3-29042 Tricuspid valve regurgitation, NOS 424.2
(T-35100) (F-32400)
Tricuspid valve insufficiency, NOS 424.2
(T-35100) (F-32400)
Tricuspid valve incompetence, NOS 424.2
(T-35100) (F-32400)
D3-29050 Pulmonary valve disorder, NOS 424.3
(T-35200)
D3-29051 Pulmonic valve stenosis, NOS 424.3
(T-35200) (M-34200)
D3-29052 Pulmonic valve regurgitation, NOS 424.3
(T-35200) (F-32400)
Pulmonic valve insufficiency, NOS 424.3
(T-35200) (F-32400)
Pulmonic valve incompetence, NOS 424.3
(T-35200) (F-32400)

SECTION 3-3 CONDUCTION DISORDERS

3-30-31 CARDIAC DYSRHYTHMIAS

D3-30000 Conduction disorder of the heart, NOS 426.9
(T-32800)
D3-30010 Cardiac dysrhythmia, NOS 427.9
Cardiac arrhythmia, NOS 427.9
D3-30220 Paroxysmal tachycardia, NOS 427.2
Bouveret-Hoffmann syndrome 427.2
Essential paroxysmal tachycardia 427.2
D3-30800 Cardiac arrest 427.5
Cardiorespiratory arrest 427.5
Cardiopulmonary arrest 427.5
D3-30900 Premature beats, NOS 427.60
Extrasystoles 427.60
Extrasystolic arrhythmia 427.60
D3-30A00 Ectopic rhythm disorder 427.89
Ectopic beats 427.60
D3-31000 Sinoatrial node dysfunction 427.81
Coronary sinus rhythm disorder 427.89
D3-31100 Sinus bradycardia 427.81
D3-31101 Severe sinus bradycardia 427.81
D3-31110 Persistent sinus bradycardia 427.81
D3-31120 Sick sinus syndrome 427.81
D3-31121 Tachycardia-bradycardia 427.81
D3-31124 Sinus tachycardia 427.81
D3-31130 Nodal rhythm disorder 427.89
D3-31140 Anomalous atrioventricular excitation 426.7
D3-31150 Pre-excitation atrioventricular conduction 426.7
D3-31300 Nonparoxysmal AV nodal tachycardia 426.89
D3-31340 Atrioventricular dissociation 426.89
Interference dissociation 426.89
Isorhythmic dissociation 426.89
D3-31350 Accelerated atrioventricular conduction 426.7
D3-31510 Atrial paroxysmal tachycardia 427.0
AV paroxysmal tachycardia 427.0
PAT 427.0
Atrioventricular paroxysmal tachycardia 427.0
Junctional paroxysmal tachycardia 427.0
Nodal paroxysmal tachycardia 427.0
D3-31520 Atrial fibrillation 427.31
D3-31530 Atrial flutter 427.32
D3-31540 Atrial premature beats 427.61
Atrial premature contractions 427.61
Atrial premature systoles 427.61
D3-31560 Wandering atrial pacemaker 427.89
D3-31700 Ventricular tachycardia, NOS 427.1
D3-31710 Paroxysmal ventricular tachycardia 427.1
D3-31720 Ventricular fibrillation 427.41
D3-31730 Ventricular flutter 427.42
D3-31740 Ventricular premature beats 427.69
Ventricular premature contractions 427.69
Ventricular premature systoles 427.69
D3-31750 Paroxysmal supraventricular tachycardia 427.0
D3-31760 Supraventricular premature beats 427.61
D3-31800 Accessory atrioventricular conduction 426.7
D3-31810 Wolff-Parkinson-White syndrome 426.7
Ventricular pre-excitation with arrhythmia, NOS 426.7
D3-31820 Lown-Ganong-Levine syndrome 426.81
Syndrome of short P-R interval, normal QRS complexes and supraventricular tachycardias 426.8

3-32-33 HEART BLOCKS

D3-32010 Sinoatrial block, NOS 426.6
Sinoauricular block, NOS 426.6
D3-32100 Heart block, NOS 426.9
(T-32800)
Atrioventricular block, NOS 426.10
AV block, NOS 426.1

3-32-33 HEART BLOCKS — Continued

D3-32102 Complete atrioventricular block 426.0
D3-32104 Stokes-Adams syndrome 426.9
D3-32106 Stokes-Adams-Morgagni syndrome 426.9
D3-32110 Incomplete atrioventricular block 426.10
  Partial atrioventricular block 426.10
D3-32111 First degree atrioventricular block 426.11
  Incomplete atrioventricular block, first degree 426.11
  Prolonged P-R interval, NOS 426.11
D3-32113 Third degree atrioventricular block 426.0
D3-32114 Mobitz type II atrioventricular block 426.12
  Mobitz type II incomplete atrioventricular block 426.12
  Second degree Mobitz type II incomplete atrioventricular block 426.12
D3-32117 Mobitz type I incomplete atrioventricular block 426.13
  Wenckebach's incomplete AV block 426.13
  Wenckebach's phenomenon 426.13
D3-32118 Incomplete atrioventricular block with atrioventricular response 426.13
D3-33000 Intraventricular block, NOS 426.6
  Intraventricular conduction defect, NOS 426.6
D3-33012 Diffuse intraventricular block 426.6
  Myofibrillar intraventricular block 426.6
D3-33100 Monofascicular block, NOS
D3-33106 Bundle branch block, NOS 426.50
D3-33110 Right bundle branch block 426.4
D3-33120 Left bundle branch block, NOS 426.3
D3-33130 Left bundle branch hemiblock, NOS 426.2
D3-33140 Left anterior fascicular block 426.2
D3-33150 Left posterior fascicular block 426.2
D3-33200 Bifascicular block, NOS 426.53
D3-33220 Complete left bundle branch block 426.3
  Anterior fascicular with posterior fascicular block 426.3
  Main stem left bundle branch block 426.3
D3-33310 Right bundle branch block and left posterior fascicular block 426.51
D3-33320 Right bundle branch block and left anterior fascicular block 426.52
D3-33340 Bilateral bundle branch block, NOS 426.53
D3-33350 Right bundle branch block with left bundle branch block 426.53
  Right bundle branch block with left main stem bundle branch block 426.53
D3-33360 Right bundle branch block and incomplete left bundle branch block 426.53
D3-33400 Trifascicular block, NOS 426.54
  Multifascicular block, NOS 426.54
D3-33410 Right bundle branch block, anterior fascicular block and posterior fascicular block 426.54
D3-33420 Right bundle blanch block, anterior fascicular block and incomplete posterior fascicular block 426.54
D3-33430 Right bundle branch block, posterior fascicular block and incomplete anterior fascicular block 426.54
D3-33440 Right branch block, incomplete anterior fascicular block and incomplete posterior fascicular block 426.54
D3-33450 Right bundle branch block, anterior fascicular block and incomplete left bundle branch block 426.54
D3-33460 Right bundle branch block, posterior fascicular block and incomplete left bundle branch block 426.54
D3-33470 Anterior fascicular block, posterior fascicular block and incomplete right bundle branch block 426.54

SECTION 3-4 DISEASES OF THE PULMONARY CIRCULATION

D3-40000 Disease of pulmonary circulation, NOS 417.9
  (T-30200)
D3-40004 Kyphoscoliotic heart disease 416.1
  (T-32000)
D3-40101 Acute pulmonary heart disease, NOS 415.-
  (T-30200) (M-32000)
D3-40103 Chronic pulmonary heart disease, NOS 416.9
  (T-32000) (T-30200)
  Chronic cardiopulmonary disease 416.9
  (T-32000) (T-30200)
D3-40111 Acute cor pulmonale 415.0
  (T-30200) (T-32000)
D3-40113 Chronic cor pulmonale, NOS 416.9
  (T-32000) (T-30200)
D3-40202 Rupture of pulmonary vessel 417.8
  (T-44000) (T-48500) (M-14400)
D3-40204 Stricture of pulmonary vessel 417.8
  (T-44000) (T-48500) (M-34260)
D3-40206 Aneurysm of pulmonary artery 417.1
  (T-44000) (M-32200)
D3-40208 Arteriovenous fistula of pulmonary vessels 417.0
  (T-44000) (M-48500) (M-39370)
D3-40210 Pulmonary infarction 415.1
  (T-28000) (M-54700)
D3-40215 Hemorrhagic pulmonary infarction 415.1
  (T-28000) (M-54730)
D3-40220 Pulmonary thrombosis 415.1
  (T-44000) (M-35100)
D3-40230 Pulmonary embolism 415.1
  (T-44000) (M-35300)
D3-40240 Pulmonary apoplexy 415.1
  (T-28000)
D3-40250 Idiopathic pulmonary arteriosclerosis 416.0
  (T-44000) (M-52000)
D3-40260 Pulmonary arteritis 417.8
  (T-44000) (M-40000)
D3-40265 Pulmonary endarteritis 417.8
  (T-44000) (M-40000)
D3-40310 Primary pulmonary hypertension 416.0
  (T-30200) (D3-02100)
  Essential pulmonary hypertension 419.0
  (T-30200) (D3-02100)

D3-40310 (cont.) Idiopathic pulmonary hypertension 416.0 (T-30200) (D3-02100)
D3-40320 Secondary pulmonary hypertension 416.8 (T-30200) (D3-02200)

SECTION 3-8 VASCULAR DISEASES
3-80 GENERAL VASCULAR DISORDERS

D3-80000 Vascular disease, NOS
Vascular disorder, NOS
D3-80100 Hemorrhage of blood vessel, NOS 459.0 (T-40000) (M-37000)
Rupture of blood vessel, NOS 459.0
Spontaneous hemorrhage, NOS 459.0
D3-80500 Peripheral vascular disease, NOS 443.9
Peripheral angiopathy, NOS 443.9
D3-80520 Intermittent claudication 443.9
D3-80522 Intermittent spinal claudication 443.9
D3-80524 Intermittent cauda equina claudication 443.9
D3-80530 Raynaud's syndrome 443.0
D3-80532 Raynaud's disease 443.0
D3-80534 Secondary Raynaud's phenomenon 443.0
D3-80536 Acrocyanosis 443.89
D3-80540 Simple acroparesthesia 443.89
Schultze's type acroparesthesia 443.89
D3-80542 Vasomotor acroparesthesia 443.89
Nothnagel's type acroparesthesia 443.89
D3-80550 Erythrocyanosis 443.89
D3-80554 Erythromelalgia 443.89
D3-80600 Shock, NOS 785.50
D3-80610 Hypovolemic shock 785.59
D3-80620 Endotoxic shock 785.59
Gram-negative shock 785.59
D3-80630 Septic shock 785.59

3-81-82 DISEASES OF THE ARTERIES

D3-81000 Disease of artery, NOS
Disorder of artery, NOS
D3-81100 Arteriosclerotic vascular disease, NOS 440.9
D3-81120 Arteriosclerosis obliterans 440.-
Senile arteriosclerosis 440.-
D3-81140 Monckeberg's medial sclerosis 440.2
D3-81150 Arterial degeneration 440-
Arteriovascular degeneration 440.-
Vascular degeneration 440.-
D3-81201 Generalized and unspecified atherosclerosis 440.9
D3-81202 Atheroma of artery, NOS 440.-
D3-81210 Atherosclerosis of renal artery 440.1
D3-81220 Atherosclerosis of arteries of the extremities 440.2
D3-81230 Atherosclerosis of other specified arteries 440.8
D3-81300 Aneurysm of artery, NOS, other than aorta 442.9
D3-81301 Ruptured aneurysm of artery, NOS 442.9
D3-81310 Dissecting aneurysm of artery, NOS 441.0
D3-81315 Cirsoid aneurysm of artery, NOS 442.9
D3-81320 False aneurysm of artery, NOS 442.9
D3-81330 Varicose aneurysm of artery, NOS 442.9
Aneurysmal varix of artery, NOS 442.9
D3-81340 Aneurysm of artery of upper extremity 442.0
D3-81345 Aneurysm of artery of lower extremity 442.3
D3-8134A Aneurysm of femoral artery 442.3
D3-81350 Aneurysm of popliteal artery 442.3
D3-81355 Aneurysm of renal artery 442.1
D3-8135A Aneurysm of iliac artery 442.2
D3-81360 Aneurysm of artery of neck 442.81
D3-81365 Aneurysm of common carotid artery 442.81
D3-8136A Aneurysm of external carotid artery 442.81
D3-81370 Aneurysm of internal carotid artery 442.81
D3-81375 Aneurysm of subclavian artery 442.82
D3-8137A Aneurysm of visceral artery, NOS 442.84
D3-81380 Aneurysm of splenic artery 442.83
D3-81385 Aneurysm of celiac artery 442.84
D3-8138A Aneurysm of gastroduodenal artery 442.84
D3-81390 Aneurysm of gastroepiploic artery 442.84
D3-81395 Aneurysm of hepatic artery 442.84
D3-8139A Aneurysm of pancreaticoduodenal artery 442.84
D3-813A0 Aneurysm of superior mesenteric artery 442.84
D3-813A5 Aneurysm of mediastinal artery 442.89
D3-813AA Aneurysm of spinal artery 442.89
D3-81400 Arterial embolism, NOS, of unspecified artery 444.9
D3-81404 Embolic infarction, NOS 444.-
D3-81410 Embolism of iliac artery 444.8
D3-81500 Arterial thrombosis, NOS, of unspecified artery 444.9
D3-81504 Thrombotic infarction, NOS 444.-
D3-81510 Thromboangiitis obliterans 443.1
Buerger's disease 443.1
Presenile gangrene 443.1
D3-81550 Thrombosis of iliac artery 444.8
D3-81560 Thrombosis of arteries of the extremities, NOS 444.2
D3-81570 Thrombosis of arteries of upper extremity 444.2
D3-81580 Thrombosis of arteries of lower extremity 444.2
D3-81582 Femoral artery thrombosis 444.2
D3-81584 Popliteal artery thrombosis 444.2
D3-81600 Arteritis, NOS 447.6
D3-81601 Endarteritis, NOS 447.6
D3-81602 Periarteritis, NOS
D3-81610 Endarteritis deformans 440.-
Endarteritis obliterans 440.-
D3-81620 Senile arteritis 440.-
D3-81621 Senile endarteritis 440.-
D3-81630 Polyarteritis nodosa 446.0
Disseminated necrotizing periarteritis 446.0
Necrotizing angiitis 446.0

3-81-82 DISEASES OF THE ARTERIES — Continued

D3-81630 (cont.) Panarteritis nodosa 446.0
Periarteritis nodosa 446.0
D3-81640 Giant cell arteritis 446.5
Cranial arteritis 446.5
Horton's disease 446.5
Temporal arteritis 446.5
Temporal giant cell arteritis 446.5
D3-81660 Acute febrile mucocutaneous lymph node syndrome 446.1
MCLS 446.1
Kawasaki disease 446.1
D3-81670 Hypersensitivity angiitis 446.2
D3-81680 Lethal midline granuloma 446.3
Malignant granuloma of face 446.3
Lethal midline granuloma of face 446.3
D3-81690 Wegener's granulomatosis 446.4
Necrotizing respiratory granulomatosis 446.4
Wegener's syndrome 446.4
D3-81692 Wegener's syndrome, limited form 446.4
Lymphomatoid granulomatosis of the lung 446.4
Lymphoid granulomatosis of the lung 446.4
D3-81900 Occlusion of artery, NOS 444.-
Arterial occlusive disease 447.1
D3-81904 Spasm of artery 443.9
D3-81910 Stricture of artery 447.1
D3-81920 Fistula of artery, NOS 447.2
D3-81930 Erosion of artery 447.2
D3-81932 Ulcer of artery 447.2
D3-81934 Necrosis of artery 447.5
D3-81936 Rupture of artery 447.2
D3-81940 Hyperplasia of renal artery 447.3
Fibromuscular hyperplasia of renal artery 447.3
D3-81950 Celiac artery compression syndrome 447.4
Celiac axis syndrome 447.4
Marable's syndrome 447.4
D3-81954 Fibromuscular hyperplasia of artery except renal 447.8

3-83 DISEASES OF THE AORTA

D3-83000 Disease of the aorta, NOS
Disorder of aorta, NOS
D3-83010 Dilatation of aorta 441.9
D3-83020 Hyaline necrosis of aorta 441.9
D3-83030 Rupture of aorta, NOS 441.5
D3-83200 Atherosclerosis of aorta 440.0
D3-83300 Aortic aneurysm, NOS 441.9
Aneurysm of aorta, NOS 441.9
D3-83310 Ruptured aortic aneurysm, NOS 441.5
D3-83312 Dissecting aortic aneurysm 441.0
D3-83320 Thoracic aortic aneurysm without mention of rupture 441.2
D3-83331 Ruptured thoracic aortic aneurysm 441.1
D3-83340 Abdominal aortic aneurysm without rupture 441.4
D3-83341 Ruptured abdominal aortic aneurysm 441.3
D3-83410 Embolism of abdominal aorta 444.0
D3-83420 Embolism of thoracic aorta 444.1
D3-83510 Thrombosis of abdominal aorta 444.0
D3-83511 Aortic bifurcation syndrome 444.0
Aortoiliac obstruction 444.0
Leriche's syndrome 444.0
Saddle embolus of abdominal aorta 444.0
D3-83520 Thrombosis of thoracic aorta 444.1
D3-83600 Aortitis, NOS 447.6
D3-83620 Takayasu's disease 446.7
Aortic arch arteritis 446.7
Pulseless disease 446.7
Raeder-Harbitz syndrome 446.6
Reverse coarctation 446.6
Young female arteritis 446.6
Martorell syndrome 446.6
Primary arteritis 446.6
Nonspecific arteritis 446.6
Idiopathic aortitis 446.6
Atypical coarctation 446.6
Takayasu's arteritis 446.6
Middle aortic syndrome 446.6
Takayasu's arteriopathy 446.6
Occlusive thromboarteriopathy 446.6
Acquired aortoarteritis 446.6
Aortitis syndrome 446.6
Idiopathic medial aortopathy and arteriopathy 446.6
Sclerosing aortitis and arteritis 446.6
Nonspecific aortoarteritis 446.6

3-85 DISEASES OF THE CAPILLARIES

D3-85000 Disease of capillaries, NOS 448.9
Capillary disease, NOS 448.9
D3-85120 Capillary hemorrhage 448.9
D3-85125 Capillary hyperpermeability 448.9
D3-85130 Capillary thrombosis 448.9
D3-85200 Non-neoplastic nevus of skin 448.1
Nevus araneus of skin 448.1
Senile nevus of skin 448.1
Spider nevus of skin 448.1
Stellar nevus of skin 448.1
Vascular spider of skin 448.1

3-87 DISEASES OF THE VEINS

D3-87000 Disease of vein, NOS
Disorder of vein, NOS
D3-87010 Portal vein obstruction, NOS 452.-
D3-87011 Budd-Chiari syndrome 453.0
D3-87020 Varicose veins of lower extremity, NOS 454.9
Phlebectasia of lower extremity, NOS 454.9
Varix of lower extremity, NOS 454.9
D3-87021 Varicose veins of lower extremity without ulcer or inflammation 454.9

D3-87022 Varicose veins of lower extremity with ulcer 454.0
Varicose ulcer of lower extremity 454.0
Varicose veins with ulcer of lower extremity 454.0
D3-87023 Varicose veins of lower extremity with inflammation 454.1
Varicose veins with inflammation of lower extremity 454.1
D3-87025 Varicose veins of lower extremity with ulcer and inflammation 454.2
D3-87200 Hemorrhoids, NOS 455.6
Piles, NOS 455.6
D3-87201 Hemorrhoids without complication 455.6
D3-87202 Bleeding hemorrhoids 455.8
D3-87203 Prolapsed hemorrhoids 455.8
D3-87204 Strangulated hemorrhoids 455.8
D3-87205 Ulcerated hemorrhoids 455.8
D3-87206 Thrombosed hemorrhoids, NOS 455.7
D3-87220 Internal hemorrhoids, NOS 455.0
D3-87221 Internal hemorrhoids without complication 455.0
D3-87222 Bleeding internal hemorrhoids 455.2
D3-87223 Prolapsed internal hemorrhoids 455.2
D3-87224 Stangulated internal hemorrhoids 455.2
D3-87225 Ulcerated internal hemorrhoids 455.2
D3-87226 Thrombosed internal hemorrhoids 455.1
D3-87240 External hemorrhoids, NOS 455.3
D3-87241 External hemorrhoids without complication 455.3
D3-87242 Bleeding external hemorrhoids 455.5
D3-87243 Prolapsed external hemorrhoids 455.5
D3-87244 Strangulated external hemorrhoids 455.5
D3-87245 Ulcerated external hemorrhoids 455.5
D3-87246 Thrombosed external hemorrhoids 455.4
D3-87250 Residual hemorrhoidal skin tags 455.9
D3-87310 Sublingual varices 456.3
D3-87314 Varicose veins of nasal septum with ulcer 456.8
D3-87320 Scrotal varices 456.4
D3-87322 Varicocele 456.4
D3-87330 Pelvic varices 456.5
D3-87332 Varices of broad ligament 456.5
D3-87340 Varices of perineum 456.6
D3-87342 Vulval varices 456.6
D3-87410 Embolism of vena cava 453.2
D3-87420 Embolism of renal vein 453.3
D3-87510 Portal vein thrombosis 452.-
D3-87520 Hepatic vein thrombosis 453.0
D3-87530 Thrombosis of vena cava 453.2
D3-87540 Thrombosis of renal vein 453.3
D3-87700 Phlebitis, NOS 451.9
Inflammation of vein, NOS 451.9
D3-87702 Endophlebitis 451.-
D3-87704 Periphlebitis 451.-
D3-87706 Suppurative phlebitis 451.-
D3-87710 Thrombophlebitis, NOS 451.9
D3-87720 Phlebitis of lower extremities, NOS 451.2
D3-87722 Thrombophlebitis of lower extremities, NOS 451.2
D3-87730 Phlebitis of superficial veins of lower extremity 451.0
D3-87731 Phlebitis of femoropopliteal vein 451.0
D3-87732 Phlebitis of saphenous vein 451.0
D3-87740 Thrombophlebitis of superficial veins of lower extremity 451.0
D3-87741 Thrombophlebitis of femoropopliteal vein 451.0
D3-87742 Thrombophlebitis of saphenous vein 451.0
D3-87750 Phlebitis of deep veins of lower extremity 451.1
D3-87751 Phlebitis of deep femoral vein 451.11
D3-87752 Phlebitis of tibial vein 451.19
D3-87753 Phlebitis of popliteal vein 451.19
D3-87754 Phlebitis of iliac vein 451.81
D3-87760 Thrombophlebitis of deep veins of lower extremity 451.1
D3-87761 Thrombophlebitis of deep femoral vein 451.11
D3-87762 Thrombophlebitis of tibial vein 451.19
D3-87763 Thrombophlebitis of popliteal vein 451.19
D3-87764 Thrombophlebitis of iliac vein 451.81
D3-87780 Thrombophlebitis of breast 451.89
Mondor's disease 451.89
D3-87790 Thrombophlebitis migrans 453.1
D3-87800 Postphlebitic syndrome 459.1
D3-87810 Compression of vein, NOS 459.2
D3-87812 Stricture of vein 459.2
D3-87820 Inferior vena cava syndrome 459.2
D3-87830 Superior vena cava syndrome 459.2
D3-87840 Peripheral venous insufficiency, NOS 459.8
Chronic venous insufficiency, NOS 459.8
D3-87850 Venous collateral circulation, any site 459.89

3-89 CEREBROVASCULAR DISEASES

D3-89000 Cerebrovascular disease, NOS 437.9
(T-40500) (M-01100)
Cerebrovascular lesion, NOS 437.9
(T-40500) (M-01100)
D3-89100 Intracranial hemorrhage, NOS 432.9
(T-D1400) (M-37000)
D3-89110 Subarachnoid hemorrhage 430.-
(T-A1500) (M-37000)
D3-89120 Meningeal hemorrhage 430.-
(T-A1110) (M-37000)
D3-89130 Hemorrhage due to ruptured congenital cerebral aneurysm, NOS 430.-
(T-45500) (M-14400) (M-24610)
Hemorrhage due to ruptured berry aneurysm 430.-
(T-45500) (M-14400) (M-24610)
D3-89140 Nontraumatic extradural hemorrhage 432.0
(T-A1300) (M-37000)
Nontraumatic epidural hemorrhage 432.0
(T-A1300) (M-37000)

3-89 CEREBROVASCULAR DISEASES — Continued

D3-89150 Nontraumatic subdural hemorrhage 432.1 (T-A1400) (M-37000)
Nontraumatic subdural hematoma 432.1 (T-A1400) (M-37000)

D3-89200 Intracerebral hemorrhage, NOS 431.- (T-A0100) (M-37000)
Rupture of blood vessel in brain 431.- (T-A0100) (M-37000)

D3-89210 Bulbar hemorrhage 431.- (T-A6700) (M-37000)

D3-89220 Basilar hemorrhage 431.- (T-45800) (M-37000)

D3-89230 Cerebellar hemorrhage 431.- (T-A6000) (M-37000)

D3-89240 Cerebral hemorrhage 431.- (T-A0100) (M-37000)

D3-89242 Cerebromeningeal hemorrhage 431.- (T-A0110) (M-A1110) (M-37000)

D3-89244 Cortical hemorrhage 431.- (T-A2020) (M-37000)

D3-89246 Internal capsule hemorrhage 431.- (T-A3700) (M-37000)

D3-89248 Subcortical hemorrhage 431.- (T-A2030) (M-37000)

D3-89250 Intrapontine hemorrhage 431.- (T-A5400) (M-37000)
Pontine hemorrhage 431.- (T-A5400) (M-37000)

D3-89260 Ventricular hemorrhage 431.- (T-A1600) (M-37000)
Intraventricular hemorrhage 431.- (T-A1600) (M-37000)

D3-89300 Stenosis of precerebral artery, NOS 433.9
Narrowing of precerebral artery, NOS 433.9

D3-89301 Obstruction of precerebral artery, NOS 433.9
Occlusion of precerebral artery, NOS 433.9

D3-89302 Thrombosis of precerebral artery, NOS 433.9

D3-89303 Embolism of precerebral artery, NOS 433.9

D3-89310 Multiple and bilateral precerebral artery stenosis 433.3

D3-89311 Multiple and bilateral precerebral artery obstruction 433.3

D3-89312 Multiple and bilateral precerebral artery thrombosis 433.3

D3-89313 Multiple and bilateral precerebral artery embolism 433.3

D3-89320 Basilar artery stenosis 433.0
Basilar artery narrowing 433.0

D3-89321 Basilar artery obstruction 433.0
Basilar artery occlusion 433.0

D3-89322 Basilar artery thrombosis 433.0

D3-89323 Basilar artery embolism 433.0

D3-89330 Carotid artery stenosis 433.1
Carotid artery narrowing 433.1

D3-89331 Carotid artery obstruction 433.1
Carotid artery occlusion 433.1

D3-89332 Carotid artery thrombosis 433.1

D3-89333 Carotid artery embolism 433.1

D3-89340 Vertebral artery stenosis 433.2
Vertebral artery narrowing 433.2

D3-89341 Vertebral artery obstruction 433.2
Vertebral artery occlusion 433.2

D3-89342 Vertebral artery thrombosis 433.2

D3-89343 Vertebral artery embolism 433.2

D3-89400 Cerebral artery occlusion, NOS 434.9
Cerebral infarction, NOS 434.9

D3-89410 Cerebral embolism 434.1

D3-89420 Cerebral thrombosis 434.0
Thrombosis of cerebral arteries 434.0

D3-89500 Transient cerebral ischemia, NOS 435.9
Impending cerebrovascular accident 435.9
Intermittent cerebral ischemia 435.9
Transient ischemic attack 435.9
TIA 435.9

D3-89508 Spasm of cerebral arteries 435.-

D3-89510 Basilar artery syndrome 435.0

D3-89520 Vertebral artery syndrome 435.1

D3-89530 Subclavian steal syndrome 435.2

D3-89550 Cerebrovascular accident, NOS 436.-
Acute ill-defined cerebrovascular disease, NOS 436.-
Apoplexy, NOS 436.-
Apoplectic attack, NOS 436.-
Cerebral apoplexy, NOS 436.-
Apoplectic seizure, NOS 436.-
Cerebral seizure, NOS 436.-
CVA, NOS 436.-
Stroke, NOS 436.-

D3-89560 Acute cerebrovascular insufficiency, NOS 437.1

D3-89565 Chronic cerebral ischemia 437.1

D3-89600 Cerebral atherosclerosis 437.0

D3-89602 Atheroma of cerebral arteries 437.0

D3-89605 Cerebral arteriosclerosis 437.0

D3-89610 Nonruptured cerebral aneurysm 437.3

D3-89620 Cerebral arteritis 437.4

D3-89630 Moyamoya disease 437.5

D3-89640 Nonpyogenic thrombosis of intracranial venous sinus 437.6

D3-89660 Hypertensive encephalopathy 437.2
Hypertensive crisis 437.2

SECTION 3-9 PERICARDIAL DISEASES

3-90 PERICARDIAL DISEASES: GENERAL CONDITIONS

D3-90000 Disease of pericardium, NOS 423.9 (T-39000)
Pericardial disorder, NOS 423.9 (T-39000)

D3-90010 Hemopericardium 423.0 (T-39000) (M-37000)

D3-90020 Pneumopyopericardium 420.99 (T-39000) (C-10130) (M-41600)

D3-90030 Pyopericardium 420.99
(T-39000) (M-41600)
D3-90040 Pneumopericardium 420.99
(T-39000)
D3-90210 Milk spots of pericardium 423.1
(T-39000) (M-78001)
Soldiers' patches 423.1
(T-39000) (M-78001)
D3-90300 Calcification of pericardium 423.8
(T-39000) (M-55400)
D3-90400 Fistula of pericardium 423.8
(T-39000) (M-39300)
D3-91000 Pericarditis, NOS 420.90
(T-39000) (M-41000)
D3-91010 Adhesive pericarditis 423.1
(T-39000) (M-45000)
Adherent pericardium 423.1
(T-39000) (M-45000)
Fibrosis of pericardium 423.1
(T-39000)
D3-91020 Obliterative pericarditis 423.1
(T-39000) (M-45100)
D3-91030 Constrictive pericarditis 423.2
(T-39000) (M-45100)
D3-91040 Concato's disease 423.2
(T-39000) (T-1A110) (M-40000)
(M-36700)
D3-91050 Pick's disease of heart and liver 423.2
(T-39000) (M-45100) (T-D4425)
(M-36700) (T-62000) (M-78000)
D3-91100 Acute pericarditis, NOS 420.90
(T-39000) (M-41000)
D3-91101 Acute mediastinopericarditis 420.-
(T-39000) (T-D3300) (M-41000)
D3-91102 Acute myopericarditis 420.-
(T-39000) (T-32020) (M-41000)
D3-91105 Acute pleuropericarditis 420.-
(T-39000) (T-29000) (M-41000)
D3-91106 Acute pneumopericarditis 420.-
(T-39000) (C-10130) (M-41000)
D3-91107 Acute pericardial effusion 420.-
(T-39000) (M-36700)
D3-91109 Pericarditis sicca 420.90
(T-39000) (M-41300)
D3-91110 Acute idiopathic pericarditis 420.91
(T-39000) (M-41000)
Acute benign pericarditis 420.91
(T-39000) (M-41000)
Acute nonspecific pericarditis 420.91
(T-39000) (M-41000)
Acute fibrinous pericarditis 420.91
(T-39000) (M-41000)
D3-91120 Acute effusive pericarditis
Acute bloody pericarditis
D3-91200 Subacute pericarditis
D3-91210 Subacute constrictive pericarditis
D3-91220 Subacute effusive constrictive pericarditis
D3-91300 Chronic pericarditis
D3-91310 Chronic constrictive pericarditis
D3-91320 Chronic effusive pericarditis
D3-91330 Chronic adhesive pericarditis
Chronic non-constrictive carditis

3-92 INFECTIOUS PERICARDITIDES

D3-92000 Infectious pericarditis, NOS 420.90
(T-39000)
D3-92200 Pyogenic pericarditis, NOS
D3-92210 Acute purulent pericarditis 420.99
(T-39000) (M-41600)
Acute suppurative pericarditis 420.99
(T-39000) (M-41600)

3-93 NON-INFECTIOUS PERICARDITIDES

D3-93000 Non-infectious pericarditis, NOS
D3-93100 Pericarditis secondary to acute myocardial infarction
D3-93200 Pericarditis secondary to uremia
D3-93300 Pericarditis secondary to neoplasia, NOS
D3-93310 Pericarditis secondary to primary tumor, NOS
D3-93311 Pericarditis secondary to benign primary tumor
D3-93312 Pericarditis secondary to malignant primary tumor
D3-93320 Pericarditis secondary to tumor metastatic to pericardium
D3-93400 Pericarditis secondary to myxedema
D3-93500 Pericarditis due to deposits of cholesterol
D3-93600 Pericarditis secondary to chylopericardium
D3-93700 Post-traumatic pericarditis
D3-93710 Pericarditis secondary to penetrating trauma
D3-93720 Pericarditis secondary to non-penetrating trauma
D3-93800 Pericarditis secondary to aortic aneurysm
D3-93810 Pericarditis secondary to aortic aneurysm with leakage into pericardial sac
D3-93900 Post-radiation pericarditis
D3-93A00 Pericarditis associated with atrial septal defect
D3-93B00 Pericarditis associated with severe chronic anemia
D3-93C00 Pericarditis associated with infectious mononucleosis
D3-93D00 Pericarditis associated with familial Mediterranean fever
D3-93E00 Familial pericarditis
D3-93E10 Pericarditis secondary to Mulibrey nanism
(D4-00203)

3-94 PERICARDITIDES RELATED TO HYPERSENSITIVITY OR AUTOIMMUNITY

D3-94200 Pericarditis secondary to collagen vascular disease, NOS
D3-94210 Pericarditis secondary to systemic lupus erythematosus

3-94 PERICARDITIDES RELATED TO HYPERSENSITIVITY OR AUTOIMMUNITY — Continued

D3-94220 Pericarditis secondary to rheumatoid arthritis
D3-94230 Pericarditis secondary to scleroderma
D3-94300 Drug-induced pericarditis, NOS
D3-94310 Procainamide-induced pericarditis
D3-94320 Hydralazine-induced pericarditis
D3-94400 Postcardiac injury pericarditis
D3-94420 Postpericardiotomy pericarditis

SECTION 3-A NON-INFECTIOUS DISORDERS OF LYMPHATICS

D3-A0000 Disorder of lymphatics, NOS
D3-A0010 Obliteration of lymphatic vessel, NOS 457.1
D3-A0020 Lymphedema praecox 457.1
D3-A0040 Lymphangitis, NOS 457.2
D3-A0042 Subacute lymphangitis 457.2
D3-A0043 Chronic lymphangitis 457.2
D3-A0050 Nonfilarial chylocele 457.8
D3-A0070 Fistula of thoracic duct 457.8
D3-A0075 Rupture of thoracic duct 457.8
D3-A0103 Chronic acquired lymphedema 457.1
  Secondary lymphedema 457.1
D3-A0110 Postmastectomy lymphedema syndrome 457.0
  Elephantiasis due to mastectomy 457.0
  Obliteration of lymphatic vessel due to mastectomy 457.0
D3-A0120 Nonfilarial elephantiasis, NOS 457.1

CHAPTER 4 — CONGENITAL DISEASES

SECTION 4-0 MULTIPLE SYSTEM MALFORMATIONS AND CHROMOSOMAL DISEASES

D4-00000 Congenital disease, NOS 759.9

4-001 Multiple System Malformation Syndromes: General Terms

D4-00100 Multiple system malformation syndrome, NOS 759.8

4-002 Multiple Malformation Syndromes, Small Stature, without Skeletal Dysplasia

D4-00200 Multiple malformation syndrome, small stature, without skeletal dysplasia, NOS 759.8
D4-00201 Rubinstein-Taybi syndrome
D4-00202 Russell-Silver syndrome
  Silver syndrome
D4-00203 Mulibrey nanism syndrome
  Perheentupa syndrome
D4-00204 Dubowitz's syndrome
D4-00205 Bloom syndrome 757.31
  Congenital telangiectatic erythema syndrome 757.31
D4-00206 DeSanctis-Cacchione syndrome
  Xerodermic idiocy
D4-00207 Johanson-Blizzard syndrome
D4-00208 Seckel syndrome
D4-00209 Hallerman-Streiff syndrome
  Oculomandibulodyscephaly with hypotrichosis syndrome
D4-00211 De Lange syndrome
  Cornelia de Lange syndrome
  Brachmann-de Lange syndrome

4-003 Multiple Malformation Syndromes, Moderate Short Stature, Facial with or without Genital Features

D4-00300 Multiple malformation syndrome, moderate short stature, facial with or without genital features, NOS 759.8
D4-00301 Williams syndrome
D4-00302 Noonan syndrome 759.8
  Turner-like syndrome
  Noonan-Ehmke syndrome
D4-00303 Aarskog syndrome
D4-00304 Robinow syndrome
  Fetal face syndrome
D4-00305 Opitz-Frias syndrome
  Opitz syndrome
  Hypertelorism-hypospadias syndrome
  G syndrome
D4-00306 Smith-Lemli-Opitz syndrome
D4-00310V Dolichocephalic dwarfism
D4-00320V Brachycephalic dwarfism
  Bull-dog calf
  Snorter dwarf

4-004 Multiple Malformation Syndromes with Senile-Like Appearance

D4-00400 Multiple malformation syndrome with senile-like appearance, NOS 759.8
D4-00401 Progeria syndrome 259.8
  Hutchinson-Gilford syndrome 259.8
  Premature senility syndrome 259.8
D4-00402 Cokayne syndrome
D4-00403 Rothmund-Thomson syndrome 757.33 (T-01000)
  Poikiloderma congenitale syndrome 757.33 (T-01000)
D4-00404 Werner syndrome 259.8
  Progeria of the adult 259.8

4-005 Multiple Malformation Syndromes with Early Overgrowth

D4-00500 Multiple malformation syndrome with early overgrowth, NOS 759.8
D4-00501 Weaver syndrome
D4-00502 Marshall-Smith syndrome
D4-00503 Beckwith-Wiedemann syndrome
  Wiedemann-Beckwith syndrome
  Exomphalos-macroglossia-gigantism syndrome
D4-00504 Fragile X syndrome
  Martin-Bell syndrome
  Marker X syndrome
D4-00505 Soto syndrome
  Cerebral gigantism syndrome

4-006 Multiple Malformation Syndromes with Unusual Brain and/or Neuromuscular Findings

D4-00600 Multiple malformation syndrome with unusual brain and/or neuromuscular findings, NOS 759.8
D4-00601 Amyoplasia congenita disruptive sequence
  Classic arthrogryposis
  Arthrogryposis multiplex congenita
  Myodystrophia fetalis deformans
  Multiple congenital articular rigidities
  Congenital arthromyodysplasia
  Myophagism congenita
  Amyoplasia congenita
  Congenital multiple arthrogryposis
D4-00602 Distal arthrogryposis syndrome
D4-00603V Inherited arthrogryposis
D4-00604 Meckel-Gruber syndrome
  Dysencephalia splanchnocystica

4-006 Multiple Malformation Syndromes with Unusual Brain And/Or Neuromuscular Findings — Continued

D4-00605 X-linked hydrocephalus syndrome
D4-00606 Sjogren-Larsson syndrome
D4-00607 Marinesco-Sjogren syndrome
D4-00608 Lethal multiple pterygium syndrome
D4-00609 Neu-Laxova syndrome
D4-00610 Miller-Dieker syndrome
  Lissencephaly syndrome
D4-00611 Pallister-Hall syndrome
D4-00612 Warburg syndrome
  Hard E syndrome
D4-00613 Ataxia-telangiectasia syndrome 334.8
  Louis-Bar syndrome 334.8
D4-00615 Prader-Willi syndrome 759.8
D4-00616 Cohen syndrome
D4-00617 Zellweger syndrome
  Cerebrohepatorenal syndrome
D4-00618 Lowe syndrome 270.8
  Oculocerebrorenal syndrome 270.8
  Lowe-Bickel syndrome 270.8
  Lowe-Terrey-MacLachlan syndrome 270.8
  Renal-oculocerebrodystrophy 270.8
D4-00619 Freeman-Sheldon syndrome
  Whistling face syndrome
D4-00621 Steinert myotonic dystrophy syndrome 359.2
  Steinert syndrome 359.2
  Dystrophia myotonica 359.2
D4-00622 Schwartz syndrome
D4-00623 Hecht syndrome
  Trismus pseudocamptodactyly syndrome
D4-00624 Angelman syndrome
  Happy puppet syndrome
D4-00626 Schwartz-Jampel syndrome
  Myotonia chondrodystrophica
D4-00627 Schinzel-Giedon syndrome
D4-00628 Pena-Shokeir phenotype
  Fetal akinesia-hypokinesia sequence
D4-00629 Cerebro-oculo-facio-skeletal syndrome
  COFS syndrome
D4-00640V Crooked calf syndrome

4-007 Multiple Malformation Syndromes with Facial Defects as Major Feature

D4-00700 Multiple malformation syndrome with facial defects as major feature, NOS 759.8
D4-00703 Cleft lip sequence
D4-00704 Van der Woude syndrome
  Lip-pit-cleft lip syndrome
D4-00705 Frontonasal dysplasia sequence
  Median cleft face syndrome
D4-00706 Fraser syndrome
  Cryptophthalmos syndrome
  Cryptophthalmos, defect of auricle and genital anomaly
D4-00707 Melnick-Fraser syndrome
  Branchio-oto-renal syndrome
  BOR syndrome
D4-00708 Waardenburg syndrome, types I and II
D4-00711 Marshall syndrome
D4-00713 Asymmetric crying face association
  Cardiofacial syndrome
D4-00714 Blepharophimosis syndrome
  Familial blepharophimosis syndrome
D4-00715 Grob's syndrome
  Dysplasia linguofacialis syndrome
D4-00716 Wildervanck's syndrome
  Cervico-oculofacial syndrome
D4-00720 First arch syndrome, NOS
D4-00721 Robin sequence
  Micrognathia-glossoptosis syndrome
  Pierre Robin syndrome
D4-00722 Treacher Collins syndrome
  Mandibulofacial dysostosis
D4-00723 Franceschetti-Klein syndrome
D4-00725V Otocephalic syndrome

4-008 Multiple Malformation Syndromes with Facial-Limb Defects as Major Feature

D4-00800 Multiple malformation syndrome with facial-limb defects as major feature, NOS 759.8
D4-00801 Nager syndrome
  Nager acrofacial dysostosis syndrome
D4-00802 Townes syndrome
D4-00803 Oral-facial-digital syndrome
  OFD syndrome type I
D4-00804 Mohr syndrome
  OFD syndrome type II
D4-00805 Shprintzen syndrome
  Velo-cardio-facial syndrome
D4-00806 Ruvalcaba syndrome
D4-00807 Mietens syndrome
D4-00808 Oculodentodigital syndrome
  Oculodentodigital dysplasia
D4-00809 Oto-palato-digital syndrome, type I
  Taybi syndrome
D4-00811 Coffin-Lowry syndrome
D4-00812 Stickler syndrome
  Hereditary arthro-ophthalmopathy
D4-00813 Oto-palato-digital syndrome, type II
D4-00814 FG syndrome
D4-00815 Larsen syndrome
D4-00816 Langer-Giedion syndrome
  Trichorhinophalangeal syndrome with exostosis
D4-00817 Trichorhinophalangeal syndrome
D4-00818 Ectrodactyly-ectodermal dysplasia-clefting syndrome
  EEC syndrome
D4-00819 Hay-Wells syndrome of ectodermal dysplasia
  Ankyloblepharon-ectodermal dysplasia-clefting syndrome
  AEC syndrome

D4-00821 Roberts-SC phocomelia syndrome
Pseudothalidomide syndrome
Hypomelia-hypotrichosis-facial hemangioma syndrome
D4-00822 Miller syndrome
Postaxial acrofacial dysostosis syndrome

4-009 Multiple Malformation Syndromes with Limb Defects as Major Feature

D4-00900 Multiple malformation syndrome with limb defect as major feature, NOS 759.8
D4-00901 Popliteal pterygium syndrome
Facio-genito-popliteal syndrome
D4-00902 Grebe syndrome
D4-00903 Escobar syndrome
Multiple pterygium syndrome
D4-00904 Limb reduction-ichthyosis syndrome
D4-00905 Femoral hypoplasia — unusual facies syndrome
D4-00906 Holt-Oram syndrome
Cardiac-limb syndrome
Atrio-digital syndrome
D4-00907 Fanconi pancytopenia syndrome 284.0
Fanconi's anemia 284.0
Pancytopenia-dysmelia syndrome 284.0
D4-00908 Radial aplasia-thrombocytopenia syndrome
Thrombocytopenia-absent radii syndrome
TAR syndrome
D4-00909 Aase syndrome
D4-00911 Polysyndactyly syndrome
D4-00912 Child syndrome
D4-00913 Adams-Oliver syndrome
D4-00914 Levy-Hollister syndrome
Lacrimo-auriculo-dento-digital syndrome
D4-00915 Poland anomaly
Poland anomalad
Unilateral defect of pectoralis muscle and syndactyly of hand
D4-00920 Nievergelt's syndrome
Nievergelt-Erb syndrome

4-00A Osteochondrodysplasia Syndromes

D4-00A10 Achondrogenesis, NOS
(T-11000) (M-21300)
D4-00A11 Achondrogenesis, type IA
D4-00A12 Achondrogenesis, type IB
D4-00A13 Achondrogenesis, type II
Langer-Saldino achondrogenesis
Hypochondrogenesis
Hypochondroplasia
D4-00A14 Jeune thoracic dystrophy
Asphyxiating thoracic dystrophy
D4-00A15 Camptomelic dysplasia
D4-00A16 Achondroplasia 756.4
Chondrodystrophia fetalis 756.4
D4-00A18 Pseudoachondroplastic spondyloepiphyseal dysplasia syndrome
SED syndrome
D4-00A19 Acromesomelic dysplasia syndrome
Acromesomelic dwarfism
D4-00A21 Spondyloepiphyseal dysplasia congenita
D4-00A22 Kniest dysplasia
D4-00A23 Kozlowski spondylometaphyseal dysplasia
D4-00A24 Metatrophic dysplasia
Metatrophic dwarfism syndrome
D4-00A25 Chondroectodermal dysplasia 756.55
Ellis-van Creveld syndrome 756.55
D4-00A26 Diastrophic dysplasia
Diastrophic nanism syndrome
D4-00A27 Thanatophoric dysplasia
Thanatophoric dwarfism syndrome
D4-00A30 Fibrochondrogenesis
D4-00A31 Atelosteogenesis
Giant cell chondrodysplasia
D4-00A32 Short rib-polydactyly syndrome, Majewski type
Short-rib syndrome, type II
D4-00A33 Short rib-polydactyly syndrome, non-Majewski type
Short-rib syndrome, type I
D4-00A34 Dyggve-Melchior-Clausen syndrome
D4-00A35 Geleophysic dysplasia
Geleophysic dwarfism syndrome
D4-00A40 Spondyloepiphyseal dysplasia tarda
X-linked spondyloepiphyseal dysplasia
D4-00A41 Multiple epiphyseal dysplasia 756.56
D4-00A42 Metaphyseal chondrodysplasia, Schmid type
Metaphyseal dysplasia, Schmid type
D4-00A43 Metaphyseal chondrodysplasia, McKusick type
Cartilage-hair hypoplasia syndrome
D4-00A51 Kenny syndrome
D4-00A53 Hajdu-Cheney syndrome
Arthro-dento-osteo dysplasia
Acroosteolysis syndrome
Familial acroosteolysis syndrome
Cheney syndrome
D4-00A54 Craniometaphyseal dysplasia
D4-00A55 Frontometaphyseal dysplasia
D4-00A56 Pyle metaphyseal dysplasia
Pyle disease
D4-00A57 Metaphyseal chondrodysplasia, Jansen type
Metaphyseal dysostosis, Jansen type
D4-00A58 Shwachman syndrome
Metaphyseal chondrodysplasia with pancreatic insufficiency and neutropenia
Shwachman-Diamond syndrome
D4-00A60 Chondrodysplasia punctata, NOS
D4-00A60V Epiphyseal dysplasia
Chondrodysplasia calcificans congenita
Chondrodysplasia punctata congenita
Chondrodysplasia calcificans
Stippled epiphyses
D4-00A61 Chondrodysplasia punctata, Conradi-Hünermann type
Conradi-Hünermann syndrome

4-00A Osteochondrodysplasia Syndromes — Continued

D4-00A61 (cont.) Conradi's syndrome

D4-00A62 Rhizomelic chondrodysplasia punctata syndrome
  Chondrodysplasia punctata, rhizomelic type

D4-00A65 Hyperphosphatasia-osteoectasia syndrome

D4-00A68 Lymphopenic agammaglobulinemia — short-limbed dwarfism syndrome

4-00B Osteochondrodysplasias with Osteopetrosis

D4-00B00 Osteochrondrodysplasia with osteopetrosis, NOS

D4-00B01 Infantile malignant osteopetrosis 756.52
  Albers-Schoenberg syndrome 756.52
  Severe osteopetrosis 756.52
  Marble bone disease 756.52
  Autosomal recessive lethal osteopetrosis 756.52
  Congenital osteopetrosis 756.52

D4-00B03 Sclerosteosis

D4-00B04 Pyknodysostosis
  Maroteaux-Lamy pyknodysostosis syndrome
  Maroteaux-Lamy syndrome II
  Stanesco's dysostosis syndrome

D4-00B05 Cleidocranial dysostosis 755.59
    (T-11100) (M-21300) (T-12310) (M-21000)
  Cleidocranial dysplasia 755.59
    (T-11100) (M-21300) (T-12310) (M-21000)

D4-00B09 Lenz-Majewski hyperostosis syndrome

4-00C Craniosynostosis Syndromes

D4-00C00 Craniosynostosis syndrome 756.0
    (T-15082) (M-20130)
  Craniostosis 756.0
    (T-15082) (M-20130)
  Craniosynostosis 756.0
    (T-15082) (M-20130)
  Premature closure of cranial sutures 756.0
    (T-15082) (M-20130)
  Congenital ossification of cranial sutures 756.0
    (T-15082) (M-20130)
  Congenital ossification of sutures of skull
    (T-11100) (T-15082) (M-20130)

D4-00C01 Saethre-Chotzen syndrome

D4-00C02 Pfeiffer syndrome
  Pfeiffer-type acrocephalosyndactyly

D4-00C04 Apert's syndrome 755.55
    (T-D1100) (M-20630) (T-D2810) (M-20100)
  Acroencephalosyndactyly 755.55
    (T-D1100) (M-20630) (T-D2810) (M-20100)
  Acrocephalosyndactyly 755.55
    (T-D1100) (M-20630) (T-D2810) (M-20100)

D4-00C05 Crouzon syndrome 756.0
    (T-11100) (T-D1200) (M-20080)
  Craniofacial dysostosis 756.0
    (T-11100) (T-D1200) (M-20080)
  Crouzon's disease 756.0
    (T-11100) (T-D1200) (M-20080)

4-00D Other Skeletal Dysplasias

D4-00D01 Multiple synostosis syndrome
  Symphalangism syndrome

D4-00D02 Multiple exostoses syndrome
  Diaphyseal aclasis, external chondromatosis syndrome

D4-00D03 Greig cephalopolysyndactyly syndrome

D4-00D04 Antley-Bixter syndrome
  Multisynostotic osteodysgenesis
  Trapezoidcephaly-multiple synostosis

D4-00D05 Baller-Gerold syndrome
  Craniosynostosis-radial aplasia syndrome

D4-00D06 Nail-patella syndrome
  Hereditary osteo-onychodysplasia

D4-00D07 Leri-Weill dyschondrosteosis

D4-00D08 Langer mesomelic dysplasia syndrome
  Homozygous Leri-Weill dyschondrosteosis syndrome

D4-00D09 Leri's pleonosteosis syndrome

D4-00D12 Brachydactyly syndrome type E

D4-00D13 Weill-Marchesani syndrome
  Brachydactyly-spherophakia syndrome

D4-00D14 Beals auriculo-osteodysplasia syndrome

D4-00D15 Acrodysostosis

D4-00D16 Melorheostosis
  Rheostosis
  Leri's disease
  Candle wax disease
  Flowing hyperostosis
  Osteopathia hyperostotica congenita

4-010 Hamartomatous Diseases

D4-01000 Hamartosis, NOS
  Hamartomatosis, NOS

D4-01005 Cowden syndrome
  Multiple hamartoma syndrome

D4-01010 Sturge-Weber sequence 759.6
  Encephalotrigeminal angiomatosis 759.6

D4-01011 Neurocutaneous melanosis sequence

D4-01012 Linear sebaceous nevus sequence
  Nevus sebaceous of Jadassohn

D4-01013 Incontinentia pigmenti syndrome
  Bloch-Sulzberger syndrome
  Incontinentia pigmenti achromians syndrome
  Ito's syndrome

D4-01015 Tuberous sclerosis syndrome 759.5
  Bourneville's disease 759.5

D4-01015 (cont.) Adenoma sebaceum syndrome 759.5
Epiloia 759.5
D4-01018 Neurofibromatosis syndrome
D4-01020 Polyostotic fibrous dysplasia of bone, NOS 756.54
(T-11000)
D4-01021 McCune-Albright syndrome 756.59
Albright syndrome 756.59
D4-01024 Von Hippel-Lindau syndrome 759.6
Familial cerebello-retinal angiomatosis 759.6
D4-01025 Klippel-Trenaunay-Weber syndrome
Cerebrofacial angiomatosis
D4-01028 Proteus syndrome
D4-01031 Maffucci syndrome
Chondroplasia angiomatosis
Maffucci's anomalad
D4-01033 Osteochondromatosis syndrome 756.4
Ollier disease 756.4
Enchondromatosis 756.4
Dyschondroplasia 756.4
Hereditary deforming chondrodysplasia 756.4
Congenital enchondromatosis 756.4
Diaphyseal aclasis 756.4
D4-01034 Juvenile polyposis syndrome
D4-01035 Peutz-Jeghers syndrome 759.6
Periorificial lentiginosis syndrome 759.6
D4-01037 Ruvalcaba-Myhre syndrome
D4-01039 Gardner syndrome
D4-01041 Osler hemorrhagic telangiectasia syndrome 448.0
Osler-Weber-Rendu disease 448.0
Hereditary hemorrhagic telangiectasia 448.0
Osler's disease 448.0
D4-01042 Turcot syndrome
D4-01046 Gorlin syndrome
Nevoid basal cell carcinoma syndrome
Basal cell carcinoma syndrome
Gorlin-Goltz syndrome
Basal cell nevus syndrome
D4-01047 Centrofacial lentiginosis syndrome
D4-01048 Multiple lentigines syndrome
LEOPARD syndrome
D4-01049 Moynahan's syndrome
Progressive cardiomyopathic lentiginosis
D4-01052 B-K mole (nevus) syndrome
D4-01054 Goltz syndrome
Focal dermal hypoplasia syndrome
Goltz-Gorlin syndrome

4-011 Ectodermal Dysplasias

D4-01100 Ectodermal dysplasia, NOS 757.31
D4-01101 Hypohidrotic ectodermal dysplasia syndrome, NOS 757.31
Anhidrotic ectodermal dysplasia syndrome 757.31
Christ-Siemens-Touraine syndrome 757.31
D4-01102 Autosomal recessive hypohidrotic ectodermal dysplasia syndrome 757.31
D4-01103 Autosomal dominant hypohidrotic ectodermal dysplasia syndrome 757.31
Rapp-Hodgkin ectodermal dysplasia syndrome 757.31
D4-01104 Hidrotic ectodermal dysplasia syndrome 757.31
Clouston syndrome
D4-01111 Tricho-dento-osseous syndrome
TDO syndrome
D4-01113 Pachyonychia congenita syndrome 757.5
(T-01600) (M-20520)
Jadassohn-Lewandowsky syndrome 757.5
(T-01600) (M-20520)
Congenital pachyonychia 757.5
(T-01600) (M-20520)
Pachyonychia congenita 757.5
(T-01600) (M-20520)
D4-01121 Pachydermoperiostosis syndrome
D4-01133 XTE syndrome
Xeroderma, talipes and enamel defect
D4-01135 Senter syndrome

4-012 Miscellaneous Multiple Malformation Syndromes

D4-01201 Coffin-Siris syndrome
D4-01202 Borjeson-Forssman-Lehmann syndrome
D4-01203 Arteriohepatic dysplasia
Alagille syndrome
Watson-Alagille syndrome
D4-01204 Melnick-Needles syndrome
D4-01205 Bardet-Biedl syndrome 759.8
Laurence-Moon-Biedl syndrome 759.8
D4-01211 Rieger eye malformation sequence 743.44
(T-AA500) (T-AA270) (M-20000)
Mesodermal dysgenesis of iris 743.44
(T-AA500) (T-AA270) (M-20000)
Goniodysgenesis 743.44
(T-AA500) (T-AA270) (M-20000)
Peter's anomaly 743.44
(T-AA500) (T-AA270) (M-20000)
Rieger's anomaly 743.44
(T-AA500) (T-AA270) (M-20000)
D4-01212 Rieger syndrome
D4-01213 Cerebro-costo-mandibular syndrome
D4-01221 Jarcho-Levin syndrome
Spondylothoracic dysplasia
D4-01224 Leprechaunism syndrome
Donohue syndrome
D4-01225 Berardinelli lipodystrophy syndrome
Lipodystrophy with muscular hypertrophy
Berardinelli's syndrome
Generalized lipodystrophy
D4-01231 Distichiasis-lymphedema syndrome
D4-01237 Hanhart's syndrome
Micrognathia with peromelia

4-012 Miscellaneous Multiple Malformation Syndromes — Continued

D4-01238 VACTEL syndrome
D4-01240 Duhamel's syndrome
  Tondury-Duhamel anomalad
D4-01242 Moore-Federman syndrome
  Familial dwarfism and stiff joints
D4-01245 Kundrat's syndrome
  Pseudotrisomy D_1 syndrome

4-013 Spectra of Defects

D4-01301 Facio-auriculo-vertebral spectrum
  First and second branchial arch syndrome
  Oculoauricular vertebral dysplasia
  Goldenhar syndrome
  Hemifacial microsomia
D4-01305 Oromandibular-limb hypogenesis spectrum
  Hypoglossia-hypodactyly syndrome
  Aglossia-adactyly syndrome
  Glossopalatine ankylosis syndrome
  Moebius syndrome
  Charlie M. syndrome
  Facial-limb disruptive spectrum
  Moebius sequence

4-014 Miscellaneous Associations

D4-01401 VATER association
  VATER anomalad
  VATER syndrome
D4-01402 MVRCS association
D4-01403 CHARGE association

4-015 Miscellaneous Sequences

D4-01510 Laterality sequence, NOS
D4-01511 Bilateral left-sidedness sequence
  Polysplenia syndrome
D4-01512 Bilateral right-sidedness sequence 759.0
    (T-C3000) (M-21000)
  Asplenia syndrome 759.0
    (T-C3000) (M-21000)
  Splenic agenesis syndrome 759.0
    (T-C3000) (M-21000)
  Ivemark syndrome 759.0
    (T-C3000) (M-21000)
  Congenital absence of spleen 759.0
    (T-C3000) (M-21000)
D4-01515 Immotile cilia syndrome 759.3
D4-01516 Kartagener syndrome 759.3
  Bronchiectasis, chronic sinusitis and dextrocardia syndrome 759.3
D4-01517 Primary ciliary dyskinesia 759.3
D4-01520 Holoprosencephaly sequence 742.2
    (T-A0101) (M-20100)
  Holoprosencephaly 742.2
    (T-A0101) (M-20100)
D4-01521 Familial alobar holoprosencephaly
    (T-A0101) (M-20100)
D4-01522 Occult spinal dysraphism sequence
  Tethered cord malformation sequence
D4-01523 Septo-optic dysplasia sequence
D4-01531 Athyrotic hypothyroidism sequence
  Hypothyroidism sequence
D4-01532 DiGeorge sequence 279.11
  Thymic hypoplasia syndrome 279.11
  Pharyngeal pouch syndrome 279.11
  Agenesis of the parathyroid and thymus glands 279.11
  Thymic-parathyroid aplasia 279.11
  DiGeorge syndrome 279.11
  Third and fourth pharyngeal arch syndrome 279.11
  Third and fourth pharyngeal pouch syndrome 279.11
D4-01537 Klippel-Feil sequence 756.16
    (T-D1600) (M-20602) (T-11600) (M-21000)
  Klippel-Feil syndrome 756.16
    (T-D1600) (M-20602) (T-11600) (M-21000)
  Klippel-Feil deformity 756.16
    (T-D1600) (M-20602) (T-11600) (M-21000)
  Cervical vertebral fusion syndrome 756.16
    (T-D1600) (M-20602) (T-11600) (M-21000)
  Cervical vertebral fusion 756.16
    (T-D1160) (M-20602) (T-11600) (M-21000)
D4-01538 Jugular lymphatic obstruction sequence
    (T-C6200) (M-20200)
D4-01541 Early urethral obstruction sequence
    (T-75000) (M-20200)
D4-01542 Exstrophy of bladder sequence 753.5
    (T-D4310) (T-74061) (M-21000) (T-74062) (M-21700)
  Exstrophy of urinary bladder 753.5
    (T-D4310) (T-74601) (M-21000) (T-74062) (M-21700)
  Ectopia vesicae 753.5
    (T-D4310) (T-74061) (M-21000) (T-74062) (M-21700)
  Congenital extroversion of urinary bladder 753.5
    (T-D4310) (T-74061) (M-21000) (T-74062) (M-21700)
D4-01543 Exstrophy of cloaca sequence
D4-01549 Rokitansky sequence
D4-01551 Oligohydramnios sequence 753.0
    (T-71800) (M-21000)
  Potter syndrome 753.0
    (T-71800) (M-21000)
  Renofacial syndrome 753.0
    (T-71800) (M-21000)
  Renal agenesis syndrome 753.0
    (T-71800) (M-21000)
  Renal agenesis 753.0
    (T-71800) (M-21000)

D4-01551 (cont.) Congenital absence of kidneys 753.0
(T-71800) (M-21000)
D4-01552 Alleman's syndrome 753.0
D4-01561 Sirenomelia sequence
Sirenomelus sequence
D4-01564 Caudal dysplasia sequence
Caudal regression syndrome
D4-01565 Early amnion rupture sequence
D4-01566 Amniotic band syndrome
Amniotic band anomalad

4-018 Multiple Malformation Syndromes Due to Non-Infectious Environmental Agents

D4-01800 Multiple malformation syndrome due to non-infectious environmental agents, NOS
D4-01801 Fetal aminopterin syndrome
(C-23820)
D4-01803 Fetal hydantoin syndrome
(C-61600)
D4-01804 Fetal trimethadione syndrome
(C-61820)
D4-01805 Fetal warfarin syndrome
(C-A6530)
D4-01806 Thalidomide embryopathy syndrome
(C-64085)
Wiedemann's syndrome
(C-64085)
Lenz's syndrome
(C-64085)
D4-01807 Fetal methyl mercury syndrome
(C-13314)
D4-01811 Hyperthermia-induced defect, NOS
D4-01821 Maternal PKV fetal effect, NOS
D4-01822 Fetal valproate syndrome
(C-61130)
D4-01824 Retinoic acid embryopathy
(C-92010)
Accutane embryopathy
(C-92010)
D4-01830 Cretinism, NOS 243.-
(C-11400) (M-27000)
Fetal iodine deficiency syndrome 243.-
(C-11400) (M-27000)
Infantile hypothyroidism 243.-
(C-11400) (M-27000)
Hypothyroid dwarfism 243.-
D4-01832 Neurologic form of cretinism 243.-
D4-01834 Myxedematous form of cretinism 243.-
Congenital myxedema 243.-
(C-11400) (M-27000)
D4-01836 Endemic cretinism 243.-
(C-11400) (M-27000)
D4-01838 Sporadic cretinism 246.1

4-02 CHROMOSOMAL DISEASES

D4-02000 Chromosomal disease, NOS 758.9
Chromosomal imbalance syndrome, NOS 758.9
Anomaly of chromosome, NOS 758.9
Chromosomopathy, NOS 758.9
Chromosomal abnormality syndrome, NOS 758.9
D4-02010 Anomaly of chromosome pair 1, NOS
D4-02011 1p partial monosomy syndrome
D4-02013 1q partial monosomy syndrome
D4-02016 1q partial trisomy syndrome
D4-02018 Ring chromosome 1 syndrome
D4-02020 Anomaly of chromosome pair 2, NOS
D4-02025 2p partial trisomy syndrome
D4-02026 2q partial trisomy syndrome
D4-02030 Anomaly of chromosome pair 3, NOS
D4-02035 3p partial trisomy syndrome
D4-02036 3q partial trisomy syndrome
D4-02040 Anomaly of chromosome pair 4, NOS
D4-02042 4p partial monosomy syndrome
Chromosome 4 short arm deletion syndrome
4p minus syndrome
Midline fusion defect syndrome
Wolff-Hirschhorn syndrome
D4-02043 4q partial monosomy syndrome
D4-02045 4p partial trisomy syndrome
Trisomy 4p syndrome
Trisomy for short arm of chromosome 4
D4-02046 4q partial trisomy syndrome
D4-02048 Ring chromosome 4 syndrome
D4-02050 Anomaly of chromosome pair 5, NOS
D4-02052 5p partial monosomy syndrome 758.3
Cri du chat syndrome 758.3
Lejeune syndrome 758.3
5p minus syndrome 758.3
Partial deletion of short arm of chromosome 5 syndrome 758.3
D4-02055 5p partial trisomy syndrome
D4-02060 Anomaly of chromosome pair 6, NOS
D4-02065 6p partial trisomy syndrome
D4-02066 6q partial trisomy syndrome
D4-02070 Anomaly of chromosome pair 7, NOS
D4-02072 7p partial monosomy syndrome
D4-02073 7q partial monosomy syndrome
D4-02075 7p partial trisomy syndrome
D4-02076 7q partial trisomy syndrome
D4-02080 Anomaly of chromosome pair 8, NOS
D4-02082 8p partial monosomy syndrome
D4-02083 8q partial monosomy syndrome
D4-02084 Complete trisomy 8 syndrome
Warkany syndrome
Trisomy 8 normal mosaicism
D4-02085 8p partial trisomy syndrome
D4-02086 8q partial trisomy syndrome
D4-02090 Anomaly of chromosome pair 9, NOS
D4-02092 9p partial monosomy syndrome
9p minus syndrome
9p monosomy syndrome
D4-02093 9q partial monosomy syndrome
D4-02094 Complete trisomy 9 syndrome
Trisomy 9 mosaic syndrome

4-02 CHROMOSOMAL DISEASES — Continued

D4-02095 9p partial trisomy syndrome
  Réthoré syndrome
  Trisomy 9p syndrome
D4-02096 9q partial trisomy syndrome
D4-02098 Ring chromosome 9 syndrome
D4-02099 Partial tetrasomy 9 syndrome
D4-02100 Anomaly of chromosome pair 10, NOS
D4-02102 10p partial monosomy syndrome
D4-02103 10q partial monosomy syndrome
D4-02104 Complete trisomy 10 syndrome
D4-02105 10p partial trisomy syndrome
D4-02106 10q partial trisomy syndrome
D4-02108 Ring chromosome 10 syndrome
D4-02110 Anomaly of chromosome pair 11, NOS
D4-02112 11p partial monosomy syndrome
  Aniridia-Wilms tumor association
D4-02113 11q partial monosomy syndrome
D4-02115 11p partial trisomy syndrome
D4-02116 11q partial trisomy syndrome
D4-02118 Ring chromosome 11 syndrome
D4-02120 Anomaly of chromosome pair 12, NOS
D4-02122 12p partial monosomy syndrome
D4-02125 12p partial trisomy syndrome
D4-02126 12q partial trisomy syndrome
D4-02129 Tetrasomy 12p
  Killian-Teschler-Nicola syndrome
  Pallister mosaic syndrome
D4-02130 Anomaly of chromosome pair 13, NOS
D4-02133 13q partial monosomy syndrome
  Orbeli syndrome
  13q minus syndrome
D4-02134 Complete trisomy 13 syndrome 758.1
  Patau syndrome 758.1
  D_1 trisomy syndrome 758.1
D4-02135 13p partial trisomy syndrome
D4-02136 13q partial trisomy syndrome
D4-02140 Anomaly of chromosome pair 14, NOS
D4-02144 Complete trisomy 14 syndrome
D4-02146 14q partial trisomy syndrome
D4-02147 14q partial proximal trisomy syndrome
D4-02148 14q partial distal trisomy syndrome
D4-02150 Anomaly of chromosome pair 15, NOS
D4-02153 15q partial monosomy syndrome
D4-02154 15q partial trisomy syndrome
D4-02160 Anomaly of chromosome pair 16, NOS
D4-02163 16q partial monosomy syndrome
D4-02164 Complete trisomy 16 syndrome
D4-02165 16p partial trisomy syndrome
D4-02166 16q partial trisomy syndrome
D4-02170 Anomaly of chromosome pair 17, NOS
D4-02175 17p partial trisomy syndrome
D4-02176 17q partial trisomy syndrome
D4-02180 Anomaly of chromosome pair 18, NOS
D4-02182 18p partial monosomy syndrome
  18p minus syndrome
D4-02183 18q partial monosomy syndrome
  18q minus syndrome
  Long arm 18 deletion syndrome
D4-02184 Complete trisomy 18 syndrome 758.2
  Edwards syndrome 758.2
D4-02185 18p partial trisomy syndrome
  Grouchy-Lamy-Thieffry syndrome
D4-02186 18q partial trisomy syndrome
  Grouchy-Lamy-Salmon-Landry syndrome
D4-02188 Ring chromosome 18 syndrome
D4-02190 Anomaly of chromosome pair 19, NOS
D4-02196 19q partial trisomy syndrome
D4-02200 Anomaly of chromosome pair 20, NOS
D4-02204 Complete trisomy 20 syndrome
D4-02205 20p partial trisomy syndrome
  Trisomy 20p syndrome
D4-02206 20q partial trisomy syndrome
D4-02208 Ring chromosome 20 syndrome
D4-02210 Anomaly of chromosome pair 21, NOS
D4-02211 Complete monosomy 21 syndrome
D4-02213 21q partial monosomy syndrome
  21q partial proximal monosomy syndrome
D4-02214 Complete trisomy 21 syndrome 758.0
  Down syndrome 758.0
  Mongolism 758.0
D4-02216 21q partial trisomy syndrome
  21q partial distal trisomy syndrome
D4-02218 Ring chromosome 21 syndrome
D4-02220 Anomaly of chromosome pair 22, NOS
D4-02223 22q partial monosomy syndrome
D4-02224 Complete trisomy 22 syndrome 758.3
  Antimongolism syndrome 758.3
D4-02226 22q partial trisomy syndrome
D4-02228 Ring chromosome 22 syndrome
D4-0222A Cat eye syndrome
  Schachenmann's syndrome
D4-02250 Anomaly of chromosome Y, NOS
D4-02252 Klinefelter syndrome 758.7
  XXY syndrome 758.7
D4-02256 Double Y syndrome
  XYY syndrome
D4-02270 Anomaly of chromosome X, NOS
D4-02272 Turner syndrome, NOS 758.6
  Pterygolymphangiectasia syndrome 758.6
  Bonnevie-Ullrich syndrome 758.6
  XO syndrome 758.6
  Gonadal dysgenesis syndrome 758.6
  45, X syndrome 758.6
D4-02274 Trisomy X syndrome 758.8
  XXX syndrome 758.8
D4-02275 Four X syndrome 758.8
  XXXX syndrome 758.8
D4-02276 Penta X syndrome 758.8
  XXXXX syndrome 758.8
  Five X syndrome 758.8
D4-02277 XXXY syndrome 758.8
D4-02278 XXXXY syndrome 758.8
D4-02320 Mixed gonadal dysgenesis 758.8
  45, X/46, XY mosaicism 758.8
D4-02330 Sex phenotype-karyotype dissociation syndrome 758.8

D4-02331 XX males 758.8
D4-02332 XY females 758.8
D4-02350 Polyploidy syndrome, NOS
D4-02351 Triploidy syndrome
D4-02355 Triploidy, diploidy, mixoploidy syndrome

SECTION 4-1 CONGENITAL ANOMALIES OF THE MUSCULOSKELETAL SYSTEM

4-10 CONGENITAL ANOMALIES OF THE MUSCULOSKELETAL SYSTEM: GENERAL TERMS

D4-10000 Congenital anomaly of musculoskeletal system, NOS 756.9
(T-10000) (M-20000)
Congenital deformity of musculoskeletal system, NOS 756.9
(T-10000) (M-20000)
D4-10100 Congenital anomaly of skeletal bone, NOS
(T-11000) (M-20000)
Congenital skeletal anomaly, NOS
(T-11000) (M-20000)
D4-10101 Ectopic bone tissue
(T-11000) (M-26000)
D4-10102 Accessory ossification center
(T-F6B72) (M-22300)
D4-10104 Bone island
(T-11022) (M-26000) (T-11032)
D4-10106 Osteopoikilosis
(T-11016) (T-11035) (M-20000) (M-78020)
D4-10110 Acephalocheiria
(T-D1100) (T-D8780) (M-21000)
Absence of head and hands
(T-D1100) (T-D8780) (M-21000)
D4-10112 Acephalorachia
(T-D1100) (T-11500) (M-21000)
Absence of head and spinal column
(T-D1100) (T-11500) (M-21000)
D4-10500 Congenital anomaly of skeletal muscle, NOS
(T-13000) (M-20000)
D4-10510 Congenital absence of skeletal muscle, NOS
(T-13000) (M-21000)
D4-10511 Accessory skeletal muscle, NOS 756.82
(T-13000) (M-22300)
D4-10520 Amyotrophia congenita 756.89
(T-13000) (M-21300)
D4-10700 Congenital anomaly of muscle and tendon, NOS
(T-13000) (T-17010) (M-20000)
D4-10710 Congenital absence of muscle and tendon, NOS 756.81
(T-13000) (T-17010) (M-21000)
D4-10711 Congenital shortening of tendon 756.89
(T-17010) (M-20601)
D4-10720V Congenital articular rigidity with myopathy
D4-10730V Congenital hyperplasia of muscle
Double muscles in cattle
Myofibrillar hyperplasia
Doppellendigkeit
Congenital muscular hypertrophy
D4-10740V Splayleg in piglets
Myofibrillar hypoplasia

4-11 CONGENITAL ANOMALIES OF THE HEAD AND NECK

D4-11000 Congenital anomaly of head and neck, NOS
(T-D1100) (T-D1600) (M-20000)
D4-11100 Congenital anomaly of skull, NOS 756.0
(T-11100) (M-20000)
D4-11102 Congenital depression in skull 754.0
(T-11100) (M-22080)
D4-11104 Dolichocephaly 754.0
(T-D1100) (M-20604)
D4-11106 Plagiocephaly 754.0
(T-D1100) (M-20650)
D4-11108 Overriding skull bones
(T-11100) (M-22160)
D4-11112 Frontal bossing
(T-11110) (M-20500)
D4-11114 Congenital hypertrophy of sphenoid bone
(T-11150) (M-20500)
D4-11200 Congenital absence of skull bones 756.0
(T-11100) (T-11000) (M-21000)
D4-11202 Acrocephaly 756.0
(T-11100) (T-15120) (T-15130) (M-20130) (M-20604)
Oxycephaly 756.0
(T-11100) (T-15120) (T-15130) (M-20130) (M-20604)
Tower skull 756.0
(T-11100) (T-15120) (T-15130) (M-20130) (M-20604)
D4-11204 Congenital deformity of forehead 756.0
(T-D1100) (M-20000)
D4-11206 Scaphocephaly
(T-11100) (T-15110) (M-20130) (M-20604)
D4-11208 Trigonocephaly 756.0
(T-15170) (M-20000)
D4-11210 Imperfect fusion of skull 756.0
(T-15082) (M-21500)
D4-11212 Platybasia 756.0
(T-11140) (T-11610) (M-21500)
Basilar impression 756.0
(T-11140) (T-11610) (M-21500)
D4-11214 Craniolacunia
(T-11100) (M-20000) (F-12100)
Lacunar skull
(T-11100) (M-20000) (F-12100)
D4-11216 Craniofenestria
(T-11100) (M-20000) (F-12100)
D4-11218 Lückenschadel
(T-11100) (M-20000) (F-12100)
D4-11220 Ocular hypertelorism 756.0
(T-AA000) (T-D1480) (M-20000)
Orbital hypertelorism 376.41
(T-AA000) (T-D1480) (M-20000)

4-11 CONGENITAL ANOMALIES OF THE HEAD AND NECK — Continued

D4-11222 Ocular hypotelorism 756.0
(T-AA000) (T-D1480) (M-20000)

D4-11230 Cranioschisis
(T-11100) (M-21500)
Cranium bifidum
(T-11100) (M-21500)

D4-11232 Diastematocrania
(T-11100) (M-21500)

D4-11300 Congenital anomaly of face bones, NOS 756.0
(T-D1200) (T-11000) (M-20000)

D4-11500 Congenital anomaly of sternocleidomastoid muscle, NOS 754.1
(T-13310) (M-20000)

D4-11502 Congenital sternomastoid torticollis 754.1
(T-13310) (M-20140)
Congenital wryneck 754.1
(T-13310) (M-20140)
Contracture of sternocleidomastoid muscle 754.1
(T-13310) (M-20140)

4-12 CONGENITAL ANOMALIES OF THE LIMBS

D4-12000 Congenital anomaly of limb, NOS 755.9
(T-D2800) (M-20000)
Congenital deformity of limb, NOS 755.9
(T-D2800) (M-20000)

D4-12010 Polymelia
(T-D2800) (M-22300)

D4-12100 Longitudinal deficiency of limb, NOS 755.4
(T-D2800) (M-20602)
Reduction deformity of limb, NOS 755.4
(T-D2800) (M-20602)

D4-12102 Amelia, NOS 755.4
(T-D2800) (M-21000)
Congenital absence of limb, NOS 755.4
(T-D2800) (M-21000)
Phocomelia, NOS 755.4
(T-D2800) (M-21000)

D4-12104 Ectromelia, NOS 755.4
(T-D2800) (T-11016) (M-20602)
(M-21070)

D4-12105 Hemimelia, NOS 755.4
(T-D2800) (M-21070) (M-20602)

D4-12108 Micromelia, NOS
(T-D2800) (M-20601) (M-20610)
Micromelus
(T-D2800) (M-20601) (M-20610)

D4-12110 Partial congenital absence of limb, NOS 755.4
(T-D2800) (M-21070)

D4-12112 Anisomelia
(T-D2800) (M-20650)

D4-12114 Dimelia
(T-D2800) (M-22360)
Congenital duplication of limb
(T-D2800) (M-22360)

D4-12200 Polydactyly, NOS 755.00
(T-D2810) (M-22300)
Hexadactyly 755.00
(T-D2810) (M-22300)

D4-12210 Congenital macrodactylia
(T-D2810) (M-20500)

D4-12212 Oligodactyly
(T-D2810) (M-20000) (M-05130)

D4-12214 Syndactyly 755.1
(T-D2810) (M-20110)
Webbing of digits 755.1
(T-D2810) (M-20110)
Mule foot

D4-12216 Polysyndactyly
(T-D2810) (M-22300) (M-20110)

D4-12220 Symphalangy 755.1
(T-D2810) (M-20100)

D4-12224 Adactylia
(T-D2810) (M-21000)

D4-12230 Ectrodactyly
(T-D2810) (M-21070)

D4-12232 Brachydactyly
(T-D8890) (T-D9890) (M-20601)

D4-12240 Brachymetapody
(T-12540) (T-12840) (M-20601)

D4-12250 Brachyphalangia
(T-11080) (M-20601)

D4-12252 Brachymegalodactyly
(T-D8890) (T-D9890) (M-20601)
(M-20500)

D4-12254 Symbrachydactyly
(T-D8890) (T-D9890) (M-20100)
(M-20601)

D4-12260 Arachnodactyly
(T-D8890) (T-D9890) (M-20604)
(M-20610)
Dolichostenomelia
(T-D8890) (T-D9890) (M-20604)
(M-20610)
Spider finger
(T-D8890) (T-D9890) (M-20604)
(M-20610)

D4-12300 Acheiropodia
(T-D8780) (T-D9780) (M-21000)
Agenesis of hands and feet
(T-D8780) (T-D9780) (M-21000)

4-13 CONGENITAL ANOMALIES OF THE UPPER LIMB

D4-13000 Congenital anomaly of upper limb, NOS 755.50
(T-D8000) (M-20000)

D4-13010 Congenital dislocation of elbow 754.89
(T-D8300) (M-22100)
Elbow dysplasia

D4-13012 Congenital dislocation of shoulder
(T-D2220) (M-22100)

D4-13014 Congenital dislocation of radial head
(T-12421) (M-22100)

D4-13016 Congenital ankylosis of elbow
(T-15430) (M-20160)

D4-13020 Congenital deformity of clavicle, NOS 755.51
(T-12310) (M-20000)

D4-13022 Congenital pseudarthrosis of clavicle
(T-12310) (M-20170)

D4-13030 Congenital elevation of scapula 755.52
(T-12280) (M-22100) (M-22205)
Sprengel's deformity 755.52
(T-12280) (M-22100) (M-22205)

D4-13040 Radioulnar synostosis 755.53
(T-1242A) (T-1243A) (M-20100)

D4-13042 Madelung's deformity 755.54
(T-1243B) (M-20500) (T-D8700)
(M-22141)

D4-13100 Reduction deformity of upper limb, NOS 755.20
(T-D8000) (M-21070) (M-20602)

D4-13101 Ectromelia of upper limb, NOS 755.20
(T-D8000) (T-11016) (M-20602)
(M-21070)

D4-13102 Hemimelia of upper limb, NOS 755.20
(T-D8500) (M-21070) (M-20602)

D4-13103 Congenital shortening of arm, NOS 755.20
(T-D8000) (M-20602)

D4-13200 Transverse deficiency of upper limb, NOS 755.21
(T-D8800) (M-21000) (M-21070)
Transverse hemimelia of upper limb 755.21
(T-D8000) (M-21000) (M-21070)

D4-13201 Amelia of upper limb 755.21
(T-D8000) (M-21000)
Congenital absence of upper limb 755.21
(T-D8000) (M-21000)
Congenital amputation of upper limb 755.21
(T-D8000) (M-21000)

D4-13202 Congenital absence of all fingers 755.21
(T-D8890) (M-21000)

D4-13203 Congenital absence of forearm with hand and fingers 755.21
(T-D8500) (T-D8700) (T-D8800)
(M-21000)

D4-13300 Longitudinal deficiency of upper limb, NOS 755.22
(T-D8000) (M-20602)

D4-13301 Phocomelia of upper limb, NOS 755.22
(T-D8000) (M-21300)
Rudimentary arm 755.22
(T-D8000) (M-21300)

D4-13302 Complete phocomelia of upper limb 755.23
(T-D8000) (M-21000)

D4-13303 Congenital absence of arm and forearm 755.23
(T-D8300) (T-D8500) (M-21000)

D4-13304 Incomplete congenital absence of arm and forearm 755.23
(T-D8200) (T-D8500) (M-21070)

D4-13310 Longitudinal deficiency of humerus, NOS 755.24
(T-12410) (M-20602)

D4-13311 Congenital absence of humerus 755.24
(T-12410) (M-21000)
Proximal phocomelia of upper limb 755.24
(T-12410) (M-21000)

D4-13330 Longitudinal deficiency of radius and ulna, NOS 755.25
(T-12420) (T-12430) (M-20602)

D4-13331 Longitudinal absence of radius and ulna 755.25
(T-12420) (T-12430) (M-21000)
Distal phocomelia of upper limb 755.25
(T-12420) (T-12430) (M-21000)

D4-13332 Longitudinal deficiency of radius, NOS 755.26
(T-12420) (M-20602)

D4-13334 Congenital absence of radius 755.26
(T-12420) (M-21000)
Agenesis of radius 755.26
(T-12420) (M-21000)

D4-13340 Longitudinal deficiency of ulna 755.27
(T-12330) (M-20602)

D4-13341 Congenital absence of ulna 755.27
(T-12430) (M-21000)
Agenesis of ulna 755.27
(T-12430) (M-21000)

D4-13342 Ulnar dimelia
(T-12430) (M-22360)

D4-13351 Longitudinal deficiency of carpal bone 755.28
(T-12440) (M-20602)

D4-13352 Longitudinal deficiency of metacarpal bone 755.28
(T-12540) (M-20602)

D4-13355V Congenital subluxation of carpus

D4-13361 Longitudinal deficiency of phalanges of hand 755.29
(T-D8800) (M-20602)

D4-13362 Complete aphalangia of upper limb 755.29
(T-D8890) (M-21000)

D4-13363 Partial aphalangia of upper limb 755.29
(T-D8800) (M-21070)

D4-13364 Congenital absence of finger 755.29
(T-D8800) (M-21000)

D4-13367 Brachymetacarpia
(T-12540) (M-20601)

D4-13375 Congenital absence of hand
(T-D8700) (M-21000)
Acheiria
(T-D8700) (M-21000)

D4-13400 Congenital anomaly of the hand, NOS
(T-D8700) (M-20000)

D4-13410 Talipomanus, NOS 754.89
(T-D8700) (M-20000) (M-02070)
Congenital clubhand 754.89
(T-D8700) (M-20000) (M-02070)

4-13 CONGENITAL ANOMALIES OF THE UPPER LIMB — Continued

D4-13412 Congenital spade-like hand 754.89
(T-D8700) (M-20630)

D4-13413 Manus vara 754.89
(T-D8700) (M-22204)
Radial clubhand 754.89
(T-D8700) (M-22204)

D4-13415 Manus valga 754.8
(T-D8700) (M-22203)
Ulnar clubhand 754.8
(T-D8700) (M-22203)

D4-13418 Manus cava 754.89
(T-D8700) (M-22142)

D4-13420 Manus extensa
(T-D8700) (M-22145)
Manus superextensa
(T-D8700) (M-22145)

D4-13422 Manus flexa
(T-D8700) (M-22146)

D4-13424 Manus plana
(T-D8700) (M-20000)

D4-13426 Mirror hands
(T-D8700) (M-22360)

D4-13500 Congenital anomaly of finger, NOS
(T-D8800) (M-20000)

D4-13510 Polydactyly of fingers 755.01
(T-D8800) (M-22300)
Accessory fingers 755.01
(T-D8800) (M-22300)

D4-13512 Syndactyly of fingers 755.11
(T-D8800) (M-20110)
Webbing of fingers 755.11
(T-D8800) (M-20110)

D4-13514 Overriding fingers
(T-D8800) (M-22160)

D4-13518 Syndactyly of fingers with fusion of bones 755.12
(T-D8800) (M-20110) (T-12610) (M-20100)

D4-13520 Bifid thumb
(T-D8810) (M-22030)

D4-13600 Accessory carpal bones 755.56
(T-12440) (M-22300)

D4-13610 Macrodactylia of fingers 755.57
(T-D8890) (M-20500)

D4-13620 Congenital cleft hand 755.58
(T-D8700) (T-12540) (M-21500)
Lobster-claw hand 755.58
(T-D8700) (T-12540) (M-21500)

D4-13622 Congenital clinodactyly
(T-D8800) (M-22141) (M-22143)

D4-13624 Congenital cubitus valgus 755.59
(T-D8300) (M-22203)

D4-13626 Congenital cubitus varus 755.59
(T-D8300) (M-22204)

4-14 CONGENITAL ANOMALIES OF THE LOWER LIMB

D4-14000 Congenital anomaly of lower limb, NOS 755.60
(T-D9000) (M-20000)

D4-14002 Congenital generalized flexion contractures of lower limb joints 754.89
(T-D9000) (T-15000) (M-20140)

D4-14010 Congenital deformity of hip joint, NOS 755.63
(T-15710) (M-20000)

D4-14011 Congenital coxa valga 755.61
(T-D2500) (T-12710) (M-22203)

D4-14012 Congenital coxa vara 755.61
(T-D2500) (T-12710) (M-22204)

D4-14013V Congenital hip dysplasia
Dysplasia of acetabulum

D4-14014 Congenital anteversion of femur 755.63
(T-12712) (M-22140)

D4-14100 Reduction deformity of lower limb, NOS 755.3
(T-D9000) (M-20602)

D4-14101 Ectromelia of lower limb, NOS 755.30
(T-D9000) (T-11016) (M-20602) (M-21070)

D4-14102 Hemimelia of lower limb, nOS 755.30
(T-D9400) (M-21070) (M-20602)

D4-14103 Congenital shortening of leg, NOS 755.30
(T-D9000) (M-20602)

D4-14200 Transverse deficiency of lower limb, NOS 755.31
(T-D9000) (M-21000) (M-21070)
Transverse hemimelia of lower limb 755.31
(T-D9000) (M-21000) (M-21070)

D4-14201 Amelia of lower limb 755.31
(T-D9000) (M-21000)
Congenital absence of lower limb 755.31
(T-D9000) (M-21000)
Congenital amputation of lower limb 755.31
(T-D9000) (M-21000)

D4-14202 Congenital absence of all toes 755.31
(T-D9890) (M-21000)

D4-14203 Congenital absence of leg with foot and toes 755.31
(T-D9400) (T-D9700) (T-D9800) (M-21000)

D4-14204 Congenital absence of foot 755.31
(T-D9700) (M-21000)

D4-14300 Longitudinal deficiency of lower limb, NOS 755.32
(T-D9000) (M-20602)

D4-14301 Phocomelia of lower limb, NOS 755.32
(T-D9000) (M-21300)
Rudimentary leg 755.32
(T-D9000) (M-21300)

D4-14302 Complete phocomelia of lower limb 755.33
(T-D9000) (M-21000)
Congenital absence of thigh and leg 755.33
(T-D9100) (T-D9400) (M-21000)

D4-14304 Incomplete congenital absence of thigh and leg 755.33
(T-D9100) (T-D9400) (M-21070)

D4-14310 Longitudinal deficiency of femur 755.34
(T-12710) (M-20602)

D4-14311 Congenital absence of femur 755.34
(T-12710) (M-21000)
Proximal phocomelia of lower limb 755.34
(T-12710) (M-21000)

D4-14330 Longitudinal deficiency of tibia and fibula 755.35
(T-12740) (T-12750) (M-20602)

D4-14331 Congenital absence of tibia and fibula 755.35
(T-12740) (T-12750) (M-21000)
Distal phocomelia of lower limb 755.35
(T-12740) (T-12750) (M-21000)

D4-14332 Longitudinal deficiency of tibia 755.36
(T-12740) (M-20602)

D4-14333 Congenital absence of tibia 755.36
(T-12740) (M-21000)
Agenesis of tibia 755.36
(T-12740) (M-21000)

D4-14334 Longitudinal deficiency of fibula 755.37
(T-12750) (M-20602)

D4-14335 Congenital absence of fibula 755.37
(T-12750) (M-21000)
Agenesis of fibula 755.37
(T-12750) (M-21000)

D4-14336 Longitudinal deficiency of tarsal bone 755.38
(T-12760) (M-20602)

D4-14337 Longitudinal deficiency of metatarsal bone 755.38
(T-12840) (M-20602)

D4-14340 Longitudinal deficiency of phalanges of foot 755.39
(T-D9890) (M-20602)

D4-14345 Complete aphalangia of lower limb 755.39
(T-D9890) (M-21000)

D4-14346 Partial aphalangia of lower limb 755.39
(T-D9890) (M-21070)

D4-14347 Congenital absence of toe 755.39
(T-D9800) (M-21000)

D4-14400 Congenital anomaly of foot, NOS
Congenital deformity of foot, NOS 754.70
(T-D9700) (M-20000)

D4-14410 Clubfoot, NOS 754.70
(T-D9700) (M-20000)
Talipes, NOS 754.70
(T-D9700) (M-20000)

D4-14420 Congenital valgus deformity of foot, NOS 754.6
(T-D9700) (M-22203)

D4-14421 Talipes valgus 754.60
(T-D9600) (M-22203)

D4-14422 Congenital pes planus 754.61
(T-12765) (T-D9750) (M-20000)
Congenital flat foot 754.61
(T-12765) (T-D9750) (M-20000)

D4-14423 Talipes calcaneovalgus 754.62
(T-D9600) (M-22203) (T-D9800) (M-22205)

D4-14424 Talipes equinovalgus 754.69
(T-D9700) (M-22203) (M-22205)

D4-14425 Talipes planovalgus 754.69
(T-D9600) (M-22203) (T-D9753) (M-22205)

D4-14428 Talipes cavus 754.71
(T-D9750) (M-22142)
Congenital cavus foot 754.71
(T-D9750) (M-22142)

D4-14429 Asymmetric talipes 754.79
(T-D9700) (M-20650)

D4-14432 Talipes calcaneus 754.79
(T-D9700) (M-22205)

D4-14434 Talipes equinus 754.79
(T-D9700) (M-22206)

D4-14450 Congenital varus deformity of foot, NOS 754.5
(T-D9700) (M-22204)
Talipes varus 754.50
(T-D9600) (M-22204)
Congenital pes varus 754.50
(T-D9600) (M-22204)

D4-14452 Talipes equinovarus 754.51
(T-D9600) (M-22204) (T-D9700) (M-22205)

D4-14454 Talipes calcaneovarus 754.59
(T-D9600) (M-22204) (T-D9800) (M-22205)

D4-14460 Metatarsus varus 754.53
(T-D9753) (M-22205)

D4-14462 Metatarsus primus varus 754.52
(T-12850) (M-22204)

D4-14464 Brachymetatarsia
(T-12840) (M-20601)

D4-14470 Astragaloscaphoid synostosis 755.67
(T-12780) (T-12800) (M-20100)
Talonavicular synostosis 755.67
(T-12780) (T-12800) (M-20100)

D4-14472 Calcaneonavicular bar 755.67
(T-12770) (T-12800) (M-20100)

D4-14474 Coalition of calcaneus 755.67
(T-12770) (T-12760) (M-20100)

D4-14476 Tarsal coalitions 755.67
(T-12760) (M-20100)

D4-14500 Congenital anomaly of toe, NOS 755.66
(T-D9800) (M-20000)

D4-14510 Macrodactylia of toes 755.65
(T-D9890) (M-20500)

D4-14512 Congenital hallux valgus 755.66
(T-D9810) (M-22203)

D4-14514 Congenital hallux varus 755.66
(T-D9810) (M-22204)

D4-14516 Congenital hammer toe 755.66
(T-D9800) (M-20140) (M-22206)

4-14 CONGENITAL ANOMALIES OF THE LOWER LIMB — Continued

D4-14520 Polydactyly of toes 755.02
(T-D9800) (M-22300)
Accessory toes 755.02
(T-D9800) (M-22300)

D4-14530 Overriding toes
(T-D9800) (M-22160)

D4-14534 Syndactyly of toes 755.13
(T-D9800) (M-20110)
Webbing of toes 755.13
(T-D9890) (M-20110)

D4-14536 Syndactyly of toes with fusion of bones 755.14
(T-D9800) (M-20110) (T-12910) (M-20100)

D4-14600 Congenital pseudarthrosis of tibia
(T-12740) (M-20170)

D4-14602 Congenital angulation of tibia 755.69
(T-12740) (M-22140)

D4-14604 Congenital deformity of ankle joint 755.69
(T-15750) (M-20000)

D4-14700 Congenital dislocation of hip, NOS 754.30
(T-D2500) (M-22100)

D4-14701 Unilateral congenital dislocation of hip 754.30
(T-D2500) (M-22101)

D4-14702 Bilateral congenital dislocation of hip 754.31
(T-D2500) (M-22102)

D4-14710 Congenital subluxation of hip, NOS 754.32
(T-D2500) (M-22105)

D4-14711 Unilateral congenital subluxation of hip 754.32
(T-D2500) (M-22106)

D4-14712 Bilateral congenital subluxation of hip 754.33
(T-D2500) (M-22107)

D4-14720 Congenital dislocation of one hip with subluxation of other 754.35
(T-D2500) (M-22100) (T-D2500) (M-22105)

D4-14730 Genu recurvatum 754.40
(T-D9200) (M-22142)

D4-14732 Congenital dislocation of knee with genu recurvatum 754.41
(T-D9200) (M-22100) (M-22142)

D4-14734 Congenital bowing of femur 754.42
(T-12710) (M-22142)

D4-14736 Congenital bowing of tibia and fibula 754.43
(T-12740) (T-12750) (M-22142)

D4-14738 Bifid patella
(T-12730) (M-22030)

D4-14740 Congenital deformity of knee joint, NOS 755.64
(T-15720) (M-20000)

D4-14742 Congenital absence of patella 755.64
(T-12730) (M-21000)

D4-14750 Congenital genu valgum 755.64
(T-D9200) (M-22203)
Congenital knock-knee 755.64
(T-D9200) (M-22203)

D4-14751 Congenital dislocation of knee
(T-D9200) (M-22100)

D4-14752 Congenital genu varum 755.64
(T-D9200) (M-22204)
Congenital bowleg 755.64
(T-D9200) (M-22204)

D4-14758 Rudimentary patella 755.64
(T-12730) (M-21300)

D4-14760 Congenital discoid meniscus 717.5
(T-15723) (M-20000) (M-02100)
Congenital discoid lateral meniscus 717.5
(T-15723) (M-20000) (M-02100)

4-15 CONGENITAL ANOMALIES OF THE SPINE

D4-15000 Congenital anomaly of spine, NOS 756.10
(T-11500) (M-20000)
Congenital anomaly of vertebral column, NOS 756.10
(T-11500) (M-20000)

D4-15007 Congenital kyphosis
(T-11700) (M-22142)

D4-15008 Congenital postural lordosis 754.2
(T-11500) (M-22142)
Congenital lordosis 754.2
(T-11500) (M-22142)

D4-15009 Congenital postural scoliosis 754.2
(T-11500) (M-22141)
Congenital scoliosis 754.2
(T-11500) (M-22141)

D4-15020 Congenital spondylolysis of lumbosacral region 756.11
(T-11A60) (T-11511) (M-21000)

D4-15021 Lumbosacral prespondylolisthesis 756.11
(T-11955) (M-21000)

D4-15022 Congenital spondylolisthesis 756.12
(T-11510) (M-22100)

D4-15040 Congenital absence of vertebra, NOS 756.13
(T-11510) (M-21000)

D4-15041 Congenital hemivertebra 756.14
(T-11510) (M-21080)

D4-15042 Congenital fusion of spine 756.15
(T-11510) (M-20100)

D4-15046 Spina bifida occulta 756.17
(T-11510) (M-21500)
Cryptomerorachischisis 756.17
(T-11510) (M-21500)

D4-15047 Platyspondylia 756.19
(T-11510) (M-20630)

D4-15048 Spondyloschisis
(T-11510) (M-21500)

D4-15049 Supernumerary vertebra 756.19
(T-11510) (M-22300)

D4-15050 Sacralization of lumbar vertebra
(T-11950) (T-11AD0) (M-20100)

D4-15060 Persistent human tail
(T-D6600) (M-26400)

D4-15100 Congenital deformity of sacroiliac joint 755.69
(T-15680) (M-20000)

D4-15110 Congenital fusion of sacroiliac joint 755.69
(T-15680) (M-20100)

D4-15120V Cervical malformation — malarticulation
Cervical stenotic myelopathy
Wobbler syndrome
Equine sensory ataxia
Enzootic equine incoordination

D4-15124V Atlanto-occipital malformation

D4-15126 Occipital dysplasia

D4-15130V Congenital lumbosacral stenosis

4-16 CONGENITAL ANOMALIES OF THE TRUNK

D4-16000 Congenital anomaly of trunk, NOS
(T-D2000) (M-20000)

D4-16100 Congenital anomaly of thoracic cage, NOS
(T-11200) (M-20000)

D4-16101 Cervical rib 756.2
(T-11300) (M-22300) (T-11600)
Supernumerary rib in cervical region 756.2
(T-11300) (M-22300) (T-11600)

D4-16102 Congenital absence of rib 756.3
(T-11300) (M-21000)

D4-16103 Congenital absence of sternum 756.3
(T-11210) (M-21000)

D4-16104 Congenital fissure of sternum 756.3
(T-11210) (M-21500)

D4-16105 Congenital fusion of ribs 756.3
(T-11300) (M-20100)

D4-16106 Sternum bifidum 756.3
(T-11210) (M-22030)

D4-16110 Congenital deformity of chest wall 754.89
(T-D3050) (M-20000)

D4-16112 Pectus excavatum 754.81
(T-11210) (M-22204)
Congenital funnel chest 754.81
(T-11210) (M-22204)

D4-16114 Pectus carinatum 754.82
(T-11210) (M-22203)
Congenital pigeon breast 754.82
(T-11210) (M-22203)

D4-16200 Congenital absence of pectoral muscle 756.81
(T-14102) (M-21000)

D4-16500 Congenital anomaly of diaphragm, NOS 756.6
(T-D3400) (M-20000)

D4-16501 Congenital absence of diaphragm 756.6
(T-D3400) (M-21000)
Aplasia of diaphragm
(T-D3400) (M-21000)

D4-16502 Congenital diaphragmatic hernia, NOS 756.6
(T-D3400) (M-21700)

D4-16503 Congenital hernia of foramen of Morgagni 756.6
(T-D3460) (M-21700)

D4-16504 Congenital hernia of foramen of Bochdalek 756.6
(T-D3450) (M-21700)

D4-16507 Congenital eventration of diaphragm 756.6
(T-D3400) (M-21700) (T-13000) (M-21000)

D4-16508 Congenital eventration of right crus of diaphragm 756.6
(T-D3402) (M-21700) (T-13000) (M-21000)

D4-16509 Congenital eventration of left crus of diaphragm
(T-D3403) (M-21700) (T-13000) (M-21000)

D4-16600 Congenital anomaly of abdominal wall, NOS 756.7
(T-D4300) (M-20000)

D4-16602 Congenital absence of abdominal muscle
(T-13000) (T-D4000) (M-21000)

D4-16610 Congenital exomphalos 756.7
(T-D4220) (M-21700)

D4-16611 Gastroschisis 756.7
(T-D4300) (M-21500) (T-50500) (M-21700)

D4-16612 Prune belly syndrome 756.7
(T-14260) (M-21000)
Triad syndrome 756.7
(T-14260) (M-21000)

D4-16613 Celoschisis
(T-D4300) (M-21500)

4-18 CONGENITAL ANOMALIES OF THE PELVIS

D4-18000 Congenital anomaly of the pelvis, NOS
(T-D6000) (M-20000)
Congenital abnormal pelvis, NOS
(T-D6000) (M-20000)

D4-18010 Assimilation pelvis, NOS
(T-D6000)

D4-18011 High assimilation pelvis
(T-D6000)

D4-18012 Low assimilation pelvis
(T-D6000)

D4-18020 Brachypellic pelvis
(T-D6000)
Transverse oval pelvis
(T-D6000)

D4-18022 Congenital contracted pelvis
(T-D6000)

D4-18024 Cordate pelvis
(T-D6000)
Cordiform pelvis
(T-D6000)
Heart-shaped pelvis
(T-D6000)

D4-18026 Robert's pelvis
(T-D6000)

4-18 CONGENITAL ANOMALIES OF THE PELVIS — Continued

D4-18028 Pelvis plana
(T-D6000)
Flat pelvis
(T-D6000)
D4-18032 Deventer's pelvis
(T-D6000)
D4-18034 Dolichopellic pelvis
(T-D6000)
Longitudinal oval pelvis
(T-D6000)
D4-18036 Dwarf pelvis
(T-D6000)
Pelvis nana
(T-D6000)
D4-18038 Pelvis justo major
(T-D6000)
Giant pelvis
(T-D6000)
D4-18042 Inverted pelvis
(T-D6000)
Split pelvis
(T-D6000)
D4-18044 Pelvis justo minor
(T-D6000)
D4-18046 Juvenile pelvis
(T-D6000)
D4-18048 Infantile pelvis
(T-D6000)
D4-18052 Funnel-shaped pelvis
(T-D6000) (M-02160)
D4-18054 Platypellic pelvis
(T-D6000) (M-02120)
Flat oval pelvis
(T-D6000) (M-02120)
D4-18056 Nagele's pelvis
(T-D6000)
D4-18058 Mesatipellic pelvis
(T-D6000) (M-02100)
Round pelvis
(T-D6000) (M-02100)
D4-18062 Oblique pelvis
(T-D6000)
D4-18064 Reniform pelvis
(T-D6000)

SECTION 4-2 CONGENITAL ANOMALIES OF THE RESPIRATORY SYSTEM

4-20 CONGENITAL ANOMALIES OF THE RESPIRATORY SYSTEM: GENERAL TERMS

D4-20000 Congenital anomaly of respiratory system, NOS 748.9
(T-20000) (M-20000)
D4-20100 Congenital anomaly of upper respiratory system, NOS 748.9
(T-20100) (M-20000)

4-21 CONGENITAL ANOMALIES OF THE NOSE AND NASAL SINUSES

D4-21100 Congenital deformity of nose, NOS 748.1
(T-21000) (M-20000)
D4-21110 Choanal atresia 748.0
(T-21350) (M-20400)
Congenital atresia of posterior nares 748.0
(T-21350) (M-20400)
D4-21111 Congenital atresia of nares 748.0
(T-21310) (M-20400)
Congenital atresia of anterior nares 748.0
(T-21310) (M-20400)
D4-21112 Congenital stenosis of choanae 748.0
(T-21350) (M-20300)
D4-21113 Congenital stenosis of nares 748.0
(T-21310) (M-20300)
D4-21114 Congenital absence of nose 748.1
(T-21000) (M-21000)
D4-21121 Accessory nose 748.1
(T-21000) (M-22300)
D4-21122 Cleft nose 748.1
(T-21000) (M-21500)
D4-21124 Congenital notching of tip of nose 748.1
(T-21130) (M-22080)
D4-21125 Congenital deviation of nasal septum 754.0
(T-21340) (M-22141)
D4-21128 Congenital bent nose 754.0
(T-21000) (M-22141)
D4-21131 Congenital deformity of wall of nasal sinus 748.1
(T-22040) (M-20000)
D4-21132 Congenital perforation of wall of nasal sinus 748.1
(T-22040) (M-21900)
D4-21140 Congenital atresia of nasopharynx 748.8
(T-23000) (M-20400)
D4-21150 Congenital enlargement of nasopharynx
(T-23000) (M-20500)

4-24 CONGENITAL ANOMALIES OF THE LARYNX

D4-24000 Congenital anomaly of larynx, NOS 748.2
(T-24100) (M-20000)
Congenital deformity of larynx, NOS 748.2
(T-24100) (M-20000)
D4-24001 Congenital web of larynx 748.2
(T-24400) (M-20110)
Congenital glottic web of larynx 748.2
(T-24400) (M-20110)
Congenital subglottic web of larynx 748.2
(T-24100) (M-20110)
D4-24002 Congenital absence of larynx 748.3
(T-24100) (M-21000)
Agenesis of larynx 748.3
(T-24100) (M-21000)
D4-24005 Congenital anomaly of cricoid cartilage 748.3
(T-24170) (M-20000)

D4-24006 Congenital anomaly of epiglottis 748.3
(T-24000) (M-20000)

D4-24007 Congenital anomaly of thyroid cartilage 748.3
(T-24160) (M-20000)

D4-24011 Congenital atresia of epiglottis 748.3
(T-24000) (M-20400)

D4-24012 Congenital atresia of glottis 748.3
(T-24440) (M-20400)

D4-24013 Congenital atresia of larynx 748.1
(T-24100) (M-20400)

D4-24019 Congenital cleft thyroid cartilage 748.3
(T-24160) (M-21500)

D4-24021 Congenital stenosis of larynx 748.3
(T-24100) (M-20300)

D4-24022 Congenital tracheocele 748.3
(T-25010) (M-21700) (T-25120)

D4-24025 Congenital fissure of epiglottis 748.3
(T-24000) (M-21500)

D4-24028 Congenital laryngocele 748.3
(T-24100) (M-21700)

D4-24029 Congenital posterior cleft of cricoid cartilage 748.3
(T-24170) (M-21500)

D4-24031 Congenital laryngeal stridor 748.3
(T-24000) (M-20500) (T-24100) (M-20200)

4-25 CONGENITAL ANOMALIES OF THE TRACHEA

D4-25000 Congenital anomaly of trachea, NOS
(T-25000) (M-20000)
Congenital deformity of trachea, NOS
(T-25000) (M-20000)

D4-25010 Congenital absence of trachea 748.3
(T-25000) (M-21000)
Agenesis of trachea 748.3
(T-25000) (M-21000)

D4-25020 Congenital atresia of trachea 748.3
(T-25000) (M-20400)

D4-25022 Congenital stenosis of trachea 748.3
(T-25000) (M-20300)

D4-25030 Congenital dilatation of trachea 748.3
(T-25000) (M-26710)

D4-25032 Congenital diverticulum of trachea 748.3
(T-25000) (M-21750)

D4-25040 Rudimentary tracheal bronchus 748.3
(T-26000) (M-21300)

D4-25050 Congenital tracheobronchiomegaly
(T-25000) (T-26000) (M-20500)

D4-25100 Congenital anomaly of tracheal cartilage 748.3
(T-25100) (M-20000)

4-26 CONGENITAL ANOMALIES OF THE BRONCHUS

D4-26000 Congenital anomaly of bronchus, NOS
(T-26000) (M-20000)
Congenital deformity of bronchus, NOS
(T-26000) (M-20000)

D4-26010 Congenital absence of bronchus 748.3
(T-26000) (M-21000)
Agenesis of bronchus 748.3
(T-26000) (M-21000)

D4-26020 Congenital atresia of bronchus
(T-26000) (M-20400)

D4-26032 Congenital diverticulum of bronchus 748.3
(T-26000) (M-21750)

D4-26040 Accessory bronchus
(T-26000) (M-22300)

4-28 CONGENITAL ANOMALIES OF THE LUNG

D4-28000 Congenital anomaly of lung, NOS 748.6
(T-28000) (M-20000)

D4-28100 Congenital cystic lung 748.4
(T-28000) (M-26700)
Congenital cystic disease of lung 748.4
(T-28000) (M-26700)
Congenital polycystic disease of lung 748.4
(T-28000) (M-26700)

D4-28110 Congenital honeycomb lung 748.4
(T-28000) (M-26700) (M-01150)

D4-28112 Congenital cystic adenomatoid malformation of lung 748.4
(T-28000) (M-26700)

D4-28200 Congenital absence of lung 748.5
(T-28000) (M-21000)
Congenital aplasia of lung 748.5
(T-28000) (M-21000)

D4-28202 Congenital absence of lobe of lung 748.5
(T-28770) (M-21000)

D4-28204 Unilobar lung
(T-28000) (M-20100)

D4-28206 Congenital hypoplasia of lung 748.5
(T-28000) (M-21300)

D4-28210 Agenesis of right lung
(T-28100) (M-21000)

D4-28220 Agenesis of left lung
(T-28500) (M-21000)

D4-28230 Congenital sequestration of lung 748.5
(T-28000) (M-26800)

D4-28232 Intralobar bronchopulmonary sequestration 748.5
(T-28000) (M-26800) (G-C006) (T-28770)

D4-28234 Extralobar bronchopulmonary sequestration 748.5
(T-28000) (M-26800) (G-A112) (T-28770)

D4-28236 Extrapulmonary subpleural pulmonary sequestration 748.5
(T-28000) (M-26800) (G-A112) (T-29020)

D4-28240 Congenital bronchopulmonary foregut malformation
(T-28000) (M-26800) (M-20700) (T-56310)

4-28 CONGENITAL ANOMALIES OF THE LUNG — Continued

D4-28300 Congenital incomplete expansion of lung
(T-28000) (M-20670)
Underexpanded lung
(T-28000) (M-20670)
Non-expanded lung
(T-28000) (M-20670)
Unexpanded lung
(T-28000) (M-20670)
Congenital atelectasis of lung
(T-28000) (M-20670)
Atelectasis neonatorum
(T-28000) (M-20670)

D4-28310 Immature lungs
(T-28000) (M-20050)

D4-28400 Accessory lung 748.6
(T-28000) (M-22300)

D4-28402 Accessory lobe of lung 748.6
(T-28770) (M-22300)

D4-28410 Bilobed right lung
(T-28100) (M-22030)

D4-28412 Trilobed left lung
(T-28500) (M-22040)

D4-28414 Azygos lobe of lung 748.6
(T-28110) (M-22300)

D4-28500 Infantile lobar overinflation of lung
(T-28000)

D4-28510 Congenital emphysema
(T-28000) (M-20671)

D4-28512 Congenital lobar emphysema
(T-28770) (M-20671)

D4-28514 Bronchial atresia with segmental pulmonary emphysema
(T-26000) (M-20400) (T-280D0) (M-20671)

D4-28520 Congenital bronchiectasis 748.6
(T-26000) (M-26710)

D4-28558 Unilateral congenital dysplasia of lung with vascular anomalies
(T-28000) (M-20020) (G-C008) (T-40000) (M-20000)

D4-28600 Congenital pulmonary lymphangiectasis
(T-28000) (M-24690)

D4-28700 Congenital anomaly of pleural folds 748.8
(T-29000) (M-20000)

D4-28710 Abnormal communication between pericardial sac and pleura 746.89
(T-39000) (T-29000) (M-20700)
Pericardial defect 746.89
(T-39000) (M-29000) (M-20700)
Congenital pericardial defect 746.89
(T-39000) (T-29000) (M-20700)

D4-28750 Congenital cyst of mediastinum 748.8
(T-D3300) (M-26500)

SECTION 4-3 CONGENITAL ANOMALIES OF THE CARDIOVASCULAR SYSTEM

4-30 CONGENITAL ANOMALIES OF THE CARDIOVASCULAR SYSTEM: GENERAL TERMS

D4-30000 Congenital anomaly of cardiovascular system, NOS 747.9
(T-30000) (M-20000)

4-31 CONGENITAL ANOMALIES OF THE HEART

D4-31000 Congenital heart disease, NOS 746.9
(T-32000) (M-20000)
Congenital anomaly of heart, NOS 746.9
(T-32000) (M-20000)

D4-31010 Complete transposition of great vessels 745.10
(T-42000) (T-44000) (M-22111)
Classical transposition of great vessels 745.10
(T-32000) (T-44000) (M-22111)

D4-31020 Double outlet left ventricle
(T-32600) (T-42000) (T-44000) (M-22112)
Origin of both great vessels from left ventricle
(T-32600) (T-42000) (T-44000) (M-22112)

D4-31030 Double outlet right ventricle 745.11
(T-32500) (T-42000) (T-44000) (M-22112)
Origin of both great vessels from right ventricle 745.11
(T-32500) (T-42000) (T-44000) (M-22112)
Taussig-Bing syndrome 745.11
(T-32500) (T-42000) (T-44000) (M-22112)
Taussig-Bing defect 745.11
(T-32500) (T-42000) (T-44000) (M-22112)
Dextratransposition of aorta 745.11
(T-32500) (T-42000) (T-44000) (M-22112)
Transposition of great vessels, interventricular septal defect and overriding aorta 745.11
(T-32500) (T-42000) (T-44000) (M-22112)

D4-31040 Corrected transposition of great vessels 745.12
(T-42000) (T-44000) (M-22114)
Transposition of great vessels with ventricular inversion 745.12
(T-42000) (T-44000) (M-22114)

D4-31100 Congenital septal defect of heart, NOS 745.9
(T-32070) (M-21900)

D4-31110 Tetralogy of Fallot 745.2
(T-32410) (M-20700) (T-35200)
(M-20300) (T-42000) (M-22110)
(T-32500) (M-20500)
Subpulmonic stenosis, ventricular septal defect, overriding aorta, and right ventricular hypertrophy 745.2
(T-32410) (M-20700) (T-35200)
(M-20300) (T-42000) (M-22110)
(T-32500) (M-20500)

D4-31120 Common ventricle 745.3
(T-32410) (M-21000)
Single ventricle 745.3
(T-32410) (M-21000)
Cor triloculare biatriatum 745.3
(T-32410) (M-21000)

D4-31150 Ventricular septal defect 745.4
(T-32410) (M-21900) (M-20700)
Interventricular septal defect 745.4
(T-32410) (M-21900) (M-20700)
Roger's disease 745.4
(T-32410) (M-21900) (M-20700)
Absence of interventricular septum 745.4
(T-32410) (M-21900) (M-20700)

D4-31160 Eisenmenger's defect 745.4
(T-32410) (M-21900) (M-20700)
(T-32500) (M-20500)
Eisenmenger's complex 745.4
(T-32410) (M-21900) (M-20700)
(T-32500) (M-20500)

D4-31164 Left ventricular-right atrial communication 745.4
(T-32410) (M-21900) (T-32200)
(T-32600) (M-20700)

D4-31200 Lutembacher's anomaly
(T-32150) (M-21900) (T-35300)
(M-20300)
Atrial septal defect and mitral stenosis
(T-32150) (M-21900) (T-35300)
(M-20300)

D4-31210 Ostium secundum type atrial septal defect 745.5
(T-32150) (M-21900) (T-32154)
(M-21500)
Ostium secundum defect 745.5
(T-32150) (M-21900) (T-32154)
(M-21500)
Fossa ovalis defect 745.5
(T-32150) (M-21900) (T-32154)
(M-21500)
Patent ostium secundum 745.5
(T-32150) (M-21900) (T-32154)
(M-21500)
Patent foramen ovale 745.5
(T-32150) (M-21900) (T-32154)
(M-21500)
Persistent ostium secundum 745.5
(T-32150) (M-21900) (T-32154)
(M-21500)
Atrial septal defect of fossa ovalis 745.5
(T-32150) (M-21900) (T-32154)
(M-21500)

D4-31300 Endocardial cushion defect, NOS 745.60
(T-F5650) (M-21500) (M-20700)

D4-31310 Atrial septal defect with endocardial cushion defect, partial type 745.61
(T-F5650) (M-21500) (T-32150)
(M-20700)

D4-31312 Ostium primum defect 745.61
(T-F5650) (M-21500) (M-20700)
(T-32153) (M-26400)
Persistent ostium primum 745.61
(T-F5650) (M-21500) (M-20700)
(T-32153) (M-26400)
Atrial septum primum defect 745.61
(T-F5650) (M-21500) (M-20700)
(T-32153)

D4-31320 Common atrium 745.69
(T-32150) (M-21000)
Congenital absence of atrial septum 745.69
(T-32150) (M-21000)
Cor triloculare biventriculare 745.69
(T-32150) (M-21000)
Atrial septal defect 745.69
(T-32150) (M-21000)
Interatrial septal defect 745.69
(T-32150) (M-21000)

D4-31322 Premature closure of foramen ovale
(T-32130) (M-20130)

D4-31330 Common atrioventricular canal 745.69
(T-F5652) (M-26400) (T-F5650)
(M-21500)
Atrioventricular canal type ventricular septal defect 745.69
(T-F5652) (M-26400) (T-F5650)
(M-21500)
Common atrioventricular valve 745.69
(T-F5652) (M-26400) (T-F5650)
(M-21500)
Ostium atrioventriculare commune 745.69
(T-F5652) (M-26400) (T-F5650)
(M-21500)
Endocardial cushion defect, complete type 745.69
(T-F5652) (M-26400) (T-F5650)
(M-21500)

D4-31340 Cor biloculare 745.7
(T-32150) (T-32410) (M-21000)
Absence of atrial and ventricular septa 745.7
(T-32150) (T-32410) (M-21000)

D4-31400 Common truncus arteriosus 745.0
(T-F5630) (M-26400)
Persistent truncus arteriosus 745.0
(T-F5630) (M-26400)

4-31 CONGENITAL ANOMALIES OF THE HEART — Continued

D4-31400 (cont.) Common aortopulmonary trunk 745.0
(T-F5630) (M-26400)

D4-31410 Truncus arteriosus, Edwards' type I 745.0
(T-F5630) (M-26400)
Common outflow, separate pulmonary artery and aorta 745.0
(T-F5630) (M-26400)

D4-31420 Truncus arteriosus, Edwards' type II 745.0
(T-F5630) (M-26400)
Main pulmonary artery arising from ascending aorta 745.0
(T-F5630) (M-26400)

D4-31430 Truncus arteriosus, Edwards' type III 745.0
(T-F5630) (M-26400)

D4-31440 Truncus arteriosus, Edwards' type IV 745.0
(T-F5630) (M-26400)
Main pulmonary artery arising from descending aorta 745.0
(T-F5630) (M-26400)

D4-31500 Cardiac valvular malformation, NOS
(T-35000) (M-20000)

D4-31502 Abnormal position of cardiac valve
(T-35000) (M-22100)

D4-31504 Double cardiac valve orifice
(T-35000) (M-22360)

D4-31510 Abnormal number of cusps, NOS
(T-35004) (M-20620) (M-05110)

D4-31511 Abnormal number of leaflets, NOS
(T-35002) (M-20620) (M-05110)

D4-31512 Monocuspid cardiac valve
(T-35000) (M-20000) (M-05130)

D4-31513 Bicuspid cardiac valve
(T-35000) (M-20000) (M-22030)

D4-31514 Quadricuspid cardiac valve
(T-35000) (M-20000) (M-05120)

D4-31516 Myxomatosis of cardiac valve
(T-35000) (M-20000) (M-50151)
Incomplete differentiation of cardiac valve
(T-35000) (M-20000) (M-50151)
Myxomatous degeneration of cardiac valve
(T-35000) (M-20000) (M-50151)

D4-31600 Pulmonary valve anomaly, NOS 746.00
(T-35200) (M-20000)

D4-31610 Congenital atresia of pulmonary valve 746.01
(T-35200) (M-20400)

D4-31612 Congenital absence of pulmonary valve 746.01
(T-35200) (M-21000)

D4-31614 Congenital stenosis of pulmonary valve 746.02
(T-35200) (M-20300)

D4-31620 Congenital supravalvular pulmonary stenosis 746.02
(T-44010) (M-20300)

D4-31622 Congenital insufficiency of pulmonary valve 746.09
(T-35200) (M-21900)

D4-31630 Fallot's triad 746.09
(T-35200) (M-20300) (T-32150) (M-21900) (T-32500) (M-20500)
Fallot's trilogy 746.09
(T-35200) (M-20300) (T-32150) (M-21900) (T-32500) (M-20500)

D4-31700 Congenital anomaly of tricuspid valve, NOS 746.1
(T-35100) (M-20000)

D4-31701 Congenital atresia of tricuspid valve 746.1
(T-35100) (M-20400)

D4-31702 Congenital stenosis of tricuspid valve 746.1
(T-35100) (M-20300)

D4-31703 Congenital hypoplasia of tricuspid valve 746.1
(T-35100) (M-21300)

D4-31704 Cleft leaflet of tricuspid valve 746.1
(T-35130) (M-21500)

D4-31710 Ebstein's anomaly 746.2
(T-35100) (M-20000)

D4-31712 Ebstein's anomaly with atrial septal defect 746.2
(T-35100) (M-20000) (T-32150) (M-21900)

D4-31800 Congenital anomaly of aortic valve, NOS 746.3
(T-35400) (M-20000)

D4-31810 Congenital stenosis of aortic valve 746.3
(T-35400) (M-20300)
Congenital aortic stenosis 746.3
(T-35400) (M-20300)

D4-31820 Congenital supravalvular aortic stenosis 747.22
(T-42000) (T-42200) (M-20200) (M-20300) (M-78003)

D4-31830 Congenital atresia of aortic valve 746.3
(T-35400) (M-20400)

D4-31832 Double aortic valve 746.3
(T-35400) (M-22360)

D4-31834 Bicuspid aortic valve 746.4
(T-35400) (M-20620)

D4-31840 Congenital insufficiency of aortic valve 746.4
(T-35400) (M-21900)
Congenital aortic insufficiency 746.4
(T-35400) (M-21900)

D4-31900 Congenital anomaly of mitral valve, NOS 746.5
(T-35300) (M-20000)

D4-31902 Congenital stenosis of mitral valve 746.5
(T-35300) (M-20300)
Congenital mitral stenosis 746.5
(T-35300) (M-20300)
Parachute deformity of mitral valve 746.5
(T-35300) (M-20300)
Parachute mitral valve 746.5
(T-35300) (M-20300)

D4-31904 Cleft leaflet of mitral valve 746.5
(T-35320) (M-21500)

D4-31906 Congenital atresia of mitral valve 746.5
(T-35300) (M-20400)
D4-31908 Supernumerary cusps of mitral valve 746.5
(T-35321) (M-22300)
D4-31910 Double mitral valve 746.5
(T-35300) (M-22360)
D4-31912 Fused commissures of mitral valve 746.5
(T-35321) (M-20100)
D4-31920 Congenital supravalvular mitral stenosis 746.5
(T-32370) (M-20300)
D4-31940 Congenital insufficiency of mitral valve 746.6
(T-35300) (M-21900)
Congenital mitral insufficiency 746.6
(T-35300) (M-21900)
D4-31A00 Hypoplastic left heart syndrome 746.7
(T-32002) (M-21300)
D4-31A02 Rudimentary left ventricle 746.7
(T-32600) (M-21300)
D4-31A20 Cor triatriatum 746.82
(T-32100) (M-22300) (T-48500) (M-24650)
Accessory atrium 746.82
(T-32100) (M-22300) (T-48500) (M-24650)
D4-31A30 Congenital subaortic stenosis 746.81
(T-32670) (M-20300)
D4-31A32 Idiopathic hypertrophic subaortic stenosis 746.81
(T-32670) (M-20500) (M-20300)
D4-31A34 Congenital subaortic stenosis of membranous type 746.81
(T-32670) (M-20300) (M-20500)
D4-31A36 Congenital subaortic stenosis of tunnel type 746.81
(T-32670) (M-20300) (M-20500)
D4-31A40 Infundibular pulmonic stenosis 746.83
(T-32550) (M-20300) (M-20500)
Subvalvular pulmonic stenosis 746.83
(T-32550) (M-20300) (M-20500)
D4-31A41 Hypoplasia of right heart 746.84
(T-32001) (M-21300)
D4-31A42 Uhl's disease 746.84
(T-32520) (M-21300) (M-26710)
Hypoplasia of right ventricle 746.84
(T-32520) (M-21300) (M-26710)
Uhl's anomaly 746.84
(T-32520) (M-21300) (M-26710)
Parchment right ventricle 746.84
(T-32520) (M-21300) (M-26710)
D4-31B00 Congenital heart block 746.86
(T-32800) (M-20030)
D4-31B02 Congenital complete atrioventricular block 746.86
(T-32820) (M-20031)
Congenital complete AV block 746.86
(T-32820) (M-20031)
D4-31B04 Congenital incomplete atrioventricular block 746.86
(T-32810) (M-20032)
Congenital incomplete AV block 746.86
(T-32820) (M-20032)
D4-31B10 Congenital malposition of heart, NOS 746.87
(T-32000) (M-22100)
Abnormal position of heart, NOS
D4-31B11 Congenital malposition of cardiac apex 746.87
(T-32004) (M-22100)
D4-31B12 Ectopia cordis 746.87
(T-32000) (M-22100) (T-.....)
Ectopic heart 746.87
(T-32000) (M-22100) (T-.....)
D4-31B14 Abdominal heart 746.87
(T-32000) (M-22100) (T-D4000)
D4-31B16 Dextrocardia 746.87
(T-32000) (M-22110) (T-D3201)
Heart in right chest 746.87
(T-32000) (M-22110) (T-D3201)
D4-31B18 Isolated dextrocardia 746.87
(T-32000) (M-22110) (T-D3201)
D4-31B20 Levocardia, NOS 746.87
(T-32000) (T-D3202)
Sinistrocardia, NOS 746.87
(T-32000) (T-D3202)
D4-31B22 Isolated levocardia 746.87
(T-32000) (M-00360) (T-D4030) (M-22110)
Isolated sinistrocardia 746.87
(T-32000) (M-00360) (T-D4030) (M-22110)
D4-31B24 Mesocardia 746.87
(T-32004) (M-22100) (T-D2002)
Heart in central chest 746.87
(T-32004) (M-22100) (T-D2002)
D4-31B50 Congenital atresia of cardiac vein 746.89
(T-48400) (M-20400)
D4-31B52 Congenital hypoplasia of cardiac vein 746.89
(T-48400) (M-21300)
D4-31B53 Chiari's network 746.89
(T-32262) (M-26300)
Remnants of valves of sinus venosus 746.89
(T-32262) (M-26300)
Atrial anomalous bands 746.89
(T-32262) (M-26300)
D4-31B54 Congenital enlargement of coronary sinus
(T-48410) (M-20500)
D4-31B56 Congenital absence of coronary sinus
(T-48410) (M-21000)
D4-31B60 Anomalous muscle bands of right ventricle
(T-32520) (M-20000)
D4-31B62 Anomalous muscle bands of left ventricle
(T-32620) (M-20000)
D4-31C00 Congenital cardiomegaly 746.89
(T-32000) (M-20500)

4-31 CONGENITAL ANOMALIES OF THE HEART — Continued

D4-31C10 Congenital diverticulum of left ventricle 746.89
(T-32600) (M-26710)

D4-31C20 Congenital rhabdomyoma of heart
(T-32000) (M-89030)
Congenital diffuse rhabdomyoma of heart
(T-32000) (M-89030)
Diffuse rhabdomyomatosis of heart
(T-32000) (M-89030)

4-32 CONGENITAL ANOMALIES OF THE AORTA AND CORONARY ARTERIES

D4-32000 Congenital anomaly of aorta, NOS 747.20
(T-42000) (M-20000)

D4-32010 Congenital anomaly of aortic arch, NOS 747.21
(T-42300) (M-20000)

D4-32012 Patent ductus arteriosus 747.0
(T-F5645) (M-26400)
Patent ductus Botalli 747.0
(T-F5645) (M-26400)
Persistent ductus arteriosus 747.0
(T-F5645) (M-26400)

D4-32014 Coarctation of aorta 747.1
(T-42000) (M-20310)

D4-32016 Preductal coarctation of aorta 747.10
(T-42340) (M-20310)
Adult-type coarctation 747.10
(T-42340) (M-20310)

D4-32018 Postductal coarctation of aorta 747.10
(T-42350) (M-20310)
Infantile type coarctation 747.10
(T-42350) (M-20310)

D4-32020 Congenital hypoplasia of aortic arch 747.10
(T-42300) (M-21300)
Tubular hypoplasia of aortic arch 747.10
(T-42300) (M-21300)

D4-32022 Congenital hypoplasia of ascending aorta 747.10
(T-42100) (M-21300)

D4-32024 Interruption of aortic arch 747.11
(T-42300) (M-20400)
Congenital atresia of aortic arch 747.11
(T-42300) (M-20400)

D4-32026 Aortic septal defect 745.0
(T-42100) (T-44000) (T-32150)
(M-20000) (M-20700)
Aorticopulmonary septal defect 745.0
(T-42100) (T-44000) (T-32150)
(M-20000) (M-20700)
Aorticopulmonary window 745.0
(T-42100) (T-44000) (T-32150)
(M-20000) (M-20700)

D4-32100 Dextraposition of aorta 747.21
(T-42000) (M-22110)
Right-sided aorta 747.21
(T-42000) (M-22110)

D4-32104 Dextraposition of ductus arteriosus 747.21
(T-F5645) (M-22110)
Right-sided ductus arteriosus 747.21
(T-F5645) (M-22110)

D4-32106 Right aortic arch 747.21
(T-43200) (M-22160) (T-26100)

D4-32110 Double aortic arch 747.21
(T-42300) (M-22360)

D4-32112 Double ductus arteriosus
(T-F5645) (M-22360)

D4-32114 Kommerell's diverticulum 747.21
(T-46110) (M-24631) (T-42300)
(M-21750)

D4-32120 Overriding aorta 747.21
(T-42300) (M-22160) (T-44000)
(T-48500)

D4-32122 Persistent convolutions of aortic arch 747.21
(T-42300) (M-20120)

D4-32124 Vascular ring of aorta 747.21
(T-42300) (M-22100) (T-56000)
(T-25000)

D4-32200 Congenital atresia of aorta 747.22
(T-42000) (M-20400)

D4-32202 Congenital stenosis of aorta 747.22
(T-42000) (M-20300)
Congenital stricture of aorta 747.22
(T-42000) (M-20300)

D4-32204 Congenital absence of aorta 747.22
(T-42000) (M-21000)
Congenital aplasia of aorta 747.22
(T-42000) (M-21000)

D4-32206 Congenital hypoplasia of aorta 747.22
(T-42000) (M-21300)

D4-32230 Congenital aneurysm of sinus of Valsalva 747.29
(T-42200) (M-24610)

D4-32232 Congenital aneurysm of aorta 747.29
(T-42000) (M-24610)

D4-32234 Congenital dilatation of aorta 747.29
(T-42000) (M-26710)

D4-32240 Aortic left ventricular tunnel
(T-42100) (T-32600) (M-20700)

D4-32500 Congenital anomaly of coronary artery, NOS 746.85
(T-43000) (M-20000)

D4-32501 Anomalous origin of coronary artery 746.85
(T-43000) (M-24631)

D4-32502 Anomalous communication of coronary artery 746.85
(T-43000) (M-24630)

D4-32503 Congenital coronary artery fistula
(T-43000) (M-24640)
Congenital coronary arteriovenous fistula
(T-43000) (M-24640)

D4-32505 Congenital absence of coronary artery 746.85
(T-43000) (M-21000)

D4-32507 Origin of left circumflex artery from right coronary artery
(T-43120) (T-43200) (M-24631)

D4-32508 Coronary artery arising from aorta 746.85
(T-43000) (M-24631) (T-42000)

D4-32511 Coronary artery arising from main pulmonary artery 746.85
(T-43000) (M-24631) (T-44000)

D4-32512 Single coronary artery 746.85
(T-43000) (M-20620)

4-33 CONGENITAL ANOMALIES OF THE PULMONARY VESSELS

D4-33100 Congenital anomaly of pulmonary artery, NOS 747.3
(T-44000) (M-20000)

D4-33110 Agenesis of pulmonary artery 747.3
(T-44000) (M-21000)
Congenital absence of pulmonary artery 747.3
(T-44000) (M-21000)

D4-33112 Congenital absence of right pulmonary artery 747.3
(T-44200) (M-21000)

D4-33114 Congenital absence of left pulmonary artery 747.3
(T-44400) (M-21000)

D4-33116 Congenital atresia of pulmonary artery 747.3
(T-44000) (M-20400)

D4-33120 Coarctation of pulmonary artery 747.3
(T-44000) (M-20310)

D4-33122 Congenital hypoplasia of pulmonary artery 747.3
(T-44000) (M-21300)

D4-33124 Congenital stenosis of pulmonary artery 747.3
(T-44000) (M-20300)

D4-33130 Anomalous origin of pulmonary artery
(T-44000) (M-24631)

D4-33140 Congenital pulmonary arteriovenous aneurysm 747.3
(T-44000) (M-24640)

D4-33500 Congenital anomaly of pulmonary veins, NOS 747.40
(T-48580) (M-20000)

D4-33510 Congenital stenosis of pulmonary veins
(T-48500) (M-20300)

D4-33600 Anomalous pulmonary venous drainage, NOS 747.41
(T-48580) (M-24660) (T-32200)

D4-33602 Total anomalous pulmonary venous return 747.41
(T-48580) (M-24660) (T-32200)
TAPVR 747.41
(T-48580) (M-24660) (T-32200)

D4-33604 Supradiaphragmatic total anomalous pulmonary venous return 747.41
(T-48580) (M-24660) (T-48300)

D4-33610 Anomalous pulmonary venous drainage to right atrium 747.41
(T-48500) (M-24660) (T-32200)

D4-33612 Anomalous pulmonary venous drainage to coronary sinus 747.41
(T-48500) (M-24660) (T-48410)

D4-33614 Anomalous pulmonary venous drainage to superior vena cava 747.41
(T-48500) (M-24660) (T-48610)

D4-33616 Subdiaphragmatic total anomalous pulmonary venous return 747.41
(T-48480) (M-24660) (M-48000) (T-D4000)

D4-33618 Anomalous pulmonary venous drainage to hepatic veins 747.41
(T-48500) (M-24660) (T-48720)

D4-33620 Anomalous pulmonary venous drainage to abdominal portion of inferior vena cava 747.41
(T-48500) (M-24660) (T-48700)

D4-33622 Partial anomalous pulmonary venous connection 747.42
(T-48500) (M-24660) (T-32200)
Partial anomalous pulmonary venous return 747.42
(T-48500) (M-24660) (T-32200)

D4-33630 Transposition of pulmonary veins, NOS 747.49
(T-48580) (M-22110)

4-34 CONGENITAL ANOMALIES OF THE VENAE CAVAE

D4-34000 Congenital anomaly of vena cava, NOS 747.40
(T-48600) (M-20000)

D4-34001 Congenital absence of vena cava 747.49
(T-48600) (M-21000)

D4-34002 Congenital stenosis of vena cava 747.49
(T-48600) (M-20300)

D4-34100 Congenital anomaly of superior vena cava, NOS 747.49
(T-48610) (M-20000)

D4-34101 Congenital absence of superior vena cava 747.49
(T-48610) (M-21000)

D4-34110 Congenital stenosis of superior vena cava 747.49
(T-48610) (M-20300)

D4-34120 Persistent left superior vena cava 747.49
(T-48611) (M-26400)

D4-34121 Scimitar syndrome 747.49
(T-48501) (M-24660) (T-48710)

D4-34500 Congenital anomaly of inferior vena cava, NOS 747.49
(T-48710) (M-20000)

D4-34501 Congenital absence of inferior vena cava 747.49
(T-48710) (M-21000)

D4-34510 Congenital stenosis of inferior vena cava 747.49
(T-48710) (M-20300)

4-36 CONGENITAL ANOMALIES OF THE ARTERIES

D4-36000 Congenital anomaly of artery, NOS 747.6
(T-41000) (M-20000)

D4-36010 Congenital absence of artery, NOS 747.6
(T-41000) (M-21000)

D4-36012 Congenital atresia of artery, NOS 747.6
(T-41000) (M-20400)

D4-36014 Congenital stricture of artery, NOS 747.6
(T-41000) (M-20300)

D4-36020 Angioectopia 747.6
(T-41000) (M-26000)
Ectopic arteries 747.6
(T-41000) (M-26000)

D4-36030 Double artery 747.6
(T-41000) (M-22360)

D4-36100 Peripheral congenital aneurysm 747.6
(T-41000) (M-24610)

D4-36110 Peripheral congenital arteriovenous aneurysm 747.6
(T-30300) (M-24640)

D4-36200 Congenital anomaly of cerebrovascular system, NOS 747.81
(T-40500) (M-20000)
Congenital anomaly of cerebral vessels, NOS 747.81
(T-40500) (M-20000)

D4-36202 Congenital anomaly of cerebral artery, NOS 747.81
(T-45510) (M-20000)

D4-36204 Congenital cerebral arteriovenous aneurysm 747.81
(T-40500) (M-24640)

D4-36210 Congenital aneurysm of anterior communicating artery 747.81
(T-45530) (M-24610)
Berry aneurysm of anterior communicating artery 747.81
(T-45530) (M-24610)

D4-36300 Congenital anomaly of umbilical artery, NOS 747.5
(T-F1810) (M-20000)

D4-36301 Single umbilical artery 747.5
(T-F1810) (M-20620)

D4-36302 Congenital absence of umbilical artery 747.5
(T-F1810) (M-21000)

D4-36303 Congenital hypoplasia of umbilical artery 747.5
(T-F1810) (M-21300)

D4-36401 Persistent omphalomesenteric artery 747.5
(T-F5610) (M-26400)

D4-36410 Anomalous origin of right subclavian artery 747.21
(T-46110) (M-24631)

D4-36414 Origin of innominate artery from left side of aortic arch 747.21
(T-46010) (T-42300) (M-24631)

D4-36501 Multiple renal arteries 747.6
(T-46600) (M-20620)

4-38 CONGENITAL ANOMALIES OF THE VEINS

D4-38000 Congenital anomaly of vein, NOS 747.6
(T-48000) (M-20000)

D4-38010 Congenital absence of vein, NOS 747.6
(T-48000) (M-21000)

D4-38020 Congenital atresia of vein, NOS 747.6
(T-48000) (M-20400)

D4-38100 Congenital phlebectasia 747.6
(T-48000) (M-26710)

D4-38110 Congenital varix 747.6
(T-48000) (M-20520) (M-26710)

D4-38120 Persistent left posterior cardinal vein 747.49
(T-F5682) (M-26400)

SECTION 4-4 CONGENITAL ANOMALIES OF THE INTEGUMENTARY SYSTEM

4-40 CONGENITAL ANOMALIES OF THE SKIN

D4-40000 Congenital anomaly of integument, NOS 757.9
(T-00000) (M-20000)
Congenital deformity of integument, NOS 757.9
(T-00000) (M-20000)

D4-40100 Congenital anomaly of skin, NOS 757.9
(T-01000) (M-20000)
Congenital cutaneous anomaly, NOS 757.9
(T-01000) (M-20000)
Genodermatosis, NOS 757.9
(T-01000) (M-20000)

D4-40102 Abnormal dermatoglyphic pattern 757.2
(T-01015) (M-20000)

D4-40104 Abnormal palmar creases 757.2
(T-01015) (T-D8740) (M-20000)

D4-40105 Congenital dermal sinus
(T-02450) (T-1151E) (T-1151F) (M-21800)

D4-40110 Congenital ichthyosis of skin, NOS 757.1
(T-01000) (M-20000) (M-59020) (M-72600)
Ichthyosis congenita 757.1
(T-01000) (M-20000) (M-59020) (M-72600)
Congenital ichthyosis 757.1
(T-01000) (M-20000) (M-59020) (M-72600)
Fish scale disease
(T-01000) (M-20000) (M-59020) (M-72600)

D4-40111 Dominant congenital ichthyosiform erythroderma 757.1
(T-01000) (M-20000) (T-59020) (M-72600)
Dominant ichthyosis vulgaris 757.1
(T-01000) (M-20000) (T-59020) (M-72600)

D4-40112 Sex-linked ichthyosis 757.1
(T-01000) (M-20000) (T-59020)
(M-72600)

D4-40114 Recessive congenital ichthyosiform erythroderma 757.1
(T-01000) (M-20000) (M-59020)
(M-72600)
Congenital non bullous ichthyosiform erythroderma 757.1
(T-01000) (M-20000) (M-59020)
(M-72600)
Lamellar ichthyosis 757.1
(T-01000) (M-20000) (M-59020)
(M-72600)

D4-40116 Erythrokeratodermia variabilis 757.1
(T-01000) (M-20000) (T-59020)
(M-72600)

D4-40118 Ichthyosis linearis circumflexa 757.1
(T-01000) (M-20000) (M-59020)
(M-72600)

D4-40120 Aplasia cutis congenita
(T-01000) (M-21000)
Epitheliogenesis imperfecta
(T-01000) (M-21000)

D4-40130 Congenital keratoderma, NOS 757.39
(T-01000) (M-72600) (M-20000)

D4-40132 Keratosis palmaris et plantaris
(T-02652) (T-02852) (M-72600)
(M-20000)
Keratoderma palmaris et plantaris
(T-02652) (T-02852) (M-72600)
(M-20000)

D4-40134 Diffuse palmoplantar keratoderma
(T-02652) (T-02852) (M-72600)
(M-20000)
Unna-Thost disease
(T-02652) (T-02852) (M-72600)
(M-20000)

D4-40140 Dyskeratosis congenita
(T-01000) (M-74430) (M-20000)
Zinsser-Cole-Engman syndrome
(T-01000) (M-74430) (M-20000)
Congenital dyskeratosis
(T-01000) (M-74430) (M-20000)

D4-40142 Hereditary benign intraepithelial dyskeratosis
(T-01000) (M-74430) (M-20000)
Witkop's disease
(T-01000) (M-74430) (M-20000)
Witkop-Von Sallmann disease
(T-01000) (M-74430) (M-20000)

D4-40160 Porokeratosis of Mibelli
(T-01000) (M-72600) (M-04200)
(M-20000)
Porokeratosis, NOS
(T-01000) (M-72600) (M-04200)
(M-20000)

D4-40162 Porokeratosis of Mibelli, plaque type
(T-01000) (M-72600) (M-04200)
(M-20000)

D4-40164 Porokeratosis of Mibelli, superficial disseminated type
(T-01000) (M-72600) (M-04200)
(M-20000)

D4-40166 Porokeratosis of Mibelli, linear unilateral type
(T-01000) (M-72600) (M-04200)
(M-20000)

D4-40168 Disseminated superficial actinic porokeratosis
(T-01000) (M-72600) (M-04200)
(M-20000)

D4-40240 Keratosis follicularis
(M-01000) (M-72600) (M-20000)
Darier's disease
(T-01000) (M-72600) (M-20000)
Dyskeratosis follicularis
(T-01000) (M-72600) (M-20000)
Darier-White disease
(T-01000) (M-72600) (M-20000)

D4-40250 Acrokeratosis verruciformis
(T-01000) (M-72600) (M-03130)
(M-20000)
Acrokeratosis verruciformis of Hopf
(T-01000) (M-72600) (M-03130)
(M-20000)

D4-40260 Familial benign pemphigus
(T-01000) (M-36750) (M-36760)
(M-20000)
Hailey-Hailey disease
(T-01000) (M-36750) (M-36760)
(M-20000)
Familial benign chronic pemphigus
(T-01000) (M-36750) (M-36760)
(M-20000)

D4-40294V Congenital skin fragility of animals

D4-40300 Vascular hamartoma of skin, NOS 757.32
(T-01000) (M-75560)

D4-40301 Birthmark of skin, NOS 757.32
(T-01000) (M-75560)

D4-40302 Port-wine stain of skin, NOS 757.32
(T-01000) (M-75560)

D4-40303 Strawberry nevus of skin, NOS 757.32
(T-01000) (M-75560)

D4-40310 Congenital cutaneous angiomatosis
(T-01000) (M-24870)

D4-40320 Connective tissue nevus of skin
(T-01000) (M-75540)
Connective tissue hamartoma of skin
(T-01000) (M-75540)

D4-40350 Congenital pigmentary anomaly of skin, NOS 757.32
(T-01000) (M-27100)

D4-40351 Congenital melanosis
(T-01000) (M-27120)

D4-40360 Congenital deficiency of pigment of skin, NOS
(T-01000) (M-27110)

D4-40366V Congenital oculocutaneous hypopigmentation
(T-01000) (T-AA000) (M-27110)

4-40 CONGENITAL ANOMALIES OF THE SKIN — Continued

D4-40370 Congenital melanocytic nevus, NOS
(T-01000) (M-87200)

D4-40372 Mongolian spot
Mongolian macula
Blue sacral spot

D4-40374 Nevus of Ito
Nevus fusoceruleus acromiodeltoideus

D4-40376 Nevus of Ota
Oculodermal malanocytosis
Nevus fusoceruleus ophthalmomaxillasis

D4-40500 Pilonidal cyst, NOS 685.-
(T-B1420) (M-26580) (M-21800)
Pilonidal fistula 685.-
(T-B1420) (M-26580) (M-21800)
Pilonidal sinus 685.-
(T-B1420) (M-26580) (M-21800)
Coccygeal fistula 685.-
(T-B1420) (M-26580) (M-21800)
Coccygeal sinus 685.-
(T-B1420) (M-26580) (M-21800)
Pilonidal cyst without mention of abscess 685.1
(T-B1420) (M-26580) (M-21800)

D4-40502 Pilonidal cyst with abscess 685.0
(T-B1420) (M-26580) (M-41610) (M-21800)

D4-40510 Congenital accessory skin tag 757.39
(T-01000) (M-76810) (M-20000)

D4-40512 Congenital scar 757.39
(T-01000) (M-78060) (M-20000)

4-41 CONGENITAL ANOMALIES OF THE HAIR AND NAILS

D4-41000 Congenital anomaly of hair, NOS 757.9
(T-01400) (M-20000)

D4-41001 Congenital alopecia 757.4
(T-01400) (M-21000)
Congenital atrichosis 757.4
(T-01400) (M-21000)
Atrichia congenita 757.4
(T-01400) (M-21000)

D4-41002 Congenital hypotrichia
(T-01400) (M-21300)

D4-41021 Congenital hypertrichosis 757.4
(T-01400) (M-20500)

D4-41031 Persistent lanugo 757.4
(T-F5495) (M-26400)

D4-41042 Monilethrix 757.4
(T-01400)
Beaded hair 757.4
(T-01400)

D4-41400 Congenital anomaly of nails, NOS 757.9
(T-01600) (M-20000)

D4-41401 Anonychia 757.5
(T-01600) (M-21000)

D4-41402 Congenital clubnail 757.5
(T-01600) (M-20630) (M-02070)

D4-41403 Congenital koilonychia 757.5
(T-01600) (M-20630) (M-02040)

D4-41404 Congenital leukonychia 757.5
(T-01600) (M-20000) (M-04020)

D4-41405 Congenital onychauxis 757.5
(T-01600) (M-20500)

D4-41407 Subungual fibroma
(T-01609) (M-88100) (M-20000)

4-42 CONGENITAL ANOMALIES OF THE SUBCUTANEOUS TISSUES

D4-42000 Congenital anomaly of subcutaneous tissue, NOS 757.9
(T-03000) (M-20000)

D4-42010 Hereditary edema of legs 757.0
(T-D9400) (M-20000) (M-36307)
(T-C6000) (M-20200)
Congenital lymphedema 757.0
(T-D9400) (M-20000) (M-36307)
(T-C6000) (M-20200)
Hereditary trophedema 757.0
(T-D9400) (M-20000) (M-36307)
(T-C6000) (M-20200)
Milroy's disease 757.0
(T-D9400) (M-20000) (M-36307)
(T-C6000) (M-20200)

D4-42020 Fordyce's disease
(T-01000) (T-01310) (M-26000)
Ectopic sebaceous gland tissue
(T-01000) (T-01310) (M-26000)
Fordyce spots
(T-01000) (T-01310) (M-26000)
Fordyce granules
(T-01000) (T-01310) (M-26000)

4-48 CONGENITAL ANOMALIES OF THE BREAST

D4-48000 Congenital anomaly of breast, NOS 757.9
(T-04000) (M-20000)

D4-48010 Congenital absence of breast 757.6
(T-04000) (M-21000)

D4-48011 Congenital absence of nipple 757.6
(T-04100) (M-21000)
Athelia 757.6
(T-04100) (M-21000)

D4-48012 Accessory breast 757.6
(T-04000) (M-22300)
Supernumerary breast 757.6
(T-04000) (M-22300)
Polymastia 757.6
(T-04000) (M-22300)

D4-48013 Accessory nipple 757.6
(T-04100) (M-22300)
Supernumerary nipple 757.6
(T-04100) (M-22300)

D4-48013 (cont.) Hyperthelia 757.6
(T-04100) (M-22300)
Polythelia 757.6
(T-04100) (M-22300)

D4-48014 Ectopic breast tissue
(T-04000) (M-26000)
Heterotopic breast tissue
(T-04000) (M-26000)

D4-48021 Congenital hypoplasia of breast 757.6
(T-04000) (M-21300)

SECTION 4-5 CONGENITAL ANOMALIES OF THE DIGESTIVE SYSTEM

4-50 CONGENITAL ANOMALIES OF THE DIGESTIVE SYSTEM: GENERAL TERMS

D4-50000 Congenital anomaly of digestive system, NOS 751.9
(T-50000) (M-20000)
Congenital deformity of digestive system, NOS 751.9
(T-50000) (M-20000)
Congenital alimentary tract anomaly, NOS 751.9
(T-50000) (M-20000)

D4-50001 Congenital absence of alimentary tract, NOS 751.8
(T-50100) (M-21000)

D4-50002 Congenital partial absence of alimentary tract, NOS 751.8
(T-50100) (M-21070)

D4-50003 Congenital duplication of digestive organs, NOS 751.8
(T-60000) (M-22360)

D4-50004 Congenital malposition of digestive organs, NOS 751.8
(T-60000) (M-22100)

D4-50020 Congenital anomaly of upper alimentary tract 750.9
(T-50110) (M-20000)
Congenital deformity of upper alimentary tract 750.9
(T-50110) (M-20000)

4-51 CONGENITAL ANOMALIES OF THE TEETH, LIPS AND PALATE

D4-51000 Congenital anomaly of teeth, NOS 520.9
(T-54010) (M-20000)

D4-51001 Dens in dente 520.2
(T-54010) (G-C006) (M-22190)
(T-54020)
Dens invaginatus 520.2
(T-54010) (G-C006) (M-22190)
(T-54020)

D4-51002 Impacted tooth 520.6
(T-54010) (M-22230)
Unerupted tooth 520.6
(T-54010) (M-22230)
Embedded tooth 520.6
(T-54010) (M-22230)

D4-51003 Hutchinson's teeth 090.5
(T-54540) (M-22080) (G-C002)
(DE-14500)
Notched incisors of Hutchinson 090.5
(T-54540) (M-22080) (G-C002)
(DE-14500)
Hutchinson's incisors 090.5
(T-54540) (M-22080) (G-C002)
(DE-14500)
Screwdriver teeth 090.5
(T-54540) (M-22080) (G-C002)
(DE-14500)

D4-51004 Mulberry molar 090.5
(T-54570) (M-20000) (G-C002)
(DE-14500)

D4-51006 Ectopic tooth 520.1
(T-54010) (M-26000)
Ectopic dentition 520.1
(T-54010) (M-26000)

D4-51007 Dentinogenesis imperfecta 520.5
(T-54890) (T-54070) (M-20020)
Odontogenesis imperfecta 520.5
(T-54890) (T-54070) (M-20020)
Dentinal dysplasia 520.5
(T-54890) (T-54070) (M-20020)

D4-51008 Shell teeth 520.5
(T-54010) (T-54070) (M-20020)

D4-51009 Amelogenesis imperfecta 520.5
(T-54890) (T-54080) (M-21300)
Congenital enamel hypoplasia 520.5
(T-54890) (T-54080) (M-21300)

D4-5100A Turner's tooth 520.4
(T-54010) (T-54080) (M-21300)

D4-51010 Anodontia, NOS 520.0
(T-54890) (M-21000)
Congenital absence of teeth, NOS 520.0
(T-54890) (M-21000)

D4-51012 Complete congenital absence of teeth 520.0
(T-54890) (M-21000)

D4-51014 Partial congenital absence of teeth 520.0
(T-54890) (M-21070)
Hypodontia 520.0
(T-54890) (M-21070)
Oligodontia 520.0
(T-54890) (M-21070)

D4-51020 Supernumerary teeth, NOS 520.1
(T-54010) (M-22300)
Supplemental teeth, NOS 520.1
(T-54010) (M-22300)
Abnormal number of teeth
(T-54010) (M-22300)

D4-51022 Distomolar 520.1
(T-54570) (M-22300)
Fourth molar 520.1
(T-54570) (M-22300)

4-51 CONGENITAL ANOMALIES OF THE TEETH, LIPS AND PALATE — Continued

D4-51022 (cont.) Paramolar 520.1
(T-54570) (M-22300)

D4-51023 Tuberculum paramolare 520.2
(T-54510) (M-22300) (M-02530)

D4-51028 Mesiodens 520.1
(T-54010) (M-22300)

D4-51030 Concrescence of teeth 520.2
(T-54010) (M-30000) (M-20000)

D4-51032 Fusion of teeth 520.2
(T-54010) (M-20100)

D4-51034 Gemination of teeth 520.2
(T-54010) (M-22300) (M-20100)

D4-51036 Dens evaginatus 520.2
(T-54010) (M-21700)

D4-51038 Enamel pearls 520.2
(T-54010) (T-54080) (M-30000)

D4-51040 Macrodontia 520.2
(T-54010) (M-02520) (M-20000)

D4-51041 Microdontia 520.2
(T-54010) (M-02530) (M-20000)

D4-51042 Peg-shaped teeth 520.2
(T-54010) (M-02010) (M-20000)
Conical teeth 520.2
(T-54010) (M-02010) (M-20000)

D4-51044 Supernumerary roots 520.2
(T-54040) (M-22300)

D4-51046 Taurodontism 520.2
(T-54570) (M-02010) (M-20000)

D4-51047 Mesotaurodontism
(T-54570) (M-02010) (M-20000)

D4-51048 Hypertaurodontism
(T-54570) (M-02010) (M-20000)

D4-51050 Mottled teeth, NOS 520.3
(T-54010) (M-01480)

D4-51051 Dental fluorosis 520.3
(T-54010) (M-01480) (G-C001)
(C-11111)

D4-51052 Mottling of enamel 520.3
(T-54080) (M-01480)

D4-51054 Non-fluoride enamel opacities 520.3
(T-54080) (M-02920) (M-20000)

D4-51060 Aplasia of cementum 520.4
(T-54090) (M-21000)

D4-51061 Hypoplasia of cementum 520.4
(T-54090) (M-21300)

D4-51062 Enamel hypoplasia 520.4
(T-54080) (M-21300)

D4-51063 Horner's teeth 520.4
(T-54540) (T-54080) (M-27000)

D4-51064 Hypocalcification of teeth 520.4
(T-54010) (M-55410)

D4-51066 Regional odontodysplasia 520.4
(T-54010) (M-20020) (G-A167)

D4-51069 Dilaceration of tooth 520.4
(T-54010) (M-14450) (M-20000)

D4-51070 Natal tooth 520.6
(T-54010) (F-51030)

D4-51072 Neonatal tooth 520.6
(T-54010) (F-51030)

D4-51074 Persistent primary tooth 520.6
(T-54890) (M-26400)
Persistent deciduous tooth 520.6
(T-54890) (M-26400)

D4-51076 Premature shedding of primary tooth 520.6
(T-54890) (F-51310)
Premature shedding of deciduous tooth 520.6
(T-54890) (F-51310)

D4-51077 Late tooth eruption 520.6
(T-54010) (F-51020)

D4-51078 Obstructed tooth eruption 520.6
(T-54010) (F-51020) (G-C008)
(M-34000)

D4-51079 Premature tooth eruption 520.6
(T-54010) (F-51030)

D4-51080 Color changes during tooth formation 520.8
(T-54010) (F-12100) (M-04010)

D4-51082 Pre-eruptive color change of tooth 520.8
(T-54010) (F-12100) (M-04010)

D4-51100 Anomaly of dental arch, NOS 524.2
(T-54150) (M-20000)

D4-51101 Malocclusion of teeth, NOS 524.4
(T-54010) (F-51160)

D4-51102 Anterior crossbite 524.2
(T-54010) (F-51160)

D4-51104 Posterior crossbite 524.2
(T-54010) (F-51160)

D4-51106 Disto-occlusion of teeth 524.2
(T-54010) (F-51170)
Distoclusion of teeth
(T-54010) (F-51170)

D4-51108 Mesio-occlusion of teeth 524.2
(T-54010) (F-51180)
Midline deviation of teeth 524.2
(T-54010) (F-51180)

D4-51110 Anterior open bite 524.2
(T-54010) (F-51180)

D4-51112 Posterior open bite 524.2
(T-54010) (F-51180)

D4-51114 Excessive overbite, NOS 524.2
(T-54010) (F-51160) (G-C008)
(M-22160)

D4-51116 Deep overbite 524.2
(T-54010) (F-51160) (G-C008)
(M-22160)

D4-51118 Horizontal overbite 524.2
(T-54010) (F-51160) (G-C008)
(M-22160)
Overjet 524.2
(T-54010) (F-51160) (G-C008)
(M-21160)

D4-51120 Vertical overbite 524.2
(T-54010) (F-51160) (G-C008)
(M-22160)

D4-51124 Posterior lingual occlusion of mandibular teeth 524.2
(T-54190) (F-51160)

D4-51126 Soft tissue impingement on teeth 524.2
(T-54010) (T-51800) (M-20500)

D4-51140 Anomaly of tooth position 524.3
(T-54010) (M-22100)

D4-51142 Crowding of teeth 524.3
(T-54010) (M-22100)

D4-51143 Diastema of teeth 524.3
(T-54010) (M-22100)
Abnormal spacing of teeth 524.3
(T-54010) (M-22100)

D4-51144 Displacement of tooth 524.3
(T-54010) (M-22110)
Transposition of tooth 524.3
(T-54010) (M-22110)

D4-51146 Rotation of tooth 524.3
(T-54010) (M-22200)

D4-51148 Impacted teeth with abnormal position 524.3
(T-54010) (M-22230) (M-22100)
Embedded teeth with abnormal position 524.3
(T-54010) (M-22230) (M-22100)

D4-51150 Congenital asymmetry of jaw, NOS 524.1
(T-D1213) (M-20000) (M-02540)

D4-51160 Congenital prognathism, NOS
(T-D1213) (M-22146)
Prognathia
(T-D1213) (M-22146)
Exognathia
(T-D1213) (M-22146)
Progenia
(T-D1213) (M-22146)

D4-51162 Mandibular prognathism 524.1
(T-11180) (M-22146)
Undershot jaw
(T-11180) (M-22146)
Prominent chin
(T-11180) (M-22146)
Bulldog jaw
(T-11180) (M-22146)

D4-51164 Maxillary prognathism 524.1
(T-11170) (M-22146)

D4-51166 Mandibular retrognathism 524.1
(T-11180) (M-22145)

D4-51168 Maxillary retrognathism 524.1
(T-11170) (M-22145)

D4-51170 Congenital macrognathism, NOS
(T-D1213) (M-20500)
Congenital macrognathia, NOS
(T-D1213) (M-20500)

D4-51172 Congenital mandibular hyperplasia 524.0
(T-11180) (M-20500)
Mandibular macrognathism 524.0
(T-11180) (M-20500)

D4-51174 Congenital maxillary hyperplasia 524.0
(T-11170) (M-20500)
Maxillary macrognathism 524.0
(T-11170) (M-20500)

D4-51180 Congenital micrognathism, NOS
(T-D1213) (M-21300)
Congenital micrognathia, NOS
(T-D1213) (M-21300)

D4-51182 Congenital mandibular hypoplasia 524.0
(T-11180) (M-21300)
Mandibular micrognathism 524.0
(T-11180) (M-21300)

D4-51183V Brachygnathism
Overshot jaw
Parrot mouth

D4-51184 Congenital maxillary hypoplasia 524.0
(T-11170) (M-21300)
Maxillary micrognathism 524.0
(T-11170) (M-21300)

D4-51300 Cleft palate, NOS 749.0
(T-51100) (M-21500)
Uranoschisis 749.0
(T-51100) (M-21500)
Palatoschisis
(T-51100) (M-21500)

D4-51301 Complete unilateral cleft palate 749.01
(T-51100) (M-21503)

D4-51302 Incomplete unilateral cleft palate 749.02
(T-51100) (M-21504)

D4-51303 Uranostaphyloschisis 749.0
(T-51120) (T-51110) (M-21500)

D4-51307 Complete bilateral cleft palate 749.03
(T-51100) (M-21505)

D4-51308 Incomplete bilateral cleft palate 749.04
(T-51100) (M-21506)

D4-51320 Congenital short hard palate
(T-51110) (M-20601)

D4-51322 Submucous cleft of hard palate
(T-51110) (M-21500)

D4-51400 Cleft lip, NOS 749.10
(T-52000) (M-21500)
Cheiloschisis 749.10
(T-52000) (M-21500)
Congenital fissure of lip 749.10
(T-52000) (M-21500)
Harelip 749.10
(T-52000) (M-21500)
Labium leporinum 749.10
(T-52000) (M-21500)

D4-51401 Complete unilateral cleft lip 749.11
(T-52000) (M-21503)

D4-51402 Incomplete unilateral cleft lip 749.11
(T-52000) (M-21504)

D4-51406 Complete bilateral cleft lip 749.11
(T-52000) (M-21505)

D4-51408 Incomplete bilateral cleft lip 749.11
(T-52000) (M-21506)

D4-51450 Cleft palate with cleft lip, NOS 749.20
(T-51100) (T-52000) (M-21500)

D4-51451 Complete unilateral cleft palate with cleft lip 749.21
(T-51100) (T-52000) (M-21503)

4-51 CONGENITAL ANOMALIES OF THE TEETH, LIPS AND PALATE — Continued

D4-51452 Incomplete unilateral cleft palate with cleft lip 749.21
(T-51100) (T-52000) (M-21504)
D4-51453 Complete bilateral cleft palate with cleft lip 749.21
(T-51100) (T-52000) (M-21505)
D4-51454 Incomplete bilateral cleft palate with cleft lip 749.21
(T-51100) (T-52000) (M-21506)
D4-51460 Cheilognathoschisis
(T-52200) (T-D1213) (M-21500)
Cleft lip and cleft jaw
(T-52200) (T-D1213) (M-21500)
D4-51461 Cheilognathopalatoschisis
(T-52100) (T-D1214) (T-51100) (M-21500)
Cheilognathouranoschisis
(T-52100) (T-D1214) (T-51100) (M-21500)
Cleft upper lip, upper jaw and palate
(T-52100) (T-D1214) (T-51100) (M-21500)
D4-51462 Cheilognathoprosoposchisis
(T-D1200) (T-52100) (T-D1214) (M-21500)
Oblique facial cleft to upper lip and upper jaw
(T-D1200) (T-52100) (T-D1214) (M-21500)
D4-51470 Congenital fistula of lip 750.25
(T-52000) (M-21800)
D4-51472 Congenital lip pits 750.25
(T-52000) (M-22080)
D4-51474 Congenital hyperplasia of sebaceous glands of lip
(T-52000) (T-01310) (M-20500)
D4-51475 Congenital macrocheilia 744.81
(T-52000) (M-20500)
Congenital hypertrophy of lip 744.81
(T-52000) (M-20500)
D4-51476 Congenital microcheilia 744.82
(T-52000) (M-20610)
D4-51478 Synchilia
(T-52000) (M-20100)
Syncheilia
(T-52000) (M-20100)
D4-51510 Gingival odontogenic cyst 523.8
(T-54910) (M-26520)
Gingival cyst 523.8
(T-54910) (M-26520)
D4-51511 Gingival cyst of newborn 523.8
(T-54910) (M-26520)
D4-51512 Gingival cyst of adult 523.8
(T-54910) (M-26520)
D4-51520 Dentigerous cyst 526.0
(T-D1213) (M-26520)
Dentigerous cyst of jaw 526.0
(T-D1213) (M-26520)
Dentigerous odontogenic cyst 526.0
(T-D1213) (M-26520)
D4-51524 Eruption cyst 526.0
(T-D1213) (M-26520)
Follicular cyst of jaw 526.0
(T-D1213) (M-26520)
Eruption cyst of jaw 526.0
(T-D1213) (M-26520)
Follicular eruption of cyst of jaw 526.0
(T-D1213) (M-26520)
Eruptive odontogenic cyst 526.0
(T-D1213) (M-26520)
D4-51525 Periodontal cyst
Periodontal odontogenic cyst
D4-51526 Lateral developmental cyst of jaw 526.0
(T-D1213) (M-26520)
Lateral periodontal cyst of jaw 526.0
(T-D1213) (M-26520)
D4-51528 Primordial cyst 526.0
(T-D1213) (M-26520)
Primordial cyst of jaw 526.0
(T-D1213) (M-26520)
Keratocyst of jaw 526.0
(T-D1213) (M-26520)
Primordial odontogenic cyst 526.0
(T-D1213) (M-26520)
D4-51532 Globulo-maxillary cyst 526.1
(T-11170) (M-26600)
Maxillary fissural cyst 526.1
(T-11170) (M-26600)
D4-51534 Naso-palatine duct cyst 526.1
(T-F6945) (M-26600)
Median anterior maxillary cyst 526.1
(T-F6945) (M-26600)
Incisive canal cyst 526.1
(T-F6945) (M-26600)
D4-51536 Median palatal cyst 526.1
(T-51110) (M-26600)
Palatine cyst of papilla 526.1
(T-51110) (M-26600)
D4-51538 Naso-labial cyst 528.4
(T-52001) (M-26600)
Naso-alveolar cyst 528.4
(T-52001) (M-26600)
D4-51539 Median mandibular cyst 526.1
(T-11180) (M-26600)
D4-51540 Epstein's pearl of mouth 528.4
(T-51110) (T-51111) (M-33420)
D4-51544V Temporal odontoma

4-52 CONGENITAL ANOMALIES OF THE TONGUE, SALIVARY GLANDS AND PHARYNX

D4-52000 Congenital anomaly of tongue, NOS 750.10
(T-53000) (M-20000)
D4-52001 Tongue tie 750.0
(T-53410) (M-20602)
Ankyloglossia 750.0
(T-53410) (M-20602)

D4-52002 Aglossia 750.11
(T-53000) (M-21000)

D4-52003 Congenital adhesions of tongue 750.12
(T-53000) (M-20130)

D4-52004 Fissure of tongue 750.13
(T-53000) (M-22080)

D4-52005 Bifid tongue 750.13
(T-53000) (M-22030)
Double tongue 750.13
(T-53000) (M-22030)

D4-52007 Trifid tongue
(T-53000) (M-22040)

D4-52011 Macroglossia 750.15
(T-53000) (M-20500)
Congenital hypertrophy of tongue 750.15
(T-53000) (M-20500)

D4-52014 Microglossia 750.16
(T-53000) (M-21300)
Congenital hypoplasia of tongue 750.16
(T-53000) (M-21300)

D4-52020 Persistent tuberculum impar 529.2
(T-F5775) (M-26400)
Glossitis rhomboidea mediana 529.2
(T-F5775) (M-26400)
Median rhomboid glossitis 529.2
(T-F5775) (M-26400)

D4-52050V Epitheliogenesis imperfecta lingua bovis
(T-53100) (T-53210) (M-21000)
Bovine smooth tongue
(T-53100) (T-53210) (M-21000)

D4-52052V Bird tongue

D4-52060V Lethal glossopharyngeal defect
(T-53000) (T-55000) (M-20000)

D4-52400 Congenital anomaly of salivary gland, NOS

D4-52401 Congenital absence of salivary gland 750.21
(T-61000) (M-21000)

D4-52402 Accessory salivary gland 750.22
(T-61000) (M-22300)

D4-52404 Atresia of salivary duct 750.23
(T-61080) (M-20400)
Imperforate salivary duct 750.23
(T-61080) (M-20400)

D4-52406 Ectopic parotid gland tissue
(T-61100) (M-26000)

D4-52408 Congenital fistula of salivary gland 750.24
(T-61080) (M-21800)

D4-52600 Congenital anomaly of pharynx, NOS
(T-55000) (M-20000)

D4-52610 Congenital absence of uvula 750.26
(T-51130) (M-21000)

D4-52612 Cleft uvula 749.02
(T-51130) (M-21500)
Bifid uvula 749.02
(T-51130) (M-21500)

D4-52620 Congenital diverticulum of pharynx 750.27
(T-55000) (M-21750)
Pharyngeal pouch 750.27
(T-55000) (M-21750)

D4-52630 Congenital atresia of pharynx 750.29
(T-55000) (M-20400)
Imperforate pharynx 750.29
(T-55000) (M-20400)

D4-52650 Rathke's pouch cyst 253.8
(T-B1410) (M-26500)

4-55 CONGENITAL ANOMALIES OF THE ESOPHAGUS AND STOMACH

D4-55000 Congenital anomaly of esophagus, NOS
(T-56000) (M-20000)

D4-55001 Congenital absence of esophagus 750.3
(T-56000) (M-21000)

D4-55002 Congenital atresia of esophagus 750.3
(T-56000) (M-20400)
Imperforate esophagus 750.3
(T-56000) (M-20400)

D4-55005 Congenital stenosis of esophagus 750.3
(T-56000) (M-20300)
Congenital esophageal ring 750.3
(T-56000) (M-20300)
Congenital stricture of esophagus 750.3
(T-56000) (M-20300)

D4-55008 Congenital web of esophagus 750.3
(T-56000) (M-20110)

D4-55011 Congenital dilatation of esophagus 750.4
(T-56000) (M-26710)

D4-55013 Congenital displacement of esophagus 750.4
(T-56000) (M-22100)

D4-55015 Congenital diverticulum of esophagus 750.4
(T-56000) (M-21750)
Esophageal pouch 750.4
(T-56000) (M-21750)

D4-55016 Congenital cyst of esophagus 750.4
(T-56000) (M-26500)

D4-55017 Congenital duplication of esophagus 750.4
(T-56000) (M-22360)

D4-55019 Giant esophagus 750.4
(T-56000) (M-20500)

D4-55100 Congenital esophagobronchial fistula 750.3
(T-56000) (T-26000) (M-21800)
Congenital bronchoesophageal fistula 750.3
(T-56000) (T-26000) (M-21800)

D4-55102 Congenital esophagotracheal fistula 750.3
(T-56000) (T-25000) (M-21800)
Congenital tracheoesophageal fistula 750.3
(T-56000) (T-25000) (M-21800)

D4-55103 H-type congenital tracheoesophageal fistula 750.3
(T-56000) (T-25000) (M-21800)

D4-55200 Vascular compression of esophagus by aberrant artery, NOS
(T-56000) (M-01460) (G-C001)
(T-41000) (M-26000)

D4-55201 Vascular compression of esophagus by aberrant right subclavian artery arising from descending aorta
(T-56000) (M-01460) (G-C001)
(T-46110) (M-26000) (G-C006)
(T-42400)

4-55 CONGENITAL ANOMALIES OF THE ESOPHAGUS AND STOMACH — Continued

D4-55500 Congenital anomaly of stomach, NOS
(T-57000) (M-20000)

D4-55510 Congenital hiatus hernia 750.6
(T-D3420) (M-21700)
Congenital displacement of cardia through esophageal hiatus 750.6
(T-57300) (T-D3420) (M-21700)

D4-55511 Congenital cardiospasm 750.7
(T-56315) (F-11310)

D4-55513 Gastric atresia
(T-57000) (M-20400)

D4-55521 Congenital hourglass stomach 750.7
(T-57122) (M-20300)

D4-55523 Congenital displacement of stomach 750.7
(T-57000) (M-22100)

D4-55525 Congenital diverticulum of stomach 750.7
(T-57000) (M-21750)

D4-55527 Congenital duplication of stomach 750.7
(T-57000) (M-22360)

D4-55528 Congenital megalogastria 750.7
(T-57000) (M-20500)

D4-55529 Congenital microgastria 750.7
(T-57000) (M-20610)
Congenital gastric hypoplasia 750.7
(T-57000) (M-20610)

D4-55530 Congenital gastric perforation
(T-57000) (M-20075) (F-88000)
Neonatal gastric perforation
(T-57000) (M-20075) (F-88000)

D4-55531 Congenital transposition of stomach 750.7
(T-57000) (M-22110)

D4-55542 Ectopic gastric tissue
(T-57000) (M-26000)
Gastric heterotopia
(T-57000) (M-26000)

D4-55543 Ectopic pancreatic tissue in stomach
(T-65000) (M-26000) (T-57000)
Pancreatic rests in stomach
(T-65000) (M-26000) (T-57000)

D4-55550 Congenital volvulus of stomach, NOS
(T-65000) (M-20200) (M-22200)

D4-55551 Congenital organoaxial volvulus of stomach
(T-65000) (M-20200) (M-22200)

D4-55552 Congenital mesenteroaxial volvulus of stomach
(T-65000) (M-20200) (M-22200)

D4-55602 Pyloric atresia
(T-57700) (M-20400)

D4-55604 Pyloric antral atresia
(T-57600) (M-20400)

D4-55610 Congenital hypertrophic pyloric stenosis 750.5
(T-57700) (M-20500) (M-20200)

D4-55612 Congenital constriction of pylorus 750.5
(T-57700) (M-20300)
Congenital stricture of pylorus 750.5
(T-57700) (M-20300)
Congenital stenosis of pylorus 750.5
(T-57700) (M-20300)
Congenital spasm of pylorus 750.5
(T-57700) (M-20300)

D4-55614 Congenital hypertrophy of pylorus 750.5
(T-57700) (M-20500)

D4-55622 Congenital pyloric membrane
(T-57700) (M-22000)

D4-55624 Congenital pyloric antral membrane
(T-57600) (M-22000)
Prepyloric septum
(T-57600) (M-22000)

4-56 CONGENITAL ANOMALIES OF THE INTESTINES

D4-56000 Congenital anomaly of lower alimentary tract 751.8
(T-50120) (M-20000)
Congenital deformity of lower alimentary tract 751.8
(T-50120) (M-20000)

D4-56001 Congenital malrotation of intestine
(T-50500) (M-22200)

D4-56002 Congenital anomaly of fixation of intestine, NOS
(T-50500) (M-22175)

D4-56004 Congenital duplication of intestine 751.5
(T-50500) (M-22360)

D4-56005 Long tubular intestinal duplication 751.5
(T-50500) (M-22360)

D4-56008 Transposition of intestine 751.5
(T-50500) (M-22110)

D4-56010 Ectopic intestinal mucosa
(T-50510) (M-26000)

D4-56100 Congenital anomaly of small intestine, NOS
(T-58000) (M-20000)

D4-56110 Congenital absence of small intestine 751.1
(T-58000) (M-21000)

D4-56112 Congenital obstruction of small intestine 751.1
(T-58000) (M-20200)

D4-56113 Congenital atresia of small intestine 751.1
(T-58000) (M-20400)

D4-56114 Congenital stenosis of small intestine 751.1
(T-58000) (M-20300)
Congenital stricture of small intestine 751.1
(T-58000) (M-20300)

D4-56120 Congenital atresia of duodenum 751.1
(T-58200) (M-20400)

D4-56122 Congenital atresia of jejunum 751.1
(T-58400) (M-20400)
Imperforate jejunum 751.1
(T-58400) (M-20400)

D4-56124 Congenital atresia of ileum 751.1
(T-58600) (M-20400)

D4-56128 Megaloduodenum 751.5
(T-58200) (M-20500)

D4-56130 Congenital omphalocele 553.1
(T-D4300) (T-D4220) (M-21500)
(T-58000) (M-21700)
Omphalocele 553.1
(T-D4300) (T-D4220) (M-21500)
(T-58000) (M-21700)

D4-56132 Omphalocele with obstruction 552.1
(T-D4300) (M-D4220) (T-21500)
(T-58000) (M-21700) (M-20200)
Incarcerated omphalocele 552.1
(T-D4300) (T-D4220) (M-21500)
(T-58000) (M-21700) (M-20200)
Irreducible omphalocele 552.1
(T-D4300) (T-D4220) (M-21500)
(T-58000) (M-21700) (M-20200)
Strangulated omphalocele 552.1
(T-D4300) (T-D4220) (M-21500)
(T-58000) (M-21700) (M-20200)

D4-56134 Gangrenous omphalocele 551.1
(T-D4300) (T-D4220) (M-21500)
(T-58000) (M-21700) (M-54600)

D4-56140 Omphalomesenteric duct cyst
(T-F1450) (M-26500)
Vitelline duct cyst
(T-F1450) (M-26500)

D4-56144 Meckel's diverticulum 751.0
(T-F1450) (M-26400) (T-58600)
Persistent omphalomesenteric duct 751.0
(T-F1450) (M-26400) (T-58600)
Persistent vitelline duct 751.0
(T-F1450) (M-26400) (T-58600)
Persistent intestinal end of vitelline duct 751.0
(T-F1450) (M-26400) (T-58600)

D4-56150 Congenital duodenal obstruction, NOS
(T-58200) (M-20200)

D4-56151 Complete congenital duodenal obstruction
(T-58200) (M-20201)

D4-56152 Partial congenital duodenal obstruction
(T-58200) (M-20202)

D4-56154 Congenital duodenal obstruction due to malrotation of intestine
(T-58200) (M-20200) (G-C001)
(T-58000) (M-22200)

D4-56155 Congenital duodenal obstruction due to annular pancreas
(T-58200) (M-20200) (G-C001)
(T-65000) (M-02100)

D4-56159 Congenital duodenal stenosis
(T-58200) (M-20300)

D4-56160 Duplication of duodenum
(T-58200) (M-22360)

D4-56500 Congenital anomaly of large intestine, NOS
(T-59000) (M-20000)

D4-56510 Congenital absence of large intestine 751.2
(T-59000) (M-21000)

D4-56512 Congenital atresia of colon 751.2
(T-59300) (M-20400)

D4-56514 Congenital obstruction of large intestine 751.2
(T-59000) (M-20200)

D4-56520 Malrotation of cecum 751.4
(T-59100) (M-22200)

D4-56522 Mobile cecum
(T-59100) (M-22200) (M-22175)

D4-56524 Failure of rotation of cecum 751.4
(T-59100) (M-22201)

D4-56525 Failure of rotation of colon 751.4
(T-59300) (M-22201)

D4-56526 Malrotation of colon 751.4
(T-59300) (M-22200)

D4-56530 Congenital diverticulum of colon 751.5
(T-59300) (M-21750)

D4-56532 Dolichocolon 751.5
(T-59300) (M-20604)

D4-56534 Congenital duplication of cecum 751.5
(T-59100) (M-22360)

D4-56535 Microcolon 751.5
(T-59300) (M-20610)

D4-56538 Transposition of colon 751.5
(T-59300) (M-22110)

D4-56539 Congenital duplication of colon

D4-56540 Congenital anomaly of appendix, NOS
(T-59200) (M-20000)

D4-56541 Congenital absence of appendix 751.2
(T-59200) (M-21000)

D4-56542 Congenital duplication of appendix 751.5
(T-59200) (M-22360)

D4-56544 Megaloappendix 751.5
(T-59200) (M-20500)

D4-56545 Transposition of appendix 751.5
(T-59200) (M-22110)

D4-56550 Congenital mesocolic hernia
(T-D4520) (M-21700)

D4-56560 Hirschsprung's disease 751.3
(T-59300) (M-26710) (T-A9840)
(M-21000)
Aganglionosis of colon 751.3
(T-59300) (M-26710) (T-A9840)
(M-21000)
Congenital megacolon 751.3
(T-59300) (M-26710) (T-A9840)
(M-21000)
Macrocolon 751.3
(T-59300) (M-26710) (T-A9840)
(M-21000)
Aganglionosis of Auerbach's plexus 751.3
(T-59300) (M-26710) (T-A9840)
(M-21000)

D4-56562 Congenital dilatation of colon 751.3
(T-59300) (M-26710)

D4-56800 Congenital anomaly of rectum, NOS

D4-56810 Congenital absence of rectum 751.2
(T-59600) (M-21000)

D4-56812 Congenital atresia of rectum 751.2
(T-59600) (M-20400)
Imperforate rectum 751.2
(T-59600) (M-20400)

4-56 CONGENITAL ANOMALIES OF THE INTESTINES — Continued

D4-56814 Congenital prolapsed rectum
(T-59600) (M-22170)

D4-56816 Congenital stricture of rectum 751.2
(T-59600) (M-20300)

D4-56820 Anorectal anomaly, NOS
(T-59600) (T-59900) (M-20000)

D4-56821 Congenital anoperineal fistula
(T-59900) (T-D2700) (M-21800)

D4-56822 Congenital anourethral fistula
(T-59900) (T-75000) (M-21800)

D4-56823 Congenital rectourethral fistula
(T-59600) (T-75000) (M-21800)

D4-56824 Congenital rectovesical fistula
(T-59600) (T-74000) (M-21800)

D4-56825 Congenital rectovestibular fistula
(T-59600) (T-81270) (M-21800)

D4-56826 Congenital rectovaginal fistula
(T-59600) (T-82000) (M-21800)

D4-56827 Congenital rectocloacal fistula
(T-59600) (T-F6630) (M-21800)

D4-56828 Anorectal agenesis
(T-59600) (T-59900) (M-21000)

D4-56829V Congenital rectovaginal constriction of Jersey cattle

D4-56830 Persistent cloaca 751.5
(T-F5430) (M-26400)

D4-56900 Congenital anomaly of anus, NOS
(T-59900) (M-20000)

D4-56910 Congenital absence of anus 751.2
(T-59900) (M-21000)

D4-56912 Congenital atresia of anus 751.2
(T-59900) (M-20400)
Imperforate anus 751.2
(T-59900) (M-20400)
Anal atresia 751.2
(T-59900) (M-20400)
Atresia ani 751.2
(T-59900) (M-20400)

D4-56914 Congenital occlusion of anus 751.2
(T-59900) (M-20200)

D4-56916 Congenital stricture of anus 751.2
(T-59900) (M-20300)
Anal stenosis 751.2
(T-59600) (M-20300)

D4-56920 Congenital duplication of anus 751.5
(T-59900) (M-22360)

D4-56922 Ectopic anus 751.5
(T-59900) (M-22100)

D4-56A10 Congenital adhesions of omentum 751.4
(T-D4600) (M-20150)

D4-56A12 Congenital adhesions of peritoneum 751.4
(T-D4400) (M-20150)

D4-56A14 Jackson's membrane 751.4
(T-50500) (M-20110) (M-20200)

D4-56A20 Universal mesentery 751.4
(T-D4500) (M-20000)

D4-56A30 Peritoneal cyst 568.89
(T-D4400) (M-26500)

D4-56A32 Mesenteric cyst 568.89
(T-D4500) (M-26500)

D4-56A34 Omental cyst 568.89
(T-D4600) (M-26500)

4-57 CONGENITAL ANOMALIES OF THE BILIARY TRACT, GALLBLADDER AND LIVER

D4-57000 Congenital anomaly of bile ducts, NOS 751.60
(T-60610) (M-20000)

D4-57010 Congenital biliary atresia 751.61
(T-60610) (M-20400)

D4-57011 Congenital atresia of extrahepatic bile duct 751.61
(T-64000) (M-20400)

D4-57012 Congenital absence of bile duct 751.61
(T-60610) (M-21000)

D4-57013 Congenital hypoplasia of bile duct 751.61
(T-60610) (M-21300)

D4-57014 Congenital hyperplasia of intrahepatic bile duct 751.61
(T-62110) (M-21300)

D4-57015 Congenital obstruction of bile duct 751.61
(T-60610) (M-20200)

D4-57016 Congenital stricture of bile duct 751.61
(T-60610) (M-20300)

D4-57017 Congenital dilatation of lobar intrahepatic bile duct
(T-62110) (M-26700)
Caroli's disease
(T-62110) (M-26700)

D4-57021 Congenital choledochal cyst 751.69
(T-64500) (M-26700)
Congenital common duct cyst 751.69
(T-64500) (M-26700)
Congenital biliary duct cyst 751.69
(T-64500) (M-26700)
Choledochocyst 751.69
(T-64500) (M-26700)
Congenital cystic dilatation of common bile duct 751.69
(T-64500) (M-26700)

D4-57022 Congenital duplication of biliary duct 751.69
(T-60610) (M-22360)

D4-57023 Congenital duplication of cystic duct 751.69
(T-64400) (M-22360)

D4-57400 Congenital anomaly of gallbladder, NOS 751.60
(T-63000) (M-20000)

D4-57410 Congenital duplication of gallbladder 751.69
(T-63000) (M-22360)

D4-57412 Congenital absence of gallbladder 751.69
(T-63000) (M-21000)

D4-57414 Congenital septation of gallbladder
(T-63000) (M-22000)
Phrygian cap
(T-63000) (M-22000)

D4-57414 (cont.) Hourglass gallbladder
(T-63000) (M-22000)

D4-57418 Multiseptate gallbladder
(T-63000) (M-22060)

D4-57420 Floating gallbladder 751.69
(T-63000) (M-22175)

D4-57440 Intrahepatic gallbladder 751.69
(T-63000) (M-22100)

D4-57442 Ectopic gallbladder
(T-63000) (M-26000)

D4-57450 Congenital hepatic fibrosis 751.62
(T-62000) (M-78000) (M-20000)

D4-57600 Congenital anomaly of liver, NOS 751.60
(T-62000) (M-20000)

D4-57610 Congenital cystic disease of liver 751.62
(T-62000) (M-26700)
Congenital polycystic disease of liver 751.62
(T-62000) (M-26700)
Fibrocystic disease of liver 751.62
(T-62000) (M-26700)

D4-57611 Congenital absence of liver 751.69
(T-62000) (M-21000)

D4-57612 Congenital absence of lobe of liver 751.69
(T-62...) (M-21000)

D4-57620 Accessory hepatic duct 751.69
(T-64000) (M-22300)

D4-57622 Accessory liver 751.69
(T-62000) (M-22300)

D4-57630 Congenital liver grooves
(T-62000) (M-22080)

D4-57640 Congenital hepatomegaly 751.69
(T-62000) (M-20500)

D4-57642 Congenital duplication of liver 751.69
(T-62000) (M-22360)

D4-57650 Floating liver 751.69
(T-62000) (M-22175)

4-58 CONGENITAL ANOMALIES OF THE PANCREAS

D4-58000 Congenital anomaly of pancreas, NOS 751.7
(T-65000) (M-20000)

D4-58001 Congenital absence of pancreas 751.7
(T-65000) (M-21000)
Agenesis of pancreas 751.7
(T-65000) (M-21000)

D4-58002 Congenital hypoplasia of pancreas 751.7
(T-65000) (M-21300)

D4-58011 Accessory pancreas 751.7
(T-65000) (M-22300)

D4-58014 Ectopic pancreas 751.7
(T-65000) (M-26000)
Pancreatic heterotopia 751.7
(T-65000) (M-26000)

D4-58015 Ectopic pancreas in duodenum
(T-65000) (M-26000) (T-58200)

D4-58021 Annular pancreas 751.7
(T-65000) (M-20000) (T-58200) (M-02100)

D4-58030 Pancreas divisum
(T-65010) (M-21500)

SECTION 4-6 CONGENITAL ANOMALIES OF THE ENDOCRINE GLANDS

4-600 Congenital Anomalies of The Endocrine Glands: General Terms

D4-60000 Congenital anomaly of endocrine gland, NOS
(T-B0000) (M-20000)
Congenital anomaly of endocrine organ, NOS
(T-B0000) (M-20000)

4-601 Congenital Anomalies of The Adrenal Glands

D4-60100 Congenital anomaly of adrenal gland, NOS 759.1
(T-B3000) (M-20000)

D4-60101 Congenital absence of adrenal gland 759.1
(T-B3000) (M-21000)
Adrenal aplasia 759.1
(T-B3000) (M-21000)

D4-60102 Accessory adrenal gland 759.1
(T-B3000) (M-22300)

D4-60103 Ectopic adrenal gland 759.1
(T-B3000) (M-26000)
Aberrant adrenal gland 759.1
(T-B3000) (M-26000)

D4-60104 Ectopic adrenal cortex
(T-B3100) (M-26000)
Adrenal rest
(T-B3100) (M-26000)

D4-60105 Accessory adrenal cortex
(T-B3100) (M-22300)

4-602 Congenital Anomalies of The Parathyroid Glands

D4-60200 Congenital anomaly of parathyroid glands, NOS
(T-B7000) (M-20000)

D4-60201 Congenital absence of parathyroid gland 759.2
(T-B7000) (M-21000)

D4-60202 Accessory parathyroid gland 759.2
(T-B7000) (M-22300)

4-603 Congenital Anomalies of The Thyroid Gland

D4-60300 Congenital anomaly of the thyroid gland, NOS
(T-B6000) (M-20000)

D4-60310 Accessory thyroid gland
(T-B6000) (M-22300)

D4-60320 Ectopic thyroid tissue
(T-B6000) (M-26000)
Aberrant thyroid tissue
(T-B6000) (M-26000)

4-603 Congenital Anomalies of The Thyroid Gland — Continued

D4-60321 Lingual thyroid
(T-B6000) (M-26000) (T-53000)

D4-60322 Cervical thyroid remnant
(T-B6000) (M-26400) (T-D1602)

D4-60330 Persistent thyroglossal duct 759.2
(T-F5785) (M-26400)
Thyrolingual fistula 759.2
(T-F5785) (M-26400)

D4-60334 Thryroglossal duct cyst 759.2
(T-F5785) (M-26500)

4-604 Congenital Anomalies of The Pituitary Gland

D4-60400 Congenital anomaly of putuitary gland, NOS
(T-B1000) (M-20000)

D4-60482 Ectopic pituitary tissue
(T-B1000) (M-26000)

D4-60483 Pharyngeal pituitary tissue
(T-B1000) (M-26000) (T-55000)

SECTION 4-7 CONGENITAL ANOMALIES OF THE URINARY SYSTEM

4-70 CONGENITAL ANOMALIES OF THE URINARY SYSTEM: GENERAL TERMS

D4-70000 Congenital anomaly of the urinary system, NOS 753.9
(T-70000) (M-20000)
Congenital anomaly of urinary tract, NOS 753.9
(T-70000) (M-20000)
Congenital deformity of urinary tract, NOS 753.9
(T-70000) (M-20000)

D4-70100 Congenital urogenital anomaly, NOS
(T-70200) (M-20000)

4-71 CONGENITAL ANOMALIES OF THE KIDNEYS

D4-71000 Congenital anomaly of the kidney, NOS
(T-71000) (M-20000)

D4-71010 Congenital atrophy of kidney 753.0
(T-71000) (M-20065)

D4-71012 Unilateral agenesis of kidney
(T-71000) (M-21080)

D4-71014 Congenital hypoplasia of kidney 753.0
(T-71000) (M-21300)

D4-71016 Ask-Upmark kidney
(T-71000) (M-21370)
Partial congenital hypoplasia of kidney
(T-71000) (M-21370)

D4-71018 Oligomeganephronic hypoplasia of kidney
(T-71000) (T-71400) (M-20500)
(M-20620) (M-05130)

D4-71040 Accessory kidney 753.3
(T-71000) (M-22300)

D4-71044 Nodular renal blastema
(T-F5370) (M-26400)

D4-71050 Congenital calculus of kidney 753.3
(T-71000) (M-20000) (M-30000)

D4-71100 Congenital malposition of kidney 753.3
(T-71000) (M-22100)

D4-71102 Pelvic kidney
(T-71000) (M-26000) (T-D6000)

D4-71110 Ectopic kidney 753.3
(T-71000) (M-26000)

D4-71112 Crossed renal ectopia 753.3
(T-71000) (M-26000)

D4-71120 Double kidney and pelvis 753.3
(T-71000) (T-72000) (M-22360)

D4-71122 Double kidney
(T-71000) (M-22360)

D4-71124 Congenital fusion of kidneys 753.3
(T-71000) (M-20100)

D4-71126 Horseshoe kidney 753.3
(T-71000) (M-20100) (M-20630)

D4-71130 Giant kidney 753.3
(T-71000) (M-20500)

D4-71132 Congenital hyperplasia of kidney 753.3
(T-71000) (M-20680)

D4-71134 Discoid kidney 753.3
(T-71000) (M-20630)

D4-71136 Congenital lobulation of kidney 753.3
(T-71000) (M-22020)
Fetal lobulation of kidney
(T-71000) (M-22020)

D4-71140 Malrotation of kidney 753.3
(T-71000) (M-22200)

D4-71300 Congenital cystic kidney disease 753.1
(T-71000) (M-26700)
Multiple congenital cysts of kidney 753.1
(T-71000) (M-26700)
Congenital fibrocystic kidney 753.1
(T-71000) (M-26700)
Congenital polycystic kidney disease 753.1
(T-71000) (M-26700)
Sponge kidney 753.1
(T-71000) (M-26700)
Multicystic dysplastic kidney 753.1
(T-71000) (M-26700)

D4-71310 Polycystic kidney disease, adult type 753.1
(T-71000) (M-26700)
Autosomal dominant adult polycystic kidney disease 753.1
(T-71000) (M-26700)

D4-71320 Polycystic kidney disease, infantile type 753.1
(T-71000) (M-26700)
Autosomal recessive infantile polycystic kidney disease 753.1
(T-71000) (M-26700)

D4-71340 Medullary cystic disease of the kidney
(T-71070) (M-26700)
Medullary cystic kidney
(T-71070) (M-26700)
Medullary sponge kidney
(T-71070) (M-26700)
Familial juvenile nephronophthisis
(T-71070) (M-26700)

D4-71346 Microcystic renal disease
(T-71000) (M-26700)

D4-71350 Congenital renal dysplasia, NOS
(T-71000) (M-20020)

D4-71500 Congenital anomaly of renal pelvis, NOS
(T-72000) (M-20000)

D4-71510 Trifid pelvis of kidney 753.3
(T-72000) (M-22040)

D4-71520 Congenital hydronephrosis 753.2
(T-72000) (M-26720)

D4-71530 Double renal pelvis
(T-72000) (M-22360)

4-73 CONGENITAL ANOMALIES OF THE URETERS

D4-73000 Congenital anomaly of ureter, NOS
(T-73000) (M-20000)

D4-73002 Congenital atresia of ureter 753.2
(T-73000) (M-20400)
Impervious ureter 753.2
(T-73000) (M-20400)

D4-73004 Congenital occlusion of ureter 753.2
(T-73000) (M-20200)

D4-73006 Congenital stricture of ureter 753.2
(T-73000) (M-20300)

D4-73010 Congenital hydroureter 753.2
(T-73000) (M-26720)

D4-73012 Congenital megaloureter 753.2
(T-73000) (M-20500)

D4-73014 Congenital dilatation of ureter 753.2
(T-73000) (M-26710)

D4-73020 Congenital absence of ureter 753.4
(T-73000) (M-21000)

D4-73022 Accessory ureter 753.4
(T-73000) (M-22300)

D4-73024 Double ureter 753.4
(T-73000) (M-22100)

D4-73026 Ectopic ureter 753.4
(T-73000) (M-26000)

D4-73030 Congenital deviation of ureter 753.4
(T-73000) (M-22100)

D4-73032 Displaced ureteric orifice 753.4
(T-74320) (M-22100)

D4-73100 Congenital stricture of ureteropelvic junction 753.2
(T-73003) (M-20300)

D4-73110 Congenital stricture of ureterovesical orifice 753.2
(T-74320) (M-20300)

D4-73112 Ureterocele 753.2
(T-73000) (M-21750) (T-74320) (M-20300)

D4-73120 Congenital hypertrophy of ureteric valve
(T-73003) (M-20500)

D4-73130 Anomalous implantation of ureter 753.4
(T-73000) (T-D4300) (M-20000)

4-74 CONGENITAL ANOMALIES OF THE BLADDER

D4-74000 Congenital anomaly of the bladder, NOS
(T-74000) (M-20000)

D4-74002 Congenital absence of bladder 753.8
(T-74000) (M-21000)

D4-74010 Congenital obstruction of bladder neck 753.6
(T-74400) (M-20200)

D4-74020 Accessory bladder 753.8
(T-74000) (M-22300)

D4-74030 Congenital diverticulum of bladder 753.8
(T-74000) (M-21750)

D4-74050 Congenital hernia of bladder 753.8
(T-74000) (M-21700)

D4-74060 Congenital prolapse of bladder 753.8
(T-74000) (M-21170)

4-75 CONGENITAL ANOMALIES OF THE URETHRA

D4-75000 Congenital anomaly of urethra, NOS
(T-75000) (M-20000)

D4-75010 Congenital obstruction of urethra 753.6
(T-75000) (M-20200)
Impervious urethra 753.6
(T-75000) (M-20200)

D4-75020 Congenital stricture of urethra 753.6
(T-75000) (M-20300)

D4-75030 Urethral valve formation 753.6
(T-75000) (M-20120)
Congenital posterior urethral valve 753.6
(T-75000) (M-20120)

D4-75040 Congenital absence of urethra 753.8
(T-71500) (M-21000)

D4-75050 Accessory urethra 753.8
(T-75000) (M-22300)

D4-75060 Double urethra 753.8
(T-75000) (M-22360)

D4-75070 Congenital prolapse of urethra 753.8
(T-75000) (M-21170)

D4-75080 Congenital stricture of vesicourethral orifice 753.6
(T-74410) (M-20300)

D4-75210 Congenital stricture of urinary meatus 753.6
(T-75180) (M-20300)

D4-75220 Atresia of urinary meatus
(T-75180) (M-20400)
Imperforate urinary meatus 753.6
(T-75180) (M-20400)
Imperforate urethral meatus
(T-75180) (M-20400)

4-75 CONGENITAL ANOMALIES OF THE URETHRA — Continued

D4-75230 Double urinary meatus 753.8
(T-75180) (M-22360)

D4-75280 Congenital urethrorectal fistula 753.8
(T-75000) (T-59600) (M-21800)

D4-75500 Congenital cyst of urachus 753.7
(T-F6625) (M-26400) (M-26500)
Congenital urachal cyst 753.7
(T-F6625) (M-26400) (M-26500)

D4-75510 Congenital fistula of urachus 753.7
(T-F6625) (M-26400) (M-21800)

D4-75520 Patent urachus 753.7
(T-F6625) (M-26400)
Persistent urachus 753.7
(T-F6625) (M-26400)
Persistent umbilical sinus 753.7
(T-F6625) (M-26400)

SECTION 4-8 CONGENITAL ANOMALIES OF THE MALE AND FEMALE GENITAL SYSTEMS

4-80 CONGENITAL ANOMALIES OF THE GENITAL SYSTEMS: GENERAL CONDITIONS

D4-80000 Congenital anomaly of genital organ, NOS 752.9
(T-70250) (T-90000) (M-20000)
Congenital deformity of genital organ, NOS 752.9
(T-70250) (T-90000) (M-20000)

D4-80001 Streak gonad, NOS
(T-70255) (M-21300)

D4-80002 Ovotestis 752.7
(T-87000) (T-94000) (M-20100)

D4-80003 Ambiguous genitalia
(T-70250) (M-00001)

D4-80024 Persistent urogenital sinus
(T-F6650) (M-26400)

D4-80100 Hermaphroditism 752.7
(T-94000) (T-87000) (M-20000)
Gynandrism 752.7
(T-94000) (T-87000) (M-20000)
True hermaphroditism 752.7
(T-94000) (T-87000) (M-20000)
Pure gonadal dysgenesis 752.7
(T-94000) (T-87000) (M-20000)

D4-80110 Pseudohermaphroditism 752.7
(T-94000) (T-87000) (M-20000)

D4-80130 Female pseudohermaphroditism 752.7
(T-70255) (T-87000) (M-20000)

D4-80140 Macrogenitosomia praecox 255.2
(T-70250) (M-20500)
Epiphyseal syndrome 255.2
(T-70250) (M-20500)
Pineal syndrome 255.2
(T-70250) (M-20500)

D4-80150 Male pseudohermaphroditism 752.7
(T-70255) (T-94000) (M-20000)

4-81-83 CONGENITAL ANOMALIES OF THE FEMALE GENITAL SYSTEM

4-810 Congenital Anomalies of The Genital System: General Terms

D4-81000 Congenital anomaly of female genital system, NOS
(T-80000) (M-20000)

D4-81020 Congenital anomaly of external female genitalia, NOS 752.40
(T-80010) (M-20000)

4-811 Congenital Anomalies of The Ovaries

D4-81100 Congenital anomaly of ovary, NOS 752.0
(T-87000) (M-20000)

D4-81101 Congenital absence of ovary 752.0
(T-87000) (M-21000)

D4-81102 Accessory ovary 752.0
(T-87000) (M-22300)
Supernumerary ovary 752.0
(T-87000) (M-22300)

D4-81103 Ectopic ovary 752.0
(T-87000) (M-26000)

D4-81104 Streak ovary 752.0
(T-87000) (M-21300)

4-813-814 Congenital Anomalies of The Fallopian Tubes and Broad Ligaments

D4-81300 Congenital anomaly of fallopian tubes, NOS 752.10
(T-88000) (M-20000)

D4-81302 Congenital absence of fallopian tube 752.19
(T-88000) (M-21000)

D4-81304 Congenital atresia of fallopian tube 752.19
(T-88000) (M-20400)

D4-81310 Accessory fallopian tube 752.19
(T-88000) (M-22300)

D4-81400 Congenital anomaly of broad ligament 752.10
(T-D6500) (M-20000)

D4-81402 Congenital absence of broad ligament 752.19
(T-D6500) (M-21000)

D4-81404 Accessory broad ligament 752.19
(T-D6500) (M-22300)

D4-81410 Congenital atresia of broad ligament 752.19
(T-D6500) (M-20400)

4-815 Cysts of Female Embryonic Structures

D4-81510 Embryonic cyst of epoophoron 752.11
(T-F6450) (M-26500) (M-26370)

D4-81520 Embryonic cyst of Gartner's duct 752.11
(T-F6460) (M-26500) (M-26370)
Gartner's duct cyst 752.11
(T-F6460) (M-26500) (M-26370)

D4-81520 (cont.) Kobelt's cyst 752.11
(T-F6460) (M-26500) (M-26370)

D4-81524 Embryonic fimbrial cyst 752.11
(T-F6450) (T-88220) (M-26500) (M-26380)
Parovarian cyst 752.11
(T-F6450) (T-88220) (M-26500) (M-26380)

4-82 CONGENITAL ANOMALIES OF THE UTERUS

D4-82000 Congenital uterine anomaly, NOS
(T-83000) (M-20000)
Anomalous uterus
(T-83000) (M-20000)
Congenital abnormal uterus, NOS
(T-83000) (M-20000)

D4-82002 Congenital absence of uterus 752.3
(T-83000) (M-21000)
Congenital aplasia of uterus 752.3
(T-83000) (M-21000)
Agenesis of uterus 752.3
(T-83000) (M-21000)

D4-82004V Segmental uterine aplasia
White heifer disease

D4-82010 Uterus arcuatus
(T-83000)
Arcuate uterus
(T-83000)

D4-82012 Uterus acollis
(T-83000)

D4-82014 Bicornuate uterus 752.3
(T-83030) (M-20000)
Bicornate uterus
(T-83030)
Uterus bicornis
(T-83030)

D4-82015 Uterus bicornuatus vetularum
(T-83030)

D4-82016 Uterus unicornis 752.3
(T-83030) (M-20620)

D4-82018 Uterus bicornis unicollis
(T-83030)

D4-82020 Uterus bicornis bicollus
(T-83030)

D4-82024 Uterus bicameratus vetularum
(T-83000)

D4-82030 Congenital duplication of uterus 752.2
(T-83000) (M-22360)
Didelphic uterus 752.2
(T-83000) (M-22360)
Uterus didelphys 752.2
(T-83000) (M-22360)

D4-82034 Uterus incudiformis
(T-83000)

D4-82038 Uterus biforus
(T-83000)

D4-82040 Cochleate uterus
(T-83000)

D4-82042 Uterus cordiformis
(T-83000)
Cordate uterus
(T-83000)

D4-82044 Fetal uterus
(T-83000)

D4-82046 Infantile uterus
(T-83000)

D4-82052 Uterus parvicollis
(T-83000)

D4-82054 Uterus bilocularis
(T-83000)
Septate uterus
(T-83000)
Bipartite uterus
(T-83000)

D4-82058 Uterus subseptus
(T-83000)
Subseptate uterus
(T-83000)

D4-82080 Congenital prolapsed uterus
(T-83000) (M-22170)

D4-82500 Congenital anomaly of cervix, NOS 752.40
(T-83200) (M-20000)

D4-82502 Congenital absence of cervix 752.49
(T-83200) (M-21000)

D4-82511 Congenital duplication of cervix 752.2
(T-83200) (M-22360)
Double cervix 752.2
(T-82300) (M-22360)

D4-82512 Congenital stenosis of cervical canal 752.49
(T-83260) (M-20300)

4-83 CONGENITAL ANOMALIES OF THE VAGINA AND VULVA

D4-83000 Congenital anomaly of vagina, NOS 752.40
(T-82000) (M-20000)

D4-83002 Congenital absence of vagina 752.49
(T-82000) (M-21000)

D4-83004 Congenital duplication of vagina 752.2
(T-82000) (M-22360)

D4-83010 Septate vagina
(T-82000) (M-22000)

D4-83020 Congenital stenosis of vagina 752.49
(T-82000) (M-20300)

D4-83030 Embryonal cyst of vagina 752.41
(T-82000) (M-26500)

D4-83040 Imperforate vagina
(T-82000) (M-20400)

D4-83500 Congenital anomaly of vulva, NOS
(T-81000) (M-20000)

D4-83510 Imperforate hymen 752.42
(T-82400) (M-20400)

D4-83520 Congenital cyst of vulva 752.41
(T-81000) (M-26500)

4-83 CONGENITAL ANOMALIES OF THE VAGINA AND VULVA — Continued

D4-83530 Congenital cyst of canal of Nuck 752.41
(T-D7061) (M-26500)

D4-83540 Congenital absence of vulva 752.49
(T-81000) (M-21000)

D4-83560 Synechia vulvae
(T-81280) (M-20100)

D4-83570 Congenital absence of clitoris 752.49
(T-81400) (M-21000)

4-85 CONGENITAL ANOMALIES OF THE MALE GENITAL SYSTEM

4-850 Congenital Anomalies of The Male Genital System: General Terms

D4-85000 Congenital anomaly of male genital system, NOS
(T-90000) (M-20000)

4-851 Congenital Anomalies of The Testes

D4-85100 Congenital anomaly of testis, NOS
(T-94000) (M-20000)

D4-85110 Undescended testis 752.5
(T-94000) (M-26000) (M-22230)
Undescended testicle 752.5
(T-94000) (M-26000) (M-22230)
Ectopic testis 752.5
(T-94000) (M-26000) (M-22230)
Cryptorchism 752.5
(T-94000) (M-26000) (M-22230)
Cryptorchidism 752.5
(T-94000) (M-26000) (M-22230)

D4-85114 Pseudocryptorchism 752.5
(T-94000) (M-26000) (M-22230)

D4-85120 Congenital hypoplasia of testis 752.8
(T-94000) (M-21300)
Streak testis 752.8
(T-94000) (M-21300)

D4-85122 Congenital absence of testis 752.8
(T-94000) (M-21000)
Anorchism 752.8
(T-94000) (M-21000)
Congenital aplasia of testis 752.8
(T-94000) (M-21000)
Anorchia 752.8
(T-94000) (M-21000)
Male agonadism 752.8
(T-94000) (M-21000)
Anorchidism 752.8
(T-94000) (M-21000)

D4-85124 Testicular regression syndrome 752.8
(T-94000) (M-21000) (T-91000) (M-21300)
Vanishing testes syndrome 752.8
(T-94000) (M-21000) (T-91000) (M-21300)

D4-85130 Congenital fusion of testis 752.8
(T-94000) (M-20100)
Synorchism 752.8
(T-94000) (M-20100)

D4-85132 Monorchism 752.8
(T-94000) (M-20620)
Monorchidism 752.8
(T-94000) (M-20620)

D4-85140 Polyorchism 752.8
(T-94000) (M-22300)
Polyorchidism 752.8
(T-94000) (M-22300)
Supernumerary testis 752.8
(T-94000) (M-22300)

D4-85150 Congenital absence of germinal epithelium of testes 752.8
(T-94120) (M-21000)
Germinal aplasia 752.8
(T-94120) (M-21000)
Sertoli-cell-only syndrome 752.8
(T-94120) (M-21000)

D4-85154 Leydig cell agenesis 752.8
(T-94210) (M-21000)
Leydig cell dysgenesis 752.8
(T-94210) (M-21000)
Gonadotropin unresponsiveness syndrome 752.8
(T-94210) (M-21000)

4-853 Congenital Anomalies of The Penis

D4-85300 Congenital anomaly of penis, NOS
(T-91000) (M-20000)

D4-85310 Congenital absence of penis 752.8
(T-91000) (M-21000)

D4-85320 Congenital hypoplasia of penis 752.8
(T-91000) (M-21300)

D4-85330 Congenital chordee 752.6
(T-91000) (M-22142)

D4-85334 Congenital lateral curvature of penis 752.8
(T-91000) (M-22141)

D4-85350 Hypospadias 752.6
(T-75050) (T-91002) (M-20000)

D4-85352 Epispadias 752.6
(T-75050) (T-91001) (M-20000)
Anaspadias 752.6
(T-75050) (T-91001) (M-20000)

D4-85354 Paraspadias 752.8
(T-75050) (T-91000) (M-20000)

4-854 Congenital Anomalies of The Prostate

D4-85400 Congenital anomaly of prostate, NOS
(T-92000) (M-20000)

D4-85410 Congenital absence of prostate 752.8
(T-92000) (M-21000)

4-855 Congenital Anomalies of The Spermatic Cords

D4-85500 Congenital anomaly of spermatic cord, NOS
(T-97000) (M-20000)

D4-85510 Congenital absence of spermatic cord 752.8
(T-97000) (M-21000)
Congenital aplasia of spermatic cord 752.8
(T-97000) (M-21000)

4-856 Congenital Anomalies of The Vasa Deferentia

D4-85600 Congenital anomaly of vas deferens, NOS
(T-96000) (M-20000)

D4-85610 Congenital absence of vas deferens 752.8
(T-96000) (M-21000)

D4-85620 Congenital atresia of vas deferens 752.8
(T-96000) (M-20400)

D4-85660 Congenital atresia of ejaculatory duct 752.8
(T-93070) (M-20400)

SECTION 4-9 CONGENITAL ANOMALIES OF THE NERVOUS SYSTEM

4-90 CONGENITAL ANOMALIES OF THE NERVOUS SYSTEM: GENERAL TERMS

D4-90000 Congenital anomaly of nervous system, NOS 742.9
(T-A0000) (M-20000)
Congenital deformity of nervous system, NOS 742.9
(T-A0000) (M-20000)
Congenital disease of nervous system, NOS 742.9
(T-A0000) (M-20000)
Congenital lesion of nervous system, NOS 742.9
(T-A0000) (M-20000)

D4-90020 Craniorachischisis 740.1
(T-11100) (T-11500) (M-21500)

D4-90024 Iniencephaly 740.2
(T-11106) (M-20500) (T-11510) (M-20000)
Iniencephalus 740.2
(T-11106) (M-20500) (T-11510) (M-20000)

D4-90028 Arnold-Chiari syndrome 741.0
(T-A6000) (T-A6700) (M-21700) (T-A7010)
Arnold-Chiari malformation 741.0
(T-A6000) (T-A6700) (M-21700) (T-A7010)

4-91 CONGENITAL ANOMALIES OF THE BRAIN

D4-91000 Congenital anomaly of brain, NOS 742.9
(T-A0100) (M-20000)
Deformity of brain, NOS 742.9
(T-A0100) (M-20000)
Congenital disease of brain, NOS 742.9
(T-A0100) (M-20000)
Congenital lesion of brain, NOS 742.9
(T-A0100) (M-20000)

D4-91002 Multiple anomalies of brain, NOS 742.4
(T-A0100) (M-20080)

D4-91010 Cerebral cortical dysgenesis
(T-A2020) (M-20000)

D4-91012 Hemicephaly 740.0
(T-A0110) (M-21000)
Hemicephalia 740.0
(T-A0110) (M-21000)
Hemicephalus 740.0
(T-A0110) (M-21000)
Congenital absence of cerebrum 740.0
(T-A0110) (M-21000)

D4-91014 Exencephaly

D4-91016 Hydranencephaly
Congenital absence of cerebral hemispheres

D4-91020 Encephalocele, NOS 742.0
(T-11100) (M-21600) (T-A0100) (M-21700)

D4-91022 Occipital encephalocele
(T-11140) (M-21600) (T-A0100) (M-21700)

D4-91024 Nasal encephalocele
(T-21000) (M-21600) (T-A0100) (M-21700)

D4-91026 Encephalomyelocele 742.0
(T-11106) (M-21600) (T-A0100) (T-A7010) (M-21700)

D4-91028 Encephalocystocele 742.0
(T-11100) (M-21600) (T-A0100) (M-21700) (M-26730)
Hydroencephalocele 742.0
(T-11100) (M-21600) (T-A0100) (M-21700) (M-26730)
Hydrencephalocele 742.0
(T-11100) (M-21600) (T-A0100) (M-21700) (M-26730)
Hydrocephalocele 742.0
(T-11100) (M-21600) (T-A0100) (M-21700) (M-26730)

D4-91032 Meningoencephalocele 742.0
(T-11100) (M-21600) (T-A0100) (T-A1112) (M-21700)
Encephalomeningocele 742.0
(T-11100) (M-21600) (T-A0100) (T-A1112) (M-21700)

D4-91040 Congenital meningocele, NOS 742.0
(T-A1110) (M-21700)

D4-91042 Congenital cerebral meningocele 742.0
(T-11100) (M-21600) (T-A1112) (M-21700)
Congenital cranial meningocele 742.0
(T-11100) (M-21600) (T-A1112) (M-21700)

4-91 CONGENITAL ANOMALIES OF THE BRAIN — Continued

D4-91044 Hydromeningocele, NOS 742.0
(T-.....) (M-21600) (T-A1110)
(M-21700) (M-26730)

D4-91046 Cranial hydromeningocele 742.0
(T-11100) (M-21600) (T-A1112)
(M-21700) (M-26730)
Hydrencephalomeningocele 742.0
(T-11100) (M-21600) (T-A1112)
(M-21700) (M-26730)

D4-91050 Microcephalus 742.1
(T-D1100) (M-20610)
Microcephaly 742.1
(T-D1100) (M-20610)
Micrencephaly 742.1
(T-D1100) (M-20610)

D4-91052 Hydromicrocephaly 742.1
(T-D1100) (M-20610) (T-A1000)
(M-26730)

D4-91054 Macrocephaly
(T-D1100) (M-20500)
Macrocephalus
(T-D1100) (M-20500)

D4-91056 Brachycephaly
(T-D1100) (M-20601)

D4-91100 Congenital absence of part of brain 742.2
(T-A0100) (M-21070)
Agenesis of part of brain 742.2
(T-A0100) (M-21070)
Congenital aplasia of part of brain 742.2
(T-A0100) (M-21070)

D4-91110 Agenesis of corpus callosum
(T-A2700) (M-21000)

D4-91112 Congenital hypoplasia of part of brain 742.2
(T-A0100) (M-21300)

D4-91150 Agyria 742.2
(T-A0100) (M-20610) (T-A2006)
(M-20000)

D4-91152 Microgyria 742.2
(T-A0100) (M-20000) (T-A2006)
(M-20610)
Polymicrogyria 742.2
(T-A0100) (M-20000) (T-A2006)
(M-20610)
Micropolygyria 742.2
(T-A0100) (M-20000) (T-A2006)
(M-20610)

D4-91160 Arhinencephaly 742.2
(T-A2900) (M-21000)

D4-91200 Hemispheric cerebral agenesis
(T-A2000) (M-21000)

D4-91210 Hemispheric cerebellar agenesis
(T-A6000) (M-21000)

D4-91220 Congenital hypoplasia of inner granular layer of cerebellum
(T-A6070) (M-21300)

D4-91222 Congenital pontocerebellar hypoplasia
(T-A5400) (T-A6000) (M-21300)

D4-91223V Cerebellar aplasia

D4-91224V Congenital cerebellar hypoplasia

D4-91225V Congenital cerebellar cortical atrophy
Daft lambs
Familial convulsions and ataxia

D4-91240 Cerebellar hemangioblastomatosis
(T-A6000) (M-24850)

D4-91242 Congenital leptomeningeal angiomatosis
(T-A1200) (M-24870)

D4-91300 Congenital hydrocephalus 742.3
(T-A1000) (M-26730)
Hydrocephalus in newborn 742.3
(T-A1000) (M-26730)

D4-91310 Aqueduct of Sylvius anomaly 742.3
(T-A1800) (M-20000)

D4-91312 Congenital obstruction of aqueduct of Sylvius 742.3
(T-A1800) (M-20200)

D4-91314 Congenital stenosis of aqueduct of Sylvius 742.3
(T-A1800) (M-20300)

D4-91316 Atresia of foramen of Magendie 742.3
(T-A1870) (M-20400)

D4-91318 Atresia of foramen of Luschka 742.3
(T-A1860) (M-20400)

D4-91320V Hereditary neuraxial edema
Congenital brain edema

D4-91400 Congenital cerebral cyst 742.4
(T-A0110) (M-26700)

D4-91410 Colloid cyst of third ventricle
(T-A1740) (M-26650)
Paraphyseal cyst
(T-A1740) (M-26650)
Neuroepithelial cyst
(T-A1740) (M-26650)

D4-91500 Macroencephaly 742.4
(T-D1100) (M-20500)
Megalencephaly 742.4
(T-D1100) (M-20500)

D4-91510 Macrogyria 742.4
(T-A2006) (M-20570)
Pachygyria 742.4
(T-A2006) (M-20570)

D4-91530 Congenital porencephaly 742.4
(T-A0100) (M-26700)
Schizencephaly 742.4
(T-A0100) (M-26700)
Congenital porencephalia 742.4
(T-A0100) (M-26700)
Congenital cerebral porosis 742.4
(T-A0100) (M-26700)
Schizencephalic porencephaly 742.4
(T-A0100) (M-26700)

D4-91534 Congenital pseudoporencephaly
(T-A0100) (M-26700)
Cystic pseudoporencephalic cavitation
(T-A0100) (M-26700)

D4-91600 Congenital ischemic atrophy of central nervous system structure
(T-A0090) (M-21310)

D4-91630 Ulegyria 742.4
(T-A2006) (M-20000)
Congenital ulegyria 742.4
(T-A2006) (M-20000)

D4-91700 Ectopic glial tissue
(T-A0400) (M-26000)
Ectopic neural glial masses
(T-A0400) (M-26000)

D4-91710 Nasal glial heterotopia
(T-A0400) (M-26000) (T-21000)
Nasal glioma
(T-A0400) (M-26000) (T-21000)

D4-91720 Ectopic neuronal tissue
(T-A2020) (M-26000)
Ectopic gray matter
(T-A2020) (M-26000)

D4-91722 Ectopic gray matter in centrum ovale
(T-A2020) (M-26000) (T-A2031)

D4-91750 Ecchordosis physaliphora
(T-F6410) (M-26000) (T-1114A)
(T-D1464)
Heterotopic notochordal tissue
(T-F6410) (M-26000) (T-1114A)
(T-D1464)

D4-91780 Sinus pericranii
(T-11100) (T-49802) (M-20700)

D4-91784 Dural arteriovenous malformation
(T-A1120) (M-24640)

4-95 CONGENITAL ANOMALIES OF THE SPINAL CORD

D4-95000 Congenital anomaly of spinal cord, NOS 742.9
(T-A7010) (M-20000)
Deformity of spinal cord, NOS 742.9
(T-A7010) (M-20000)
Congenital disease of spinal cord, NOS 742.9
(T-A7010) (M-20000)
Congenital lesion of spinal cord, NOS 742.9
(T-A7010) (M-20000)

D4-95030V Spinal cord dysplasia

D4-95100 Spina bifida, NOS 741.-
(T-11500) (M-21600) (T-A7010)
(T-A1115) (M-21700)

D4-95110 Spina bifida aperta 741.-
(T-11500) (M-21600) (T-A7010)
(T-A1115) (M-21700)
Spina bifida cystica 741.-
(T-11500) (M-21600) (T-A7010)
(T-A1115)

D4-95120 Spina bifida without hydrocephalus 741.9
(T-11500) (M-21600) (T-A7010)
(T-A1115) (M-21700)

D4-95122 Spina bifida of cervical region 741.1
(T-11600) (M-21600) (T-A7010)
(T-A1115) (M-21700)

D4-95124 Spina bifida of dorsal region 741.2
(T-11700) (M-21600) (T-A7010)
(T-A1115) (M-21700)

D4-95126 Spina bifida of lumbar region 741.3
(T-11900) (M-21600) (T-A7010)
(T-A1115) (M-21700)

D4-95130 Spina bifida with hydrocephalus 741.0
(T-11500) (M-21600) (T-A7010)
(T-A1112) (M-21700) (M-26730)

D4-95140 Hydromeningomyelocele
(T-11500) (M-21600) (T-A7010)
(T-A1115) (M-21700) (M-26730)
Hydromyelomeningocele
(T-11500) (M-21600) (T-A7010)
(T-A1115) (M-21700) (M-26730)

D4-95142 Hydromyelocele 741.9
(T-11500) (M-21600) (T-A7010)
(M-21700) (M-26730)

D4-95150 Congenital spinal hydromeningocele 741.9
(T-11500) (M-21600) (T-A1115)
(M-21700) (M-26730)

D4-95152 Congenital spinal meningocele 741.9
(T-11500) (M-21600) (T-A1115)
(M-21700) (M-26730)

D4-95160 Myelocele 741.9
(T-11500) (M-21600) (T-A7010)
(M-21700)
Syringomyelocele 741.9
(T-11500) (M-21600) (T-A7010)
(M-21700)
Syringocele 741.9
(T-11500) (M-21600) (T-A7010)
(M-21700)

D4-95170 Meningomyelocele 741.9
(T-11500) (M-21600) (T-A7010)
(T-A1115) (M-21700)
Myelocystocele 741.9
(T-11500) (M-21600) (T-A7010)
(T-A1115) (M-21700)
Myelomeningocele 741.9
(T-11500) (M-21600) (T-A7010)
(T-A1115) (M-21700)

D4-95200 Myeloschisis
(T-A7010) (M-21500)
Diplomyelia
(T-A7010) (M-21500)

D4-95210 Rachischisis 741.9
(T-11500) (M-21500)

D4-95220 Diastematomyelia 742.51
(T-A7010) (M-21500) (T-11000)
(M-21700)

D4-95230 Hydromyelia 742.51
(T-A7010) (M-26730)

D4-95234 Hydrorhachis 742.53
(T-11500) (M-26730)

4-95 CONGENITAL ANOMALIES OF THE SPINAL CORD — Continued

D4-95300 Amyelia 742.59
(T-A7010) (M-21000)

D4-95310 Atelomyelia 742.59
(T-A7010) (M-21300)
Congenital hypoplasia of spinal cord 742.59
(T-A7010) (M-21300)

D4-95350 Hemimyelia
(T-A7010) (M-21070)

D4-95370 Defective development of cauda equina 742.59
(T-A7900) (M-20000)

D4-95380 Myelatelia 742.59
(T-A7010) (M-21300)

D4-95386 Myelodysplasia 742.59
(T-A7010) (M-20020)

D4-95390 Congenital anomaly of spinal meninges, NOS 742.59
(T-A1115) (M-20000)

4-96 CONGENITAL ANOMALIES OF THE PERIPHERAL NERVOUS SYSTEM

D4-96000 Congenital anomaly of the peripheral nervous system, NOS
(T-A0140) (M-20000)

D4-96100 Congenital anomaly of nerve, NOS
(T-A9001) (M-20000)

D4-96110 Agenesis of nerve, NOS 742.8
(T-A9001) (M-21000)

D4-96200 Developmental displacement of brachial plexus 742.8
(T-A9090) (M-22100)

D4-96300 Familial dysautonomia 742.8
(T-A9600) (M-20000)
Riley-Day syndrome 742.8
(T-A9600) (M-20000)

D4-96304V Feline dysautonomia
Key-Gaskell syndrome
Feline autonomic polyganglionopathy

D4-96310 Jaw-winking syndrome 742.8
(T-AA810) (M-22170)
Marcus-Gunn syndrome 742.8
(T-AA810) (M-22170)

D4-96400 Aganglionosis of parasympathetic nerve ganglia, NOS
(T-A9902) (M-21000)
Congenital absence of parasympathetic ganglion cells, NOS
(T-A9902) (M-21000)

D4-96420V Hypomyelinogenesis congenita

SECTION 4-A CONGENITAL ANOMALIES OF THE EYE

D4-A0000 Congenital anomaly of eye, NOS 743.9
(T-AA000) (M-20000)
Congenital deformity of eye, NOS 743.9
(T-AA000) (M-20000)

D4-A0010 Anophthalmos, NOS 743.00
(T-AA000) (M-21000)
Clinical anophthalmos, NOS 743.00
(T-AA000) (M-21000)
Agenesis of eye 743.00
(T-AA000) (M-21000)
Congenital absence of eye 743.00
(T-AA000) (M-21000)
Anophthalmia 743.00
(T-AA000) (M-21000)

D4-A0012 Congenital cystic eyeball 743.03
(T-AA000) (M-26700)

D4-A0014 Cryptophthalmos 743.06
(T-AA000) (T-10000) (M-20500)
Cryptophthalmia 743.06
(T-AA000) (T-10000) (M-20500)

D4-A0016 Microphthalmos, NOS 743.10
(T-AA000) (M-20610)
Simple microphthalmos 743.11
(T-AA000) (M-20610)
Microphthalmia 743.10
(T-AA000) (M-20610)

D4-A0017 Microphthalmos associated with other anomalies of eye and adnexa 743.12
(T-AA000) (M-20610)

D4-A0018 Dysplasia of eye 743.1
(T-AA000) (M-20020)

D4-A0021 Hypoplasia of eye 743.1
(T-AA000) (M-21300)
Rudimentary eye 743.1
(T-AA000) (M-21300)

D4-A0050 Buphthalmos, NOS 743.20
(T-AA100) (M-20520)
Hydrophthalmos 743.20
(T-AA100) (M-20520)
Simple buphthalmos 743.21
(T-AA100) (M-20520)
Buphthalmia 743.20
(T-AA100) (M-20520)
Congenital glaucoma 743.2
(T-AA100) (T-AA200) (M-20520)
Newborn glaucoma 743.2
(T-AA100) (T-AA200) (M-20520)

D4-A0052 Buphthalmos with congenital keratoglobus 743.22
(T-AA100) (M-20520) (T-AA200) (M-20631)

D4-A0054 Buphthalmos with megalocornea 743.22
(T-AA100) (M-20520) (T-AA200) (M-20500)
Buphthalmos with macrocornea 743.22
(T-AA100) (M-20520) (T-AA200) (M-20500)

D4-A0060 Macrocornea
(T-AA200) (M-20500)
Megalocornea
(T-AA200) (M-20500)

D4-A0100 Congenital cataract, NOS 743.30
(T-AA700) (M-20520)

D4-A0102 Congenital capsular cataract 743.31
(T-AA710) (M-20520)

D4-A0104 Congenital subcapsular cataract 743.31
(T-AA701) (M-20520)

D4-A0106 Congenital cortical cataract 743.32
(T-AA720) (M-20521)

D4-A0108 Congenital zonular cataract 743.32
(T-AA730) (M-20521)
Congenital lamellar cataract 743.32
(T-AA730) (M-20521)

D4-A0110 Embryonal nuclear cataract 743.33
(T-AA702) (M-20520)

D4-A0112 Congenital total cataract 743.34
(T-AA700) (M-20520)
Congenital complete cataract 743.34
(T-AA700) (M-20520)

D4-A0116 Congenital subtotal cataract 743.34
(T-AA700) (M-20522)

D4-A0150 Congenital ectopic lens 743.37
(T-AA700) (M-26000)
Ectopia lentis 743.37
(T-AA700) (M-26000)

D4-A0154 Congenital aphakia 743.35
(T-AA700) (M-21000)
Congenital absence of lens 743.35
(T-AA700) (M-21000)

D4-A0160 Congenital anomaly of lens shape 743.36
(T-AA700) (M-20630)

D4-A0162 Microphakia 743.36
(T-AA700) (M-20610)

D4-A0164 Spherophakia 743.36
(T-AA700) (M-20631)

D4-A0180 Persistent tunica vasculosa lentis
(T-F5841) (M-26400)

D4-A0210 Microcornea 743.41
(T-AA200) (M-20610)

D4-A0220 Congenital corneal opacity interfering with vision 743.42
(T-AA200) (M-20520)

D4-A0222 Congenital corneal opacity not interfering with vision 743.43
(T-AA200) (M-20520)

D4-A0250 Congenital anomaly of anterior chamber of eye 743.44
(T-AA050) (M-20000)

D4-A0260 Axenfeld's anomaly 743.44
(T-AA500) (T-AA740) (M-20000)

D4-A0310 Aniridia 743.45
(T-AA500) (M-21000)
Irideremia 743.45
(T-AA500) (M-21000)

D4-A0314 Congenital anisocoria 743.46
(T-AA530) (M-20650)

D4-A0316 Atresia of pupil 743.46
(T-AA530) (M-20400)

D4-A0320 Congenital coloboma of iris 743.46
(T-AA500) (M-21500)

D4-A0322 Pseudocoloboma of iris
(T-AA500) (M-78060)

D4-A0326 Corectopia 743.46
(T-AA530) (M-22100)

D4-A0400 Congenital anomaly of sclera, NOS 743.47
(T-AA110) (M-20000)

D4-A0500 Congenital anomaly of vitreous body, NOS 743.51
(T-AA081) (M-20000)

D4-A0502 Congenital opacity of vitreous body 743.51
(T-AA081) (M-20520)

D4-A0504 Fundus coloboma 743.52
(T-AA635) (M-20000)
Retinochoroidal coloboma 743.52
(T-AA635) (M-20000)

D4-A0510 Persistent primary vitreous
(T-F5890) (M-26400)

D4-A0530 Congenital chorioretinal degeneration 743.53
(T-AA310) (T-AA610) (M-20070)

D4-A0550 Congenital fold of posterior segment of eye 743.54
(T-AA070) (M-20120)

D4-A0560 Congenital cyst of posterior segment of eye 743.54
(T-AA070) (M-26500)

D4-A0610 Retinal hemangioblastomatosis
(T-AA610) (M-24850)

D4-A0620 Congenital anomaly of macula, NOS 743.55
(T-AA620) (M-20000)

D4-A0630 Congenital anomaly of retina, NOS 743.56
(T-AA610) (M-20000)

D4-A0650 Congenital anomaly of optic disc 743.57
(T-AA630) (M-20000)

D4-A0654 Congenital coloboma of optic disc 743.57
(T-F5810) (M-21500)

D4-A0680 Persistent hyaloid artery
(T-F5840) (M-26400)

D4-A0684 Vestigial remnants of canal of Cloquet
(T-AA083) (M-26400)
Vestigial remnants of hyaloid canal
(T-AA083) (M-26400)

D4-A0700 Congenital vascular anomaly of eye, NOS 743.58
(T-AA000) (M-24600)

D4-A0710 Congenital retinal aneurysm 743.58
(T-AA380) (M-24610)

D4-A0800 Congenital anomaly of eyelid, NOS 743.6
(T-AA810) (M-20000)

D4-A0810 Congenital ptosis of upper eyelid 743.61
(T-AA820) (M-22170)

D4-A0820 Ablepharon 743.62
(T-AA810) (M-21000)
Complete ablepharon 743.62
(T-AA810) (M-21000)
Congenital absence of eyelid 743.62
(T-AA810) (M-21000)

SECTION 4-A CONGENITAL ANOMALIES OF THE EYE — Continued

D4-A0822 Partial ablepharon 743.62
(T-AA810) (M-21070)

D4-A0830 Accessory eyelid 743.62
(T-AA810) (M-22300)

D4-A0840 Congenital ectropion 743.62
(T-AA810) (M-22203)

D4-A0842 Congenital entropion 743.62
(T-AA810) (M-22204)

D4-A0850 Congenital ankyloblepharon
(T-AA810) (M-20100)
Ankyloblepharon totale
(T-AA810) (M-20100)

D4-A0882 Congenital absence of cilia 743.63
(T-01530) (M-21000)
Agenesis of cilia 743.63
(T-01530) (M-21000)

D4-A0900 Congenital anomaly of lacrimal system, NOS 743.6
(T-AA900) (M-20000)

D4-A0910 Congenital absence of lacrimal apparatus 743.65
(T-AA900) (M-21000)
Agenesis of lacrimal apparatus 743.65
(T-AA900) (M-21000)

D4-A0912 Congenital anomaly of lacrimal gland 743.64
(T-AA910) (M-20000)

D4-A0914 Congenital absence of punctum lacrimale 743.65
(T-AA931) (M-21000)

D4-A0916 Accessory lacrimal canal 743.65
(T-AA920) (M-22300)

D4-A0918 Accessory lacrimal gland
(T-AA910) (M-22300)

D4-A0A00 Congenital anomaly of orbit, NOS 743.66
(T-D1480) (M-20000)

D4-A0A20 Accessory eye muscle 743.69
(T-13170) (M-22300)

SECTION 4-B CONGENITAL ANOMALIES OF THE EAR, NECK AND FACE

4-B0 CONGENITAL ANOMALIES OF THE EAR

D4-B0000 Congenital anomaly of ear, NOS 744.3
(T-AB000) (M-20000)
Congenital deformity of ear, NOS 744.3
(T-AB000) (M-20000)

D4-B0001 Congenital absence of ear, NOS 744.09
(T-AB000) (M-21000) (M-20030)

D4-B0005 Pleonotia
(T-AB000) (M-22300) (T-B1600)

D4-B0010 Congenital anomaly of ear with impairment of hearing 744.00
(T-AB000) (M-20000) (G-C008)
(M-20030) (F-F5000)

D4-B0011 Congenital absence of external ear 744.01
(T-AB100) (M-21000) (G-C008)
(M-20030) (F-F5000)

D4-B0013 Congenital absence of external auditory canal 744.01
(T-AB200) (M-21000) (G-C008)
(M-20030) (F-F5000)

D4-B0014 Congenital absence of auricle with atresia of auditory canal 744.01
(T-AB105) (M-21000) (G-C008)
(T-AB200) (M-20400)

D4-B0016 Congenital absence of auricle with stenosis of auditory canal 744.01
(T-AB105) (M-21000) (G-C008)
(T-AB200) (M-20300)

D4-B0018 Congenital stricture of external auditory canal 744.02
(T-AB200) (M-20300)

D4-B0021 Congenital atresia of external auditory canal 744.02
(T-AB200) (M-20400)

D4-B0022 Double auditory canal
(T-AB200) (M-22360)

D4-B0023 Congenital anomaly of middle ear 744.03
(T-AB300) (M-20000)

D4-B0025 Congenital atresia of osseous meatus of middle ear 744.03
(T-11134) (M-20400)

D4-B0027 Congenital stricture of osseous meatus of middle ear 744.03
(T-11134) (M-20300)

D4-B0031 Congenital anomaly of ossicles of ear 744.04
(T-AB400) (M-20000)

D4-B0032 Congenital fusion of ossicles of ear 744.04
(T-AB400) (M-20100)
Congenital fixation of auditory ossicles 744.04
(T-AB400) (M-20100)

D4-B0033 Congenital absence of ossicles of ear
(T-AB400) (M-21000)

D4-B0034 Congenital anomaly of inner ear 744.05
(T-AB700) (M-20000)

D4-B0035 Congenital aplasia of inner ear
(T-AB700) (M-21000)

D4-B0036 Congenital anomaly of membranous labyrinth 744.05
(T-AB710) (M-20000)

D4-B0037 Congenital absence of membranous labyrinth
(T-AB710) (M-21000)

D4-B0038 Incomplete development of membranous labyrinth
(T-AB710) (M-21300)

D4-B0041 Congenital anomaly of organ of Corti 743.05
(T-AB840) (M-20000)

D4-B0050 Accessory auricle of ear 744.1
(T-AB105) (M-22300)

D4-B0051 Accessory tragus of ear 744.1
(T-AB130) (M-22300)
Preauricular appendage 744.1
(T-AB130) (M-22300)

D4-B0052 Congenital preauricular fistula
(T-D1156) (M-21800)
Fistula auris congenita
(T-D1156) (M-21800)

D4-B0053 Preauricular dimple
(T-D1156) (M-22080)
Congenital preauricular pit
(T-D1156) (M-22080)

D4-B0054 Polyotia 744.1
(T-AB000) (M-22300)

D4-B0055 Supernumerary external ear 744.1
(T-AB100) (M-22300)

D4-B0058 Supernumerary ear lobule 744.1
(T-AB150) (M-22300)

D4-B0061 Congenital absence of ear lobe 744.21
(T-AB150) (M-21000)

D4-B0062 Macrotia 744.22
(T-AB100) (M-20500)

D4-B0063 Microtia 744.23
(T-AB100) (M-21300)

D4-B0065 Bat ear 744.29
(T-AB100) (M-20000)

D4-B0066 Darwin's tubercle 744.29
(T-AB113) (M-20000)

D4-B0070 Congenital absence of eustachian tube 744.24
(T-AB600) (M-21000)

4-B1 CONGENITAL ANOMALIES OF THE FACE

D4-B1000 Congenital anomaly of face, NOS 744.9
(T-D1200) (M-20000)
Congenital deformity of face, NOS 744.9
(T-D1200) (M-20000)

D4-B1001 Asymmetry of face 754.0
(T-D1200) (M-20650)
Compression facies 754.0
(T-D1200) (M-20650)

D4-B1002 Potter's facies 754.0
(T-D1200) (M-20000)

D4-B1021 Congenital macrostomia 744.82
(T-51000) (M-20500)

D4-B1022 Unilateral congenital macrostomia
(T-51000) (M-20501)

D4-B1023 Bilateral congenital macrostomia
(T-51000) (M-20502)

D4-B1025 Microstomia 744.82
(T-51000) (M-20610)

4-B2 CONGENITAL ANOMALIES OF THE NECK

D4-B2000 Congenital anomaly of neck, NOS 744.9
(T-D1600) (M-20000)
Congenital deformity of neck, NOS 744.9
(T-D1600) (M-20000)

D4-B2010 Branchial cleft cyst 744.42
(T-F5500) (M-26500)
Branchial cyst 744.42
(T-F5500) (M-26500)

D4-B2011 Branchial cleft sinus 744.41
(T-F5500) (M-21800)
Branchial cleft fistula 744.41
(T-F5500) (M-21800)
Branchial vestige 744.41
(T-F5500) (M-21800)
Branchial fistula 744.41
(T-F5500) (M-21800)

D4-B2015 Cervical auricle 744.43
(T-D1606) (M-20500) (T-F5500) (M-21500)

D4-B2021 Preauricular sinus 744.46
(T-D1156) (M-21800)
Preauricular fistula 744.46
(T-D1156) (M-21800)

D4-B2022 Preauricular cyst 744.47
(T-F5510) (T-F5520) (M-21500) (M-26500)

D4-B2025 Congenital fistula of auricle 744.49
(T-AB100) (M-21800)

D4-B2026 Congenital cervicoaural fistula 744.49
(T-AB100) (T-D1600) (M-21800)

D4-B2050 Pterygium colli 744.5
(T-D1600) (T-D2220) (M-20110)
Congenital webbing of neck 744.5
(T-D1600) (T-D2220) (M-20110)

D4-B2052 Fistula colli congenita
(T-D1600) (T-55000) (M-21800)
Congenital fistula of neck
(T-D1600) (T-55000) (M-21800)

SECTION 4-C CONGENITAL ANOMALIES OF THE HEMATOPOIETIC SYSTEM

4-C0 CONGENITAL ANOMALIES OF THE HEMATOPOIETIC SYSTEM: GENERAL TERMS

D4-C0000 Congenital anomaly of the hematopoietic system, NOS

4-C1 CONGENITAL ANOMALIES OF THE SPLEEN

D4-C1000 Congenital anomaly of spleen, NOS 759.0
(T-C3000) (M-20000)

D4-C1002 Accessory spleen 759.0
(T-C3000) (M-22300)
Polysplenia 759.0
(T-C3000) (M-22300)

D4-C1003 Ectopic spleen 759.0
(T-C3000) (M-26000)
Aberrant spleen 759.0
(T-C3000) (M-26000)

D4-C1004 Ectopic splenic tissue 759.0
(T-C3000) (M-26000)

D4-C1010 Congenital splenomegaly 759.0
(T-C3000) (M-20500)

D4-C1012 Congenital lobulation of spleen 759.0
(T-C3000) (M-21500)

4-C1 CONGENITAL ANOMALIES OF THE SPLEEN — Continued

D4-C1015 Splenogonadal fusion
(T-C3000) (T-70255) (M-20100)

4-C2 CONGENITAL ANOMALIES OF THE THYMUS

D4-C2000 Congenital anomaly of the thymus, NOS
D4-C2005 Ectopic thymic tissue
(T-C8000) (M-26000)
D4-C2006 Accessory thymic tissue
(T-C8000) (M-22300)
D4-C2007 Cervical thymic remnant
(T-C8000) (M-26400) (T-D1602)

SECTION 4-D REGIONAL CONGENITAL ANOMALIES

D4-D0050 Situs ambiguus
(T-D0010)
D4-D0100 Situs inversus viscerum
(T-04030) (T-D3030) (M-22111)
Visceral inversion
(T-04030) (T-D3030) (M-22111)
D4-D0150 Situs inversus abdominalis 759.3
(T-D4030) (M-22111)
Transposition of abdominal viscera 759.3
(T-D4030) (M-22111)
Transposition of abdominal organs 759.3
(T-D4030) (M-22111)
D4-D0180 Situs inversus thoracis 759.3
(T-D3030) (M-22111)
Transposition of thoracic viscera 759.3
(T-D3030) (M-22111)
Transposition of thoracic organs 759.3
(T-D3030) (M-22111)

SECTION 4-F CONGENITAL ANOMALIES OF THE FETUS AND AFTERBIRTH

4-F0 CONGENITAL ANOMALIES OF THE FETUS

D4-F0000 Congenital anomalies of fetus, NOS
(T-F1000) (M-20000)
D4-F0010 Blighted ovum 631.-
(T-87500) (M-20000)
Pathologic ovum 631.-
(T-87500) (M-20000)
D4-F0050 Nodular embryo
(T-F5010)
D4-F0060 Cylindrical embryo
(T-F5010)
D4-F0070 Stunted embryo
(T-F5010) (M-21300)
D4-F0100 Abnormal fetus, NOS
(T-F5000) (M-20000)
D4-F0110 Fetus papyraceus 646.0
(T-F5000) (M-20000)
Fetus compressus 646.0
(T-F5000) (M-20000)
D4-F0120 Lithopedion 656.8
(T-F5000) (M-20000) (F-12100)
Osteopedion
(T-F5000) (M-20000) (F-12100)
Calcified fetus
(T-F5000) (M-20000) (F-12100)
D4-F0130 Mummified fetus
(T-F5000) (M-20000) (M-54360)
D4-F0140 Frog fetus
(T-F5000) (M-20000)
D4-F0150 Harlequin fetus 757.1
(T-F5000) (T-01000) (M-20000)
(M-59020)
Collodion baby 757.1
(T-F5000) (T-01000) (M-20000)
(M-59020)
D4-F0160 Immature fetus
(T-F5000) (M-20050)
D4-F0200 Macerated fetus
(T-F5000) (M-54315)
Macerated stillbirth
(T-F5000) (M-54315)
Fetus sanguinolentus
(T-F5000) (M-54315)

4-F1 MONSTERS

D4-F1000 Monster, NOS 759.7
(T-F5000) (M-20000)
Teratism, NOS 759.7
(T-F5000) (M-20000)
D4-F1010 Autositic monster, NOS
(T-F5000) (M-20000)
D4-F1020 Parasitic monster, NOS
(T-F5000) (M-20000)
D4-F1030 Triplet monster, NOS
(T-F5000) (M-20000)
D4-F1040 Polysomatous monster, NOS
(T-F5000) (M-20000)
D4-F1050 Abnormal fetal duplication, NOS
(T-F5000) (M-22360)
Abnormal twins, NOS
(T-F5000) (M-22360)
Abnormal twinning, NOS
(T-F5000) (M-22360)
D4-F1055 Notomelus
(T-F5000) (T-D2800) (M-22300)
(T-D2100)
D4-F1080 Ectopic fetus
(T-F5000) (M-26000)
Ectopic fetal tissue
(T-F5000) (M-26000)
D4-F1100 Single monster, NOS
(T-F5000) (M-20000)
D4-F1110 Sirenoform monster
(T-F5000) (M-20000)
Siren
(T-F5000) (M-20000)

D4-F1110 (cont.) Symmelia
(T-F5000) (M-20000)
Sympodia
(T-F5000) (M-20000)
Sympus
(T-F5000) (M-20000)
Syrenomelus
(T-F5000) (M-20000)
Sympus apus
(T-F5000) (M-20000)
Symmelus
(T-F5000) (M-20000)

D4-F1120 Cyclopic monster, NOS
(T-F5000) (M-20000)
Cyclops
(T-F5000) (M-20000)
Cyclocephaly
(T-F5000) (M-20000)
Cyclopia
(T-F5000) (M-20000)
Synophthalmus
(T-F5000) (M-20000)

D4-F1122 Cyclops hypognathus
(T-F5000) (M-20000)

D4-F1124 Opocephalus
(T-F5000) (M-20000)

D4-F1130 Acraniate monster, NOS 740.0
(T-F5000) (T-11100) (M-21000)
Acranius 740.0
(T-F5000) (T-11100) (M-21000)
Acrania 740.0
(T-F5000) (T-11100) (M-21000)

D4-F1132 Podencephalus 740.0
(T-F5000) (T-11100) (M-21000)

D4-F1134 Anencephalus 740.0
(T-F5000) (T-11100) (T-A2000) (M-21000)
Anencephaly 740.0
(T-F5000) (T-11100) (T-A2000) (M-21000)
Anencephalic monster 740.0
(T-F5000) (T-11100) (T-A2000) (M-21000)

D4-F1135 Hemianencephaly 740.0
(T-F5000) (T-11100) (T-A2000) (M-21080)
Hemicrania 740.0
(T-F5000) (T-11100) (T-A2000) (M-21080)
Incomplete anencephaly 740.0
(T-F5000) (T-11100) (T-A2000) (M-21080)

D4-F1137 Amyelencephalus 740.0
(T-A0100) (T-A7010) (M-21000)

D4-F1140 Monster with cranial anomalies, NOS
(T-F5000) (T-11100) (M-20000)

D4-F1141 Cranial duplication
(T-F5000) (T-11100) (M-22360)
Craniodidymus
(T-F5000) (T-11100) (M-22360)

D4-F1142 Atretocephalus
(T-F5000) (T-11100) (M-22360)

D4-F1143 Agnathus
(T-F5000) (M-20000)

D4-F1144 Synotus
(T-F5000) (M-20000)
Synotia
(T-F5000) (M-20000)

D4-F1146 Derencephalus
(T-F5000) (M-20000)

D4-F1148 Cebocephalus
(T-F5000) (M-20000)
Cebocephaly
(T-F5000) (M-20000)

D4-F1152 Ethmocephalus
(T-F5000) (M-20000)

D4-F1154 Omocephalus
(T-F5000) (M-20000)

D4-F1160 Celosomial monster, NOS
(T-F5000) (M-20000)
Celosomus
(T-F5000) (M-20000)
Celosomia
(T-F5000) (M-20000)

D4-F1162 Cryptodidymus
(T-F5000) (M-20000)

D4-F1164 Fetus in fetu
(T-F5000) (M-26000) (T-F5000)

D4-F1170 Double monster, NOS 759.4
(T-F5000) (M-22360)
Twin monster, NOS 759.4
(T-F5000) (M-22360)

D4-F1171 Anadidymus, NOS
(T-F5000) (M-20000)

D4-F1172 Cephalodymus
(T-F5000) (M-20000)

D4-F1174 Dipygus
(T-F5000) (M-20000)

D4-F1177 Cephalothoracopagus
(T-F5000) (M-20000)

D4-F1178 Thoracodelphus
(T-F5000) (M-20000)
Thoradelphus
(T-F5000) (M-20000)

D4-F1181 Pygodidymus
(T-F5000) (M-20000)

D4-F1190 Craniopagus, NOS 759.4
(T-F5000) (M-20000)
Cephalopagus, NOS 759.4
(T-F5000) (M-20000)

D4-F1192 Craniopagus occipitalis
(T-F5000) (M-20000)

D4-F1194 Craniopagus parietalis
(T-F5000) (M-20000)

D4-F1200 Monocephalus, NOS
(T-F5000) (M-20000)

D4-F1202 Monocephalus tetrapus dibrachius
(T-F5000) (M-20000)

4-F1 MONSTERS — Continued

D4-F1204 Monocephalus tripus dibrachius
(T-F5000) (M-20000)

D4-F1206 Syncephalus
(T-F5000) (M-20000)
Synencephalus
(T-F5000) (M-20000)
Synencephaly
(T-F5000) (M-20000)

D4-F1208 Deradelphus
(T-F5000) (M-20000)

D4-F1212 Janiceps
(T-F5000) (M-20000)
Janus
(T-F5000) (M-20000)

D4-F1230 Anakatadidymus, NOS 759.4
(T-F5000) (M-20000)
Dicephalus dipygus 759.4
(T-F5000) (M-20000)

D4-F1234 Gastrothoracopagus
(T-F5000) (M-20000)

D4-F1240 Thoracodidymus, NOS
(T-F5000) (M-20000)

D4-F1242 Thoracopagus 759.4
(T-F5000) (M-20000)
Synthorax 759.4
(T-F5000) (M-20000)

D4-F1244 Thoracopagus parasiticus
(T-F5000) (M-20000)

D4-F1245 Thoracopagus epigastricus
(T-F5000) (M-20000)

D4-F1246 Thoracoparacephalus
(T-F5000) (M-20000)

D4-F1248 Omphalopagus
(T-F5000) (M-20000)
Monomphalus
(T-F5000) (M-20000)

D4-F1252 Omphaloangiopagus
(T-F5000) (M-20000)
Allantoidoangiopagus
(T-F5000) (M-20000)

D4-F1254 Ischiopagus
(T-F5000) (M-20000)

D4-F1256 Pygopagus 759.4
(T-F5000) (M-20000)

D4-F1270 Katadidymus, NOS
(T-F5000) (M-20000)

D4-F1272 Heterodymus
(T-F5000) (M-20000)
Heterodidymus
(T-F5000) (M-20000)

D4-F1275 Dicephalus dipus tetrabrachius 759.4
(T-F5000) (M-20000)

D4-F1276 Dicephalus dipus tribrachius 759.4
(T-F5000) (M-20000)

D4-F1277 Dicephalus tripus tribrachius 759.4
(T-F5000) (M-20000)

D4-F1290 Acardiac monster, NOS
(T-F5000) (T-32000) (M-21000)
Acardius
(T-F5000) (T-32000) (M-21000)
Acardiacus
(T-F5000) (T-32000) (M-21000)
Acardiac twins, NOS
(T-F5000) (T-32000) (M-21000)

D4-F1412 Holoacardius
(T-F5000) (T-32000) (M-21000)

D4-F1414 Holoacardius amorphus
(T-F5000) (T-32000) (M-21000)
Fetus anideus
(T-F5000) (T-32000) (M-21000)

D4-F1416 Acardiacus anceps
(T-F5000) (T-32000) (M-21000)
Hemiacardius
(T-F5000) (T-32000) (M-21000)

D4-F1422 Holoacardius acephalus
(T-F5000) (T-32000) (M-21000)

D4-F1424 Holoacardius acormus
(T-F5000) (T-32000) (M-21000)

D4-F1450 Compound monster, NOS
(T-F5000) (M-20000)
Incomplete conjoined twins, NOS
(T-F5000) (M-20000)

D4-F1452 Desmiognathus
(T-F5000) (M-20000)
Dicephalus parasiticus
(T-F5000) (M-20000)

D4-F1454 Epignathus
(T-F5000) (M-20000)

D4-F1456 Thoracomelus
(T-F5000) (M-20000)

D4-F1458 Ischiomelus
(T-F5000) (M-20000)

D4-F1462 Pygomelus
(T-F5000) (M-20000)

D4-F1466 Gastrothoracopagus dipygus
(T-F5000) (M-20000)
Dipygus parasiticus
(T-F5000) (M-20000)

D4-F1469 Dicheirus
(T-F5000) (M-20000)

D4-F1480 Diprosopus, NOS
(T-F5000) (M-20000)
Monocephalus diprosopus
(T-F5000) (M-20000)

D4-F1482 Diprosopus tetrophthalmus
(T-F5000) (M-20000)

D4-F1484 Cephalodiprosopus
(T-F5000) (M-20000)

D4-F1486 Opodidymus
(T-F5000) (M-20000)
Opodymus
(T-F5000) (M-20000)

D4-F1488 Dicephalus 759.4
(T-F5000) (M-20000)
Derodidymis 759.4
(T-F5000) (M-20000)

D4-F1492 Dicephalus dipus dibrachius
(T-F5000) (M-20000)
D4-F1494 Dipodia
(T-F5000) (M-20000)
D4-F1496 Diplopodia
(T-F5000) (M-20000)
D4-F1498 Pygoamorphus
(T-F5000) (M-20000)
D4-F1500 Conjoined twins, NOS 749.4
(T-F5000) (M-22360)
Siamese twins, NOS 759.4
(T-F5000) (M-22360)
D4-F1510 Symmetrical conjoined twins, NOS
(T-F5000) (M-22360)
Equal conjoined twins, NOS
(T-F5000) (M-22360)
Diplopagus
(T-F5000) (M-22360)
Duplicitas symmetros
(T-F5000) (M-22360)
D4-F1514 Xiphopagus 759.4
(T-F5000) (M-22360)
D4-F1550 Asymmetrical conjoined twins, NOS
(T-F5000) (M-22360)
Heteradelphus
(T-F5000) (M-22360)
Unequal conjoined twins, NOS
(T-F5000) (M-22360)
D4-F1552 Heteropagus
(T-F5000) (M-22360)
D4-F1600 Chimera, NOS
D4-F1601 Heterologous chimera
D4-F1602 Homologous chimera
D4-F1603 Isologous chimera
D4-F1604 Radiation chimera
D4-F1630V Freemartin

4-F3 ANOMALIES OF THE PLACENTA

D4-F3000 Anomaly of placenta, NOS
(T-F1100) (M-20000)
Abnormal placenta, NOS
(T-F1100) (M-20000)
D4-F3010 Immature abnormal placenta
(T-F1100) (M-20050)
D4-F3011 Premature abnormal placenta
(T-F1100) (M-20050)
D4-F3012 Mature abnormal placenta
(T-F1100) (M-20000)
D4-F3013 Postmature abnormal placenta
(T-F1100) (M-20000)
D4-F3015 Ectopic placenta
(T-F1100) (M-26000)
D4-F3016 Annular placenta
(T-F1100) (M-02100)
Zonary placenta
(T-F1100) (M-02100)
D4-F3030 Twin placenta, NOS
(T-F1100) (M-22360)
D4-F3031 Twin monochorionic diamniotic placenta
(T-F1100) (M-22360)
D4-F3032 Twin monochorionic monoamniotic placenta
(T-F1100) (M-22360)
D4-F3033 Twin dichorionic diamniotic placenta
(T-F1100) (M-22360)
D4-F3038 Placenta of multiple birth higher than twin
(T-F1100) (M-22360)
D4-F3041 Chorioallantoic placenta
(T-F1100)
D4-F3043 Choriovitelline placenta
(T-F1100)
D4-F3045 Placenta extrachorales
(T-F1100)
D4-F3047 Tubal-cornual placenta
(T-F1100)
D4-F3048 Placenta cirsoides
(T-F1100)
D4-F3060 Placenta previa, NOS
(T-F1100) (M-22100) (T-83050)
D4-F3061 Placenta previa marginalis
(T-F1100) (M-22100) (T-83050)
Marginal placenta previa
(T-F1100) (M-22100) (T-83050)
D4-F3062 Placenta previa centralis
(T-F1100) (M-22100) (T-83050)
Total placenta previa
(T-F1100) (M-22100) (T-83050)
D4-F3063 Placenta previa partialis
(T-F1100) (M-22100) (T-83050)
Partial placenta previa
(T-F1100) (M-22100) (T-83050)
D4-F3070 Placenta accreta, NOS
(T-F1100) (M-20150) (T-83600)
D4-F3071 Placenta increta
(T-F1100) (M-20150) (T-83600)
D4-F3072 Placenta percreta
(T-F1100) (M-20150) (T-83600)
D4-F3080 Placenta bipartita
(T-F1100) (M-22030)
Placenta duplex
(T-F1100) (M-22030)
Bilobate placenta
(T-F1100) (M-22030)
D4-F3081 Placenta tripartita
(T-F1100) (M-22040)
Trilobate placenta
(T-F1100) (M-22040)
Placenta triplex
(T-F1100) (M-22040)
D4-F3082 Placenta multipartita
(T-F1100) (M-22060)
Multilobate placenta
(T-F1100) (M-22060)
D4-F3083 Placenta circumvallata
(T-F1100)
Circumvallate placenta
(T-F1100)

4-F3 ANOMALIES OF THE PLACENTA — Continued

D4-F3083 (cont.) Placenta nappiformis
(T-F1100)

D4-F3084 Placenta marginalis
(T-F1100)
Marginal placenta
(T-F1100)
Placenta marginata
(T-F1100)

D4-F3085 Placenta reflexa
(T-F1100)

D4-F3086 Placenta membranacea
(T-F1100)
Placenta diffusa
(T-F1100)

D4-F3087 Placenta succenturiata
(T-F1100) (M-22300)
Accessory placenta
(T-F1100) (M-22300)
Supernumerary placenta
(T-F1100) (M-22300)

D4-F3088 Placenta spuria
(T-F1100)

D4-F3089 Placenta fenestrata
(T-F1100)

D4-F3090 Tenney changes of placenta
(T-F1100)

D4-F3095 Trapped placenta
(T-F1100)

D4-F3096 Adherent placenta
(T-F1100) (M-20150)

4-F4 ANOMALIES OF THE AMNION

D4-F4000 Abnormal amnion, NOS
(T-F1300) (M-20000)

D4-F4010 Abnormal amniotic fluid, NOS
(T-F1320) (M-20000)

D4-F4020 Abnormal yolk sac
(T-F1400) (M-20000)

D4-F4035 Amniotic band
(T-F1300) (M-78400)
Amniotic adhesion
(T-F1300) (M-78400)

D4-F4036 Incomplete amnion
(T-F1300)

D4-F4050 Allantoic cyst
(T-F1840) (M-26500)
Urachal cyst
(T-F1840) (M-25600)

4-F5 ANOMALIES OF THE UMBILICAL CORD

D4-F5000 Abnormal umbilical cord, NOS
(T-F1800) (M-20000)

D4-F5004 Short cord 663.4
(T-F1800)
Excessively short umbilical cord 663.4
(T-F1800)
Short umbilical cord 663.4
(T-F1800)

D4-F5006 Excessively long umbilical cord
(T-F1800)

D4-F5010 Marginal insertion of umbilical cord
(T-F1800)
Battledore placenta
(T-F1800)

D4-F5016 One vessel umbilical cord
(T-F1800)

D4-F5020 Velamentous insertion of umbilical cord 663.5
(T-F1800) (M-20700) (T-F1100)
Velamentous placenta 663.5
(T-F1800) (M-20700) (T-F1100)

D4-F5034 False knot of umbilical cord
(T-F1800)

D4-F5035 True knot of umbilical cord
(T-F1800)

D4-F5040 Vascular anomaly of umbilical cord
(T-F1800) (M-24600)

D4-F5041 Arterial anomaly of umbilical cord
(T-F1800) (M-20000) (T-41000)

D4-F5042 Venous anomaly of umbilical cord
(T-F1800) (M-20000) (T-48000)

D4-F5045 Single artery and vein of umbilical cord
(T-F1800)

D4-F5048 Single vessel of umbilical cord, NOS
(T-F1800)

D4-F5051 Compression of umbilical cord
(T-F1800) (M-01460) (M-20000)

D4-F5055 Umbilical cord of intertwined twins
(T-F1800)

D4-F5056 Umbilical polyp
(T-F1800) (M-26400)

CHAPTER 5 — DISEASES OF THE DIGESTIVE SYSTEM

SECTION 5-0 DISEASES OF THE DIGESTIVE SYSTEM: GENERAL CONDITIONS

D5-00000 Disease of digestive system, NOS
(T-50000) (DF-00000)

D5-00010 Disease of digestive tract, NOS
(T-50100) (DF-00000)

D5-00020 Disease of upper digestive tract, NOS
(T-50110) (DF-00000)

D5-00030 Disease of lower digestive tract, NOS
(T-50120) (DF-00000)

D5-00040 Disease of digestive organ, NOS
(T-60000) (DF-00000)

D5-00100 Gastrointestinal hemorrhage, NOS 578.9
(T-50100) (M-37000)
Gastrointestinal bleeding, NOS 578.9
(T-50100) (M-37000)

D5-00110 Upper gastrointestinal hemorrhage
(T-50110) (M-37000)
Upper gastrointestinal bleeding
(T-50110) (M-37000)

D5-00112 Acute upper gastrointestinal hemorrhage
(T-50110) (M-37001)
Acute upper gastrointestinal bleeding
(T-50110) (M-37001)

D5-00114 Chronic upper gastrointestinal hemorrhage
(T-50110) (M-37003)
Chronic upper gastrointestinal bleeding
(T-50110) (M-37003)

D5-00120 Hematemesis 578.0
(T-50110) (F-52770) (T-C2000)
Vomiting of blood 578.0
(T-50110) (F-52770) (T-C2000)

D5-00130 Lower gastrointestinal hemorrhage
(T-50120) (M-37000)
Lower gastrointestinal bleeding
(T-50120) (M-37000)

D5-00132 Acute lower gastrointestinal hemorrhage
(T-50120) (M-37001)
Acute lower gastrointestinal bleeding
(T-50120) (M-37001)

D5-00134 Chronic lower gastrointestinal hemorrhage
(T-50120) (M-37003)
Chronic lower gastrointestinal bleeding
(T-50120) (M-37003)

D5-00140 Hematochezia
(T-50120) (T-C2000) (T-59666) (M-37000)
Passage of bloody stools
(T-50120) (T-C2000) (T-59666) (M-37000)

D5-00150 Melena 578.1
(T-50100) (T-C2000) (T-59666)
Blood in stool 578.1
(T-50100) (T-C2000) (T-59666)

D5-00152 Occult blood in stools
(T-50120) (T-59666) (M-37007)
Guaiac-positive stools
(T-50120) (T-59666) (M-37007)

D5-00300 Gastrointestinal food allergy, NOS
(T-50100) (F-C3000) (C-E0000)
Gastrointestinal food sensitivity, NOS
(T-50100) (F-C3000) (C-E0000)

D5-00301 Cow's milk protein sensitivity
(T-50100) (F-C3000) (C-E0410)

D5-00302 Soy protein sensitivity
(T-50100) (F-C3000) (C-E0130)

D5-00303 Transient gluten sensitivity
(T-50100) (F-C3000) (C-E0120)

D5-00350 Eosinophilic gastroenteropathy, NOS
(T-50100) (M-43040)

D5-00352 Eosinophilic gastroenteropathy with predominant mucosal disease
(T-50130) (M-43040)

D5-00354 Eosinophilic gastroenteropathy with predominant muscle layer disease
(T-50133) (M-43040)

D5-00356 Eosinophilic gastroenteropathy with predominant subserosal disease
(T-50136) (M-43040)

D5-00360 Eosinophilic gastroenteropathy with collagen vascular disease
(T-50100) (M-43040) (G-C002) (D1-10000)

D5-00362 Eosinophilic gastroenteropathy with food sensitivity
(T-50100) (M-43040) (G-C002) (F-C3000) (C-E0000)

D5-00364 Gastrointestinal eosinophilic granuloma
(T-50100) (M-44050)

D5-01000 Primary chronic pseudo-obstruction of gastrointestinal tract, NOS
(T-50100) (M-34060) (G-A332)

D5-01001 Primary chronic pseudo-obstruction of esophagus
(T-56000) (M-34060) (G-A332)

D5-01002 Primary chronic pseudo-obstruction of stomach
(T-57000) (M-34060) (G-A332)

D5-01004 Primary chronic pseudo-obstruction of small intestine
(T-58000) (M-34060) (G-A332)

D5-01006 Primary chronic pseudo-obstruction of large intestine
(T-59000) (M-34060) (G-A332)

D5-01008 Primary chronic pseudo-obstruction of colon
(T-59300) (M-34060) (G-A332)
Ogilvie's syndrome
(T-59300) (M-34060) (G-A332)

D5-01020 Secondary intestinal pseudo-obstruction, NOS
(T-50500) (M-34060) (G-A570)

SECTION 5-0 DISEASES OF THE DIGESTIVE SYSTEM: GENERAL CONDITIONS — Continued

D5-01030 Diffuse dysfunction of smooth muscle of gastrointestinal tract, NOS
(T-50100) (T-50133) (F-01100)

D5-01032 Hereditary hollow viscus myopathy
(T-50100) (T-50133) (M-50000) (M-78000)
Familial visceral myopathy
(T-50100) (T-50133) (M-50000) (M-78000)

D5-01034 Familial visceral neuropathy
(T-50100) (T-A9840) (M-50000)

D5-02000 Acute abdomen, NOS
(T-D4000) (F-50861)
Acute abdominal pain syndrome, NOS
(T-D4000) (F-50861)

D5-02004 Abdominal mass, NOS 789.3
(T-D4000) (M-03000)
Abdominal lump, NOS 789.3
(T-D4000) (M-03000)
Abdominal swelling, NOS 789.3
(T-D4000) (M-03000)

D5-02010 Infantile colic
(T-D4000) (F-01330)

D5-02020 Endemic colic
(T-D4000) (F-01330) (DF-00120)

D5-03000 Gastrointestinal fistula, NOS
(T-50100) (M-39300)

D5-03002 Internal gastrointestinal fistula
(T-50100) (M-39301)

D5-03004 External gastrointestinal fistula
(T-50100) (M-39302)

D5-03006 High-output external gastrointestinal fistula
(T-50100) (M-39303)

D5-03008 Low-output external gastrointestinal fistula
(T-50100) (M-39304)

SECTION 5-1 DISEASES OF THE TEETH AND SUPPORTING STRUCTURES

D5-10000 Disease of teeth, NOS 525.9
(T-54010) (DF-00000)
Nondevelopmental disease of teeth, NOS 525.9
(T-54010) (DF-00000)

D5-10010 Teething syndrome 520.7
(T-54600) (F-51010)

D5-10100 Disease of hard tissues of teeth, NOS 521.9
(T-54010) (DF-00000)

D5-10110 Dental caries, NOS 521.0
(T-54010) (M-54210)

D5-10120 Arrested dental caries 521.0
(T-54010) (M-54210)

D5-10130 Cementum caries 521.0
(T-54090) (M-54210)

D5-10140 Dentin caries, NOS 521.0
(T-54070) (M-54210)

D5-10141 Acute dentin caries 521.0
(T-54070) (M-54210)

D5-10142 Chronic dentin caries 521.0
(T-54070) (M-54210)

D5-10200 Enamel caries, NOS 521.0
(T-54080) (M-54210)

D5-10201 Acute enamel caries 521.0
(T-54080) (M-54210)

D5-10202 Chronic enamel caries 521.0
(T-54080) (M-54210)

D5-10230 Incipient enamel caries 521.0
(T-54080) (M-54210)

D5-10300 Infantile melanodontia 521.0
(T-54010) (M-57200)

D5-10320 White spot lesions of teeth 521.0
(T-54010) (M-01100) (M-04170)

D5-10400 Excessive attrition of teeth, NOS 521.1
(T-54010) (F-51042)
Excessive dental attrition, NOS 521.1
(T-54010) (F-51042)

D5-10401 Approximal wear of teeth 521.1
(T-54010) (F-51042)

D5-10402 Occlusal wear of teeth 521.1
(T-54010) (F-51042)

D5-10420V Irregularities of wear of tooth
(T-54010) (F-51052) (G-A402)

D5-10421V Sharp tooth
(T-54010)

D5-10422V Shear mouth
(T-54010)

D5-10423V Wave mouth
(T-54010)

D5-10424V Step mouth
(T-54010)

D5-10425V Smooth mouth
(T-54010)

D5-10450 Abrasion of teeth, NOS 521.2
(T-54010) (M-14700)

D5-10451 Dentifrice abrasion of teeth 521.2
(T-54010) (M-14700) (C-22660)

D5-10452 Habitual abrasion of teeth 521.2
(T-54010) (M-14700)

D5-10453 Occupational abrasion of teeth 521.2
(T-54010) (M-14700) (G-C001) (J-00000)

D5-10454 Ritual abrasion of teeth 521.2
(T-54010) (M-14700) (G-C002) (F-93640)

D5-10455 Traditional abrasion of teeth 521.2
(T-54010) (M-14700)

D5-10456 Wedge defect of teeth, NOS 521.2
(T-54010) (M-01130) (M-02260)

D5-10500 Erosion of teeth, NOS 521.3
(T-54010) (M-01140)

D5-10501 Erosion of teeth due to medicine 521.3
(T-54010) (M-01140) (C-50000)

D5-10502 Erosion of teeth due to persistent vomiting 521.3
(T-54010) (M-01140) (F-52820)

D5-10503 Idiopathic erosion of teeth 521.3
(T-54010) (M-01140)

D5-10504 Occupational erosion of teeth 521.3
(T-54010) (M-01140) (G-C001)
(J-00000)

D5-10505 Perimylolysis
(T-54013) (T-54011) (M-38350)
(G-C001) (F-52883)
Perimolysis
(T-54013) (T-54011) (M-38350)
(G-C001) (F-52883)

D5-10550 Pathological resorption of tooth, NOS 521.4
(T-54010) (F-51140)

D5-10552 External resorption of tooth 521.4
(T-54010) (F-51143)

D5-10553 External resorption of root of tooth 521.4
(T-54040) (F-51143)

D5-10554 Internal resorption of tooth 521.4
(T-54010) (F-51142)

D5-10555 Internal resorption of root of tooth 521.4
(T-54040) (F-51142)

D5-10570 Hypercementosis 521.5
(T-54090) (M-72000)
Cementation hyperplasia 521.5
(T-54090) (M-72000)
Cementum hyperplasia 521.5
(T-54090) (M-72000)
Cementosis 521.5
(T-54090) (M-72000)

D5-10572 Ankylosis of tooth 521.6
(T-54010) (M-13500)

D5-10577 Irradiated enamel 521.8
(T-54080) (M-11600)

D5-10578 Sensitive dentin 521.8
(T-54070) (F-A2620)

D5-10600 Posteruptive color change of tooth, NOS 521.7
(T-54010) (M-04010)
Posteruptive staining of tooth, NOS 521.7
(T-54010) (M-04010)
Posteruptive discoloration of tooth, NOS 521.7
(T-54010) (M-04010)

D5-10610 Posteruptive tooth staining due to drug, NOS 521.7
(T-54010) (M-04010) (G-C001)
(C-50000)

D5-10611 Posteruptive tooth staining due to tetracycline
(T-54010) (M-04010) (G-C001)
(C-55000)
Tetracycline staining of tooth
(T-54010) (M-04010) (G-C001)
(C-55000)

D5-10620 Posteruptive tooth staining due to metal 521.7
(T-54010) (M-04010) (G-C001)
(C-11800)

D5-10630 Posteruptive tooth staining due to pulpal bleeding 521.7
(T-54010) (M-04010) (G-C001)
(T-54060) (M-37000)

D5-10650 Accretion on teeth, NOS 523.6
(T-54010) (M-30420)
Deposition on teeth, NOS 523.6
(T-54010) (M-30420)

D5-10651 Dental plaque 523.6
(T-54010) (M-01470)

D5-10652 Supragingival dental plaque 523.6
(T-54010) (M-01470)

D5-10653 Soft deposit on teeth 523.6
(T-54010) (M-30420) (M-02711)
Materia alba on teeth 523.6
(T-54010) (M-30420) (M-02711)

D5-10654 Tobacco deposit on teeth 523.6
(T-54010) (M-30420) (L-D9871)

D5-10655 Betel deposit on teeth 523.6
(T-54010) (M-30420) (L-DB301)

D5-10660 Dental calculus, NOS 523.6
(T-54010) (M-30000)
Tartar 523.6
(T-54010) (M-30000)
Odontolith 523.6
(T-54010) (M-30000)

D5-10661 Subgingival dental calculus 523.6
(T-54990) (T-54010) (M-30000)

D5-10662 Supragingival dental calculus 523.6
(T-54020) (T-54010) (M-30000)

D5-10700 Disease of pulp of tooth, NOS 522.9
(T-54060) (DF-00000)
Endodontic disease, NOS 522.9
(T-54060) (DF-00000)

D5-10710 Pulpitis, NOS 522.0
(T-54060) (M-40000)

D5-10711 Acute pulpitis 522.0
(T-54060) (M-41000)

D5-10712 Suppurative pulpitis 522.0
(T-54060) (M-41600)

D5-10713 Pulpal abscess 522.0
(T-54060) (M-41610)

D5-10720 Chronic pulpitis 522.0
(T-54060) (M-43000)

D5-10721 Chronic hyperplastic pulpitis 522.0
(T-54060) (M-43800)

D5-10722 Chronic ulcerative pulpitis 522.0
(T-54060) (M-43750)

D5-10723 Pulpal polyp 522.0
(T-54060) (M-76820)

D5-10724 Internal granuloma of pulp 521.4
(T-54060) (M-44000)

D5-10730 Necrosis of the pulp 522.1
(T-54060) (M-54000)

D5-10731 Pulp gangrene 522.1
(T-54060) (M-54600)

D5-10740 Pulp degeneration 522.2
(T-54060) (M-50000)

SECTION 5-1 DISEASES OF THE TEETH AND SUPPORTING STRUCTURES — Continued

D5-10741 Denticles 522.2
(T-54060) (M-30000)
Pulp calcification 522.2
(T-54060) (M-30000)
Pulp stone 522.2
(T-54060) (M-30000)

D5-10745 Abnormal hard tissue formation in pulp 522.3
(T-54060) (M-02712)

D5-10746 Secondary dentin 522.3
(T-54070) (F-510B0) (G-A402)
Irregular dentin 522.3
(T-54070) (F-510B0) (G-A402)

D5-10750 Disease of periapical tissues of tooth, NOS 522.9
(T-54990) (DF-00000)

D5-10752 Acute apical periodontitis of pulpal origin 522.4
(T-54990) (M-41000) (G-C001)
(T-54060) (M-41000)

D5-10754 Periapical abscess without sinus tract 522.5
(T-54990) (M-41610) (G-D009)
(M-39300)
Dental abscess 522.5
(T-54990) (M-41610) (G-D009)
(M-39300)
Dentoalveolar abscess 522.5
(T-54990) (M-41610) (G-D009)
(M-39300)

D5-10755V Carnassial abscess
(T-545A1) (M-41610)
Abscess at the root of a carnassial tooth
(T-545A1) (M-41610)
Malar abscess of a carnassial tooth
(T-545A1) (M-41610)
Facial abscess of a carnassial tooth
(T-545A1) (M-41610)

D5-10760 Apical periodontitis, NOS 522.6
(T-54990) (M-41000)

D5-10764 Chronic apical periodontitis 522.6
(T-54990) (M-43000)

D5-10770 Apical granuloma 522.6
(T-54041) (M-44000)
Periapical granuloma 522.6
(T-54041) (M-44000)
Dental granuloma 522.6
(T-54041) (M-44000)

D5-10772 Periapical abscess with sinus tract 522.7
(T-54990) (M-41610) (G-C008)
(M-39300)
Alveolar process fistula 522.7
(T-54990) (M-41610) (G-C008)
(M-39300)
Dental fistula 522.7
(T-54990) (M-41610) (G-C008)
(M-39300)

D5-10780 Radicular cyst 522.8
(T-54041) (M-33400)
Apical cyst 522.8
(T-54041) (M-33400)
Periapical cyst 522.8
(T-54041) (M-33400)
Radiculodental cyst 522.8
(T-54041) (M-33400)
Residual radicular cyst 522.8
(T-54041) (M-33400)

D5-10800 Disease of supporting structures of teeth, NOS 525.9
(T-54900) (DF-00000)

D5-10805 Gingival disease, NOS 523.9
(T-54910) (DF-00000)

D5-10810 Gingivitis, NOS 523.1
(T-54910) (M-40000)

D5-10812 Acute gingivitis 523.0
(T-54910) (M-41000)

D5-10814 Chronic gingivitis 523.1
(T-54910) (M-43000)

D5-10815 Desquamative gingivitis 523.1
(T-54910) (M-40000) (F-41500)

D5-10816 Hyperplastic gingivitis 523.1
(T-54910) (M-43900)

D5-10817 Simple marginal gingivitis 523.1
(T-54914) (M-40000)

D5-10818 Ulcerative gingivitis 523.1
(T-54910) (M-40750)

D5-10820 Gingivostomatitis 523.1
(T-54910) (T-51004) (M-40000)

D5-10825 Leukoplakia of gingiva 528.6
(T-54910) (M-72830)

D5-10830 Gingival recession, NOS 523.2
(T-54910) (M-31150)

D5-10831 Generalized gingival recession 523.2
(T-54910) (M-31151)

D5-10832 Localized gingival recession 523.2
(T-54910) (M-31152)

D5-10833 Postinfective gingival recession 523.2
(T-54910) (M-31150) (F-06050)

D5-10834 Postoperative gingival recession 523.2
(T-54910) (M-31150) (F-06030)

D5-10850 Giant cell epulis 523.8
(T-54910) (M-44110)
Peripheral giant cell granuloma 523.8
(T-54910) (M-44110)

D5-10860 Gingival enlargement, NOS 523.8
(T-54910) (M-71000)
Gingival hyperplasia 523.8
(T-54910) (M-71000)

D5-10861 Gingival fibromatosis 523.8
(T-54910) (M-78800)

D5-10862 Gingival polyp 523.8
(T-54910) (M-76820)

D5-10870V Gingival hair impaction
(T-54910) (M-33100) (G-C001)
(T-01400)

D5-10872V Gingival food impaction
(T-54910) (M-33100) (G-C001)
(C-F0000)

D5-10900 Periodontal disease, NOS 523.9
(T-54990) (DF-00000)

D5-10910 Periodontitis, NOS 523.4
(T-54990) (M-40000)

D5-10920 Acute periodontitis 523.3
(T-54990) (M-41000)
Acute pericementitis 523.3
(T-54990) (M-41000)

D5-10922 Periodontal abscess 523.3
(T-54990) (M-41610)
Paradontal abscess 523.3
(T-54990) (M-41610)

D5-10924 Pericoronitis 523.3
(T-54914) (M-40000)

D5-10930 Chronic periodontitis 523.4
(T-54990) (M-43000)
Chronic pericementitis 523.4
(T-54990) (M-43000)

D5-10934 Chronic pericoronitis 523.4
(T-54914) (M-43000)

D5-10940 Marginal periodontitis 523.4
(T-54990) (M-43600)
Periodontitis simplex 523.4
(T-54990) (M-43600)
Alveolar pyorrhea 523.4
(T-54990) (M-43600)
Simple periodontitis 523.4
(T-54990) (M-43600)
Chronic suppurative pericementitis 523.4
(T-54990) (M-43600)
Fauchard's disease 523.4
(T-54990) (M-43600)
Pyorrhea 523.4
(T-54990) (M-43600)
Pyorrhea alveolaris 523.4
(T-54990) (M-43600)
Riggs' disease 523.4
(T-54990) (M-43600)
Alveolar periostitis 523.4
(T-54990) (M-43600)

D5-10946 Chronic ossifying alveolar periostitis 523.4
(T-54990) (M-43600) (G-C008)
(F-12100)

D5-10947 Acute suppurative alveolar periostitis 523.4
(T-54990) (M-41600)

D5-10950 Juvenile periodontitis 523.5
(T-54990) (M-40000) (DF-00220)
Periodontosis 523.5
(T-54990) (M-40000) (DF-00220)
Paradentosis 523.5
(T-54990) (M-40000) (DF-00220)

D5-10954 Prepubertal periodontitis
(T-54990) (M-40000)

D5-10960 Rapidly progressive periodontitis
(T-54990) (M-41000) (G-A494)

D5-10970 Adult periodontitis
(T-54990) (M-43000) (DF-00230)

D5-10980 Necrotizing ulcerative gingivoperiodontitis
(T-54910) (T-54990) (M-41700)
(M-41750)

D5-10990 Periodontal lesion due to traumatic occlusion 523.8
(T-54990) (M-01100) (G-C001)
(M-10000) (F-51150)

D5-11000 Dentofacial functional anomaly, NOS 524.9
(T-54010) (T-D1213) (F-01100)

D5-11100 Abnormal jaw closure, NOS 524.5
(T-D1213) (F-01100)
Malocclusion of jaws 524.5
(T-D1213) (F-01100)

D5-11101 Malocclusion due to abnormal swallowing 524.5
(T-54010) (F-51160) (F-51702)

D5-11102 Malocclusion due to mouth breathing 524.5
(T-54010) (F-51160) (F-20160)

D5-11103 Malocclusion due to tongue habits 524.5
(T-54010) (F-51160) (G-C001)
(T-53000) (F-93450)

D5-11104 Malocclusion due to lip habits 524.5
(T-54010) (F-51160) (G-C001)
(T-52000) (F-93450)

D5-11105 Malocclusion due to finger habits 524.5
(T-54010) (F-51160) (G-C001)
(T-D8800) (F-93450)

D5-11110V Mandibular neuropraxia
(T-D1213) (M-31050)
Dropped jaw
(T-D1213) (M-31050)

D5-12000 Temporomandibular joint disorder, NOS 524.6
(T-15290) (DF-00000)

D5-12010 Ankylosis of temporomandibular joint 524.6
(T-15290) (M-13500)

D5-12020 Derangement of temporomandibular joint 524.6
(T-15290) (M-31000)

D5-12022 Temporomandibular luxation 524.6
(T-15290) (M-13010)

D5-12024 Temporomandibular subluxation 524.6
(T-15290) (M-13020)

D5-12030 Temporomandibular joint-pain-dysfunction syndrome 524.6
(T-15290) (F-01100) (F-A2600)
TMJ syndrome 524.6
(T-15290) (F-01100) (F-A2600)
Costen's complex 524.6
(T-15290) (F-01100) (F-A2600)
Costen's syndrome 524.6
(T-15290) (F-01100) (F-A2600)
Snapping jaw 524.6
(T-15290) (F-01100) (F-A2600)

D5-12031 Jaw claudication 524.6
(T-D1213) (F-18010)

SECTION 5-1 DISEASES OF THE TEETH AND SUPPORTING STRUCTURES — Continued

D5-12040V Temporomandibular dysplasia
(T-15290) (M-74000)

D5-13000 Acquired absence of teeth, NOS 525.1
(T-54010) (M-16000)
Loss of teeth, NOS 525.1
(T-54010) (M-16000)

D5-13002 Avulsion of tooth
(T-54010) (M-14120)

D5-13100 Exfoliation of teeth due to systemic disease 525.0
(T-54010) (M-16000) (G-C001) (DF-00100)

D5-13110 Loss of teeth due to accident 525.1
(T-54010) (M-16000) (G-C001) (A-A1000)

D5-13112 Fracture of tooth
(T-54010) (M-12000)

D5-13113V Fracture of fissure of tooth
(T-54010) (M-12000)

D5-13115V Luxation of tooth
(T-54010) (M-13010)

D5-13120 Loss of teeth due to extraction 525.1
(T-54010) (M-16000) (G-C001) (P.-.....)

D5-13130 Loss of teeth due to local periodontal disease 525.1
(T-54010) (M-16000) (G-C001) (T-54990) (DF-00280)

D5-13141 Atrophy of edentulous maxillary alveolar ridge 525.2
(T-11177) (T-54010) (M-16000) (M-58000)

D5-13142 Atrophy of edentulous mandibular alveolar ridge 525.2
(T-1118B) (T-54010) (M-16000) (M-58000)

D5-13150 Retained dental root 525.3
(T-54040) (M-33000)

D5-13160 Enlargement of alveolar ridge, NOS 525.8
(T-1118B) (T-11177) (M-71000)

D5-13170 Irregular alveolar process 525.8
(T-1118B) (T-11177) (M-01000)

D5-14000 Disease of jaw, NOS 526.9
(T-D1213) (DF-00000)

D5-14100 Cyst of jaw, NOS 526.2
(T-D1213) (M-33400)

D5-14110 Aneurysmal cyst of jaw 526.2
(T-D1213) (M-33640)

D5-14120 Hemorrhagic cyst of jaw 526.2
(T-D1213) (M-33540)

D5-14130 Traumatic cyst of jaw 526.2
(T-D1213) (M-33400) (M-10000)

D5-14180 Central giant cell reparative granuloma of jaw 526.3
(T-D1213) (M-44110)

D5-14200 Abscess of jaw, NOS 526.4
(T-D1213) (M-41610)
Acute abscess of jaw 526.4
(T-D1213) (M-41610)
Suppurative abscess of jaw 526.4
(T-D1213) (M-41610)

D5-14202 Chronic abscess of jaw 526.4
(T-D1213) (M-43610)

D5-14300 Nonsuppurative osteitis of jaw, NOS 526.4
(T-D1213) (M-40000)

D5-14301 Acute nonsuppurative osteitis of jaw 526.4
(T-D1213) (M-41000)

D5-14302 Chronic nonsuppurative osteitis of jaw 526.4
(T-D1213) (M-43000)
Sclerosing osteitis 526.4
(T-D1213) (M-43000)

D5-14400 Osteomyelitis of jaw, NOS 526.4
(T-D1213) (T-11000) (M-40000)

D5-14401 Acute osteomyelitis of jaw 526.4
(T-D1213) (T-11000) (M-41000)

D5-14402 Chronic osteomyelitis of jaw 526.4
(T-D1213) (T-11000) (M-43000)

D5-14410 Suppurative osteomyelitis of jaw 526.4
(T-D1213) (T-11000) (M-41600)

D5-14420 Neonatal osteomyelitis of jaw 526.4
(T-D1213) (T-11000) (M-40000) (DF-00200)

D5-14500 Periostitis of jaw, NOS 526.4
(T-D1213) (T-11020) (M-40000)

D5-14501 Acute periostitis of jaw 526.4
(T-D1213) (T-10020) (M-41000)

D5-14502 Chronic periostitis of jaw 526.4
(T-D1213) (T-11020) (M-43000)

D5-14510 Suppurative periostitis of jaw 526.4
(T-D1213) (T-11020) (M-41600)

D5-14580 Sequestrum of jaw bone 526.4
(T-D1213) (T-11000) (M-39100)

D5-14600 Alveolitis of jaw, NOS 526.5
(T-D1213) (T-54970) (M-40000)
Alveolar osteitis 526.5
(T-D1213) (T-54970) (M-40000)
Dry socket 526.5
(T-D1213) (T-54970) (M-40000)
Alveolitis sicca dolorosa 526.5
(T-D1213) (T-54970) (M-40000)

D5-14610 Alveolitis of mandible 526.5
(T-11180) (T-54972) (M-40000)
Mandibular osteitis 526.5
(T-11180) (T-54972) (M-40000)

D5-14620 Alveolitis of maxilla 526.5
(T-11170) (T-54971) (M-40000)
Maxillary osteitis 526.5
(T-11170) (T-54971) (M-40000)

D5-14700 Exostosis of jaw, NOS 526.81
(T-D1213) (M-71450)

D5-14710 Torus mandibularis 526.81
(T-11180) (M-03150)

D5-14720 Torus palatinus 526.81
(T-51100) (M-03150)

D5-14800 Cherubism 526.89
(T-11189) (M-74600) (DF-00190)
Familial fibrous dysplasia of jaw 526.89
(T-11189) (M-74600) (DF-00190)

D5-14810 Fibrous dysplasia of jaw 526.89
(T-D1213) (M-74600)
D5-14820 Latent bone cyst of jaw 526.89
(T-D1213) (M-33630)
D5-14830 Osteoradionecrosis of jaw 526.89
(T-D1213) (M-11660)
D5-14840 Unilateral condylar hyperplasia of mandible 526.89
(T-11185) (M-72001)
D5-14850 Unilateral condylar hypoplasia of mandible 526.89
(T-11185) (M-75301)

SECTION 5-2 DISEASES OF THE SALIVARY GLANDS AND ORAL CAVITY

5-20 DISEASES OF THE SALIVARY GLANDS

D5-20000 Disease of salivary gland, NOS 527.9
(T-61000) (DF-00000)
D5-20110 Atrophy of salivary gland 527.0
(T-61000) (M-58000)
D5-20115 Hypertrophy of salivary gland 527.1
(T-61000) (M-71000)
D5-20120 Sialoadenitis, NOS 527.2
(T-61000) (M-40000)
Sialoangitis, NOS 527.2
(T-61000) (M-40000)
D5-20130 Sialodochitis 527.2
(T-61080) (M-40000)
D5-20150 Parotitis, NOS 527.2
(T-61100) (M-40000)
D5-20152 Allergic parotitis 527.2
(T-61100) (M-40000) (F-C3000)
D5-20153 Toxic parotitis 527.2
(T-61100) (M-40000) (F-06150)
D5-20200 Abscess of salivary gland 527.3
(T-61000) (M-41610)
D5-20210 Fistula of salivary gland 527.4
(T-61000) (M-39300)
D5-20220 Sialolithiasis 527.5
(T-61000) (M-30000)
Calculus of salivary gland 527.5
(T-61000) (M-30000)
Stone of salivary gland 527.5
(T-61000) (M-30000)
D5-20230 Sialodocholithiasis 527.5
(T-61080) (M-30000)
Calculus of salivary duct 527.5
(T-61080) (M-30000)
Stone of salivary duct 527.5
(T-61080) (M-30000)
D5-20240 Mucocele of salivary gland 527.6
(T-61000) (M-33560)
Retention cyst of salivary gland 527.6
(T-61000) (M-33560)
Salivary cyst 527.6
(T-61000) (M-33560)
Sialocele 527.6
(T-61000) (M-33560)
Ptyalocele 527.6
(T-61000) (M-33560)
D5-20242 Extravasation cyst of salivary gland 527.6
(T-61000) (M-36600) (M-33400)
D5-20244 Ranula 527.6
(T-61000) (M-33560)
Ranula of salivary gland of floor of mouth 527.6
(T-61000) (M-33560)
Ranula of floor of mouth 527.6
(T-61000) (M-33560)
Sublingual cyst 527.6
(T-61000) (M-33560)
D5-20300 Disturbance of salivary secretion, NOS 527.7
(T-61000) (T-61083) (F-57102)
D5-20302 Hyposecretion of salivary gland 527.7
(T-61000) (T-61083) (F-57102)
Hyposalivation 527.7
(T-61000) (T-61083) (F-57102)
D5-20304 Ptyalism 527.7
(T-61000) (T-61083) (F-57102)
Sialorrhea 527.7
(T-61000) (T-61083) (F-57102)
Sialosis 527.8
(T-61000) (T-61083) (F-57102)
Hypersalivation 527.7
(T-61000) (T-61083) (F-57102)
Polysialia 527.7
(T-61000) (T-61083) (F-57102)
Sialism 527.7
(T-61000) (T-61083) (F-57102)
Sialismus 527.7
(T-61000) (T-61083) (F-57102)
Ptyalorrhea 527.7
(T-61000) (T-61083) (F-57102)
Hypersecretion of salivary gland 527.7
(T-61000) (T-61083) (F-57102)
Hypersecretion of saliva 527.7
(T-61000) (T-61083) (F-57102)
D5-20305V Pseudoptyalism
(T-61083) (M-33000) (G-C001)
(D5-30250)
D5-20306 Aptyalism 527.7
(T-61000) (T-61083) (F-57102)
Xerostomia 527.7
(T-61000) (T-61083) (F-57102)
Absent salivary secretion 527.7
(T-61000) (T-61083) (F-57102)
Aptyalia 527.7
(T-61000) (T-61083) (F-57102)
Asialia 527.7
(T-61000) (T-61083) (F-57102)
D5-20308 Continuous salivary secretion 527.7
(T-61000) (T-61083) (F-57102)
D5-20350 Benign lymphoepithelial lesion of salivary gland 527.8
(T-61000) (M-72240)

5-20 DISEASES OF THE SALIVARY GLANDS — Continued

D5-20360 Sialectasia 527.8
(T-61080) (M-32000)

D5-20380 Stenosis of salivary duct 527.8
(T-61080) (M-34200)
Stricture of salivary duct 527.8
(T-61080) (M-34200)

5-21 DISEASES OF THE ORAL SOFT TISSUES

D5-21000 Disease of the oral soft tissues, NOS 528.-
(T-51800) (DF-00000)

D5-21100 Stomatitis, NOS 528.0
(T-51030) (M-40000)

D5-21110 Ulcerative stomatitis 528.0
(T-51004) (M-40750)

D5-21120 Vesicular stomatitis 528.0
(T-51004) (M-40210)

D5-21140V Granular stomatitis
(T-51030) (M-40000)

D5-21200 Cancrum oris 528.1
(T-51030) (M-40700)
Gangrenous stomatitis 528.1
(T-51030) (M-40700)
Noma 528.1
(T-51030) (M-40700)

D5-21240 Oral aphthae, NOS 528.2
(T-51030) (M-38000)
Aphthous stomatitis 528.2
(T-51030) (M-38000)
Canker sore 528.2
(T-51030) (M-38000)
Stomatitis herpetiformis 528.2
(T-51030) (M-38000)
Aphthous ulcer
(T-51030) (M-38000)

D5-21250 Recurrent aphthous ulcer 528.2
(T-51030) (M-38000) (M-78060)
Periadenitis mucosa necrotica recurrens 528.2
(T-51030) (M-38000) (M-78060)
Mikulicz's aphthae 528.2
(T-51030) (M-38000) (M-78060)
Recurring scarring aphthae 528.2
(T-51030) (M-38000) (M-78060)
Sutton's disease 528.2
(T-51030) (M-38000) (M-78060)

D5-21300 Cellulitis of oral soft tissues, NOS 528.3
(T-51800) (M-41650)

D5-21310 Abscess of oral tissue, NOS 528.3
(T-51800) (M-41610)

D5-21320 Cellulitis of floor of mouth 528.3
(T-51200) (M-41650)
Ludwig's angina 528.3
(T-51200) (M-41650)

D5-21340 Oral fistula 528.3
(T-51004) (M-39300)

D5-21400 Dermoid cyst of mouth 528.4
(T-51004) (M-33410)
Epidermoid cyst of mouth 528.4
(T-51004) (M-33410)

D5-21404 Lymphoepithelial cyst of mouth 528.4
(T-51004) (T-C2000) (M-33410)

D5-21500 Leukoplakia of oral mucosa, NOS 528.6
(T-51030) (M-72830)
Leukokeratosis of oral mucosa 528.6
(T-51050) (M-72830)

D5-21510 Erythroplakia of mouth 528.7
(T-51030) (M-80802)
Erythroplasia of Queyrat of oral mucosa 528.7
(T-51030) (M-80802)

D5-21512 Focal epithelial hyperplasia of mouth 528.7
(T-51030) (M-72151)

D5-21514 Leukoedema of mouth 528.7
(T-51030) (M-72820)

D5-21520 Oral submucosal fibrosis 528.8
(T-51030) (M-78000)

D5-21610 Denture stomatitis 528.9
(T-51030) (M-40000) (F-A2600) (G-C001) (A-04220)
Denture sore mouth 528.9
(T-51030) (M-40000) (F-A2600) (G-C001) (A-04220)

D5-21620 Hemorrhage from mouth
(T-51030) (M-37000)
Bleeding from mouth
(T-51030) (M-37000)

D5-21630 Melanoplakia 528.9
(T-51030) (M-04200) (M-57200)

D5-21640 Papillary hyperplasia of palate 528.9
(T-51100) (M-72050)

D5-21642V Lampas
(T-51110) (M-40000)
Palatitis
(T-51110) (M-40000)
Lampers
(T-51110) (M-40000)

D5-21650 Eosinophilic granuloma of oral mucosa 528.9
(T-51030) (M-44050)

D5-21652V Feline eosinophilic granuloma
(T-51030) (M-44050)
Feline rodent ulcer
(T-51030) (M-44050)

D5-21660 Irritative hyperplasia of oral mucosa 528.9
(T-51030) (M-72000) (G-C001) (M-14700)

D5-21670 Pyogenic granuloma of oral mucosa 528.9
(T-51030) (M-44020)

D5-21680 Traumatic ulcer of oral mucosa 528.9
(T-51030) (M-38000) (G-C001) (M-10000)

D5-21682V Plant awn stomatitis
(T-51030) (M-40000) (G-C001) (L-D0006)

5-22 DISEASES OF THE LIPS

D5-22000 Disease of lips, NOS 528.5
(T-52000) (DF-00000)
D5-22010 Abscess of lip 528.5
(T-52000) (M-41610)
D5-22020 Cellulitis of lip 528.5
(T-52000) (M-41650)
D5-22030 Fistula of lip 528.5
(T-52000) (M-39300)
D5-22040 Hypertrophy of lip 528.5
(T-52000) (M-71000)
D5-22050 Cheilitis, NOS 528.5
(T-52000) (M-40000)
D5-22060 Cheilosis 528.5
(T-52000) (M-59020) (M-01560)
D5-22070 Cheilodynia 528.5
(T-52000) (F-A2600)
Painful lips
(T-52000) (F-A2600)
D5-22080 Leukoplakia of lips 528.6
(T-52000) (M-72830)
D5-22100V Avulsion of lip
(T-52000) (M-14120)
D5-22110V Chronic lip fold dermatitis
(T-52000) (T-01000) (M-43000)
D5-22120V Granuloma of lip
(T-52000) (M-44000)
D5-22130V Ulcer of lip
(T-52000) (M-38000)
D5-22150 Cheilitis glandularis, NOS 528.5
(T-52200) (M-71000) (M-31314)
(G-C008) (T-61400) (M-40000)
D5-22151 Simple cheilitis glandularis 528.5
(T-52200) (M-71000) (M-31314)
(G-C008) (T-61400) (M-40000)
D5-22152 Cheilitis glandularis, superficial suppurative type 528.5
(T-52200) (M-71000) (M-31314)
(G-C008) (T-61400) (M-40600)
Baelz's disease 528.5
(T-52200) (M-71000) (M-31314)
(G-C008) (T-61400) (M-40600)
D5-22153 Cheilitis glandularis, deep suppurative type 528.5
(T-52200) (M-71000) (M-31314)
(G-C008) (T-61400) (M-41600)
(M-39300)
Apostematous cheilitis glandularis 528.5
(T-52200) (M-71000) (M-31314)
(G-C008) (T-61400) (M-41600)
(M-39300)
D5-22160 Cheilitis granulomatosa of Mescher-Melkersson-Rosenthal
(T-52200) (M-44000)

5-23 DISEASES OF THE TONGUE

D5-23000 Disease of tongue, NOS 529.9
(T-53000) (DF-00000)
D5-23100 Glossitis, NOS 529.0
(T-53000) (M-40000)
D5-23110 Abscess of tongue 529.0
(T-53000) (M-41610)
D5-23120 Traumatic ulceration of tongue 529.0
(T-53000) (M-38000) (G-C001)
(M-10000)
D5-23150 Glossitis due to oil of cinnamon
(T-53000) (M-40000) (G-C001)
(C-31129)
D5-23180 Leukoplakia of tongue 528.6
(T-53000) (M-72830)
D5-23188 Hairy leukoplakia of tongue
(T-53000) (M-72830)
D5-23200 Geographic tongue 529.1
(T-53000) (M-40000) (G-C008)
(T-53230) (F-41500) (M-02100)
Benign migratory glossitis 529.1
(T-53000) (M-40000) (G-C008)
(T-53230) (F-41500) (M-02100)
Glossitis areata exfoliativa 529.1
(T-53000) (M-40000) (G-C008)
(T-53230) (F-41500) (M-02100)
D5-23210 Hypertrophy of tongue papillae 529.3
(T-53210) (M-71000)
D5-23220 Black hairy tongue 529.3
(T-53210) (M-71000) (M-04110)
Lingua villosa nigra 529.3
(T-53210) (M-71000) (M-04110)
Melanoglossia 529.3
(T-53210) (M-71000) (M-04110)
D5-23230 Coated tongue 529.3
(T-53000) (T-00250) (F-41500)
(M-04170)
D5-23240 Hypertrophy of foliate papillae 529.3
(T-53260) (M-71000)
D5-23300 Atrophy of tongue papillae 529.4
(T-53210) (M-58000)
Smooth atrophic tongue 529.4
(T-53210) (M-58000)
D5-23320 Atrophic glossitis 529.4
(T-53000) (M-43000) (F-A2600)
(G-C002) (DC-12300)
Hunter's glossitis 529.4
(T-53000) (M-43000) (F-A2600)
(G-C002) (DC-12300)
D5-23330 Moeller's glossitis 529.4
(T-53000) (M-43000) (M-38350)
Bald tongue 529.4
(T-53000) (M-43000) (M-38350)
Glazed tongue 529.4
(T-53000) (M-43000) (M-38350)
Glossodynia exfoliativa 529.4
(T-53000) (M-43000) (M-38350)
D5-23400 Plicated tongue 529.5
(T-53120) (M-01560)
Fissured tongue 529.5
(T-53120) (M-01560)

5-23 DISEASES OF THE TONGUE — Continued

D5-23400 (cont.) Furrowed tongue 529.5
(T-53120) (M-01560)
Scrotal tongue 529.5
(T-53120) (M-01560)

D5-23500 Glossodynia 529.6
(T-53000) (F-A2600)
Painful tongue 529.6
(T-53000) (F-A2600)

D5-23510 Glossopyrosis 529.6
(T-53000) (F-A260A)
Burning tongue 529.6
(T-53000) (F-A260A)

D5-23600 Atrophy of tongue 529.8
(T-53000) (M-58000)

D5-23610 Crenated tongue 529.8
(T-53000) (M-01450)

D5-23620 Enlargement of tongue 529.8
(T-53000) (M-71000)
Hypertrophy of tongue 528.9
(T-53000) (M-71000)

D5-23630 Glossocele 529.8
(T-53000) (M-31400) (M-02570)

D5-23640 Glossoptosis 529.8
(T-53000) (M-31050)

D5-23650 Paralysis of tongue, NOS
(T-53000) (F-A0840)
Glossoplegia, NOS
(T-53000) (F-A0840)

D5-23651 Unilateral paralysis of tongue
(T-53000) (F-A0842)

D5-23652 Bilateral paralysis of tongue
(T-53000) (F-A0844)

D5-23660 Erythroplakia of tongue 528.7
(T-53000) (M-80802)

D5-23670 Focal epithelial hyperplasia of tongue 528.7
(T-53000) (M-72151)

D5-23680 Leukoedema of tongue 528.7
(T-53000) (M-72820)

D5-23710 Leukokeratosis nicotina palati 528.7
(T-51100) (M-72830) (G-C001)
(C-30384)

D5-23750 Palatal myoclonus
(T-51120) (F-11150)
Palatal nystagmus
(T-51120) (F-11150)

SECTION 5-3 DISEASES OF THE ESOPHAGUS, STOMACH AND DUODENUM

5-30 DISEASES OF THE ESOPHAGUS

D5-30000 Disease of esophagus, NOS 530.9
(T-56000) (DF-00000)

D5-30100 Esophagitis, NOS 530.1
(T-56000) (M-40000)

D5-30120 Abscess of esophagus 530.1
(T-56000) (M-41610)

D5-30130 Chemical esophagitis 530.1
(T-56000) (M-40000) (G-C001)
(C-10030)

D5-30140 Gastroesophageal reflux disease 530.1
(T-56000) (M-40000) (G-C001)
(F-50530)
Esophageal reflux 530.1
(T-56000) (M-40000) (G-C001)
(F-50530)
Reflux esophagitis 530.1
(T-56000) (M-40000) (G-C001)
(F-50530)

D5-30142 Peptic reflux disease 530.1
(T-56000) (M-40000) (G-C001)
(F-50530) (F-52300)
Peptic esophagitis 530.1
(T-56000) (M-40000) (G-C001)
(F-50530) (F-52300)
Peptic reflux esophagitis 530.1
(T-56000) (M-40000) (G-C001)
(F-50530) (F-52300)

D5-30144 Alkaline reflux disease 530.1
(T-56000) (M-40000) (G-C001)
(F-50530) (F-52310)
Alkaline reflux esophagitis 530.1
(T-56000) (M-40000) (G-C001)
(F-50530) (F-52310)

D5-30150 Postoperative esophagitis 530.1
(T-56000) (M-40000) (F-06030)

D5-30152 Regurgitant esophagitis 530.1
(T-56000) (M-40000) (F-52880)

D5-30200 Esophageal motor disorder, NOS
(T-56000) (F-A0810)

D5-30202 Achalasia of esophagus 530.0
(T-56000) (F-50510)

D5-30204 Disorder of upper esophageal sphincter
(T-56100) (F-A0810)
Disorder of cervical esophageal region
(T-56100) (F-A0810)

D5-30210 Cricopharyngeus muscle dysfunction
(T-1357B) (F-A0810)

D5-30212 Spasm of the cricopharyngeus muscle
(T-1357B) (F-50510) (F-11310)
Achalasia of the cricopharyngeus muscle
(T-1357B) (F-50510) (F-11310)
Cricopharyngeal achalasia
(T-1357B) (F-50510) (F-11310)
Cricopharyngeal dysphagia
(T-1357B) (F-50510) (F-11310)

D5-30215 Spastic disorder of smooth muscle segment of esophagus
(T-56000) (T-1A500) (F-11310)

D5-30220 Cardiospasm, NOS 530.0
(T-56315) (F-50510)
Achalasia of cardia 530.0
(T-56315) (F-50510)
Lack of reflex relaxation of lower esophageal sphincter 530.0
(T-56315) (F-50510)

D5-30220 (cont.) Hypertensive lower esophageal sphincter
(T-56315) (F-50510)

D5-30224 Chalasia of lower esophageal sphincter
(T-56315) (F-50500)
Hypotensive lower esophageal sphincter
(T-56315) (F-50500)
Chalasia of cardia
(T-56315) (F-50500)
Cardio-esophageal relaxation
(T-56315) (F-50500)
Cardiochalasia
(T-56315) (F-50500)
Relaxation of lower esophageal sphincter
(T-56315) (F-50500)

D5-30230 Aperistalsis of esophagus 530.0
(T-56000) (F-50505)

D5-30234 Megaesophagus 530.0
(T-56000) (M-71000)

D5-30236 Dilatation of esophagus
(T-56000) (M-32000)

D5-30238V Canine idiopathic megaesophagus
(T-56000) (M-71000)

D5-30250 Dysphagia, NOS 787.2
(T-56000) (F-51702)
Difficulty in swallowing 787.2
(T-56000) (F-51702)

D5-30251 Constant low-grade dysphagia
(T-56000) (F-51702)

D5-30252 Intermittent dysphagia
(T-56000) (F-51702)

D5-30253 Oropharyngeal dysphagia
(T-56000) (F-51710) (F-51720)
Transfer dysphagia
(T-56000) (F-51710) (F-51720)
Pharyngeal dysphagia
(T-56000) (F-51710) (F-51720)

D5-30254 Esophageal dysphagia
(T-56000) (F-51730)

D5-30258 Dysphagia lusoria
(T-56000) (F-51702)

D5-30260 Odynophagia
(T-56000) (F-51700) (F-A2600)
Painful swallowing
(T-56000) (F-51700) (F-A2600)
Pain on swallowing
(T-56000) (F-51700) (F-A2600)

D5-30300 Ulcer of esophagus, NOS 530.2
(T-56000) (M-38000)

D5-30310 Fungal ulcer of esophagus 530.2
(T-56000) (M-38000) (G-C001)
(L-40000)

D5-30320 Peptic ulcer of esophagus 530.2
(T-56000) (M-40000) (G-C001)
(F-52300)

D5-30360 Esophagogastric ulcer
(T-56000) (T-57000) (M-38000)

D5-30400 Stricture of esophagus 530.3
(T-56000) (M-34260)

D5-30402 Stenosis of esophagus 530.3
(T-56000) (M-34200)

D5-30410 Compression of esophagus 530.3
(T-56000) (M-01460)

D5-30420 Obstruction of esophagus 530.3
(T-56000) (M-34000)
Thoracic choke
(T-56000) (M-34000)

D5-30440 Esophageal web, NOS
(T-56000) (M-01570)

D5-30442 Upper esophageal web
(T-56110) (M-01570)

D5-30444 Esophageal body web
(T-56210) (M-01570)

D5-30448 Terminal esophageal web
(T-56310) (M-01570)
Terminal esophageal ring
(T-56310) (M-01570)
Schatzki's ring
(T-56310) (M-01570)

D5-30500 Perforation of esophagus 530.4
(T-56000) (M-39210)

D5-30510 Spontaneous rupture of esophagus 530.4
(T-56000) (M-14400)
Boerhaave's syndrome 530.4
(T-56000) (M-14400)

D5-30600 Dyskinesia of esophagus 530.5
(T-56000) (F-A4230)

D5-30610 Corkscrew esophagus 530.5
(T-56000) (M-02010)

D5-30620 Curling esophagus 530.5
(T-56000) (M-02010)

D5-30630 Esophagospasm 530.5
(T-56000) (F-11310)
Spasm of esophagus 530.5
(T-56000) (F-11310)
Esophagism
(T-56000) (F-11310)

D5-30632 Diffuse spasm of esophagus 530.5
(T-56000) (F-11319)

D5-30700 Acquired diverticulum of esophagus 530.6
(T-56000) (M-32700)

D5-30710 Acquired pharyngoesophageal diverticulum 530.6
(T-55300) (M-32700)
Zenker's diverticulum 530.6
(T-55300) (M-32700)
Hypopharyngeal diverticulum 530.6
(T-55300) (M-32700)

D5-30720 Acquired subdiaphragmatic diverticulum of esophagus 530.6
(T-56000) (M-32700) (T-D4440)
Acquired epiphrenic diverticulum of esophagus 530.6
(T-56000) (M-32700) (T-D4440)

D5-30730 Acquired pulsion diverticulum of esophagus 530.6
(T-56000) (M-32720)

5-30 DISEASES OF THE ESOPHAGUS — Continued

D5-30740 Acquired traction diverticulum of esophagus 530.6
(T-56000) (M-32730)

D5-30750 Acquired esophagocele 530.6
(T-56050) (M-31500)
Acquired esophageal pouch 530.6
(T-56050) (M-31500)

D5-30770 Intramural diverticulosis of esophagus
(T-56000) (M-32790)
Pseudodiverticulosis of esophagus
(T-56000) (M-32790)

D5-30800 Mallory-Weiss syndrome 530.7
(T-56350) (M-14400) (M-37000)
Gastroesophageal laceration-hemorrhage syndrome 530.7
(T-56350) (M-14400) (M-37000)

D5-30810 Hemorrhage of esophagus 530.8
(T-56000) (M-37000)

D5-30812 Intramural esophageal hematoma
(T-56000) (M-35060)

D5-30820 Aorto-esophageal fistula
(T-56000) (T-42000) (M-39300)

D5-30830 Esophageal varices, NOS 456.1
(T-56000) (M-32600)

D5-30831 Esophageal varices without bleeding 456.1
(T-56000) (M-32600) (G-C009)
(M-37000)

D5-30832 Bleeding esophageal varices 456.0
(T-56000) (M-32601)

D5-30840 Gastroesophageal intussusception
(T-56000) (M-31430) (T-57000)

D5-30850 Esophageal fistula
(T-56000) (M-39300)

D5-30852 Esophagobronchial fistula
(T-56000) (T-26000) (M-39300)

D5-30900 Leukoplakia of esophagus 530.8
(T-56000) (M-72830)

D5-30910 Barrett's esophagus
(T-56000) (M-73330)
Gastric metaplasia of esophagus
(T-56000) (M-73330)
Barrett's syndrome
(T-56000) (M-73330)
Barrett's ulcer
(T-56000) (M-73330)

D5-30930 Esophageal injury, NOS
(T-56000) (M-10000)

D5-30932 Caustic esophageal injury
(T-56000) (M-10000) (G-C001)
(C-10300)

D5-30950 Pill esophagitis, NOS
(T-56000) (M-40000) (G-C001)
(C-50701)

D5-30952 Pill esophagitis due to tetracycline
(T-56000) (M-40000) (G-C001)
(C-50701) (C-55000)

D5-30954 Pill esophagitis due to quinidine
(T-56000) (M-40000) (G-C001)
(C-50701) (C-80460)

D5-30956 Pill esophagitis due to potassium chloride
(T-56000) (M-40000) (G-C001)
(C-50701) (C-71063)

D5-30960 Ulcer of esophagus due to ingestion of chemicals, NOS 530.2
(T-56000) (M-38000) (G-C001)
(F-50440) (C-10030)

D5-30970 Ulcer of esophagus due to ingestion of medicines, NOS 530.2
(T-56000) (M-38000) (G-C001)
(F-50440) (C-50000)

D5-30972 Ulcer of esophagus due to ingestion of aspirin 530.2
(T-56000) (M-38000) (G-C001)
(F-50440) (C-60320)

D5-30A00V Ingluvitis
(T-56500) (M-40000)

D5-30A10V Crop impaction
(T-56500) (M-33100)
Crop bound
(T-56500) (M-33100)
Pendulous crop
(T-56500) (M-33100)

D5-30A12V Crop stasis
(T-56500) (M-33350)

5-32-33 DISEASES OF THE STOMACH

D5-32000 Disease of stomach, NOS 537.9
(T-57000) (DF-00000)

D5-32010 Gastric polyp, NOS
(T-57000) (M-76800)

D5-32018 Gastric polyposis
(T-57000) (M-76900)

D5-32020 Gastric dysplasia, NOS
(T-57000) (M-74000)

D5-32100 Gastric ulcer, NOS 531.-
(T-57000) (M-38000)
Stomach ulcer, NOS 531.-
(T-57000) (M-38000)
Peptic ulcer of stomach 531.-
(T-57000) (M-38090)

D5-32110 Acute gastric mucosal erosion, NOS 531.-
(T-57010) (M-38351)
Acute erosion of stomach 531.-
(T-57010) (M-38351)

D5-32112 Stress ulcer, NOS 533.-
(T-57010) (M-38350) (G-C002)
(F-06300)
Stress ulcers of stomach, NOS 533.-
(T-57010) (M-38350) (G-C002)
(F-06300)

D5-32114 Curling's ulcers 533.-
(T-57010) (M-38351) (G-C002)
(M-11100)
Acute gastric erosion associated with severe burns 533.-
(T-57010) (M-38351) (G-C002)
(M-11100)

D5-32116 Cushing's ulcers 533.-
(T-57010) (M-38351) (G-C002)
(T-A0090) (M-10000)
Acute gastric erosion associated with central nervous system trauma 533.-
(T-57010) (M-38351) (G-C002)
(T-A0090) (M-10000)

D5-32118 Acute gastric erosion associated with drug ingestion
(T-57010) (M-38351) (G-C002)
(F-50440) (C-50000)

D5-32120 NSAID-associated gastropathy
(T-57000) (DF-00000) (G-C002)
(C-60300)
Nonsteroidal anti-inflammatory drug-associated gastropathy
(T-57000) (DF-00000) (G-C002)
(C-60300)

D5-32140 Prepyloric ulcer 531.-
(T-57520) (M-38000)

D5-32150 Pyloric ulcer 531.-
(T-57700) (M-38000)

D5-32200 Gastric ulcer, NOS with hemorrhage 531.4
(T-57000) (M-38000) (G-C008)
(M-37000)

D5-32202 Gastric ulcer, NOS with hemorrhage but without obstruction 531.40
(T-57000) (M-38000) (G-C008)
(M-37000) (G-C009) (M-34000)

D5-32204 Gastric ulcer, NOS with hemorrhage and obstruction 531.41
(T-57000) (M-38000) (G-C008)
(M-37000) (M-34000)

D5-32210 Gastric ulcer, NOS with perforation 531.5
(T-57000) (M-38000) (G-C008)
(M-39210)

D5-32212 Gastric ulcer, NOS with perforation but without obstruction 531.50
(T-57000) (M-38000) (G-C008)
(M-39210) (G-C009) (M-34000)

D5-32214 Gastric ulcer, NOS with perforation and obstruction 531.51
(T-57000) (M-38000) (G-C008)
(M-39210) (M-34000)

D5-32220 Acute gastric ulcer with hemorrhage 531.0
(T-57000) (M-38010) (G-C008)
(M-37000)
Acute gastric ulcer with bleeding 531.0
(T-57000) (M-38010) (G-C008)
(M-37000)

D5-32222 Acute gastric ulcer with hemorrhage but without obstruction 531.00
(T-57000) (M-38010) (G-C008)
(M-37000) (G-C009) (M-34000)

D5-32224 Acute gastric ulcer with hemorrhage and obstruction 531.01
(T-57000) (M-38010) (G-C008)
(M-37000) (M-34000)

D5-32230 Acute gastric ulcer with perforation 531.1
(T-57000) (M-38010) (G-C008)
(M-39210)

D5-32232 Acute gastric ulcer with perforation but without obstruction 531.10
(T-57000) (M-38010) (G-C008)
(M-39210) (G-C009) (M-34000)

D5-32234 Acute gastric ulcer with perforation and obstruction 531.11
(T-57000) (M-38010) (G-C008)
(M-39210) (M-34000)

D5-32240 Acute gastric ulcer with hemorrhage and perforation 531.2
(T-57000) (M-38010) (G-C008)
(M-37000) (M-39210)

D5-32242 Acute gastric ulcer with hemorrhage and perforation but without obstruction 531.20
(T-57000) (M-38010) (G-C008)
(M-37000) (M-39210) (G-C009)
(M-34000)

D5-32244 Acute gastric ulcer with hemorrhage and perforation and with obstruction 531.21
(T-57000) (M-38010) (G-C008)
(M-37000) (M-39210) (M-34000)

D5-32250 Acute gastric ulcer without hemorrhage or perforation 531.3
(T-57000) (M-38010) (G-C009)
(M-37000) (M-39210)

D5-32252 Acute gastric ulcer without hemorrhage or perforation and without obstruction 531.30
(T-57000) (M-38010) (G-C009)
(M-37000) (M-39210) (M-34000)

D5-32254 Acute gastric ulcer without hemorrhage or perforation but with obstruction 531.31
(T-57000) (M-38010) (G-C009)
(M-37000) (M-39210) (G-C008)
(M-34000)

D5-32300 Chronic gastric ulcer with hemorrhage 531.4
(T-57000) (M-38020) (G-C008)
(M-37000)

D5-32302 Chronic gastric ulcer with hemorrhage but without obstruction 531.40
(T-57000) (M-38020) (G-C008)
(M-37000) (G-C009) (M-34000)

D5-32304 Chronic gastric ulcer with hemorrhage and obstruction 531.41
(T-57000) (M-38020) (G-C008)
(M-37000) (M-34000)

D5-32310 Chronic gastric ulcer with perforation 531.5
(T-57000) (M-38020) (G-C008)
(M-39210)

D5-32312 Chronic gastric ulcer with perforation but without obstruction 531.50
(T-57000) (M-38020) (G-C008)
(M-39210) (G-C009) (M-34000)

D5-32314 Chronic gastric ulcer with perforation and obstruction 531.51
(T-57000) (M-38020) (G-C008)
(M-39210) (M-34000)

5-32-33 DISEASES OF THE STOMACH — Continued

D5-32320 Chronic gastric ulcer with hemorrhage and perforation 531.6
(T-57000) (M-38000) (G-C008) (M-37000) (M-39210)

D5-32322 Chronic gastric ulcer with hemorrhage and perforation but without obstruction 531.60
(T-57000) (M-38020) (G-C008) (M-37000) (M-39210) (G-C009) (M-34000)

D5-32324 Chronic gastric ulcer with hemorrhage and perforation and with obstruction 531.61
(T-57000) (M-38020) (G-C008) (M-37000) (M-39210) (M-34000)

D5-32330 Chronic gastric ulcer without hemorrhage or perforation 531.7
(T-57000) (M-38020) (G-C009) (M-37000) (M-39210)

D5-32332 Chronic gastric ulcer without hemorrhage or perforation and without obstruction 531.70
(T-57000) (M-38020) (G-C009) (M-37000) (M-39210) (M-34000)

D5-32334 Chronic gastric ulcer without hemorrhage or perforation but with obstruction 531.71
(T-57000) (M-38020) (G-C009) (M-37000) (M-39210) (G-C008) (M-34000)

D5-32410 Gastric ulcer, NOS with hemorrhage and perforation 531.6
(T-57000) (M-38000) (G-C008) (M-37000) (M-39210)

D5-32412 Gastric ulcer, NOS with hemorrhage and perforation but without obstruction 531.60
(T-57000) (M-38000) (G-C008) (M-37000) (M-39210) (G-C009) (M-34000)

D5-32414 Gastric ulcer, NOS with hemorrhage and perforation and with obstruction 531.61
(T-57000) (M-38000) (G-C008) (M-37000) (M-39210) (M-34000)

D5-32420 Gastric ulcer, NOS without hemorrhage or perforation 531.9
(T-57000) (M-38000) (G-C009) (M-37000) (M-39210)

D5-32422 Gastric ulcer, NOS without hemorrhage or perforation and without obstruction 531.90
(T-57000) (M-38000) (G-C009) (M-37000) (M-39210) (M-34000)

D5-32424 Gastric ulcer, NOS without hemorrhage or perforation but with obstruction 531.91
(T-57000) (M-38000) (G-C009) (M-37000) (M-39210) (G-C008) (M-34000)

D5-32500 Gastritis, NOS 535.5
(T-57000) (M-40000)
Gastric catarrh
(T-57000) (M-40000)

D5-32510 Acute gastritis 535.0
(T-57000) (M-41000)

D5-32511 Phlegmonous gastritis
(T-56000) (M-41650)

D5-32512 Acute hemorrhagic gastritis
(T-57000) (M-41000) (M-38000)

D5-32514 Idiopathic erosive/hemorrhagic gastritis
(T-57000) (M-40000) (M-38350) (M-37000)

D5-32516 Chronic erosive gastritis
(T-57000) (M-43000) (G-C008) (M-38350)
Diffuse varioliform gastritis
(T-57000) (M-43000) (G-C008) (M-38350)

D5-32520 Atrophic gastritis 535.1
(T-57000) (M-45100)
Chronic atrophic gastritis 535.1
(T-57000) (M-45100)

D5-32522 Atrophic-hyperplastic gastritis 535.1
(T-57000) (M-45100) (M-45200)

D5-32528 Atrophic fundic gland gastritis
(T-57000) (M-40000) (G-C001) (T-57040) (M-58000)

D5-32530 Hypertrophic gastritis 535.2
(T-57010) (M-71000)
Gastric mucosal hypertrophy 535.2
(T-57010) (M-71000)
Ménétrier's disease 535.2
(T-57010) (M-71000)
Hypertrophic gastropathy 535.2
(T-57010) (M-71000)
Chronic hypertrophic gastritis 535.2
(T-57010) (M-71000)
Giant rugal gastritis 535.2
(T-57010) (M-71000)
Gastritis hypertrophic gigantica 535.2
(T-57010) (M-71000)

D5-32534 Chronic hypertrophic pyloric gastropathy
(T-57010) (T-57700) (M-71000)

D5-32535V Focal cystic hypertrophic gastropathy
(T-57010) (M-71000) (M-33400)

D5-32536V Hypertrophic gastritis of Basenji dogs
(T-57010) (M-71000)

D5-32537V Hypertrophic glandular gastritis
(T-57010) (T-57040) (M-71000)

D5-32550 Allergic gastritis 535.4
(T-57000) (M-40000) (F-C3000)

D5-32554 Eosinophilic gastritis
(T-57A10) (M-43040)

D5-32560 Postgastrectomy gastritis
(T-57000) (M-40000) (F-06090) (P1-02000) (T-57000)

D5-32564 Emphysematous gastritis
(T-57000) (M-40000) (M-33900)
Gastric emphysema
(T-57000) (M-40000) (M-33900)

D5-32570 Irritant gastritis 535.4
(T-57000) (G-C001) (M-14700)
D5-32572 Alcoholic gastritis 535.3
(T-57000) (M-40000) (G-C001)
(C-21005)
D5-32574V Reflux gastritis
(T-57000) (M-40000) (G-C001)
(F-50530)
D5-32576 Bile-induced gastritis 535.4
(T-57000) (M-40000) (G-C001)
(T-60650)
D5-32580 Superficial gastritis 535.4
(T-57010) (M-40000)
D5-32582 Nonerosive nonspecific gastritis, NOS
(T-57000) (M-40000)
D5-32584 Superficial nonerosive nonspecific gastritis
(T-57010) (M-40000)
D5-32586 Atrophic nonerosive nonspecific gastritis
(T-57010) (M-45100)
D5-32590 Toxic gastritis 535.4
(T-57000) (G-C001) (C-00220)
D5-32592 Caustic injury gastritis
(T-57000) (M-40000) (G-C001)
(M-10000) (C-10300)
D5-325A0 Gastroduodenitis 535.5
(T-57000) (T-58200) (M-40000)
D5-32600 Disorder of function of stomach, NOS 536.-
(T-57000) (F-01100)
Functional gastric disorder, NOS 536.-
(T-57000) (F-01100)
Functional gastric disturbance, NOS 536.-
(T-57000) (F-01100)
Functional gastric irritation, NOS 536.-
(T-57000) (F-01100)
D5-32602 Dyspepsia, NOS 536.8
(T-57000) (F-50002) (F-50818)
Indigestion, NOS 536.8
(T-57000) (F-50002) (F-50818)
Mild dietary indigestion 536.8
(T-57000) (F-50002) (F-50818)
D5-32604 Nonulcer dyspepsia
(T-57000) (F-50002) (F-50818)
(G-C009) (M-38000)
D5-32606V Vagus indigestion
(T-57000) (F-50002) (F-50818)
D5-32620 Acute dilatation of stomach 536.1
(T-57000) (M-32008)
Acute distention of stomach 536.1
(T-57000) (M-32008)
Gastric tympany 536.1
(T-57000) (M-32008)
D5-32630 Achlorhydria 536.0
(T-57000) (F-52300) (G-A201)
Gastric anacidity
(T-57000) (F-52300) (G-A201)
Absent gastric acidity
(T-57000) (F-52300) (G-A201)
D5-32634 Hyperchlorhydria 536.8
(T-57000) (F-52300) (G-A317)
Gastric hyperacidity 536.8
(T-57000) (F-52300) (G-A317)
Increased gastric acidity 536.8
(T-57000) (F-52300) (G-A317)
D5-32636 Hypochlorhydria 536.8
(T-57000) (F-52300) (G-A316)
Gastric hypoacidity 536.8
(T-57000) (F-52300) (G-A316)
Decreased gastric acidity 536.8
(T-57000) (F-52300) (G-A316)
D5-32640 Achylia gastrica 536.8
(T-57000) (F-52300) (F-52360)
(G-A201)
D5-32650 Idiopathic gastric stasis
(T-57000) (M-33350)
D5-32660 Cyclical vomiting syndrome
(T-57000) (F-52770) (G-A487)
Periodic vomiting
(T-57000) (F-52770) (G-A487)
Cyclical vomiting
(T-57000) (M-52770) (G-A487)
D5-32661 Habit vomiting 536.2
(T-57000) (F-52770) (G-A538)
D5-32662 Persistent vomiting 536.2
(T-57000) (F-52770) (G-A480)
Uncontrollable vomiting 536.2
(T-57000) (F-52770) (G-A480)
D5-32664 Vomiting in infants and children
(T-57000) (F-52770)
D5-32666 Projectile vomiting
(T-57000) (F-52770)
D5-32670 Gastric motor function disorder, NOS
(T-57000) (F-A0810)
Gastric motor dysfunction, NOS
(T-57000) (F-A0810)
Idiopathic gastric motility disorder
(T-57000) (F-A0810)
D5-32680 Gastroparesis syndrome, NOS
(T-57000) (F-A0850) (F-11195)
Gastric atony
(T-57000) (F-A0850) (F-11195)
Gastric stasis
(T-57000) (F-A0850) (F-11195)
D5-32681 Nondiabetic gastroparesis
(T-57000) (F-11195) (G-C009)
(DB-61000)
D5-32682 Diabetic gastroparesis
(T-57000) (F-11195) (G-C008)
(DB-61000)
D5-32700 Acquired hypertrophic pyloric stenosis 537.0
(T-57700) (M-34200) (M-71000)
Adult hypertrophic pyloric stenosis 537.0
(T-57700) (M-34200) (M-71000)
Acquired gastric outlet stenosis 537.0
(T-57700) (M-34200) (M-71000)

5-32-33 DISEASES OF THE STOMACH — Continued

D5-32710 Acquired nonhypertrophic constriction of pylorus 537.0
(T-57700) (M-34260)
Acquired stricture of pylorus 537.0
(T-57700) (M-34260)

D5-32720 Acquired obstruction of pylorus 537.0
(T-57700) (M-34000)

D5-32730 Gastric diverticulum 537.1
(T-57000) (M-32700)

D5-32740 Gastrocolic fistula 537.4
(T-57000) (T-59300) (M-39300)

D5-32750 Gastrojejunocolic fistula 537.4
(T-57000) (T-58400) (T-59300) (M-39300)

D5-32760 Gastroptosis 537.5
(T-57000) (M-31050)
Gastric prolapse 537.5
(T-57000) (M-31050)
Prolapse gastropathy 537.5
(T-57000) (M-31050)

D5-32765 Hourglass contraction of stomach 536.8
(T-57000) (M-34200)
Hourglass stricture of stomach 537.6
(T-57000) (M-34200)
Hourglass stenosis of stomach 537.6
(T-57000) (M-34200)

D5-32768 Cascade stomach 537.6
(T-57000) (M-34200)

D5-32770 Gastric rupture 537.89
(T-57000) (M-14400)

D5-32774 Stenosis of stomach 537.6
(T-57000) (M-34200)

D5-32776 Pyloric antral stenosis 537.6
(T-57600) (M-34200)

D5-32780 Pylorospasm 537.81
(T-57700) (F-11310)

D5-32790 Intestinal metaplasia of gastric mucosa 537.89
(T-57010) (M-73320)

D5-32800 Passive congestion of stomach 537.89
(T-57000) (M-36140)

D5-32810 Malakoplakia of stomach
(T-57000) (M-44170)

D5-32820 Gastric volvulus, NOS
(T-57000) (M-34110) (M-34000)

D5-32822 Organoaxial gastric volvulus
(T-57000) (M-34110) (M-34000)

D5-32824 Mesenteroaxial gastric volvulus
(T-57000) (M-34110) (M-34000)

D5-32826 Mixed gastric volvulus
(T-57000) (M-34110) (M-34000)

D5-32830 Acute gastric volvulus
(T-57000) (M-34110) (M-34000)

D5-32840 Chronic gastric volvulus
(T-57000) (M-34110) (M-34000)

D5-32842 Chronic torsion of stomach
(T-57000) (M-34110) (M-34000)

D5-32844V Gastric dilatation-volvulus-torsion syndrome
(T-57000) (M-32000) (M-34110) (M-34000)
GDVT syndrome
(T-57000) (M-32000) (M-34110) (M-34000)

D5-32850 Gastric foreign body, NOS
(T-57000) (M-30400)

D5-32852 Postgastrectomy phytobezoar
(T-58000) (M-30470) (F-06090) (P1-02000) (T-58000)

D5-32853V Phytobezoariasis
(L-D6550)

D5-32854 Gastric concretion
(T-57000) (M-30000)

D5-32856 Gastrointestinal fungal ball
(T-50100) (M-30490) (L-40000)

D5-32858V Chronic trichobezoar formation
(T-50100) (M-30460)
Gastric hairball
(T-50100) (M-30460)

D5-32910 Drug-induced nausea and vomiting, NOS
(T-57000) (F-52760) (F-52770) (G-C001) (F-50550) (C-50000)

D5-32B00 Lymphoid hyperplasia of stomach
(T-57000) (M-72200)
Gastric pseudolymphoma
(T-57000) (M-72200)

D5-32B10 Isolated idiopathic granuloma of stomach
(T-57000) (M-44000)

D5-32B12 Isolated idiopathic granuloma of stomach, foreign body type
(T-57000) (M-44140)

D5-32B14 Inflammatory fibroid polyps of stomach
(T-57000) (M-76820)

D5-33010 Gastric hemorrhage, NOS 578.9
(T-57000) (M-37000)
Gastric bleeding, NOS 578.9
(T-57000) (M-37000)

D5-33020 Gastric varices
(T-57000) (M-32600)

D5-33022 Bleeding gastric varices
(T-57000) (M-32601)

D5-33030 Pyloric antral vascular ectasia
(T-57600) (T-40050) (M-32000)

D5-33032 Watermelon stomach
(T-57600) (T-40050) (M-32000)

D5-33500V Disease of ruminant stomach, NOS
(T-57A10) (DF-00000)
Disorder of ruminant stomach, NOS
(T-57A10) (DF-00000)

D5-33510V Rumenitis, NOS
(T-57A10) (M-40000)

D5-33520V Reticulitis, NOS
(T-57A20) (M-40000)

D5-33522V Traumatic reticuloperitonitis
(T-57A20) (T-D4400) (M-40000) (G-C001) (M-10000)
Hardware disease
(T-57A20) (T-D4400) (M-40000) (G-C001) (M-10000)

D5-33524V Traumatic reticulopericarditis
(T-57A20) (T-39000) (M-40000)
(G-C001) (M-10000)

D5-33526V Traumatic reticulopleurisy
(T-57A20) (T-29000) (M-40000)
(G-C001) (M-10000)

D5-33528V Traumatic reticulosplenitis
(T-57A20) (T-C3000) (M-40000)
(G-C001) (M-10000)

D5-33530V Ruminal parakeratosis
(T-57A10) (M-74470)

D5-33540V Grain overload
(T-57A10) (G-C001) (F-61900)
Lactic acidosis secondary to grain overload
(T-57A10) (G-C001) (F-61900)
Carbohydrate engorgement
(T-57A10) (G-C001) (F-61900)
Rumen impaction
(T-57A10) (G-C001) (F-61900)
Rumen overload
(T-57A10) (G-C001) (F-61900)

D5-33542V Ruminal stasis
(T-57A10) (M-33350)

D5-33544V Ruminal atony
(T-57A10) (F-11195)

D5-33546V Impaction of the stomach
(T-57A10) (M-33100)

D5-33548V Ruminal ulcer
(T-57A10) (M-38000)

D5-33560V Ruminal tympany
(T-57A10) (F-54150)
Bloat in ruminants
(T-57A10) (F-54150)

D5-33562V Primary ruminal tympany
(T-57A10) (F-54150)
Frothy bloat
(T-57A10) (F-54150)

D5-33564V Secondary ruminal tympany
(T-57A10) (F-54150)
Free gas bloat
(T-57A10) (F-54150)

D5-33570V Omasitis, NOS
(T-57A30) (M-40000)

D5-33574V Omasul impaction
(T-57A30) (M-33100)

D5-33610V Abomasitis, NOS
(T-57A40) (M-40000)

D5-33620V Abomasul ulcer, NOS
(T-57A40) (M-38000)

D5-33621V Abomasul ulcer, type I
(T-57A40) (M-38000)

D5-33622V Abomasul ulcer, type II
(T-57A40) (M-38000)

D5-33623V Abomasul ulcer, type III
(T-57A40) (M-38000)

D5-33624V Abomasul ulcer, type IV
(T-57A40) (M-38000)

D5-33630V Abomasul atony
(T-57A40) (F-11195)
Atony of abomasum
(T-57A40) (F-11195)

D5-33632V Abomasul dilatation
(T-57A40) (M-32000)

D5-33634V Abomasul bloat
(T-57A40) (M-32008)
Acute distention of abomasum
(T-57A40) (M-32008)

D5-33636V Rattle belly in lambs
Watery mouth of lambs
Slavers
Slavery mouth

D5-33638V Abomasul rupture
(T-57A40) (M-14400)

D5-33640V Dietary abomasul impaction
(T-57A40) (M-33100) (G-C001)
(C-F2000)

D5-33644V Abomasul trichobezoars
(T-57A40) (M-30460)

D5-33650V Left-sided displacement of abomasum
(T-57A40) (M-31070)
LDA
(T-57A40) (M-31070)

D5-33654V Right-sided displacement of abomasum
(T-57A40) (M-31070)
RDA
(T-57A40) (M-31070)

D5-33656V Abomasul torsion
(T-57A40) (M-34110)

D5-33700V Disease of avian stomach, NOS
(T-57000) (L-82000) (DF-00000)
Disorder of avian stomach, NOS
(T-57000) (L-82000) (DF-00000)

D5-33710V Disease of proventriculus, NOS
(T-57A00) (L-82000) (DF-00000)
Disorder of proventriculus, NOS
(T-57A00) (L-82000) (DF-00000)

D5-33750V Disease of ventriculus, NOS
(T-57000) (L-82000) (DF-00000)
Disorder of ventriculus, NOS
(T-57000) (L-82000) (DF-00000)

D5-33752V Ventriculitis, NOS
(T-57000) (L-82000) (M-40000)

D5-33756V Erosion of gizzard
(T-57000) (L-82000) (M-38350)

5-34 DISEASES OF THE DUODENUM

D5-34000 Disease of duodenum, NOS 537.9
(T-58200) (DF-00000)

D5-34010 Acute erosion of duodenum 532.-
(T-58200) (M-38351)

D5-34040 Postpyloric ulcer 532.-
(T-58260) (M-38090)
Postbulbar duodenal ulcer 532.-
(T-58260) (M-38090)

5-34 DISEASES OF THE DUODENUM — Continued

D5-34050 Duodenal ulcer disease, NOS
(T-58200) (M-38000) (DF-00000)

D5-34060 Duodenal ulcer, NOS 532.-
(T-58200) (M-38090)
Peptic ulcer of duodenum, NOS 532.-
(T-58200) (M-38090)
Common duodenal ulcer, NOS 532.-
(T-58200) (M-38090)

D5-34062 Duodenal ulcer with increased serum pepsinogen I
(T-58200) (M-38000) (G-C008)
(F-52360) (G-A317)

D5-34064 Normopepsinogenemic familial duodenal ulcer
(T-58200) (M-38000) (G-C008)
(F-52360) (G-A460) (DF-00190)

D5-34066 Familial duodenal ulcer associated with rapid gastric emptying
(T-58200) (M-38000) (G-C008)
(F-52630) (DF-00190)

D5-34068 Familial hypergastrinemic duodenal ulcer
(T-58200) (M-38000) (G-C008)
(F-B6100) (DF-00190)

D5-34070 Childhood duodenal ulcer
(T-58200) (M-38000) (DF-00220)

D5-34080 Combined gastric and duodenal ulcer
(T-57000) (T-58200) (M-38000)

D5-34082 Giant duodenal ulcer
(T-58200) (M-38000) (G-A368)

D5-34084 Pyloric channel ulcer
(T-57601) (M-38000)

D5-34100 Acute duodenal ulcer with hemorrhage 532.0
(T-58200) (M-38010) (G-C008)
(M-37000)

D5-34102 Acute duodenal ulcer with hemorrhage but without obstruction 532.00
(T-58200) (M-38010) (G-C008)
(M-37000) (G-C009) (M-34000)

D5-34104 Acute duodenal ulcer with hemorrhage and obstruction 532.01
(T-58200) (M-38010) (G-C008)
(M-37000) (M-34000)

D5-34110 Acute duodenal ulcer with perforation 532.1
(T-58200) (M-38010) (G-C008)
(M-39210)

D5-34112 Acute duodenal ulcer with perforation but without obstruction 532.10
(T-58200) (M-38010) (G-C008)
(M-39210) (G-C009) (M-34000)

D5-34114 Acute duodenal ulcer with perforation and obstruction 532.11
(T-58200) (M-38010) (G-C008)
(M-39210) (M-34000)

D5-34120 Acute duodenal ulcer with hemorrhage and perforation 532.2
(T-58200) (M-38010) (G-C008)
(M-37000) (M-39210)

D5-34122 Acute duodenal ulcer with hemorrhage and perforation but without obstruction 532.20
(T-58200) (M-38010) (G-C008)
(M-37000) (M-39210) (G-C009)
(M-34000)

D5-34124 Acute duodenal ulcer with hemorrhage and perforation and with obstruction 532.21
(T-58200) (M-38010) (G-C008)
(M-37000) (M-39210) (M-34000)

D5-34130 Acute duodenal ulcer without hemorrhage or perforation 532.3
(T-58200) (M-38010) (G-C009)
(M-37000) (M-39210)

D5-34132 Acute duodenal ulcer without hemorrhage or perforation and without obstruction 532.30
(T-58200) (M-38010) (G-C009)
(M-37000) (M-39210) (M-34000)

D5-34134 Acute duodenal ulcer without hemorrhage or perforation but with obstruction 532.31
(T-58200) (M-38010) (G-C009)
(M-37000) (M-39210) (G-C008)
(M-34000)

D5-34140 Chronic duodenal ulcer with hemorrhage 532.4
(T-58200) (M-38020) (G-C008)
(M-37000)

D5-34142 Chronic duodenal ulcer with hemorrhage but without obstruction 532.40
(T-58200) (M-38020) (G-C008)
(M-37000) (G-C009) (M-34000)

D5-34144 Chronic duodenal ulcer with hemorrhage and obstruction 532.41
(T-58200) (M-38020) (G-C008)
(M-37000) (M-34000)

D5-34150 Duodenal ulcer, NOS with hemorrhage 532.4
(T-58200) (M-38000) (G-C008)
(M-37000)

D5-34152 Duodenal ulcer, NOS with hemorrhage but without obstruction 532.40
(T-58200) (M-38000) (G-C008)
(M-37000) (G-C009) (M-34000)

D5-34154 Duodenal ulcer, NOS with hemorrhage and obstruction 532.41
(T-58200) (M-38000) (G-C008)
(M-37000) (M-34000)

D5-34160 Chronic duodenal ulcer with perforation 532.5
(T-58200) (M-38020) (G-C008)
(M-39210)

D5-34162 Chronic duodenal ulcer with perforation but without obstruction 532.50
(T-58200) (M-38020) (G-C008)
(M-39210) (G-C009) (M-34000)

D5-34164 Chronic duodenal ulcer with perforation and obstruction 532.51
(T-58200) (M-38020) (G-C008)
(M-39210) (M-34000)

D5-34170 Duodenal ulcer, NOS with perforation 532.5
(T-58200) (M-38000) (G-C008)
(M-39210)

D5-34172 Duodenal ulcer, NOS with perforation but without obstruction 532.50
(T-58200) (M-38000) (G-C008)
(M-39210) (G-C009) (M-34000)

D5-34174 Duodenal ulcer, NOS with perforation and obstruction 532.51
(T-58200) (M-38000) (G-C008)
(M-39210) (M-34000)

D5-34180 Chronic duodenal ulcer with hemorrhage and perforation 532.6
(T-58200) (M-38020) (G-C008)
(M-37000) (M-39210)

D5-34182 Chronic duodenal ulcer with hemorrhage and perforation but without obstruction 532.60
(T-58200) (M-38020) (G-C008)
(M-37000) (M-39210) (G-C009)
(M-34000)

D5-34184 Chronic duodenal ulcer with hemorrhage and perforation and with obstruction 532.61
(T-58200) (M-38020) (G-C008)
(M-37000) (M-39210) (M-34000)

D5-34190 Duodenal ulcer, NOS with hemorrhage and perforation 532.6
(T-58200) (M-38000) (G-C008)
(M-37000) (M-39210)

D5-34192 Duodenal ulcer, NOS with hemorrhage and perforation but without obstruction 532.60
(T-58200) (M-38000) (G-C008)
(M-37000) (M-39210) (G-C009)
(M-34000)

D5-34194 Duodenal ulcer, NOS with hemorrhage and perforation and with obstruction 532.61
(T-58200) (M-38000) (G-C008)
(M-37000) (M-39210) (M-34000)

D5-34200 Chronic duodenal ulcer without hemorrhage or perforation 532.7
(T-58200) (M-38020) (G-C009)
(M-37000) (M-39210)

D5-34202 Chronic duodenal ulcer without hemorrhage or perforation and without obstruction 532.70
(T-58200) (M-38020) (G-C009)
(M-37000) (M-39210) (M-34000)

D5-34204 Chronic duodenal ulcer without hemorrhage or perforation but with obstruction 532.71
(T-58200) (M-38020) (G-C009)
(M-37000) (M-39210) (G-C008)
(M-34000)

D5-34210 Duodenal ulcer, NOS without hemorrhage or perforation 532.9
(T-58200) (M-38000) (G-C009)
(M-37000) (M-39120)

D5-34212 Duodenal ulcer, NOS without hemorrhage or perforation and without obstruction 532.90
(T-58200) (M-38000) (G-C009)
(M-37000) (M-39210) (M-34000)

D5-34214 Duodenal ulcer, NOS without hemorrhage or perforation but with obstruction 532.91
(T-58200) (M-38000) (G-C009)
(M-37000) (M-39210) (G-C008)
(M-34000)

D5-34300 Peptic ulcer, NOS 533.-
(T-57000) (T-58200) (M-38090)
(G-C001) (F-52300)
Gastroduodenal ulcer, NOS 533.-
(T-57000) (T-58200) (M-38090)
(G-C001) (F-52300)

D5-34310 Acute peptic ulcer with hemorrhage 533.0
(T-57000) (T-58200) (M-38091)
(G-C008) (M-37000)

D5-34312 Acute peptic ulcer with hemorrhage but without obstruction 533.00
(T-57000) (T-58200) (M-38091)
(G-C008) (M-37000) (G-C009)
(M-34000)

D5-34314 Acute peptic ulcer with hemorrhage and obstruction 533.01
(T-57000) (T-58200) (M-38091)
(G-C008) (M-37000) (M-34000)

D5-34320 Acute peptic ulcer with perforation 533.1
(T-57000) (T-58200) (M-38091)
(G-C008) (M-39210)

D5-34322 Acute peptic ulcer with perforation but without obstruction 533.10
(T-57000) (T-58200) (M-38091)
(G-C008) (M-39210) (G-C009)
(M-34000)

D5-34324 Acute peptic ulcer with perforation and obstruction 533.11
(T-57000) (T-58200) (M-38091)
(G-C008) (M-39210) (M-34000)

D5-34330 Acute peptic ulcer with hemorrhage and perforation 533.2
(T-57000) (T-58200) (M-38091)
(G-C008) (M-37000) (M-39210)

D5-34332 Acute peptic ulcer with hemorrhage and perforation but without obstruction 533.20
(T-57000) (T-58200) (M-39091)
(G-C008) (M-37000) (M-39210)
(G-C009) (M-34000)

D5-34334 Acute peptic ulcer with hemorrhage and perforation and with obstruction 533.21
(T-57000) (T-58200) (M-38091)
(G-C008) (M-37000) (M-39210)
(M-34000)

D5-34340 Acute peptic ulcer without hemorrhage and perforation 533.3
(T-57000) (T-58200) (M-38091)
(G-C009) (M-37000) (M-39210)

D5-34342 Acute peptic ulcer without hemorrhage and perforation and without obstruction 533.30
(T-57000) (T-58200) (M-38091)
(G-C009) (M-37000) (M-39210)
(M-34000)

5-34 DISEASES OF THE DUODENUM — Continued

D5-34344 Acute peptic ulcer without hemorrhage and perforation but with obstruction 533.31
(T-57000) (T-58200) (M-38091) (G-C009) (M-37000) (M-39210) (G-C008) (M-34000)

D5-34350 Chronic peptic ulcer with hemorrhage 533.4
(T-57000) (T-58200) (M-38093) (G-C008) (M-37000)

D5-34352 Chronic peptic ulcer with hemorrhage but without obstruction 533.40
(T-57000) (T-58200) (M-38093) (G-C008) (M-37000) (G-C009) (M-34000)

D5-34354 Chronic peptic ulcer with hemorrhage and obstruction 533.41
(T-57000) (T-58200) (M-38093) (G-C008) (M-37000) (M-34000)

D5-34360 Peptic ulcer, NOS with hemorrhage 533.4
(T-57000) (T-58200) (M-38090) (G-C008) (M-37000)

D5-34362 Peptic ulcer, NOS with hemorrhage but without obstruction 533.40
(T-57000) (T-58200) (M-38090) (G-C008) (M-37000) (G-C009) (M-34000)

D5-34364 Peptic ulcer, NOS with hemorrhage and obstruction 533.41
(T-57000) (T-58200) (M-38090) (G-C008) (M-37000) (M-34000)

D5-34370 Chronic peptic ulcer with perforation 533.5
(T-57000) (T-58200) (M-38093) (G-C008) (M-39210)

D5-34372 Chronic peptic ulcer with perforation but without obstruction 533.50
(T-57000) (T-58200) (M-38093) (G-C008) (M-39210) (G-C009) (M-34000)

D5-34374 Chronic peptic ulcer with perforation and obstruction 533.51
(T-57000) (T-58200) (M-38093) (G-C008) (M-39210) (M-34000)

D5-34380 Peptic ulcer, NOS with perforation 533.5
(T-57000) (T-58200) (M-38090) (G-C008) (M-39210)

D5-34382 Peptic ulcer, NOS with perforation but without obstruction 533.50
(T-57000) (T-58200) (M-39090) (G-C008) (M-39210) (G-C009) (M-34000)

D5-34384 Peptic ulcer, NOS with perforation and obstruction 533.51
(T-57000) (T-58200) (M-38090) (G-C008) (M-39210) (M-34000)

D5-34390 Chronic peptic ulcer with hemorrhage and perforation 533.6
(T-57000) (T-58200) (M-38093) (G-C008) (M-37000) (M-39210)

D5-34392 Chronic peptic ulcer with hemorrhage and perforation but without obstruction 533.60
(T-57000) (T-58200) (M-38093) (G-C008) (M-37000) (M-39210) (G-C009) (M-34000)

D5-34394 Chronic peptic ulcer with hemorrhage and perforation and with obstruction 533.61
(T-57000) (T-58200) (M-38093) (G-C008) (M-37000) (M-39210) (M-34000)

D5-34400 Peptic ulcer, NOS with hemorrhage and perforation 533.6
(T-57000) (T-58200) (M-38090) (G-C008) (M-37000) (M-39210)

D5-34402 Peptic ulcer, NOS with hemorrhage and perforation but without obstruction 533.60
(T-57000) (T-58200) (M-38090) (G-C008) (M-37000) (M-39210) (G-C009) (M-34000)

D5-34404 Peptic ulcer, NOS with hemorrhage and perforation and with obstruction 533.61
(T-57000) (T-58200) (M-38090) (G-C008) (M-37000) (M-39210) (M-34000)

D5-34410 Chronic peptic ulcer without hemorrhage or perforation 533.7
(T-57000) (T-58200) (M-38090) (G-C009) (M-37000) (M-39210)

D5-34412 Chronic peptic ulcer without hemorrhage or perforation and without obstruction 533.70
(T-57000) (T-58200) (M-38093) (G-C009) (M-37000) (M-39210) (M-34000)

D5-34414 Chronic peptic ulcer without hemorrhage and perforation but with obstruction 533.71
(T-57000) (T-58200) (M-38093) (G-C009) (M-37000) (M-39210) (G-C008) (M-34000)

D5-34420 Peptic ulcer, NOS without hemorrhage or perforation 533.9
(T-57000) (T-58200) (M-38090) (G-C009) (M-37000) (M-39210)

D5-34422 Peptic ulcer, NOS without hemorrhage or perforation and without obstruction 533.90
(T-57000) (T-58200) (M-38090) (G-C009) (M-37000) (M-39210) (M-34000)

D5-34424 Peptic ulcer, NOS without hemorrhage or perforation but with obstruction 533.91
(T-57000) (T-58200) (M-38090) (G-C009) (M-37000) (M-39210) (G-C008) (M-34000)

D5-34500 Gastrointestinal ulcer, NOS 534.-
(T-57000) (T-58000) (M-38000)

D5-34504 Anastomotic ulcer, NOS 534.-
(T-57000) (T-58000) (M-18200) (G-C008) (M-38000)

D5-34510 Gastrojejunal ulcer, NOS 534.-
(T-57000) (T-58400) (M-18200)
(G-C008) (M-38000)
Marginal ulcer 534.-
(T-57000) (T-58400) (M-18200)
(G-C008) (M-38000)
Stomal ulcer 534.-
(T-57000) (T-58400) (M-18200)
(G-C008) (M-38000)

D5-34520 Gastrocolic ulcer 534.-
(T-57000) (T-59300) (M-18200)
(G-C008) (M-38000)

D5-34600 Acute gastrojejunal ulcer with hemorrhage 534.0
(T-57000) (T-58400) (M-18200)
(G-C008) (M-38010) (M-37000)

D5-34602 Acute gastrojejunal ulcer with hemorrhage but without obstruction 534.00
(T-57000) (T-58400) (M-18200)
(G-C008) (M-38010) (M-37000)
(G-C009) (M-34000)

D5-34604 Acute gastrojejunal ulcer with hemorrhage and obstruction 534.01
(T-57000) (T-58300) (M-18200)
(G-C008) (M-38010) (M-37000)
(M-34000)

D5-34610 Acute gastrojejunal ulcer with perforation 534.1
(T-57000) (T-58400) (M-18200)
(G-C008) (M-39210)

D5-34612 Acute gastrojejunal ulcer with perforation but without obstruction 534.10
(T-57000) (T-58400) (M-18200)
(G-C008) (M-38010) (M-39210)
(G-C009) (M-34000)

D5-34614 Acute gastrojejunal ulcer with perforation and obstruction 534.11
(T-57000) (T-58200) (M-18200)
(G-C008) (M-38010) (M-39210)
(M-34000)

D5-34620 Acute gastrojejunal ulcer with hemorrhage and perforation 534.2
(T-57000) (T-58400) (M-18200)
(G-C008) (M-38010) (M-37000)
(M-39210)

D5-34622 Acute gastrojejunal ulcer with hemorrhage and perforation but without obstruction 534.20
(T-57000) (T-58400) (M-18200)
(G-C008) (M-38010) (M-37000)
(M-39210) (G-C009) (M-34000)

D5-34624 Acute gastrojejunal ulcer with hemorrhage and perforation and with obstruction 534.21
(T-57000) (T-58400) (M-18200)
(G-C008) (M-38010) (M-37000)
(M-39210) (M-34000)

D5-34630 Acute gastrojejunal ulcer without hemorrhage or perforation 534.3
(T-57000) (T-58400) (M-18200)
(G-C008) (M-38010) (G-C009)
(M-37000) (M-39210)

D5-34632 Acute gastrojejunal ulcer without hemorrhage or perforation and without obstruction 534.30
(T-57000) (T-58400) (M-18200)
(G-C008) (M-38010) (G-C009)
(M-37000) (M-39210) (M-34000)

D5-34634 Acute gastrojejunal ulcer without hemorrhage or perforation but with obstruction 534.31
(T-57000) (T-58400) (M-18200)
(G-C008) (M-38010) (G-C009)
(M-37000) (M-39210) (G-C008)
(M-34000)

D5-34640 Chronic gastrojejunal ulcer with hemorrhage 534.4
(T-57000) (T-58400) (M-18200)
(G-C008) (M-38020) (M-37000)

D5-34642 Chronic gastrojejunal ulcer with hemorrhage but without perforation 534.40
(T-57000) (T-58400) (M-18200)
(G-C008) (M-38020) (M-37000)
(G-C009) (M-39210)

D5-34644 Chronic gastrojejunal ulcer with hemorrhage and obstruction 534.41
(T-57000) (T-58400) (M-18200)
(G-C008) (M-38020) (M-37000)
(M-34000)

D5-34650 Gastrojejunal ulcer, NOS with hemorrhage 534.4
(T-57000) (T-58400) (M-18200)
(G-C008) (M-38000) (M-37000)

D5-34652 Gastrojejunal ulcer, NOS with hemorrhage but without obstruction 534.40
(T-57000) (T-58400) (M-18200)
(G-C008) (M-38000) (M-37000)
(G-C009) (M-34000)

D5-34654 Gastrojejunal ulcer, NOS with hemorrhage and obstruction 534.41
(T-57000) (T-58400) (M-18200)
(G-C008) (M-38000) (M-37000)
(M-34000)

D5-34660 Chronic gastrojejunal ulcer with perforation 534.5
(T-57000) (T-58400) (M-18200)
(G-C008) (M-38020) (M-39210)

D5-34662 Chronic gastrojejunal ulcer with perforation but without obstruction 534.50
(T-57000) (T-58400) (M-18200)
(G-C008) (M-38020) (M-39210)
(G-C008) (M-34000)

D5-34664 Chronic gastrojejunal ulcer with perforation and with obstruction 534.51
(T-57000) (T-58400) (M-18200)
(G-C008) (M-38020) (M-39210)
(M-34000)

D5-34670 Gastrojejunal ulcer, NOS with perforation 534.5
(T-57000) (T-58400) (M-18200)
(G-C008) (M-38000) (M-39210)

5-34 DISEASES OF THE DUODENUM — Continued

D5-34672 Gastrojejunal ulcer, NOS with perforation but without obstruction 534.50
(T-57000) (T-58400) (M-18200) (G-C008) (M-38000) (M-39210) (G-C009) (M-34000)

D5-34674 Gastrojejunal ulcer, NOS with perforation and obstruction 534.51
(T-57000) (T-58400) (M-18200) (G-C008) (M-38000) (M-39210) (M-34000)

D5-34680 Chronic gastrojejunal ulcer with hemorrhage and perforation 535.6
(T-57000) (T-58400) (M-18200) (G-C008) (M-38020) (M-37000) (M-39210)

D5-34682 Chronic gastrojejunal ulcer with hemorrhage and perforation but without obstruction 534.60
(T-57000) (T-58400) (M-18200) (G-C008) (M-38020) (M-37000) (M-39210) (G-C009) (M-34000)

D5-34684 Chronic gastrojejunal ulcer with hemorrhage and perforation and with obstruction 534.61
(T-57000) (T-58400) (M-18200) (G-C008) (M-38020) (M-37000) (M-39210) (M-34000)

D5-34690 Gastrojejunal ulcer, NOS with hemorrhage and perforation 534.6
(T-57000) (T-58400) (M-18200) (G-C008) (M-38000) (M-37000) (M-39210)

D5-34692 Gastrojejunal ulcer, NOS with hemorrhage and perforation but without obstruction 534.60
(T-57000) (T-58400) (M-18200) (G-C008) (M-38000) (M-37000) (M-39210) (G-C009) (M-34000)

D5-34694 Gastrojejunal ulcer, NOS with hemorrhage and perforation and with obstruction 534.61
(T-57000) (T-58400) (M-18200) (G-C008) (M-38000) (M-37000) (M-39210) (M-34000)

D5-34700 Chronic gastrojejunal ulcer without hemorrhage or perforation 534.7
(T-57000) (T-58400) (M-18200) (G-C008) (M-38020) (G-C009) (M-37000) (M-39210)

D5-34702 Chronic gastrojejunal ulcer without hemorrhage or perforation and without obstruction 534.70
(T-57000) (T-58400) (M-18200) (G-C008) (M-38020) (G-C009) (M-37000) (M-39210) (M-34000)

D5-34704 Chronic gastrojejunal ulcer without hemorrhage or perforation but with obstruction 534.71
(T-57000) (T-58400) (M-18200) (G-C008) (M-38020) (G-C009) (M-37000) (M-39210) (G-C008) (M-34000)

D5-34710 Gastrojejunal ulcer, NOS without hemorrhage or perforation 534.9
(T-57000) (T-58400) (M-18200) (G-C008) (M-38000) (G-C009) (M-37000) (M-39210)

D5-34712 Gastrojejunal ulcer, NOS without hemorrhage or perforation and without obstruction 534.90
(T-57000) (T-58400) (M-18200) (G-C008) (M-38000) (G-C009) (M-37000) (M-39210) (M-34000)

D5-34714 Gastrojejunal ulcer, NOS without hemorrhage or perforation but with obstruction 534.91
(T-57000) (T-58400) (M-18200) (G-C008) (M-38000) (G-C009) (M-37000) (M-39210) (G-C008) (M-34000)

D5-34800 Duodenitis, NOS 535.6
(T-58200) (M-40000)

D5-34810 Chronic duodenal ileus 537.2
(T-58200) (M-34002)

D5-34820 Cicatrix of duodenum 537.3
(T-58200) (M-78060)

D5-34830 Stenosis of duodenum 537.3
(T-58200) (M-34200)

D5-34835 Stricture of duodenum 535.3
(M-58200) (M-34260)

D5-34840 Volvulus of duodenum 537.3
(T-58200) (M-34110) (M-34000)

D5-34850 Duodenal prolapse 537.89
(T-58200) (M-31050)

D5-34860 Duodenal rupture 537.89
(T-58200) (M-14400)

SECTION 5-4 DISEASES OF THE SMALL AND LARGE INTESTINES

5-40-45 DISEASES OF THE INTESTINAL TRACT

D5-40000 Disease of intestine, NOS 569.9
(T-50500) (DF-00000)

D5-40010 Abscess of intestine, NOS 569.5
(T-50500) (M-41610)

D5-40100 Malakoplakia of ileum
(T-58600) (M-44170)

D5-40150 Small intestinal stasis syndrome, NOS
(T-58000) (M-33350)

D5-40200 Angiodysplasia of intestinal tract, NOS
(T-50500) (M-74800) (M-32420)
Localized arteriovenous malformations of intestinal tract, NOS
(T-50500) (M-74800) (M-32420)

D5-40210 Vascular ectasia of small intestine, NOS
(T-50500) (M-74800) (M-32420)

D5-40212 Vascular ectasia of cecum
(T-59100) (M-74800) (M-32420)

D5-40214 Vascular ectasia of colon
(T-59300) (M-74800) (M-32420)

D5-40220 Acquired telangiectasia of small and large intestines, NOS
(T-58000) (T-59000) (M-32440)

D5-40240 Primary intestinal lymphangiectasia
(T-50500) (M-32450) (M-34000)
Intestinal lymphatic obstruction
(T-50500) (M-32450) (M-34000)

D5-40250 Intestinal hemorrhage, NOS 578.9
(T-50500) (M-37000)
Intestinal bleeding, NOS 578.9
(T-50500) (M-37000)

D5-40990 Inflammatory bowel disease, NOS
(T-58000) (T-59000) (M-40000)

D5-409A0 Idiopathic chronic inflammatory bowel disease
(T-58000) (T-59000) (M-43000)
Idiopathic colitis
(T-58000) (T-59000) (M-43000)

D5-409A2 Chronic colitis
(T-59300) (M-43000)

D5-41000 Crohn's disease, NOS 555.9
(T-50500) (M-44000)
Regional enteritis, NOS 555.9
(T-50500) (M-44000)
Granulomatous enteritis, NOS 555.9
(T-50500) (M-44000)

D5-41010 Crohn's disease of small intestine 555.0
(T-58000) (M-44000)
Regional enteritis of small intestine 555.0
(T-58000) (M-44000)
Regional ileitis of small intestine 555.0
(T-58000) (M-44000)
Segmental ileitis of small intestine 555.0
(T-58000) (M-44000)
Terminal ileitis of small intestine 555.0
(T-58000) (M-44000)

D5-41020 Crohn's disease of duodenum 555.0
(T-58200) (M-44000)

D5-41022 Crohn's disease of pylorus 555.0
(T-57700) (M-44000)

D5-41024 Crohn's disease of pyloric antrum 555.0
(T-57600) (M-44000)

D5-41030 Crohn's disease of jejunum 555.0
(T-58400) (M-44000)

D5-41040 Crohn's disease of ileum 555.0
(T-58600) (M-44000)

D5-41050 Crohn's disease of large bowel 555.1
(T-59000) (M-44000)

D5-41052 Crohn's disease of colon 555.1
(T-59300) (M-44000)
Regional colitis 555.1
(T-59300) (M-44000)
Granulomatous colitis 555.1
(T-59300) (M-44000)

D5-41060 Crohn's disease of rectum 555.1
(T-59600) (M-44000)
Regional enteritis of rectum 555.1
(T-59600) (M-44000)

D5-41080 Crohn's disease of small and large intestines 555.2
(T-58000) (T-59000) (M-44000)
Regional ileocolitis 555.2
(T-58000) (T-59000) (M-44000)

D5-41100 Idiopathic proctocolitis 556.-
(T-59300) (T-59600) (M-40000)

D5-41110 Chronic ulcerative colitis, NOS 556.-
(T-59300) (M-43750)
Colitis gravis, NOS 556.-
(T-59300) (M-43750)

D5-41112 Mild chronic ulcerative colitis 556.-
(T-59300) (M-43750) (G-A001)

D5-41114 Moderate chronic ulcerative colitis 556.-
(T-59300) (M-43750) (G-A002)

D5-41116 Severe chronic ulcerative colitis 556.-
(T-59300) (M-43750) (G-A003)
Fulminant ulcerative colitis 556.-
(T-58000) (M-43750) (G-A003)

D5-41120 Chronic ulcerative enterocolitis 556.-
(T-58000) (T-59300) (M-43750)

D5-41122 Chronic ulcerative ileocolitis 556.-
(T-58600) (T-59300) (M-43750)

D5-41130 Chronic ulcerative rectosigmoiditis 556.-
(T-59470) (T-59600) (M-43750)

D5-41140 Chronic ulcerative proctitis 556.-
(T-59600) (M-43750)

D5-41150 Toxic megacolon 556.-
(T-59300) (M-32000)

D5-41160 Pseudopolyposis of colon 556.-
(T-59300) (M-76820)
Inflammatory polyps of colon 556.-
(T-59300) (M-76820)

D5-41170 Polyp of colon, NOS
(T-59300) (M-76800)

D5-41180 Inflammatory pseudotumor of colon
(T-59300) (M-76890)
Fibroid polyp of colon
(T-59300) (M-76890)

D5-41200 Vascular insufficiency of intestine, NOS 557.9
(T-50500) (F-39300)
Ischemic bowel disease, NOS 557.9
(T-50500) (F-39300)

D5-41202 Nonocclusive intestinal infarction 557.9
(T-50500) (M-54700) (G-C009) (M-34000)

D5-41210 Ischemic colitis, NOS 557.9
(T-59300) (M-40000) (G-C001) (F-39340)

D5-41220 Ischemic enteritis, NOS 557.9
(T-58000) (M-40000) (G-C001) (F-39340)

D5-41230 Ischemic enterocolitis, NOS 557.9
(T-58000) (T-59300) (M-40000) (G-C001) (F-39340)

D5-41240 Alimentary tract pain due to vascular insufficiency 557.9
(T-50100) (F-A2600) (G-C001) (F-39300)

5-40-45 DISEASES OF THE INTESTINAL TRACT — Continued

D5-41300 Acute vascular insufficiency of intestine, NOS 557.0
(T-50500) (F-39310) (F-39340)
Acute intestinal ischemic syndrome, NOS 557.0
(T-50500) (F-39310) (F-39340)

D5-41310 Acute ischemic colitis 557.0
(T-59300) (M-41000) (G-C001) (F-39310) (F-39340)

D5-41320 Acute ischemic enteritis 557.0
(T-58000) (M-41000) (G-C001) (F-39310) (F-39340)

D5-41330 Enterocolitis, NOS
(T-50500) (T-59300) (M-40000)

D5-41332 Acute hemorrhagic enterocolitis 557.0
(T-58000) (T-59300) (M-41790)
Hemorrhagic enteritis
(T-58000) (T-59300) (M-41790)

D5-41334 Acute ischemic enterocolitis 557.0
(T-58000) (T-59300) (M-41000) (G-C001) (F-39310) (F-39340)

D5-41338 Fulminant enterocolitis 557.0
(T-58000) (T-59300) (M-41000)

D5-41350 Massive necrosis of intestine 557.0
(T-50500) (M-54008)

D5-41360 Hemorrhagic necrosis of intestine 557.0
(T-50500) (M-54040)

D5-41370 Acute bowel infarction 557.0
(T-50500) (M-54720)
Acute intestinal infarction 557.0
(T-50500) (M-54720)

D5-41390 Intestinal gangrene 557.0
(T-50500) (M-54600)

D5-41400 Mesenteric infarction, NOS 557.0
(T-D4500) (M-54700)

D5-41402 Embolic mesenteric infarction 557.0
(T-D4500) (M-54700) (G-C001) (M-35300)
Mesenteric arterial embolization 557.0
(T-D4500) (M-54700) (G-C001) (M-35300)

D5-41404 Thrombotic mesenteric infarction 557.0
(T-D4500) (M-54700) (G-C001) (M-35100)

D5-41410 Terminal hemorrhagic enteropathy 557.0
(T-50500) (M-41790) (G-A023)

D5-41420 Thrombosis of mesenteric artery 557.0
(T-46500) (M-35100)
Acute mesenteric arterial occlusion 557.0
(T-46500) (M-35100)

D5-41430 Embolism of mesenteric artery 557.0
(T-46500) (M-35300)

D5-41450 Mesenteric venous thrombosis
(T-48840) (T-48910) (M-35100)

D5-41500 Chronic vascular insufficiency of intestine, NOS 557.1
(T-50500) (M-39320) (F-39340)
Chronic intestinal ischemic syndrome, NOS 557.1
(T-50500) (M-39320) (F-39340)

D5-41510 Chronic ischemic colitis 557.1
(T-59300) (M-43000) (G-C001) (F-39340) (F-39320)

D5-41520 Chronic ischemic enteritis 557.1
(T-58000) (M-43000) (G-C001) (F-39340) (F-39320)

D5-41530 Chronic ischemic enterocolitis 557.1
(T-58000) (T-59300) (M-43000) (G-C001) (F-39340) (F-39320)

D5-41540 Ischemic stricture of intestine 557.1
(T-58000) (F-39340) (G-C001) (M-34260)

D5-41550 Mesenteric vascular insufficiency 557.1
(T-46510) (F-39300) (G-C008) (F-37100)
Superior mesenteric artery syndrome 557.1
(T-46510) (F-39300) (G-C008) (F-37100)
Mesenteric angina 557.1
(T-46510) (F-39300) (G-C008) (F-37100)
Abdominal angina 557.1
(T-46510) (F-39300) (G-C008) (F-37100)
Intestinal angina 557.1
(T-46510) (F-39300) (G-C008) (F-37100)

D5-41600 Noninfectious gastroenteritis, NOS 558.9
(T-57000) (T-50500) (M-40000)

D5-41601 Allergic gastroenteritis 558.9
(T-57000) (T-50500) (M-40000) (G-C001) (F-C3000)

D5-41602 Dietetic gastroenteritis 558.9
(T-57000) (T-50500) (M-40000) (G-C001) (C-E2000)

D5-41610 Noninfectious enteritis, NOS 558.9
(T-50500) (M-40000)

D5-41611 Allergic enteritis 558.9
(T-50500) (M-40000) (G-C001) (F-C3000)

D5-41612 Dietetic enteritis 558.9
(T-50500) (M-40000) (G-C001) (C-F2000)

D5-41620 Noninfectious jejunitis, NOS 558.9
(T-58400) (M-40000)

D5-41621 Allergic jejunitis 558.9
(T-58400) (M-40000) (G-C001) (F-C3000)

D5-41622 Dietetic jejunitis 558.9
(T-58400) (M-40000) (G-C001) (C-F2000)

D5-41630 Noninfectious ileitis, NOS 558.9
(T-58600) (M-40000)

D5-41631 Allergic ileitis 558.9
(T-58600) (M-40000) (G-C001) (F-C3000)

D5-41632 Dietetic ileitis 558.9
(T-58600) (M-40000) (G-C001)
(C-F2000)

D5-41640 Noninfectious colitis, NOS 558.9
(T-59300) (M-40000)

D5-41641 Allergic colitis 558.9
(T-59300) (M-40000) (G-C001)
(F-C3000)

D5-41642 Dietetic colitis 558.9
(T-59300) (M-40000) (G-C001)
(C-F2000)

D5-41650 Noninfectious sigmoiditis, NOS 558.9
(T-59470) (M-40000)

D5-41651 Allergic sigmoiditis 558.9
(T-59470) (M-40000) (G-C001)
(F-C3000)

D5-41652 Dietetic sigmoiditis 558.9
(T-59470) (M-40000) (G-C001)
(C-F2000)

D5-41660 Noninfectious diarrhea, NOS 558.9
(T-50500) (F-54400)

D5-41661 Allergic diarrhea 558.9
(T-50500) (F-54400) (G-C001)
(F-C3000)

D5-41662 Dietetic diarrhea 558.9
(T-50500) (F-54400) (G-C001)
(C-F2000)

D5-41670 Toxic gastroenteritis 558.2
(T-57000) (T-50500) (M-40000)

D5-41674 Toxic colitis 558.2
(T-59300) (M-40000) (G-C001)
(C-00220)

D5-41680 Gastroenteritis due to radiation 558.1
(T-57000) (T-50500) (M-40000)
(G-C001) (A-81000)

D5-41682 Colitis due to radiation 558.1
(T-59300) (M-40000) (G-C001)
(A-81000)

D5-41684 Enteritis due to radiation 558.1
(T-58000) (M-40000) (G-C001)
(A-81000)

D5-41690V Canine hemorrhagic gastroenteritis
(T-57000) (T-50500) (M-41790)

D5-41700 Colitis, NOS 009.1
(T-59300) (M-40000)

D5-41704 Enteritis, NOS 009.1
(T-58000) (M-40000)

D5-41706 Gastroenteritis, NOS 009.1
(T-57000) (T-50500) (M-40000)

D5-41710V Lymphocytic-plasmacytic colitis
(T-59300) (M-43010) (M-43060)

D5-41712V Eosinophilic colitis
(T-59300) (M-43040)

D5-41714V Suppurative colitis
(T-59300) (M-41600)

D5-41716V Eosinophilic ulcerative colitis
(T-59300) (M-43040) (M-43750)

D5-41718V Histiocytic ulcerative colitis of Boxer dogs
(T-59300) (M-43750) (G-C008)
(M-47070)

D5-41724V Purulent enteritis
(T-58000) (M-40600)

D5-41726V Fibrinous enteritis
(T-58000) (M-40300)

D5-41728V Necrotic enteritis
(T-58000) (M-40700)

D5-41730V Chronic proliferative enteritis
(T-58000) (M-45200)

D5-41732V Villous atrophy of intestine
(T-58040) (M-58000)

D5-41734V Granulomatous enteritis, non-Crohn's disease
(T-58000) (M-44000)

D5-41736V Pyogranulomatous enteritis
(T-58000) (M-44030)

D5-41738V Pyogranulomatous serositis
(T-1A110) (M-44030)

D5-41740V Chronic inflammatory small bowel disease
(T-58000) (T-43000)

D5-41742V Proliferative ileitis in hamsters
(T-58600) (M-45200)

D5-42000 Intestinal obstruction, NOS 560.9
(T-50500) (M-34000)
Intestinal occlusion, NOS 560.9
(T-50500) (M-34000)
Ileus, NOS 560.9
(T-50500) (M-34000)

D5-42002 Mechanical ileus 560.9
(T-50500) (M-34000) (G-C001)
(M-78400)

D5-42003 Dynamic ileus
(T-50500) (M-34000) (G-C001)
(F-11310)

D5-42004 Obturation obstruction of intestine
(T-50500) (M-34005)

D5-42006 Strangulation obstruction of intestine
(T-50500) (M-34000) (G-C001)
(M-01460) (F-39200)

D5-42008 Recurrent intestinal obstruction
(T-50500) (M-34000) (G-A500)

D5-42010 Stenosis of intestine 560.9
(T-50500) (M-34200)
Enterostenosis 560.9
(T-50500) (M-34200)

D5-42012 Stricture of intestine 560.9
(T-50500) (M-34260)

D5-42020 Obstruction of colon 560.9
(T-59300) (M-34000)
Occlusion of colon 560.9
(T-59300) (M-34000)

D5-42030 Stenosis of colon 560.9
(T-59300) (M-34200)

D5-42032 Stricture of colon 560.9
(T-59300) (M-34260)

D5-42100 Intussusception of intestine 560.0
(T-50500) (M-31430)
Invagination of intestine 560.0
(T-50500) (M-31430)

5-40-45 DISEASES OF THE INTESTINAL TRACT — Continued

D5-42110 Intussusception of colon 560.0
(T-59300) (M-31430)
Invagination of colon 560.0
(T-59300) (M-31430)

D5-42120 Intussusception of rectum 560.0
(T-59600) (M-31430)
Invagination of rectum 560.0
(T-59600) (M-31430)

D5-42130 Intestinal volvulus, NOS 560.2
(T-50500) (M-34000) (G-C001)
(M-34110)
Twisting of intestine on mesenteric axis 560.2
(T-50500) (M-34000) (G-C001)
(M-34110)

D5-42132 Torsion of intestine, NOS 560.2
(T-50500) (M-34000) (G-C001)
(M-34110)
Twisting of intestine on long axis
(T-50500) (M-34000) (G-C001)
(M-34110)

D5-42134 Strangulation of intestine, NOS 560.2
(T-50500) (M-34000) (G-C001)
(M-01460) (F-39200)

D5-42140 Volvulus of colon 560.2
(T-59300) (M-34000) (G-C001)
(M-34110)
Twisting of colon on mesenteric axis 560.2
(T-59300) (M-34000) (G-C001)
(M-34110)

D5-42142 Torsion of colon 560.2
(T-59300) (M-34000) (G-C001)
(M-34110)
Twisting of colon on long axis 560.2
(T-59300) (M-34000) (G-C001)
(M-34110)

D5-42144 Strangulation of colon 560.2
(T-59300) (M-34000) (G-C001)
(M-01460) (F-39200)

D5-42150 Paralytic ileus 560.1
(T-50500) (M-34000) (G-C001)
(F-53952)
Adynamic ileus 560.1
(T-50500) (M-34000) (G-C001)
(F-53952)
Paralysis of intestine 560.1
(T-50500) (M-34000) (G-C001)
(F-53952)

D5-42152 Paralysis of colon 560.1
(T-59300) (M-34000) (G-C001)
(F-53952)

D5-42300 Impaction of intestine, NOS 560.30
(T-50500) (M-33100)

D5-42310 Impaction of colon 560.30
(T-59300) (M-33100)

D5-42320 Gallstone ileus 560.31
(T-50500) (M-34000) (G-C001)
(T-63000) (M-30000)
Obstruction of intestine by gallstone 560.31
(T-50500) (M-34000) (G-C001)
(T-63000) (M-30000)

D5-42330 Concretion of intestine 560.39
(T-50500) (M-30000)
Enterolith 560.39
(T-50500) (M-30000)

D5-42350 Fecal impaction of colon 560.39
(T-59300) (M-33110)

D5-42360 Fecal impaction of rectum 560.39
(T-59600) (M-33110)

D5-42370 Intestinal adhesions with obstruction 560.81
(T-50500) (M-78400) (G-C008)
(M-34000)

D5-42380 Peritoneal adhesions with obstruction 560.81
(T-D4400) (M-78400) (G-C008)
(M-34000)

D5-42390 Mural thickening of intestine causing obstruction 560.89
(T-50500) (M-34000) (G-C001)
(M-02520)

D5-42500 Fistula of intestine, NOS 569.81
(T-50500) (M-39300)

D5-42510 Fistula of intestine to abdominal wall 569.81
(T-D4300) (M-39300)

D5-42520 Enterocolic fistula 569.81
(T-50500) (M-59300) (M-39300)

D5-42530 Enteroenteric fistula 569.81
(T-50500) (T-50500) (M-39300)

D5-42540 Ileorectal fistula 569.81
(T-58600) (T-59600) (M-39300)

D5-42560 Arterial-enteric fistula
(T-41000) (T-50500) (M-39300)

D5-42600 Perforation of intestine, NOS 569.83
(T-50500) (M-39210)

D5-42610 Ulceration of intestine, NOS 569.82
(T-50500) (M-38000)
Primary ulcer of intestine, NOS 569.82
(T-50500) (M-38000)

D5-42612 Jejunal ulcer 534.-
(T-58400) (M-38000)

D5-42620 Ulceration of colon 569.82
(T-59300) (M-38000)

D5-42630 Granuloma of intestine, NOS 569.89
(T-50500) (M-44000)

D5-42640 Prolapse of intestine, NOS 569.89
(T-50500) (M-31050)
Enteroptosis 569.89
(T-50500) (M-31050)

D5-42645 Visceroptosis 569.89
(T-D4030) (M-31050)
Splanchnoptosis 569.89
(T-D4030) (M-31050)

D5-42650 Pericolitis 569.89
(T-59390) (M-40000)
D5-42660 Perisigmoiditis 569.89
(T-59390) (M-40000)
D5-43000 Diverticula of intestine, NOS 562.-
(T-50500) (M-32700)
D5-43010 Meckel's diverticulitis
(T-58600) (T-F1450) (M-26400)
(M-40000)
D5-43100 Diverticulosis of small intestine, NOS 562.00
(T-58000) (M-32700)
D5-43110 Diverticulosis of duodenum without diverticulitis 562.00
(T-58200) (M-32700) (G-C009)
(M-40000)
D5-43120 Diverticulosis of jejunum without diverticulitis 562.00
(T-58400) (M-32700) (G-C009)
(M-40000)
D5-43130 Diverticulosis of ileum without diverticulitis 562.00
(T-58600) (M-32700) (G-C009)
(M-40000)
D5-43140 Diverticulitis of small intestine, NOS 562.01
(T-58000) (M-32700) (M-40000)
D5-43150 Diverticulitis of duodenum 562.01
(T-58200) (M-32700) (M-40000)
D5-43160 Diverticulitis of jejunum 562.01
(T-58400) (M-32700) (M-40000)
D5-43170 Diverticulitis of ileum 562.01
(T-58600) (M-32700) (M-40000)
D5-43200 Diverticulosis of large intestine without diverticulitis 562.10
(T-59000) (M-32700) (G-C009)
(M-40000)
D5-43202 Diverticulosis of colon without diverticulitis 562.10
(T-59300) (M-32700) (G-C009)
(M-40000)
Diverticular disease of colon 562.10
(T-59300) (M-32700) (G-C009)
(M-40000)
D5-43210 Diverticulitis of large intestine 562.11
(T-59000) (M-32700) (M-40000)
D5-43220 Diverticulitis of colon 562.11
(T-59300) (M-32700) (M-40000)
D5-43300 Colitis cystica profunda
(T-59300) (M-40000) (G-C008)
(M-33440)
D5-43320 Pneumatosis cystoides intestinalis
(T-50510) (M-33960)
D5-44000 Functional disorder of intestine, NOS 564.9
(T-50500) (F-01100)
D5-44010 Constipation 564.0
(T-59300) (T-59600) (F-54222)
D5-44012 Chronic idiopathic constipation 564.0
(T-59300) (T-59600) (F-54222)
D5-44014 Colonic constipation 564.0
(T-59300) (F-54222) (G-C001)
(F-54142)
Constipation by delayed colonic transit 564.0
(T-59300) (F-54222) (G-C001)
(F-54142)
Slow transit constipation 564.0
(T-59300) (F-54222) (G-C001)
(F-54142)
D5-44016 Constipation by outlet obstruction 564.0
(T-59600) (F-54222) (G-C001)
(M-34000) (T-59900)
D5-44018 Drug-induced constipation 564.0
(T-59600) (F-54222) (G-C001)
(C-50000)
D5-44019 Obstipation 564.0
(T-59600) (F-54222)
Intractable constipation 564.0
(T-59600) (F-54222)
D5-44020 Functional diarrhea 564.5
(T-59300) (F-54400)
D5-44030 Anal spasm 564.6
(T-59900) (F-11310)
D5-44050 Megacolon, not Hirschsprung's 564.7
(T-59300) (M-32000)
Dilatation of colon 564.7
(T-59300) (M-32000)
Acquired megacolon 564.7
(T-59300) (M-32000)
Idiopathic megacolon 564.7
(T-59300) (M-32000)
D5-44052 Acquired megacolon in children 564.7
(T-59300) (M-32000) (DF-00210)
Idiopathic megacolon in children 564.7
(T-59300) (M-32000) (DF-00210)
D5-44054 Acquired megacolon in adults 564.7
(T-59300) (M-32000) (DF-00230)
Idiopathic megacolon in adults 564.7
(T-59300) (M-32000) (DF-00230)
D5-44060 Intestinal autonomic neuropathy, NOS
(T-50500) (T-A9600) (F-01100)
D5-44070 Anal pain 569.42
(T-59900) (F-A2600)
D5-44072 Chronic idiopathic anal pain 569.2
(T-59900) (F-A2950)
D5-44080 Rectal pain 569.42
(T-59600) (F-A2600)
D5-44085 Proctalgia fugax 564.6
(T-59900) (T-59600) (F-11310)
Anorectal spasm 564.6
(T-59900) (T-59600) (F-11310)
Paroxysmal proctalgia 564.6
(T-59900) (T-59600) (F-11310)
Levator syndrome 564.6
(T-59900) (T-59600) (F-11310)
D5-44090 Atony of colon 564.8
(T-59300) (F-11950)

5-40-45 DISEASES OF THE INTESTINAL TRACT — Continued

D5-44100 Irritable colon 564.1
(T-59300) (M-40000) (F-11310) (F-54400)
Adaptive colitis 564.1
(T-59300) (M-40000) (F-11310) (F-54400)
Membranous colitis 564.1
(T-59300) (M-40000) (F-11310) (F-54400)
Spastic colon 564.1
(T-59900) (M-40000) (F-11310) (F-54400)
Irritable bowel syndrome 564.1
(T-59300) (M-40000) (F-11310) (F-54400)
Mucous colitis 564.1
(T-59300) (M-40000) (F-11310) (F-54400)

D5-44104 Enterospasm 564.1
(T-58000) (F-11310)

D5-44106 Colonospasm 564.1
(T-59300) (F-11310)

D5-44120 Chemical colitis
(T-59900) (M-40000) (G-C001) (C-10030)

D5-44122 Soap colitis
(T-59300) (M-40000) (G-C001) (C-22640)

D5-44124 Cathartic colon
(T-59300) (M-40000) (G-C001) (C-84801)

D5-44130 Collagenous colitis
(T-59300) (F-62840)

D5-44150 Melanosis coli
(T-59300) (M-57210)

D5-44200 Postgastric surgery syndrome 564.2
(DF-00000) (G-C003) (P1-02000) (T-57000) (G-C008) (F-52463) (F-52633)
Dumping syndrome 564.2
(DF-00000) (G-C003) (P1-02000) (T-57000) (G-C008) (F-52463) (F-52633)
Jejunal syndrome 564.2
(DF-00000) (G-C003) (P1-02000) (T-57000) (G-C008) (F-52463) (F-52633)
Postgastrectomy syndrome 564.2
(DF-00000) (G-C003) (P1-02000) (T-57000) (G-C008) (F-52463) (F-52633)

D5-44220 Bilious vomiting following gastrointestinal surgery 564.3
(T-57000) (F-52780) (G-C003) (P1-00000) (T-50500)

D5-44230 Diarrhea following gastrointestinal surgery 564.4
(T-50500) (F-54400) (G-C003) (P1-00000) (T-50500)

D5-44240 Enterostomy malfunction 569.6
(T-58000) (M-18000) (F-01100)

D5-44250 Colostomy malfunction 569.6
(T-59300) (M-18000) (F-01100)

D5-44262 Small stomach syndrome
(DF-00000) (G-C001) (T-57000) (M-02530)

D5-44264 Afferent loop syndrome
(T-58200) (T-58400) (M-32000) (M-34000) (G-C001) (P1-02000) (T-57000)

D5-44268 Chronic partial afferent loop obstruction
(T-58200) (T-58400) (M-32000) (M-34006) (G-C001) (P1-02000) (T-57000)

D5-44270 Retained antrum syndrome
(DF-00000) (G-C001) (T-57600) (M-33000)

D5-44280 Diversion colitis
(T-59300) (M-40000) (G-C001) (M-18000)

D5-44300 Ulcer of cecum
(T-59100) (M-38000)
Cecal ulcer
(T-59100) (M-38000)

D5-44310 Proximal colon ulcer
(T-59420) (M-38000)

D5-44320 Sigmoid colon ulcer
(T-59470) (M-38000)

D5-44360 Malakoplakia of colon
(T-59300) (M-44170)

D5-44400 Typhlitis, NOS
(T-59100) (M-40000)
Cecitis, NOS
(T-59100) (M-40000)

D5-44410 Neutropenic typhlitis
(T-59100) (M-40000) (G-C009) (T-C1260)

D5-44420V Typhlocolitis
(T-59100) (T-59300) (M-40000)

D5-44430V Typhlolithiasis
(T-59100) (M-30000)

D5-44432V Impaction of cecum
(T-59100) (M-33100)

D5-44440V Dilatation of cecum
(T-59100) (M-32000)
Typhlectasis
(T-59100) (M-32000)

D5-44442V Tympanites of cecum
(T-59100) (F-54150)

D5-44450V Intussusception of cecum
(T-59100) (M-31430)

D5-44452V Cecocolic intussusception
(T-59100) (T-59300) (M-31430)
Cecal inversion
(T-59100) (T-59300) (M-31430)

D5-44454V Ileocolic intussusception
(T-58600) (T-59300) (M-31430)

D5-44458V Intestinal trichobezoar
(T-50500) (M-30460)
Intestinal hairball
(T-50500) (M-30460)

D5-44460V Colitis-X
(T-59300) (M-40000)

D5-44462V Bacterial overgrowth syndrome
(T-50500) (G-C008) (G-A317)
(L-10000)

D5-44470V Immunoproliferative enteropathy of Basenjis
(T-50500) (M-97603)

D5-44474V Canine eosinophilic gastroenteritis
(T-50100) (M-43040)

D5-44478V Feline hypereosinophilic syndrome
(DF-00000) (T-C2000) (G-C008)
(DC-45010)

D5-44480V Lymphocytic-plasmacytic enteritis
(T-50500) (M-43010) (M-43060)

D5-44490 Osmotic diarrhea
(T-59000) (F-54450)
Permeability diarrhea
(T-59000) (F-54450)

D5-44491 Secretory diarrhea
(T-59000) (F-54460)

D5-44493 Drug and toxin-induced diarrhea
(T-59000) (F-54400) (G-C001)
(C-30310) (C-50000)

D5-45000 Disease of rectum, NOS
(T-59600) (DF-00000)

D5-45010 Disease of anus, NOS
(T-59900) (DF-00000)

D5-45100 Anal fissure 565.0
(T-59900) (M-01560)
Nontraumatic tear of anus 565.0
(T-59900) (M-01560)

D5-45110 Anal fistula 565.1
(T-59900) (M-39300)

D5-45114 Perianal fistula
(T-59990) (M-39300)

D5-45115 Anal furunculosis
(T-59900) (M-41718)

D5-45120 Anorectal fistula 565.1
(T-59900) (T-59600) (M-39300)

D5-45130 Rectal fistula 565.1
(T-59600) (M-39300)

D5-45140 Rectum to skin fistula 565.1
(T-59600) (T-02507) (M-39300)

D5-45200 Ischiorectal abscess 566.-
(T-18965) (M-41610)

D5-45210 Perianal abscess 566.-
(T-59990) (M-41610)

D5-45212 Hidradenitis suppurativa of anus
(T-01320) (T-59900) (M-43600)

D5-45220 Perirectal abscess 566.-
(T-59690) (M-41610)

D5-45225 Anorectal abscess 566.-
(T-59900) (T-59600) (M-41610)

D5-45230 Anal cellulitis 566.-
(T-59900) (M-41650)

D5-45240 Perirectal cellulitis 566.-
(T-59690) (M-41650)

D5-45250 Rectal cellulitis 566.-
(T-59600) (M-41650)

D5-45260 Ischiorectal fistula 566.-
(T-18965) (M-39300)

D5-45270 Proctitis, NOS 569.49
(T-59600) (M-40000)

D5-45274 Nonspecific ulcerative proctitis
(T-59600) (M-40750)

D5-45310 Anal polyp 590.0
(T-59900) (M-76800)

D5-45315 Hypertrophy of anal papillae 569.49
(T-59600) (T-F6640) (M-26400)
(M-71000)

D5-45320 Rectal polyp 569.0
(T-59600) (M-76800)

D5-45325 Granuloma of rectum 569.49
(T-59600) (M-44000)

D5-45330 Rectal prolapse 569.1
(T-59610) (M-31050)
Rectal mucosa prolapse 569.1
(T-59610) (M-31050)
Procidentia of rectum 569.1
(T-59610) (M-31050)

D5-45332 Incomplete rectal prolapse
(T-59600) (M-31050) (G-A381)
Partial rectal prolapse
(T-59600) (M-31050) (G-A381)

D5-45334 Complete rectal prolapse with displacement of anal sphincter
(T-59600) (M-31050) (G-A290)
(G-C008) (M-31000) (T-14330)

D5-45336 Complete rectal prolapse with no displacement of anal muscles
(T-59600) (M-31050) (G-A290)
(G-C009) (T-14310)

D5-45338 Internal complete rectal prolapse with intussusception of rectosigmoid
(T-59600) (M-31050) (G-A290)
(G-C008) (M-31430) (T-59670)

D5-45340 Proctoptosis 569.1
(T-59910) (M-31050)
Anal canal prolapse 569.1
(T-59910) (M-31050)
Procidentia of anus 569.1
(T-59910) (M-31050)

D5-45350 Stenosis of rectum 569.2
(T-59600) (M-34200)

D5-45352 Stricture of rectum 569.2
(T-59600) (M-34260)

D5-45354 Anorectal stricture 569.2
(T-59900) (T-59600) (M-34260)

5-40-45 DISEASES OF THE INTESTINAL TRACT — Continued

D5-45360 Stenosis of anus 569.2
(T-59900) (M-34200)

D5-45362 Stricture of anus 569.2
(T-59900) (M-34260)

D5-45370 Stricture of anal canal 569.2
(T-59910) (M-34260)

D5-45380 Malakoplakia of rectum
(T-59600) (M-44170)

D5-45400 Ulcer of anus 569.41
(T-59900) (M-38000)
Solitary ulcer of anus 569.41
(T-59900) (M-38000)

D5-45410 Stercoral ulcer of anus 569.41
(T-59900) (M-38160)

D5-45414V Pseudocoprostasis
(T-01000) (T-D2701) (T-01400)
(T-59666) (G-C008) (M-34000)

D5-45420 Ulcer of rectum 569.41
(T-59600) (M-38000)
Solitary ulcer of rectum 569.41
(T-59600) (M-38000)

D5-45430 Stercoral ulcer of rectum 569.41
(T-59600) (M-38160)

D5-45440 Hemorrhage of anus 569.3
(T-59900) (M-37000)

D5-45450 Hemorrhage of rectum 569.3
(T-59600) (M-37000)

D5-45460 Rupture of rectum 569.49
(T-59600) (M-14400)
Rectal tear 569.49
(T-59600) (M-14400)

D5-45470 Megarectum
(T-59600) (M-32000)

D5-45480 Nonfamilial multiple polyposis syndrome
(T-59000) (M-76808)

D5-45490 Familial multiple polyposis syndrome
(T-59000) (M-76808) (DF-00190)

D5-45500 Cronkhite-Canada syndrome
(T-50100) (M-76808)
Gastrointestinal multiple polyposis syndrome
(T-50100) (M-76808)

D5-45540 Anismus
(T-D6236) (F-11310)
Spastic pelvic floor syndrome
(T-D6236) (F-11310)
Sphinteric disobedience syndrome
(T-D6236) (F-11310)
Rectosphincteric dyssynergia
(T-D6236) (F-11310)

D5-45550 Descending perineum syndrome

D5-45570 Sigmoidorectal intussusception
(T-59600) (T-59470) (M-31430)

D5-45800V Anal sac disease, NOS
(T-59915) (DF-00000)

D5-45810V Anal sac infection
(T-59915) (M-40000)

D5-45814V Anal sac abscessation
(T-59915) (M-41610)

D5-45820V Anal sac impaction
(T-59915) (M-33100)

D5-45830V Squamous metaplasia of rectal mucosa
(T-59610) (M-73220)

D5-45900V Cloacal disease, NOS
(T-F6630) (DF-00000)

D5-45910V Cloacal prolapse
(T-F6630) (M-31050)

D5-45920V Cloacitis
(T-F6630) (M-40000)

5-46 DISEASES OF THE APPENDIX

D5-46000 Disease of appendix, NOS 543.9
(T-59200) (DF-00000)

D5-46100 Appendicitis, NOS 541.-
(T-59200) (M-40000)

D5-46110 Chronic appendicitis 542.-
(T-59200) (M-43000)

D5-46120 Recurrent appendicitis 542.-
(T-59200) (M-40000) (G-A500)

D5-46130 Relapsing appendicitis 542.-
(T-59200) (M-40000) (G-A501)

D5-46140 Subacute appendicitis 542.-
(T-59200) (M-42000)

D5-46150 Atypical appendicitis
(T-59200) (M-40000) (G-A248)

D5-46152 Retrocecal appendicitis
(T-59200) (T-D4952) (M-40000)

D5-46154 Retroileal appendicitis
(T-59200) (T-58692) (M-40000)

D5-46156 Pelvic appendicitis
(T-59200) (M-40000) (T-D6221)

D5-46200 Acute appendicitis without peritonitis 540.9
(T-59200) (M-41000) (G-C009)
(T-D4400) (M-40000)
Inflamed acute appendicitis without peritonitis 540.9
(T-59200) (M-41000) (G-C009)
(T-D4400) (M-40000)

D5-46210 Acute appendicitis, NOS 540.9
(T-59200) (M-41000)

D5-46220 Acute fulminating appendicitis 540.9
(T-59200) (M-41000)

D5-46230 Acute gangrenous appendicitis 540.9
(T-59200) (M-41700)

D5-46240 Acute obstructive appendicitis 540.9
(T-59200) (M-41000) (G-C008)
(M-34000)

D5-46250 Acute cecitis 540.9
(T-59100) (M-41000)

D5-46300 Acute appendicitis with generalized peritonitis 540.0
(T-59200) (M-41000) (G-C008)
(T-D4400) (M-41000) (G-A366)

D5-46310 Rupture of appendix 540.0
(T-59200) (M-14400)

D5-46320 Acute fulminating appendicitis with perforation and peritonitis 540.0
(T-59200) (M-41000) (G-C008) (M-39210) (T-D4400) (M-40000)

D5-46330 Acute gangrenous appendicitis with perforation and peritonitis 540.0
(T-59200) (M-41700) (G-C008) (M-39210) (T-D4400) (M-40000)

D5-46340 Acute obstructive appendicitis with perforation and peritonitis 540.0
(T-59200) (M-41000) (G-C008) (M-34000) (M-39210) (T-D4400) (M-40000)

D5-46350 Acute cecitis with perforation and peritonitis 540.0
(T-59100) (M-41000) (G-C008) (M-39210) (T-D4400) (M-40000)

D5-46360 Acute appendicitis with peritoneal abscess 540.1
(T-59200) (M-41000) (G-C008) (T-D4400) (M-41610)

D5-46370 Abscess of appendix 540.1
(T-59200) (M-40000)

D5-46400 Lymphoid hyperplasia of appendix 543.0
(T-59200) (M-72200)

D5-46410 Appendiceal colic 543.9
(T-59200) (F-01330)

D5-46420 Concretion of appendix 543.9
(T-59200) (M-30000)

D5-46430 Fistula of appendix 543.9
(T-59200) (M-39300)

D5-46440 Diverticulum of appendix 543.9
(T-59200) (M-32700)

D5-46450 Fecalith of appendix 543.9
(T-59200) (M-30280)
Stercolith of appendix 543.9
(T-59200) (M-30280)

D5-46460 Mucocele of appendix 543.9
(T-59200) (M-33440)

D5-46470 Intussusception of appendix 543.9
(T-59200) (M-31430)

5-47 MALABSORPTION SYNDROMES

D5-47000 Malabsorption syndrome, NOS 579.9
(T-50500) (F-53202)
Intestinal malabsorption, NOS 579.9
(T-50500) (F-53202)
Malabsorption, NOS 579.9
(T-50500) (F-53202)

D5-47100 Celiac disease 579.0
(T-50500) (F-53202) (G-C001) (F-50440) (C-F0120)
Celiac crisis 579.0
(T-50500) (F-53202) (G-C001) (F-50440) (C-F0120)
Celiac rickets 579.0
(T-50500) (F-53202) (G-C001) (F-50440) (C-F0120)
Gee-Herter disease 579.0
(T-50500) (F-53202) (G-C001) (F-50440) (C-F0120)
Gluten enteropathy 579.0
(T-50500) (F-53202) (G-C001) (F-50440) (C-F0120)
Idiopathic steatorrhea 579.0
(T-50500) (F-53202) (G-C001) (F-50440) (C-F0120)
Nontropical sprue 579.0
(T-50500) (F-53202) (G-C001) (F-50440) (C-F0120)
Celiac sprue 579.0
(T-50500) (F-53202) (G-C001) (F-50440) (C-F0120)
Wheat-sensitive enteropathy 579.0
(T-50500) (F-53202) (G-C001) (F-50440) (C-F0120)

D5-47104 Celiac disease with diffuse intestinal ulceration 579.0
(T-50500) (F-53202) (G-C001) (F-50440) (C-F0120) (G-C008) (M-38350)

D5-47110 Celiac infantilism 579.0
(T-50500) (F-53202) (G-C001) (F-50440) (C-F0120)

D5-47150 Tropical sprue 579.1
(T-50500) (F-53202)
Tropical steatorrhea 579.1
(T-50500) (F-53202)

D5-47160 Exudative enteropathy 579.8

D5-47170 Protein-losing enteropathy 579.8

D5-47180 Chronic steatorrhea 579.8

D5-47190 Idiopathic diffuse ulcerative nongranulomatous enteritis
Unclassified sprue

D5-47200 Diffuse ulcerations of jejunum and ileum
(T-58400) (T-58600) (M-38000)
Idiopathic small intestinal ulcers
(T-58400) (T-58600) (M-38000)

D5-47210 Malabsorption in the elderly
(T-50500) (F-53202)

D5-47220 Drug-induced malabsorption
(T-50500) (F-53202) (G-C001) (C-50000)

D5-47300 Blind loop syndrome, NOS 579.2

D5-47310 Postoperative blind loop syndrome 579.2

D5-47350 Hypoglycemia following gastrointestinal surgery 579.3

D5-47360 Malnutrition following gastrointestinal surgery 579.3

D5-47500 Bile acid malabsorption syndrome, NOS

D5-47502 Bile acid malabsorption syndrome type I

D5-47504 Bile acid malabsorption syndrome type II

D5-47506 Bile acid malabsorption syndrome type III

5-47 MALABSORPTION SYNDROMES — Continued

D5-47610 Postcholecystectomy diarrhea
D5-47620 Postvagotomy diarrhea 564.2
(DF-00000) (G-C003) (P1-01000)
(T-A8640) (G-C008) (F-54400)
Postvagotomy syndrome 564.2
(DF-00000) (G-C003) (P1-01000)
(T-A8640) (F-54400)
D5-47630 Diarrhea in diabetes
D5-47640 Diarrhea due to alcohol intake
D5-47650 Raw-milk associated diarrhea
D5-47660 Chronic diarrhea of infants and young children
D5-47670 Congenital secretory diarrhea, NOS
D5-47672 Congenital secretory diarrhea, chloride type
Congenital chloridorrhea
Defective Cl^-/HCO_3^- exchange in ileum and colon
D5-47674 Congenital secretory diarrhea, sodium type
Defective Na^+/H^+ exchange in jejunum and ileum
Congenital sodium diarrhea
D5-47680 Chronic diarrhea of unknown origin
D5-47780 Short bowel syndrome
(DF-00000) (G-C001) (T-58000)
(P1-02000) (G-C008) (F-54400)
(F-54600)

SECTION 5-6 HERNIAS OF THE ABDOMINAL CAVITY

D5-60000 Hernia of abdominal cavity, NOS 553.9
(T-D4010) (M-31500)
D5-60002 Intestinal hernia, NOS 553.9
(T-50500) (M-31500)
D5-60004 Intra-abdominal hernia, NOS 553.9
(T-D4010) (M-31500)
D5-60006 Interstitial hernia 553.9
(T-D4300) (M-31500)
D5-60010 Hernia, NOS, with gangrene 551.9
(T-.....) (M-31500) (G-C008) (M-54600)
D5-60020 Hernia, NOS, with obstruction 552.9
(T-.....) (M-31500) (G-C008) (M-34000)
D5-60030 Rupture of hernia, NOS 553.9
(T-.....) (M-31500) (M-14400)
D5-60100 Inguinal hernia, NOS 550.9
(T-D7040) (M-31500) (G-C009)
(M-34000) (M-54600)
Inguinal hernia without obstruction or gangrene 550.9
(T-D7040) (M-31500) (G-C009)
(M-34000) (M-54600)
Bubonocele, NOS 550.9
(T-D7040) (M-31500) (G-C009)
(M-34000) (M-54600)
D5-60101 Unilateral inguinal hernia 550.90
(T-D7040) (M-31500) (G-A103)
D5-60102 Unilateral recurrent inguinal hernia 550.91
(T-D7040) (M-31500) (G-A500)
(G-A103)
D5-60103 Bilateral inguinal hernia 550.92
(T-D7040) (M-31500) (G-A102)
D5-60104 Bilateral recurrent inguinal hernia 550.93
(T-D7040) (M-31500) (G-A500)
(G-A102)
D5-60110 Inguinal hernia with gangrene 550.0
(T-D7040) (M-31500) (G-C008)
(M-54600)
D5-60111 Unilateral inguinal hernia with gangrene 550.00
(T-D7040) (M-31500) (G-C008)
(M-54600) (G-A103)
D5-60112 Unilateral recurrent inguinal hernia with gangrene 550.01
(T-D7040) (M-31500) (G-C008)
(M-54600) (G-A500) (G-A103)
D5-60113 Bilateral inguinal hernia with gangrene 550.02
(T-D7040) (M-31500) (G-C008)
(M-54600) (G-A102)
D5-60114 Bilateral recurrent inguinal hernia with gangrene 550.03
(T-D7040) (M-31500) (G-C008)
(M-54600) (G-A500) (G-A102)
D5-60120 Inguinal hernia with gangrene and obstruction 550.0
(T-D7040) (M-31500) (G-C008)
(M-54600) (M-34000)
D5-60121 Unilateral inguinal hernia with gangrene and obstruction 550.00
(T-D7040) (M-31500) (G-C008)
(M-54600) (M-34000) (G-A103)
D5-60122 Unilateral recurrent inguinal hernia with gangrene and obstruction 550.01
(T-D7040) (M-31500) (G-C008)
(M-54600) (M-34000) (G-A500)
(G-A103)
D5-60123 Bilateral inguinal hernia with gangrene and obstruction 550.02
(T-D7040) (M-31500) (G-C008)
(M-54600) (M-34000) (G-A102)
D5-60124 Bilateral recurrent inguinal hernia with gangrene and obstruction 550.03
(T-D7040) (M-31500) (G-C008)
(M-54600) (M-34000) (G-A500)
(G-A102)
D5-60130 Inguinal hernia with obstruction but no gangrene 550.1
(T-D7040) (M-31500) (G-C008)
(M-34000) (G-C009) (M-54600)
Inguinal hernia with incarceration 550.1
(T-D7040) (M-31500) (G-C008)
(M-34000) (G-C009) (M-54600)
Inguinal hernia with irreducibility 550.1
(T-D7040) (M-31500) (G-C008)
(M-34000) (G-C009) (M-54600)
Inguinal hernia with strangulation 550.1
(T-D7040) (M-31500) (G-C008)
(M-34000) (G-C009) (M-54600)

D5-60131 Unilateral inguinal hernia with obstruction but no gangrene 550.10
(T-D7040) (M-31500) (G-C008) (M-34000) (G-C009) (M-54600) (G-A103)

D5-60132 Unilateral recurrent inguinal hernia with obstruction but no gangrene 550.11
(T-D7040) (M-31500) (G-C008) (M-34000) (G-C009) (M-54600) (G-A500) (G-A103)

D5-60133 Bilateral inguinal hernia with obstruction but no gangrene 550.12
(T-D7050) (M-31500) (G-C008) (M-34000) (G-C009) (M-54600) (G-A102)

D5-60134 Bilateral recurrent inguinal hernia with obstruction but no gangrene 550.13
(T-D7040) (M-31500) (G-C008) (M-34000) (G-C009) (M-54600) (G-A500) (G-A102)

D5-60150 Direct inguinal hernia 550.-
(T-D7040) (T-18745) (M-31500)
Internal inguinal hernia 550.-
(T-D7040) (T-18745) (M-31500)

D5-60152 Indirect inguinal hernia 550.-
(T-D7040) (T-18745) (M-31500)
External inguinal hernia 550.-
(T-D7040) (T-18745) (M-31500)
Oblique inguinal hernia 550.-
(T-D7040) (T-18745) (M-31500)

D5-60160 Scrotal hernia 550.-
(T-98000) (M-31500)

D5-60200 Femoral hernia, NOS 553.0
(T-18920) (M-31500)
Femoral hernia without obstruction or gangrene 553.0
(T-18920) (M-31500) (G-C009) (M-34000) (M-54600)

D5-60201 Unilateral femoral hernia without obstruction or gangrene 553.00
(T-18920) (M-31500) (G-C009) (M-34000) (M-54600) (G-A103)

D5-60202 Unilateral recurrent femoral hernia without obstruction or gangrene 553.01
(T-18920) (M-31500) (G-C009) (M-34000) (M-54600) (G-A500) (G-A103)

D5-60203 Bilateral femoral hernia without obstruction or gangrene 553.02
(T-18920) (M-31500) (G-C009) (M-34000) (M-54600) (G-A102)

D5-60204 Bilateral recurrent femoral hernia without obstruction or gangrene 553.03
(T-18920) (M-31500) (G-C009) (M-34000) (M-54600) (G-A500) (G-A102)

D5-60210 Femoral hernia with gangrene 551.0
(T-18920) (M-31500) (G-C008) (M-54600)

D5-60211 Unilateral femoral hernia with gangrene 551.00
(T-18920) (M-31500) (G-C008) (M-54600) (G-A103)

D5-60212 Unilateral recurrent femoral hernia with gangrene 551.01
(T-18920) (M-31500) (G-C008) (M-54600) (G-A500) (G-A103)

D5-60213 Bilateral femoral hernia with gangrene 551.02
(T-18920) (M-31500) (G-C008) (M-54600) (G-A102)

D5-60214 Bilateral recurrent femoral hernia with gangrene 551.03
(T-18920) (M-31500) (G-C008) (M-54600) (G-A500) (G-A102)

D5-60220 Femoral hernia with gangrene and obstruction 551.0
(T-18920) (M-31500) (G-C008) (M-54600) (M-34000)

D5-60221 Unilateral femoral hernia with gangrene and obstruction 551.00
(T-18920) (M-31500) (G-C008) (M-54600) (M-34000) (G-A103)

D5-60222 Unilateral recurrent femoral hernia with gangrene and obstruction 551.01
(T-18920) (M-31500) (G-C008) (M-54600) (M-34000) (G-A500) (G-A103)

D5-60223 Bilateral femoral hernia with gangrene and obstruction 551.02
(T-18920) (M-31500) (G-C008) (M-54600) (M-34000) (G-A102)

D5-60224 Bilateral recurrent femoral hernia with gangrene and obstruction 551.03
(T-18920) (M-31500) (G-C008) (M-54600) (M-34000) (G-A500) (G-A102)

D5-60230 Femoral hernia with obstruction but no gangrene 552.0
(T-18920) (M-31500) (G-C008) (M-34000) (G-C009) (M-54600)

D5-60231 Unilateral femoral hernia with obstruction but no gangrene 552.00
(T-18920) (M-31500) (G-C008) (M-34000) (G-C009) (M-54600) (G-A103)

D5-60232 Unilateral recurrent femoral hernia with obstruction but no gangrene 552.01
(T-18920) (M-31500) (G-C008) (M-34000) (G-C009) (M-54600) (G-A500) (G-A103)

D5-60233 Bilateral femoral hernia with obstruction but no gangrene 552.02
(T-18920) (M-31500) (G-C008) (M-34000) (G-C009) (M-54600) (G-A102)

SECTION 5-6 HERNIAS OF THE ABDOMINAL CAVITY — Continued

D5-60234 Bilateral recurrent femoral hernia with obstruction but no gangrene 552.03
(T-18920) (M-31500) (G-C008) (M-34000) (G-C009) (M-54600) (G-A500) (G-A102)

D5-60300 Umbilical hernia, NOS 553.1
(T-D4220) (M-31500)
Exomphalos
(T-D4220) (M-31500)

D5-60301 Umbilical hernia without obstruction or gangrene 553.1
(T-D4220) (M-31500) (G-C009) (M-34000) (M-54600)

D5-60302 Paraumbilical hernia, NOS 553.1
(T-D4230) (M-31500)

D5-60310 Umbilical hernia with gangrene 551.1
(T-D4220) (M-31500) (G-C008) (M-54600)

D5-60312 Paraumbilical hernia with gangrene 551.1
(T-D4230) (M-31500) (G-C008) (M-54600)

D5-60320 Umbilical hernia with gangrene and obstruction 551.1
(T-D4220) (M-31500) (G-C008) (M-54600) (M-34000)

D5-60322 Paraumbilical hernia with gangrene and obstruction 551.1
(T-D4230) (M-31500) (G-C008) (M-54600) (M-34000)

D5-60330 Umbilical hernia with obstruction but no gangrene 552.1
(T-D4220) (M-31500) (G-C008) (M-34000) (G-C009) (M-54600)
Incarcerated umbilical hernia 552.1
(T-D4220) (M-31500) (G-C008) (M-34000) (G-C009) (M-54600)
Irreducible umbilical hernia 552.1
(T-D4220) (M-31500) (G-C008) (M-34000) (G-C009) (M-54600)
Strangulated umbilical hernia 552.1
(T-D4220) (M-31500) (G-C008) (M-43000) (G-C009) (M-54600)

D5-60340V Hepatomphalocele
(T-D4220) (M-31500) (G-C008) (M-31400) (T-62000)
Umbilical hernia with liver in the sac
(T-D4220) (M-31500) (G-C008) (M-31400) (T-62000)

D5-60400 Ventral hernia, NOS 553.20
(T-D4300) (M-31500)

D5-60401 Ventral hernia without obstruction or gangrene 553.20
(T-D4300) (M-31500) (G-C009) (M-34000) (M-54600)

D5-60410 Ventral hernia with gangrene 551.20
(T-D4300) (M-31500) (G-C008) (M-54600)

D5-60420 Ventral hernia with gangrene and obstruction 551.20
(T-D4300) (M-31500) (G-C008) (M-54600) (M-34000)

D5-60430 Ventral hernia with obstruction but no gangrene 552.20
(T-D4300) (M-31500) (G-C008) (M-34000) (G-C009) (M-54600)
Incarcerated ventral hernia 552.20
(T-D4300) (M-31500) (G-C008) (M-34000) (G-C009) (M-54600)
Irreducible ventral hernia 552.20
(T-D4300) (M-31500) (G-C008) (M-34000) (G-C008) (M-54600)
Strangulated ventral hernia 552.20
(T-D4300) (M-31500) (G-C008) (M-34000) (G-C009) (M-54600)

D5-60450 Epigastric hernia 553.29
(T-D4200) (T-D4330) (M-31500)
Spigelian hernia 553.29
(T-D4200) (T-D4330) (M-31500)

D5-60460 Gangrenous epigastric hernia 551.29
(T-D4200) (T-D4330) (M-31500) (G-C008) (M-54600)

D5-60470 Epigastric hernia with gangrene and obstruction 551.29
(T-D4200) (T-D4330) (M-31500) (G-C008) (M-54600) (M-34000)

D5-60480 Epigastric hernia with obstruction but no gangrene 552.29
(T-D4200) (T-D4330) (M-31500) (G-C008) (M-34000) (G-C009) (M-54600)
Incarcerated epigastric hernia 552.29
(T-D4200) (T-D4330) (M-31500) (G-C008) (M-34000) (G-C009) (M-54600)
Irreducible epigastric hernia 552.29
(T-D4200) (T-D4330) (M-31500) (G-C008) (M-34000) (G-C009) (M-54600)
Strangulated epigastric hernia 552.29
(T-D4200) (T-D4330) (M-31500) (G-C008) (M-34000) (G-C009) (M-54600)

D5-60500 Incisional hernia, NOS 553.21
(T-D4300) (P1-01000) (M-31500)

D5-60502 Recurrent ventral hernia 553.21
(T-D4300) (M-31500) (G-A500)

D5-60504 Postoperative incisional hernia 553.21
(T-D4300) (P1-01000) (M-31500) (F-06030)

D5-60510 Incisional hernia with gangrene 551.21
(T-D4300) (P1-01000) (M-31500) (G-C008) (M-54600)

D5-60512 Gangrenous recurrent ventral hernia 551.21
(T-D4300) (M-31500) (G-C008) (M-54600) (G-A500)

D5-60514 Gangrenous postoperative incisional hernia 551.21
(T-D4300) (P1-01000) (M-31500) (G-C008) (M-54600) (F-06030)

D5-60520 Incisional hernia with gangrene and obstruction 551.21
(T-D4300) (P1-01000) (M-31500) (G-C008) (M-54600) (M-34000)

D5-60530 Incisional hernia with obstruction but no gangrene 552.21
(T-D4300) (P1-01000) (M-31500) (G-C008) (M-34000) (G-C009) (M-54600)
Incarcerated incisional hernia 552.21
(T-D4300) (P1-01000) (M-31500) (G-C008) (M-34000) (G-C009) (M-54600)
Irreducible incisional hernia 552.21
(T-D4300) (P1-01000) (M-31500) (G-C008) (M-34000) (G-C009) (M-54600)
Strangulated incisional hernia 552.21
(T-D4300) (P1-01000) (M-31500) (G-C008) (M-34000) (G-C009) (M-54600)

D5-60532 Recurrent ventral hernia with obstruction 552.21
(T-D4300) (M-31500) (G-C008) (M-34000) (G-A500)

D5-60534 Postoperative incisional hernia with obstruction 552.21
(T-D4300) (P1-01000) (M-31500) (G-C008) (M-34000) (F-06030)

D5-60600 Diaphragmatic hernia, NOS 553.3
(T-D3400) (M-31500)

D5-60602 Hiatal hernia 553.3
(T-D3420) (M-31500)
Esophageal hiatal hernia 553.3
(T-D3420) (M-31500)

D5-60604 Paraesophageal hernia 553.3
(T-D3420) (M-31500) (G-C008) (T-57000) (G-A113) (T-D3000)
Thoracic stomach 553.3
(T-D3420) (M-31500) (G-C008) (T-57000) (G-A113) (T-D3000)

D5-60610 Diaphragmatic hernia with gangrene 551.3
(T-D3400) (M-31500) (G-C008) (M-54600)

D5-60612 Gangrenous hiatal hernia 551.3
(T-D3420) (M-31500) (G-C008) (M-54600)

D5-60614 Gangrenous paraesophageal hernia 551.3
(T-D3420) (M-31500) (G-C008) (T-57000) (G-A113) (T-D3000) (G-C008) (M-54600)
Gangrenous thoracic stomach 551.3
(T-D3420) (M-31500) (G-C008) (T-57000) (G-A113) (T-D3000) (G-C008) (M-54600)

D5-60620 Diaphragmatic hernia with gangrene and obstruction 551.3
(T-D3400) (M-31500) (G-C008) (M-54600) (M-34000)

D5-60622 Hiatal hernia with gangrene and obstruction 551.3
(T-D3420) (M-31500) (G-C008) (M-54600) (M-34000)

D5-60624 Paraesophageal hernia with gangrene and obstruction 551.3
(T-D3420) (M-31500) (G-C008) (T-57000) (G-A113) (T-D3000) (G-C008) (M-54600) (M-34000)
Gangrenous thoracic stomach with obstruction 551.3
(T-D3420) (M-31500) (G-C008) (T-57000) (G-A113) (T-D3000) (G-C008) (M-54600) (M-34000)

D5-60630 Diaphragmatic hernia with obstruction but no gangrene 552.3
(T-D3400) (M-31500) (G-C008) (M-34000) (G-C009) (M-54600)

D5-60632 Hiatal hernia with obstruction but no gangrene 552.3
(T-D3420) (M-31500) (G-C008) (M-34000) (G-C009) (M-54600)
Incarcerated hiatal hernia 552.3
(T-D3420) (M-31500) (G-C008) (M-34000) (G-C009) (M-54600)
Irreducible hiatal hernia 552.3
(T-D3420) (M-31500) (G-C008) (M-34000) (G-C009) (M-54600)
Strangulated hiatal hernia 552.3
(T-D3420) (M-31500) (G-C008) (M-34000) (G-C009) (M-54600)

D5-60634 Paraesophageal hernia with obstruction but no gangrene 552.3
(T-D3420) (M-31500) (T-57000) (G-A113) (T-D3000) (G-C008) (M-34000) (G-C009) (M-54600)
Thoracic stomach with obstruction but no gangrene 552.3
(T-D3420) (M-31500) (T-57000) (G-A113) (T-D3000) (G-C008) (M-34000) (G-C009) (M-54600)
Incarcerated paraesophageal hernia 552.3
(T-D3420) (M-31500) (T-57000) (G-A113) (T-D3000) (G-C008) (M-34000) (G-C009) (M-54600)
Irreducible paraesophageal hernia 552.3
(T-D3420) (M-31500) (T-57000) (G-A113) (T-D3000) (G-C008) (M-34000) (G-C009) (M-54600)
Strangulated paraesophageal hernia 552.3
(T-D3420) (M-31500) (T-57000) (G-A113) (T-D3000) (G-C008) (M-34000) (G-C009) (M-54600)

SECTION 5-6 HERNIAS OF THE ABDOMINAL CAVITY — Continued

D5-60800 Ischiatic hernia 553.8
(T-15704) (M-31500)
Sciatic hernia 553.8
(T-15704) (M-31500)

D5-60801 Ischiatic hernia with gangrene 551.8
(T-15704) (M-31500) (G-C008)
(M-54600)

D5-60802 Ischiatic hernia with obstruction 552.8
(T-15704) (M-31500) (G-C008)
(M-34000)

D5-60810 Ischiorectal hernia 553.8
(T-D2700) (M-31500)
Perineal hernia
(T-D2700) (M-31500)

D5-60811 Ischiorectal hernia with gangrene 551.8
(T-D2700) (M-31500) (G-C008)
(M-54600)

D5-60812 Ischiorectal hernia with obstruction 552.8
(T-D2700) (M-31500) (G-C008)
(M-34000)

D5-60820 Lumbar hernia 553.8
(T-D2305) (T-D2306) (M-31500)

D5-60821 Lumbar hernia with gangrene 551.8
(T-D2305) (T-D2306) (M-31500)
(G-C008) (M-54600)

D5-60822 Lumbar hernia with obstruction 552.8
(T-D2305) (T-D2306) (M-31500)
(G-C008) (M-34000)

D5-60830 Obturator hernia 553.8
(T-12371) (M-31500)

D5-60831 Obturator hernia with gangrene 551.8
(T-12371) (M-31500) (G-C008)
(M-54600)

D5-60832 Obturator hernia with obstruction 552.8
(T-12371) (M-31500) (G-C008)
(M-34000)

D5-60840 Pudendal hernia 553.8
(T-81000) (M-31500)

D5-60841 Pudendal hernia with gangrene 551.8
(T-81000) (M-31500) (G-C008)
(M-54600)

D5-60842 Pudental hernia with obstruction 552.8
(T-81000) (M-31500) (G-C008)
(M-34000)

D5-60850 Retroperitoneal hernia 553.8
(T-D4464) (M-31500) (T-50500)
Treitz's hernia
(T-D4464) (M-31500) (T-50500)

D5-60851 Retroperitoneal hernia with gangrene 551.8
(T-D4464) (M-31500) (T-50500)
(G-C008) (M-54600)

D5-60852 Retroperitoneal hernia with obstruction 552.8
(T-D4464) (M-31500) (T-50500)
(G-C008) (M-34000)

D5-60900 Enterocele 553.9
(T-50500) (M-31500)

D5-60910 Epiplocele 553.9
(T-D4600) (M-31500)

D5-60920 Sarcoepiplocele 553.9
(T-D4600) (M-31500)

D5-60930 Mesenteric hernia
(T-D4500) (M-31500)

SECTION 5-7 DISEASES OF THE PERITONEUM

D5-70000 Disease of peritoneum, NOS 568.9
(T-D4400) (DF-00000)

D5-70100 Peritonitis, NOS 567.9
(T-D4400) (M-40000)
Peritonitis of undetermined cause 567.9
(T-D4400) (M-40000)

D5-70110 Acute generalized peritonitis 567.2
(T-D4400) (M-41000) (G-A366)

D5-70112 Acute suppurative peritonitis 567.2
(T-D4400) (M-41600)

D5-70116 Subphrenic peritonitis 567.2
(T-D4440) (M-40000)

D5-70118 Male pelvic peritonitis 567.2
(T-D6020) (M-40000)

D5-70200 Abdominal abscess, NOS
(T-D4010) (M-41610)

D5-70202 Abscess of peritoneum, NOS 567.2
(T-D4425) (M-41610)
Intraperitoneal abscess, NOS 567.2
(T-D4425) (M-41610)

D5-70204 Abdominal visceral abscess
(T-D4030) (M-41610)

D5-70206 Midabdominal abscess
(T-D4003) (M-41610)

D5-70210 Abscess of omentum 567.2
(T-D4600) (M-41610)

D5-70220 Abdominopelvic abscess 567.2
(T-D4010) (T-D6221) (M-41610)

D5-70222 Pelvic abscess
(T-D6221) (M-41610)

D5-70230 Mesenteric abscess 567.2
(T-D4500) (M-41610)

D5-70240 Retrocecal abscess 567.2
(T-59265) (M-41610)

D5-70250 Retroperitoneal abscess 567.2
(T-D4900) (M-41610)

D5-70260 Subdiaphragmatic abscess 567.2
(T-D4440) (M-41610)
Subphrenic abscess 567.2
(T-D4440) (M-41610)

D5-70270 Subhepatic abscess 567.2
(T-62460) (M-41610)

D5-70300 Chronic peritonitis, NOS 567.8
(T-D4400) (M-43000)

D5-70310 Chronic proliferative peritonitis 567.8
(T-D4400) (M-43000) (M-45200)

D5-70312 Granulomatous peritonitis
(T-D4400) (M-44000)

D5-70314 Sclerosing peritonitis
(T-D4400) (M-45100)
D5-70320 Fat necrosis of peritoneum 567.8
(T-D4400) (M-54110)
D5-70330 Mesenteric saponification 567.8
(T-D4500) (M-54110)
D5-70334 Mesenteric hematoma
(T-D4500) (M-35060)
D5-70340 Bile peritonitis 567.8
(T-D4400) (M-40000) (G-C001)
(T-60650)
D5-70350 Urine peritonitis 567.8
(T-D4400) (M-40000) (G-C001)
(T-70060)
Uroperitonitis 567.8
(T-D4400) (M-40000) (G-C001)
(T-70060)
D5-70360 Retractile mesenteritis
(T-D4500) (M-40000) (M-02595)
D5-70370 Retroperitoneal fibrosis
(T-D4900) (M-78000)
D5-70400 Ascites, NOS 789.5
(T-D4425) (M-36710)
Hydroperitoneum 789.5
(T-D4425) (M-36710)
D5-70410 Pancreatic ascites
(T-65000) (M-36710)
D5-70420 Bile ascites
(T-D4425) (M-36630)
D5-70430 Chylous ascites 457.8
(T-D4425) (M-36740)
D5-70440 Urine ascites
(T-D4425) (M-36620)
D5-70442 Urine ascites of the neonate
(T-D4425) (M-36620) (F-88000)
D5-70444 Dialysis-associated ascites
(T-D4500) (M-36710) (G-C001) (P.-.....)
D5-71000 Peritoneal adhesion, NOS 568.0
(T-D4400) (M-78400)
Adhesive peritoneal band, NOS 568.0
(T-D4400) (M-78400)
D5-71010 Adhesion of abdominal wall 568.0
(T-D4300) (M-78400)
D5-71030 Adhesion of intestine 568.0
(T-50500) (M-78400)
D5-71040 Adhesion of male pelvis 568.0
(T-D6020) (M-78400)
D5-71050 Adhesion of mesentery 568.0
(T-D4500) (M-78400)
D5-71060 Adhesion of omentum 568.0
(T-D4600) (M-78400)
D5-71062 Omental torsion
(T-D4600) (M-34110)
D5-71064 Omental infarction
(T-D4600) (M-54700)
D5-71070 Adhesion of stomach 568.0
(T-57000) (M-78400)
D5-71200 Nontraumatic hemoperitoneum 568.81
(T-D4425) (M-37000)
D5-71220 Chronic peritoneal effusion 568.82
(T-D4425) (M-36700)
D5-71260 Peritoneal granuloma 568.89
(T-D4400) (M-44000)
D5-71280 Mesenteric arteriovenous fistula, NOS
(T-46500) (T-48910) (M-39370)
D5-71282 Mesenteric-portal fistula
(T-46500) (T-48810) (M-39370)
D5-71290 Mesenteric varices
(T-48840) (T-48910) (M-32600)

SECTION 5-8 DISEASES OF THE LIVER AND BILIARY SYSTEM
5-80-81 DISEASES OF THE LIVER

D5-80000 Disease of liver, NOS 573.9
(T-62000) (DF-00000)
Hepatopathy
(T-62000) (DF-00000)
D5-80100 Hepatic necrosis 570.-
(T-62000) (M-54000)
D5-80110 Acute hepatic necrosis 570.-
(T-62000) (M-54001) (M-58010)
Massive hepatic necrosis 570.-
(T-62000) (M-54001) (T-58010)
Acute yellow atrophy of liver 570.-
(T-62000) (M-54001) (M-58010)
D5-80114 Diffuse hepatic necrosis 570.-
(T-62000) (M-54006) (M-58010)
D5-80120 Subacute hepatic necrosis 570.-
(T-62000) (M-54002) (M-58010)
Subacute yellow atrophy of liver 570.-
(T-62000) (M-54002) (M-58010)
D5-80130 Parenchymatous degeneration of liver 570.-
(T-62260) (M-50050)
D5-80140 Acute hepatitis, NOS 570.-
(T-62000) (M-41000)
D5-80141 Acute noninfective hepatitis 570.-
(T-62000) (M-41000)
D5-80142 Subacute noninfective hepatitis 570.-
(T-62000) (M-42000)
D5-80310 Focal hepatic necrosis
(T-62000) (M-54004)
D5-80311V Sawdust liver
(T-62000) (M-54004)
D5-80312 Peripheral hepatic necrosis
(T-62230) (M-54120)
D5-80314 Midzonal hepatic necrosis
(T-62220) (M-54120)
D5-80316 Centrilobular hepatic necrosis
(T-62210) (M-54120)
Paracentral hepatic necrosis
(T-62210) (M-54120)
D5-80320 Acute red atrophy of liver
(T-62000) (M-41000) (M-58010)

5-80-81 DISEASES OF THE LIVER — Continued

D5-80400 Alcoholic liver damage, NOS 571.3
(T-62000) (M-01150) (G-C001)
(C-21005)

D5-80410 Alcoholic fatty liver 571.0
(T-62000) (M-50080) (G-C001)
(C-21005)

D5-80420 Acute alcoholic liver disease 571.1
(T-62000) (M-41000) (G-C001)
(C-21005)
Acute alcoholic hepatitis 571.1
(T-62000) (M-41000) (G-C001)
(C-21005)

D5-80430 Alcoholic cirrhosis of liver 571.2
(T-62000) (M-78000) (G-C001)
(C-21005)
Laennec's cirrhosis 571.2
(T-62000) (M-78000) (G-C001)
(C-21005)
Portal cirrhosis, NOS 571.5
(T-62000) (M-78000) (G-C001)
(C-21005)

D5-80450 Florid cirrhosis 571.2
(T-62000) (M-78000) (G-C001)
(C-21005)

D5-80500 Chronic hepatitis, NOS 571.40
(T-62000) (M-43000)

D5-80510 Chronic persistent hepatitis 571.41
(T-62000) (M-43000) (G-A480)

D5-80520 Chronic active hepatitis 571.49
(T-62000) (M-43000)
Chronic aggressive hepatitis 571.49
(T-62000) (M-43000)
Recurrent hepatitis 571.49
(T-62000) (M-43000)

D5-80550V Chronic lobular hepatitis
(T-62200) (M-43000)

D5-80600 Cirrhosis of liver, NOS 571.5
(T-62000) (M-78000)
Cirrhosis of liver without mention of alcohol 571.5
(T-62000) (M-78000)

D5-80602 Cryptogenic cirrhosis 571.5
(T-62000) (M-78000)

D5-80610 Macronodular cirrhosis 571.5
(T-62000) (M-78000) (G-C008)
(M-79944)

D5-80620 Micronodular cirrhosis 571.5
(T-62000) (M-78000) (G-C008)
(M-79942)

D5-80630 Posthepatitic cirrhosis 571.5
(T-62000) (M-78000) (G-C003)
(D5-80140)

D5-80640 Postnecrotic cirrhosis 571.5
(T-62000) (M-78000) (G-C003)
(M-54000)
Healed yellow atrophy of liver 571.5
(T-62000) (M-78000) (G-C003)
(M-54000)

D5-80650 Pigment cirrhosis
(T-62000) (M-78000) (M-55800)

D5-80660 Parasitic cirrhosis
(T-62000) (M-78000) (G-C001)
(L-50000)

D5-80670V Glissonian cirrhosis
(T-62030) (M-78000)

D5-80700 Biliary cirrhosis 571.6
(T-62000) (M-78000) (G-C001)
(T-60600) (M-34000)
Cholangitic cirrhosis 571.6
(T-62000) (M-78000) (G-C001)
(T-60600) (M-34000)
Cholestatic cirrhosis 571.6
(T-62000) (M-78000) (G-C001)
(T-60600) (M-34000)
Chronic nonsuppurative destructive cholangitis 571.6
(T-62000) (M-78000) (G-C001)
(T-60600) (M-34000)

D5-80800 Chronic nonalcoholic liver disease, NOS 571.9
(T-62000) (DF-00003) (G-C009)
(C-21005)

D5-80810 Chronic yellow atrophy of liver 571.8
(T-62000) (M-54003) (M-58000)

D5-80820 Nonalcoholic fatty liver 571.8
(T-62000) (M-50080) (G-C009)
(C-21005)
Hepatic lipidosis
(T-62000) (M-50080) (G-C009)
(C-21005)
Fatty liver
(T-62000) (M-50080) (G-C009)
(C-21005)

D5-81000 Abscess of liver, NOS 572.0
(T-62000) (M-41610)
Hepatic abscess, NOS
(T-62000) (M-41610)

D5-81010 Phlebitis of portal vein 572.1
(T-48810) (M-40000)
Pylephlebitis 572.1
(T-48810) (M-40000)

D5-81012 Portal pyemia 572.1
(T-48810) (M-40600)
Suppurative pylephlebitis 572.1
(T-48810) (M-40600)

D5-81020 Portal thrombophlebitis 572.1
(T-48810) (M-40000) (G-C008)
(M-35100)
Pylethrombophlebitis 572.1
(T-48810) (M-40000) (G-C008)
(M-35100)

D5-81100 Hepatic failure, NOS
(T-62000) (F-00150)
Hepatic insufficiency, NOS
(T-62000) (F-00150)

D5-81100 (cont.) Liver function failure, NOS
(T-62000) (F-00150)

D5-81110 Hepatic encephalopathy 572.2
(DA-13000) (G-C001) (T-62000) (DF-00000)
Portal-systemic encephalopathy 572.2
(DA-13000) (G-C001) (T-62000) (DF-00000)

D5-81120 Hepatic coma 572.2
(T-A0100) (F-A5640) (G-C001) (T-62000) (DF-00000)
Hepatocerebral intoxication 572.2
(T-A0100) (F-A5640) (G-C001) (T-62000) (DF-00000)

D5-81200 Portal hypertension 572.3
(T-48800) (D3-02000)

D5-81210 Hepatic congestion
(T-62000) (M-36100)

D5-81212 Chronic passive congestion of liver 573.0
(T-62000) (M-36142)
Nutmeg liver
(T-62000) (M-36142)

D5-81220 Hepatomegaly 789.1
(T-62000) (M-71000)

D5-81230 Hepatorenal syndrome 572.4
(T-71000) (F-00150) (G-C001) (T-62000)

D5-81240 Cardiac cirrhosis, NOS
(T-62000) (M-78000) (G-C001) (D3-16010)

D5-81250 Hepatic infarction 573.4
(T-62000) (M-54700)

D5-81280 Hepatoptosis 573.8
(T-62000) (M-31050)

D5-81400 Hepatitis, NOS 573.3
(T-62000) (M-40000)

D5-81410 Toxic noninfectious hepatitis 573.3
(T-62000) (M-40000) (G-C001) (C-00220)

D5-81412 Acute toxic hepatitis
(T-62000) (M-41000) (G-C001) (C-00220)

D5-81420V Lobular dissecting hepatitis
(T-62200) (M-40000) (G-A356)

D5-81430V Copper-associated hepatitis in Bedlington terriers
(T-62000) (M-40000) (G-C002) (C-12700)

D5-81450 Pyogenic hepatic abscess
(T-62000) (M-41610)

D5-81460 Microhepatia
(T-62000) (M-02530)

D5-81470 Hepatic fibrosis, NOS
(T-62000) (M-78000)

D5-81500 Acquired portal-systemic shunt
(T-48810) (T-48710) (F-39370)

D5-81510 Acquired arteriovenous fistula of liver
(T-62000) (M-39370)

D5-81520 Peliosis hepatis
(T-62000) (M-32440)
Telangiectasis of liver
(T-62000) (M-32440)

D5-81530 Hepatic cyst
(T-62000) (M-33400)

D5-81540 Torsion of liver lobe
(T-62200) (M-34110)

D5-81800V Cholangitis-cholangiohepatitis syndrome in cats
(T-62000) (T-60610) (M-40000)

D5-81810V Chronic lymphocytic cholangitis-cholangiohepatitis
(T-62000) (T-60610) (M-43010)

D5-81840 Hepatic amyloidosis
(T-62000) (M-55100)

5-85-86 DISEASES OF THE GALLBLADDER AND BILE DUCTS

D5-85000 Disease of gallbladder, NOS 575.9
(T-63000) (DF-00000)

D5-85050 Disease of biliary tract, NOS 576.9
(T-60610) (DF-00000)

D5-85100 Cholecystitis, NOS 575.1
(T-63000) (M-40000)

D5-85102 Cholecystitis, NOS without calculus 575.1
(T-63000) (M-40000) (G-C009) (M-30000)

D5-85110 Acute cholecystitis 575.0
(T-63000) (M-41000)

D5-85112 Acute cholecystitis without calculus 575.0
(T-63000) (M-41000) (G-C009) (M-30000)
Acute acalculous cholecystitis 575.0
(T-63000) (M-41000) (G-C009) (M-30000)

D5-85120 Acute gangrenous cholecystitis 575.0
(T-63000) (M-41700)

D5-85124 Acute suppurative cholecystitis 575.0
(T-63000) (M-41600)

D5-85128 Acute emphysematous cholecystitis 575.0
(T-63000) (M-41000) (G-C008) (M-33900)

D5-85130 Angiocholecystitis 575.0
(T-63000) (T-40000) (M-40000)

D5-85140 Abscess of gallbladder 575.0
(T-63000) (M-41610)

D5-85142 Pericholecystic abscess 575.0
(T-63000) (M-41610)

D5-85145 Empyema of gallbladder 575.0
(T-63000) (M-40620)

D5-85150 Gangrene of gallbladder 575.0
(T-63000) (M-54600)

D5-85160 Chronic cholecystitis, NOS 575.1
(T-63000) (M-43000)

D5-85162 Chronic cholecystitis without calculus 575.1
(T-63000) (M-43000) (G-C009) (M-30000)

5-85-86 DISEASES OF THE GALLBLADDER AND BILE DUCTS — Continued

D5-85200 Calculus of gallbladder with cholecystitis, NOS 574.1
(T-63000) (M-40000) (G-C008) (M-30000)
Biliary calculus with cholecystitis, NOS 574.1
(T-63000) (M-40000) (G-C008) (M-30000)
Cholelithiasis with cholecystitis, NOS 574.1
(T-63000) (M-40000) (G-C008) (M-30000)

D5-85210 Calculus of cystic duct with cholecystitis, NOS 574.1
(T-63000) (M-40000) (G-C008) (T-64400) (M-30000)

D5-85220 Cholelithiasis and cholecystitis without obstruction 574.10
(T-63000) (M-40000) (G-C001) (M-30000) (G-C009) (M-34000)

D5-85230 Cholelithiasis and cholecystitis with obstruction 574.11
(T-63000) (M-40000) (G-C008) (M-30000) (M-34000)

D5-85300 Calculus of gallbladder with acute cholecystitis 574.0
(T-63000) (M-41000) (G-C008) (M-30000)
Biliary calculus with acute cholecystitis 574.0
(T-63000) (M-41000) (G-C008) (M-30000)
Cholelithiasis with acute cholecystitis 574.0
(T-63000) (M-41000) (G-C008) (M-30000)

D5-85310 Calculus of cystic duct with acute cholecystitis 574.0
(T-63000) (M-41000) (G-C008) (T-64400) (M-30000)

D5-85320 Cholelithiasis and acute cholecystitis without obstruction 574.00
(T-63000) (M-41000) (G-C008) (M-30000) (G-C009) (M-34000)

D5-85330 Cholelithiasis and acute cholecystitis with obstruction 574.01
(T-63000) (M-41000) (G-C008) (M-30000) (M-34000)

D5-85340V Hyperplastic cholecystitis
(T-63000) (M-45200)

D5-85500 Biliary calculus, NOS 574.2
(T-63000) (M-30000)
Cholelithiasis, NOS 574.2
(T-63000) (M-30000)
Gallstone, NOS 574.2
(T-63000) (M-30000)

D5-85502 Cholelithiasis without obstruction 574.20
(T-63000) (M-30000) (G-C009) (M-34000)

D5-85504 Cholelithiasis with obstruction 574.21
(T-63000) (M-30000) (G-C008) (M-34000)

D5-85510 Calculus of cystic duct 574.2
(T-64400) (M-30000)

D5-85512 Calculus of cystic duct without obstruction 574.20
(T-64400) (M-30000) (G-C009) (M-34000)

D5-85514 Calculus of cystic duct with obstruction 574.21
(T-64400) (M-30000) (G-C008) (M-34000)

D5-85520 Impacted gallstone of gallbladder 574.2
(T-63000) (M-30000) (M-33100)

D5-85530 Impacted gallstone of cystic duct 574.2
(T-64400) (M-30000) (M-33100)

D5-85550 Biliary colic 574.2
(T-64400) (M-34000) (F-01330)

D5-85552 Recurrent biliary colic 574.2
(T-64400) (M-34000) (F-01330) (G-A500)

D5-85600 Calculus of bile duct, NOS 574.5
(T-64400) (M-30000)

D5-85602 Calculus of bile duct without obstruction 574.50
(T-64400) (M-30000) (G-C009) (M-34000)

D5-85604 Calculus of bile duct with obstruction 574.51
(T-64400) (M-30000) (G-C008) (M-34000)

D5-85610 Calculus of common duct 574.5
(T-64500) (M-30000)
Choledocholithiasis 574.5
(T-64500) (M-30000)

D5-85612 Calculus of common duct without obstruction 574.50
(T-64500) (M-30000) (G-C009) (M-34000)

D5-85614 Calculus of common duct with obstruction 574.51
(T-64500) (M-30000) (G-C008) (M-34000)

D5-85620 Calculus of hepatic duct 574.5
(T-64100) (M-30000)
Hepatic lithiasis 574.5
(T-64100) (M-30000)

D5-85622 Calculus of hepatic duct without obstruction 574.50
(T-64100) (M-30000) (G-C009) (M-34000)

D5-85624 Calculus of hepatic duct with obstruction 574.51
(T-64100) (M-30000) (G-C008) (M-34000)

D5-85650 Hepatic colic 574.5
(T-64100) (M-34000) (F-01330)
D5-85652 Recurrent hepatic colic 574.5
(T-64100) (M-34000) (F-01330)
(G-A500)
D5-85700 Calculus of bile duct with cholecystitis, NOS 574.4
(T-60610) (M-30000) (G-C008)
(T-63000) (M-40000)
D5-85710 Calculus of bile duct with chronic cholecystitis 574.4
(T-60610) (M-30000) (G-C008)
(T-63000) (M-43000)
D5-85712 Calculus of bile duct with chronic cholecystitis without obstruction 574.40
(T-60610) (M-30000) (G-C008)
(T-63000) (M-43000) (G-C009)
(M-34000)
D5-85714 Calculus of bile duct with chronic cholecystitis with obstruction 574.41
(T-60610) (M-30000) (G-C008)
(T-63000) (M-43000) (G-C008)
(M-34000)
D5-85720 Calculus of common bile duct with chronic cholecystitis 574.4
(T-64500) (M-30000) (G-C008)
(M-63000) (M-43000)
Choledocholithiasis with chronic cholecystitis 574.4
(T-64500) (M-30000) (G-C008)
(T-63000) (M-43000)
D5-85722 Calculus of common bile duct with chronic cholecystitis without obstruction 574.40
(T-64500) (M-30000) (G-C008)
(T-63000) (M-43000) (G-C009)
(M-34000)
D5-85724 Calculus of common bile duct with chronic cholecystitis with obstruction 574.41
(T-64500) (M-30000) (G-C008)
(T-63000) (M-43000) (G-C008)
(M-34000)
D5-85750 Calculus of bile duct with acute cholecystitis 574.3
(T-60610) (M-30000) (G-C008)
(T-63000) (M-41000)
D5-85752 Calculus of bile duct with acute cholecystitis without obstruction 574.30
(T-60610) (M-30000) (G-C008)
(T-63000) (M-41000) (G-C009)
(M-34000)
D5-85754 Calculus of bile duct with acute cholecystitis with obstruction 574.31
(T-60610) (M-30000) (G-C008)
(T-63000) (M-41000) (G-C008)
(M-34000)
D5-85760 Calculus of common bile duct with acute cholecystitis 574.3
(T-64500) (M-30000) (G-C008)
(T-63000) (M-41000)
Choledocholithiasis with acute cholecystitis 574.3
(T-64500) (M-30000) (G-C008)
(T-63000) (M-41000)
D5-85762 Calculus of common bile duct with acute cholecystitis without obstruction 574.30
(T-64500) (M-30000) (G-C008)
(T-63000) (M-41000) (G-C009)
(M-34000)
D5-85764 Calculus of common bile duct with acute cholecystitis with obstruction 574.31
(T-64500) (M-30000) (G-C008)
(T-63000) (M-41000) (G-C008)
(M-34000)
D5-86000 Obstruction of gallbladder 575.2
(T-63000) (M-34000)
Occlusion of gallbladder 575.2
(T-63000) (M-34000)
D5-86020 Stenosis of gallbladder 575.2
(T-63000) (M-34200)
D5-86022 Stricture of gallbladder 575.2
(T-63000) (M-34260)
D5-86030 Hydrops of gallbladder 575.3
(T-63000) (M-36010)
D5-86031 Acute hydrops of gallbladder 575.3
(T-63000) (M-36011)
D5-86040 Mucocele of gallbladder 575.3
(T-63000) (M-33440)
D5-86050 Perforation of gallbladder 575.4
(T-63000) (M-39210)
D5-86055 Rupture of gallbladder 575.4
(T-62000) (M-14400)
D5-86060 Fistula of gallbladder, NOS 575.5
(T-63000) (M-39300)
D5-86062 Cholecystoduodenal fistula 575.5
(T-63000) (T-58200) (M-39300)
D5-86064 Cholecystoenteric fistula 575.5
(T-63000) (T-58000) (M-39300)
D5-86066 Vascular-biliary fistula
(T-60610) (T-40000) (M-39300)
D5-86070 Cholesterolosis of gallbladder 575.6
(T-63000) (M-55250)
Strawberry gallbladder 575.6
(T-63000) (M-55250)
D5-86100 Adhesion of gallbladder 575.8
(T-63000) (M-78400)
D5-86105 Adhesion of cystic duct 575.8
(T-64400) (M-78400)
D5-86110 Atrophy of gallbladder 575.8
(T-63000) (M-58000)
D5-86115 Atrophy of cystic duct 575.8
(T-64400) (M-58000)
D5-86120 Cyst of gallbladder 575.8
(T-63000) (M-33400)
D5-86125 Cyst of cystic duct 575.8
(T-64400) (M-33400)
D5-86130 Hypertrophy of gallbladder 575.8
(T-63000) (M-71000)
D5-86132V Cystic mucinous hypertrophy of gallbladder
(T-63000) (M-71000) (G-C008)
(M-33440)

5-85-86 DISEASES OF THE GALLBLADDER AND BILE DUCTS — Continued

D5-86135 Hypertrophy of cystic duct 575.8
(T-64400) (M-71000)
D5-86140 Ulcer of gallbladder 575.8
(T-63000) (M-38000)
D5-86145 Ulcer of cystic duct 575.8
(T-64400) (M-38000)
D5-86150 Nonfunctioning gallbladder 575.8
(T-63000) (F-60955)
D5-86155 Nonfunctioning cystic duct 575.8
(T-64400) (F-60955)
D5-86160 Biliary dyskinesia 575.8
(T-63000) (F-A4230)
Atony of gallbladder 575.8
(T-63000) (F-A4230)
D5-86170 Biliary achalasia
(T-63000) (F-50510)
D5-86180 Postcholecystectomy syndrome 576.0
(T-D4000) (F-A2600) (M-57610)
(F-06030) (G-C003) (P1-02000)
(T-63000)
D5-86400 Cholangitis, NOS 576.1
(T-60610) (M-40000)
D5-86410 Acute cholangitis 576.1
(T-60610) (M-41000)
D5-86420 Chronic cholangitis 576.1
(T-60610) (M-43000)
D5-86430 Ascending cholangitis 576.1
(T-64100) (M-40000)
D5-86440 Primary cholangitis 576.1
(T-60610) (M-40000) (G-A332)
D5-86442 Recurrent pyogenic cholangitis 576.1
(T-60610) (M-40600) (G-A500)
D5-86444 Oriental cholangiohepatitis 576.1
(T-60610) (M-40000) (G-A332)
D5-86450 Recurrent cholangitis 576.1
(T-60610) (M-40000) (G-A500)
D5-86460 Primary sclerosing cholangitis 576.1
(T-60610) (M-43000) (G-A332)
(G-C008) (M-78020)
D5-86470 Secondary cholangitis 576.1
(T-60610) (M-40000) (G-A570)
D5-86480 Stenosing cholangitis 576.1
(T-60610) (M-43000) (G-C008)
(M-34200)
D5-86490 Suppurative cholangitis 576.1
(T-60610) (M-40600)
D5-86600 Obstruction of bile duct, NOS 576.2
(T-60610) (M-34000)
Occlusion of bile duct, NOS 576.2
(T-60610) (M-34000)
D5-86610 Stenosis of bile duct 576.2
(T-60610) (M-34200)
D5-86611 Postoperative biliary stricture
(T-60610) (M-34260) (F-06030)
D5-86612 Stricture of bile duct 576.2
(T-60610) (M-34260)
D5-86620 Perforation of bile duct 576.3
(T-60610) (M-39210)
D5-86630 Rupture of bile duct 576.3
(T-60610) (M-14400)
D5-86640 Fistula of bile duct, NOS 576.4
(T-60610) (M-39300)
D5-86650 Choledochoduodenal fistula 576.4
(T-64500) (T-58200) (M-39300)
D5-86700 Spasm of sphincter of Oddi 576.5
(T-64710) (F-11310)
D5-86710 Adhesion of bile duct 576.5
(T-60610) (M-78400)
D5-86720 Atrophy of bile duct 576.5
(T-60610) (M-58000)
D5-86730 Cyst of bile duct 576.5
(T-60610) (M-33400)
D5-86740 Hypertrophy of bile duct 576.5
(T-60610) (M-71000)
D5-86750 Stasis of bile duct 576.5
(T-60610) (M-33360)
D5-86760 Ulcer of bile duct 576.5
(T-60610) (M-38000)
D5-86765 Hemobilia
(T-60650) (M-37000)
Hemorrhage in bile
(T-60650) (M-37000)
Hematobilia
(T-60650) (M-37000)
D5-86800 Extrahepatic obstructive biliary disease
(T-64000) (M-34000)

SECTION 5-9 DISEASES OF THE PANCREAS

D5-90000 Disease of pancreas, NOS 577.9
(T-65000) (DF-00000)
D5-90100 Pancreatitis, NOS 577.0
(T-65000) (M-40000)
D5-90110 Acute pancreatitis 577.0
(T-65000) (M-41000)
Idiopathic acute pancreatitis 577.0
(T-65000) (M-41000)
D5-90120 Recurrent acute pancreatitis 577.0
(T-65000) (M-41000) (G-A500)
D5-90130 Subacute pancreatitis 577.0
(T-65000) (M-42000)
D5-90140 Suppurative pancreatitis 577.0
(T-65000) (M-40600)
D5-90150 Acute hemorrhagic pancreatitis 577.0
(T-65000) (M-41790)
D5-90152 Acute necrotizing pancreatitis
(T-65000) (M-41700)
D5-90160 Apoplectic pancreatitis 577.-
(T-65000) (M-41790) (G-C001)
(DA-00000)
D5-90200 Abscess of pancreas 577.0
(T-65000) (M-41610)
D5-90204 Phlegmon of pancreas
(T-65000) (M-41650)

D5-90240 Pancreatic fistula
(T-65000) (M-39300)

D5-90300 Chronic pancreatitis, NOS 577.1
(T-65000) (M-43000)
Painless pancreatitis 577.1
(T-65000) (M-43000)
Recurrent pancreatitis 577.1
(T-65000) (M-43000)

D5-90304 Chronic fibrosing pancreatitis
(T-65000) (M-43000) (G-C008)
(M-78003)

D5-90310 Infectious pancreatitis 577.1
(T-65000) (M-40000) (G-C001)
(L-10000)

D5-90320 Interstitial pancreatitis 577.1
(T-65500) (M-40000)

D5-90330 Relapsing pancreatitis 577.1
(T-65000) (M-40000) (G-A501)

D5-90340 Hereditary pancreatitis
(T-65000) (M-40000) (DF-00180)

D5-90350 Metabolic pancreatitis
(T-65000) (M-40000) (G-C002)
(F-60000)

D5-90360 Cyst of pancreas 577.2
(T-65000) (M-33400)

D5-90370 Pseudocyst of pancreas 577.2
(T-65000) (M-33980)

D5-90400 Atrophy of pancreas 577.8
(T-65000) (M-58000)

D5-90404V Pancreatic degenerative atrophy
(T-65000) (M-58000) (G-C008)
(M-50000)
Juvenile atrophy of the pancreas
(T-65000) (M-58000) (G-C008)
(M-50000)

D5-90410 Calculus of pancreas 577.8
(T-65000) (M-30000)
Pancreatolithiasis 577.8
(T-65000) (M-30000)

D5-90420 Fibrosis of pancreas 577.8
(T-65000) (M-78000)
Cirrhosis of pancreas 577.8
(T-65000) (M-78000)

D5-90430 Necrosis of pancreas 577.0
(T-65000) (M-54000)
Pancreatic necrosis 577.8
(T-65000) (M-54000)

D5-90432 Fat necrosis of pancreas 577.8
(T-65000) (M-54110)

D5-90434 Aseptic necrosis of pancreas 577.8
(T-65000) (M-54030)

D5-90440 Acute necrosis of pancreas 577.0
(T-65000) (M-54001)
Acute pancreatic necrosis 577.0
(T-65000) (M-54001)

D5-90442 Infective necrosis of pancreas 577.0
(T-65000) (M-54000) (G-C001)
(L-10000)

D5-90444 Subacute pancreatic necrosis
(T-65000) (M-54002)

D5-90446 Relapsing pancreatic necrosis
(T-65000) (M-54000) (G-A501)

D5-90460 Pancreatic infantilism 577.8
(D5-90000) (G-C008) (M-70110)

D5-90480 Pancreatic steatorrhea 579.4
(T-59666) (F-63600) (G-C001)
(D5-90000)

D5-90490 Pancreatic insufficiency, NOS
(T-65000) (F-00160)

D5-90510 Congenital deficiency of pancreatic lipase
(T-65000) (M-27000) (F-6A120)

D5-90520 Congenital pancreatic trypsin deficiency
(T-65000) (M-27000) (F-6AC98)

D5-90530 Congenital pancreatic enterokinase deficiency
(T-65000) (M-27000) (F-6ACB8)

D5-90550V Exocrine pancreatic insufficiency
(T-65000) (F-00160)
EPI
(T-65000) (F-00160)

D5-90560V Pancreatic acinar atrophy
(T-65090) (M-58000)
PAA
(T-65090) (M-58000)

D5-90600 Pseudopancreatic cholera syndrome

D5-90620 Pancreatic pleural effusion
(T-29000) (M-36700) (G-C001)
(D5-90000)

CHAPTER 6 — NUTRITIONAL AND METABOLIC DISEASES

SECTION 6-0 NUTRITIONAL AND METABOLIC DISEASES: GENERAL TERMS

D6-00000 Metabolic disease, NOS 277.9
Metabolic disorder, NOS 277.9
D6-00010 Localized metabolic disorder
D6-00020 Generalized metabolic disorder
D6-00050 Enzymopathy, NOS 277.9
D6-00100 Inborn error of metabolism, NOS 277.9
D6-00200 Storage disease, NOS 277.9

SECTION 6-1 NUTRITIONAL DISORDERS

6-100 Nutritional Disorders: General Terms

D6-10000 Nutritional disorder, NOS 269.9
(F-60500)
Nutritional disease, NOS 269.9
(F-60500)

6-101-109 Nutritional Deficiencies

D6-10100 Nutritional deficiency, NOS 269.9
(F-60500)
Nutritional deficiency disorder, NOS 269.9
(F-60500)
D6-10110 Nutritional deficiency, NEC 269.8
D6-10200 Starvation, NOS 994.2
(F-60500)
Effects of hunger 994.2
(F-60500)
Deprivation of food 994.2
(F-60500)
Starvation due to lack of food 994.2
(F-60500)
Inanition due to lack of food 994.2
(F-60500)
Nutrition deficiency due to insufficient food 994.2
(F-60500)
D6-10202 Nutrition deficiency due to a particular kind of food 263.9
(F-60500)
D6-10220 Semi-starvation, NOS 994.2
(F-60500)
D6-10230 Undernutrition, NOS 994.2
(F-60500)
Undernutrition syndrome, NOS 994.2
(F-60500)
D6-10240 Cachexia, NOS 799.4
Wasting disease, NOS 799.4
D6-10300 Protein-energy malnutrition, NOS 263.9
Protein-calorie malnutrition, NOS 263.9
Malnutrition (calorie), NOS 263.9
Dystrophy due to malnutrition 263.9
Protein-calorie undernutrition 263.9
D6-10310 Malnutrition of mild degree (Gomez: 75% to less than 90% of standard weight) 263.1
D6-10320 Malnutrition of moderate degree (Gomez: 60% to less than 75% of standard weight) 263.0
D6-10330 Arrested development following protein-calorie malnutrition 263.2
Nutritional dwarfism 263.2
Physical retardation due to malnutrition 263.2
D6-10340 Severe protein-calorie malnutrition (Gomez: less than 60% of standard weight) 262.-
Nutritional edema without dyspigmentation of skin and hair 262.-
D6-10400 Nutritional marasmus 261.-
Severe malnutrition, NOS 261.-
Nutritional atrophy 261.-
Athrepsia 261.-
Infantile atrophy 261.-
Marasmus infantilis 261.-
Marcor 261.-
Marasmus lactantium 261.-
Parrot atrophy of the newborn 261.-
Pedatrophia 261.-
Pedatrophy 261.-
Primary infantile atrophy 261.-
D6-10500 Kwashiorkor 260.-
Nutritional edema with dyspigmentation of skin and hair 260.-
Deposed child syndrome 260.-
Fatty liver of Brahmin children 260.-
Malignant malnutrition 260.-
Protein malnutrition 260.-
D6-10700 Failure to thrive syndrome 783.4
D6-10800 Nutritional desexing syndrome 994.2
Inanition desexing syndrome 994.2
KZ syndrome 994.2
Castration syndrome in starved POWs 994.2
D6-10900 Protein-energy malnutrition, NEC 263.8

6-110-111 Hyperalimentation and Obesity

D6-11000 Hyperalimentation, NOS 783.6
Excessive eating, NOS 783.6
Polyphagia 783.6
Hyperphagia 783.6
Gluttony 783.6
D6-11100 Obesity, NOS 278.0
Adiposis 278.0
Adiposity 278.0
Simple obesity 278.0
D6-11110 Constitutional obesity 278.0
Exogenous obesity 278.0
Familial obesity 278.0

D6-11110 (cont.) Alimentary obesity 278.0
D6-11130 Obesity of endocrine origin, NOS 259.9
D6-11170 Localized adiposity 278.1
Fat pad 278.1
Fatty tissue hyperplasia 278.1
Lipohyperplasia 278.1
D6-11180 Steatopygia 278.1

SECTION 6-2 DISORDERS OF FLUID, ELECTROLYTE AND ACID-BASE BALANCE

6-20-21 FLUID AND ELECTROLYTE DISORDERS

D6-20000 Disorder of fluid or electrolyte, NOS 276.-
D6-20100 Fluid volume disorder, NOS 276.9
D6-20200 Hypovolemia 276.5
Fluid volume depletion 276.5
Volume depletion 276.5
Depletion of volume of plasma or extracellular fluid 276.5
D6-20210 Volume depletion, renal, due to effector loss (hormonal deficit) 276.5
D6-20220 Volume depletion, renal, due to output loss (renal deficit) 276.5
D6-20230 Volume depletion, extrarenal loss 276.5
D6-20240 Volume depletion, gastrointestinal loss 276.5
D6-20300 Hypervolemia 276.6
Fluid volume excess 276.6
Volume excess 276.6
Fluid overload 276.6
Fluid excess 276.6
D6-20302 Fluid retention 276.6
D6-20310 Volume excess, disturbed Starling forces 276.6
D6-20320 Volume excess, primary hormone excess 276.6
D6-20330 Volume excess, primary renal sodium retention 276.6
D6-20400 Osmolality disturbance, NOS 276.9
(F-60710)
D6-20500 Hyposmolality, NOS 276.1
(F-60710)
Hypotonic disorder, NOS 276.1
(F-60710)
Hyposmolality syndrome, NOS 276.1
(F-60710)
D6-20510 Hyponatremia, NOS 276.1
(C-15500)
Na deficiency, NOS 276.1
(C-15500)
D6-20520 Acute hyponatremia 276.1
(C-15500)
Acute low salt syndrome 276.1
(C-15500)
Schroeder's syndrome 276.1
(C-15500)
D6-20530 Chronic hyponatremia 276.1
(C-15500)
D6-20540 Water intoxication syndrome 276.1
(C-10120)
D6-20600 Hyperosmolality, NOS 276.0
(F-60170)
Hypertonic disorder, NOS 276.0
(F-60710)
Hyperosmolality syndrome, NOS 276.0
(F-60710)
D6-20610 Hypernatremia, NOS 276.0
(C-15500)
Na overload 276.0
(C-15500)
Na excess 276.0
(C-15500)
D6-20620 Acute hypernatremia 276.0
(C-15500)
D6-20630 Chronic hypernatremia 276.0
(C-15500)
D6-20640 Essential hypernatremia 276.0
(C-15500)
D6-20650 Dehydration 276.5
(C-10120)
Pure water depletion syndrome 276.5
(C-10120)
D6-20700 Deprivation of water 994.3
(C-10120)
Effects of thirst 994.3
(C-10120)
D6-21000 Potassium disorder, NOS 276.9
(C-13500)
D6-21100 Hypokalemia 276.8
(C-13500)
Potassium depletion 276.8
(C-13500)
K deficiency 276.8
(C-13500)
Hypopotassemia syndrome 276.8
(C-13500)
Hypokalemic syndrome 276.8
(C-13500)
D6-21110 Acute hypokalemia 276.8
(C-13500)
D6-21120 Chronic hypokalemia 276.8
(C-13500)
Chronic hypopotassemia 276.8
(C-13500)
D6-21130 Hypokalemia, inadequate intake 276.8
(C-13500)
D6-21140 Hypokalemia, excessive renal losses 276.8
(C-13500)
D6-21150 Hypokalemia, gastrointestinal losses 276.8
(C-13500)
D6-21160 Hypokalemia, ECF to ICF shifts 276.8
(C-13500)
D6-21200 Hyperkalemia 276.7
(C-13500)
Potassium excess 276.7
(C-13500)

6-20-21 FLUID AND ELECTROLYTE DISORDERS — Continued

D6-21200 (cont.) Hyperkalemic syndrome 276.7
(C-13500)
K overload 276.7
(C-13500)
K excess 276.7
(C-13500)
Hyperpotassemia 276.7
(C-13500)

D6-21204 Potassium intoxication 276.7
(C-13500)

D6-21210 Acute hyperkalemia 276.7
(C-13500)

D6-21220 Chronic hyperkalemia 276.7
(C-13500)

D6-21230 Hyperkalemia, diminished renal excretion 276.7
(C-13500)

D6-21240 Hyperkalemia, transcellular shifts 276.7
(C-13500)

D6-21300 Chloride disorder, NOS 276.9
(C-11220)

D6-21310 Hypochloremia 276.9

D6-21320 Hyperchloremia 276.9

D6-21480 Electrolyte and fluid disorder, NEC 276.9
(C-10010)
Electrolyte imbalance, NOS 276.9
(C-10010)

6-23-24 ACID-BASE BALANCE DISORDERS

D6-23000 Disorder of acid-base balance, NOS 276.9
(F-602A0)
Disturbance of acid-base balance, NOS 276.9
(F-602A0)

D6-23100 Acidosis, NOS 276.2
(F-602A0)

D6-23110 Compensated acidosis, NOS 276.2
(F-602A0)

D6-23200 Metabolic acidosis, NOS 276.2
(F-602A0)

D6-23210 Compensated metabolic acidosis 276.2
(F-602A0)

D6-23220 Metabolic acidosis, normal anion gap (NAG), NOS 276.2
(F-602A0)

D6-23230 Metabolic acidosis, NAG, bicarbonate losses 276.2
(F-602A0)

D6-23240 Metabolic acidosis, NAG, failure of bicarbonate regeneration 276.2
(F-602A0)

D6-23250 Metabolic acidosis, NAG, acidifying salts 276.2
(F-602A0)
Hyperchloremic acidosis 276.2
(F-602A0)

D6-23260 Metabolic acidosis, increased anion gap (IAG), NOS 276.2
(F-602A0)

D6-23270 Metabolic acidosis, IAG, reduced excretion of inorganic acids 276.2
(F-602A0)

D6-23280 Metabolic acidosis, IAG, accumulation of organic acids 276.2
(F-602A0)

D6-23300 Lactic acidosis 276.2
(F-602A0) (F-61750)

D6-23400 Ketoacidosis, NOS 276.2
(F-602A0) (F-64040)

D6-23402 Alcoholic ketoacidosis 276.2
(F-602A0) (F-64040)

D6-23404 Starvation ketoacidosis 276.2
(F-602A0) (F-64040)

D6-23500 Metabolic acidosis due to ingestion of drugs or chemicals 276.2
(F-602A0) (C-10030) (C-50000)

D6-23501 Metabolic acidosis due to salicylate 276.2
(F-602A0) (C-60311)

D6-23502 Metabolic acidosis due to paraldehyde 276.2
(F-602A0) (C-64304)

D6-23503 Metabolic acidosis due to methanol 276.2
(F-602A0) (C-21002)

D6-23504 Metabolic acidosis due to ethylene glycol 176.2
(F-602A0) (C-21301)

D6-23600 Respiratory acidosis, NOS 276.2
(F-602A0)

D6-23610 Compensated respiratory acidosis 276.2
(F-602A0)

D6-23620 Acute respiratory acidosis 276.2
(F-602A0)

D6-23630 Chronic respiratory acidosis 276.2
(F-602A0)

D6-24000 Alkalosis, NOS 276.3
(F-602A0)

D6-24010 Compensated alkalosis, NOS 276.3
(F-602A0)

D6-24020 Altitude alkalosis 276.3
(F-602A0)

D6-24100 Metabolic alkalosis 276.3
(F-602A0)

D6-24110 Compensated metabolic alkalosis 276.3
(F-602A0)

D6-24120 Hypokalemic alkalosis 276.3
(F-602A0)

D6-24200 Respiratory alkalosis, NOS 276.3
(F-602A0)

D6-24210 Compensated respiratory alkalosis 276.3
(F-602A0)

D6-24220 Acute respiratory alkalosis 276.3
(F-602A0)
Acute hyperventilation syndrome 276.3
(F-602A0)

D6-24220 (cont.) Acute hyperventilation 276.3
(F-602A0)

D6-24230 Chronic respiratory alkalosis 276.3
(F-602A0)
Chronic hyperventilation syndrome 275.3
(F-602A0)
Chronic hyperventilation 276.3
(F-602A0)

D6-24700 Mixed acid-base balance disorder 276.4
(F-602A0)

D6-24710 Hypercapnia with mixed acid-base disorder 276.4
(F-602A0)

D6-24720 Hypercapnia, NOS
Hypercapnemia, NOS
Hypercarbia, NOS

D6-24730 Hypocapnia, NOS
Hypocapnemia, NOS

SECTION 6-3 DISORDERS OF MINERAL METABOLISM

6-30 DISORDERS OF MINERAL METABOLISM: GENERAL TERMS

D6-30000 Disorder of mineral metabolism, NOS 275.9
(C-20100)

D6-30010 Mineral deficiency, NEC 275.8

D6-30500 Other disorder of mineral metabolism, NEC 275.8

6-31 DISORDERS OF IRON METABOLISM

D6-31000 Disorder of iron metabolism, NOS 275.0
(C-13000)

D6-31100 Iron deficiency, NOS 275.0

D6-31200 Iron overload, NOS 275.0
Iron excess 275.0
Increased storage iron 275.0

D6-31210 Hemochromatosis, NOS 275.0
Iron storage disease, NOS 275.0
Bronzed cirrhosis 275.0
Pigmentary cirrhosis of liver 275.0
von Recklinghausen-Appelbaum disease 275.0

D6-31212 Hereditary hemochromatosis 275.0
Primary hemochromatosis 275.0
Idiopathic hemochromatosis 275.0
Familial hemochromatosis

D6-31214 Neonatal hemochromatosis 275.0

D6-31215 Juvenile hemochromatosis 275.0

D6-31218 Precirrhotic hemochromatosis
Latent hemochromatosis

D6-31220 Secondary hemochromatosis, NOS 275.0

D6-31222 Erythropoietic hemochromatosis
Hemochromatosis secondary to erythropoietic disorder

D6-31230 African nutritional hemochromatosis
Bantu siderosis

D6-31250 Hemosiderosis, NOS 275.0

D6-31252 Transfusion hemosiderosis 275.0 —999.8*

D6-31253 Focal hemosiderosis 275.0

D6-31260 Idiopathic pulmonary hemosiderosis 275.0 —516.1*
(T-28000) (M-55700) (F-D5340) (G-C002) (M-37000)
Brown induration of lung 275.0 —516.1*
(T-28000) (M-55700) (F-D5340) (G-C002) (M-37000)

D6-31266 Hepatic hemosiderosis

D6-31268 Renal hemosiderosis 275.0

D6-31280 Secondary hemosiderosis, NOS 275.0

D6-31290 Shunt hemosiderosis 275.0

6-32 DISORDERS OF COPPER METABOLISM

D6-32000 Disorder of copper metabolism, NOS 275.1
(C-12700)

D6-32100 Hypocupremia, NOS 275.1
Chronic copper deficiency 275.1

D6-32102V Nutritional myelopathy of pigs

D6-32110 Menkes kinky-hair syndrome 275.1
Congenital hypocupremia 275.1
X-linked copper deficiency 275.1
Copper transport disease 275.1
Steely-hair syndrome 275.1
Menkes disease 275.1
Trichopoliodystrophy 275.1

D6-32300 Hypercupremia, NOS 275.1

D6-32310 Wilson's disease 275.1
Hepatolenticular degeneration syndrome 275.1
Copper storage disease 275.1
Cerebral pseudosclerosis 275.1
Westphal-Strümpell syndrome 275.1

D6-32330 Familial hypoceruloplasminemia 275.1

D6-32350 Indian childhood cirrhosis 275.1

D6-32380V Swayback
(D6-10100) (C-12700)
Enzootic ataxia
(D6-10100) (C-12700)

6-33 DISORDERS OF MAGNESIUM METABOLISM

D6-33000 Disorder of magnesium metabolism, NOS 275.2
(C-14800)

D6-33010 Hypomagnesemia 275.2
Magnesium deficiency syndrome 275.2

D6-33012 Neonatal hypomagnesemia 275.2

D6-33050 Hypermagnesemia 275.2

6-34 DISORDERS OF PHOSPHORUS AND CALCIUM METABOLISM

D6-34100 Disorder of phosphorus metabolism, NOS 275.3
(C-10600)

6-34 DISORDERS OF PHOSPHORUS AND CALCIUM METABOLISM — Continued

D6-34110 Hypophosphatemia, NOS 275.3
D6-34130 Familial x-linked hypophosphatemic vitamin D refractory rickets 275.3
Familial hypophosphatemia 275.3
Familial hypophosphatemic rickets 275.3
Familial hypophosphatemic osteomalacia 275.3
Vitamin D-resistant rickets 275.3
Vitamin D-resistant osteomalacia 275.3
VDRR 275.3
XLH 275.3
D6-34180 Autosomal recessive hypophosphatemic vitamin D refractory rickets 275.3
Autosomal hypophosphatemic bone disease 275.3
D6-34600 Disorder of calcium metabolism, NOS 275.4
(C-14300)
D6-34610 Hypocalcemia 275.4
Hypocalcemia syndrome 275.4
D6-34700 Hypercalcemia 275.4
Hypercalcemia syndrome 275.4
D6-34710 Idiopathic hypercalcemia of infancy 275.4
D6-34720 Hypercalciuria 275.4
D6-34730 Calcinosis 275.4
D6-34732 Nephrocalcinosis 275.4
D6-34750 Pseudogout, NOS 275.4 —712.3*
Chondrocalcinosis articularis 275.4 —712.3*
Idiopathic articular chondrocalcinosis 275.4 —712.3*
Chondrocalcinosis due to pyrophosphate crystals 275.4 —712.2*
Calcium pyrophosphate deposition disease 275.4 —712.2*
CPDD 275.4 —712.2*
Chondrocalcinosis 275.4 —712.2*
D6-34752 Chondrocalcinosis due to calcium hydroxyapatite crystals 275.4 —712.1*
Hydroxyapatite arthropathy 275.4 —712.1*

6-38 DISORDERS OF TRACE MINERAL METABOLISM

D6-38000 Disorder of trace mineral metabolism, NOS 275.8
D6-38100 Disorder of zinc metabolism, NOS 275.8
(C-14100)
D6-38110 Acute zinc deficiency 275.8
D6-38120 Chronic zinc deficiency 275.8
D6-38130 Hereditary acrodermatitis enterohepatica 275.8
Primary zinc malabsorption syndrome 275.8
Brandt syndrome 275.8
Danbolt-Closs syndrome 275.8
D6-38140 Acquired acrodermatitis enterohepatica
D6-38200 Disorder of manganese metabolism, NOS 275.8
(C-14900)
D6-38210 Manganese deficiency 275.8
D6-38220V Perosis
(D6-10100) (C-14900)
Chondrodystrophy due to manganese deficiency
(D6-10100) (C-14900)
Slipped tendon
(D6-10100) (C-14900)
D6-38300 Disorder of chromium metabolism, NOS 275.8
(C-12900)
D6-38310 Chromium deficiency 275.8
D6-38400 Disorder of selenium metabolism, NOS 275.8
(C-11600)
D6-38410 Selenium deficiency 275.8
D6-38420 Keshan disease 275.8
Congestive cardiomyopathy due to selenium deficiency 275.8
D6-38440V Dietary deficiency of selenium and vitamin E, NOS
(C-11600) (C-A5100)
D6-38442V Nutritional muscular degeneration
Nutritional muscular dystrophy
D6-38444V Nutritional myopathy of lambs and calves
White muscle disease
Stiff lamb disease
Enzootic muscular dystrophy
D6-38446V Dietetic microangiopathy
D6-38448V Mulberry heart disease
D6-38500V Hepatosis dietetica
Toxic liver dystrophy of swine
Dietary hepatic necrosis

SECTION 6-4 DISORDERS OF PURINE AND PYRIMIDINE METABOLISM

6-40 DISORDERS OF PURINE METABOLISM

D6-40000 Disorder of purine metabolism, NOS 277.2
(F-65500)
D6-40200 Gout, NOS 274.9
(F-65500)
D6-40210 Acute gouty arthritis 274.0 —712.0*
(T-15000)
Acute gouty arthropathy 274.0 —712.0*
(T-15000)
D6-40212 Interval gout
(T-15000)
Intercritical gout
(T-15000)
D6-40220 Chronic gouty arthritis 274.10 —583.8*
(T-15000)
D6-40230 Chronic tophaceous gout
D6-40232 Gouty tophi of ear 274.81 —380.8*
(T-A0000)

D6-40236 Gouty tophi of heart 274.82 —425.7*
(T-32000)

D6-40240 Gouty iritis 274.89 —364.11*
(T-AA500)

D6-40250 Gouty neuritis 274.89 —357.4*
(T-A9001)

D6-40260 Primary gout

D6-40270 Familial juvenile gout
Familial gout nephropathy
Precocious adolescent gout

D6-40280 Gout with other manifestation, NEC 274.89

D6-40290V Visceral gout

D6-40400 Hypoxanthine-guanine phosphoribosyltransferase deficiency, NOS 277.2
(M-27000) (F-68BB0)
HGPRT deficiency
(M-27000) (F-68BB0)

D6-40410 Lesch-Nyhan syndrome 277.2
(M-27000) (F-68BB0)
Complete HGPRT deficiency 277.2
(M-27000) (F-68BB0)
Choreoathetosis self-mutilation syndrome 277.2
(M-27000) (F-68BB0)
Total HGPRT deficiency 277.2
(M-27000) (F-68BB0)

D6-40420 X-linked hyperuricemia 277.2
(M-27000) (F-68BB0)
Partial HGPRT deficiency 277.2
(M-27000) (F-68BB0)

D6-40500 Hereditary xanthinuria, NOS
(M-27000) (F-667F8)

D6-40510 Isolated xanthine oxidase deficiency 277.2
(M-27000) (F-667F8)
Hereditary xanthinuria, type I 277.2
(M-27000) (F-667F8)
Classical xanthinuria 277.2
(M-27000) (F-667F8)

D6-40520 Combined molybdoflavoprotein enzyme deficiency 277.2
(M-27000) (F-667F8) (F-66FF0)
Deficiency of molybdenum cofactor 277.2
(M-27000) (F-667F8) (F-66FF0)
Hereditary xanthinuria, type 2 277.2
(M-27000) (F-667F8) (F-66FF0)
Xanthine oxidase-sulfite oxidase deficiency 277.2
(M-27000) (F-667F8) (F-66FF0)

D6-40600 Adenine phosphoribosyltransferase deficiency 277.2
(M-27000) (F-68BA8)
APRT deficiency 277.2
(M-27000) (F-68BA8)
2,8-Dihydroxyadenine urolithiasis 277.2
(M-27000) (F-68BA8)

D6-40604 APRT deficiency, Japanese type 277.2

D6-40660 Ribose-phosphate pyrophosphokinase overactivity 277.2
(F-69460)
Phosphoribosyl pyrophosphate synthetase overactivity 277.2
(F-69460)
PRPPS overactivity 277.2
(F-69460)
PRPS overactivity 277.2
(F-69460)

D6-40700 Muscle AMP deaminase deficiency 277.2
(M-27000) (F-6B3C0)
Myoadenylate deaminase deficiency 277.2
(M-27000) (F-6B3C0)
Myoadenylate deaminase deficiency myopathy 277.2
(M-27000) (F-6B3C0)
Muscle adenylate deaminase deficiency 277.2
(M-27000) (F-6B3C0)

D6-40800 Adenosine deaminase deficiency 277.2
(M-27000) (F-6B3B0)
ADA deficiency 277.2
(M-27000) (F-6B3B0)
Adenosine aminohydrolase deficiency 277.2
(M-27000) (F-6B3B0)

D6-40900 Purine-nucleoside phosphorylase deficiency 277.2
(M-27000) (F-68B78)
PNP deficiency 277.2
(M-27000) (F-68B78)
NP deficiency 277.2
(M-27000) (F-68B78)
Nucleoside phophorylase deficiency 277.2
(M-27000) (F-68B78)

D6-40A00 Adenylosuccinate lyase deficiency
(M-27000) (F-6C860)
Adenylosuccinate deficiency
(M-27000) (F-6C860)
Succinyladenosinuria
(M-27000) (F-6C860)
Succinylpurinemic autism
(M-27000) (F-6C860)

6-44 DISORDERS OF PYRIMIDINE METABOLISM

D6-44000 Disorder of pyrimidine metabolism, NOS 277.2
(F-65510)

D6-44100 Orotic aciduria, NOS
(T-7A100) (F-61370)

D6-44110 Secondary orotic aciduria 281.4
(T-7A100) (F-61370)

D6-44200 Hereditary orotic aciduria, NOS 281.4

D6-44210 Hereditary orotic aciduria, type 1 281.4
(M-27000) (F-68BC0) (F-6C1B0)
UMP synthase deficiency 281.4
(M-27000) (F-68BC0) (F-6C1B0)

6-44 DISORDERS OF PYRIMIDINE METABOLISM — Continued

D6-44210 (cont.) OPRT and OMP decarboxylase deficiency 281.4
(M-27000) (F-68BC0) (F-6C1B0)
Orotidylic pyrophosphorylase orotidylic decarboxylase deficiency 281.4
(M-27000) (F-68BC0) (F-6C1B0)

D6-44220 Hereditary orotic aciduria, type 2 281.4
(M-27000) (F-6C1B0)
OMP decarboxylase deficiency 281.4
(M-27000) (F-6C1B0)
Orotidine-5'-phosphate decarboxylase deficiency 281.4
(M-27000) (F-6C1B0)

D6-44230 Dihydrouracil dehydrogenase ($NADP^+$) deficiency
(M-27000) (F-66A98)
Dihydropyrimidine dehydrogenase deficiency
(M-27000) (F-66A98)
Dihydrothymine dehydrogenase deficiency
(M-27000) (F-66A98)
DPD deficiency
(M-27000) (F-66A98)
Familial pyrimidinemia
(M-27000) (F-66A98)
Hereditary thymine-uraciluria
(M-27000) (F-66A78)
Sensitivity to fluorouracil toxicity
(M-27000) (F-66A98)

D6-44300 beta-Aminoisobutyricaciduria 277.2
(T-7A100) (F-64140)

D6-44500 Deficiency of DNA repair, NOS

D6-44510 Xeroderma pigmentosum, NOS 757.33
(T-01000)
Angioma pigmentosum atrophicum 757.33
(T-01000)
Atrophoderma pigmentosum 757.33
(T-01000)
Kaposi dermatosis 757.33
(T-01000)
Melanosis lenticularis progressiva 757.33
(T-01000)
Pigmented epitheliomatosis 757.33
(T-01000)
Xeroderma of Kaposi 757.33
(T-01000)

D6-44511 Xeroderma pigmentosum, group A 757.33
(T-01000)

D6-44512 Xeroderma pigmentosum, group B 757.33
(T-01000)

D6-44513 Xeroderma pigmentosum, group C 757.33
(T-01000)

D6-44514 Xeroderma pigmentosum, group D 757.33
(T-01000)

D6-44515 Xeroderma pigmentosum, group E 757.33
(T-01000)

D6-44516 Xeroderma pigmentosum, group F 757.33
(T-01000)

D6-44517 Xeroderma pigmentosum, group G 757.33
(T-01000)

D6-4451C Xeroderma pigmentosum, variant form 757.33
(T-01000)

D6-44520 Neurologic xeroderma pigmentosum, NOS 757.33
(T-01000)

D6-44530 Non-neurologic xeroderma pigmentosum, NOS 757.33
(T-01000)

SECTION 6-5 DISORDERS OF CARBOHYDRATE METABOLISM AND TRANSPORT

6-50 DISORDERS OF CARBOHYDRATE METABOLISM

D6-50000 Disorder of carbohydrate metabolism, NOS 271.9
(F-61900)

D6-50200 Glycogen storage disease, NOS 271.0
(F-61C00)
Glycogenosis, NOS 271.0
(F-61C00)

D6-50300 Glycogen storage disease, hepatic form, NOS 271.0
(F-61C00)

D6-50310 Glycogen storage disease, type I 271.0
(F-61C00) (M-27000) (F-6A338)
Hepatorenal glycogen storage disease 271.0
(F-61C00) (M-27000) (F-6A338)
Glucose-6-phosphatase deficiency 271.0
(F-61C00) (M-27000) (F-6A338)
von Gierke's disease 271.0
(F-61C00) (M-27000) (F-6A338)
GSD I 271.0
(F-61C00) (M-27000) (F-6A338)

D6-50314 Glucose-6-phosphate transport defect 271.0
(F-6A338)

D6-50320 Glycogen storage disease, type III 271.0
(F-61C00) (M-27000) (F-6A7E0)
Cori's disease 271.0
(F-61C00) (M-27000) (F-6A7E0)
Amylo-1,6-glucosidase deficiency 271.0
(F-61C00) (M-27000) (F-6A7E0)
Debrancher deficiency glycogen storage disease 271.0
(F-61C00) (M-27000) (F-6A7E0)
Limit dextrinosis 271.0
(F-61C00) (M-27000) (F-6A7E0)
GSD III 271.0
(F-61C00) (M-27000) (F-6A7E0)

D6-50330 Glycogen storage disease, type IV 271.0
(F-61C00) (M-27000) (F-687D0)
1,4,alpha-glucan 6-alpha-glucosyltransferase deficiency 271.0
(F-61C00) (M-27000) (F-687D0)

D6-50330 (cont.) Brancher deficiency glycogen storage disease 271.0
(F-61C00) (M-27000) (F-687D0)
Amylopectinosis 271.0
(F-61C00) (M-27000) (F-687D0)
Andersen's disease 271.0
(F-61C00) (M-27000) (F-687D0)
Branching-transferase deficiency glycogenosis
(F-61C00) (M-27000) (F-687D0)
GSD IV 271.0
(F-61C00) (M-27000) (F-687D0)

D6-50340 Glycogen storage disease, type VI 271.0
(F-61C00) (M-27000) (F-68728)
Hepatic phosphorylase deficiency 271.0
(F-61C00) (M-27000) (F-68728)
Hers disease 271.0
(F-61C00) (M-27000) (F-68728)
GSD VI 271.0
(F-61C00) (M-27000) (F-68728)
Hepatic glycogen phosphorylase deficiency 271.0
(F-61C00) (M-27000) (F-68728)

D6-50344 Glycogen storage disease, type IX 271.0
(F-61C00) (M-27000) (F-690E0)
Hepatic glycogen phophorylase kinase deficiency 271.0
(F-61C00) (M-27000) (F-690E0)
GSD IX 271.0
(F-61C00) (M-27000) (F-690E0)

D6-50346 Glycogen storage disease type VIII
(F-61C00) (F-68728)
Glycogenosis due to inactive phosphorylase
(F-61C00) (F-68728)
GSD VIII
(F-61C00) (F-68728)
Glycogenosis due to inactive hepatic glycogen phosphorylase
(F-61C00) (F-68728)

D6-50400 Glycogen storage disease, muscular form, NOS 271.0
(F-61C00) (F-6A788)

D6-50410 Glycogen storage disease, type II 271.0
(F-61C00) (M-27000) (F-6A788)
alpha-1,4-Glucosidase deficiency 271.0
(F-61C00) (M-27000) (F-6A788)
Acid maltase deficiency 271.0
(F-61C00) (M-27000) (F-6A788)
Generalized glycogen storage disease of infants 271.0
(F-61C00) (M-27000) (F-6A788)
Pompe's disease 271.0
(F-61C00) (M-27000) (F-6A788)
alpha-Glucosidase deficiency 271.0
(F-61C00) (M-27000) (F-6A788)
Glycogen heart disease 271.0
(F-61C00) (M-27000) (F-6A788)

D6-50420 Glycogen storage disease, type V 271.0
(F-61C00) (M-27000) (F-68728)
Myophosphorylase deficiency glycogenosis 271.0
(F-61C00) (M-27000) (F-68728)
McArdle's disease 271.0
(F-61C00) (M-27000) (F-68728)
GSD V 271.0
(F-61C00) (M-27000) (F-68728)
Muscle glycogen phosphorylase deficiency 271.0
(F-61C00) (M-27000) (F-68728)

D6-50430 Glycogen storage disease, type VII 271.0
(F-61C00) (M-27000) (F-69008)
Muscle phosphofructokinase deficiency 271.0
(F-61C00) (M-27000) (F-69008)
Tarui's disease 271.0
(F-61C00) (M-27000) (F-69008)
GSD VII 271.0
(F-61C00) (M-27000) (F-69008)

D6-50440 Glycogen storage disease type X 271.0
(F-61C00) (F-68728) (F-690E0)
Glycogenosis due to inactive phosphorylase and kinase 271.0
(F-61C00) (F-68728) (F-690E0)
GSD X 271.0
(F-61C00) (F-68728) (F-690E0)

D6-50450 Glycogenosis with glucoaminophosphaturia
(F-61C00)
Fanconi-Bickel syndrome
(F-61C00)
Hepatic glycogenosis with de Toni-Debré-Fanconi syndrome
(F-61C00)
Pseudo-phlorizin diabetes
(F-61C00)
Renal glucose-losing syndrome
(F-61C00)

D6-50500 Galactosemia, NOS 271.1
(F-61A00)

D6-50510 Classical galactosemia 271.1
(F-61A00) (M-27000) (F-694D0)
Galactose-1-phosphate uridyltransferase deficiency 271.1
(F-61A00) (M-27000) (F-694D0)
Transferase deficiency galactosemia 271.1
(F-61A00) (M-27000) (F-694D0)
UTP-hexose-1-phosphate uridyltransferase deficiency 271.1
(F-61A00) (M-27000) (F-694D0)
GALT 271.1
(F-61A00) (M-27000) (F-694D0)

D6-50512 Classical galactosemia, homozygous Duarte-type 371.1
(F-61A00) (M-27000) (F-694D0)

D6-50513 Classical galactosemia, homozygous Negro-type 271.1
(F-61A00) (M-27000) (F-694D0)

6-50 DISORDERS OF CARBOHYDRATE METABOLISM — Continued

D6-50515 Classical galactosemia, heterozygous type 271.1
(F-61A00) (M-27000) (F-694D0)

D6-50520 Galactokinase deficiency galactosemia 271.1
(F-61A00) (M-27000) (F-68FE8)
Galactosemia II 271.1
(F-61A00) (M-27000) (F-68FE8)
GALK 271.1
(F-61A00) (M-27000) (F-68FE8)

D6-50530 UDPglucose-4-epimerase deficiency 271.1
(F-61A00) (M-27000) (F-6D1B0)
Galactose epimerase deficiency 271.1
(F-61A00) (M-27000) (F-6D1B0)
UDPgalactose-4-epimerase deficiency 271.1
(F-61A00) (M-27000) (F-6D1B0)
Uridine diphosphate galactose-4 epimerase deficiency 271.1
(F-61A00) (M-27000) (F-6D1B0)
GALE 271.1
(F-61A00) (M-27000) (F-6D1B0)
Galactosemia III 271.1
(F-61A00) (M-27000) (F-6D1B0)

D6-50580 Galactosuria 271.1
(T-7A100) (F-61A00)

D6-50600 Fructose disorder, NOS 271.2
(F-61950)

D6-50601 Fructosemia 271.2
(T-0A000) (F-61950)
Fructose intolerance, NOS 271.2
(T-0A000) (F-61950)

D6-50602 Fructosuria 271.2
(T-7A100) (F-61950)

D6-50610 Essential benign fructosuria 271.2
(F-61950) (M-27000) (F-68FD8)
Essential fructosuria 271.2
(F-61950) (M-27000) (F-68FD8)
Hepatic fructokinase deficiency 271.2
(F-61950) (M-27000) (F-68FD8)
Fructokinase deficiency 271.2
(F-61950) (M-27000) (F-68FD8)
Benign fructosemia 271.2
(F-61950) (M-27000) (F-68FD8)
Essential fructosemia 271.2
(F-61950) (M-27000) (F-68FD8)

D6-50620 Hereditary fructosuria 271.2
(F-61950) (M-27000) (F-6C348)
Hereditary fructose intolerance 271.2
(F-61950) (M-27000) (F-6C348)
Fructose-1-phosphate aldolase deficiency 271.2
(F-61950) (M-27000) (F-6C348)
Fructose-biphosphate aldolase B deficiency 271.2
(F-61950) (M-27000) (F-6C348)
ALDB deficiency 271.2
(F-61950) (M-27000) (F-6C348)
Aldolase B deficiency 271.2
(F-61950) (M-27000) (F-6C348)

D6-50630 Fructose-biphosphatase deficiency 271.2
(F-61950) (M-27000) (F-6A348)
Fructose-1,6-diphosphatase deficiency 271.2
(F-61950) (M-27000) (F-6A348)
Hereditary fructose-1,6-phosphatase deficiency 271.2
(F-61950) (M-27000) (F-6A348)

D6-50700 Pentose disorder, NOS 271.8
(F-61B20)

D6-50710 Essential benign pentosuria 271.8
(M-27000) (F-66158)
Pentosuria 271.8
(M-27000) (F-66158)
Xylitol dehydrogenase deficiency 271.8
(M-27000) (F-66158)
L-xylulose reductase deficiency 271.8
(M-27000) (F-66158)
L-xylulosuria 271.8
(M-27000) (F-66158)

D6-50720 Xylosuria, NOS 271.8

D6-50800 Primary hyperoxaluria, NOS 271.8
Primary oxalosis, NOS 271.8

D6-50810 Primary hyperoxaluria, type I 271.8
(M-27000) (F-68F00)
Glycolic aciduria 271.8
(M-27000) (F-68F00)
Alanine-glyoxylate aminotransferase deficiency 271.8
(M-27000) (F-68F00)
PH I 271.8
(M-27000) (F-68F00)

D6-50820 Primary hyperoxaluria, type II 271.8
(M-27000) (F-661F0) (F-661D8)
Glyoxylate reductase deficiency 271.8
(M-27000) (F-661F0) (F-661D8)
Glyceric dehydrogenase deficiency 271.8
(M-27000) (F-661F0) (F-661D8)
L-glyceric aciduria 271.8
(M-27000) (F-661F0) (F-661D8)
Glycerate dehydrogenase deficiency 271.8
(M-27000) (F-661F0) (F-661D8)

D6-50870 Secondary hyperoxaluria 271.8
Acquired hyperoxaluria 271.8
Acquired hyperoxaluric state 271.8
Secondary hyperoxaluric state 271.8

D6-50872 Enteric hyperoxaluria 271.8

D6-50874 Antifreeze oxalosis 271.8
(C-21301)

D6-50900 Pancreatic alpha-amylase deficiency
(M-27000) (F-6A720)

D6-50910 Muscle phosphoglycerate mutase deficiency
(M-27000) (F-6D3A0)
Phosphoglucomutase deficiency
(M-27000) (F-6D3A0)

D6-50920 Muscle D-lactate dehydrogenase deficiency
(M-27000) (F-661E8)
Lactic acid dehydrogenase deficiency
(M-27000) (F-661E8)

D6-50930 Muscle L-lactate dehydrogenase deficiency
(M-27000) (F-661E0)

6-54 DISORDERS OF CARBOHYDRATE TRANSPORT

D6-54000 Disorder of carbohydrate transport, NOS 271.9
(F-61900)

D6-54100 Syndrome of carbohydrate intolerance, NOS 271.3
(F-61900)

D6-54110 Acquired monosaccharide malabsorption
(F-61910)
Secondary monosaccharide malabsorption
(F-61910)

D6-54190 Nonglucosuric melituria 271.8
(F-61910)
Non glucose melituria 271.8
(F-61910)

D6-54200 Intestinal disaccharidase deficiency, NOS 271.3
(F-61B80)
Disaccharide malabsorption, NOS 271.3
(F-61B80)

D6-54202 Disacchariduria, NOS 271.3
(F-61B80)

D6-54210 Congenital lactase deficiency 271.3
(F-61990) (M-27000) (F-6AA20)
Congenital lactose intolerance 271.3
(F-61990) (M-27000) (F-6AA20)
Congenital lactose malabsorption 271.3
(F-61990) (M-27000) (F-6AA20)
Congenital alactasia syndrome
(F-61990) (M-27000) (F-6AA20)
Disaccharide intolerance II 271.3
(F-61990) (M-27000) (F-6AA20)

D6-54214 Hereditary gastrogenic lactose intolerance
(F-61990) (M-27000) (F-6AA20)
Severe familial lactose intolerance
(F-61990) (M-27000) (F-6AA20)

D6-54220 Nonpersistence of intestinal lactase 271.3
(F-61990) (M-27000) (F-6AA20)
Delayed-onset isolated lactase deficiency 271.3
(F-61990) (M-27000) (F-6AA20)
Primary hypolactasia 271.3
(F-61990) (M-27000) (F-6AA20)
Disaccharide intolerance III 271.3
(F-61990) (M-27000) (F-6AA20)
Late-onset lactose intolerance 271.3
(F-61990) (M-27000) (F-6AA20)

D6-54230 Lactose intolerance in children without lactase deficiency 271.3
(F-61990)

D6-54240 Acquired lactase deficiency
(F-6AA20)
Acquired lactose intolerance
(F-6AA20)
Secondary lactase deficiency
(F-6AA20)
Secondary lactose intolerance
(F-6AA20)

D6-54250 Lactase deficiency in diseases other than of the small intestine 271.3
(F-6AA20)

D6-54300 Sucrase-isomaltase deficiency 271.3
(M-27000) (F-6A758)
Congenital sucrose intolerance 271.3
(M-27000) (F-6A758)
Congenital sucrose malabsorption 271.3
(M-27000) (F-6A758)
Intestinal sucrase-a-dextrinase deficiency 271.3
(M-27000) (F-6A758)
Invertase deficiency 271.3
(M-27000) (F-6A758)
Disaccharide intolerance I 271.3
(M-27000) (F-6A758)

D6-54320 Congenital glucose-galactose malabsorption 271.3
(F-61920) (F-61A00)
Congenital glucose-galactose intolerance 271.3
(F-61920) (F-61A00)

D6-54340 alpha, alpha-Trehalase deficiency 271.3
(M-27000) (F-6A7C0)
Trehalose intolerance 271.3
(M-27000) (F-6A7C0)

D6-54400 Renal glucosuria, NOS 271.4
(F-61920)
Renal glycosuria, NOS 271.4
(F-61920)
Familial renal glucosuria 271.4
(F-61920)

D6-54410 Renal glucosuria, type A 271.4
(F-61920)

D6-54420 Renal glucosuria, type B 271.4
(F-61920)

D6-54430 Renal glucosuria, type O
(F-61920)

D6-54500 Other disorder of carbohydrate metabolism or transport, NEC 271.8
(F-61900)

6-58 DISORDERS OF PYRUVATE METABOLISM

D6-58000 Inborn error of pyruvate metabolism, NOS 277.8
(F-61040)

D6-58100 Pyruvate dehydrogenase complex deficiency 277.8
(F-61040)
PDH deficiency 277.8
(F-61040)

6-58 DISORDERS OF PYRUVATE METABOLISM — Continued

D6-58100 (cont.) Ataxia with lactic acidosis I 277.8
(F-61040)

D6-58110 Pyruvate carboxylase deficiency 277.8
(M-27000) (F-6E3B0)
PC deficiency 277.8
(M-27000) (F-6E3B0)
Ataxia with lactic acidosis II 277.8
(M-27000) (F-6E3B0)

D6-58130 Dihydrolipoamide dehydrogenase deficiency
(M-27000) (F-66FE0)
Maple syrup urine disease with lactic acidosis
(M-27000) (F-66FE0)
Congenital infantile lactic acidosis due to LAD deficiency
(M-27000) (F-66FE0)

D6-58150 Phosphoenolpyruvate carboxykinase (GTP) deficiency
(M-27000) (F-6C1E8)

SECTION 6-6 DISORDERS OF LIPOPROTEIN AND LIPID METABOLISM

D6-60000 Disorder of lipoprotein and lipid metabolism, NOS 272.9
(F-63500) (F-63600)

D6-60010 Hyperlipidemia, NOS 272.4
(F-63600)

D6-60020 Hyperlipoproteinemia, NOS 272.4
(F-63500)

D6-60030 Hypercholesterolemia, NOS 272.4
(F-63980)

D6-60100 Inborn error of lipoprotein metabolism, NOS 272.9
(F-63500)

D6-60200 Familial lipoprotein deficiency, NOS 272.5
(M-27000) (F-63500)

D6-60210 Abetalipoproteinemia 272.5
(M-27000) (F-63560)
Bassen-Kornzweig disease 272.5
(M-27000) (F-63560)
Abetalipoproteinemia neuropathy 272.5
(M-27000) (F-63560)
Acanthocytosis 272.5
(M-27000) (F-63560)
Apolipoprotein B deficiency 272.5
(M-27000) (F-63560)

D6-60220 Familial hypobetalipoproteinemia 272.5
(F-63560)

D6-60230 Familial hypoalphalipoproteinemia 272.5
(F-63570)
Tangier disease 272.5
(F-63570)
Familial HDL deficiency 272.5
(F-63570)
Familial high density lipoprotein deficiency 272.5
(F-63570)
Alphalipoproteinemia neuropathy 272.5
(F-63570)
Cholesterol thesaurismosis 272.5
(F-63570)

D6-60400 Familial lipoprotein lipase deficiency 272.3
(M-27000) (F-6A1F8)
Familial LPL deficiency 272.3
(M-27000) (F-6A1F8)
Primary hyperchylomicronemia 272.3
(M-27000) (F-6A1F8)
Familial hyperlipoproteinemia, type I 272.3
(M-27000) (F-6A1F8)
Burger-Grutz syndrome 272.3
(M-27000) (F-6A1F8)
Endogenous hypertriglyceridemia 272.3
(M-27000) (F-6A1F8)
Familial fat-induced hypertriglyceridemia 272.3
(M-27000) (F-6A1F8)
Familial hyperchylomicronemia 272.3
(M-27000) (F-6A1F8)
Hepatosplenomegalic lipoidosis 272.3
(M-27000) (F-6A1F8)
Hypercholesterinemic xanthomatosis 272.3
(M-27000) (F-6A1F8)

D6-60420 Familial apolipoprotein C-II deficiency 272.3
(F-63530)
Apo-c-II deficiency 272.3
(F-63530)
Anapolipoproteinemia 272.3
(F-63530)

D6-60430 Familial hypercholesterolemia 272.0
(F-63980)
Essential familial hypercholesterolemia 272.0
(F-63980)
Low density lipoprotein catabolic defect 272.0
(F-63980)
Familial hyperbetalipoproteinemia 272.0
(F-63980)
LDL receptor disorder 272.0
(F-63980)

D6-60450 Familial combined hyperlipidemia 272.4
Familial multiple lipoprotein-type hyperlipidemia 272.4
Multiple-type hyperlipidemia 272.4

D6-60460 Familial type 3 hyperlipoproteinemia 272.2
Familial dysbetalipoproteinemia 272.2
Remnant hyperlipoproteinemia 272.2
Xanthoma tuberosum 272.2
Tubo-eruptive xanthoma 272.2
Broad-beta disease 272.2
Floating beta disease 272.2

D6-60470 Familial hypertriglyceridemia 272.4

D6-60480 Familial type 5 hyperlipoproteinemia
D6-64000 Familial disease with storage of sterols (other than cholesterol), NOS 272.8
(F-63970)
D6-64010 Cholestanol storage disease 272.7
Cerebrotendinous xanthomatosis 272.7
Cerebral cholesterinosis 272.7
van Bogaert-Scherer-Epstein syndrome 272.7
D6-64020 Sitosterolemia with xanthomatosis 272.7
(F-63A30)
Sitosterolemic xanthomatosis 272.7
(F-63A30)
beta-Sitosterolemia 272.7
(F-63A30)
D6-64700 Hoffa's disease 272.8
Liposynovitis prepatellaris 272.8
D6-64800 Launois-Bensaude's lipomatosis 272.8
D6-64900 Lipoid dermatoarthritis 272.8
Multicentric reticulohistiocytosis 272.8
Nicolau-Balus syndrome 272.8

SECTION 6-7 DISORDERS OF LYSOSOMAL ENZYMES

D6-70000 Disorder of lysosomal enzyme, NOS
D6-70100 Mucopolysaccharidosis, NOS 277.5
D6-70110 Mucopolysaccharidosis, MPS-I 277.5
(M-27000) (F-6A928)
MPS I 277.5
(M-27000) (F-6A928)
L-iduronidase deficiency, NOS
(M-27000) (F-6A928)
D6-70112 Mucopolysaccharidosis, MPS-I-H 277.5
(M-27000) (F-6A928)
Hurler's syndrome 277.5
(M-27000) (F-6A928)
L-iduronidase deficiency, Hurler type 277.5
(M-27000) (F-6A928)
Gargoylism 277.5
(M-27000) (F-6A928)
Lipochondrodystrophy 277.5
(M-27000) (F-6A928)
Hurler-Pfaundler syndrome 277.5
(M-27000) (F-6A928)
Dysostosis multiplex syndrome 277.5
(M-27000) (F-6A928)
D6-70114 Mucopolysaccharidosis, MPS-I-S 277.5
(M-27000) (F-6A928)
Scheie's syndrome 277.5
(M-27000) (F-6A928)
L-iduronidase deficiency, Scheie type 277.5
(M-27000) (F-6A928)
D6-70116 Mucopolysaccharidosis, MPS-I-H/S 277.5
(M-27000) (F-6A928)
Hurler-Scheie syndrome 277.5
(M-27000) (F-6A928)
L-iduronidase deficiency, Hurler-Scheie type 277.5
(M-27000) (F-6A928)
D6-70220 Mucopolysaccharidosis, MPS-II 277.5
(M-27000) (F-6A5A8)
Hunter's syndrome 277.5
(M-27000) (F-6A5A8)
Sulfoiduronidate sulfatase deficiency 277.5
(M-27000) (F-6A5A8)
Iduronate 2-sulfatase deficiency
(M-27000) (F-6A5A8)
D6-70222 Hunter's syndrome, severe form 277.5
(M-27000) (F-6A5A8)
D6-70224 Hunter's syndrome, mild form 277.5
(M-27000) (F-6A5A8)
D6-70230 Sanfilippo syndrome, NOS
D6-70231 Mucopolysaccharidosis, MPS-III-A 277.5
(M-27000) (F-6B630)
Sanfilippo syndrome, type A 277.5
(M-27000) (F-6B630)
Heparan sulfate sulfatase deficiency 277.5
(M-27000) (F-6B630)
N-sulfoglucosamine sulfohydrolase deficiency 277.5
(M-27000) (F-6B630)
D6-70232 Mucopolysaccharidosis, MPS-III-B 277.5
(M-27000) (F-68AF8)
Sanfilippo syndrome, type B 277.5
(M-27000) (F-68AF8)
alpha-N-acetylglucosaminidase deficiency 277.5
(M-27000) (F-68AF8)
D6-70233 Mucopolysaccharidosis, MPS-III-C 277.5
(M-27000) (F-68678)
Sanfilippo syndrome, type C 277.5
(M-27000) (F-68678)
Acetyl-CoA: heparan-alpha-D-glucosaminide N-acetyltransferase deficiency 277.5
(M-27000) (F-68678)
Heparan-alpha-glucosaminide acetyltransferase deficiency 277.5
(M-27000) (F-68678)
D6-70234 Mucopolysaccharidosis, MPS-III-D 277.5
(M-27000) (F-6A5B0)
Sanfilippo syndrome, type D 277.5
(M-27000) (F-6A5B0)
N-acetylglucosamine-6-sulfatase deficiency 277.5
(M-27000) (F-6A5B0)
D6-70240 Morquio syndrome, NOS 277.5
(F-62820)
Brailsford-Morquio syndrome 277.5
(F-62820)
Familial osteochondrodystrophy 277.5
(F-62820)
Chondrodystrophia tarda 277.5
(F-62820)

SECTION 6-7 DISORDERS OF LYSOSOMAL ENZYMES — Continued

D6-70240 (cont.) Chondro-osteodystrophy 277.5
(F-62820)
Familial osseous dystrophy 277.5
(F-62820)
Hereditary enchondral dysostosis 277.5
(F-62820)
Keratan sulfaturia 277.5
(F-62820)
Morquio disease, NOS 277.5
(F-62820)
Morquio-Suarez syndrome 277.5
(F-62820)
Morquio-Ullrich disease 277.5
(F-62820)
Osteochondrodystrophia deformans 277.5
(F-62820)
Atypical chondrodystrophy 277.5
(F-62820)

D6-70242 Mucopolysaccharidosis, MPS-IV-A 277.5
(M-27000) (F-6A568)
Morquio's syndrome, classic form 277.5
(M-27000) (F-6A568)
N-acetylgalactosamine-6-sulfatase deficiency 277.5
(M-27000) (F-6A568)
Morquio A syndrome 277.5
(M-27000) (F-6A568)

D6-70244 Mucopolysaccharidosis, MPS-IV-B 277.5
(M-27000) (F-6A7A0)
Morquio-like syndrome 277.5
(M-27000) (F-6A7A0)
beta-Galactosidase deficiency 277.5
(M-27000) (F-6A7A0)
Morquio B syndrome 277.5
(M-27000) (F-6A7A0)

D6-70250 Maroteaux-Lamy syndrome, NOS 277.5
(M-27000) (F-6A5A0)
Mucopolysaccharidosis, MPS-VI 277.5
(M-27000) (F-6A5A0)
N-acetylgalactosamine-4-sulfatase deficiency 277.5
(M-27000) (F-6A5A0)
Polydystrophic dwarfism 277.5
(M-27000) (F-6A5A0)
Arylsulfatase B deficiency 277.5
(M-27000) (F-6A5A0)
Maroteaux-Lamy disease 277.5
(M-27000) (F-6A5A0)
ARSB deficiency 277.5
(M-27000) (F-6A5A0)
Mucopolysaccharidosis chondroitin sulfate B 277.5
(M-27000) (F-6A5A0)

D6-70252 Maroteaux-Lamy syndrome, severe form 277.5
(M-27000) (F-6A5A0)

D6-70254 Maroteaux-Lamy syndrome, intermediate form
(M-27000) (F-6A5A0)

D6-70256 Maroteaux-Lamy syndrome, mild form 277.5
(M-27000) (F-6A5A0)

D6-70260 Mucopolysaccharidosis, MPS-VII 277.5
(M-27000) (F-6A7D0)
Sly syndrome 277.5
(M-27000) (F-6A7D0)
beta-Glucuronidase deficiency 277.5
(M-27000) (F-6A7D0)
GUSB deficiency 277.5
(M-27000) (F-6A7D0)
GUS deficiency 277.5
(M-27000) (F-6A7D0)

D6-72000 Lipid storage disease, NOS 272.7
(F-63600)
Lipidosis, NOS 272.7
(F-63600)

D6-72010 Chemically-induced lipidosis 272.7
(F-63600)

D6-72100 Glycoprotein storage disorder, NOS 271.8
(F-625A0)

D6-72200 I-cell disease 272.7
(M-27000) (F-69688)
Mucolipidosis II 272.7
(M-27000) (F-69688)
N-acetylglucosamine-1-phosphotransferase deficiency 272.7
(M-27000) (F-69688)

D6-72220 Pseudo-Hurler polydystrophy
(M-27000) (F-69688)
Mucolipidosis III 272.7
(M-27000) (F-69688)
Pseudo-Hurler disease 272.7
(M-27000) (F-69688)

D6-72300 Fucosidosis, NOS 271.8
(M-27000) (F-6A868)
Fucosidase deficiency 271.8
(M-27000) (F-6A868)
alpha-L-fucosidase deficiency 271.8
(M-27000) (F-6A868)

D6-72302 Infantile fucosidosis 272.8
(M-27000) (F-6A868)
Fucosidosis, type I 271.8
(M-27000) (F-6A868)
Fucosidosis, fatal infantile type 271.8
(M-27000) (F-6A868)

D6-72304 Juvenile fucosidosis 271.8
(M-27000) (F-6A868)
Fucosidosis, type II 271.8
(M-27000) (F-6A868)
Fucosidosis, juvenile form 271.8
(M-27000) (F-6A868)
Adult fucosidosis 271.8
(M-27000) (F-6A868)
Childhood fucosidosis 271.8
(M-27000) (F-6A868)

D6-72400 Mannosidosis, NOS 271.8
(M-27000) (F-6A7A8)
alpha-Mannosidase deficiency 271.8
(M-27000) (F-6A7A8)

D6-72410 Mannosidosis, type I 271.8
(M-27000) (F-6A7A8)
Mannosidosis infantile onset 271.8
(M-27000) (F-6A7A8)
Mannosidosis, severe form 271.8
(M-27000) (F-6A7A8)

D6-72420 Mannosidosis, type II 271.8
(M-27000) (F-6A7A8)
Mannosidosis, juvenile-adult onset 271.8
(M-27000) (F-6A7A8)
Mannosidosis, mild form 271.8
(M-27000) (F-6A7A8)

D6-72500 Aspartylglucosaminuria 270.8
(M-27000) (F-6AA88)
Aspartylglycosaminuria 270.8
(M-27000) (F-6AA88)
Aspartylglucosaminidase deficiency 270.8
(M-27000) (F-6AA88)

D6-72550 alpha-1-Antitrypsin deficiency 277.6
(F-62110)
alpha-1-Proteinase inhibitor deficiency 277.6
(F-62110)

D6-72600 Sialidosis
(M-27000) (F-6A780)
Neuroaminidase deficiency
(M-27000) (F-6A780)
Mucolipidosis I
(M-27000) (F-6A780)
Sialidase deficiency
(M-27000) (F-6A780)

D6-72610 Normosomatic sialidosis
(M-27000) (F-6A780)
Sialidosis, type 1
(M-27000) (F-6A780)
Cherry-red-spot myoclonus syndrome
(M-27000) (F-6A780)

D6-72620 Dysmorphic sialidosis
(M-27000) (F-6A780)
Sialidosis, type 2
(M-27000) (F-6A780)

D6-72622 Dysmorphic sialidosis, juvenile form
(M-27000) (F-6A780)

D6-72623 Dysmorphic sialidosis, infantile form
(M-27000) (F-6A780)

D6-72624 Dysmorphic sialidosis, congenital form
(M-27000) (F-6A780)

D6-72628 Dysmorphic sialidosis with renal involvement
(M-27000) (F-6A780)
Nephrosialidosis
(M-27000) (F-6A780)

D6-72630 Combined deficiency of sialidase and beta galactosidase
(M-27000) (F-6A780) (F-6A7A0)
Galactosialidosis
(M-27000) (F-6A780) (F-6A7A0)
Goldberg syndrome
(M-27000) (F-6A780) (F-6A7A0)
Neuraminidase deficiency with beta-galactosidase deficiency
(M-27000) (F-6A780) (F-6A7A0)

D6-72640 Salla disease
Sialuria, Finnish type

D6-72642 Sialic acid storage disease, severe infantile type
Sialuria, French type
Sialuria, infantile type

D6-72700 Acid lipase deficiency, NOS
(M-27000) (F-6A120)

D6-72710 Wolman's disease 272.7
(M-27000) (F-6A120) (F-6A160)
Primary familial xanthomatosis with adrenal calcification 272.7
(M-27000) (F-6A120) (F-6A160)
Familial visceral xanthomatosis 272.7
(M-27000) (F-6A120) (F-6A160)
Lysosomal acid lipase deficiency 272.7
(M-27000) (F-6A120) (F-6A160)
Deficiency of cholesterol esterase and triacylglycerol lipase
(M-27000) (F-6A120) (F-6A160)
LIPA deficiency 272.7
(M-27000) (F-6A120) (F-6A160)

D6-72720 Cholesterol ester storage disease 272.7
(F-63990)

D6-72730 Cytochrome-c oxidase deficiency
(M-27000) (F-67050)

D6-72740 Triglyceride storage disease with ichthyosis
(F-63610)
Chanarin-Dorfman disease
(F-63610)
Chanarin-Miranda syndrome
(F-63610)
Ichthyosiform erythroderma with leukocyte vacuolation
(F-63610)
Ichthyotic neutral lipid storage disease
(F-63610)
Lipid storage myopathy and congenital ichthyosis
(F-63610)
Neutral lipid storage disease
(F-63610)

D6-72750 Phosphatidylcholine-sterol acyltransferase deficiency 272.5
(M-27000) (F-68550)
Familial lecithin-cholesterol acyltransferase deficiency 272.5
(M-27000) (F-68550)
LCAT deficiency 272.5
(M-27000) (F-68550)
Norum's disease 272.5
(M-27000) (F-68550)

SECTION 6-7 DISORDERS OF LYSOSOMAL ENZYMES — Continued

D6-72760 Pancreatic triacylglycerol lipase deficiency
(T-65000) (M-27000) (F-6A120)
Congenital absence of pancreatic lipase
(T-65000) (M-27000) (F-6A120)
Isolated lipase deficiency
(T-65000) (M-27000) (F-6A120)

D6-72764 Pancreatic colipase deficiency
(T-65000)

D6-74000 Sphingomyelin/cholesterol lipidosis, NOS 272.7
(M-27000) (F-6A4C0)
Niemann-Pick disease, NOS 272.7
(M-27000) (F-6A4C0)
Sphingomyelin lipidosis, NOS 272.7
(M-27000) (F-6A4C0)
Sphingomyelinase deficiency 272.7
(M-27000) (F-6A4C0)
Neuronal cholesterol lipidosis, NOS 272.7
(M-27000) (F-6A4C0)

D6-74010 Niemann-Pick disease, type A 272.7
(M-27000) (F-6A4C0)
Niemann-Pick disease, acute neuropathic form 272.7
(M-27000) (F-6A4C0)
Classical Niemann-Pick disease 272.7
(M-27000) (F-6A4C0)
Niemann-Pick disease, acute neurovisceral form 272.7
(M-27000) (F-6A4C0)

D6-74020 Niemann-Pick disease, type B 272.7
(M-27000) (F-6A4C0)
Niemann-Pick disease, chronic non-neuronopathic 272.7
(M-27000) (F-6A4C0)

D6-74030 Niemann-Pick disease, type C 272.7
(M-27000) (F-6A4C0)

D6-74032 Niemann-Pick disease, type C, acute form
(M-27000) (F-6A4C0)

D6-74034 Niemann-Pick disease, type C, subacute form 272.7
(M-27000) (F-6A4C0)

D6-74036 Niemann-Pick disease, type C, chronic form
(M-27000) (F-6A4C0)

D6-74040 Niemann-Pick disease, type D 272.7
(M-27000) (F-6A4C0)
Niemann-Pick disease, Nova Scotian 272.7
(M-27000) (F-6A4C0)

D6-74050 Niemann-Pick disease, type E 272.7
(M-27000) (F-6A4C0)
Niemann-Pick disease, adult non-neuronopathic 272.7
(M-27000) (F-6A4C0)

D6-74100 Gaucher's disease, NOS 272.7
(M-27000) (F-6A838)
Glucosylceramidase deficiency 272.7
(M-27000) (F-6A838)
Kerasin histiocytosis 272.7
(M-27000) (F-6A838)
Kerasin lipoidosis
(M-27000) (F-6A838)
Glucocerebrosidosis 272.7
(M-27000) (F-6A838)
Kerasin thesaurismosis 272.7
(M-27000) (F-6A838)
Gaucher splenomegaly 272.7
(M-27000) (F-6A838)
Gaucher syndrome 272.7
(M-27000) (F-6A838)

D6-74110 Chronic non-neuropathic Gaucher's disease 272.7
(M-27000) (F-6A838)
Chronic adult Gaucher's disease 272.7
(M-27000) (F-6A838)
Noncerebral juvenile Gaucher's disease
(M-27000) (F-6A838)
Glucosylceramidase deficiency, chronic type 272.7
(M-27000) (F-6A838)
Gaucher's disease, type I 272.7
(M-27000) (F-6A838)

D6-74120 Acute neuronopathic Gaucher's disease 272.7
(M-27000) (F-6A838)
Infantile Gaucher's disease 272.7
(M-27000) (F-6A838)
Infantile cerebral Gaucher's disease 272.7
(M-27000) (F-6A838)
Gaucher's disease, type II
(M-27000) (F-6A838)
Acute cerebral Gaucher's disease 272.7
(M-27000) (F-6A838)
Glucosylceramidase deficiency, acute type 272.7
(M-27000) (F-6A838)

D6-74130 Subacute neuronopathic Gaucher's disease 272.7
(M-27000) (F-6A838)
Juvenile Gaucher's disease 272.7
(M-27000) (F-6A838)
Glucosylceramidase deficiency, subacute type 272.7
(M-27000) (F-6A838)
Gaucher's disease, type III 272.7
(M-27000) (F-6A838)

D6-74200 Globoid cell leukodystrophy, early onset 330.0
(M-27000) (F-6A7A0)
Galactosylceramide lipidosis 330.0
(M-27000) (F-6A7A0)
Krabbe's disease 330.0
(M-27000) (F-6A7A0)
Galactocerebroside beta-galactosidase deficiency 330.0
(M-27000) (F-6A7A0)

D6-74200 (cont.) Diffuse globoid body sclerosis 330.0
(M-27000) (F-6A7A0)
Diffuse globoid cell cerebral sclerosis 330.0
(M-27000) (F-6A7A0)
Familial infantile diffuse brain sclerosis 330.0
(M-27000) (F-6A7A0)
Krabbe's leukodystrophy 330.0
(M-27000) (F-6A7A0)

D6-74210 Globoid cell leukodystrophy, late-onset 330.0
(M-27000) (F-6A7A0)
Adult-type globoid cell leukodystrophy 330.0
(M-27000) (F-6A7A0)
Adult-type Krabbe's disease 330.0
(M-27000) (F-6A7A0)

D6-74220 Pelizaeus-Merzbacher disease 330.0
Sudanophilic leukodystrophy 330.0

D6-74222 Pelizaeus-Merzbacher disease, classic form 330.0

D6-74224 Pelizaeus-Merzbacher disease, connatal variant 330.0

D6-74230 Leukodystrophy, NOS 330.0

D6-74240 Farber's lipogranulomatosis 272.7
(M-27000) (F-6B1E0)
Acid ceramidase deficiency 272.7
(M-27000) (F-6B1E0)
Farber's disease 272.7
(M-27000) (F-6B1E0)
Acylsphingosine deacylase deficiency 272.7
(M-27000) (F-6B1E0)
Farber-Uzman syndrome 272.7
(M-27000) (F-6B1E0)
Disseminated lipogranulomatosis 272.7
(M-27000) (F-6B1E0)

D6-74400 Metachromatic leukodystrophy, NOS 330.0
(M-27000) (F-6A550)
Sulfatide lipidosis, NOS 330.0
(M-27000) (F-6A550)
Arylsulfatase A deficiency 330.0
(M-27000) (F-6A550)
Familial progressive cerebral sclerosis 330.0
(M-27000) (F-6A550)
Greenfield disease 330.0
(M-27000) (F-6A550)
Metachromatic leukoencephaly 330.0
(M-27000) (F-6A550)
Scholz-Bielschowsky-Henneberg diffuse cerebral sclerosis
(M-27000) (F-6A550)
Scholz cerebral sclerosis 330.0
(M-27000) (F-6A550)
van Bogaert-Nijssen disease 330.0
(M-27000) (F-6A550)
Severe deficiency of arylsulfatase 330.0
(M-27000) (F-6A550)
MLD, NOS 330.0
(M-27000) (F-6A550)

D6-74410 Metachromatic leukodystrophy, congenital type 330.0
(M-27000) (F-6A550)

D6-74420 Metachromatic leukodystrophy, late infantile type 330.0
(M-27000) (F-6A550)

D6-74430 Metachromatic leukodystrophy, juvenile type 330.0
(M-27000) (F-6A550)

D6-74440 Metachromatic leukodystrophy, adult type 330.0

D6-74450 Metachromatic leukodystrophy without arylsulfatase deficiency 330.0

D6-74460 Arylsulfatase deficiency without MLD 330.0
(M-27000) (F-6A550)

D6-74470 Sphingolipid activator protein 1 deficiency 330.0
(F-63780)

D6-74500 Multiple sulfatase deficiency, NOS 272.7
Juvenile sulfatidosis, Austin type 272.7
Mucosulfatidosis 272.7

D6-74510 Deficiency of cerebroside-sulfatase 272.7
(M-27000) (F-6A580)

D6-74511 Deficiency of N-acetylgalactosamine-4-sulfatase 272.7
(M-27000) (F-6A5A0)

D6-74512 Deficiency of N-acetylgalactosamine-6-sulfatase 272.7
(M-27000) (F-6A568)

D6-74513 Deficiency of N-acetylglucosamine-6-sulfatase 272.7
(M-27000) (F-6A5B0)

D6-74514 Deficiency of steryl-sulfatase 272.7
(M-27000) (F-6A558)

D6-74516 Deficiency of iduronate-2-sulfatase 272.7
(M-27000) (F-6A5A8)

D6-74600 Fabry's disease 272.7
(M-27000) (F-6A798)
alpha-Galactosidase-A deficiency 272.7
(M-27000) (F-6A798)
Angiokeratoma corporis diffusum universale 272.7
(M-27000) (F-6A798)
Anderson-Fabry disease 272.7
(M-27000) (F-6A798)
Cardiovasorenal syndrome 272.7
(M-27000) (F-6A798)
GLA deficiency 272.7
(M-27000) (F-6A798)
Hereditary dystopic lipidosis 272.7
(M-27000) (F-6A798)
Ruiter-Pompen syndrome 272.7
(M-27000) (F-6A798)

SECTION 6-7 DISORDERS OF LYSOSOMAL ENZYMES — Continued

D6-74600 (cont.) Sweeley-Klionsky disease 272.7
(M-27000) (F-6A798)
Thesaurismosis hereditaria 272.7
(M-27000) (F-6A798)
Thesaurismosis lipoidica 272.7
(M-27000) (F-6A798)
Ceramide trihexosidase deficiency 272.7
(M-27000) (F-6A798)

D6-76000 Gangliosidosis, NOS 330.1
Ganglioside storage disease, NOS 330.1
Ganglioside accumulation in nervous tissue lysosomes 330.1

D6-76010 GM_1 gangliosidosis, NOS 330.1
(M-27000) (F-6A7A0)
beta-Galactosidase isoenzyme deficiency 330.1
(M-27000) (F-6A7A0)

D6-76020 Infantile GM_1 gangliosidosis 330.1
(M-27000) (F-6A7A0)
GM_1 gangliosidosis, type 1 330.1
(M-27000) (F-6A7A0)
Generalized gangliosidosis 330.1
(M-27000) (F-6A7A0)
Infantile gangliosidosis with bony involvement 330.1
(M-27000) (F-6A7A0)
Deficiency of beta-galactosidase isoenzymes A, B and C 330.1
(M-27000) (F-6A7A0)

D6-76030 Juvenile GM_1 gangliosidosis 330.1
(M-27000) (F-6A7A0)
GM_1 gangliosidosis, type 2 330.1
(M-27000) (F-6A7A0)

D6-76040 Adult GM_1 gangliosidosis 330.1
(M-27000) (F-6A7A0)
GM_1 gangliosidosis, type 3 330.1
(M-27000) (F-6A7A0)

D6-76060 Ganglioside sialidase deficiency
(M-27000) (F-6A780)
Mucolipidosis IV 272.7
(M-27000) (F-6A780)

D6-76100 GM_2 gangliosidosis, NOS 330.1
(M-27000) (F-6A870)
Deficiency of beta-N-acetylhexosaminidase isoenzymes 330.1
(M-27000) (F-6A870)

D6-76110 Sandhoff disease 272.7
(M-27000) (F-6A870)
Hexosaminidase A and B deficiency 272.7
(M-27000) (F-6A870)
GM_2 gangliosidosis, type 2 272.7
(M-27000) (F-6A870)

D6-76130 Tay-Sachs disease 330.1
(M-27000) (F-6A870)
Severe hexosaminidase A deficiency 330.1
(M-27000) (F-6A870)
TSD 330.1
(M-27000) (F-6A870)
Amaurotic familial idiocy 330.1
(M-27000) (F-6A870)
Infantile amaurotic familial disease 330.1
(M-27000) (F-6A870)
GM_2 gangliosidosis, type 1 330.1
(M-27000) (F-6A870)

D6-76134 Tay-Sachs disease, variant AB 330.1
(M-27000) (F-6A870)
GM_2 gangliosidosis, type AB 330.1
(M-27000) (F-6A870)
Hexosaminidase activator deficiency 330.1
(M-27000) (F-6A870)

D6-76140 Juvenile GM_2 gangliosidosis 330.1
(M-27000) (F-6A870)
GM_2 gangliosidosis, type 3 330.1
(M-27000) (F-6A870)

D6-76150 Adult chronic GM_2 gangliosidosis 330.1
(M-27000) (F-6A870)

D6-76160 Infantile GM_2 gangliosidosis 330.1
(M-27000) (F-6A870)

D6-77000 Lipofuscinosis, NOS 330.1

D6-77010 Intestinal lipofuscinosis 330.1
Brown bowel syndrome 330.1

D6-77100 Neuronal ceroid lipofuscinosis 330.1
(F-62B30)
Cerebromacular degeneration 330.1
Cerebromacular dystrophy 330.1
Pigmentary retinal lipoid neuronal heredodegeneration 330.1

D6-77110 Infantile neuronal ceroid lipofuscinosis 330.1
Hagberg-Santavuori disease 330.1
Santavuori disease 330.1
Neuronal ceroid lipofuscinosis, infantile Finnish type 330.1
Polyunsaturated acid lipidosis 330.1

D6-77120 Late-infantile neuronal ceroid lipofuscinosis 330.1
Bielschowsky-Jansky disease 330.1
Amaurotic idiocy, early juvenile type 330.1
Amaurotic idiocy, late infantile type
Dollinger-Bielschowsky syndrome 330.1

D6-77140 Juvenile neuronal ceroid lipofuscinosis 330.1
Batten-Mayou disease 330.1
Spielmeyer-Vogt disease 330.1
Amaurotic idiocy, juvenile type 330.1
Cerebral lipidosis, myoclonic variant 330.1
Batten-Spielmeyer-Vogt disease 330.1

D6-77150 Adult neuronal ceroid lipofuscinosis 330.1
Kufs' disease 330.1
Adult-type amaurotic idiocy 330.1
Late familial amaurotic idiocy 330.1

D6-77160 Cerebral lipidosis, NOS 330.1

SECTION 6-8 DISORDERS OF STEROID, BILIRUBIN AND PORPHYRIN METABOLISM
6-80 DISORDERS OF STEROID METABOLISM

D6-80000 Disorder of steroid metabolism, NOS

D6-80100 Congenital adrenal cortical hyperplasia, NOS 255.2
- Congenital adrenal hyperplasia, NOS 255.2
- Adrenogenital syndrome 255.2
- Adrenal virilism 255.2
- Androgenital syndrome 255.2
- Apert-Gallais syndrome 255.2
- Wilkins disease 255.2

D6-80110 Cholesterol monooxygenase (side-chain cleaving) deficiency 255.2
(M-27000) (F-67400)
- Cholesterol desmolase deficiency 255.2
(M-27000) (F-67400)
- 20,22-Desmolase deficiency 255.2
(M-27000) (F-67400)
- Congenital lipoid hyperplasia of adrenal cortex with male pseudohermaphroditism 255.2
(M-27000) (F-67400)

D6-80120 Steroid 17 alpha-monooxygenase deficiency 255.2
(M-27000) (F-67480)
- 17 alpha-Hydroxylase deficiency 255.2
(M-27000) (F-67480)
- Adrenogenital disorder due to 17 alpha-hydroxylase deficiency 255.2
(M-27000) (F-67480)
- Congenital adrenal hyperplasia, type 5 255.2
(M-27000) (F-67480)

D6-80130 3 beta-Hydroxysteroid dehydrogenase deficiency 255.2
(M-27000) (F-662A0)
- 3 beta-HSD deficiency 255.2
(M-27000) (F-662A0)
- Congenital adrenal hyperplasia, type 4 255.2
(M-27000) (F-662A0)

D6-80140 Steroid 21-monooxygenase deficiency, simple virilizing type 255.2
(M-27000) (F-67488)
- Steroid 21-hydroxylase deficiency 255.2
(M-27000) (F-67488)
- Simple virilizing adrenal hyperplasia 255.2
(M-27000) (F-67488)
- Adrenogenital disorder due to 21-hydroxylase deficiency 255.2
(M-27000) (F-67488)
- Congenital adrenal hyperplasia, type 1 255.2
(M-27000) (F-67488)

D6-80142 Mild steroid 21-hydroxylase deficiency 255.2
(M-27000) (F-67488)

D6-80144 Moderate steroid 21-hydroxylase deficiency 255.2
(M-27000) (F-67488)

D6-80146 Severe steroid 21-hydroxylase deficiency 255.2
(M-27000) (F-67488)

D6-80150 Steroid 21-monooxygenase deficiency, salt wasting type 255.2
(M-27000) (F-67488)
- Congenital adrenal hyperplasia, type 2 255.2
(M-27000) (F-67488)

D6-80160 Steroid 11 beta-monooxygenase deficiency 255.2
(M-27000) (F-673F0)
- 11 beta-hydroxylase deficiency 255.2
(M-27000) (F-673F0)
- Adrenogenital disorder due to 11 beta-hydroxylase deficiency 255.2
(M-27000) (F-673F0)
- Congenital adrenal hyperplasia, type 3 255.2
(M-27000) (F-673F0)
- Hypertensive congenital adrenal hyperplasia 255.2
(M-27000) (F-673F0)

D6-80170 Corticosterone 18-monooxygenase deficiency 255.2
(M-27000) (F-673F8)
- 18-Hydroxylase deficiency 255.2
(M-27000) (F-673F8)
- Aldosterone deficiency due to 18-hydroxylase defect 255.2
(M-27000) (F-673F8)
- Corticosterone methyl oxidase type I deficiency 255.2
(M-27000) (F-673F8)
- CMO I deficiency 255.2
(M-27000) (F-673F8)

D6-80180 18-Hydroxycorticosterone dehydrogenase deficiency 255.2
- Aldosterone deficiency due to 18-hydroxysteroid dehydrogenase deficiency 255.2
- CMO II deficiency 255.2
- Corticosterone methyl oxidase type II deficiency 255.2

D6-80190 17 alpha-Hydroxyprogesterone aldolase deficiency 255.2
(M-27000) (F-6C3D0)
- Steroid 17,20-lyase deficiency 255.2
(M-27000) (F-6C3D0)
- Male pseudohermaphroditism due to testicular 17,20-desmolase deficiency 255.2
(M-27000) (F-6C3D0)

6-80 DISORDERS OF STEROID METABOLISM — Continued

D6-801A0 Testosterone 17-beta-dehydrogenase deficiency 255.2
(M-27000) (F-66308)
17B-HSD deficiency 255.2
(M-27000) (F-66308)
17-Ketosteroid reductase deficiency 255.2
(M-27000) (F-66308)
17-KSR deficiency 255.2
(M-27000) (F-66308)
Neutral 17-beta-hydroxysteroid oxidoreductase deficiency 255.2
(M-27000) (F-66308)
D6-80300 Androgen resistance syndrome, NOS 255.2
Androgen insensitivity syndrome 255.2
D6-80310 3-Oxo-5 alpha-steroid delta 4-dehydrogenase deficiency 255.2
(M-27000) (F-66C08)
Steroid 5a-reductase deficiency 255.2
(M-27000) (F-66C08)
Pseudovaginal perineoscrotal hypospadias 255.2
(M-27000) (F-66C08)
Familial incomplete male pseudohermaphroditism, type 2 255.2
(M-27000) (F-66C08)
PPSH 255.2
(M-27000) (F-66C08)
D6-80400 Disorder of androgen receptor, NOS 255.2
D6-80410 Testicular feminization, NOS 257.8
Goldberg-Maxwell syndrome 257.8
Goldberg-Morris syndrome 257.8
Hairless woman syndrome 257.8
Syndrome of feminizing testes 257.8
D6-80412 Complete testicular feminization syndrome 255.2
D6-80414 Incomplete testicular feminization syndrome 255.2
D6-80420 Reifenstein syndrome 255.2
Lubs syndrome 255.2
Gilbert-Dreyfuss syndrome 255.2
Rosewater syndrome 255.2
Familial incomplete male pseudohermaphroditism, type 1 255.2
D6-80430 Infertile male syndrome 255.2
D6-80450 Receptor-positive androgen resistance syndrome, NOS 255.2
(M-27000) (F-66C08)
D6-80600 Steryl-sulfatase deficiency 255.2
(M-27000) (F-6A558)
Steroid sulfatase deficiency 255.2
(M-27000) (F-6A558)
X-linked ichthyosis 255.2
(M-27000) (F-6A558)
Placental sulfatase deficiency 255.2
(M-27000) (F-6A558)
Placental steroidal sulfatase deficiency 255.2
(M-27000) (F-6A558)
SSDD 255.2
(M-27000) (F-6A558)
Steroid sulfatase deficiency disease 255.2
(M-27000) (F-6A558)
STS 255.2
(M-27000) (F-6A558)

6-84-85 DISORDERS OF BILIRUBIN METABOLISM

D6-84000 Disorder of bilirubin metabolism, NOS 277.4
(F-65000)
D6-84100 Unconjugated hyperbilirubinemia, NOS 277.4
(F-65010)
D6-84200 Conjugated hyperbilirubinemia, NOS
(F-65020)
D6-84340 Cyclic premenstrual unconjugated hyperbilirubinemia 277.4
(F-65010)
D6-84380 Acquired hyperbilirubinemia, NOS 277.4
(F-65000)
D6-85000 Inherited disorder of bilirubin metabolism, NOS 277.4
(F-65000)
D6-85100 Gilbert's syndrome 277.4
(F-65010)
Benign unconjugated bilirubinemia syndrome 277.4
(F-65010)
Cholemia familiaris simplex 277.4
(F-65010)
Chronic intermittent juvenile jaundice 277.4
(F-65010)
Congenital familial cholemia 277.4
(F-65010)
Constitutional hepatic dysfunction 277.4
(F-65010)
Familial nonhemolytic bilirubinemia 277.4
(F-65010)
Familial nonhemolytic jaundice 277.4
(F-65010)
Gilbert's disease 277.4
(F-65010)
Gilbert-Lereboullet syndrome 277.4
(F-65010)
Hereditary nonhemolytic jaundice 277.4
(F-65010)
Low-grade chronic hyperbilirubinemia syndrome 277.4
(F-65010)
Meulengracht syndrome 277.4
(F-65010)
D6-85200 Crigler-Najjar syndrome, NOS 277.4
D6-85210 Crigler-Najjar syndrome, type I 277.4
(M-27000) (F-68798)
Deficiency of glucuronosyltransferase 277.4
(M-27000) (F-68798)

D6-85210 (cont.) Glucuronyltransferase deficiency 277.4
(M-27000) (F-68798)
UDP glucuronyl transferase deficiency 277.4
(M-27000) (F-68798)

D6-85220 Crigler-Najjar syndrome, type II 277.4
(M-27000) (F-68798)

D6-85500 Dubin-Johnson syndrome 277.4
(M-27000) (F-68798)
Black liver-jaundice syndrome 277.4
(M-27000) (F-68798)
Chronic idiopathic jaundice with pigmented liver 277.4
(M-27000) (F-68798)
Dubin-Sprinz syndrome 277.4
(M-27000) (F-68798)
Spinz-Nelson syndrome 277.4
(M-27000) (F-68798)
Icterus-hepatic pigmentation syndrome 277.4
(M-27000) (F-68798)

D6-85550 Rotor syndrome 277.4

D6-85600 Progressive intrahepatic cholestasis
Byler syndrome
Familial intrahepatic cholestasis
Fatal intrahepatic cholestasis

D6-85610 North American Indian intrahepatic cholestasis

D6-85620 Benign recurrent intrahepatic cholestasis
Benign familial recurrent cholestasis
Benign recurrent cholestasis

D6-85650 Cholestasis-edema syndrome, Norwegian type
Aagenaes syndrome
Cholestasis-lymphedema syndrome
Cholestatic jaundice with hereditary lymphedema
Norwegian cholestasis

D6-85680 Intrahepatic cholestasis of pregnancy
Cholestasis of pregnancy
Pruritus of pregnancy
Recurrent jaundice of pregnancy
Recurrent intrahepatic cholestasis of pregnancy
RICP

6-88 DISORDERS OF PORPHYRIN METABOLISM

D6-88000 Disorder of porphyrin metabolism, NOS 277.1
(F-64800)

D6-88100 Porphyria, NOS 277.1
Porphyrinopathy, NOS 277.1

D6-88200 Erythropoietic porphyria, NOS 277.1

D6-88210 Congenital erythropoietic porphyria 277.1
(M-27000) (F-6C730)
Gunther's disease 277.1
(M-27000) (F-6C730)
Congenital photosensitive porphyria 277.1
(M-27000) (F-6C730)
Congenital porphyria 277.1
(M-27000) (F-6C730)
Hematoporphyria congenita 277.1
(M-27000) (F-6C730)
Porphyria erythropoietica 277.1
(M-27000) (F-6C730)

D6-88220 Erythropoietic protoporphyria 277.1
(M-27000) (F-6C908)
EPP 277.1
(M-27000) (F-6C908)
Erythrohepatic protoporphyria 277.1
(M-27000) (F-6C908)
Heme synthase deficiency 277.1
(M-27000) (F-6C908)
Magnus syndrome 277.1
(M-27000) (F-6C908)

D6-88300 Hepatic porphyria, NOS 277.1

D6-88310 Acute intermittent porphyria 277.1
(M-27000) (F-6C828)
Pyrroloporphyria 277.1
(M-27000) (F-6C828)
Intermittent acute porphyria syndrome 277.1
(M-27000) (F-6C828)
PBGD deficiency 277.1
(M-27000) (F-6C828)
Porphobilinogen deaminase deficiency 277.1
(M-27000) (F-6C828)
Uroporphyrinogen 1 synthase deficiency 277.1
(M-27000) (F-6C828)
Swedish porphyria 277.1
(M-27000) (F-6C828)

D6-88320 Hereditary coproporphyria 277.1
(M-27000) (F-66BC0)
Berger-Goldberg syndrome 277.1
(M-27000) (F-66BC0)
CPO deficiency 277.1
(M-27000) (F-66BC0)
CPRO deficiency 277.1
(M-27000) (F-66BC0)
Porphyria hepatica II 277.1
(M-27000) (F-66BC0)
Watson syndrome 277.1
(M-27000) (F-66BC0)

D6-88330 Variegate porphyria 277.1
(M-27000) (F-66BC8)
South African porphyria 277.1
(M-27000) (F-66BC8)
South African genetic porphyria 277.1
(M-27000) (F-66BC8)
Protocoproporphyria 277.1
(M-27000) (F-66BC8)
Dean-Barnes syndrome 277.1
(M-27000) (F-66BC8)

6-88 DISORDERS OF PORPHYRIN METABOLISM — Continued

D6-88330 (cont.) Mixed porphyria 277.1
(M-27000) (F-66BC8)
D6-88336 Chester-type porphyria
D6-88340 Porphyria cutanea tarda, NOS 277.1
(M-27000) (F-6C210)
Symptomatic porphyria 277.1
(M-27000) (F-6C210)
Cutaneous hepatic porphyria 277.1
(M-27000) (F-6C210)
PCT 277.1
(M-27000) (F-6C210)
Porphyria cutanea tarda symptomatica 277.1
(M-27000) (F-6C210)
Porphyria, hepatocutaneous type 277.1
(M-27000) (F-6C210)
Urocoproporphyria 277.1
(M-27000) (F-6C210)
UROD deficiency 277.1
(M-27000) (F-6C210)
D6-88342 Familial porphyria cutanea tarda 277.1
Hereditary porphyria cutanea tarda 277.1
PCT, type II 277.1
D6-88344 Homozygous porphyria cutanea tarda 277.1
Hepatoerythropoietic porphyria 277.1
D6-88400 Secondary porphyria, NOS 277.1
D6-88410 Toxic porphyria, NEC 277.1
D6-88412 Drug-induced porphyria, NOS 277.1
D6-88420 Porphyruria 277.1
Porphyrinuria 277.1
Hematoporphyrinuria 277.1
Pink tooth
D6-88500 Porphobilinogen synthase deficiency 277.1
(M-27000) (F-6C5B0)
ALA dehydratase deficiency porphyria 277.1
(M-27000) (F-6C5B0)
ALAD deficiency 277.1
(M-27000) (F-6C5B0)
ALADH deficiency 277.1
(M-27000) (F-6C5B0)
delta-Aminolevulinate dehydrase deficiency 277.1
(M-27000) (F-6C5B0)
Hereditary delta-aminolevulinic aciduria 277.1
(M-27000) (F-6C5B0)
delta-Aminolevulinic acid dehydratase deficiency 277.1
(M-27000) (F-6C5B0)

SECTION 6-9 OTHER METABOLIC DISEASES

6-90 METABOLIC DISEASES OF COLLAGEN

D6-90000 Metabolic disease of collagen, NOS 756.8
D6-90100 Ehlers-Danlos syndrome, NOS 756.83
Cutis elastica 756.83
Cutis hyperelastica 756.83
Cutis hyperelastica dermatorrhexis 756.83
Danlos disease 756.83
Dermatorrhexis with dermatochalasis and arthrochalasis 756.83
Dystrophia mesodermalis congenita 756.83
Fibrodysplasia elastica generalisata 756.83
India rubber skin 756.83
Meekeren-Ehlers-Danlos syndrome 756.83
Cutaneous asthenia in dogs and cats
Hereditary collagen dysplasia
Dermatosparaxis in cattle and sheep
D6-90110 Ehlers-Danlos syndrome, type 1 756.83
Ehlers-Danlos syndrome, gravis 756.83
Ehlers-Danlos syndrome, severe classic form 756.83
D6-90120 Ehlers-Danlos syndrome, type 2 756.83
Ehlers-Danlos syndrome, mitis 756.83
Ehlers-Danlos syndrome, mild classic form 756.83
D6-90130 Ehlers-Danlos syndrome, type 3 756.83
Benign hypermobility syndrome 756.83
Ehlers-Danlos syndrome, benign hypermobile form 756.83
D6-90140 Ehlers-Danlos syndrome, type 4 756.83
Sack syndrome 756.83
Sack-Barabas syndrome 756.83
D6-90142 Ehlers-Danlos syndrome, dominant type 4
D6-90144 Ehlers-Danlos syndrome, recessive type 4
D6-90150 Ehlers-Danlos syndrome, type 5 756.83
Ehlers-Danlos syndrome, mild x-linked
D6-90160 Ehlers-Danlos syndrome, hydroxylysine-deficient 756.83
(M-27000) (F-672A0)
Hydroxylysine-deficient collagen disease 756.83
(M-27000) (F-672A0)
Ehlers-Danlos syndrome, lysyl hydroxylase deficient 756.83
(M-27000) (F-672A0)
Protocollagen lysyl hydroxylase deficiency 756.83
(M-27000) (F-672A0)
D6-90162 Ehlers-Danlos syndrome, non hydroxylysine deficient ocular type
D6-90166 Corneal fragility keratoglobus, blue sclerae and joint hypermobility
Fragilitas oculi with joint hyperextensibility
Ehlers-Danlos syndrome, type 6 phenotype with macrocephaly
D6-90170 Ehlers-Danlos syndrome, procollagen proteinase deficient
(M-27000) (F-6B068)
Ehlers-Danlos syndrome, autosomal recessive type 7 756.83
(M-27000) (F-6B068)

D6-90170 (cont.) Procollagen peptidase deficiency 756.83 (M-27000) (F-6B068)
Procollagen protease deficiency (M-27000) (F-6B068)
Procollagen aminoprotease deficiency (M-27000) (F-6B068)
Arthrochalasis multiplex congenita (M-27000) (F-6B068)

D6-90174 Ehlers-Danlos syndrome, procollagen proteinase resistant
Ehlers-Danlos syndrome, autosomal dominant type 7
Ehlers-Danlos syndrome, mutant procollagen type 7

D6-90180 Ehlers-Danlos syndrome, type 8 756.83
Ehlers-Danlos syndrome, periodontitis type 756.83

D6-901A0 Ehlers-Danlos syndrome, dysfibronectinemic 756.83
Ehlers-Danlos syndrome, type 10 756.83
Ehlers-Danlos syndrome with platelet dysfunction 756.83

D6-901B0 Ehlers-Danlos syndrome, familial joint laxity type 756.83
Ehlers-Danlos syndrome, type 11 756.83
Familial generalized articular hypermobility 756.83
Familial joint instability syndrome 756.83
Familial joint laxity 756.83

D6-90300 Cutis laxa, NOS 756.83

D6-90310 Cutis laxa, autosomal dominant 756.83

D6-90320 Cutis laxa, autosomal recessive 756.83

D6-90324 Hemolytic anemia with emphysema and cutis laxa

D6-90330 Cutis laxa, x-linked 756.83
Ehlers-Danlos syndrome, mental retardation type 756.83
Ehlers-Danlos syndrome, occipital horn type 756.83
Ehlers-Danlos syndrome, type 9 756.83
Ehlers-Danlos syndrome, x-linked skeletal type 756.83

D6-90340 Cutis laxa-corneal clouding-oligophrenia syndrome 756.83
Cutis laxa, corneal clouding and mental retardation 756.83
de Barsey-Moens-Dierckx syndrome 756.83
de Barsey syndrome 756.83
Progeroid syndrome of de Barsey 756.83

D6-90350 Cutis laxa with osteodystrophy
Cutis laxa with bone dystrophy
Cutis laxa with joint laxity and retarded development

D6-90500 Osteogenesis imperfecta, NOS 756.51
Fragilitas ossium 756.51
Osteopsathyrosis 756.51
Brittle bone syndrome 756.51

D6-90510 Osteogenesis imperfecta with blue sclerae
Osteogenesis imperfecta, type I 756.51
Blue sclerae syndrome
Eddowes syndrome
Ekman syndrome
Ekman-Lobstein syndrome
Fragilitas ossium-blue sclerae-otosclerosis syndrome
Fragilitas ossium hereditaria tarda
Lobstein disease
OI type 1
Osteogenesis imperfecta psathyrotica
Osteogenesis imperfecta tarda
Osteopsathyrosis idiopathica tarda
Spurway-Eddowes syndrome
van der Hoeve syndrome with deafness

D6-90512 Osteogenesis imperfecta with blue sclerae and normal teeth
Osteogenesis imperfecta, type IB 756.51

D6-90516 Osteogenesis imperfecta with blue sclerae and dentinogenesis imperfecta
Osteogenesis imperfecta, type IA
Osteogenesis imperfecta with opalescent teeth

D6-90520 Osteogenesis imperfecta, perinatal lethal 756.51
Aplasia ossea microplastica 756.51
Aplasia periostealis 756.51
Fragilitas ossium congenita 756.51
Osteogenesis imperfecta letalis 756.51
Osteogenesis imperfecta, neonatal lethal 756.51
Osteogenesis imperfecta, type II
Fetal osteoporosis 756.51
Osteopsathyrosis congenita 756.51
Fetal osteopsathyrosis
Congenital periosteal dysplasia 756.51

D6-90522 Osteogenesis imperfecta, dominant perinatal lethal
Neonatal lethal osteogenesis imperfecta congenita
Osteogenesis imperfecta type II, dominant form

D6-90526 Osteogenesis imperfecta, recessive perinatal lethal
Osteogenesis imperfecta, type II, recessive form
Osteogenesis imperfecta, Vrolik type
Porak-Durante syndrome
Vrolik disease

D6-90528 Osteogenesis imperfecta, recessive perinatal lethal, with microcephaly and cataracts

D6-90530 Osteogenesis imperfecta with progressive deformity and normal sclerae
Osteogenesis imperfecta, type III 756.51
Progressively deforming osteogenesis imperfecta with normal sclerae

D6-90540 Osteogenesis imperfecta with normal sclerae, dominant form
Osteogenesis imperfecta, type IV A 756.51

6-90 METABOLIC DISEASES OF COLLAGEN — Continued

D6-90540 (cont.) Osteogenesis imperfecta, type IV B 756.51
  Osteogenesis imperfecta, type IV
D6-90800 Marfan's syndrome 759.8
  Marfan's disease 759.8
D6-90810 Marfanoid mental retardation syndrome
D6-90812 Marfanoid joint hypermobility syndrome
D6-90820 Pseudoxanthoma elasticum 757.39
  (T-01000) (T-1A240) (M-50010)
  Nevus elasticus 757.39
  (T-01000) (T-1A240) (M-50010)
D6-90822 Gronblad-Strandberg syndrome 757.39
D6-90840 Systemic elastorrhexis 757.3
D6-90900 Epidermolysis bullosa, NOS 757.39
  Acantholysis bullosa 757.39
  Acanthosis bullosa 757.39
  Bullous recurrent eruption 757.39
  Dermatitis bullosa hereditaria 757.39
  Fox disease 757.39
  Keratolysis bullosa hereditaria 757.39
D6-90910 Recessive dystrophic epidermolysis bullosa
  Dysplastic epidermolysis bullosa dystrophica
  Polydysplastic epidermolysis bullosa
D6-90912 Progressive recessive dystrophic epidermolysis bullosa
  Epidermolysis bullosa dystrophica neurotrophica
  EBR 3
  Epidermolysis bullosa progressiva with congenital deafness
  Goldscheider disease
D6-90920 Dominant dystrophic epidermolysis bullosa
  Epidermolysis bullosa dystrophica dominans
  Hyperplastic epidermolysis bullosa
D6-90922 Dominant dystrophic epidermolysis bullosa, albopapular type
  Epidermolysis bullosa dystrophica, Parsini type
D6-90926 Dominant dystrophic epidermolysis bullosa with absence of skin
  Epidermolysis bullosa dystrophica, Bart type
D6-90930 Junctional epidermolysis bullosa, NOS
D6-90932 Congenital junctional epidermolysis bullosa
  Epidermolysis bullosa hereditaria letalis
  Epidermolysis bullosa, junctional Herlitz-Pearson type
D6-90934 Congenital junctional epidermolysis bullosa-pyloric atresia syndrome
  Epidermolysis bullosa letalis with pyloric atresia
D6-90936 Adult junctional epidermolysis bullosa
  Epidermolysis bullosa junctionalis, Disentis type
D6-90940 Epidermolysis bullosa simplex
D6-90942 Generalized epidermolysis bullosa simplex
  Epidermolysis bullosa simplex, Kobner type
  Kobner disease
D6-90946 Epidermolysis bullosa simplex of the hands and feet
  DEBS-WC
  Dominant epidermolysis bullosa simplex, Weber-Cockayne type
  Epidermolysis bullosa, Cockayne-Touraine type
  Weber-Cockayne syndrome
D6-90947 Autosomal dominant epidermolysis bullosa simplex
  Epidermolysis bullosa simplex, Ogna type
  EBS 1
D6-90948 Pretibial epidermolysis bullosa

6-94-96 MISCELLANEOUS METABOLIC DISEASES

D6-94000 Metabolic disease, NEC 277.8
D6-94400 Serum cholinesterase defect 277.8
  (M-27000) (F-6A148)
  Pseudocholinesterase deficiency 277.8
  (M-27000) (F-6A148)
  Suxamethonium paralysis 277.8
  (M-27000) (F-6A148)
  Suxamethonium sensitivity 277.8
  (M-27000) (F-6A148)
D6-94450 Periodic disease 277.3
  Periodic fever 277.3
  Familial Mediterranean fever 277.3
  Paroxysmal polyserositis 277.3
  Familial recurrent polyserositis 277.3
D6-94500 Amyloidosis, NOS 277.3
D6-94510 Systemic amyloidosis, NOS
D6-94520 AA amyloidosis 277.3
  Secondary amyloidosis 277.3
  Reactive systemic amyloidosis 277.3
  Amyloid of familial Mediterrean fever 277.3
D6-94530 AL amyloidosis 277.3
  Primary amyloidosis 277.3
  Idiopathic amyloidosis 277.3
  Myeloma associated amyloidosis 277.3
D6-94540 Amyloid nephropathy 277.3
  Lardaceous kidney 277.3
  Soapy kidney 277.3
  Waxy kidney 277.3
  Renal amyloidosis 277.3
D6-94550 Familial amyloid polyneuropathy, NOS 277.3
  Hereditary amyloidosis 277.3
  AF type amyloidosis 277.3
  Familial polyneuropathic amyloidosis 277.3
D6-94551 Familial amyloid polyneuropathy, type VI 277.3
  Familial amyloid polyneuropathy, 60 Ala-for-Thr 277.3

D6-94551 (cont.) Familial amyloid polyneuropathy, Appalachian type 277.3

D6-94552 Amyloidosis, type I 277.3
Familial amyloid polyneuropathy, 30 Met-for-Val 277.3
Andrade syndrome 277.3
Corino de Andrade paramyloidosis 277.3
Familial amyloid neuropathy, Andrade type 277.3
Familial amyloid neuropathy, Portuguese type 277.3
Familial amyloid neuropathy, type I 277.3
Portuguese polyneuritic amyloidosis 277.3
Hereditary neuropathic amyloidosis, type I 277.3
Wohlwill-Corino Andrade syndrome 277.3
Hereditary amyloid polyneuropathy Portuguese type 277.3

D6-94553 Familial amyloid polyneuropathy, Jewish type 277.3
Familial amyloid polyneuropathy, 33 Ile-for-Phe 277.3

D6-94554 Familial amyloid polyneuropathy, type II 277.3
Familial amyloid polyneuropathy, 84 Ser-for-Ile 277.3
Familial amyloid polyneuropathy, Indiana-Swiss type 277.3
Amyloidosis, Indiana-Maryland type 277.3
Hereditary neuropathic amyloidosis, type II 277.3

D6-94555 Familial amyloid polyneuropathy, Iowa type 277.3
Iowa type amyloidosis 277.3
van Allen type amyloidosis 277.3

D6-94556 Familial amyloid neuropathy, Finnish type 277.3
Finnish type amyloidosis 277.3
Meretoja type amyloidosis 277.3

D6-94570 Familial visceral amyloidosis, Ostertag type 277.3
Amyloid nephropathy of Ostertag 277.3
Amyloidosis VIII 277.3
Familial renal amyloidosis 277.3
German type amyloidosis 277.3

D6-94576 Familial amyloid nephropathy with urticaria and deafness 277.3
Muckle-Wells syndrome 277.3
Muckle-Wells type amyloidosis 277.3

D6-94580 Danish type familial amyloid cardiomyopathy 277.3
Familial amyloid heart disease, 111 Met-for-Leu 277.3
Danish type amyloidosis 277.3
Denmark type amyloidosis 277.3

D6-94600 Localized amyloidosis, NOS 277.3

D6-94610 Hereditary cerebral amyloid angiopathy, Icelandic type 277.3
Amyloidosis VI 277.3
Autosomal dominant cerebrovascular amyloidosis 277.3
Iceland type amyloidosis 277.3
Familial cerebral hemorrhage, amyloid type 277.3
Hereditary cerebral hemorrhage with amyloidosis 277.3
HCHWA 277.3
Hereditary cerebral angiopathic amyloidosis 277.3

D6-94612 Hereditary cerebral amyloid angiopathy, Dutch type 277.3

D6-94620 Hereditary oculoleptomeningeal amyloid angiopathy 277.3
Amyloidosis VII 277.3
Ohio type amyloidosis 277.3

D6-94630 Isolated atrial amyloid 277.3

D6-94640 Primary localized cutaneous amyloidosis 277.3
Amyloidosis cutis 277.3
Lichen amyloidosis 277.3
Primary cutaneous amyloidosis 277.3
Amyloidosis of dermis 277.3
AD type amyloidosis 277.3

D6-94642 Dominant primary localized cutaneous amyloidosis 277.3
Amyloidosis IX 277.3
Familial amyloidosis cutis 277.3
Familial lichen amyloidosis 277.3
Familial generalized dyschromic amyloidosis cutis 277.3

D6-94648 Bullous cutaneous amyloidosis 277.3

D6-94650 Ocular amyloid deposit 277.3

D6-94652 Isolated corneal amyloidosis 277.3

D6-94654 Conjunctival amyloidosis 277.3

D6-94660 Other localized amyloid deposit 277.3

D6-94662 Gingival amyloidosis 277.3

D6-94680 Hemodialysis-associated amyloidosis 277.3
beta-2-Microglobulin amyloidosis 277.3
AH type amyloidosis 277.3

D6-94700 Age-related amyloidosis, NOS 277.3
AS type amyloidosis 277.3
Senile amyloidosis, NOS 277.3

D6-94710 Senile cardiac amyloidosis 277.3
AS transthyretin amyloidosis 277.3

D6-94720 Senile brain amyloidosis 277.3
AS beta protein amyloidosis 277.3

D6-94800 Cystic fibrosis 277.0
Mucoviscidosis 277.0
Fibrocystic disease of the pancreas 277.0
CF 277.0

D6-94802 Cystic fibrosis without meconium ileus 277.00

D6-94810 Cystic fibrosis with meconium ileus 277.01
Meconium ileus of the newborn 277.02
Meconium obstruction of intestine in mucoviscidosis 277.02

6-94-96 MISCELLANEOUS METABOLIC DISEASES — Continued

D6-95100 Acid phosphatase deficiency
(M-27000) (F-6A300)

D6-95200 Hypophosphatasia, NOS 275.3
(M-27000) (F-6A2F8)
Alkaline phosphatase deficiency 275.3
(M-27000) (F-6A2F8)
Rathbun syndrome 275.3
(M-27000) (F-6A2F8)

D6-95210 Infantile hypophosphatasia 275.3
Hypophosphatasia, infantile type 275.3
Congenital hypophosphatasia 275.3
Fetal hypophosphatasia 275.2

D6-95220 Childhood hypophosphatasia 275.3
Hypophosphatasia, childhood type 275.3
Juvenile hypophosphatasia 275.3

D6-95230 Adult hypophosphatasia 275.3
Hypophosphatasia, adult type 275.3

D6-95250 Hyperphosphatasemia with bone disease
Chronic congenital idiopathic hyperphosphatasemia
Familial idiopathic hyperphosphatasemia
Familial osteoectasia
Hyperostosis corticalis deformans juvenilis
Juvenile Paget disease
Osteochalasia desmalis familiaris

D6-95252 Hyperphosphatasemia tarda
van Buchem's syndrome
Hyperostosis corticalis generalisata
Hyperphosphatasia tarda
Leontiasis ossea generalisata

D6-95254 Hyperphosphatasemia with mental retardation

D6-95300 Intestinal enteropeptidase deficiency
(M-27000) (F-6ACB8)
Intestinal enterokinase deficiency
(M-27000) (F-6ACB8)
Intestinal pseudo-trypsinogen deficiency
(M-27000) (F-6ACB8)

D6-95310 Pancreatic trypsinogen deficiency
Congenital trypsinogen deficiency

D6-95360 Glycerol kinase deficiency
(M-27000) (F-690A0)
Familial hyperglycerolemia
(M-27000) (F-690A0)
GK1 deficiency
(M-27000) (F-690A0)
Hyperglycerolemia
(M-27000) (F-690A0)

D6-95400 Acatalasia 277.8
(M-27000) (F-670D8)
Acatalasemia 277.8
(M-27000) (F-670D8)
Takahara disease 277.8
(M-27000) (F-670D8)

D6-95420 Familial arthrogryposis-cholestatic hepatorenal syndrome
Lethal familial cholestatic and pigmentary liver disease

D6-95450 Cytochrome-b reductase deficiency
(M-27000) (F-66E80)
Diaphorase deficiency
(M-27000) (F-66E80)
DPNH methemoglobin reductase deficiency
(M-27000) (F-66E80)
Chronic familial methemoglobin reductase deficiency
(M-27000) (F-66E80)

D6-95800 Ethanolaminosis 270.8
(M-27000) (F-69230)
Ethanolamine kinase deficiency 270.8
(M-27000) (F-69230)
Ethanolaminuria 270.8
(M-27000) (F-69230)

D6-96300 Alstrom syndrome 759.8

D6-96900 Rowley-Rosenberg syndrome 270.8

6-98-99 MISCELLANEOUS METABOLIC DISORDERS OF TRANSPORT, NEC

D6-98000 Disorder of transport, NEC

D6-98100 Renal tubular acidosis, NOS 588.8
RTA, NOS 588.8

D6-98110 Hypokalemic distal renal tubular acidosis 588.8
Renal tubular acidosis, type 1 588.8
Classical renal tubular acidosis 588.8

D6-98112 San Francisco RTA syndrome 588.8

D6-98113 Atlanta RTA syndrome 588.8

D6-98114 Philadelphia RTA syndrome 588.8

D6-98115 Oklahoma City RTA syndrome 588.8

D6-98120 Hyperkalemic distal renal tubular acidosis 588.8
Renal tubular acidosis, type 4 588.8

D6-98130 Proximal renal tubular acidosis 588.8
Renal tubular acidosis, type 2 588.8
Bicarbonate reabsorption defect 588.8
Renal tubular acidosis, rate type 588.8

D6-98150 Pseudohypoaldosteronism, NOS 588.8
Pseudohypoadrenocorticalism 588.8

D6-98160 Pseudohypoaldosteronism, type 1 588.8

D6-98162 Pseudohypoaldosteronism, type 1, dominant form 588.8
Classic pseudohypoaldosteronism 588.8

D6-98164 Pseudohypoaldosteronism, type 1, recessive form 588.8
Pseudohypoaldosteronism, Persian-Jewish type 588.8

D6-98170 Pseudohypoaldosteronism, type 2 588.8

D6-98190 Glucoaminophosphaturia syndrome 270.8
Amino acid-glucose defective tubular absorption 270.8
Glucoaminophosphate diabetes 270.8
Luder-Sheldon syndrome 270.8

D6-98194 Glucoaminophosphaturia syndrome with rickets

D6-98196 Fanconi syndrome, NOS 270.0 —588.8*

D6-98300 Hereditary nephrogenic diabetes insipidus, NOS 588.1
Familial nephrogenic diabetes insipidus 588.1
ADH-resistant diabetes insipidus 588.1
Adiuretin-resistant diabetes insipidus 588.1
Renal diabetes insipidus 588.1
Vasopressin-resistant diabetes insipidus 588.1
Vasopressin-unresponsiveness hyposthenuria 588.1
Vasopressin-resistant hyposthenuria 588.1
D6-98310 Secondary nephrogenic diabetes insipidus
D6-98320 Acquired nephrogenic diabetes insipidus 588.1
D6-98420 Familial hypokalemic alkalosis, Gullner type
Familial hypokalemia
Gullner syndrome
D6-98500 Familial periodic paralysis, NOS 359.3
Cavarre disease 359.3
Familial myoplegia 359.3
Familial recurrent paralysis 359.3
Myoplegic dystrophy 359.3
Periodic myotonia 359.3
Westphal disease 359.3
Periodic paralysis 359.3
Periodic paralysis I 359.3
D6-98510 Familial hypokalemic periodic paralysis 359.3
Hypokalemic periodic paralysis 359.3
D6-98520 Familial hyperkalemic periodic paralysis 359.3
Adynamia episodica hereditaria 359.3
Gamstorp disease 359.3
Hyperkalemic periodic paralysis 359.3
Periodic paralysis II 359.3
D6-98530 Familial normokalemic periodic paralysis 359.3
Sodium-responsive periodic paralysis 359.3
Normokalemic periodic paralysis 359.3
Periodic paralysis III 359.3
D6-98540 Thyrotoxic periodic paralysis
Hashitoxic periodic paralysis
D6-98700 Primary hypomagnesemia
D6-98710 Isolated familial renal hypomagnesemia
D6-98720 Familial hypokalemia-hypomagnesemia
Gitelman syndrome
D6-98730 Familial hypomagnesemia-hypercalciuria
D6-98740 Isolated familial intestinal hypomagnesemia
Magnesium malabsorption

SECTIONS 6-A-B DISORDERS OF AMINO ACID METABOLISM

6-A0 DISORDERS OF AMINO ACID METABOLISM: GENERAL TERMS

D6-A0000 Disorder of amino acid metabolism, NOS 270.9
Amino acidopathy, NOS 270.9
Amino acid disorder, NOS 270.9
D6-A0100 Inborn error of amino acid metabolism, NOS 270.9
Hyperaminoaciduria, NOS 270.9
D6-A0200 Disorder of amino acid transport, NOS 270.9
D6-A0300 Benign neonatal hyperaminoaciduria, NOS 775.8

6-A1 DISORDERS OF PHENYLALANINE AND TRYPTOPHAN METABOLISM

6-A10-A11 Disorders of Phenylalanine Metabolism

D6-A1000 Disorder of phenylalanine metabolism, NOS
D6-A1110 Hyperphenylalaninemia, NOS 270.1
D6-A1120 Classical phenylketonuria 270.1
(M-27000) (F-67408)
Phenylalanine hydroxylase deficiency 270.1
(M-27000) (F-67408)
Folling's syndrome 270.1
(M-27000) (F-67408)
PKU 270.1
(M-27000) (F-67408)
PAH deficiency 270.1
(M-27000) (F-67408)
Hyperphenylalaninemia, type I 270.1
(M-27000) (F-67408)
Imbecilitus phenylpyruvica 270.1
(M-27000) (F-67408)
Oligophrenia phenylpyruvica 270.1
(M-27000) (F-67408)
D6-A1130 Persistent hyperphenylalaninemia
(M-27000) (F-67408)
Essential hyperphenylalaninemia
(M-27000) (F-67408)
Hyperphenylalaninemia, type II
(M-27000) (F-67408)
D6-A1140 Transient hyperphenylalaninemia 775.8
(M-27000) (F-67408)
Neonatal hyperphenylalaninemia 775.8
(M-27000) (F-67408)
Transient mild hyperphenylalaninemia 775.8
(M-27000) (F-67408)
Hyperphenylalaninemia, type III 775.8
(M-27000) (F-67408)
D6-A1150 Dihydropteridine reductase deficiency 270.1
(M-27000) (F-66F60)
Atypical phenylketonuria 270.1
(M-27000) (F-66F60)
Hyperphenylalaninemia, type IV 270.1
(M-27000) (F-66F60)
Atypical PKU 270.1
(M-27000) (F-66F60)
DHPR deficiency 270.1
(M-27000) (F-66F60)

6-A10-A11 Disorders of Phenylalanine Metabolism — Continued

D6-A1150 (cont.) Phenylketonuria II 270.1
(M-27000) (F-66F60)
D6-A1160 Tetrahydrobiopterin synthesis defect, NOS
Hyperphenylalaninemia, type V
D6-A1162 GTP cyclohydrolase I deficiency
(M-27000) (F-6B410)
Hyperphenylalaninemia with neopterin deficiency
(M-27000) (F-6B410)
D6-A1164 Sepiapterin reductase deficiency
(M-27000) (F-66598)
Biopterin deficiency
(M-27000) (F-66598)
7,8-Dihydrobiopterin synthetase deficiency
(M-27000) (F-66598)
D6-A1170 Persistent hyperphenylalaninemia and tyrosinemia 270.1
Hyperphenylalaninemia, type VI 270.1

6-A14 Disorders of Tryptophan Metabolism

D6-A1400 Disorder of tryptophan metabolism, NOS
D6-A1410 Tryptophanuria, NOS
D6-A1420 Tryptophanuria with dwarfism
D6-A1430 Hydroxykynureninuria 270.2
D6-A1440 Xanthurenic aciduria
D6-A1450 Kynureninase deficiency 270.2
(M-27000) (F-6B5E0)
D6-A1460 Indicanuria 270.2

6-A2 DISORDERS OF TYROSINE METABOLISM AND ALBINISM

6-A20-A21 Disorders of Tyrosine Metabolism

D6-A2000 Disturbance of tyrosine metabolism, NOS 270.2
D6-A2100 Hypertyrosinemia, NOS 270.2
Elevated tyrosine blood level 270.2
D6-A2110 Tyrosinosis, NOS
Excessive accumulation of tyrosine in tissue
D6-A2120 Transient neonatal hypertyrosinemia 775.8
Neonatal tyrosinemia 775.8
D6-A2130 Hereditary hypertyrosinemia, NOS
D6-A2140 Hypertyrosinemia, Richner-Hanhart type 270.2
Tyrosinemia, type II 270.2
Richner-Hanhart syndrome 270.2
Hereditary hypertyrosinemia, type II 270.2
Hypertyrosinemia, Oregon type 270.2
Keratosis palmoplantaris with corneal dystrophy 270.2
Persistent hypertyrosinemia 270.2
Richner syndrome 270.2
Oculocutaneous tyrosinemia 270.2
Tyrosinemia without hepatorenal dysfunction 270.2
Tyrosine transaminase deficiency 270.2
D6-A2150 Fumarylacetoacetase deficiency, acute type
(M-27000) (F-6B5D8)
Subacute tyrosinosis
(M-27000) (F-6B5D8)
Tyrosinemia, type I
(M-27000) (F-6B5D8)
D6-A2160 Fumarylacetoacetase deficiency, chronic type
(M-27000) (F-6B5D8)
Chronic tyrosinosis
(M-27000) (F-6B5D8)
Tyrosinemia with hepatorenal dysfunction
(M-27000) (F-6B5D8)
Hereditary hypertyrosinemia, type I
(M-27000) (F-6B5D8)
D6-A2180 Alkaptonuria 270.2
(M-27000) (F-67138)
Homogentisic acid oxidase deficiency 270.2
(M-27000) (F-67138)
Homogentisicaciduria 270.2
(M-27000) (F-67138)
Homogentisate 1,2-dioxygenase deficiency 270.2
(M-27000) (F-67138)
D6-A2182 Ochronosis 270.2
Alkaptonuric ochronosis 270.2
D6-A2185 Ochronotic arthritis 270.2 —713.0*

6-A24-A26 Albinism

D6-A2400 Albinism, NOS 270.2
Albinismus, NOS 270.2
D6-A2410 Oculocutaneous albinism, NOS 270.2
Complete perfect albinism 270.2
Albinismus totalis 270.2
Albinismus universalis 270.2
Total albinism 270.2
Complete universal albinism 270.2
D6-A2412 Tyrosinase-negative oculocutaneous albinism 270.2
(M-27000) (F-67440)
D6-A2414 Tyrosinase-positive oculocutaneous albinism 270.2
D6-A2420 Hermansky-Pudlak syndrome 270.2
Albinism with hemorrhagic diathesis 270.2
D6-A2430 Chédiak-Higashi syndrome 270.2
Congenital gigantism of peroxidase granules 270.2
Granulation anomaly of leukocytes 270.2
Hereditary gigantism of cytoplasmic organelles 270.2
Béguez César disease 270.2
Chédiak anomaly 270.2
Chédiak-Steinbrinck anomaly 270.2
Hereditary leukomelanopathy 270.2
Steinbrinck anomaly 270.2
D6-A2440 Cross syndrome 270.2
Oculocerebral-hypopigmentation syndrome 270.2

D6-A2440 (cont.) Hypopigmentation and microphthalmia 270.2
Gingival fibromatosis, hypopigmentation, microphthalmia, oligophrenia and athetosis 270.2
D6-A2450 Brown oculocutaneous albinism 270.2
Brown albinism 270.2
D6-A2456 Rufous albinism 270.2
Red-skin albinism 270.2
D6-A2460 Autosomal dominant oculocutaneous albinism 270.2
D6-A2470 Yellow mutant oculocutaneous albinism 270.2
Amish albinism 270.2
Xanthos albinism 270.2
Yellow-type albinism 270.2
D6-A2480 Black locks, oculocutaneous albinism, and deafness of the sensorineural type 270.2
BADS syndrome 270.2
D6-A2500 Ocular albinism, NOS 270.2 —743.8*
D6-A2510 X-linked ocular albinism, Nettleship type 270.2 —743.8*
D6-A2520 Autosomal recessive ocular albinism 270.2 —743.8*
D6-A2530 Ocular albinism-lentigines-deafness syndrome 270.2 —743.8*
D6-A2540 Forsius-Eriksson syndrome 270.2 —743.8*
Aland eye disease and ocular albinism 270.2 —743.8*
D6-A2600 Albinoidism, NOS 270.2
D6-A2610 Oculocutaneous albinoidism 270.2
D6-A2614 Punctate oculocutaneous albinoidism 270.2
D6-A2620 Hypopigmentation-immunodeficiency disease 270.2
Giscelli syndrome 270.2
D6-A2630 Partial albinism 270.2
Piebaldism 270.2
D6-A2640 Woolf's syndrome 270.2
D6-A2650 Waardenburg's syndrome 270.2

6-A3 DISORDERS OF HISTIDINE METABOLISM AND OF THE GAMMA-GLUTAMYL CYCLE

D6-A3100 Disorder of histidine metabolism, NOS 270.5
D6-A3102 Neonatal hyperhistidinemia 775.8
D6-A3110 Histidine ammonia-lyase deficiency
(M-27000) (F-6C800)
Histidinemia 270.5
(M-27000) (F-6C800)
D6-A3120 Urocanate hydratase deficiency
(M-27000) (F-6C670)
Urocanase deficiency 270.5
(M-27000) (F-6C670)
Urocanic aciduria 270.5
(M-27000) (F-6C670)
D6-A3130 Aminoacyl-histidine dipeptidase deficiency
(M-27000) (F-6AB78)
Serum carnosinase deficiency 270.5
(M-27000) (F-6AB78)
Carnosinuria 270.5
(M-27000) (F-6AB78)
Carnosinemia
(M-27000) (F-6AB78)
Carnosinase deficiency
(M-27000) (F-6AB78)
Hyper-beta-carnosinemia
(M-27000) (F-6AB78)
D6-A3190 Imidazole aminoaciduria 270.5
D6-A3500 Disorder of the gamma-glutamyl cycle, NOS 270.8
D6-A3505 Inborn error of glutathione metabolism, NOS 270.8
D6-A3510 Glutathione synthase deficiency with 5-oxoprolinuria
(M-27000) (F-6E278)
5-Oxoprolinuria 270.8
(M-27000) (F-6E278)
Pyroglutamic aciduria 270.8
(M-27000) (F-6E278)
D6-A3520 Glutathione synthase deficiency without 5-oxoprolinuria 270.8
(M-27000) (F-6E278)
D6-A3530 Glutathione S-transferase deficiency
(M-27000) (F-68D30)
D6-A3550 Glutamate-cysteine ligase deficiency
(M-27000) (F-6E270)
gamma-Glutamylcysteine synthetase deficiency 270.8
(M-27000) (F-6E270)
D6-A3560 gamma-Glutamyltransferase deficiency
(M-27000) (F-686C8)
gamma-Glutamyl transpeptidase deficiency 270.8
(M-27000) (F-686C8)
Glutathioninuria
(M-27000) (F-686C8)
D6-A3570 5-Oxoprolinase deficiency 270.8
Pyroglutamate hydrolase deficiency 270.8

6-A4 DISORDERS OF PROLINE AND HYDROXYPROLINE METABOLISM

D6-A4000 Disorder of proline and hydroxyproline metabolism, NOS 270.8
Iminoacidopathy, NOS 270.8
D6-A4100 Hyperprolinemia, NOS 270.8
D6-A4110 Proline dehydrogenase deficiency 270.8
(M-27000) (F-66E70)
Hyperprolinemia, type I 270.8
(M-27000) (F-66E70)
Proline oxidase deficiency 270.8
(M-27000) (F-66E70)
D6-A4120 Pyrroline-5-carboxylate reductase deficiency
(M-27000) (F-66D78)
Hyperprolinemia, type II 270.8
(M-27000) (F-66D78)

6-A4 DISORDERS OF PROLINE AND HYDROXYPROLINE METABOLISM — Continued

D6-A4120 (cont.) delta'-Pyrroline-5-carboxylate dehydrogenase deficiency
(M-27000) (F-66D78)

D6-A4130 Hyperhydroxyprolinemia 270.8
Hydroxyprolinemia 270.8

D6-A4140 Proline dipeptidase deficiency 270.8
(M-27000) (F-6ABA8)
Prolidase deficiency with hyperimidodipeptiduria 270.8
(M-27000) (F-6ABA8)
Prolidase deficiency 270.8
(M-27000) (F-6ABA8)
Iminodipeptiduria 270.8
(M-27000) (F-6ABA8)
Hyperimidodipeptiduria 270.8
(M-27000) (F-6ABA8)

D6-A4150 Hyperdicarboxylicaminoaciduria and hyperprolinemia 270.8

D6-A4170 Prolinuria 270.8

D6-A4172 Glycoprolinuria 270.8

D6-A4174 Glucoglycinuria 270.8

D6-A4190 Pipecolic acidemia 270.7

6-A5 DISORDERS OF THE UREA CYCLE METABOLISM

D6-A5000 Disorder of the urea cycle metabolism, NOS 270.6

D6-A5100 Hyperornithinemia, NOS 270.6

D6-A5110 Gyrate atrophy of the choroid and retina 270.6
(M-27000) (F-68E18)
Ornithine-delta-aminotransferase deficiency 270.6
(M-27000) (F-68E18)
Ornithine-oxo-acid amino acid transferase deficiency 270.6
(M-27000) (F-68E18)
OAT deficiency 270.6
(M-27000) (F-68E18)
OKT deficiency 270.6
(M-27000) (F-68E18)
Ornithinemia with gyrate atrophy 270.6
(M-27000) (F-68E18)
Ornithine ketoacid transaminase deficiency 270.6
(M-27000) (F-68E18)

D6-A5120 Hyperornithinemia-hyperammonemia-homocitrullinuria syndrome 270.6
(M-27000) (F-6C180)

D6-A5200 Hyperammonemia, NOS 270.6

D6-A5210 Congenital hyperammonemia, type I 270.6
(M-27000) (F-6E380)
Carbomyl-phosphate synthethase deficiency 270.6
(M-27000) (F-6E380)
CPS deficiency 270.6
(M-27000) (F-6E380)
CPS I deficiency 270.6
(M-27000) (F-6E380)

D6-A5220 Ornithine carbamoyltransferase deficiency 270.6
(M-27000) (F-683C8)
Ornithine transcarbamylase deficiency 270.6
(M-27000) (F-683C8)
OCTD 270.6
(M-27000) (F-683C8)
OCT deficiency 270.6
(M-27000) (F-683C8)

D6-A5230 Hyperammonemia, type III 270.6
(M-27000) (F-68410)
N-acetylglutamate synthetase deficiency 270.6
(M-27000) (F-68410)
Amino acid acetyltransferase deficiency 270.6
(M-27000) (F-68410)
N-acetylglutamate transferase deficiency 270.6
(M-27000) (F-68410)
AGA deficiency 270.6
(M-27000) (F-68410)
Congenital AGA deficiency 270.6
(M-27000) (F-68410)

D6-A5300 Citrullinemia 270.6
(M-27000) (F-6E328)
Arginosuccinate synthetase deficiency 270.6
(M-27000) (F-6E328)
Argininosuccinate synthase deficiency 270.6
(M-27000) (F-6E328)
Argininosuccinase deficiency 270.6
(M-27000) (F-6E328)
ASAS deficiency 270.6
(M-27000) (F-6E328)
ASA synthase deficiency 270.6
(M-27000) (F-6E328)
ASS deficiency 270.6
(M-27000) (F-6E328)
Citrullinuria 270.6
(M-27000) (F-6E328)

D6-A5301 Citrullinemia, neonatal type

D6-A5302 Citrullinemia, subacute type 270.6

D6-A5303 Citrullinemia, late-onset type 270.6

D6-A5310 Argininosuccinate lyase deficiency 270.6
(M-27000) (F-6C858)
Argininosuccinic aciduria 270.6
(M-27000) (F-6C858)
ASAL deficiency 270.6
(M-27000) (F-6C858)
ASL deficiency 270.6
(M-27000) (F-6C858)

D6-A5320 Arginase deficiency 270.6
(M-27000) (F-6B318)
Argininemia 270.6
(M-27000) (F-6B318)
Hyperargininemia 270.6
(M-27000) (F-6B318)
ARGI deficiency 270.6
(M-27000) (F-6B318)

D6-A5400 Transient hyperammonemia in infancy 775.8

6-A6 DISORDERS OF LYSINE, HYDROXYLYSINE AND GLYCINE METABOLISM

6-A61 Disorders of Lysine and Hydroxylysine Metabolism

D6-A6100 Disorder of lysine and hydroxylysine metabolism, NOS

D6-A6110 Hyperlysinemia, NOS 270.7

D6-A6120 Persistent hyperlysinemia 270.7
Persistent hyperlysinemia without hyperammonemia 270.7

D6-A6130 Periodic hyperlysinemia 270.7
Periodic hyperlysinemia with hyperammonemia 270.7
Lysine intolerance 270.7
Hyperlysinuria with hyperammonemia 270.7

D6-A6150 Saccharopinuria 270.7

6-A64 Disorders of Glycine Metabolism

D6-A6400 Disorder of glycine metabolism, NOS

D6-A6410 Hyperglycinemia, NOS 270.7

D6-A6412 Transient neonatal hyperglycinemia

D6-A6420 Glycine dehydrogenase (decarboxylating) deficiency 270.7
(M-27000) (F-66D48)
Nonketotic hyperglycinemia, type I 270.7
(M-27000) (F-66D48)
Glycine decarboxylase deficiency 270.7
(M-27000) (F-66D48)
P-protein deficiency 270.7
(M-27000) (F-66D48)

D6-A6430 Aminomethyltransferase deficiency
(M-27000) (F-683A8)
Nonketotic hyperglycinemia, type II
(M-27000) (F-683A8)
T-protein deficiency
(M-27000) (F-683A8)
Tetrahydrofolate aminomethyltransferase deficiency
(M-27000) (F-683A8)

D6-A6450 Sarcosine dehydrogenase deficiency 270.8
(M-27000) (F-66E38)
Hypersarcosinemia 270.8
(M-27000) (F-66E38)
Sarcosinemia 270.8
(M-27000) (F-66E38)
Sarcosinuria 270.8
(M-27000) (F-66E38)
Deficiency of the sarcosine dehydrogenase complex 270.8
(M-27000) (F-66E38)
Demethylation defect of N-methylglycine 270.8
(M-27000) (F-66E38)

D6-A6480 Renal glycinuria 270.0

6-B0 DISORDERS OF BRANCHED-CHAIN AMINO ACID AND ORGANIC ACID METABOLISM

D6-B0000 Disturbance of branched-chain amino acid and organic acid metabolism, NOS 270.3
Branched-chain hyperaminoacidemia, NOS 270.3

D6-B0010 Intermittent branched-chain ketonuria 270.3

D6-B0100 Maple syrup urine disease, NOS 270.3
(M-27000) (F-66A60)
Branched-chain alpha-keto acid dehydrogenase deficiency 270.3
(M-27000) (F-66A60)
BCKD deficiency 270.3
(M-27000) (F-66A60)
MSUD 270.3
(M-27000) (F-66A60)
Ketoacid decarboxylase deficiency
(M-27000) (F-66A60)

D6-B0110 Classical maple syrup urine disease 270.3

D6-B0120 Intermittent maple syrup urine disease 270.3
Intermittent branched-chain ketoaciduria 270.3

D6-B0124 Mild maple syrup urine disease 270.3

D6-B0140 Thiamin-responsive maple syrup urine disease

D6-B0150 Maple syrup urine disease, multiple dehydrogenase form 270.3
Maple syrup urine disease, E3 deficiency 270.3

D6-B0200 Hypervalinemia 270.3
Valine transaminase deficiency 270.3
Valinemia 270.3

D6-B0210 Hyperleucine-isoleucinemia 270.3

D6-B0230 Isovaleryl-CoA dehydrogenase deficiency 270.3
(M-27000) (F-66C30)
Isovaleric acidemia 270.3
(M-27000) (F-66C30)
Isovaleric acid CoA dehydrogenase deficiency 270.3
(M-27000) (F-66C30)

D6-B0250 Hyperleucinemia 270.3
Leucinosis 270.3

6-B1 DISORDERS OF PROPIONATE AND METHYMALONATE METABOLISM

D6-B1000 Disorder of propionate and methylmalonate metabolism, NOS 270.3
D6-B1400 Propionic acidemia, NOS 270.3
D6-B1410 Propionyl-CoA carboxylase deficiency 270.3
(M-27000) (F-6E3C0)
Propionic acidemia, type I 270.3
(M-27000) (F-6E3C0)
Propionic acidemia, type II 270.3
(M-27000) (F-6E3C0)
Hyperglycinemia with ketosis and leukopenia, types I and II 270.3
(M-27000) (F-6E3C0)
Ketotic glycinemia, types I and II 270.3
(M-27000) (F-6E3C0)
D6-B1420 Biotin-(propionyl-CoA-carboxylase) ligase deficiency 270.3
(M-27000) (F-6E350)
Neonatal multiple carboxylase deficiency 270.3
(M-27000) (F-6E350)
Neonatal biotin-responsive multiple carboxylase deficiency 270.3
(M-27000) (F-6E350)
Holocarboxylase synthetase deficiency
(M-27000) (F-6E350)
D6-B1500 Methylmalonic acidemia, NOS 270.3
D6-B1510 Methylmalonyl-CoA mutase deficiency 270.3
D6-B1530 Adenosylcobalamin synthesis defect, NOS
Methylmalonic aciduria, type II
D6-B1532 Cobalamin A disease
D6-B1536 Cobalamin B disease
D6-B1550 Adenosylcobalamin and methylcobalamin synthesis defect, NOS
D6-B1552 Cobalamin C disease
D6-B1556 Cobalamin D disease
D6-B1580 Inherited methylmalonic acidemia and homocystinuria 270.3

6-B2 NON-AMINO ORGANIC ACIDEMIAS AND ACIDURIAS

D6-B2000 Non-amino organic acidemia and aciduria, NOS
D6-B2100 Glutaric aciduria, NOS
D6-B2110 Glutaric aciduria, type 1
(M-27000) (F-66C18)
Glutaric acidemia, type 1
(M-27000) (F-66C18)
GA I
(M-27000) (F-66C18)
D6-B2120 Glutaric aciduria, type 2 270.3
(M-27000) (F-66BE8)
Ethylmalonic-adipicaciduria 270.3
(M-27000) (F-66BE8)
ACAD 270.3
(M-27000) (F-66BE8)
EMA 270.3
(M-27000) (F-66BE8)
Glutaric acidemia, type 2 270.3
(M-27000) (F-66BE8)
GA II 270.3
(M-27000) (F-66BE8)
D6-B2122 X-linked glutaric aciduria, type 2 270.3
GA II A 270.3
D6-B2124 Autosomal recessive glutaric aciduria, type 2 270.3
GA II B 270.3
D6-B2200 Methylcrotonic aciduria, NOS 270.3
D6-B2210 Methylcrotonyl-CoA carboxylase deficiency 270.3
(M-27000) (F-6E3C8)
BMCC deficiency 270.3
(M-27000) (F-6E3C8)
MCC deficiency 270.3
(M-27000) (F-6E3C8)
3-Methylcrotonylglycinuria, type 1 270.3
(M-27000) (F-6E3C8)
D6-B2230 Biotinidase deficiency
(M-27000) (F-6B188)
Juvenile multiple carboxylase deficiency
(M-27000) (F-6B188)
Late-onset multiple carboxylase deficiency
(M-27000) (F-6B188)
D6-B2240 Hydroxymethylglutaryl-CoA lyase deficiency
(M-27000) (F-6C3F8)
HMG-CoA lyase deficiency 270.3
(M-27000) (F-6C3F8)
Hydroxymethylglutaric aciduria
(M-27000) (F-6C3F8)
D6-B2250 Acetyl-CoA: acyltransferase deficiency 270.3
(M-27000) (F-68450)
3-Ketothiolase deficiency 270.3
(M-27000) (F-68450)
alpha-Methylacetoacetic aciduria 270.3
(M-27000) (F-68450)
3-Methylhydroxybutyric acidemia 270.3
(M-27000) (F-68450)
D6-B2260 Acetyl-CoA: carboxylase deficiency
(M-27000) (F-6E3B8)
ACC deficiency
(M-27000) (F-6E3B8)

6-B3 INHERITED DISORDERS OF FOLATE METABOLISM

D6-B3000 Inherited disorder of folate metabolism, NOS 270.8
D6-B3100 Congenital defect of folate absorption 270.8
Folic acid transport defect 270.8
Congenital malabsorption of folic acid 270.8
D6-B3110 Dihydrofolate reductase deficiency 270.8
(M-27000) (F-66D80)
D6-B3120 Glutamate formiminotransferase deficiency 270.8
FIGLUria 270.8

D6-B3120 (cont.) Formiminoglutamic aciduria 270.8

D6-B3130 Methylene THF reductase deficiency and homocystinuria 270.8
(M-27000) (F-68170)

D6-B3140 Tetrahydrofolate methyltransferase deficiency 270.8
THF methyltransferase deficiency 270.8

6-B4 DISORDERS OF SULPHUR-BEARING AMINO ACID METABOLISM

D6-B4000 Disorder of sulphur-bearing amino acid metabolism, NOS 270.4
Disorder of transsulfuration, NOS 270.4

D6-B4100 Homocystinuria, NOS 270.4

D6-B4110 Cystathionine beta-synthase deficiency 270.4
(M-27000) (F-6C5A8)
CBS deficiency 270.4
(M-27000) (F-6C5A8)

D6-B4120 5,10-Methylenetetrahydrofolate reductase deficiency
(M-27000) (F-66FC8)

D6-B4130 Cystathionine gamma-lyase deficiency
(M-27000) (F-6C870)
gamma-Cystathionase deficiency 270.4
(M-27000) (F-6C870)

D6-B4180 Homocystinemia, NOS

D6-B4182 Cystathioninuria, NOS 270.4

D6-B4184 Cystathioninemia, NOS 270.4

D6-B4300 Hypermethioninemia, NOS 270.4

D6-B4302 Neonatal hypermethioninemia 775.8

D6-B4310 Hepatic methionine adenosyltransferase deficiency 270.4
(M-27000) (F-68CE8)
MAT deficiency 270.4
(M-27000) (F-68CE8)

D6-B4320 Familial methionine malabsorption 270.2
Methionine malabsorption syndrome 270.2
Oast-house urine disease 270.2
Beery-baby syndrome 270.2
Oast-house disease 270.2
Smith-Strang disease 270.2

D6-B4400 4-Hydroxyphenylpyruvate dioxygenase deficiency
(M-27000) (F-671E0)
Hawkinsinuria
(M-27000) (F-671E0)

D6-B4900 Sulfite oxidase deficiency syndrome 277.8
(M-27000) (F-66FF0)
Sulfocysteinuria 277.8
(M-27000) (F-66FF0)

6-B5 CYSTINOSIS

D6-B5300 Cystinosis, NOS 270.0
Cystine storage disease 270.0
Cystine diathesis 270.0
Cystine disease 270.0

D6-B5310 Infantile nephropathic cystinosis 270.0
Nephropathic cystinosis 270.0

D6-B5320 Juvenile nephropathic cystinosis 270.0
Adolescent cystinosis 270.0
Late-onset cystinosis 270.0
Intermediate cystinosis 270.0
Cystinosis, type II 270.0
Juvenile cystinosis 270.0

D6-B5330 Benign adult cystinosis 270.0
Benign cystinosis 270.0

6-B6 DISORDERS OF BETA-ALANINE, CARNOSINE AND HOMOCARNOSINE METABOLISM

D6-B6000 Disorder of beta alanine, carnosine and homocarnosine metabolism, NOS 270.8

D6-B6100 Hyper-beta-alaninemia 270.8
Hyperalaninemia 270.8

D6-B6110 Succinate-semialdehyde dehydrogenase deficiency 270.8
(M-27000) (F-66950)
gamma-Hydroxybutyric aciduria 270.8
(M-27000) (F-66950)
GABAuria 270.8
(M-27000) (F-66950)
GABA metabolic defect 270.8
(M-27000) (F-66950)

D6-B6220 Homocarnosinase deficiency 270.8
(M-27000) (F-6ABC8)
Homocarnosinosis 270.5
(M-27000) (F-6ABC8)

6-B7 DISORDERS OF FATTY ACID METABOLISM

D6-B7000 Disorder of fatty acid metabolism, NOS

D6-B7100 Acyl-CoA dehydrogenase deficiency, NOS
(M-27000) (F-66BF8)

D6-B7200 Phytanic acid storage disease 356.3
(F-61580)
Refsum's disease 356.3
(F-61580)
Refsum syndrome 356.3
(F-61580)
Refsum-Thiébaut disease 356.3
(F-61580)
Heredoataxia hemeralopica polyneuritiformis 356.3
(F-61580)
Heredopathia atactica polyneuritiformis 356.3
(F-61580)

D6-B7300 Muscle carnitine deficiency

D6-B7310 Renal carnitine transport defect
Systemic carnitine deficiency

D6-B7340 Carnitine palmitoyltransferase deficiency
(M-27000) (F-684B0)

6-B8 AMINO ACID TRANSPORT DISORDERS

D6-B8000 Amino acid transport disorder, NOS
D6-B8100 Histidine transport defect
Histidinuria
Hyperhistidinuria
Renal histidinuria
D6-B8200 Cystinuria, NOS 270.0
D6-B8210 Cystinuria, type 1 270.0
Recessive cystinuria 270.0
D6-B8220 Cystinuria, type 2 270.0
D6-B8230 Cystinuria, type 3 270.0
D6-B8240 Isolated cystinuria 270.0
Hypercystinuria 270.0
D6-B8300 Lysinuric protein intolerance, NOS 270.6
Hyperdibasic aminoaciduria, NOS 270.6
Congenital lysinuria 270.6
Dibasic aminoaciduria 270.6
D6-B8302 Neonatal cystine-lysinuria 775.8
D6-B8310 Lysinuric protein intolerance, type 1 270.6
D6-B8320 Lysinuric protein intolerance, type 2 270.6
D6-B8400 Neutral 1 amino acid transport defect 270.0
Hartnup disease 270.0
Hartnup disorder 270.0
D6-B8410 Hartnup disorder, renal type 270.0
D6-B8420 Hartnup disorder, renal/jejunal type 270.0
D6-B8500 Iminoglycinuria, NOS 270.8
D6-B8502 Neonatal iminoglycinuria 775.8
D6-B8510 Familial renal iminoglycinuria 270.8

SECTION 6-C VITAMIN-RELATED DISORDERS

D6-C0000 Vitamin disease, NOS
(F-BB000)
D6-C0100 Vitamin deficiency, NOS 269.2
(F-BB000)
Hypovitaminosis, NOS 269.2
(F-BB000)
D6-C0200 Vitamin A deficiency, NOS 264.9
(F-BB010)
Hypovitaminosis A, NOS 264.9
D6-C0202 Vitamin A deficiency with conjunctival xerosis 264.0 —372.5*
D6-C0204 Vitamin A deficiency with Bitot's spot and conjunctival xerosis 264.1 —372.5*
D6-C0210 Vitamin A deficiency with corneal xerosis 264.2 —371.4*
D6-C0212 Vitamin A deficiency with corneal ulceration and xerosis 264.3 —371.4*
D6-C0214 Vitamin A deficiency with keratomalacia 264.4 —371.4*
D6-C0220 Vitamin A deficiency with night blindness 264.5 —368.6*
D6-C0222 Vitamin A deficiency with xerophthalmia 264.7 —372.5*
D6-C0224 Vitamin A deficiency with xerophthalmic scars of cornea 264.6 —371.0*
D6-C0230 Vitamin A deficiency with xeroderma 264.8 —701.1*
D6-C0240 Vitamin A deficiency with follicular keratosis 264.8 —701.1*
D6-C0280 Vitamin A deficiency with other ocular manifestations 264.7
D6-C0300 Hypervitaminosis A 278.2
D6-C0310 Hypercarotinemia 278.3
D6-C0312 Carotenosis cutis 278.3
D6-C1000 Vitamin B deficiency, NOS 266.9
Vitamin B-complex deficiency, NOS 266.9
D6-C1100 Thiamin deficiency, NOS 265.1
(F-BB310)
Vitamin B1 deficiency, NOS 265.1
(F-BB310)
D6-C1110 Beriberi, NOS 265.0
D6-C1120 Wet beriberi 265.0
D6-C1130 Dry beriberi 265.0
D6-C1200 Pellagra 265.2
(F-BB430)
Niacin deficiency 265.2
(F-BB430)
Nicotinamide deficiency 265.2
(F-BB430)
Nicotinic acid deficiency 265.2
(F-BB430)
Vitamin PP deficiency 265.2
(F-BB430)
D6-C1210 Alcoholic pellagra 265.2
D6-C1300 Nicotinamide toxicity 963.5
D6-C1400 Vitamin B6 deficiency (non anemic) 266.1
(F-BB350)
Pyridoxine deficiency 266.1
(F-BB350)
Pyridoxamine deficiency 266.1
(F-BB350)
Pyridoxal deficiency 266.1
(F-BB350)
D6-C1500 Pyridoxine toxicity 963.5
D6-C1550 Pyridoxine dependency syndrome
D6-C1600 Ariboflavinosis 266.0
Riboflavin deficiency 266.0
Vitamin B2 deficiency 266.0
D6-C1650V Avian curley toe paralysis
Curled toe paralysis
Crooked toe disease
D6-C1700 Folic acid deficiency (non anemic) 266.2
(F-BB390)
D6-C1800 Vitamin B12 deficiency (non anemic) 266.2
(F-BB360)
Cyanocobalamine deficiency (non anemic) 266.2
(F-BB360)
D6-C1900 Other B-complex deficiencies 266.2
D6-C2000 Ascorbic acid deficiency 267.-
(F-BB370)
Vitamin C deficiency 267.-
(F-BB370)
Scurvy 267.-
(F-BB370)

D6-C2200 Ascorbic acid toxicity 963.5
D6-C3000 Vitamin K deficiency 269.0
(F-BB180)
D6-C3200 Vitamin E deficiency 269.1
(F-BB170)
D6-C3250V Nutritional steatitis
Yellow fat disease
Nutritional panniculitis
Pansteatitis
D6-C3300 Vitamin P deficiency 269.1
D6-C4000 Vitamin D deficiency, NOS 268.9
(F-BB070)
Avitaminosis D, NOS 268.9
(F-BB070)
D6-C4100 Vitamin D-dependent rickets, NOS 268.0
Active rickets 268.0
VDDR 268.0
D6-C4110 Vitamin D-dependent rickets, type 1 268.0
(M-27000) (F-67358)
Calcidiol 1-monooxygenase defect 268.0
(M-27000) (F-67358)
Pseudo-vitamin-D-deficient rickets 268.0
(M-27000) (F-67358)
VDDRI 268.0
(M-27000) (F-67358)
D6-C4120 Vitamin D-dependent rickets, type 2 268.0
Calcitriol receptor defect
D6-C4190 Late effects of rickets (one year or more)
268.1
D6-C4300 Osteomalacia 268.2
D6-C4800 Hypervitaminosis D 278.4

CHAPTER 7 — DISEASES OF THE GENITOURINARY SYSTEMS

D7-00000 Disease of the genitourinary system, NOS
Disorder of genitourinary system, NOS
Syndrome of the genitourinary system, NOS

SECTION 7-1 DISEASES AND SYNDROMES OF THE URINARY TRACT

7-10 URINARY TRACT DISEASES: GENERAL TERMS

D7-10000 Disease of urinary tract, NOS 599.9
Disorder of urinary tract, NOS 599.9
Syndrome of urinary tract, NOS 599.9
D7-10030 Urinary tract infectious disease, NOS 590.9 (T-70000) (DE-00000)
Urinary tract infection, NOS 590.9 (T-70000) (DE-00000)
D7-10040 Urinary tract obstruction, NOS 599.6
Obstructive uropathy, NOS 599.6
D7-10041 Partial obstruction of the urinary tract
D7-10042 Complete obstruction of the urinary tract
D7-10044 Urolith, NOS
Urinary calculus
Urinary stone
Urolithiasis, NOS
D7-10048V Feline urological syndrome
FUS
Feline urolithiasis
Fat lazy cat syndrome
D7-10050 Hematuria syndrome, NOS 599.7
D7-10052 Benign hematuria 599.7
Essential hematuria 599.7
D7-10054 Idiopathic myoglobinuria
Spontaneous myoglobinuria
Meyer-Betz disease
D7-10060 Urinary fistula, NOS 599.1

7-11 GENERAL CONDITIONS OF THE KIDNEY AND URETER

D7-11000 Kidney disease, NOS 593.9
Nephropathy, NOS 593.9
Renal disease, NOS 593.9
D7-11010 Renal failure syndrome, NOS 586.-
Renal insufficiency syndrome, NOS 586.-
D7-11011 Acute renal failure syndrome, NOS 584.9
D7-11013 Chronic renal failure syndrome, NOS 585.-
D7-11020 Uremia, NOS 586.-
D7-11022 Uremic acidosis 586.-
D7-11023 Chronic uremia 585.-
D7-11024 Uremic encephalopathy 585.-
D7-11026 Uremic neuropathy 585.-
D7-11028 Prerenal uremia syndrome 586.-
Extrarenal uremia syndrome 586.-
Blum's syndrome 586.-
Prerenal azotemia 586.-
D7-11050 End stage renal disease
End stage kidney disease
D7-11060 Nephrolithiasis, NOS 592.0
Kidney stone 592.0
D7-11200 Renal tubular defect, NOS
D7-11250 Proteinuria syndrome, NOS
Isolated non-nephrotic proteinuria
D7-11252 Benign postural proteinuria 593.6
D7-11270 Loin pain-hematuria syndrome
D7-11280 Nephrotic syndrome, NOS
D7-11282 Congenital nephrotic syndrome
Familial nephrotic syndrome
D7-11288 Nephrotic-nephritic syndrome
D7-11600 Small kidney, NOS 589.9
Small kidney of unknown cause 589.-
D7-11602 Unilateral small kidney 589.0
D7-11604 Bilateral small kidney 589.1
D7-11610 Nephroptosis 593.0
Floating kidney 593.0
Mobile kidney 593.0
D7-11620 Hypertrophy of kidney 593.1
D7-11700 Acute pyelitis
D7-11702 Acute pyelitis without renal medullary necrosis 590.10
D7-11704 Acute pyelitis with renal medullary necrosis 590.11
D7-11710 Acute pyonephrosis without renal medullary necrosis 590.10
D7-11712 Acute pyonephrosis with renal medullary necrosis 590.11
D7-11750 Renal abscess 590.2
Renal carbuncle 590.2
D7-11760 Perirenal abscess 590.2
D7-11800 Pyeloureteritis cystica 590.3
Ureteritis cystica 590.3
D7-11810 Calculous pyelonephritis 592.9
D7-11910 Dysuria-frequency syndrome
D7-11930 Ureterolithiasis 592.1
Ureteric stone 592.1
D7-11940 Stricture of ureter 593.3
D7-11942 Postoperative kinking of ureter 593.3
Postoperative angulation of ureter 593.3
D7-11946 Stricture of pelviureteric junction 593.3
D7-11950 Idiopathic retroperitoneal fibrosis 593.4
D7-11960 Occlusion of ureter, NOS 593.4
D7-11962 Occlusion of ureter due to calculus 592.1
D7-11970 Hydroureter, NOS 593.5
D7-11980 Pyoureter

7-12 RENAL GLOMERULAR AND TUBULOINTERSTITIAL DISEASES

7-120-123 Renal Glomerular Diseases

D7-12000 Renal glomerular disease, NOS
Renal glomerular syndrome, NOS
Renal glomerular disorder, NOS

D7-12010 Nephritic syndrome, NOS
D7-12020 Acute nephritis, NOS 580.9
D7-12030 Acute nephropathy, NOS 580.9
D7-12100 Acute glomerulonephritis, NOS 580.9
D7-12110 Acute post-streptococcal glomerulonephritis 580.0
D7-12120 Idiopathic crescentic glomerulonephritis, NOS 583.4
D7-12122 Idiopathic crescentic glomerulonephritis, type I 583.4
D7-12124 Idiopathic crescentic glomerulonephritis, type II 583.4
D7-12126 Idiopathic crescentic glomerulonephritis, type III 583.4
D7-12130 Primary IgA nephropathy
  Berger's disease
D7-12140 Minimal change disease
  Nil disease
D7-12150 Mesangial proliferative glomerulonephritis
D7-12160 Focal glomerular sclerosis
D7-12170 Membranous glomerulonephritis
D7-12180 Mesangiocapillary glomerulonephritis, NOS
D7-12182 Mesangiocapillary glomerulonephritis, type I
D7-12184 Mesangiocapillary glomerulonephritis, type II
D7-12190 Focal and segmental proliferative glomerulonephritis
D7-12200 Diffuse crescentic glomerulonephritis
D7-12210 Diffuse endocapillary proliferative glomerulonephritis
D7-12220 Diffuse mesangial sclerosis
D7-12230 Fibrillary glomerulonephritis
D7-12300 Chronic glomerulonephritis, NOS
D7-12310 Acute benign hemorrhagic glomerulonephritic syndrome
  Recurrent hematuria syndrome
  Idiopathic benign hematuria of childhood
D7-12320 Hereditary nephritis
  Alport's syndrome
  Familial nephritis
  Familial hematuria
D7-12330 Focal embolic nephritis syndrome
D7-12340 Goodpasture's syndrome 446.2
  Pulmonary-renal syndrome 446.2
  Lung purpura with nephritis syndrome 446.2
  Pulmonary hemorrhage with glomerulonephritis 446.2
  Hemorrhagic pneumonia and glomerulonephritis 446.2
  Pulmonary hemosiderosis with glomerulonephritis 446.2
  Anti-GBM nephritis with pulmonary hemorrhage 446.2
D7-12350 Shunt nephritis
D7-12380 SLE glomerulonephritis syndrome, NOS
D7-12381 SLE glomerulonephritis syndrome, WHO class I
  SLE with normal kidneys
D7-12382 SLE glomerulonephritis syndrome, WHO class II
  SLE with mesangial proliferative glomerulonephritis
D7-12383 SLE glomerulonephritis syndrome, WHO class III
  SLE with focal and segmental proliferative glomerulonephritis
D7-12384 SLE glomerulonephritis syndrome, WHO class IV
  SLE with diffuse proliferative glomerulonephritis
D7-12385 SLE glomerulonephritis syndrome, WHO class V
  SLE with membranous glomerulonephritis
  Membranous lupus glomerulonephritis
D7-12386 SLE glomerulonephritis syndrome, WHO class VI
  SLE with advanced sclerosing glomerulonephritis
  Lupus with glomerular sclerosis

7-124-126 Tubulointerstitial Diseases

D7-12400 Interstitial nephritis, NOS
  Tubulointerstitial nephropathy, NOS
  T.I.N., NOS
D7-12410 Acute interstitial nephritis, NOS
  Acute T.I.N., NOS
  Acute tubulointerstitial disease, NOS
D7-12419 Acute tubular necrosis, NOS
D7-12420 Chronic interstitial nephritis, NOS
  Chronic T.I.N., NOS
  Chronic tubulointerstitial nephritis, NOS
D7-12430 Acute infectious tubulointerstitial nephritis, NOS
D7-12432 Acute bacterial tubulointerstitial nephritis 590.1
  Acute bacterial T.I.N. 590.1
  Acute pyelonephritis 590.1
D7-12434 Acute fungal tubulointerstitial nephritis
  Acute fungal T.I.N.
D7-12436 Acute viral tubulointerstitial nephritis
  Acute viral T.I.N.
D7-12438 Acute tubulointerstitial nephritis associated with systemic infection
D7-12440 Acute drug-induced tubulointerstitial nephritis
  Acute tubulointerstitial nephritis due to hypersensitivity to drugs
D7-12450 Chronic drug-induced tubulointerstitial nephritis, NOS
  Chronic drug-induced T.I.N., NOS
  Toxic nephropathy, NOS
D7-12452 Analgesic nephropathy
D7-12454 Lithium nephropathy
D7-12456 Cis-platinum nephropathy
D7-12458 Methyl CCNU nephropathy
D7-12460 Chronic gouty nephropathy 274.10 —583.8*
  Urate nephropathy 274.10 —583.8*

7-124-126 Tubulointerstitial Diseases — Continued

D7-12462 Uric acid nephropathy 274.11 —592.0*
  Uric acid nephrolithiasis 274.11 —592.0*
D7-12470 Oxalate nephropathy, NOS
D7-12471 Oxalate nephropathy, type I
D7-12472 Oxalate nephropathy, type II
D7-12474 Secondary oxalosis, NOS
D7-12480 Hypercalcemic nephropathy
D7-12490 Hypokalemic nephropathy 588.8
D7-12494 Heavy metal nephropathy
D7-12495 Radiographic contrast agent nephropathy
D7-12500 Immunologic mediated T.I.N., NOS
D7-12502 Anti-GBM T.I.N.
D7-12510 Idiopathic chronic interstitial nephritis
D7-12514V White spotted kidney disease
  Focal nonsuppurative interstitial nephritis in calves
D7-12520 Idiopathic acute interstitial nephritis
D7-12530 Balkan nephropathy
D7-12540 Idiopathic granulomatous interstitial nephropathy, NOS
D7-12542 Granulomatous sarcoid nephropathy
D7-12560 Light chain nephropathy
D7-12562 Myeloma kidney 593.9
D7-12570 Salt-losing nephropathy 593.9
  Salt-losing nephritis 593.9
  Pseudo-Addison's disease
  Thorn's syndrome
D7-12572 Salt-wasting syndrome of infancy
D7-12600 Pyelonephritis, NOS 590.80
D7-12610 Pyelitis, NOS 590.80
D7-12620 Reflux nephropathy
  Nephropathy associated with vesicoureteral reflux
D7-12630 Obstructive nephropathy, NOS
D7-12640 Hereditary tubulointerstitial disorder, NOS
D7-12650 Familial interstitial nephritis

7-13 RENAL VASCULAR DISORDERS

D7-13000 Renal vascular disorder, NOS
D7-13010 Thromboembolism of renal arteries
D7-13020 Atheroembolism of renal arteries
D7-13030 Renal vein thrombosis
D7-13100 Hemolytic uremic syndrome, NOS
D7-13104 Hemolytic uremic syndrome of childhood
  HUS, childhood type
D7-13106 Hemolytic uremic syndrome, adult type
  HUS, adult type
D7-13120 Arteriolar nephrosclerosis, NOS
D7-13124 Benign arteriolar nephrosclerosis
D7-13128 Malignant arteriolar nephrosclerosis
D7-13140 Sickle-cell nephropathy
D7-13150 Renal infarction
D7-13160 Papillary necrosis
  Renal medullary necrosis
D7-13170 Radiation nephritis

7-14 ACQUIRED RENAL CYSTIC DISEASES

D7-14010 Simple renal cyst 593.2
D7-14012 Solitary multilocular cyst
D7-14020 Acquired polycystic kidney disease 593.2
D7-14030 Peripelvic lymphatic cyst 593.2
D7-14100 Hydronephrosis 591.-
D7-14110 Hydrocalycosis 591.-
D7-14120 Hydroureteronephrosis 591.-

7-15 MISCELLANEOUS METABOLIC RENAL DISEASES

D7-15030 Renal phosphaturia
  Phosphate diabetes
D7-15040 Pseudohyperparathyroidism
D7-15050 Secondary hyperparathyroidism of renal origin 588.8
D7-15220 Milk alkali syndrome 999.9
  Burnett's syndrome 999.9
D7-15221 Acute milk alkali syndrome 999.9
D7-15222 Subacute milk alkali syndrome 999.9
D7-15223 Chronic milk alkali syndrome 999.9
D7-15240 Scriver-Goldbloom-Roy syndrome
D7-15350 Renal osteodystrophy
  Renal rickets
D7-15354 Renal dwarfism 588.0
D7-15356V Renal secondary osteodystrophia fibrosa
  Rubber jaw syndrome
D7-15360 Dialysis disequilibrium syndrome
D7-15370 Dialysis dementia
D7-15404 Dipsogenic diabetes insipidus
  Primary polydipsia
D7-15406 Nephrogenic diabetes insipidus 588.1
D7-15408 Polyuric state, NOS
D7-15610 Hyponatremia with extracellular fluid depletion
D7-15612 Hyponatremia with excess extracellular fluid volume
D7-15614 Hyponatremia with normal extracellular fluid volume

SECTION 7-2 DISEASES OF THE LOWER URINARY TRACT

7-20 DISEASES OF THE LOWER URINARY TRACT: GENERAL CONDITIONS

D7-20000 Disease of the lower urinary tract, NOS
  Disorder of the lower urinary tract, NOS
  Syndrome of the lower urinary tract, NOS

7-21 DISEASES OF THE BLADDER

D7-21000 Disease of bladder, NOS 596.9
  Disorder of bladder, NOS 596.9
D7-21100 Cystitis, NOS 595.9
D7-21110 Acute cystitis 595.0
D7-21120 Chronic interstitial cystitis 595.1
  Panmural fibrosis of bladder 595.1
  Submucous cystitis 595.1

D7-21126 Hunner's ulcer 595.1
D7-21130 Chronic cystitis, NOS 595.2
D7-21140 Subacute cystitis, NOS 595.2
D7-21160 Trigonitis, NOS 595.3
D7-21170 Acute trigonitis 595.3
D7-21180 Chronic trigonitis 595.3
D7-21190 Follicular cystitis 595.3
D7-211A0 Urethrotrigonitis 595.3
D7-21200 Cystitis with actinomycosis 595.4 —038.8!
D7-21202 Cystitis with amebiasis 595.4 —006.8!
D7-21204 Cystitis with bilharziasis 595.4 —120.9!
D7-21206 Cystitis with Echinococcus infestation 595.4 —122.6!
D7-21210 Cystitis cystica 595.81
D7-21220 Irradiation cystitis 595.82
D7-21230 Bullous cystitis 595.89
D7-21234 Emphysematous cystitis 595.89
D7-21240 Cystitis glandularis 595.89
D7-21250 Abscess of bladder 595.89
D7-21260 Malakoplakia of bladder 596.8
D7-21400 Bladder neck obstruction, NOS 596.0
  Acquired bladder neck obstruction, NOS 596.0
  Vesicourethral orifice obstruction, NOS 596.0
D7-21410 Acquired contracture of bladder neck 596.0
D7-21420 Acquired stenosis of bladder neck 596.0
D7-21500 Bladder fistula, NOS 596.2
D7-21510 Vesicocolic fistula 596.1
D7-21520 Vesicorectal fistula 596.1
D7-21530 Intestinovesical fistula 596.1
  Enterovesical fistula 596.1
  Vesicoenteric fistula 596.1
D7-21540 Urethrovesical fistula 596.2
D7-21550 Vesicocutaneous fistula 596.2
D7-21560 Vesicoperineal fistula 596.2
D7-21580 Diverticulum of bladder 596.3
  Acquired diverticulum of bladder 596.3
  False diverticulum of bladder 596.3
D7-21590 Diverticulitis of bladder 596.3
D7-21600 Atony of bladder 596.4
  Hypotonicity of bladder 596.4
  Inertia of bladder 596.4
  High compliance bladder 596.4
D7-21610 Hypertonicity of bladder 596.5
  Low compliance bladder 596.5
D7-21620 Paralysis of bladder 596.5
D7-21622 Detrusor instability of bladder 596.5
  Detrusor dyssynergia 596.5
D7-21700 Nontraumatic rupture of bladder 596.6
D7-21704 Ruptured bladder with uroperitoneum
D7-21710 Hemorrhage into bladder wall 596.7
D7-21720 Hyperemia of bladder 596.7
D7-21730 Calcification of bladder 596.8
  Calcified bladder 596.8
D7-21740 Contracted bladder 596.8
D7-21750 Hypertrophy of bladder 596.8
D7-21760 Hemorrhage into bladder lumen 596.8
D7-21800 Calculus of lower urinary tract, NOS 594.9
D7-21810 Urinary bladder stone 594.1
D7-21820 Calculus in diverticulum of bladder 594.0

7-23 DISEASES OF THE URETHRA

D7-23000 Disease of urethra, NOS 599.9
  Disorder of urethra, NOS 599.9
D7-23100 Urethritis, NOS 597.80
D7-23110 Urethral syndrome, NOS 597.81
D7-23120 Skene's gland adenitis 597.89
D7-23130 Cowperitis 597.89
D7-23140 Urethral meatitis 597.89
D7-23150 Urethral ulcer 597.89
D7-23160 Verumontanitis 597.89
D7-23200 Urethral abscess, NOS 597.0
  Urethral gland abscess, NOS 597.0
D7-23210 Abscess of Cowper's gland 597.0
  Abscess of bulbourethral gland 597.0
D7-23220 Abscess of Littré's glands 597.0
D7-23230 Periurethral abscess 597.0
D7-23240 Periurethral cellulitis 597.0
D7-23300 Urethral stricture, NOS 598.9
D7-23310 Pinhole meatus 598.9
  Stricture of urethral meatus 598.9
D7-23320 Urethral stricture due to infection, NOS 598.00
D7-23322 Urethral stricture due to gonococcal infection 598.01 —098.2!
D7-23324 Urethral stricture due to schistosomiasis 598.01 —120.9!
D7-23326 Urethral stricture due to syphilis 598.1 —095.8!
D7-23330 Traumatic urethral stricture 598.1
D7-23340 Postobstetric urethral stricture 598.1
D7-23350 Postoperative urethral stricture 598.2
D7-23360 Postcatheterization urethral stricture 598.2
D7-23370 Calculus in urethra 594.2
  Urethral stone 594.2
D7-23510 Urethral fistula, NOS 599.1
D7-23520 Urethroperineal fistula 599.1
D7-23530 Urethrorectal fistula 599.1
D7-23540 Urethral diverticulum 599.2
D7-23550 Urethral caruncle 599.3
D7-23554 Polyp of urethra 599.3
D7-23560 Urethral false passage 599.4
D7-23570 Prolapse of urethra 599.5
  Urethrocele 599.5
D7-23630 Nontraumatic rupture of urethra 599.8
D7-23640 Urethral cyst 599.8
D7-23650 Urethral granuloma 599.8

SECTION 7-5 DISEASES OF THE MALE GENITAL ORGANS

7-50 DISEASES OF THE MALE GENITAL ORGANS: GENERAL TERMS

D7-50000 Disease of male genital organs, NOS 608.9
D7-50010 Edema of male genital organs 608.86

7-51 DISEASES OF THE PROSTATE

D7-51000 Disease of prostate, NOS 602.9
Disorder of prostate, NOS 602.9
D7-51010 Prostatitis, NOS 601.9
D7-51020 Acute prostatitis 601.0
D7-51030 Chronic prostatitis 601.1
D7-51040 Abscess of prostate 601.2
D7-51050 Prostatocystitis 601.3
D7-51060 Cavitary prostatitis 601.8
D7-51062 Diverticular prostatitis 601.8
D7-51066 Granulomatous prostatitis 601.8
D7-51070 Prostatitis in disease classified elsewhere 601.4
D7-51080 Other specified inflammation of prostate 601.8
D7-51200 Hyperplasia of prostate, NOS 600.-
Benign enlargement of prostate, NOS 600.-
Benign prostatic hyperplasia, NOS 600.-
BPH 600.-
Adenofibromatous hypertrophy of prostate, NOS 600.-
D7-51210 Benign adenoma of prostate 600.-
D7-51212 Fibroma of prostate 600.-
D7-51214 Fibroadenoma of prostate 600.-
D7-51216 Median bar of prostate 600.-
D7-51218 Myoma of prostate 600.-
D7-51220 Prostatic obstruction, NOS 600.-
D7-51224 Calculus of prostate 602.0
Prostatic stone 602.0
D7-51230 Congestion of prostate 602.1
D7-51240 Hemorrhage of prostate 602.1
D7-51250 Atrophy of prostate 602.2
D7-51300 Fistula of prostate 602.8
D7-51310 Infarction of prostate 602.8
D7-51320 Stricture of prostate 602.8
D7-51330 Periprostatic adhesions 602.8

7-52 DISEASES OF THE SEMINAL VESICLES

D7-52000 Disease of seminal vesicle, NOS
Disorder of seminal vesicle, NOS
D7-52010 Seminal vesiculitis 608.0
D7-52012 Abscess of seminal vesicle 608.0
D7-52014 Cellulitis of seminal vesicle 608.0
D7-52020 Nontraumatic hematoma of seminal vesicle 608.83
D7-52024 Hemorrhage of seminal vesicle 608.83
D7-52028 Thrombosis of seminal vesicle 608.83
D7-52030 Atrophy of seminal vesicle 608.89
D7-52034 Fibrosis of seminal vesicle 608.89
D7-52040 Hypertrophy of seminal vesicle 608.89
D7-52050 Ulcer of seminal vesicle 608.89

7-53 DISEASES OF THE VASA DEFERENTIA

D7-53000 Disease of the vas deferens, NOS
Disorder of the vas deferens, NOS
D7-53010 Vasitis, NOS 608.4
D7-53020 Abscess of vas deferens 608.4
D7-53024 Cellulitis of vas deferens 608.4
D7-53026 Boil of vas deferens 608.4
D7-53028 Carbuncle of vas deferens 608.4
D7-53030 Hematoma of vas deferens 608.83
D7-53034 Hemorrhage of vas deferens 608.83
D7-53036 Thrombosis of vas deferens 608.83
D7-53040 Stricture of vas deferens 608.85
D7-53044 Fibrosis of vas deferens 608.89
D7-53050 Atrophy of vas deferens 608.89
D7-53060 Hypertrophy of vas deferens 608.89
D7-53070 Ulcer of vas deferens 608.89

7-54 DISEASES OF THE SCROTUM

D7-54000 Disease of scrotum, NOS
Disorder of scrotum, NOS
D7-54100 Hydrocele, NOS 603.9
D7-54102 Infected hydrocele 603.1
D7-54103 Hydrocele of tunica vaginalis 603.-
D7-54110 Encysted hydrocele 603.0
D7-54112 Hydrocele of spermatic cord 603.-
D7-54114 Hydrocele of testis 603.-
D7-54118 Other hydrocele, NEC 603.8
D7-54120 Chylocele of tunica vaginalis 608.84
D7-54130 Torsion of spermatic cord 608.2
D7-54132 Stricture of tunica vaginalis 608.85
D7-54134 Stricture of spermatic cord 608.85
D7-54140 Abscess of scrotum 608.4
D7-54142 Boil of scrotum 608.4
D7-54144 Carbuncle of scrotum 608.4
D7-54148 Cellulitis of scrotum 608.4
D7-54150 Abscess of spermatic cord 608.4
D7-54152 Boil of spermatic cord 608.4
D7-54154 Carbuncle of spermatic cord 608.4
D7-54158 Cellulitis of spermatic cord 608.4
D7-54160 Abscess of tunica vaginalis 608.4
D7-54162 Boil of tunica vaginalis 608.4
D7-54164 Carbuncle of tunica vaginalis 608.4
D7-54168 Cellulitis of tunica vaginalis 608.4
D7-54170 Hematoma of scrotum 608.83
D7-54172 Hemorrhage of scrotum 608.83
D7-54174 Thrombosis of scrotum 608.83
D7-54180 Hematoma of spermatic cord 608.83
D7-54182 Hemorrhage of spermatic cord 608.83
D7-54184 Thrombosis of spermatic cord 608.83
D7-54190 Hematoma of tunica vaginalis 608.83
D7-54192 Hemorrhage of tunica vaginalis 608.83
D7-54194 Thrombosis of tunica vaginalis 603.83
D7-54200 Atrophy of scrotum 608.89
D7-54202 Fibrosis of scrotum 608.89
D7-54204 Hypertrophy of scrotum 608.89
D7-54206 Ulcer of scrotum 608.89
D7-54210 Atrophy of spermatic cord 608.89
D7-54212 Fibrosis of spermatic cord 608.89
D7-54214 Hypertrophy of spermatic cord 608.89
D7-54216 Ulcer of spermatic cord 608.89
D7-54220 Atrophy of tunica vaginalis 608.89

D7-54222 Fibrosis of tunica vaginalis 608.89
D7-54224 Hypertrophy of tunica vaginalis 608.89
D7-54226 Ulcer of tunica vaginalis 608.89

7-55 DISEASES OF THE TESTES AND EPIDIDYMIDES

D7-55000 Disease of testis, NOS
  Disorder of testis, NOS
D7-55100 Orchitis, NOS 604.90
D7-55101 Acute orchitis
D7-55103 Chronic orchitis
D7-55105 Orchitis without abscess 604.9
D7-55110 Orchitis with abscess 604.0
  Abscess of testis 604.0
D7-55120 Epididymitis, NOS 604.90
D7-55122 Epididymitis without abscess 604.9
D7-55124 Epididymitis with abscess 604.0
D7-55126 Abscess of epididymis 604.0
D7-55140 Epididymo-orchitis, NOS 604.9
D7-55142 Epididymo-orchitis without abscess 604.9
D7-55144 Epididymo-orchitis with abscess 604.0
D7-55150 Orchitis in disease classified elsewhere 604.91
D7-55160 Epididymitis in disease classified elsewhere 604.91
D7-55170 Spermatocele 608.1
D7-55174 Torsion of testis 608.2
  Torsion of testicle 608.2
D7-55176 Torsion of epididymis 608.2
D7-55180 Nontraumatic hematoma of testis 608.83
D7-55182 Hemorrhage of testis 608.83
D7-55184 Thrombosis of testis 608.83
D7-55185 Male hematocele 608.83
D7-55190 Atrophy of testis 608.3
D7-55192 Fibrosis of testis 608.89
D7-55194 Hypertrophy of testis 608.89
D7-55196 Ulcer of testis 608.89

7-56 MALE INFERTILITY DISORDERS

D7-56000 Male infertility, NOS 606.9
D7-56010 Infertility due to azoospermia 606.0
  Absolute male infertility 606.0
  Primary male infertility 606.0
D7-56014 Infertility due to germinal cell aplasia 606.0
D7-56016 Infertility due to complete spermatogenic arrest 606.0
D7-56020 Infertility due to oligospermia 606.1
  Infertility due to hypospermatogenesis 606.1
D7-56024 Infertility due to germinal cell desquamation 606.1
D7-56026 Infertility due to incomplete spermatogenic arrest 606.1
D7-56040 Infertility due to extratesticular cause 606.8
D7-56042 Infertility due to drug therapy 606.8
D7-56044 Infertility due to infection 606.8
D7-56046 Infertility due to radiation 606.8
D7-56048 Infertility due to systemic disease 606.8
D7-56052 Infertility due to obstruction of efferent ducts 606.8

7-57 DISEASES OF THE PENIS

D7-57000 Disease of penis, NOS 607.9
  Disorder of penis, NOS 607.9
D7-57100 Balanoposthitis 607.1
D7-57110 Balanitis 607.1
D7-57130 Lichen sclerosus et atrophicus of glans penis and prepuce 607.81
    (T-01000) (T-91300) (T-91320)
  Balanitis xerotica obliterans 607.81
    (T-01000) (T-91300) (T-91330)
D7-57132 Leukoplakia of penis 607.0
  Kraurosis of penis 607.0
D7-57136 Induratio penis plastica 607.81
D7-57140 Edema of penis 607.83
D7-57150 Priapism 607.3
  Pathologic erection 607.3
D7-57154 Chordee
  Mentulagra 607.3
  Gryposis penis
D7-57160 Redundant prepuce and phimosis 605.-
D7-57162 Adherent prepuce 605.-
D7-57164 Phimosis 605.-
  Tight foreskin 605.-
D7-57166 Paraphimosis 605.-
D7-57168V Prolapse of prepuce
D7-57200 Cavernitis of penis 607.2
D7-57210 Abscess of penis 607.2
D7-57212 Boil of penis 607.2
D7-57214 Carbuncle of penis 607.2
D7-57216 Cellulitis of penis 607.2
D7-57220 Abscess of corpus cavernosum 607.2
D7-57222 Boil of corpus cavernosum 607.2
D7-57224 Carbuncle of corpus cavernosum 607.2
D7-57226 Cellulitis of corpus cavernosum 607.2
D7-57230 Nontraumatic hematoma of penis 607.82
D7-57232 Hemorrhage of penis 607.82
D7-57234 Thrombosis of penis 607.82
D7-57236 Embolism of penis 607.82
D7-57240 Nontraumatic hematoma of corpus cavernosum 607.82
D7-57242 Hemorrhage of corpus cavernosum 607.82
D7-57244 Thrombosis of corpus cavernosum 607.82
D7-57246 Embolism of corpus cavernosum 607.82
D7-57260 Atrophy of penis 607.89
D7-57262 Fibrosis of penis 607.89
D7-57266 Hypertrophy of penis 607.89
D7-57268 Chronic ulcer of penis 607.89
D7-57270 Atrophy of corpus cavernosum 607.89
D7-57272 Fibrosis of corpus cavernosum 607.89
D7-57276 Hypertrophy of corpus cavernosum 607.89
D7-57278 Chronic ulcer of corpus cavernosum 607.89
D7-57300V Deviation of penis
D7-57310V Corkscrew penis

SECTION 7-7 DISEASES OF THE FEMALE GENITAL ORGANS
7-70 DISEASES OF THE FEMALE GENITAL ORGANS: GENERAL TERMS

D7-70000 Disease of female genital organs, NOS 629.9
  Disorder of female genital organs, NOS 629.9

7-71 INFLAMMATORY DISEASES OF THE FEMALE PELVIC ORGANS AND TISSUES

D7-71000 Inflammatory disease of female pelvic organs and tissues, NOS 614.9
  Pelvic inflammatory disease 614.9
  Female pelvic inflammation 614.9
  PID 614.9
D7-71010 Acute pelvic inflammatory disease of the female pelvic organs and tissues 614.3
  Acute pelvic inflammatory disease 614.3
  Acute PID 614.3
  Acute parametritis 614.3
  Acute female pelvic cellulitis 614.3
D7-71020 Chronic pelvic inflammatory disease of the female pelvic organs and tissues 614.4
  Chronic pelvic inflammatory disease 614.4
  Chronic PID 614.4
  Chronic parametritis 614.4
  Chronic female pelvic cellulitis 614.4
D7-71030 Abscess of female pelvis, NOS 614.4
D7-71031 Chronic abscess of female pelvis 614.4
D7-71032 Abscess of parametrium, NOS 614.4
D7-71033 Chronic abscess of parametrium 614.4
D7-71034 Abscess of broad ligament, NOS 614.4
D7-71035 Chronic abscess of broad ligament 614.4
D7-71036 Abscess of pouch of Douglas, NOS 614.4
D7-71037 Chronic abscess of pouch of Douglas 614.4
D7-71040 Female pelvic peritonitis, NOS 614.5
D7-71042 Acute female pelvic peritonitis 614.5
D7-71044 Chronic female pelvic peritonitis 614.7
D7-71048 Female pelvic peritoneal adhesions 614.6
D7-71100 Oophoritis, NOS 614.2
D7-71110 Acute oophoritis 614.0
D7-71112 Abscess of ovary 614.2
D7-71120 Subacute oophoritis 614.0
D7-71130 Chronic oophoritis 614.1
D7-71140 Perioophoritis, NOS 614.2
D7-71200 Salpingitis, NOS 614.2
D7-71210 Acute salpingitis 614.0
D7-71211 Pyosalpingitis
  Pyosalpinx
D7-71212 Abscess of fallopian tube 614.2
D7-71220 Subacute salpingitis 614.0
D7-71230 Chronic salpingitis 614.1
D7-71232 Hydrosalpinx 614.1
D7-71234 Salpingitis follicularis 614.1
D7-71236 Salpingitis isthmica nodosa 614.1
D7-71240 Perisalpingitis, NOS 614.2
D7-71250 Peritubal adhesions 614.6
D7-71300 Tubo-ovarian inflammatory disease 614.2
  Salpingo-oophoritis 614.2
D7-71310 Tubo-ovarian abscess 614.2
D7-71320 Tubo-ovarian adhesions 614.6
D7-71400 Inflammatory disease of the uterus, NOS 615.9
D7-71410 Metritis, NOS 615.9
D7-71412 Acute metritis 615.0
D7-71414 Chronic metritis 615.1
D7-71420 Endometritis, NOS 615.9
D7-71422 Acute endometritis 615.0
D7-71424 Chronic endometritis 615.1
D7-71430 Endomyometritis, NOS 615.9
D7-71432 Acute endomyometritis 615.0
D7-71434 Chronic endomyometritis 615.1
D7-71440 Myometritis, NOS 615.9
D7-71442 Acute myometritis 615.0
D7-71444 Chronic myometritis 615.1
D7-71450 Perimetritis, NOS 615.9
D7-71452 Acute perimetritis 615.0
D7-71454 Chronic perimetritis 615.1
D7-71460 Pyometra 615.9
D7-71470 Uterine abscess 615.9
D7-71500 Inflammatory disease of the uterine cervix 616.9
  Inflammatory disease of the cervix 616.9
D7-71510 Cervicitis, NOS 616.0
D7-71512 Acute cervicitis 616.0
D7-71514 Chronic cervicitis 616.0
D7-71520 Cervicitis with erosion 616.0
D7-71522 Cervicitis with ectropion 616.0
D7-71524 Chronic cervicitis with erosion 616.0
D7-71526 Chronic cervicitis with ectropion 616.0
D7-71530 Endocervicitis, NOS 616.0
D7-71532 Acute endocervicitis 616.0
D7-71534 Chronic endocervicitis 616.0
D7-71540 Endocervicitis with erosion 616.0
D7-71542 Endocervicitis with ectropion 616.0
D7-71544 Chronic endocervicitis with erosion
D7-71546 Chronic endocervicitis with ectropion 616.0
D7-71550 Nabothian gland cyst 616.0
  Nabothian follicles 616.0
  Naboth's follicles 616.0
  Nabothian cyst 616.0
D7-71600 Inflammatory disease of vagina and vulva, NOS 616.9
D7-71610 Vaginitis, NOS 616.10
D7-71612 Acute vaginitis 616.10
D7-71613V Mucopurulent vaginitis
D7-71614 Chronic vaginitis 616.10
D7-71615V Granular vaginitis
D7-71616 Postirradiation vaginitis 616.10
D7-71618 Ulcer of vagina 616.8
D7-71619 Caruncle of vagina 616.8
D7-71620 Vulvovaginitis, NOS 616.10

D7-71622 Acute vulvovaginitis 616.10
D7-71624 Chronic vulvovaginitis 616.10
D7-71626 Vulvar vestibulitis
D7-71630 Vulvitis, NOS 616.10
D7-71632 Acute vulvitis 616.10
D7-71634 Chronic vulvitis 616.10
D7-71636 Cyclic vulvovaginitis
D7-71650 Abscess of vulva 616.4
D7-71652 Furuncle of vulva 616.4
D7-71654 Carbuncle of vulva 616.4
D7-71658 Ulceration of vulva, NOS 616.50
D7-71660 Cyst of Bartholin's gland 616.2
Bartholin's gland cyst 616.2
D7-71662 Cyst of Bartholin's duct 616.2
Bartholin's duct cyst 616.2
D7-71668 Abscess of Bartholin's gland 616.3
Vulvovaginal gland abscess 616.3
D7-71670 Caruncle of labium 616.8
D7-71674V Vaginal hyperplasia
D7-71680 Ulceration of vulva in disease classified elsewhere 616.51
D7-71682 Vaginitis in disease classified elsewhere 616.11
D7-71684 Vulvitis in disease classified elsewhere 616.11
D7-71686 Vulvovaginitis in disease classified elsewhere 616.11
D7-71700 Essential vulvodynia
D7-71710 Idiopathic vulvodynia
D7-71750 Vestibular papillomatosis

7-72 ENDOMETRIOSES

D7-72000 Endometriosis, NOS 617.9
D7-72010 Endometriotic cyst
Endometrioma
D7-72020 External endometriosis
D7-72022 Implanted endometriosis
D7-72030 Deciduomatosis
D7-72040 Chorioblastosis
D7-72100 Endometriosis of uterus, NOS 617.0
Internal endometriosis 617.0
Endometriosis of myometrium 617.0
Adenomyosis 617.0
D7-72106 Endometriosis of cervix 617.0
D7-72110 Endometriosis of ovary 617.1
Endometrial cystoma of ovary 617.1
Chocolate cyst of ovary 617.1
D7-72114 Endometriosis of fallopian tube 617.2
D7-72120 Endometriosis of parametrium 617.3
D7-72122 Endometriosis of broad ligament 617.3
D7-72124 Endometriosis of round ligament 617.3
D7-72126 Endometriosis of the cul-de-sac 617.3
Endometriosis of the pouch of Douglas 617.3
D7-72130 Endometriosis of rectovaginal septum 617.4
D7-72132 Endometriosis of vagina 617.4
D7-72134 Endometriosis of vulva 617.8
D7-72140 Endometriosis of intestine, NOS 617.5
D7-72142 Endometriosis of appendix 617.5
D7-72144 Endometriosis of colon 617.5
D7-72146 Endometriosis of rectum 617.5
D7-72160 Endometriosis in scar of skin 617.6
D7-72170 Endometriosis of bladder 617.8
D7-72180 Endometriosis of lung 617.8
D7-72190 Endometriosis of umbilicus 617.8

7-73 PROLAPSE OF THE FEMALE GENITAL ORGANS

D7-73000 Prolapse of female genital organs, NOS 618.9
Genital prolapse, NOS 618.9
D7-73100 Prolapse of vaginal walls without uterine prolapse 618.0
D7-73110 Vaginal prolapse without uterine prolapse 618.0
D7-73120 Cystocele without uterine prolapse 618.0
D7-73130 Cystourethrocele without uterine prolapse 618.0
D7-73140 Female proctocele without uterine prolapse 618.0
D7-73150 Female rectocele without uterine prolapse 618.0
D7-73160 Female urethrocele without uterine prolapse 618.0
D7-73200 Uterine prolapse, NOS 618.1
Descensus uteri 618.1
D7-73202 Uterine prolapse without vaginal wall prolapse 618.1
D7-73210 Complete uterine prolapse 618.1
D7-73220 First degree uterine prolapse 618.1
D7-73230 Second degree uterine prolapse 618.1
D7-73240 Third degree uterine prolapse 618.1
D7-73300 Uterovaginal prolapse, NOS 618.4
Vaginal and cervical prolapse
D7-73310 Complete uterovaginal prolapse 618.3
D7-73320 Incomplete uterovaginal prolapse 618.2
D7-73330 Prolapse of vaginal vault after hysterectomy 618.5
D7-73340 Acquired vaginal enterocele 618.6
D7-73344 Acquired pelvic enterocele 618.6
D7-73350 Old laceration of muscles of pelvic floor 618.7
D7-73360 Incompetence of pelvic fundus 618.8
Weakening of pelvic fundus 618.8
D7-73364 Relaxation of vaginal outlet or pelvis 618.8

7-74 FISTULAS OF THE FEMALE GENITAL ORGANS

D7-74000 Fistula of the female genital organs, NOS 619.9
Fistula of the female genital tract, NOS 619.9
D7-74100 Female urinary-genital tract fistula, NOS 619.0
D7-74110 Cervicovesical fistula 619.0
D7-74120 Ureterovaginal fistula 619.0

7-74 FISTULAS OF THE FEMALE GENITAL ORGANS — Continued

D7-74130 Urethrovaginal fistula 619.0
D7-74140 Urethrovesicovaginal fistula 619.0
D7-74150 Uteroureteric fistula 619.0
D7-74160 Uterovesical fistula 619.0
D7-74170 Vesicocervicovaginal fistula 619.0
D7-74180 Vesicovaginal fistula 619.0
D7-74200 Female digestive-genital tract fistula, NOS 619.1
D7-74210 Intestinouterine fistula 619.1
D7-74220 Intestinovaginal fistula 619.1
D7-74230 Rectovaginal fistula 619.1
(T-59600) (T-82000) (M-39300)
D7-74240 Rectovulval fistula 619.1
D7-74250 Sigmoidovaginal fistula 619.1
D7-74260 Uterorectal fistula 619.1
D7-74300 Female genital tract-skin fistula, NOS 619.2
D7-74310 Uterus to abdominal wall fistula 619.2
D7-74320 Vaginoperineal fistula 619.2
D7-74410 Fistula of cervix 619.8
D7-74420 Fistula of cul-de-sac 619.8
Fistula of pouch of Douglas 619.8
D7-74430 Fistula of uterus 619.8
D7-74440 Fistula of vagina 618.9
D7-74480 Other specified fistula involving female genital tract, NEC 619.8

7-75 NONINFLAMMATORY DISORDERS OF THE FEMALE GENITAL ORGANS

D7-75000 Noninflammatory disorder of the female genital organs, NOS
D7-75010 Pelvic mass, NOS 789.3
Pelvic swelling, NOS 789.3
Pelvic lump, NOS 789.3
D7-75080 Female hematocele, NOS 629.0
D7-75100 Noninflammatory disorder of ovary, NOS 620.9
D7-75110 Ovarian cyst, NOS 620.2
Ovarian retention cyst, NOS 620.2
D7-75120 Follicular cyst of ovary 620.0
Cyst of graafian follicle 620.0
Follicular cystic ovary disease
D7-75122 Rupture of follicular cyst of ovary
D7-75130 Corpus luteum cyst 610.1
Lutein cyst 620.1
Luteal cystic ovary disease 620.1
Luteinized follicular cyst 610.1
D7-75132 Rupture of corpus luteum cyst 620.1
Hemorrhage of corpus luteum cyst 620.1
D7-75136V Retained corpus luteum
D7-75140 Germinal inclusion cyst of ovary
Germinal epithelial inclusion cyst of ovary
D7-75150 Theca-lutein cyst of ovary 620.2
D7-75160 Corpus albicans cyst of ovary 620.2
D7-75200 Acquired atrophy of ovary 620.3
Senile involution of ovary 620.3
D7-75210 Prolapse of ovary 620.4
Downward displacement of ovary 620.4
D7-75220 Hernia of ovary 620.4
D7-75230 Torsion of ovary 620.5
D7-75234 Torsion of ovarian pedicle 620.5
D7-75236 Infarction of ovary 620.8
D7-75238 Rupture of ovary 620.8
D7-75400 Noninflammatory disorder of fallopian tube, NOS 620.9
D7-75410 Acquired atrophy of fallopian tube 620.3
D7-75420 Prolapse of fallopian tube 620.4
Downward displacement of fallopian tube 620.4
D7-75424 Hernia of fallopian tube 620.4
Salpingocele 620.4
D7-75430 Torsion of fallopian tube 620.5
D7-75432 Torsion of accessory fallopian tube 620.5
D7-75434 Torsion of hydatid of Morgagni 620.5
D7-75440 Infarction of fallopian tube 620.8
D7-75450 Rupture of fallopian tube 620.8
D7-75460 Hematosalpinx 620.8
D7-75470 Cyst of fallopian tube 620.8
D7-75474 Polyp of fallopian tube 620.8
D7-75500 Noninflammatory disorder of broad ligament, NOS 620.9
D7-75510 Broad ligament laceration syndrome 620.6
Masters-Allen syndrome 620.6
D7-75520 Hematoma of broad ligament 620.7
D7-75524 Hematocele of broad ligament 620.7
D7-75530 Polyp of broad ligament 620.8
D7-75534 Cyst of broad ligament 620.8
D7-75600 Noninflammatory disorder of uterus, NOS 621.9
D7-75610 Hypertrophy of uterus 621.2
Enlarged uterus 612.2
D7-75620 Endometrial cystic hyperplasia 621.3
Adenomatous endometrial hyperplasia 621.3
Glandular endometrial hyperplasia 621.3
D7-75626 Polyp of corpus uteri 621.0
Endometrial polyp 621.0
D7-75630 Hematometra 621.4
Hemometra 621.4
D7-75640 Chronic subinvolution of uterus 621.1
D7-75650 Intrauterine synechiae 621.5
Adhesions of uterus 621.5
Bands of uterus 621.5
D7-75654 Fibrosis of uterus 621.8
D7-75658 Old postpartum laceration uterus 621.8
D7-75660 Malposition of uterus, NOS 621.6
D7-75661 Anteversion of uterus 621.6
D7-75662 Retroversion of uterus 621.6
D7-75664 Retroflexion of uterus 621.6
D7-75668 Chronic inversion of uterus 621.7
D7-75670 Acquired atrophy of uterus 621.8
D7-75680 Cyst of uterus 621.8
D7-75700 Noninflammatory disorder of cervix, NOS 622.9

D7-75710 Erosion of cervix 622.0
Superficial ulcer of cervix 622.0
D7-75712 Ectropion of cervix 622.0
Eversion of cervix 622.0
D7-75720 Dysplasia of cervix 622.1
D7-75722 Squamous metaplasia of cervix 622.1
D7-75724 Epidermidization of cervix 622.1
D7-75726 Cervical atypism 622.1
D7-75728 Anaplasia of cervix 622.1
D7-75730 Leukoplakia of cervix 622.2
D7-75740 Old laceration of cervix 622.3
D7-75742 Postpartum cicatrix of cervix 622.3
D7-75744 Adhesions of cervix 622.3
Bands of cervix 622.3
D7-75750 Occlusion of cervix 622.4
Acquired atresia of cervix 622.4
D7-75752 Pinpoint os uteri 622.4
D7-75754 Stenosis of cervix 622.4
D7-75756 Stricture of cervix 622.4
D7-75758 Contracture of cervix 622.4
D7-75760 Incompetence of cervix 622.5
D7-75770 Hypertrophic elongation of cervix 622.6
D7-75780 Polyp of cervix, NOS 622.7
D7-75784 Mucous polyp of cervix 622.7
D7-75788 Cyst of cervix 622.8
D7-75790 Fibrosis of cervix 622.8
D7-75794 Senile atrophy of cervix 622.8
D7-75798 Hemorrhage of cervix 622.8
D7-75800 Noninflammatory disorder of the vagina, NOS 623.9
D7-75810 Dysplasia of vagina 623.0
D7-75820 Leukoplakia of vagina 623.1
D7-75830 Occlusion of vagina 623.2
Acquired atresia of vagina 623.2
D7-75832 Stenosis of vagina 623.2
D7-75834 Stricture of vagina 623.2
D7-75840 Adhesions of vagina, NOS 623.2
D7-75842 Postoperative adhesions of vagina 623.2
D7-75844 Postradiation adhesions of vagina 623.2
D7-75850 Tight hymenal ring 623.3
Rigid hymen 623.3
Tight introitus 623.3
D7-75860 Old vaginal laceration 623.4
D7-75880 Vaginal hematoma 623.6
D7-75884 Vaginal hemorrhage 623.8
D7-75890 Polyp of vagina 623.7
D7-75894 Cyst of vagina 623.8
D7-75900 Noninflammatory disorder of vulva, NOS 624.9
D7-75910 Dystrophy of vulva 624.0
D7-75920 Lichen sclerosus et atrophicus of the vulva 624.0
D7-75922 Kraurosis vulvae 624.0
Kraurosis of vulva 624.0
Leukoplakia of vulva 624.0
Leukokraurosis 624.0
Leukoplakic vulvitis 624.0
Breisky's disease
D7-75930 Atrophy of vulva 624.1
D7-75940 Hypertrophy of vulva, NOS 624.3
Hypertrophy of labia, NOS 624.3
D7-75942 Hypertrophy of clitoris 624.2
D7-75950 Polyp of vulva, NOS 624.6
D7-75952 Polyp of labia, NOS 624.6
D7-75960 Cyst of vulva 624.8
D7-75964 Edema of vulva 624.8
D7-75966 Stricture of vulva 624.8
D7-75968 Hematoma of vulva 624.5
D7-75970 Old laceration of vulva 624.4
Scarring of vulva 624.4
D7-75980 Hydrocele of canal of Nuck 629.1
D7-75982 Acquired cyst of canal of Nuck 629.1

7-76 DISORDERS ASSOCIATED WITH MENSTRUATION AND THE MENOPAUSE

D7-76000 Premenstrual tension syndrome, NOS 625.4
D7-76010 Menstrual migraine 625.4
D7-76100 Pelvic congestion syndrome 625.5
Taylor's syndrome 625.5
Congestion-fibrosis syndrome 625.5
D7-76150 Senile atrophic vaginitis 627.3
Postmenopausal atrophic vaginitis 627.3
D7-76200 Postartificial menopausal syndrome 627.4

7-79 FEMALE INFERTILITY DISORDERS

D7-79000 Female infertility, NOS 628.9
D7-79002 Primary female infertility 628.9
D7-79004 Secondary female infertility 628.9
D7-79010 Female infertility associated with anovulation 628.0
Anovulatory cycle 628.0
D7-79020 Female infertility of pituitary-hypothalamic origin 628.1
D7-79030 Female infertility of tubal origin, NOS 628.2
D7-79032 Female infertility due to congenital anomaly of fallopian tube 628.2
D7-79034 Female infertility due to occlusion of fallopian tube 628.2
Female infertility due to block of fallopian tube 628.2
D7-79036 Female infertility due to acquired stenosis of fallopian tube 628.2
D7-79040 Female infertility of uterine origin, NOS 628.3
D7-79042 Female infertility associated with congenital anomaly of uterus 628.3
D7-79044 Female infertility due to nonimplantation 628.3
D7-79050 Female infertility of cervical origin, NOS 628.4
D7-79052 Female infertility due to structural congenital anomaly of cervix 628.4
D7-79054 Female infertility associated with anomaly of cervical mucus 628.4
Female infertility associated with dysmucorrhea 628.4

7-79 FEMALE INFERTILITY DISORDERS — Continued

D7-79060 Female infertility of vaginal origin, NOS 628.4
D7-79062 Female infertility due to structural congenital anomaly of vagina 628.4

SECTION 7-9 DISEASES OF THE BREAST

D7-90000 Disease of breast, NOS 611.9
  Disorder of breast, NOS 611.9
D7-90100 Mastitis, NOS 611.0
D7-90102 Nonpuerperal mastitis, NOS 611.0
D7-90110 Acute mastitis 611.0
D7-90120 Subacute mastitis 611.0
D7-90130 Retromammary mastitis 611.0
  Submammary mastitis 611.0
D7-90140 Infective mastitis 611.0
D7-90150 Abscess of breast, NOS 611.0
D7-90152 Nonpuerperal abscess of breast 611.0
D7-90160 Acute abscess of breast 611.0
D7-90162 Acute abscess of areola 611.0.
D7-90170 Chronic abscess of breast 611.0
D7-90172 Chronic abscess of areola 611.0
D7-90180 Mammary fistula 611.0
D7-90300 Benign mammary dysplasia, NOS 610.9
D7-90310 Fibrocystic disease of breast 610.1
  Cystic disease of breast 610.1
  Chronic cystic mastitis 610.1
  Diffuse cystic mastopathy 610.1
D7-90330 Fibroadenosis of breast, NOS 610.2
D7-90331 Chronic fibroadenosis of breast 610.2
D7-90332 Cystic fibroadenosis of breast 610.2
D7-90334 Diffuse fibroadenosis of breast 610.2
D7-90336 Periodic fibroadenosis of breast 610.2
D7-90338 Segmental fibroadenosis of breast 610.2
D7-90350 Fibrosclerosis of breast 610.3
D7-90360 Cyst of breast, NOS 610.0
  Simple cyst of breast, NOS 610.0
  Blue dome cyst, NOS 610.0
  Benign retention cyst of breast, NOS 610.0
D7-90364 Lactocele
  Milk cyst
  Galactocele
  Lacteal cyst
D7-90370 Mammary duct ectasia 610.4
  Duct ectasia of breast 610.4
  Comedomastitis 610.4
D7-90372 Periductal mastitis 610.4
D7-90374 Plasma cell mastitis 610.4
D7-90380 Mazoplasia 610.8
D7-90382 Sebaceous cyst of skin of breast 610.8
D7-90390 Other benign mammary dysplasia, NEC 610.8
D7-90400 Hypertrophy of breast, NOS 611.1
D7-90410 Massive pubertal hypertrophy of breast 611.1
D7-90420 Gynecomastia 611.1
  Hypertrophy of male breast 611.1
D7-90430 Fissure of nipple 611.2
D7-90434 Fat necrosis of breast 611.3
D7-90436 Atrophy of breast 611.4
D7-90440 Galactocele not associated with childbirth 611.5
D7-90444 Galactorrhea not associated with childbirth 611.6
D7-90450 Nontraumatic hematoma of breast 611.8
D7-90452 Infarction of breast 611.8
D7-90454 Occlusion of breast duct 611.8
D7-90530 Lump in breast 611.72
  Mass in breast 611.72
D7-90540 Induration of breast 611.79
D7-90550 Inversion of nipple 611.79
D7-90554 Retraction of nipple 611.79
D7-90556 Nipple discharge 611.79
D7-90560 Peau d'orange over breast 611.79

CHAPTER 8 — DIAGNOSES RELATED TO PREGNANCY AND THE PERINATAL PERIOD

SECTION 8-0 ABNORMAL PRODUCTS OF CONCEPTION, ABORTIONS AND RELATED COMPLICATIONS

8-00 ABNORMAL PRODUCTS OF CONCEPTION

D8-00100 Abnormal products of conception, NOS 631.-
D8-00110 Molar pregnancy, NOS 631.-
D8-00112 Mole, NOS 631.-
D8-00114 Carneous mole 631.-
  Fleshy mole 631.-
D8-00115 Stone mole 631.-
D8-00130 Missed abortion 632.-
  Fetal death before 22 weeks with retention of dead fetus 632.-
D8-00140 Molar pregnancy with hydatidiform mole 630.-
    (T-83000) (F-84002) (M-91000)
  Molar pregnancy with vesicular mole 630.-
    (T-83000) (F-84002) (M-91000)
  Molar pregnancy with hydatid mole 630.-
    (T-83000) (F-84002) (M-91000)
D8-00150 Molar pregnancy with invasive hydatidiform mole 236.1
    (T-83000) (F-84002) (M-91001)
  Molar pregnancy with chorioadenoma destruens 236.1
    (T-83000) (F-84002) (M-91001)
  Molar pregnancy with malignant hydatidiform mole 236.1
    (T-83000) (F-84002) (M-91001)
  Molar pregnancy with invasive mole 236.1
    (T-83000) (F-84002) (M-91001)
  Molar pregnancy with chorioadenoma 235.1
    (T-83000) (F-84002) (M-91001)
D8-00160 Molar pregnancy with choriocarcinoma 181.-
  Molar pregnancy with chorionepithelioma 181.-
  Molar pregnancy with chorioepithelioma 181.-
D8-00180 Trophoblastic disease, NOS 630.-
D8-00190 Retained products of conception, NOS 632.-
  Retained products of conception not following abortion 632.-
D8-00192 Retained products of conception following abortion, NEC 637.-

8-02 ECTOPIC PREGNANCIES

D8-02000 Ectopic pregnancy, NOS 633.9
D8-02004 Ruptured ectopic pregnancy 633.9
D8-02010 Abdominal pregnancy 633.0
D8-02014 Intraperitoneal pregnancy 633.0
D8-02020 Tubal pregnancy 633.1
  Fallopian pregnancy 633.1
D8-02024 Ruptured tubal pregnancy 633.1
  Tubal abortion 633.1
D8-02030 Ovarian pregnancy 633.2
D8-02040 Cervical pregnancy 633.8
D8-02050 Cornual pregnancy 633.8
D8-02060 Mural pregnancy 633.8
D8-02070 Intraligamentous pregnancy 633.8
D8-02074 Mesometric pregnancy 633.8
D8-02100 Other ectopic pregnancy, NEC 633.8
D8-02120 Combined pregnancy 633.8
  Simultaneous intrauterine and extrauterine pregnancies 633.8

8-03 COMPLICATIONS FOLLOWING ECTOPIC AND MOLAR PREGNANCIES

D8-03000 Unspecified complication following molar or ectopic pregnancy 639.9
D8-03010 Genital tract and pelvic infection following molar or ectopic pregnancy 639.0
D8-03011 Endometritis following molar or ectopic pregnancy 639.0
D8-03012 Parametritis following molar or ectopic pregnancy 639.0
D8-03013 Pelvic peritonitis following molar or ectopic pregnancy 639.0
D8-03014 Salpingitis following molar or ectopic pregnancy 639.0
D8-03015 Salpingo-oophoritis following molar or ectopic pregnancy 639.0
D8-03016 Sepsis, NOS, following molar or ectopic pregnancy 639.0
D8-03017 Septicemia, NOS, following molar or ectopic pregnancy 639.0
D8-03020 Delayed or excessive hemorrhage following molar or ectopic pregnancy 639.1
D8-03022 Afibrinogenemia following molar or ectopic pregnancy 639.1
D8-03023 Defibrination syndrome following molar or ectopic pregnancy 639.1
D8-03024 Intravascular hemolysis following molar or ectopic pregnancy 639.1
D8-03030 Damage to pelvic organs and tissues following molar or ectopic pregnancy 639.2
D8-03031 Damage to bladder following molar or ectopic pregnancy 639.2
D8-03033 Damage to bowel following molar or ectopic pregnancy 639.2
D8-03035 Damage to broad ligament following molar or ectopic pregnancy 639.2
D8-03037 Damage to cervix following molar or ectopic pregnancy 639.2
D8-03039 Damage to periurethral tissue following molar or ectopic pregnancy 639.2
D8-0303B Damage to uterus following molar or ectopic pregnancy 639.2

8-03 COMPLICATIONS FOLLOWING ECTOPIC AND MOLAR PREGNANCIES — Continued

D8-0303D Damage to vagina following molar or ectopic pregnancy 639.2
D8-03050 Renal failure following molar or ectopic pregnancy 639.3
D8-03051 Oliguria following molar or ectopic pregnancy 639.3
D8-03052 Acute renal failure following molar or ectopic pregnancy 639.3
Renal shutdown following molar or ectopic pregnancy 636.3
D8-03054 Renal tubular necrosis following molar or ectopic pregnancy 639.3
D8-03056 Uremia following molar or ectopic pregnancy 639.3
D8-03060 Metabolic disorder following molar or ectopic pregnancy 639.4
D8-03062 Electrolyte imbalance following molar or ectopic pregnancy 639.4
D8-03070 Shock following molar or ectopic pregnancy 639.5
Circulatory collapse following molar or ectopic pregnancy 639.5
D8-03072 Postoperative shock following molar or ectopic pregnancy 639.5
D8-03073 Septic shock following molar or ectopic pregnancy 639.5
D8-03080 Embolism, NOS, following molar or ectopic pregnancy 639.6
D8-03082 Air embolism following molar or ectopic pregnancy 639.6
D8-03083 Amniotic fluid embolism following molar or ectopic pregnancy 639.6
D8-03084 Blood clot embolism following molar or ectopic pregnancy 639.6
D8-03085 Fat embolism following molar or ectopic pregnancy 639.6
D8-03086 Pulmonary embolism following molar or ectopic pregnancy 639.6
D8-03087 Pyemic embolism following molar or ectopic pregnancy 639.6
D8-03088 Septic embolism following molar or ectopic pregnancy 639.6
D8-03089 Soap embolism following molar or ectopic pregnancy 639.6
D8-03090 Specified complication following molar or ectopic pregnancy, NEC 639.8
D8-03091 Acute yellow atrophy of liver following molar or ectopic pregnancy 639.8
Acute necrosis of liver following molar or ectopic pregnancy 639.8
D8-03092 Cardiac arrest or heart failure following molar or ectopic pregnancy 639.8
D8-03094 Cerebral anoxia following molar or ectopic pregnancy 639.8
D8-03096 Urinary tract infection following molar or ectopic pregnancy 639.8

8-04 ABORTIONS

8-040 Unspecified Abortions with Complications

D8-04000 Abortion, NOS 637.-
Unspecified abortion 637.-
D8-04004 Unspecified abortion without complication 637.9
D8-04006 Unspecified abortion with unspecified complication 637.8
D8-04010 Unspecified abortion complicated by genital-pelvic infection, NOS 637.0
D8-04011 Unspecified abortion with endometritis 637.0
D8-04012 Unspecified abortion with parametritis 637.0
D8-04013 Unspecified abortion with pelvic peritonitis 637.0
D8-04014 Unspecified abortion with salpingitis 637.0
D8-04015 Unspecified abortion with salpingo-oophoritis 637.0
D8-04016 Unspecified abortion with sepsis 637.0
D8-04017 Unspecified abortion with septicemia 637.0
D8-04020 Unspecified abortion complicated by delayed or excessive hemorrhage 637.1
D8-04022 Unspecified abortion with afibrinogenemia 637.1
D8-04023 Unspecified abortion with defibrination syndrome 637.1
D8-04024 Unspecified abortion with intravascular hemolysis 637.1
D8-04030 Unspecified abortion complicated by damage to pelvic organs and tissues 637.2
D8-04031 Unspecified abortion with laceration of bladder 637.2
Unspecified abortion with tear of bladder 637.2
D8-04032 Unspecified abortion with perforation of bladder 637.2
D8-04033 Unspecified abortion with laceration of bowel 637.2
Unspecified abortion with tear of bowel 637.2
D8-04034 Unspecified abortion with perforation of bowel 637.2
D8-04035 Unspecified abortion with laceration of broad ligament 637.2
Unspecified abortion with tear of broad ligament 637.2
D8-04036 Unspecified abortion with perforation of broad ligament 637.2
D8-04037 Unspecified abortion with laceration of cervix 637.2
Unspecified abortion with tear of cervix 637.2
D8-04038 Unspecified abortion with perforation of cervix 637.2
D8-04039 Unspecified abortion with laceration of periurethral tissue 637.2
Unspecified abortion with tear of periurethral tissue 637.2

D8-0403A Unspecified abortion with perforation of periurethral tissue 637.2
D8-0403B Unspecified abortion with laceration of uterus 637.2
  Unspecified abortion with tear of uterus 637.2
D8-0403C Unspecified abortion with perforation of uterus 637.2
D8-0403D Unspecified abortion with laceration of vagina 637.2
  Unspecified abortion with tear of vagina 637.2
D8-0403E Unspecified abortion with perforation of vagina 637.2
D8-04050 Unspecified abortion complicated by renal failure 637.3
D8-04051 Unspecified abortion with oliguria 637.3
D8-04052 Unspecified abortion with acute renal failure 637.3
  Unspecified abortion with renal shutdown 637.3
D8-04054 Unspecified abortion with renal tubular necrosis 637.3
D8-04056 Unspecified abortion with uremia 637.3
D8-04060 Unspecified abortion complicated by metabolic disorder 637.4
D8-04062 Unspecified abortion with electrolyte imbalance 637.4
D8-04070 Unspecified abortion complicated by shock 637.5
  Unspecified abortion with circulatory collapse 637.5
D8-04072 Unspecified abortion with postoperative shock 637.5
D8-04073 Unspecified abortion with septic shock 637.5
D8-04080 Unspecified abortion complicated by embolism 637.6
D8-04082 Unspecified abortion with air embolism 637.6
D8-04083 Unspecified abortion with amniotic fluid embolism 637.6
D8-04084 Unspecified abortion with blood-clot embolism 637.6
D8-04085 Unspecified abortion with fat embolism 637.6
D8-04086 Unspecified abortion with pulmonary embolism 637.6
D8-04087 Unspecified abortion with pyemic embolism 637.6
D8-04088 Unspecified abortion with septic embolism 637.6
D8-04089 Unspecified abortion with soap embolism 637.6
D8-04090 Unspecified abortion with specified complication, NEC 637.7
D8-04091 Unspecified abortion with acute yellow atrophy of liver 637.7
  Unspecified abortion with acute necrosis of liver 637.7
D8-04092 Unspecified abortion with cardiac arrest or failure 637.7
D8-04094 Unspecified abortion with cerebral anoxia 637.7
D8-04096 Unspecified abortion with urinary tract infection 637.7

8-041 Spontaneous Abortions with Complications

D8-04100 Spontaneous abortion, NOS 634.-
  Miscarriage, NOS 634.-
D8-04101 Spontaneous abortion in first trimester
D8-04102 Spontaneous abortion in second trimester
D8-04103 Spontaneous abortion in third trimester
D8-04104 Spontaneous abortion without complication 634.9
D8-04106 Spontaneous abortion with unspecified complication 634.8
D8-04110 Spontaneous abortion complicated by genital-pelvic infection, NOS 634.0
D8-04111 Spontaneous abortion with endometritis 634.0
D8-04112 Spontaneous abortion with parametritis 634.0
D8-04113 Spontaneous abortion with pelvic peritonitis 634.0
D8-04114 Spontaneous abortion with salpingitis 634.0
D8-04115 Spontaneous abortion with salpingo-oophoritis 634.0
D8-04116 Spontaneous abortion with sepsis 634.0
D8-04117 Spontaneous abortion with septicemia 634.0
D8-04120 Spontaneous abortion complicated by delayed or excessive hemorrhage 634.1
D8-04122 Spontaneous abortion with afibrinogenemia 634.1
D8-04123 Spontaneous abortion with defibrination syndrome 634.1
D8-04124 Spontaneous abortion with intravascular hemolysis 634.1
D8-04130 Spontaneous abortion complicated by damage to pelvic organs and tissues 634.2
D8-04131 Spontaneous abortion with laceration of bladder 634.2
  Spontaneous abortion with tear of bladder 634.2
D8-04132 Spontaneous abortion with perforation of bladder 634.2
D8-04133 Spontaneous abortion with laceration of bowel 634.2
  Spontaneous abortion with tear of bowel 634.2
D8-04134 Spontaneous abortion with perforation of bowel 634.2
D8-04135 Spontaneous abortion with laceration of broad ligament 634.2
  Spontaneous abortion with tear of broad ligament 634.2
D8-04136 Spontaneous abortion with perforation of broad ligament 634.2
D8-04137 Spontaneous abortion with laceration of cervix 634.2
  Spontaneous abortion with tear of cervix 634.2

8-041 Spontaneous Abortions with Complications — Continued

D8-04138 Spontaneous abortion with perforation of cervix 634.2
D8-04139 Spontaneous abortion with laceration of periurethral tissue 634.2
  Spontaneous abortion with tear of periurethral tissue 634.2
D8-0413A Spontaneous abortion with perforation of periurethral tissue 634.2
D8-0413B Spontaneous abortion with laceration of uterus 634.2
  Spontaneous abortion with tear of uterus 634.2
D8-0413C Spontaneous abortion with perforation of uterus 634.2
D8-0413D Spontaneous abortion with laceration of vagina 634.2
  Spontaneous abortion with tear of vagina 634.2
D8-0413E Spontaneous abortion with perforation of vagina 634.2
D8-04150 Spontaneous abortion complicated by renal failure 634.3
D8-04151 Spontaneous abortion with oliguria 634.3
D8-04152 Spontaneous abortion with acute renal failure 634.3
  Spontaneous abortion with renal shutdown 634.3
D8-04154 Spontaneous abortion with renal tubular necrosis 634.3
D8-04156 Spontaneous abortion with uremia 634.3
D8-04160 Spontaneous abortion complicated by metabolic disorder 634.4
D8-04162 Spontaneous abortion with electrolyte imbalance 634.4
D8-04170 Spontaneous abortion complicated by shock 634.5
  Spontaneous abortion with circulatory collapse 634.5
D8-04172 Spontaneous abortion with postoperative shock 634.5
D8-04173 Spontaneous abortion with septic shock 634.5
D8-04180 Spontaneous abortion complicated by embolism 634.6
D8-04182 Spontaneous abortion with air embolism 634.6
D8-04183 Spontaneous abortion with amniotic fluid embolism 634.6
D8-04184 Spontaneous abortion with blood-clot embolism 634.6
D8-04185 Spontaneous abortion with fat embolism 634.6
D8-04186 Spontaneous abortion with pulmonary embolism 634.6
D8-04187 Spontaneous abortion with pyemic embolism 634.6
D8-04188 Spontaneous abortion with septic embolism 634.6
D8-04189 Spontaneous abortion with soap embolism 634.6
D8-04190 Spontaneous abortion with specified complication, NEC 634.7
D8-04191 Spontaneous abortion with acute yellow atrophy of liver 634.7
  Spontaneous abortion with acute necrosis of liver 634.7
D8-04192 Spontaneous abortion with cardiac arrest or failure 634.7
D8-04194 Spontaneous abortion with cerebral anoxia 634.7
D8-04196 Spontaneous abortion with urinary tract infection 634.7

8-042 Legally Induced Abortions with Complications

D8-04200 Legally induced abortion 635.-
  Legal abortion 635.-
D8-04201 Elective abortion 635.-
D8-04202 Therapeutic abortion 635.-
D8-04204 Legal abortion without complication 635.9
D8-04206 Legal abortion with unspecified complication 635.8
D8-04210 Legal abortion complicated by genital-pelvic infection, NOS 635.0
D8-04211 Legal abortion with endometritis 635.0
D8-04212 Legal abortion with parametritis 635.0
D8-04213 Legal abortion with pelvic peritonitis 635.0
D8-04214 Legal abortion with salpingitis 635.0
D8-04215 Legal abortion with salpingo-oophoritis 635.0
D8-04216 Legal abortion with sepsis 635.0
D8-04217 Legal abortion with septicemia 635.0
D8-04220 Legal abortion complicated by delayed or excessive hemorrhage 635.1
D8-04222 Legal abortion with afibrinogenemia 635.1
D8-04223 Legal abortion with defibrination syndrome 635.1
D8-04224 Legal abortion with intravascular hemolysis 635.1
D8-04230 Legal abortion complicated by damage to pelvic organs and tissues 635.2
D8-04231 Legal abortion with laceration of bladder 635.2
  Legal abortion with tear of bladder 635.2
D8-04232 Legal abortion with perforation of bladder 635.2
D8-04233 Legal abortion with laceration of bowel 635.2
  Legal abortion with tear of bowel 635.2
D8-04234 Legal abortion with perforation of bowel 635.2
D8-04235 Legal abortion with laceration of broad ligament 635.2
  Legal abortion with tear of broad ligament 635.2
D8-04236 Legal abortion with perforation of broad ligament 635.2

D8-04237 Legal abortion with laceration of cervix 635.2
Legal abortion with tear of cervix 635.2
D8-04238 Legal abortion with perforation of cervix 635.2
D8-04239 Legal abortion with laceration of periurethal tissue 635.2
Legal abortion with tear of periurethral tissue 635.2
D8-0423A Legal abortion with perforation of periurethral tissue 635.2
D8-0423B Legal abortion with laceration of uterus 635.2
Legal abortion with tear of uterus 635.2
D8-0423C Legal abortion with perforation of uterus 635.2
D8-0423D Legal abortion with laceration of vagina 635.2
Legal abortion with tear vagina 635.2
D8-0423E Legal abortion with perforation of vagina 635.2
D8-04250 Legal abortion complicated by renal failure 635.3
D8-04251 Legal abortion with oliguria 635.3
D8-04252 Legal abortion with acute renal failure 635.3
Legal abortion with renal shutdown 635.3
D8-04254 Legal abortion with renal tubular necrosis 635.3
D8-04256 Legal abortion with uremia 635.3
D8-04260 Legal abortion complicated by metabolic disorder 635.4
D8-04262 Legal abortion with electrolyte imbalance 635.4
D8-04270 Legal abortion complicated by shock 635.5
Legal abortion with circulatory collapse 635.5
D8-04272 Legal abortion with postoperative shock 635.5
D8-04273 Legal abortion with septic shock 635.5
D8-04280 Legal abortion complicated by embolism 635.6
D8-04282 Legal abortion with air embolism 635.6
D8-04283 Legal abortion with amniotic fluid embolism 635.6
D8-04284 Legal abortion with blood-clot embolism 635.6
D8-04285 Legal abortion with fat embolism 635.6
D8-04286 Legal abortion with pulmonary embolism 635.6
D8-04287 Legal abortion with pyemic embolism 635.6
D8-04288 Legal abortion with septic embolism 635.6
D8-04289 Legal abortion with soap embolism 635.6
D8-04290 Legal abortion with specified complication, NEC 635.7
D8-04291 Legal abortion with acute yellow atrophy of liver 635.7
Legal abortion with acute necrosis of liver 635.7
D8-04292 Legal abortion with cardiac arrest or failure 635.7
D8-04294 Legal abortion with cerebral anoxia 635.7
D8-04296 Legal abortion with urinary tract infection 635.7

8-043 Illegally Induced Abortions with Complications

D8-04300 Illegally induced abortion 636.-
Criminal abortion 636.-
Illegal abortion 636.-
D8-04301 Self-induced abortion 636.-
D8-04304 Illegal abortion without complication 636.9
D8-04306 Illegal abortion with unspecified complication 636.8
D8-04310 Illegal abortion complicated by genital-pelvic infection, NOS 636.0
D8-04311 Illegal abortion with endometritis 636.0
D8-04312 Illegal abortion with parametritis 636.0
D8-04313 Illegal abortion with pelvic peritonitis 636.0
D8-04314 Illegal abortion with salpingitis 636.0
D8-04315 Illegal abortion with salpingo-oophoritis 636.0
D8-04316 Illegal abortion with sepsis 636.0
D8-04317 Illegal abortion with septicemia 636.0
D8-04320 Illegal abortion complicated by delayed or excessive hemorrhage 636.1
D8-04322 Illegal abortion with afibrinogenemia 636.1
D8-04323 Illegal abortion with defibrination syndrome 636.1
D8-04324 Illegal abortion with intravascular hemolysis 636.1
D8-04330 Illegal abortion complicated by damage to pelvic organs and tissues 636.2
D8-04331 Illegal abortion with laceration of bladder 636.2
Illegal abortion with tear of bladder 636.2
D8-04332 Illegal abortion with perforation of bladder 636.2
D8-04333 Illegal abortion with laceration of bowel 636.2
Illegal abortion with tear of bowel 636.2
D8-04334 Illegal abortion with perforation of bowel 636.2
D8-04335 Illegal abortion with laceration of broad ligament 636.2
Illegal abortion with tear of broad ligament 636.2
D8-04336 Illegal abortion with perforation of broad ligament 636.2
D8-04337 Illegal abortion with laceration of cervix 636.2
Illegal abortion with tear of cervix 636.2
D8-04338 Illegal abortion with perforation of cervix 636.2
D8-04339 Illegal abortion with laceration of periurethral tissue 636.2
Illegal abortion with tear of periurethral tissue 636.2
D8-0433A Illegal abortion with perforation of periurethral tissue 636.2
D8-0433B Illegal abortion with laceration of uterus 636.2
Illegal abortion with tear of uterus 636.2

8-043 Illegally Induced Abortions with Complications — Continued

D8-0433C Illegal abortion with perforation of uterus 636.2
D8-0433D Illegal abortion with laceration of vagina 636.2
Illegal abortion with tear of vagina 636.2
D8-0433E Illegal abortion with perforation of vagina 636.2
D8-04350 Illegal abortion complicated by renal failure 636.3
D8-04351 Illegal abortion with oliguria 636.3
D8-04352 Illegal abortion with acute renal failure 636.3
Illegal abortion with renal shutdown 636.3
D8-04354 Illegal abortion with renal tubular necrosis 636.3
D8-04356 Illegal abortion with uremia 636.3
D8-04360 Illegal abortion complicated by metabolic disorder 636.4
D8-04362 Illegal abortion with electrolyte imbalance 636.4
D8-04370 Illegal abortion complicated by shock 636.5
Illegal abortion with circulatory collapse 636.5
D8-04372 Illegal abortion with postoperative shock 636.5
D8-04373 Illegal abortion with septic shock 636.5
D8-04380 Illegal abortion complicated by embolism 636.6
D8-04382 Illegal abortion with air embolism 636.6
D8-04383 Illegal abortion with amniotic fluid embolism 636.6
D8-04384 Illegal abortion with blood-clot embolism 636.6
D8-04385 Illegal abortion with fat embolism 636.6
D8-04386 Illegal abortion with pulmonary embolism 636.6
D8-04387 Illegal abortion with pyemic embolism 636.6
D8-04388 Illegal abortion with septic embolism 636.6
D8-04389 Illegal abortion with soap embolism 636.6
D8-04390 Illegal abortion with specified complication, NEC 636.7
D8-04391 Illegal abortion with acute yellow atrophy of liver 636.7
Illegal abortion with acute necrosis of liver 636.7
D8-04392 Illegal abortion with cardiac arrest or failure 636.7
D8-04394 Illegal abortion with cerebral anoxia 636.7
D8-04396 Illegal abortion with urinary tract infection 636.7

8-044 Failed Attempted Abortions with Complications

D8-04400 Failed attempted abortion 638.-
Failed attempted legal abortion 638.-
Failure of attempted induction of legal abortion 638.-
D8-04404 Failed attempted abortion without complication 638.9
D8-04406 Failed attempted abortion with unspecified complication 638.8
D8-04410 Failed attempted abortion complicated by genital-pelvic infection, NOS 638.0
D8-04411 Failed attempted abortion with endometritis 638.0
D8-04412 Failed attempted abortion with parametritis 638.0
D8-04413 Failed attempted abortion with pelvic peritonitis 638.0
D8-04414 Failed attempted abortion with salpingitis 638.0
D8-04415 Failed attempted abortion with salpingo-oophoritis 638.0
D8-04416 Failed attempted abortion with sepsis 638.0
D8-04417 Failed attempted abortion with septicemia 638.0
D8-04420 Failed attempted abortion complicated by delayed or excessive hemorrhage 638.1
D8-04422 Failed attempted abortion with afibrinogenemia 638.1
D8-04423 Failed attempted abortion with defibrination syndrome 638.1
D8-04424 Failed attempted abortion with intravascular hemolysis 638.1
D8-04430 Failed attempted abortion complicated by damage to pelvic organs and tissues 638.2
D8-04431 Failed attempted abortion with laceration of bladder 638.2
Failed attempted abortion with tear of bladder 638.2
D8-04432 Failed attempted abortion with perforation of bladder 638.2
D8-04433 Failed attempted abortion with laceration of bowel 638.2
Failed attempted abortion with tear of bowel 638.2
D8-04434 Failed attempted abortion with perforation of bowel 638.2
D8-04435 Failed attempted abortion with laceration of broad ligament 638.2
Failed attempted abortion with tear of broad ligament 638.2
D8-04436 Failed attempted abortion with perforation of broad ligament 638.2
D8-04437 Failed attempted abortion with laceration of cervix 638.2
Failed attempted abortion with tear of cervix 638.2
D8-04438 Failed attempted abortion with perforation of cervix 638.2
D8-04439 Failed attempted abortion with laceration of periurethral tissue 638.2
Failed attempted abortion with tear of periurethral tissue 638.2
D8-0443A Failed attempted abortion with perforation of periurethral tissue 638.2

D8-0443B Failed attempted abortion with laceration of uterus 638.2
Failed attempted abortion with tear of uterus 638.2

D8-0443C Failed attempted abortion with perforation of uterus 638.2

D8-0443D Failed attempted abortion with laceration of vagina 638.2
Failed attempted abortion with tear of vagina 638.2

D8-0443E Failed attempted abortion with perforation of vagina 638.2

D8-04450 Failed attempted abortion complicated by renal failure 638.3

D8-04451 Failed attempted abortion with oliguria 638.3

D8-04452 Failed attempted abortion with acute renal failure 638.3
Failed attempted abortion with renal shutdown 638.3

D8-04454 Failed attempted abortion with renal tubular necrosis 638.3

D8-04456 Failed attempted abortion with uremia 638.3

D8-04460 Failed attempted abortion complicated by metabolic disorder 638.4

D8-04462 Failed attempted abortion with electrolyte imbalance 638.4

D8-04470 Failed attempted abortion complicated by shock 638.5
Failed attempted abortion with circulatory collapse 638.5

D8-04472 Failed attempted abortion with postoperative shock 638.5

D8-04473 Failed attempted abortion with septic shock 638.5

D8-04480 Failed attempted abortion complicated by embolism 638.6

D8-04482 Failed attempted abortion with air embolism 638.6

D8-04483 Failed attempted abortion with amniotic fluid embolism 638.6

D8-04484 Failed attempted abortion with blood-clot embolism 638.6

D8-04485 Failed attempted abortion with fat embolism 638.6

D8-04486 Failed attempted abortion with pulmonary embolism 638.6

D8-04487 Failed attempted abortion with pyemic embolism 638.6

D8-04488 Failed attempted abortion with septic embolism 638.6

D8-04489 Failed attempted abortion with soap embolism 638.6

D8-04490 Failed attempted abortion with specified complication, NEC 638.7

D8-04491 Failed attempted abortion with acute yellow atrophy of liver 638.7
Failed attempted abortion with acute necrosis of liver 638.7

D8-04492 Failed attempted abortion with cardiac arrest or failure 638.7

D8-04494 Failed attempted abortion with cerebral anoxia 638.7

D8-04496 Failed attempted abortion with urinary tract infection 638.7

SECTION 8-1 COMPLICATIONS RELATED TO PREGNANCY
8-10 HEMORRHAGIC COMPLICATIONS OF PREGNANCY

D8-10000 Complication related to pregnancy, NOS 646.9
Complicated pregnancy, NOS 646.9

D8-10100 Hemorrhage in early pregnancy, NOS 640.9
Hemorrhage before 22 weeks gestation, NOS 640.9

D8-10102 Unspecified hemorrhage in early pregnancy, unspecified as to episode of care 640.90

D8-10104 Unspecified hemorrhage in early pregnancy, delivered, with or without antepartum condition 640.91

D8-10106 Unspecified hemorrhage in early pregnancy, antepartum condition or complication 640.93

D8-10120 Threatened abortion, NOS 640.0

D8-10121 Threatened abortion in first trimester

D8-10122 Threatened abortion in second trimester

D8-10123 Threatened abortion in third trimester

D8-10124 Threatened abortion, delivered, with or without antepartum condition 640.01

D8-10126 Threatened abortion, antepartum condition or complication 640.03

D8-10128 Threatened abortion, unspecified as to episode of care 640.00

D8-10140 Other specified hemorrhage in early pregnancy, NEC 640.8

D8-10142 Other specified hemorrhage in early pregnancy, unspecified as to episode of care 640.80

D8-10144 Other specified hemorrhage in early pregnancy, delivered, with or without antepartum condition 640.81

D8-10146 Other specified hemorrhage in early pregnancy, antepartum condition or complication 640.83

D8-10200 Hemorrhage of pregnancy, NOS 641.9

D8-10202 Antepartum hemorrhage, NOS 641.9

D8-10204 Intrapartum hemorrhage, NOS 641.9

D8-10210 Placenta previa without hemorrhage 641.0
Low implantation of placenta without hemorrhage 641.0
Placenta previa found during pregnancy without hemorrhage 641.0

D8-10212 Placenta previa found before labor and delivery by cesarean section without hemorrhage 641.0

D8-10220 Hemorrhage from placenta previa 641.1
Low-lying placenta with intrapartum hemorrhage 641.1

8-10 HEMORRHAGIC COMPLICATIONS OF PREGNANCY — Continued

D8-10222 Marginal placenta previa with intrapartum hemorrhage 641.1

D8-10224 Partial placenta previa with intrapartum hemorrhage 641.1
Incomplete placenta previa with intrapartum hemorrhage 641.1

D8-10226 Total placenta previa with intrapartum hemorrhage 641.1

D8-10300 Premature separation of placenta 641.2
Ablatio placentae 641.2
Abruptio placentae 641.2
Accidental antepartum hemorrhage 641.2
Premature detachment of placenta 641.2
Premature detachment of normally implanted placenta 641.2

D8-10304 Couvelaire uterus 641.2
Uteroplacental apoplexy 641.2

D8-10400 Antepartum hemorrhage associated with coagulation defects 641.3

D8-10402 Parturient hemorrhage associated with afibrinogenemia 641.2

D8-10404 Parturient hemorrhage associated with hyperfibrinolysis 641.3

D8-10406 Parturient hemorrhage associated with hypofibrinogenemia 641.3

D8-10420 Ante or intrapartum hemorrhage associated with trauma 641.8

D8-10430 Ante or intrapartum hemorrhage associated with leiomyoma 641.8

D8-10480 Other antepartum hemorrhage, NEC 641.8

8-11 HYPERTENSION AND VOMITING COMPLICATING PREGNANCY, CHILDBIRTH AND THE PUERPERIUM

D8-11000 Hypertension in the obstetric context, NOS 642.9
Unspecified hypertension complicating pregnancy, childbirth or puerperium 642.9
Hypertension without albuminuria or edema in the obstetric context, NOS 642.9

D8-11100 Benign essential hypertension in obstetric context, NOS 642.0

D8-11102 Benign essential hypertension complicating or reason for care during pregnancy 642.0

D8-11104 Benign essential hypertension complicating or reason for care during childbirth 642.0

D8-11106 Benign essential hypertension complicating or reason for care during puerperium 642.0

D8-11110 Pre-existing hypertension in obstetric context, NOS 642.0

D8-11112 Pre-existing hypertension, NOS, complicating or reason for care during pregnancy 642.0

D8-11114 Pre-existing hypertension, NOS, complicating or reason for care during childbirth 642.0

D8-11116 Pre-existing hypertension, NOS, complicating or reason for care during puerperium 642.0

D8-11120 Chronic hypertension in obstetric context, NOS 642.0

D8-11122 Chronic hypertension complicating or reason for care during pregnancy 642.0

D8-11124 Chronic hypertension complicating or reason for care during childbirth 642.0

D8-11126 Chronic hypertension complicating or reason for care during puerperium 642.0

D8-11130 Essential hypertension in obstetric context, NOS 642.0

D8-11132 Essential hypertension complicating or reason for care during pregnancy 642.0

D8-11134 Essential hypertension complicating or reason for care during childbirth 642.0

D8-11136 Essential hypertension complicating or reason for care during puerperium 642.0

D8-11150 Malignant hypertension in obstetric context, NOS 642.2

D8-11152 Malignant hypertension complicating or reason for care during pregnancy 642.2

D8-11154 Malignant hypertension complicating or reason for care during childbirth 642.2

D8-11156 Malignant hypertension complicating or reason for care during puerperium 642.2

D8-11160 Hypertensive heart and renal disease in obstetric context, NOS

D8-11162 Hypertensive heart and renal disease complicating or reason for care during pregnancy 642.2

D8-11164 Hypertensive heart and renal disease complicating or reason for care during childbirth 642.2

D8-11166 Hypertensive heart and renal disease complicating or reason for care during puerperium 642.2

D8-11170 Hypertensive heart disease in obstetric context, NOS 642.2

D8-11172 Hypertensive heart disease complicating or reason for care during pregnancy 642.2

D8-11174 Hypertensive heart disease complicating or reason for care during childbirth 642.2

D8-11176 Hypertensive heart disease complicating or reason for care during puerperium 642.2

D8-11180 Hypertensive renal disease in obstetric context, NOS 642.2

D8-11182 Hypertensive renal disease complicating or reason for care during pregnancy 642.2

D8-11184 Hypertensive renal disease complicating or reason for care during childbirth 642.2

D8-11186 Hypertensive renal disease complicating or reason for care during puerperium 642.2

D8-11190 Hypertension secondary to renal disease in obstetric context, NOS 642.1

D8-11192 Hypertension secondary to renal disease complicating or reason for care during pregnancy 642.1

D8-11194 Hypertension secondary to renal disease complicating or reason for care during childbirth 642.1

D8-11196 Hypertension secondary to renal disease complicating or reason for care during puerperium 642.1
D8-11200 Transient hypertension of pregnancy 642.3
  Gestational hypertension 642.3
D8-11205 Toxemia of pregnancy, NOS 624.-
D8-11206V Pregnancy toxemia of ewes
  Ovine ketosis
D8-11210 Pre-eclampsia, NOS 624.4
  Pre-eclamptic toxemia, NOS 642.4
D8-11212 Mild pre-eclampsia 642.4
  Mild pre-eclamptic toxemia 642.4
D8-11220 Severe pre-eclampsia 642.5
  Hypertension with albuminuria 642.5
  Severe edema 642.5
  Severe pre-eclamptic toxemia 642.5
D8-11250 Eclampsia 642.6
  Eclamptic toxemia 642.6
  Toxemia with convulsions 642.6
D8-11270 Pre-eclampsia added to pre-existing hypertension 642.7
D8-11272 Eclampsia added to pre-existing hypertension 642.7
D8-11500 Vomiting of pregnancy, NOS 643.9
  Vomiting as reason for care in pregnancy, NOS 643.9
D8-11510 Excessive vomiting in pregnancy 643.9
  Hyperemesis arising during pregnancy 643.9
  Persistent or vicious vomiting arising during pregnancy 643.9
  Hyperemesis gravidarum 643.9
D8-11512 Mild hyperemesis gravidarum 643.0
  Mild hyperemesis before end of 22 weeks of gestation 643.0
D8-11520 Hyperemesis gravidarum with metabolic disturbance, NOS 643.1
D8-11522 Hyperemesis gravidarum before end of 22 week gestation with carbohydrate depletion 643.1
D8-11524 Hyperemesis gravidarum before end of 22 week gestation with dehydration 643.1
D8-11526 Hyperemesis gravidarum before end of 22 week gestation with electrolyte imbalance 643.1
D8-11540 Late vomiting of pregnancy 643.2
  Excessive vomiting after 22 weeks of gestation 643.2
D8-11560 Vomiting due to organic disease during pregnancy, NOS 643.8
D8-11580 Other vomiting complicating pregnancy, NEC 643.8

8-12 EARLY LABOR AND PROLONGED PREGNANCY

D8-12000 Threatened premature labor 644.0
  Premature labor after 22 weeks but before 37 completed weeks of gestation without delivery 644.0
D8-12020 Threatened labor, NOS, without delivery 644.1
  False labor, NOS, without delivery 644.1
  False labor after 37 weeks of gestation without delivery 644.1
D8-12040 Early onset of delivery before 37 weeks 644.2
  Premature labor, onset of delivery before 37 weeks of gestation 644.2
D8-12200 Prolonged pregnancy 645.-
  Post term pregnancy 645.-
  Pregnancy beyond 42 weeks of gestation 645.-
  Prolonged gestation 645.-

8-14 OTHER COMPLICATIONS OF PREGNANCY

D8-14000 Other complication of pregnancy, NEC 646.-
  Other specified complication of pregnancy, NEC 646.8
D8-14100 Gestational edema without mention of hypertension 646.1
D8-14110 Maternal obesity syndrome 646.1
  Maternal obesity without hypertension 646.1
D8-14120 Habitual aborter 646.3
D8-14150 Renal disease, NOS, in pregnancy or puerperium without hypertension 646.2
  Nephropathy, NOS, in pregnancy or puerperium without hypertension 646.2
D8-14152 Gestational proteinuria 646.2
D8-14154 Albuminuria in pregnancy without hypertension 646.2
D8-14160 Peripheral neuritis in pregnancy 646.4
D8-14170 Asymptomatic bacteriuria in pregnancy 646.5
D8-14180 Infection of genitourinary tract in pregnancy, NOS 646.6
D8-14200 Liver disorder in pregnancy, NOS 646.7
D8-14202 Necrosis of liver of pregnancy 646.7
D8-14206 Icterus gravis of pregnancy 646.7
  Acute yellow atrophy of liver during pregnancy 646.7
D8-14210 Fatigue during pregnancy 646.8
D8-14214 Insufficient weight gain of pregnancy 646.8
D8-14220 Herpes gestationis 646.8
  Dermatitis herpetiformis of pregnancy 646.8
D8-14300 Diabetes mellitus in mother complicating pregnancy, childbirth or puerperium 648.0
D8-14306 Abnormal glucose tolerance in mother complicating pregnancy, childbirth or puerperium 648.8
D8-14310 Thyroid disease in mother complicating pregnancy, childbirth or puerperium 648.1
D8-14320 Anemia in mother complicating pregnancy, childbirth or puerperium 648.2
D8-14330 Drug dependence in mother complicating pregnancy, childbirth or puerperium 648.3

8-14 OTHER COMPLICATIONS OF PREGNANCY — Continued

D8-14340 Emotional or mental disease in mother complicating pregnancy, childbirth or puerperium 648.4
D8-14350 Congenital cardiovascular disorder in mother complicating pregnancy, childbirth or puerperium 648.5
D8-14360 Heart disease, NOS, in mother complicating pregnancy, childbirth or puerperium 648.6
D8-14370 Bone and joint disorder of back in mother complicating pregnancy, childbirth or puerperium 648.7
D8-14380 Bone and joint disorder of pelvis in mother complicating pregnancy, childbirth or puerperium 648.7
D8-14390 Bone and joint disorder of lower extremities in mother complicating pregnancy, childbirth or puerperium 648.7

SECTION 8-2 MATERNAL AND FETAL CONDITIONS AFFECTING LABOR AND DELIVERY

8-20 DELIVERY AND MATERNAL CONDITIONS AFFECTING MANAGEMENT

D8-20000 Delivery of fetus, completely normal case 650.-
D8-20100 Multiple gestation, NOS 651.9
Multiple pregnancy, NOS 651.9
D8-20102 Twin pregnancy 651.0
D8-20103 Triplet pregnancy 651.1
D8-20104 Quadruplet pregnancy 651.2
D8-20105 Quintuplet pregnancy 651.8
D8-20106 Sextuplet pregnancy 651.8
D8-20107 Septuplet pregnancy 651.8
D8-20110 Other specified multiple gestation, NEC 651.8
D8-20200 Malposition of fetus, NOS 652.9
D8-20204 Unstable lie of fetus 652.0
D8-20210 Malpresentation of fetus, NOS 652.9
D8-20212 Cephalic version, NOS 652.1
D8-20214 Breech malpresentation successfully converted to cephalic presentation 652.1
D8-20216 Other malpresentation successfully converted to cephalic presentation 652.1
D8-20220 Spontaneous breech delivery, NOS 652.2
Breech presentation, no version 652.2
Assisted breech delivery, NOS 652.2
D8-20224 Transverse or oblique presentation of fetus 652.3
D8-20225 Oblique lie of fetus 652.3
D8-20226 Transverse lie of fetus 652.3
D8-20230 Face or brow presentation of fetus 652.4
D8-20232 Mentum presentation of fetus 652.4
D8-20236 High fetal head at term 652.5
Failure of fetal head to enter pelvic brim 652.5
D8-20240 Multiple gestation with one or more fetal malpresentations 652.6
D8-20250 Presentation of prolapsed arm of fetus 652.7
D8-20254 Compound presentation of fetus 652.8
D8-20280 Other specific malposition or malpresentation of fetus, NEC 652.8
D8-20300 Disproportion between fetal head and pelvis, NOS 653.9
D8-20310 Major abnormality of bony pelvis, NOS 653.0
D8-20312 Pelvic deformity, NOS 653.0
D8-20313 Contracted pelvis, NOS 651.1
Generally contracted pelvis 651.1
D8-20315 Inlet contraction of pelvis 651.2
D8-20316 Outlet contraction of pelvis 651.3
D8-20320 Cephalopelvic disproportion, NOS 653.4
Fetopelvic disproportion, NOS 653.4
Disproportion of mixed maternal and fetal origin with normally formed fetus 653.4
D8-20330 Fetal disproportion, NOS 653.5
Very large fetus causing disproportion, NOS 653.5
D8-20332 Hydrocephalic fetus causing disproportion 653.6
D8-20340 Conjoined twins causing disproportion 653.7
D8-20342 Fetal ascites causing disproportion 653.7
D8-20344 Fetal hydrops causing disproportion 653.7
D8-20346 Fetal myelomeningocele causing disproportion 653.7
D8-20347 Fetal sacral teratoma causing disproportion 653.7
D8-20348 Fetal congenital tumor causing disproportion 653.7
D8-20380 Disproportion of other origin, NEC 653.8
D8-20400 Abnormality of organs and soft tissues of pelvis affecting pregnancy, NOS 654.9
D8-20410 Congenital abnormality of uterus, NOS, affecting pregnancy 654.0
D8-20412 Double uterus affecting pregnancy 654.0
D8-20414 Uterus bicornis affecting pregnancy 654.0
D8-20420 Tumor of body of uterus affecting pregnancy 654.1
D8-20422 Uterine fibroids affecting pregnancy 654.1
D8-20430 Uterine scar from previous surgery affecting pregnancy 654.2
D8-20432 Previous cesarean section, NOS 654.2
D8-20440 Retroverted gravid uterus 654.3
D8-20442 Incarcerated gravid uterus 654.3
D8-20450 Other shape or position of gravid uterus and adjacent structures affecting pregnancy 654.4
D8-20452 Cystocele affecting pregnancy 654.4
D8-20454 Rectocele affecting pregnancy 654.4
D8-20456 Prolapse of gravid uterus 654.4
Hernial protrusion of gravid uterus through abdominal rectus muscle 654.4
D8-20458 Pendulous abdomen 654.4
D8-20460 Healed pelvic floor repair affecting pregnancy 654.4

D8-20462 Rigid pelvic floor affecting pregnancy 654.4
D8-20470 Cervical incompetence 654.5
  Abnormal dilatation of cervix before onset of labor 654.5
D8-20474 Presence of Shirodkar suture with or without cervical incompetence 654.5
D8-20480 Other congenital or acquired abnormality of cervix affecting pregnancy, NEC 654.6
D8-20481 Cicatrix of cervix affecting pregnancy 654.6
D8-20482 Polyp of cervix affecting pregnancy 654.6
D8-20483 Previous operation to cervix affecting pregnancy 654.6
D8-20485 Rigid cervix uteri affecting pregnancy 654.6
D8-20486 Stenosis or stricture of cervix affecting pregnancy 654.6
D8-20488 Tumor of cervix affecting pregnancy 654.6
D8-20500 Congenital or acquired abnormality of vagina affecting pregnancy, NEC 654.7
D8-20501 Previous surgery to vagina affecting pregnancy 654.7
D8-20502 Septate vagina affecting pregnancy 654.7
D8-20503 Congenital stenosis of vagina affecting pregnancy 654.7
D8-20504 Acquired stenosis of vagina affecting pregnancy 654.7
D8-20506 Stricture of vagina affecting pregnancy 654.7
D8-20507 Tumor of vagina affecting pregnancy 654.7
D8-20530 Congenital or acquired abnormality of vulva affecting pregnancy, NEC 654.8
D8-20531 Fibrosis of perineum affecting pregnancy 654.8
D8-20532 Persistent hymen affecting pregnancy 654.8
D8-20534 Previous surgery to perineum or vulva affecting pregnancy 654.8
D8-20536 Rigid perineum affecting pregnancy 654.8
D8-20538 Tumor of vulva affecting pregnancy 654.8

8-21 FETAL CONDITIONS AFFECTING OBSTETRICAL CARE OF MOTHER

D8-21000 Known or suspected fetal abnormality affecting management of mother, NOS 655.9
D8-21100 Central nervous system malformation in fetus affecting obstetrical care 655.0
D8-21102 Fetal or suspected fetal anencephaly affecting obstetrical care 655.0
D8-21104 Fetal or suspected fetal hydrocephalus affecting obstetrical care 655.0
D8-21106 Fetal or suspected fetal spina bifida with myelomeningocele affecting obstetrical care 655.0
D8-21110 Chromosomal abnormality in fetus affecting obstetrical care 655.1
D8-21120 Hereditary disease in family possibly affecting fetus 655.2
D8-21130 Suspected damage to fetus from viral disease in the mother 655.3
D8-21132 Suspected damage to fetus from maternal rubella 655.3
D8-21140 Suspected damage to fetus from maternal drug use 655.5
D8-21142 Suspected damage to fetus from maternal alcohol addiction 655.4
D8-21148 Suspected damage to fetus from environmental toxin 655.8
D8-21152 Suspected damage to fetus from maternal listeriosis 655.4
D8-21154 Suspected damage to fetus from maternal toxoplasmosis 655.4
D8-21156 Suspected damage to fetus from intrauterine contraceptive device 655.8
  Suspected damage to fetus from IUD 655.8
D8-21160 Suspected damage to fetus from radiation 655.6
D8-21168 Suspected damage to fetus from disease in the mother, NEC 655.4
D8-21180 Other known or suspected fetal abnormality, NEC, affecting obstetrical care 655.8
D8-21400 Fetal and placental disorder affecting management of mother, NOS 656.9
  Feto-placental disorder affecting management of mother, NOS 656.9
D8-21410 Fetal-maternal hemorrhage 656.0
  Leakage of fetal blood into maternal circulation 656.0
D8-21420 Rhesus isoimmunization affecting pregnancy 656.1
  Rh incompatibility affecting pregnancy 656.1
D8-21422 ABO isoimmunization affecting pregnancy 656.2
D8-21430 Isoimmunization from other and unspecified blood-group incompatibility affecting pregnancy 656.2
D8-21500 Fetal distress affecting management of mother 656.3
  Abnormal fetal heart rate or rhythm affecting management of mother 656.3
D8-21502 Fetal bradycardia affecting management of mother 656.3
D8-21504 Fetal tachycardia affecting management of mother 656.3
D8-21510 Abnormal acid-base balance affecting management of mother 656.3
D8-21512 Fetal acidemia affecting management of mother 656.3
  Fetal acidosis affecting management of mother 656.3
D8-21520 Meconium in amniotic fluid affecting management of mother 656.3
D8-21550 Fetal death, NOS, affecting management of mother 656.4
D8-21554 Intrauterine death affecting management of mother 656.4
  Fetal death after 22 week gestation affecting management of mother 656.4

8-21 FETAL CONDITIONS AFFECTING OBSTETRICAL CARE OF MOTHER — Continued

D8-21554 (cont.) Late fetal death affecting management of mother 656.4
Missed delivery affecting management of mother 656.4
D8-21600 Poor fetal growth affecting management of mother 656.5
Light for dates affecting management of mother 656.5
Placental insufficiency affecting management of mother 656.5
Small for dates affecting management of mother 656.5
D8-21620 Excessive fetal growth affecting management of mother 656.6
Large for dates affecting management of mother 656.6
D8-21700 Abnormal placenta affecting management of mother 656.7
D8-21710 Placental infarct affecting management of mother 656.7
D8-21780 Other placental condition, NEC, affecting management of mother 656.7

8-22 CONDITIONS OF THE AMNIOTIC CAVITY AND MEMBRANES

D8-22000 Disorder of amniotic cavity or membrane, NOS 658.9
D8-22100 Polyhydramnios 657.-
Hydramnios 657.-
D8-22110 Oligohydramnios, NOS 658.0
D8-22112 Oligohydramnios without rupture of membranes 658.0
D8-22118 Ruptured amnion, NOS
Rupture of membranes, NOS
D8-22120 Premature rupture of membranes 658.1
Rupture of amniotic sac under 24 hours before onset of labor 658.1
D8-22122 Prolonged rupture of membranes 658.2
Delayed delivery after spontaneous or unspecified rupture of membranes 658.2
Rupture of amniotic sac 24 or more hours before labor 658.2
D8-22124 Delayed delivery after artificial rupture of membranes 658.3
D8-22200 Infection of amniotic cavity, NOS 658.4
Amnionitis 658.4
D8-22202 Chorioamnionitis 658.4
Membranitis 658.4
D8-22206 Placentitis 658.4
D8-22210 Amnion nodosum 658.8
D8-22220 Amniotic cyst 658.8

8-23 INDICATIONS FOR CARE OR INTERVENTION DURING LABOR OR DELIVERY

D8-23000 Indication for care or intervention in labor or delivery, NOS 659.9
D8-23100 Failed induction of labor, NOS 659.1
D8-23110 Failed mechanical induction 659.0
Failure of induction of labor by surgical or other instrumental method 659.0
D8-23120 Failed medical induction of labor 659.1
D8-23122 Failure of induction of labor by oxytocic drugs 659.1
D8-23200 Maternal pyrexia during labor, NOS 659.2
D8-23210 Generalized infection during labor 659.3
D8-23212 Septicemia during labor 659.3
D8-23300 Grand multiparity 659.4
D8-23320 Elderly primigravida 659.5
D8-23380 Other specified indication for action related to labor and delivery, NEC 659.8

SECTION 8-3 COMPLICATIONS IN THE COURSE OF LABOR AND DELIVERY

8-30 PELVIC DYSTOCIAS AND UTERINE DISORDERS

D8-30000 Complication of labor and delivery, NOS 669.9
D8-30100 Dystocia, NOS 660.9
Obstructed labor, NOS 660.9
Unspecified obstructed labor 660.9
D8-30102 Fetal dystocia, NOS 660.9
D8-30104 Maternal dystocia, NOS 660.9
D8-30108V Avian dystocia
Egg bound
D8-30110 Obstruction caused by position of fetus at onset of labor 660.0
D8-30120 Obstruction by bony pelvis 660.1
D8-30130 Obstruction by abnormal pelvic soft tissues 660.2
D8-30132 Prolapse of anterior lip of cervix obstructing labor 660.2
D8-30140 Deep transverse arrest 660.3
D8-30141 Persistent occipitoposterior position 660.3
D8-30142 Shoulder girdle dystocia 660.4
Impacted shoulders 660.4
D8-30150 Locked twins obstructing labor 660.5
D8-30160 Failed trial of labor, NOS 660.6
D8-30170 Failed forceps 660.7
D8-30174 Failed vacuum extractor 660.7
D8-30176 Failed ventouse application 660.7
D8-30180 Other cause of obstructed labor, NEC 660.8
D8-30200 Abnormality of forces of labor, NOS 661.9
D8-30210 Uterine inertia, NOS 661.2
D8-30212 Primary uterine inertia 661.0
Primary hypotonic uterine dysfunction 661.0
Prolonged latent phase of labor 661.0
D8-30214 Failure of cervical dilation 661.0

D8-30220 Secondary uterine inertia 661.1
Secondary hypotonic uterine dysfunction 661.1
D8-30222 Arrested active phase of labor 661.1
D8-30230 Other uterine inertia, NEC 661.2
D8-30231 Atony of uterus 661.2
D8-30232 Desultory labor 661.2
D8-30233 Irregular labor 661.2
D8-30234 Poor labor contractions 661.2
D8-30236 Slow slope active phase of labor 661.2
D8-30240 Precipitate labor 661.3
D8-30250 Abnormal uterine contraction, NOS 661.4
Uterine dystocia, NOS 661.4
D8-30251 Cervical spasm 661.4
D8-30252 Contraction ring dystocia 661.4
Hourglass contraction of uterus 661.4
D8-30253 Dyscoordinate labor 661.4
Incoordinate uterine action 661.4
D8-30254 Retraction ring dystocia 661.4
Bandl's ring dystocia 661.4
Bandl's ring 661.4
Uterine retraction ring 661.4
D8-30255 Tetanic contractions of uterus 661.4
D8-30256 Uterine spasm 661.4
D8-30257 Hypertonic uterine dysfunction 661.4
D8-30400 Prolonged labor, NOS 662.1
Long labor, NOS 662.1
D8-30402 Prolonged first stage of labor 662.0
D8-30404 Prolonged second stage of labor 662.2
D8-30420 Delayed delivery of second of multiple births 662.3

8-31 UMBILICAL CORD COMPLICATIONS

D8-31000 Umbilical cord complication, NOS 663.9
D8-31010 Prolapse of cord 663.0
(T-F1800) (M-22170)
Presentation of cord 663.0
(T-F1800) (M-22170)
D8-31100 Cord entanglement, NOS 663.2
Umbilical cord around fetal part 663.2
D8-31110 Cord around neck with compression 663.1
Cord tightly around neck 663.1
D8-31120 Knot in cord with compression 663.2
D8-31130 Entanglement of cords of twins in monoamniotic sac 663.2
D8-31150 Cord entanglement without compression 663.3
D8-31190 Rupture of cord
(T-F1800) (M-14400)
D8-31200 Vasa previa 663.5
D8-31220 Vascular lesion of cord, NOS 663.6
D8-31222 Bruising of cord 663.6
D8-31224 Hematoma of cord 663.6
D8-31226 Thrombosis of vessels of cord 663.6
D8-31280 Other umbilical cord complication, NEC 663.8

8-33 TRAUMATIC LESIONS DURING DELIVERY

D8-33000 Traumatic lesion during delivery, NOS 665.9
Obstetrical trauma, NOS 665.9
D8-33100 Trauma to perineum during delivery, NOS 664.9
D8-33104 Trauma to vulva during delivery, NOS 664.9
D8-33106 Trauma from instrument during delivery 664.9
D8-33108 Traumatic extension of episiotomy 664.9
D8-33110 First degree perineal laceration, NOS 664.0
Laceration of superficial layers of perineal structures 664.0
D8-33111 Perineal laceration involving fourchette 664.0
D8-33112 Perineal laceration involving hymen 664.0
D8-33113 Perineal laceration involving labia 664.0
D8-33114 Perineal laceration involving skin 664.0
D8-33115 Perineal laceration involving vagina 664.0
D8-33116 Perineal laceration involving vulva 664.0
D8-33130 Second degree perineal laceration, NOS 664.1
Laceration of inner and muscular layers of perineal structures 664.1
D8-33132 Perineal laceration involving pelvic floor 664.1
D8-33134 Perineal laceration involving perineal muscles 664.1
D8-33136 Perineal laceration involving vaginal muscles 664.1
D8-33150 Third degree perineal laceration, NOS 664.2
Laceration of tissues between vaginal and perineal muscular layers and rectal mucosa 664.2
D8-33152 Perineal laceration involving anal sphincter 664.2
D8-33154 Perineal laceration involving rectovaginal septum 664.2
D8-33170 Fourth degree perineal laceration, NOS 664.3
D8-33172 Fourth degree perineal laceration involving anal mucosa 664.3
D8-33174 Fourth degree perineal laceration involving rectal mucosa 664.3
D8-33180 Perineal laceration during delivery, NOS 664.4
D8-33182 Central laceration during delivery 664.4
D8-33190 Vulval hematoma during delivery 664.5
D8-33192 Perineal hematoma during delivery 664.5
D8-33198 Other specified trauma to perineum and vulva during delivery, NEC 664.8
D8-33300 Obstetrical rupture of uterus, NOS 665.1
D8-33310 Rupture of uterus before onset of labor 665.0
D8-33320 Rupture of uterus during and after labor 665.1
D8-33330 Inversion of uterus during delivery 665.2
D8-33340 Obstetrical laceration of cervix 665.3
D8-33344 High vaginal obstetrical laceration 665.4
Laceration of vaginal wall or sulcus without perineal laceration during delivery 665.4

8-33 TRAUMATIC LESIONS DURING DELIVERY — Continued

D8-33350 Obstetrical trauma to bladder 665.5
D8-33352 Obstetrical trauma to urethra 665.5
D8-33358 Other obstetrical injury to pelvic organ, NEC 665.5
D8-33400 Damage to pelvic joints and ligaments during delivery, NOS 665.6
D8-33410 Avulsion of inner symphyseal cartilage during delivery 665.6
D8-33414 Separation of symphysis pubis during delivery 665.5
D8-33420 Damage to coccyx during delivery 665.6
D8-33510 Pelvic hematoma during delivery 665.7
D8-33514 Hematoma of vagina during delivery 665.7
D8-33580 Other specified obstetrical trauma, NEC 665.8

8-34 POSTPARTUM HEMORRHAGE

D8-34000 Postpartum hemorrhage, NOS 666.-
  Hemorrhage after delivery of fetus, NOS 666.-
D8-34010 Third stage hemorrhage 666.0
  Hemorrhage with retained, trapped or adherent placenta 666.0
D8-34020 Atonic postpartum hemorrhage, NOS 666.1
  Immediate postpartum hemorrhage 666.1
  Hemorrhage within 24 hours following delivery of placenta 666.1
D8-34030 Delayed or secondary postpartum hemorrhage 666.2
  Hemorrhage after first 24 hours following delivery of placenta 666.2
  Postpartum hemorrhage specified as delayed or secondary 666.2
D8-34040 Retained products of conception, NOS, following delivery with hemorrhage 666.2
  Hemorrhage from retained portion of placenta or membranes 666.2
D8-34100 Postpartum coagulation defect with hemorrhage, NOS 666.3
D8-34110 Postpartum afibrinogenemia with hemorrhage 666.3
D8-34120 Postpartum fibrinolysis with hemorrhage 666.3
D8-34200 Retained placenta, NOS, without hemorrhage 667.0
  Retained total placenta without hemorrhage 667.0
D8-34210 Placenta accreta without hemorrhage 667.0
D8-34212 Retained portions of placenta or membranes without hemorrhage 667.1
  Retained portions of products of conception following delivery without hemorrhage 667.1

8-36 OBSTETRICAL COMPLICATIONS OF ANESTHESIA AND SEDATION

D8-36000 Obstetrical complication of anesthesia or sedation, NOS 668.9
D8-36010 Obstetrical complication of anesthesia, NOS 668.9
D8-36012 Obstetrical complication of general anesthesia 668.9
D8-36014 Obstetrical complication of local anesthesia 668.9
D8-36020 Obstetrical complication of sedation, NOS 668.9
D8-36100 Obstetrical pulmonary complication of anesthesia or sedation 668.0
D8-36110 Aspiration of stomach contents after anesthesia or sedation in labor or delivery 668.0
  Mendelson's syndrome after anesthesia or sedation in labor or delivery 668.0
  Pulmonary acid aspiration syndrome after anesthesia or sedation in labor or delivery 668.0
D8-36120 Pressure collapse of lung after anesthesia or sedation in labor or delivery 668.0
D8-36130 Obstetrical cardiac complication of anesthesia or sedation 668.1
  Cardiac disorder following anesthesia or sedation in labor and delivery 668.1
D8-36132 Cardiac arrest or failure following anesthesia or sedation in labor or delivery 668.1
D8-36140 Obstetrical central nervous system complication of anesthesia or sedation 668.2
D8-36142 Cerebral anoxia following anesthesia or sedation in labor and delivery 668.2
D8-36180 Other complication of anesthesia or sedation in labor and delivery, NEC 668.8

8-37 OTHER MATERNAL COMPLICATIONS OF LABOR AND DELIVERY

D8-37000 Other complication of labor and delivery, NEC 669.8
D8-37100 Maternal distress 669.0
D8-37110 Metabolic disturbance in labor and delivery 669.0
D8-37120 Shock during or following labor and delivery 669.1
  Obstetric shock 669.1
D8-37124 Maternal hypotension syndrome 669.2
D8-37130 Acute renal failure following labor and delivery 669.3
D8-37200 Complication of obstetrical surgery or procedure, NOS 669.4
D8-37210 Cardiac arrest after obstetrical surgery or other procedure including delivery 669.4
D8-37212 Cardiac failure after obstetrical surgery or other procedure including delivery 669.4

D8-37220 Cerebral anoxia after obstetrical surgery or other procedure including delivery 669.4
D8-37300 Forceps or vacuum extraction delivery without mention of indication 669.5
D8-37310 Breech extraction without indication 669.6
D8-37320 Cesarean delivery without indication 669.7

SECTION 8-4 COMPLICATIONS OF THE PUERPERIUM AND RELATED BREAST DISORDERS

8-40 COMPLICATIONS OF THE PUERPERIUM

D8-40000 Complication of the puerperium, NOS 674.9
D8-40100 Major puerperal infection, NOS 670.-
D8-40102 Puerperal endometritis 670.-
D8-40104 Puerperal salpingitis 670.-
D8-40110 Puerperal pelvic cellulitis 670.-
D8-40112 Puerperal pelvic sepsis 670.-
D8-40120 Puerperal peritonitis 670.-
D8-40130 Puerperal septicemia 670.-
D8-40140 Puerperal fever 670.-
D8-40160V Postparturient hemoglobinuria
D8-40162V Parturient paresis
  Milk fever
  Bovine parturient hypocalcemia
D8-40170V Lactation tetany, NOS
D8-40172V Lactation tetany of mares
  Transit tetany of mares
  Eclampsia of mares
D8-40173V Lactation tetany of ruminants
  Hypomagnesemic tetany of ruminants
  Grass tetany
  Grass staggers
D8-40176V Transport tetany of ruminants
  Railroad disease
  Railroad sickness
D8-40178V Puerperal tetany of canines
  Canine parturient hypocalcemia
D8-40180V Ruminant ketosis
  Ruminant acetonemia
  Fat cow syndrome
D8-40200 Venous complication in pregnancy or the puerperium, NOS 671.9
D8-40210 Varicose veins, NOS, complicating pregnancy or puerperium 671.0
D8-40212 Varicose veins of legs complicating pregnancy or puerperium 671.0
D8-40214 Varicose veins of vulva and perineum complicating pregnancy or puerperium 671.1
D8-40216 Hemorrhoids complicating pregnancy or puerperium 671.8
D8-40220 Phlebitis, NOS, complicating pregnancy or puerperium 671.9
D8-40222 Superficial thrombophlebitis complicating pregnancy or puerperium 671.2
D8-40250 Thrombosis, NOS, complicating pregnancy or puerperium 671.9
D8-40251 Antepartum deep phlebothrombosis 671.3
  Antepartum deep vein thrombosis 671.3
D8-40254 Postpartum deep phlebothrombosis 671.4
  Postpartum deep vein thrombosis 671.4
D8-40256 Postpartum pelvic thrombophlebitis 671.4
D8-40257 Puerperal phlegmasia alba dolens 671.4
D8-40260 Cerebral venous thrombosis of pregnancy or puerperium 671.5
D8-40264 Thrombosis of intracranial venous sinus of pregnancy or puerperium 671.5
D8-40268 Phlebitis or thrombosis, NEC, complicating pregnancy or puerperium 671.5
D8-40270 Other venous complication of pregnancy or puerperium, NEC 671.8
D8-40300 Puerperal pyrexia, NOS 672.-
  Pyrexia of unknown origin during the puerperium 672.-
D8-40400 Obstetrical pulmonary embolism, NOS 673.2
  Pulmonary embolism in pregnancy childbirth or puerperium, NOS 673.2
  Puerperal pulmonary embolism, NOS 673.2
D8-40402 Obstetrical blood clot embolism 673.2
D8-40410 Obstetrical air embolism 673.0
D8-40420 Amniotic fluid embolism 673.1
D8-40430 Obstetrical pyemic or septic embolism 673.3
D8-40450 Obstetrical pulmonary fat embolism 673.8
D8-40460 Other obstetrical pulmonary embolism, NEC 673.8
D8-40470 Cerebrovascular disorder in the puerperium, NOS 674.0
D8-40500 Complication of obstetrical surgical wound, NOS 674.3
D8-40510 Disruption of cesarean wound in the puerperium 674.1
  Dehiscence or disruption of uterine wound in the puerperium 674.1
D8-40520 Disruption of perineal wound in the puerperium 674.2
  Breakdown of perineum in the puerperium 674.2
D8-40522 Disruption of episiotomy wound in the puerperium 674.2
D8-40523 Disruption of perineal laceration repair in the puerperium 674.2
D8-40524 Secondary perineal tear in the puerperium 674.2
D8-40530 Hematoma of cesarean section or perineal wound 674.3
D8-40534 Hemorrhage of cesarean section or perineal wound 674.3
D8-40540 Infection of cesarean section or perineal wound 674.3
D8-40610 Placental polyp 674.4
D8-40620 Hepatorenal syndrome following delivery 674.8
D8-40630 Postpartum cardiomyopathy 674.8
D8-40640 Postpartum subinvolution of uterus 674.8
D8-40650 Postpartum uterine hypertrophy 674.8
D8-40670 Other and unspecified complication of the puerperium, NEC 674

8-40 COMPLICATIONS OF THE PUERPERIUM — Continued

D8-40680 Sudden death of unknown cause during the puerperium 674.9

8-41 DISORDERS OF THE BREAST ASSOCIATED WITH CHILDBIRTH

D8-41000 Disorder of breast associated with childbirth, NOS 676.3

D8-41100 Infection of the breast and nipple during childbirth, NOS 675.9

D8-41110 Infection of nipple, NOS, associated with childbirth 675.0

D8-41112 Abscess of nipple associated with childbirth 675.0

D8-41120 Abscess of breast, NOS, associated with childbirth 675.1
  Mammary abscess associated with childbirth 676.1

D8-41122 Subareolar abscess associated with childbirth 675.1

D8-41124 Retromammary abscess associated with childbirth 675.1

D8-41126 Submammary abscess associated with childbirth 675.1

D8-41130 Mastitis, NOS, associated with childbirth 675.2

D8-41131 Purulent mastitis associated with childbirth 675.1

D8-41132 Nonpurulent mastitis associated with childbirth 675.2

D8-41134 Interstitial mastitis associated with childbirth 675.2

D8-41140 Parenchymatous mastitis associated with childbirth 675.2

D8-41142 Retromammary mastitis associated with childbirth 675.1

D8-41144 Submammary mastitis associated with childbirth 675.1

D8-41150 Lymphangitis of breast associated with childbirth 675.2

D8-41180 Other specified infection of the breast and nipple, NEC, associated with childbirth 675.8

D8-41210 Retracted nipple associated with childbirth 676.0

D8-41212 Cracked nipple associated with childbirth 676.1
  Fissure of nipple associated with childbirth 676.1

D8-41220 Engorgement of breasts associated with childbirth 676.2

D8-41230 Disorder of lactation, NOS 676.9

D8-41240 Failure of lactation 676.4
  Agalactia 676.4

D8-41241 Suppressed lactation 676.5

D8-41242 Polygalactia 676.8

D8-41250 Galactorrhea associated with childbirth 676.6
  Persistent secretion of milk associated with childbirth 676.6

D8-41260 Galactocele associated with childbirth 676.8

D8-41280 Other disorder of lactation, NEC 676.8

SECTION 8-6 MATERNAL CAUSES OF PERINATAL MORBIDITY AND MORTALITY

8-60 GENERAL MATERNAL CONDITIONS AFFECTING FETUS OR NEWBORN

D8-60000 Fetus or newborn affected by maternal condition, NOS 760.9
  Fetus or newborn affected by maternal condition which may be unrelated to present pregnancy 760.9
  Unspecified maternal condition affecting fetus or newborn 760.9

D8-60010 Fetus or newborn affected by maternal hypertensive disorder 760.0

D8-60020 Fetus or newborn affected by maternal renal and urinary tract disease 760.1

D8-60030 Fetus or newborn affected by maternal infectious disease, NOS 760.2
  Fetus or newborn affected by maternal infection, NOS 760.2

D8-60040 Fetus or newborn affected by chronic maternal respiratory disease 760.3

D8-60044 Fetus or newborn affected by chronic maternal circulatory disease 760.3

D8-60050 Fetus or newborn affected by maternal nutritional disorder, NOS 760.4
  Fetus or newborn affected by maternal malnutrition, NOS 760.4

D8-60060 Fetus or newborn affected by maternal injury 760.5

D8-60070 Fetus or newborn affected by surgical operation on mother 760.6

D8-60100 Fetus or newborn affected by noxious substance transmitted via placenta 760.70

D8-60104 Fetus or newborn affected by noxious substance transmitted via breast milk 760.70

D8-60110 Fetus or newborn affected by alcohol transmitted via placenta or breast milk 760.71
    (C-21005)
  Fetal alcohol syndrome 760.71
    (C-21005)

D8-60120 Fetus or newborn affected by narcotic transmitted via placenta or breast milk 760.72

D8-60130 Fetus or newborn affected by hallucinogenic agent transmitted via placenta or breast milk 760.73

D8-60140 Fetus or newborn affected by anti-infective agent transmitted via placenta or breast milk 760.74

D8-60142 Fetus or newborn affected by antibiotic transmitted via placenta or breast milk 760.74

D8-60150 Fetus or newborn affected by immune serum transmitted via placenta or breast milk 760.79

D8-60160 Fetus or newborn affected by medicinal agents, NEC, transmitted via placenta or breast milk 760.79

D8-60170 Fetus or newborn affected by toxic substance, NEC, transmitted via placenta or breast milk 760.79

D8-60180 Other specified maternal condition affecting fetus or newborn, NEC 760.8

8-61 MATERNAL COMPLICATIONS OF PREGNANCY AFFECTING THE FETUS OR NEWBORN

D8-61000 Fetus or newborn affected by maternal complication of pregnancy, NOS 761.9
  Unspecified complication of pregnancy affecting fetus or newborn 761.9

D8-61020 Fetus or newborn affected by incompetent cervix 761.0

D8-61030 Fetus or newborn affected by premature rupture of membranes 761.1

D8-61040 Fetus or newborn affected by oligohydramnios 761.2

D8-61050 Fetus or newborn affected by polyhydramnios 761.3
  Fetus or newborn affected by hydramnios 761.3

D8-61052 Fetus or newborn affected by acute hydramnios 761.3

D8-61054 Fetus or newborn affected by chronic hydramnios 761.3

D8-61060 Fetus or newborn affected by ectopic pregnancy, NOS 761.4

D8-61062 Fetus or newborn affected by abdominal pregnancy 761.4

D8-61064 Fetus or newborn affected by intraperitoneal pregnancy 761.4

D8-61066 Fetus or newborn affected by tubal pregnancy 761.4

D8-61070 Fetus or newborn affected by multiple pregnancy, NOS 761.5

D8-61072 Fetus or newborn affected by twin pregnancy 761.5

D8-61073 Fetus or newborn affected by triplet pregnancy 761.5

D8-61080 Fetus or newborn affected by maternal death 761.6

D8-61100 Fetus or newborn affected by malpresentation before labor, NOS 761.7

D8-61101 Fetus or newborn affected by breech presentation before labor 761.7

D8-61102 Fetus or newborn affected by external version before labor 761.7

D8-61104 Fetus or newborn affected by oblique lie before labor 761.7

D8-61106 Fetus or newborn affected by transverse lie before labor 761.9

D8-61108 Fetus or newborn affected by unstable lie before labor 761.7

D8-61120 Fetus or newborn affected by spontaneous abortion 761.8

D8-61180 Other specified maternal complication affecting fetus or newborn, NEC 761.8

D8-61300 Fetus or newborn affected by complication of placenta, cord or membranes 762.-

D8-61310 Fetus or newborn affected by placental separation and hemorrhage 762.1

D8-61320 Fetus or newborn affected by placenta previa 762.0

D8-61330 Fetus or newborn affected by premature separation of placenta 762.1
  Fetus or newborn affected by abruptio placenta 762.1
  Fetus or newborn affected by antepartum hemorrhage 762.1

D8-61350 Fetus or newborn affected by maternal blood loss 762.1

D8-61370 Fetus or newborn affected by rupture of marginal sinus 762.1

D8-61380 Fetus or newborn affected by damage to placenta from amniocentesis 762.1

D8-61382 Fetus or newborn affected by damage to placenta from cesarean section 762.1

D8-61384 Fetus or newborn affected by damage to placenta from surgical induction 762.1

D8-61400 Fetus or newborn affected by unspecified morphologic abnormality of placenta 762.2

D8-61410 Fetus or newborn affected by unspecified functional abnormality of placenta 762.2

D8-61420 Fetus or newborn affected by placental dysfunction 762.2

D8-61430 Fetus or newborn affected by placental infarction 762.2

D8-61440 Fetus or newborn affected by placental insufficiency 762.2

D8-61450 Fetus or newborn affected by placental transfusion syndrome 762.3
  Fetus or newborn affected by placental and cord abnormality causing twin-to-twin transplacental transfusion 762.3

D8-61500 Fetus or newborn affected by condition of umbilical cord, NOS 762.6

D8-61510 Fetus or newborn affected by compression of umbilical cord, NOS 762.5

D8-61512 Fetus or newborn affected by prolapsed cord 762.4
  Fetus or newborn affected by cord presentation 762.4

D8-61513 Fetus or newborn affected by cord around neck 762.5

D8-61514 Fetus or newborn affected by entanglement of cord 762.5

D8-61515 Fetus or newborn affected by knot in cord 762.5

D8-61516 Fetus or newborn affected by torsion of cord 762.5

8-61 MATERNAL COMPLICATIONS OF PREGNANCY AFFECTING THE FETUS OR NEWBORN — Continued

D8-61530 Fetus or newborn affected by short cord 762.6

D8-61540 Fetus or newborn affected by thrombosis of umbilical cord 762.6

D8-61550 Fetus or newborn affected by varices of umbilical cord 762.6

D8-61560 Fetus or newborn affected by velamentous insertion of umbilical cord 762.6

D8-61570 Fetus or newborn affected by vasa previa 762.6

D8-61600 Fetus or newborn affected by abnormality of chorion, NOS 762.9

D8-61610 Fetus or newborn affected by abnormality of amnion, NOS 762.9

D8-61620 Fetus or newborn affected by chorioamnionitis 762.7

D8-61630 Fetus or newborn affected by amnionitis 762.7

D8-61640 Fetus or newborn affected by membranitis 762.7

D8-61650 Fetus or newborn affected by placentitis 762.7

D8-61670 Fetus or newborn affected by other specified abnormality of chorion, NEC 762.8

D8-61680 Fetus or newborn affected by other specified abnormality of amnion, NEC 762.8

D8-61700 Complication of labor or delivery affecting fetus or newborn, NOS 763.9

D8-61710 Fetus or newborn affected by malpresentation, malposition or disproportion during labor and delivery 763.1

D8-61720 Fetus or newborn affected by breech delivery and extraction 763.0

D8-61730 Fetus or newborn affected by abnormality of bony pelvis 763.1

D8-61732 Fetus or newborn affected by contracted pelvis 763.1

D8-61734 Fetus or newborn affected by persistent occipitoposterior position 763.1

D8-61736 Fetus or newborn affected by shoulder presentation 763.1

D8-61738 Fetus or newborn affected by transverse lie 763.1

D8-61740 Fetus or newborn affected by forceps delivery 763.2

Fetus or newborn affected by forceps extraction 763.2

D8-61750 Fetus or newborn affected by delivery by vacuum extractor 763.3

D8-61760 Fetus or newborn affected by cesarean delivery 763.4

D8-61770 Fetus or newborn affected by maternal anesthesia or analgesia 763.5

Fetus or newborn affected by reaction or intoxication from maternal opiate or tranquilizer during labor and delivery 763.5

D8-61780 Fetus or newborn affected by precipitate delivery 763.6

Fetus or newborn affected by rapid second stage of labor 763.6

D8-61800 Fetus or newborn affected by abnormal uterine contraction, NOS 763.7

D8-61802 Fetus or newborn affected by contraction ring 763.7

D8-61803 Fetus or newborn affected by hypertonic labor 763.7

D8-61804 Fetus or newborn affected by hypotonic uterine dysfunction 763.7

Fetus or newborn affected by uterine inertia or dysfunction 763.7

D8-61810 Other specified complication of labor and delivery affecting fetus or newborn, NEC 763.8

D8-61820 Fetus or newborn affected by abnormality of maternal soft tissues 763.8

D8-61830 Fetus or newborn affected by destructive operation on live fetus to facilitate delivery 762.8

D8-61840 Fetus or newborn affected by medical induction of labor 763.8

D8-61850 Fetus or newborn affected by previous surgery to uterus or pelvic organs 763.8

D8-61880 Fetus or newborn affected by other condition or procedure used in labor and delivery, NEC 763.8

SECTION 8-7 FETAL OR NEWBORN CONDITIONS ARISING IN THE PERINATAL PERIOD

8-70 CONDITIONS OF FETAL GROWTH AND MALNUTRITION

D8-70000 Condition in fetus originating in the perinatal period, NOS 779.9

D8-70008 Condition in fetus originating in the perinatal period, NEC 779.8

D8-70010 Congenital debility of fetus, NOS 779.9

D8-70100 Slow fetal growth and fetal malnutrition, NOS 764.-

D8-70110 Fetal growth retardation, NOS 764.9

Intrauterine growth retardation, NOS 764.9

Microsomia 764.9

Microsomic baby 764.9

Poor fetal growth state 764.9

D8-70120 Light-for-dates without mention of fetal malnutrition 764.0

Infant underweight for gestational age 764.0

Fetus small-for-dates 764.0

D8-70130 Light-for-dates with signs of fetal malnutrition 764.1

Infant light-for-dates with dry peeling skin and loss of subcutaneous tissue 764.1

D8-70140 Fetal malnutrition without mention of light-for-dates 764.2

Infant not underweight for age showing signs of fetal malnutrition as dry peeling skin and loss of subcutaneous tissue 764.2

D8-70140 (cont.) Intrauterine malnutrition 764.2

D8-70200 Disorder relating to short gestation and unspecified low birthweight 765.-

D8-70210 Extreme immaturity of fetus 765.0
  Fetus with birthweight less than 1000 grams and gestation less than 28 weeks 765.0

D8-70220 Prematurity of fetus, NOS 765.1
  Preterm infant, NOS 765.1
  Fetus with birthweight of 1000-2499 grams and gestation of 28-37 weeks 765.1

D8-70300 Disorder relating to long gestation and high birthweight 766.-

D8-70310 Exceptionally large baby 766.0
  Birth weight 4500 grams or more 766.0
  Macrosomia 766.0
  Macrosomic baby 766.0

D8-70320 Heavy-for-dates infant regardless of gestation period 766.1
  Large-for-dates infant regardless of gestation period 766.1

D8-70330 Post-term infant, not heavy-for-dates 766.2
  Fetus or newborn with 42 weeks or more gestation and not heavy for dates 766.2

D8-70350 Postmaturity, NOS 766.2

8-71 BIRTH TRAUMA

D8-71000 Birth trauma, NOS 767.9
  Birth injury, NOS 767.9

D8-71100 Cerebral hemorrhage in fetus or newborn, NOS 767.0

D8-71102 Cerebral hemorrhage due to birth trauma 767.0

D8-71104 Cerebral hemorrhage due to intrapartum anoxia of hypoxia 767.0

D8-71110 Subdural hemorrhage in fetus or newborn, NOS 767.0
  Subdural hemorrhage due to birth trauma 767.0

D8-71114 Subdural hemorrhage due to intrapartum anoxia or hypoxia 767.0

D8-71120 Local subdural hematoma as birth trauma 767.0

D8-71130 Tentorial tear as birth trauma 767.0

D8-71140 Birth injury to scalp, NOS 767.1

D8-71142 Caput succedaneum 767.1
  Swelling edema of scalp during labor 767.1

D8-71144 Cephalhematoma 767.1

D8-71146 Chignon from vacuum extraction 767.1

D8-71150 Massive epicranial subaponeurotic hemorrhage as birth trauma 767.1

D8-71200 Injury to skeleton, NOS, as birth trauma 767.3

D8-71210 Fracture of clavicle as birth trauma 767.2

D8-71220 Fracture of long bone, NOS, as birth trauma 767.3

D8-71230 Fracture of skull as birth trauma 767.3

D8-71300 Injury of spine and spinal cord, NOS, as birth trauma 767.4

D8-71310 Dislocation of spine due to birth trauma 767.4

D8-71320 Fracture of spine due to birth trauma 767.4

D8-71330 Laceration of spinal cord due to birth trauma 767.4
  Rupture of spinal cord due to birth trauma 767.4

D8-71400 Cranial nerve injury as birth trauma 767.7

D8-71410 Peripheral nerve injury as birth trauma 767.7

D8-71420 Facial nerve injury as birth trauma 767.5

D8-71422 Facial palsy as birth trauma 767.5

D8-71430 Injury to brachial plexus as birth trauma 767.6

D8-71432 Brachial palsy as birth trauma 767.6

D8-71434 Erb-Duchenne palsy as birth trauma 767.6

D8-71436 Klumpke-Déjérine paralysis as birth trauma 767.6

D8-71440 Phrenic nerve paralysis as birth trauma 767.7

D8-71500 Other specified birth trauma, NEC 767.8

D8-71510 Subcapsular hematoma of liver as birth trauma 767.8

D8-71512 Rupture of liver as birth trauma 767.8

D8-71520 Hematoma of testis as birth trauma 767.8

D8-71524 Hematoma of vulva as birth trauma 767.8

D8-71530 Rupture of spleen as birth trauma 767.8

D8-71540 Eye damage as birth trauma 767.8

D8-71542 Glaucoma as birth trauma 767.8

D8-71580 Scalpel wound as birth trauma 767.8

8-72 HYPOXIA, ASPHYXIA AND OTHER RESPIRATORY CONDITIONS OF THE FETUS AND NEWBORN

D8-72000 Intrauterine hypoxia or birth asphyxia, NOS 768.-

D8-72010 Anoxia, NOS,in liveborn infant 768.9
  Hypoxia, NOS,in liveborn infant 768.9

D8-72020 Asphyxia, NOS,in liveborn infant 768.9

D8-72100 Fetal death from asphyxia or anoxia, not clear if noted before or after onset of labor 768.0

D8-72110 Fetal distress, NOS, in liveborn infant 768.4
  Fetal intrauterine distress, not clear if noted before or after onset of labor in liveborn infant 768.4

D8-72120 Abnormal fetal heart beat, not clear if noted before or after onset of labor in liveborn infant 768.4

D8-72130 Fetal or intrauterine acidosis, not clear if noted before or after onset of labor in liveborn infant 768.4

D8-72140 Fetal or intrauterine anoxia or hypoxia not clear if noted before or after onset of labor in liveborn infant 768.4

D8-72144 Fetal or intrauterine asphyxia, not clear if noted before or after onset of labor in liveborn infant 768.4

8-72 HYPOXIA, ASPHYXIA AND OTHER RESPIRATORY CONDITIONS OF THE FETUS AND NEWBORN — Continued

D8-72150 Meconium in amniotic fluid, not clear if noted before or after onset of labor in liveborn infant 768.4
  Passage of meconium, not clear if noted before or after onset of labor in liveborn infant 768.4
D8-72170 Fetal or intrauterine hypercapnia, not clear if noted before or after onset of labor in liveborn infant 768.4
D8-72200 Fetal death from asphyxia or anoxia before onset of labor 768.0
D8-72210 Fetal intrauterine distress noted before labor in liveborn infant 768.2
D8-72220 Abnormal fetal heart beat noted before labor in liveborn infant 768.2
D8-72230 Fetal or intrauterine acidosis noted before labor in liveborn infant 768.2
D8-72240 Fetal or intrauterine anoxia or hypoxia noted before labor in liveborn infant 768.2
D8-72244 Fetal or intrauterine asphyxia noted before labor in liveborn infant 768.2
D8-72250 Meconium in amniotic fluid noted before labor in liveborn infant 768.2
D8-72270 Fetal or intrauterine hypercapnia noted before labor in liveborn infant 768.2
D8-72300 Fetal death from asphyxia or anoxia during labor 768.1
D8-72310 Fetal intrauterine distress first noted during labor or delivery in liveborn infant 768.3
D8-72320 Abnormal fetal heart beat first noted during labor or delivery in liveborn infant 768.3
D8-72330 Fetal or intrauterine acidosis first noted during labor or delivery in liveborn infant 768.3
D8-72340 Fetal or intrauterine anoxia or hypoxia first noted during labor or delivery in liveborn infant 768.3
D8-72350 Meconium in amniotic fluid first noted during labor or delivery in liveborn infant 768.3
D8-72370 Fetal or intrauterine hypercapnia first noted during labor or delivery in liveborn infant 768.3
D8-72400 Severe birth asphyxia 768.5
  Birth asphyxia with 1 minute Apgar score 0-3 768.5
  White asphyxia 768.5
D8-72410 Mild to moderate birth asphyxia 768.-
  Birth asphyxia with 1 minute Apgar score 4-7 768.-
  Blue asphyxia 768.-
D8-72500 Respiratory condition of fetus or newborn, NOS 770.9
D8-72502 Perinatal apneic spells, NOS 770.8
D8-72504 Perinatal cyanotic attacks, NOS 770.8
D8-72506 Perinatal respiratory distress, NOS 770.8
D8-72508 Perinatal respiratory failure, NOS 770.8
D8-72510 Respiratory distress syndrome in the newborn 769.-
  Cardiorespiratory distress syndrome of newborn 769.-
  Idiopathic respiratory distress syndrome of newborn 769.-
  Pulmonary hypoperfusion syndrome of newborn 769.-
  IRDS of newborn 769.-
  RDS of newborn 769.-
  Congenital alveolar dysplasia 769.-
  Wet lung disease of newborn 769.-
D8-72520 Hyaline membrane disease 769.-
D8-72530 Congenital pneumonia, NOS 770.0
D8-72532 Infective pneumonia acquired prenatally, NOS 770.0
D8-72540 Massive aspiration syndrome, NOS 770.1
  Aspiration of contents of birth canal, NOS 770.1
D8-72544 Fetal aspiration pneumonitis 770.1
D8-72550 Meconium aspiration syndrome 770.1
D8-72554 Meconium pneumonitis 770.1
D8-72600 Perinatal interstitial emphysema 770.2
D8-72610 Perinatal pneumomediastinum 770.2
D8-72612 Perinatal pneumopericardium 770.2
D8-72614 Perinatal pneumothorax 770.2
D8-72630 Pulmonary hemorrhage, NOS, in fetus or newborn 770.3
D8-72632 Perinatal lung alveolar hemorrhage 770.3
  Perinatal lung intra-alveolar hemorrhage 770.3
D8-72638 Perinatal massive pulmonary hemorrhage 770.3
D8-72640 Primary atelectasis, NOS, in perinatal period 770.4
  Pulmonary immaturity, NOS 770.4
D8-72650 Perinatal atelectasis, NOS 770.5
D8-72652 Perinatal partial atelectasis 770.5
D8-72654 Perinatal secondary atelectasis 770.5
D8-72656 Perinatal pulmonary collapse 770.5
D8-72700 Transitory tachypnea of newborn 770.6
  Idiopathic tachypnea of newborn 770.6
  Tachypnea resolving about 6 hours postnatally 770.6
D8-72800 Chronic respiratory disease in perinatal period, NOS 770.7
D8-72810 Interstitial pulmonary fibrosis of prematurity 770.7
D8-72820 Bronchopulmonary dysplasia of newborn 770.7
D8-72830 Wilson-Mikity syndrome 770.7

8-73 CERTAIN INFECTIONS OF THE PERINATAL PERIOD

D8-73000 Infection specific to the perinatal period, NOS 771.-
D8-73010 TORCH syndrome 771.8
  Toxoplasma, rubella, cytomegalovirus and herpes simplex mixed infection 771.8

D8-73040 Omphalitis of the newborn 771.4
D8-73041V Omphalophlebitis
D8-73042 Infection of navel cord 771.4
D8-73044 Infection of umbilical stump 771.4
D8-73050 Neonatal infective mastitis 771.5
D8-73100 Ophthalmia neonatorum, NOS 771.6
D8-73102 Neonatal conjunctivitis, NOS 771.6
D8-73104 Neonatal dacryocystitis, NOS 771.6
D8-73200 Intra-amniotic infection of fetus, NOS 771.8
D8-73210 Intrauterine sepsis of fetus 771.8
D8-73220 Septicemia of newborn 771.8
D8-73300 Neonatal urinary tract infection 771.8

8-74 NEONATAL HEMORRHAGE AND HEMOLYTIC DISEASE OF THE NEWBORN

D8-74000 Hemorrhage of newborn, NOS 772.9
  Fetal or neonatal hemorrhage, NOS 772.9
D8-74010 Fetal blood loss from cut end of co-twin's cord 772.0
D8-74020 Fetal blood loss from ruptured cord 772.0
D8-74030 Fetal blood loss from vasa previa 772.0
D8-74040 Fetal blood loss from placenta 772.0
D8-74050 Fetal hemorrhage into co-twin 772.0
D8-74060 Fetal hemorrhage into mother's circulation 772.0
D8-74080 Fetal exsanguination 772.0
D8-74100 Perinatal intraventricular hemorrhage 772.1
  Intraventricular hemorrhage from any perinatal cause 772.1
D8-74104 Perinatal subarachnoid hemorrhage 772.2
  Subarachnoid hemorrhage from any perinatal cause 772.2
D8-74110 Umbilical hemorrhage after birth 772.3
D8-74112 Slipped umbilical ligature with hemorrhage 772.3
D8-74120 Perinatal gastrointestinal hemorrhage 772.4
D8-74130 Perinatal adrenal hemorrhage 772.5
D8-74160 Perinatal cutaneous hemorrhage, NOS 772.6
D8-74162 Petechiae in fetus or newborn 772.6
D8-74164 Ecchymoses in fetus or newborn 772.6
D8-74166 Bruising in fetus or newborn 772.6
D8-74168 Superficial hematoma in fetus or newborn 772.6
D8-74180 Other specified hemorrhage of fetus or newborn, NEC 772.8
D8-74300 Hemolytic disease of fetus or newborn, NOS 773.2
  Erythroblastosis fetalis, NOS 773.2
  Erythroblastosis neonatorum, NOS 773.2
D8-74310 Hemolytic disease of fetus or newborn due to isoimmunization, NOS 773.2
D8-74320 Hemolytic disease of fetus or newborn due to Rh isoimmunization 773.0
  Hemolytic disease due to Rh isoimmunization 773.0
  Anemia due to Rh isoimmunization 773.0
  Erythroblastosis fetalis due to Rh isoimmunization 773.0
  Jaundice due to Rh isoimmunization of the newborn 773.0
  Rh hemolytic disease of the newborn 773.0
  Rh isoimmunization of the newborn 773.0
D8-74340 Hemolytic disease of fetus or newborn due to ABO immunization 773.1
  Hemolytic disease due to ABO isoimmunization 773.1
  ABO hemolytic disease of the newborn 773.1
  ABO isoimmunization of the newborn 773.1
  Anemia due to ABO incompatibility in the newborn 773.1
  Erythroblastosis fetalis due to ABO isoimmunization 773.1
  Jaundice due to ABO isoimmunization of the newborn 773.1
D8-74380 Hemolytic disease due to other isoimmunization, NEC 773.2
D8-74410 Hydrops fetalis due to isoimmunization 773.3
D8-74420 Kernicterus due to isoimmunization 773.4
D8-74430 Late anemia due to isoimmunization 773.5
D8-74500 Fetal and neonatal jaundice, NOS 774.6
  Physiologic jaundice in newborn, NOS 774.6
  Neonatal hyperbilirubinemia, NOS 774.6
D8-74510 Transient familial neonatal hyperbilirubinemia 774.6
  Icterus neonatorum 774.6
  Arias syndrome 774.6
  Lucey-Arias syndrome 774.6
D8-74520 Kernicterus of newborn, NOS 774.7
  Kernicterus not due to isoimmunization 774.7
  Bilirubin encephalopathy 774.7
D8-74530 Perinatal jaundice from hereditary hemolytic anemia 774.0
D8-74540 Perinatal jaundice from excessive hemolysis, NOS 774.1
D8-74541 Fetal or neonatal jaundice from bruising 774.1
D8-74542 Fetal or neonatal jaundice from drugs or toxins transmitted from mother 774.1
D8-74543 Lucey-Driscoll syndrome 774.1
D8-74544 Fetal or neonatal jaundice from infection 774.1
D8-74546 Fetal or neonatal jaundice from polycythemia 774.1
D8-74548 Fetal or neonatal jaundice from swallowed maternal blood 774.1
D8-74550 Neonatal jaundice associated with preterm delivery 774.2
  Hyperbilirubinemia of prematurity 774.2
  Jaundice due to delayed conjugation associated with preterm delivery 774.2
D8-74560 Neonatal jaundice due to delayed conjugation, NOS 774.30

8-74 NEONATAL HEMORRHAGE AND HEMOLYTIC DISEASE OF THE NEWBORN — Continued

D8-74562 Neonatal jaundice due to delayed conjugation in diseases classified elsewhere 774.31
D8-74564 Neonatal jaundice due to delayed conjugation from delayed development of conjugating system 774.39
D8-74566 Neonatal jaundice due to delayed conjugation from breast milk inhibitors 774.39
Breast milk jaundice 774.39
D8-74610 Perinatal jaundice to due to hepatocellular damage 774.4
D8-74612 Perinatal jaundice due to fetal or neonatal hepatitis 774.4
Perinatal jaundice due to giant cell hepatitis 774.4
D8-74616 Perinatal jaundice due to inspissated bile syndrome 774.4
D8-74630 Perinatal jaundice from causes classified elsewhere 774.5

8-75 ENDOCRINE, METABOLIC AND HEMATOLOGIC DISORDERS SPECIFIC TO THE FETUS OR NEWBORN

D8-75000 Endocrine or metabolic disorder specific to the fetus or newborn, NOS 775.9
D8-75100 Syndrome of infant of diabetic mother 775.0
Maternal diabetes mellitus with hypoglycemia affecting fetus or newborn 775.0
D8-75110 Neonatal diabetes mellitus 775.1
Diabetes mellitus syndrome in newborn infant 775.1
D8-75120 Neonatal myasthenia gravis 775.2
D8-75130 Neonatal thyrotoxicosis 775.3
D8-75132 Neonatal transient hyperthyroidism 775.3
D8-75140 Hypocalcemia and hypomagnesemia of newborn 775.4
D8-75142 Cow's milk hypocalcemia of newborn 775.4
D8-75144 Neonatal hypocalcemic tetany 775.4
D8-75145 Phosphate-loading hypocalcemia 775.4
D8-75146V Hypomagnesemic tetany in calves
D8-75150 Neonatal hypoparathyroidism 775.4
D8-75160 Transitory neonatal electrolyte disturbance, NOS 775.5
D8-75164 Neonatal dehydration 775.5
D8-75170 Neonatal hypoglycemia 775.6
D8-75176V Hypoglycemia of piglets
D8-75180 Late metabolic acidosis of newborn 775.7
D8-75200 Transitory neonatal endocrine or metabolic disorder, NOS 775.8
D8-75210 Transitory amino acid metabolic disorder, NOS 775.8
D8-75500 Hematologic disorder specific to fetus or newborn, NOS 776.9
D8-75510 Hemorrhagic disease of the newborn due to vitamin K deficiency 776.0
Hemorrhagic diathesis of newborn 776.0
Vitamin K deficiency of newborn 776.0
Neonatal vitamin K deficiency 776.0
D8-75520 Transient neonatal thrombocytopenia, NOS 776.1
D8-75522 Neonatal thrombocytopenia due to exchange transfusion 776.1
D8-75524 Neonatal thrombocytopenia due to idiopathic maternal thrombocytopenia 776.1
D8-75526 Neonatal thrombocytopenia due to isoimmunization 776.1
D8-75530 Disseminated intravascular coagulation in newborn 776.2
DIC in newborn 776.2
D8-75540 Transient neonatal disorder of coagulation, NOS 776.3
Transient coagulation defect of newborn 776.3
D8-75600 Polycythemia neonatorum 776.4
Plethora of newborn 776.4
D8-75602 Polycythemia due to donor twin transfusion 776.4
D8-75604 Polycythemia due to maternal-fetal transfusion 776.4
D8-75620 Congenital anemia, NOS 776.5
D8-75622 Anemia following fetal blood loss 776.5
D8-75630 Anemia of prematurity 776.6
D8-75650 Transient neonatal neutropenia 776.7
D8-75652 Isoimmune neutropenia 776.7
D8-75654 Maternal transfer neutropenia 776.7
D8-75680 Transient hematological disorder, NEC 776.8

8-76 DIGESTIVE DISORDERS SPECIFIC TO THE FETUS OR NEWBORN

D8-76000 Disorder of digestive system specific to fetus or newborn, NOS 777.9
Perinatal disorder of digestive system, NOS 777.9
D8-76100 Meconium obstruction 777.1
Delayed passage of meconium 777.1
Meconium plug syndrome 777.1
D8-76110 Congenital fecaliths 777.1
D8-76120 Intestinal obstruction by inspissated milk in newborn 777.2
D8-76130 Transitory ileus of newborn 777.4
D8-76150 Hematemesis and melena due to swallowed maternal blood 777.3
Swallowed blood syndrome in newborn 777.3
D8-76200 Necrotizing enterocolitis in fetus or newborn 777.5
Pseudomembranous enterocolitis in newborn 777.5
D8-76220 Perinatal intestinal perforation 777.6
D8-76224 Meconium peritonitis 777.6
D8-76280 Specified perinatal disorder of digestive system, NEC 777.8

8-77 DISORDERS OF INTEGUMENT AND TEMPERATURE REGULATION IN THE FETUS OR NEWBORN

D8-77000 Conditions involving the integument and temperature regulation of fetus or newborn, NOS 778.9
D8-77100 Idiopathic hydrops fetalis 778.0
 Hydrops fetalis not due to isoimmunization 778.0
D8-77110 Sclerema neonatorum 778.1
 (T-03000) (M-54110) (F-88000)
 Subcutaneous fat necrosis of newborn 778.1
 (T-03000) (M-54110) (F-88000)
D8-77200 Disturbance of temperature regulation of newborn, NOS 778.4
D8-77210 Hypothermia of newborn, NOS 778.3
D8-77214 Cold injury syndrome of newborn 778.2
D8-77230 Dehydration fever in newborn 778.4
D8-77232 Environmentally-induced pyrexia in newborn 778.4
D8-77234 Hyperthermia in newborn 778.4
D8-77236 Transitory fever of newborn 778.4
D8-77300 Edema of newborn, NOS 778.5
 Edema neonatorum 778.5
D8-77310 Congenital hydrocele, NOS 778.6
 Congenital hydrocele of tunica vaginalis 778.6
D8-77330 Breast engorgement in newborn 778.7
D8-77334 Noninfective mastitis of newborn 778.7
D8-77340 Urticaria neonatorum 778.8
D8-77380 Disorder involving the integument of fetus or newborn, NEC 778.8

8-78 MISCELLANEOUS DISORDERS IN THE FETUS OR NEWBORN

D8-78100 Central nervous system dysfunction in the newborn 779.2
 CNS dysfunction in the newborn, NOS 779.2
D8-78110 Cerebral irritability in newborn, NOS 779.1
D8-78120 Cerebral depression in newborn 779.2
D8-78122 Coma in the newborn 779.2
D8-78126 Abnormal cerebral signs in the newborn 779.2
D8-78130 Convulsions in the newborn 779.0
 Seizures in the newborn 779.0
 Fits in the newborn 779.0
D8-78200 Feeding problem in newborn, NOS 779.3
D8-78210 Regurgitation of food in newborn 779.3
D8-78220 Slow feeding in newborn 779.3
D8-78230 Vomiting in newborn 779.3
D8-78300 Drug reaction or intoxication specific to newborn 779.4
D8-78310 Gray syndrome from chloramphenicol administration in newborn 779.4
D8-78330 Drug withdrawal syndrome in newborn 779.5
 Drug withdrawal syndrome in infant of dependent mother 779.5
D8-78400 Fetal death due to termination of pregnancy, NOS 779.6
 Fetal death due to induced abortion, NOS 779.6

CHAPTER 9 — MENTAL DISORDERS

SECTION 9-0 GENERAL CONVENIENCE TERMS

D9-00000 Mental disorder, NOS 300.90
D9-00005 Neurosis, NOS 300.90
  Nonpsychotic mental disorder, NOS 300.90
D9-00010 No diagnosis on Axis I V71.09
  No condition on Axis I V71.09
D9-00015 Deferred diagnosis on Axis I 799.90
  Deferred condition on Axis I 799.90
D9-00020 No diagnosis on Axis II V71.09
  No condition on Axis II V71.09
D9-00025 Deferred diagnosis on Axis II 799.90
  Deferred condition on Axis II 799.90
D9-00030 No diagnosis on Axis III
  No condition on Axis III
D9-00035 Deferred diagnosis on Axis III
  Deferred condition on Axis III
D9-00040 No diagnosis on Axis IV
  No condition on Axis IV
  No psychosocial stressor on Axis IV
D9-00045 Deferred diagnosis on Axis IV
  Deferred psychosocial stressor evaluation on Axis IV
D9-00050 No diagnosis on Axis V
  No assessment on Axis V
D9-00055 Deferred diagnosis on Axis V
  Deferred assessment on Axis V
D9-00110 Axis I diagnosis, NOS
D9-00120 Axis II diagnosis, NOS
D9-00130 Axis III diagnosis, NOS
D9-00140 Axis IV diagnosis, NOS
D9-00150 Axis V diagnosis, NOS

SECTION 9-1 DISORDERS USUALLY FIRST EVIDENT IN INFANCY, CHILDHOOD OR ADOLESCENCE

D9-10000 Disorder usually first evident in infancy, childhood or adolescence, NOS
D9-10001 Disorder in infancy, NOS
D9-10002 Disorder in childhood, NOS
D9-10003 Disorder in adolescence, NOS

9-10 MISCELLANEOUS DISORDERS OF INFANCY, CHILDHOOD OR ADOLESCENCE

D9-10110 Elective mutism 313.23
D9-10120 Identity disorder 313.82
D9-10130 Reactive attachment disorder, NOS 313.89
D9-10131 Reactive attachment disorder of infancy or early childhood 313.89
D9-10132 Reactive attachment disorder of infancy 313.89
D9-10133 Reactive attachment disorder of early childhood 313.89
D9-10140 Stereotypy habit disorder 307.30
D9-10150 Undifferenciated attention deficit disorder 314.00
D9-10200 Psychosocial dwarfism
  Emotional deprivation syndrome

9-11 DISRUPTIVE BEHAVIOR DISORDERS

D9-11000 Disruptive behavior disorder, NOS 312.90
D9-11100 Conduct disorder, undifferentiated type 312.90
D9-11110 Conduct disorder, group type 312.20
D9-11120 Conduct disorder, solitary aggressive type 312.00
D9-11200 Attention deficit hyperactivity disorder 314.01
D9-11300 Oppositional defiant disorder 313.81
D9-11400 Emancipation disorder of adolescent

9-12 ANXIETY DISORDERS OF CHILDHOOD OR ADOLESCENCE

D9-12000 Anxiety disorder of childhood or adolescence, NOS
D9-12010 Anxiety disorder of childhood, NOS
D9-12020 Anxiety disorder of adolescence, NOS
D9-12100 Separation anxiety disorder of childhood 309.21
D9-12200 Avoidant disorder of childhood or adolescence 313.21
D9-12210 Avoidant disorder of childhood 313.21
  Withdrawing reaction of childhood 313.21
D9-12211 Shyness disorder of childhood 313.21
D9-12220 Avoidant disorder of adolescence 313.21
D9-12300 Overanxious disorder of childhood 313.00

9-13 EATING DISORDERS

D9-13000 Eating disorder, NOS 307.50
D9-13100 Anorexia nervosa 307.10
D9-13200 Bulimia nervosa 307.51
D9-13300 Pica 307.52
  Abnormal craving 307.52
D9-13400 Rumination disorder, NOS 307.53
D9-13410 Rumination disorder of infancy 307.53

9-14 GENDER IDENTITY DISORDERS

D9-14000 Gender identity disorder, NOS 302.85
D9-14100 Gender identity disorder of childhood 302.60
D9-14200 Gender identity disorder of adolescence, NOS 302.85
D9-14210 Gender identity disorder of adolescence, previously asexual 302.85
D9-14220 Gender identity disorder of adolescence, previously homosexual 302.85
D9-14230 Gender identity disorder of adolescence, previously heterosexual 302.85

D9-14300 Gender identity disorder of adulthood, NOS
D9-14310 Gender identity disorder of adulthood, previously asexual 302.85
D9-14320 Gender identity disorder of adulthood, previously homosexual 302.85
D9-14330 Gender identity disorder of adulthood, previously heterosexual 302.85
D9-14400 Transsexualism, NOS 302.50
D9-14410 Transsexualism, previously asexual 302.50
D9-14420 Transsexualism, previously homosexual 302.50
D9-14430 Transsexualism, previously heterosexual 302.50

9-15 TIC DISORDERS

D9-15000 Tic disorder, NOS 307.20
D9-15110 Chronic motor tic disorder 307.22
D9-15120 Chronic vocal tic disorder 307.22
D9-15200 Transient tic disorder, NOS 307.21
D9-15210 Transient tic disorder, single episode 307.21
D9-15220 Recurrent transient tic disorder 307.21
D9-15300 Tourette's disorder 307.23
D9-15400 Atypical tic disorder

9-16 ELIMINATION DISORDERS

D9-16000 Elimination disorder, NOS
D9-16100 Functional encopresis, NOS 307.70
Encopresis, NOS 787.6
D9-16110 Primary functional encopresis 307.70
D9-16120 Secondary functional encopresis 307.70
D9-16200 Functional enuresis, NOS 307.60
D9-16210 Primary functional enuresis 307.60
D9-16220 Secondary functional enuresis 307.60
D9-16230 Nocturnal only enuresis 307.60
D9-16240 Diurnal only enuresis 307.60
D9-16250 Nocturnal and diurnal enuresis 307.60

9-18 DEVELOPMENTAL DISORDERS

D9-18000 Developmental disorder, NOS 315.90
D9-18100 Pervasive developmental disorder, NOS 299.80
D9-18110 Autistic disorder, NOS 299.00
D9-18111 Autistic disorder of childhood onset 299.00
D9-18200 Specific developmental disorder, NOS 315.90
D9-18210 Developmental academic disorder, NOS
Academic skill disorder, NOS
D9-18212 Developmental arithmetic disorder 315.10
D9-18213 Developmental expressive writing disorder 315.80
D9-18214 Developmental reading disorder 315.00
D9-18220 Developmental language disorder, NOS
D9-18221 Developmental speech disorder, NOS
D9-18222 Developmental expressive language disorder 315.31
D9-18223 Developmental receptive language disorder 315.31
D9-18224 Developmental articulation disorder 315.39
D9-18230 Motor skill disorder, NOS
D9-18231 Developmental coordination disorder 315.40
D9-18300 Mental retardation, NOS
D9-18310 Mild mental retardation (I.Q. 50-70) 317.00
Moron (mental age 8-12 years) 317.00
D9-18320 Moderate mental retardation (I.Q. 35-49) 318.00
Imbecile (mental age 2-7 years) 318.00
D9-18330 Severe mental retardation (I.Q. 20-34) 318.10
D9-18340 Profound mental retardation (I.Q. below 20) 318.20
Idiot (mental age less than 2 years) 318.20
D9-18350 Borderline mental retardation (I.Q. 70-85)
D9-18360 Idiot savant

SECTION 9-2 ORGANIC MENTAL DISORDERS

9-20 ORGANIC MENTAL DISORDERS OF UNKNOWN ETIOLOGY

D9-20000 Organic mental disorder, NOS 294.80
D9-20100 Delirium, NOS 293.00
D9-20200 Dementia, NOS 294.10
D9-20300 Amnestic disorder, NOS 294.00
D9-20400 Organic delusional disorder, NOS 293.81
D9-20500 Organic hallucinosis, NOS 293.81
D9-20600 Organic mood disorder, NOS 293.83
D9-20610 Organic mood disorder of manic type 293.83
D9-20620 Organic mood disorder of depressed type 293.83
D9-20630 Organic mood disorder of mixed type 293.83
D9-20700 Organic anxiety disorder 294.80
D9-20800 Organic personality disorder, NOS 310.10
D9-20810 Explosive type organic personality disorder 310.10

9-22 DEMENTIAS IN THE SENIUM AND PRESENIUM

D9-22000 Dementia arising in the senium and presenium, NOS
D9-22010 Senile dementia, NOS 290.00
D9-22020 Presenile dementia, NOS 290.10
D9-22100 Primary degenerative dementia of the Alzheimer type, senile onset, uncomplicated 290.00
(DA-20020)
D9-22110 Primary degenerative dementia of the Alzheimer type, senile onset, with delirium 290.30
(DA-20020)
D9-22120 Primary degenerative dementia of the Alzheimer type, senile onset, with delusions 290.20
(DA-20020)
D9-22130 Primary degenerative dementia of the Alzheimer type, senile onset, with depression 290.21
(DA-20020)

9-22 DEMENTIAS IN THE SENIUM AND PRESENIUM — Continued

D9-22200 Primary degenerative dementia of the Alzheimer type, presenile onset, uncomplicated 290.10
(DA-20020)

D9-22210 Primary degenerative dementia of the Alzheimer type, presenile onset, with delirium 290.11
(DA-20020)

D9-22220 Primary degenerative dementia of the Alzheimer type, presenile onset, with delusions 290.12
(DA-20020)

D9-22230 Primary degenerative dementia of the Alzheimer type, presenile onset, with depression 290.13
(DA-20020)

D9-22300 Multi-infarct dementia, NOS 290.4

D9-22310 Multi-infarct dementia, uncomplicated 290.40

D9-22320 Multi-infarct dementia with delirium 290.41

D9-22330 Multi-infarct dementia with delusions 290.42

D9-22340 Multi-infarct dementia with depression 290.43

9-23 PSYCHOACTIVE SUBSTANCE-INDUCED ORGANIC MENTAL DISORDERS

D9-23000 Psychoactive substance-induced organic mental disorder, NOS 292.90

D9-23010 Psychoactive substance-induced organic intoxication 305.90

D9-23020 Psychoactive substance-induced organic withdrawal 292.00

D9-23030 Psychoactive substance-induced organic delirium 292.81

D9-23040 Psychoactive substance-induced organic dementia 292.82

D9-23050 Psychoactive substance-induced organic amnestic disorder 292.83

D9-23060 Psychoactive substance-induced organic delusional disorder 292.11

D9-23070 Psychoactive substance-induced organic hallucinosis 292.12

D9-23080 Psychoactive substance-induced organic mood disorder 292.84

D9-23090 Psychoactive substance-induced organic anxiety disorder 292.89

D9-230A0 Psychoactive substance-induced organic personality disorder 292.89

D9-23100 Alcohol-induced organic mental disorder, NOS

D9-23110 Alcohol intoxication 303.00

D9-23120 Idiosyncratic intoxication 291.40

D9-23130 Uncomplicated alcohol withdrawal 291.80

D9-23140 Alcohol withdrawal delirium 291.00

D9-23150 Alcohol hallucinosis 291.30

D9-23160 Alcohol amnestic disorder 291.10

D9-23170 Dementia associated with alcoholism 291.20

D9-23200 Amphetamine-induced organic mental disorder, NOS

D9-23210 Amphetamine intoxication 305.70

D9-23220 Amphetamine withdrawal 292.00

D9-23230 Amphetamine delirium 292.81

D9-23240 Amphetamine delusional disorder 292.11

D9-23300 Caffeine-induced organic mental disorder, NOS

D9-23310 Caffeine intoxication 305.90

D9-23400 Cannabis-induced organic mental disorder, NOS

D9-23410 Cannabis intoxication 305.20

D9-23420 Cannabis delusional disorder 292.11

D9-23500 Cocaine-induced organic mental disorder, NOS

D9-23510 Cocaine intoxication 305.60

D9-23520 Cocaine withdrawal 292.00

D9-23530 Cocaine delirium 292.81

D9-23540 Cocaine delusional disorder 292.11

D9-23600 Hallucinogen-induced organic mental disorder, NOS

D9-23610 Hallucinogen hallucinosis 305.30

D9-23620 Hallucinogen delusional disorder 292.11

D9-23630 Hallucinogen mood disorder 292.84

D9-23640 Posthallucinogen perception disorder 292.89

D9-23700 Inhalant-induced organic mental disorder, NOS

D9-23710 Inhalant intoxication 305.90

D9-23800 Nicotine-induced organic mental disorder, NOS

D9-23810 Nicotine withdrawal 292.00

D9-23900 Opioid-induced organic mental disorder, NOS

D9-23910 Opioid intoxication 305.50

D9-23920 Opioid withdrawal 292.00

D9-23A00 Phencyclidine-induced mental disorder, NOS 292.90
PCP-induced organic mental disorder, NOS 292.90
Arylcyclohexylamine-induced organic mental disorder, NOS 292.90

D9-23A10 PCP intoxication 305.90

D9-23A20 PCP delirium 292.81

D9-23A30 PCP delusional disorder 292.11

D9-23A40 PCP mood disorder 292.84

D9-23B00 Sedative-induced organic mental disorder, NOS
Hypnotic-induced organic mental disorder, NOS
Anxiolytic-induced organic mental disorder, NOS

D9-23B10 Sedative intoxication 305.40
Hypnotic intoxication 305.40
Anxiolytic intoxication 305.40

D9-23B20 Uncomplicated sedative, hypnotic or anxiolytic withdrawal 292.00

D9-23B30 Sedative withdrawal delirium 292.00

D9-23B40 Sedative amnestic disorder 292.83

SECTION 9-3 PSYCHOACTIVE SUBSTANCE USE DISORDERS

D9-30000 Psychoactive substance use disorder, NOS
D9-30010 Psychoactive substance abuse, NOS 305.90
D9-30020 Psychoactive substance dependence, NOS 304.90
D9-30030 Polysubstance dependence 304.90
D9-30100 Alcohol abuse 305.00
D9-30110 Alcohol dependence 303.90
D9-30120 Alcoholism, NOS
D9-30170 Nicotine dependence 305.10
D9-30200 Amphetamine abuse 305.70
D9-30210 Amphetamine dependence 304.40
D9-30300 Cannabis abuse 305.20
D9-30310 Cannabis dependence 304.30
D9-30400 Cocaine abuse 305.60
D9-30410 Cocaine dependence 304.20
D9-30500 Hallucinogen abuse 305.30
D9-30510 Hallucinogen dependence 304.50
D9-30600 Inhalant abuse 305.90
D9-30610 Inhalant dependence 304.60
D9-30800 Opioid abuse 305.50
D9-30810 Opioid dependence 304.00
D9-30900 PCP abuse 305.90
D9-30910 PCP dependence 304.50
D9-30A00 Sedative abuse 305.40
D9-30A10 Sedative dependence 304.10

SECTION 9-4 SCHIZOPHRENIAS

D9-40000 Schizophrenia, NOS
D9-40010 Subchronic schizophrenia, NOS
D9-40011 Subchronic schizophrenia with acute exacerbations, NOS
D9-40020 Chronic schizophrenia, NOS
D9-40021 Chronic schizophrenia with acute exacerbations, NOS
D9-40030 Schizophrenia in remission, NOS
D9-40100 Catatonic schizophrenia, NOS 295.20
  Catatonia, NOS
D9-40108 Stauder's lethal catatonia
  Bell's disease
D9-40110 Subchronic catatonic schizophrenia 295.21
D9-40111 Subchronic catatonic schizophrenia with acute exacerbations 295.23
D9-40120 Chronic catatonic schizophrenia 295.22
D9-40121 Chronic catatonic schizophrenia with acute exacerbations 295.24
D9-40130 Catatonic schizophrenia in remission 295.25
D9-40200 Disorganized schizophrenia, NOS 295.10
D9-40210 Subchronic disorganized schizophrenia 295.11
D9-40211 Subchronic disorganized schizophrenia with acute exacerbations 295.13
D9-40220 Chronic disorganized schizophrenia 295.12
D9-40221 Chronic disorganized schizophrenia with acute exacerbations 295.14
D9-40230 Disorganized schizophrenia in remission 295.15
D9-40300 Paranoid schizophrenia, NOS 295.30
D9-40310 Subchronic paranoid schizophrenia 295.31
D9-40311 Subchronic paranoid schizophrenia with acute exacerbations 295.33
D9-40320 Chronic paranoid schizophrenia 295.32
D9-40321 Chronic paranoid schizophrenia with acute exacerbations 295.34
D9-40330 Paranoid schizophrenia in remission 295.35
D9-40400 Undifferentiated schizophrenia, NOS 295.90
D9-40410 Subchronic undifferentiated schizophrenia 295.91
D9-40411 Subchronic undifferentiated schizophrenia with acute exacerbations 295.93
D9-40420 Chronic undifferentiated schizophrenia 295.92
D9-40421 Chronic undifferentiated schizophrenia with acute exacerbations 295.94
D9-40430 Undifferentiated schizophrenia in remission 295.95
D9-40500 Residual schizophrenia, NOS 295.60
D9-40510 Subchronic residual schizophrenia 295.61
D9-40511 Subchronic residual schizophrenia with acute exacerbations 295.63
D9-40520 Chronic residual schizophrenia 295.62
D9-40521 Chronic residual schizophrenia with acute exacerbations 295.64
D9-40530 Residual schizophrenia in remission 295.65

SECTION 9-5 MOOD DISORDERS

9-50 UNSPECIFIED MOOD DISORDERS

D9-50000 Mood disorder, NOS
D9-50010 Mild mood disorder
D9-50020 Moderate mood disorder
D9-50030 Severe mood disorder without psychotic features
D9-50040 Severe mood disorder with psychotic features
D9-50041 Severe mood disorder with psychotic features, mood-congruent
D9-50042 Severe mood disorder with psychotic features, mood-incongruent
D9-50051 Mood disorder in partial remission
D9-50052 Mood disorder in full remission

9-51 BIPOLAR DISORDERS

D9-51000 Bipolar disorder, NOS 296.70
D9-51010 Mild bipolar disorder 296.71
D9-51020 Moderate bipolar disorder 296.72
D9-51030 Severe bipolar disorder without psychotic features 296.73
D9-51040 Severe bipolar disorder with psychotic features 296.74
D9-51041 Severe bipolar disorder with psychotic features, mood-congruent 296.74
D9-51042 Severe bipolar disorder with psychotic features, mood-incongruent 296.76
D9-51050 Bipolar disorder in remission 296.76

9-51 BIPOLAR DISORDERS — Continued

D9-51051 Bipolar disorder in partial remission 296.75
D9-51052 Bipolar disorder in full remission 296.76
D9-51100 Mixed bipolar disorder, NOS 296.60
D9-51110 Mild mixed bipolar disorder 296.61
D9-51120 Moderate mixed bipolar disorder 296.62
D9-51130 Severe mixed bipolar disorder without psychotic features 296.63
D9-51140 Severe mixed bipolar disorder with psychotic features 296.64
D9-51141 Severe mixed bipolar disorder with psychotic features, mood-congruent 296.64
D9-51142 Severe mixed bipolar disorder with psychotic features, mood-incongruent 296.64
D9-51150 Mixed bipolar disorder in remission 296.66
D9-51151 Mixed bipolar disorder in partial remission 296.65
D9-51152 Mixed bipolar disorder in full remission 296.66
D9-51200 Manic bipolar disorder, NOS 296.40
D9-51210 Mild manic bipolar disorder 296.41
D9-51220 Moderate manic bipolar disorder 296.42
D9-51230 Severe manic bipolar disorder without psychotic features 296.43
D9-51240 Severe manic bipolar disorder with psychotic features 296.44
D9-51241 Severe manic bipolar disorder with psychotic features, mood-congruent 296.44
D9-51242 Severe manic bipolar disorder with psychotic features, mood-incongruent 296.44
D9-51250 Manic bipolar disorder in remission 296.46
D9-51251 Manic bipolar disorder in partial remission 296.45
D9-51252 Manic bipolar disorder in full remission 296.46
D9-51300 Depressed bipolar disorder, NOS 296.50
D9-51310 Mild depressed bipolar disorder 296.51
D9-51320 Moderate depressed bipolar disorder 296.52
D9-51330 Severe depressed bipolar disorder without psychotic features 296.53
D9-51340 Severe depressed bipolar disorder with psychotic features 296.54
D9-51341 Severe depressed bipolar disorder with psychotic features, mood-congruent 296.54
D9-51342 Severe depressed bipolar disorder with psychotic features, mood-incongruent 296.54
D9-51350 Depressed bipolar disorder in remission 296.56
D9-51351 Depressed bipolar disorder in partial remission 296.55
D9-51352 Depressed bipolar disorder in full remission 296.56
D9-51360 Cyclothymia 301.13

9-52 DEPRESSIVE DISORDERS

D9-52000 Depressive disorder, NOS 311.00
Major depression, NOS
D9-52010 Mild major depression
D9-52020 Moderate major depression
D9-52030 Severe major depression without psychotic features
D9-52040 Severe major depression with psychotic features, NOS
D9-52041 Severe major depression with psychotic features, mood-congruent
D9-52042 Severe major depression with psychotic features, mood-incongruent
D9-52050 Major depression in remission, NOS
D9-52051 Major depression in partial remission
D9-52052 Major depression in complete remission
D9-52100 Major depression, single episode, NOS 296.20
D9-52110 Mild major depression, single episode 296.21
D9-52120 Moderate major depression, single episode 296.22
D9-52130 Severe major depression, single episode, without psychotic features 296.23
D9-52141 Severe major depression, single episode, with psychotic features, mood-congruent 296.24
D9-52142 Severe major depression, single episode, with psychotic features, mood-incongruent 296.24
D9-52151 Major depression single episode, in partial remission 296.25
D9-52152 Major depression, single episode, in complete remission 296.26
D9-52200 Recurrent major depression, NOS 296.30
D9-52210 Mild recurrent major depression 296.31
D9-52220 Moderate recurrent major depression 296.32
D9-52230 Severe recurrent major depression without psychotic features 296.33
D9-52240 Severe recurrent major depression with psychotic features 296.34
D9-52241 Severe recurrent major depression with psychotic features, mood-congruent 296.34
D9-52242 Severe recurrent major depression with psychotic features, mood-incongruent 296.34
D9-52250 Recurrent major depression in remission 296.36
D9-52251 Recurrent major depression in partial remission 296.35
D9-52252 Recurrent major depression in complete remission 296.36
D9-52300 Dysthymia, NOS 300.40
Depressive neurosis 300.40
D9-52301 Early onset dysthymia 300.40
D9-52302 Late onset dysthymia 300.40
D9-52310 Primary dysthymia, NOS 300.40
D9-52311 Primary dysthymia early onset 300.40
D9-52312 Primary dysthymia late onset 300.40
D9-52320 Secondary dysthymia, NOS 300.40
D9-52321 Secondary dysthymia early onset 300.40
D9-52332 Secondary dysthymia late onset 300.40
D9-52410V Agitated depression
D9-52412V Stuporous depression

SECTION 9-6 PERSONALITY DISORDERS

D9-60000 Personality disorder, NOS 301.90

9-61 CLUSTER A PERSONALITY DISORDERS

D9-61000 Cluster A personality disorder, NOS
D9-61100 Paranoid personality disorder 301.00
D9-61200 Schizoid personality disorder 301.20
D9-61300 Schizotypal personality disorder 301.22

9-62 CLUSTER B PERSONALITY DISORDERS

D9-62000 Cluster B personality disorder, NOS
D9-62100 Antisocial personality disorder 301.70
D9-62200 Borderline personality disorder 301.83
D9-62300 Histrionic personality disorder 301.50
D9-62400 Narcissistic personality disorder 301.81

9-63 CLUSTER C PERSONALITY DISORDERS

D9-63000 Cluster C personality disorder, NOS
D9-63100 Avoidant personality disorder 301.82
D9-63200 Dependent personality disorder 301.60
D9-63300 Obsessive compulsive personality disorder 301.40
D9-63400 Passive aggressive personality disorder 301.84

SECTIONS 9-7-8 OTHER MENTAL DISORDERS
9-71 DELUSIONAL DISORDERS

D9-71000 Delusional disorder, NOS 297.10
  Paranoid disorder, NOS 297.10
D9-71010 Erotomanic delusion disorder 297.10
D9-71020 Grandiose delusion disorder 297.10
D9-71030 Jealous delusion disorder 297.10
D9-71040 Persecutory delusion disorder 297.10
D9-71050 Somatic delusion disorder 297.10
  Somatic delusion 297.10

9-72 PSYCHOTIC DISORDERS NOT ELSEWHERE CLASSIFIED

D9-72000 Psychotic disorder, NOS 298.90
  Psychosis, NOS 298.90
  Atypical psychosis 298.90
D9-72010 Brief reactive psychosis 298.80
D9-72020 Schizophreniform disorder, NOS 295.40
D9-72021 Schizophreniform disorder without good prognostic features 295.40
D9-72022 Schizophreniform disorder with good prognostic features 295.40
D9-72030 Schizoaffective disorder, NOS 295.70
D9-72031 Schizoaffective disorder, bipolar type 295.70
D9-72032 Schizoaffective disorder, depressive type 295.70
D9-72040 Induced psychotic disorder 297.30

9-73 PSYCHOSEXUAL DISORDERS

D9-73000 Psychosexual disorder, NOS 302.90
D9-73100 Paraphilia, NOS 302.90
  Sexual perversion, NOS 302.90
  Sexual aberration, NOS 302.90
  Sexual deviation, NOS 302.90
D9-73110 Necrophilia 302.90
D9-73120 Zoophilia 302.90
D9-73121 Erotic zoophilia 302.90
D9-73130 Coprophilia 302.90
D9-73140 Urophilia 302.90
D9-73150 Klismaphilia 302.90
D9-73160 Exhibitionism 302.40
D9-73161 Compulsive exhibitionism 302.40
D9-73162 Symptomatic exhibitionism 302.40
D9-73170 Fetishism 302.81
D9-73171 True compulsive fetishism 302.81
D9-73172 Symptomatic fetishism 302.81
D9-73180 Frotteurism 302.89
  Frottage 302.89
D9-73190 Telephone scatologia 302.90
  Obscene telephone call 302.90
D9-73200 Pedophilia, NOS 302.20
D9-73201 Pedophilia, same sex 302.20
D9-73202 Pedophilia, opposite sex 302.20
D9-73203 Pedophilia, same and opposite sex 302.20
D9-73204 Pedophilia, limited to incest 302.20
D9-73205 Pedophilia, exclusive type 302.20
D9-73206 Pedophilia, nonexclusive type 302.20
D9-73207 Compulsive pedophilia 302.20
D9-73208 Symptomatic pedophilia 302.20
D9-73209 Pederasty 302.20
D9-73218 Flagellantism
D9-73220 Sexual masochism 302.83
D9-73221 Compulsive sexual masochism 302.83
D9-73223 Symptomatic sexual masochism 302.83
D9-73230 Sexual sadism 302.84
D9-73231 Compulsive sexual sadism 302.84
D9-73232 Symptomatic sexual sadism 302.84
D9-73233 Necrosadism 302.84
D9-73240 Transvestic fetishism 302.30
  Transvestism 302.30
D9-73241 Primary transvestism 302.30
D9-73242 Secondary transvestism 302.30
D9-73250 Voyeurism 302.82
D9-73252 Ecouteurism
  Ecoutage
D9-73260 Sodomy
  Bestiality
D9-73264 Partialism 302.90
D9-73270 Lecherism
D9-73280 Sexual pyromania
D9-73290 Erotic vomiting
D9-73300 Pygmalionism
D9-73500 Sexual dysfunction, NOS 302.70
D9-73510 Sexual desire disorder, NOS
D9-73511 Hypoactive sexual desire disorder 302.71
D9-73512 Situational hypoactive sexual desire disorder 302.71

9-73 PSYCHOSEXUAL DISORDERS — Continued

D9-73520 Sexual arousal disorder, NOS
D9-73521 Female sexual arousal disorder 302.72
D9-73522 Male erectile disorder 302.72
D9-73530 Orgasm disorder, NOS
D9-73531 Inhibited female orgasm 302.73
D9-73532 Inhibited male orgasm 302.74
D9-73533 Premature ejaculation 302.75
  Ejaculatio praecox 302.75
D9-73540 Sexual pain disorder, NOS
D9-73541 Psychologic dyspareunia 302.76
  Psychologic painful sexual act of female 302.76
D9-73542 Psychologic vaginismus 306.51

9-74 SLEEP DISORDERS

D9-74000 Sleep disorder, NOS
D9-74100 Dyssomnia, NOS 307.40
D9-74110 Insomnia, NOS 307.42
  Hyposomnia, NOS
  Sleeplessness
D9-74111 Primary insomnia 307.42
D9-74112 Insomnia disorder related to another mental disorder 307.42
D9-74113 Insomnia disorder related to known organic factor 780.50
D9-74115 Initial insomnia
  Vesperal insomnia
D9-74116 Middle insomnia
D9-74117 Terminal insomnia
  Matutinal insomnia
D9-74118 Mixed insomnia
D9-74119 Rebound insomnia
D9-74120 Hypersomnia, NOS 780.54
D9-74121 Primary hypersomnia 780.54
D9-74122 Hypersomnia disorder related to another mental disorder 307.44
D9-74123 Hypersomnia disorder related to a known organic factor 780.50
D9-74130 Sleep-wake schedule disorder, NOS 307.45
D9-74131 Sleep-wake schedule disorder, advanced phase type 307.45
D9-74132 Sleep-wake schedule disorder, delayed phase type 307.45
D9-74133 Sleep-wake schedule disorder, disorganized type 307.45
D9-74134 Sleep-wake schedule disorder, frequently changing type 307.45
D9-74140 Insomnia with sleep apnea 780.51
D9-74144 Hypersomnia with sleep apnea 780.53
D9-74200 Parasomnia, NOS 307.40
D9-74210 Dream anxiety disorder 307.47
  Nightmare disorder 307.47
  Nightmare, NOS 307.47
D9-74220 Sleep terror disorder 307.46
D9-74222 Pavor diurnus
  Day terrors
D9-74224 Pavor nocturnus
  Night terrors
D9-74230 Sleep walking disorder 307.46
  Somnanbulism
D9-74250 Narcolepsy 347.-
  Paroxysmal sleep 347.-
  Gelineau's syndrome 347.-
D9-74260 Cataplexy 347.-

9-75 IMPULSE CONTROL DISORDERS

D9-75000 Impulse control disorder, NOS 312.39
D9-75010 Intermittent explosive disorder 312.34
D9-75020 Kleptomania 312.32
D9-75030 Pathological gambling 312.31
  Compulsive gambling 312.31
D9-75040 Pyromania 312.33
D9-75050 Trichotillomania 312.39
  Hair plucking 312.39
  Trichologia

9-81 ANXIETY DISORDERS

D9-81000 Anxiety disorder, NOS 300.00
  Anxiety neurosis 300.00
  Phobic neurosis 300.00
D9-81010 Generalized anxiety disorder 300.02
D9-81100 Panic disorder with agoraphobia, NOS 300.21
D9-81110 Panic disorder with agoraphobia and mild panic attacks, NOS 300.21
D9-81111 Panic disorder with agoraphobia, mild agoraphobic avoidance and mild panic attacks 300.21
D9-81112 Panic disorder with agoraphobia, moderate agoraphobic avoidance and mild panic attacks 300.21
D9-81113 Panic disorder with agoraphobia, severe agoraphobic avoidance and mild panic attacks 300.21
D9-81114 Panic disorder with agoraphobia, agoraphobic avoidance in partial remission and mild panic attacks 300.21
D9-81115 Panic disorder with agoraphobia, agoraphobic avoidance in full remission and mild panic attacks 300.21
D9-81120 Panic disorder with agoraphobia and moderate panic attacks, NOS 300.21
D9-81121 Panic disorder with agoraphobia, mild agoraphobic avoidance and moderate panic attacks 300.21
D9-81122 Panic disorder with agoraphobia, moderate agoraphobic avoidance and moderate panic attacks 300.21
D9-81123 Panic disorder with agoraphobia, severe agoraphobic avoidance and moderate panic attacks 300.21
D9-81124 Panic disorder with agoraphobia, agoraphobic avoidance in partial remission and moderate panic attacks 300.21
D9-81125 Panic disorder with agoraphobia, agoraphobic avoidance in full remission and moderate panic attacks 300.21

D9-81130 Panic disorder with agoraphobia and severe panic attacks, NOS 300.21
D9-81131 Panic disorder with agoraphobia, mild agoraphobic avoidance and severe panic attacks 300.21
D9-81132 Panic disorder with agoraphobia, moderate agoraphobic avoidance and severe panic attacks 300.21
D9-81133 Panic disorder with agoraphobia, severe agoraphobic avoidance and severe panic attacks 300.21
D9-81134 Panic disorder with agoraphobia, agoraphobic avoidance in partial remission and severe panic attacks 300.21
D9-81135 Panic disorder with agoraphobia, agoraphobic avoidance in full remission and severe panic attacks 300.21
D9-81140 Panic disorder with agoraphobia and panic attacks in partial remission, NOS 300.21
D9-81141 Panic disorder with agoraphobia, mild agoraphobic avoidance and panic attacks in partial remission 300.21
D9-81142 Panic disorder with agoraphobia, moderate agoraphobic avoidance and panic attacks in partial remission 300.21
D9-81143 Panic disorder with agoraphobia, severe agoraphobic avoidance and panic attacks in partial remission 300.21
D9-81144 Panic disorder with agoraphobia, agoraphobic avoidance in partial remission and panic attacks in partial remission 300.21
D9-81145 Panic disorder with agoraphobia, agoraphobic avoidance in full remission and panic attacks in partial remission 300.21
D9-81150 Panic disorder with agoraphobia and panic attacks in full remission, NOS 300.21
D9-81151 Panic disorder with agoraphobia, mild agoraphobic avoidance and panic attacks in full remission 300.21
D9-81152 Panic disorder with agoraphobia, moderate agoraphobic avoidance and panic attacks in full remission 300.21
D9-81153 Panic disorder with agoraphobia, severe agoraphobic avoidance and panic attacks in full remission 300.21
D9-81154 Panic disorder with agoraphobia, agoraphobic avoidance in partial remission and panic attacks in full remission 300.21
D9-81155 Panic disorder with agoraphobia, agoraphobic avoidance in full remission and panic attacks in full remission 300.21
D9-81200 Panic disorder without agoraphobia, NOS 300.01
D9-81210 Panic disorder without agoraphobia with mild panic attacks 300.01
D9-81220 Panic disorder without agoraphobia with moderate panic attacks 300.01
D9-81230 Panic disorder without agoraphobia with severe panic attacks 300.01
D9-81240 Panic disorder without agoraphobia with panic attacks in partial remission 300.01
D9-81250 Panic disorder without agoraphobia with panic attacks in full remission 300.01
D9-81300 Agoraphobia, NOS
Fear of open places
D9-81310 Agoraphobia without history of panic disorder, NOS 300.22
D9-81311 Agoraphobia without history of panic disorder with limited symptom attacks 300.22
D9-81312 Agoraphobia without history of panic disorder without limited symptom attacks 300.22
D9-81400 Social phobia, NOS 300.23
D9-81401 Generalized social phobia 300.23
D9-81410 Simple phobia 300.29
D9-81500 Obsessive compulsive disorder, NOS 300.30
Obsessive compulsive neurosis 300.30
D9-81600 Posttraumatic stress disorder, NOS 309.89
D9-81610 Posttraumatic stress disorder, delayed onset 309.89
D9-81650V Porcine stress syndrome
(T-D0010) (F-A4600) (F-11320) (F-03003)
Herztod
(T-D0010) (F-A4600) (F-11320) (F-03003)
Pale soft exudative pork
(T-D0010) (F-A4600) (F-11320) (F-03003)
Malignant hyperthermia of pigs
(T-D0010) (F-A4600) (F-11320) (F-03003)

9-82 SOMATOFORM DISORDERS

D9-82000 Somatoform disorder, NOS 300.70
D9-82010 Undifferentiated somatoform disorder 300.70
D9-82020 Body dysmorphic disorder 300.70
D9-82030 Conversion disorder, NOS 300.11
Hysterical neurosis, conversion type 300.11
D9-82031 Conversion disorder, single episode 300.11
D9-82032 Recurrent conversion disorder 300.11
D9-82034 Hysterical blindness
D9-82035 Hysterical deafness
D9-82036 Hysterical paralysis
D9-82040 Hypochondriasis 300.70
Hypochondriacal neurosis 300.70
Hypochondria
D9-82050 Somatization disorder 300.81
D9-82060 Somatoform pain disorder 307.80
D9-82100V Farrowing hysteria

9-83 DISSOCIATIVE DISORDERS

D9-83000 Dissociative disorder, NOS 300.15
Hysterical neurosis, dissociative type 300.15
D9-83100 Multiple personality disorder 301.14
D9-83200 Psychogenic fugue 300.13
Hysterical fugue

9-83 DISSOCIATIVE DISORDERS — Continued

D9-83300 Psychogenic amnesia 300.12
D9-83400 Depersonalization disorder 300.60
Depersonalization neurosis

9-84 FACTITIOUS DISORDERS

D9-84000 Factitious disorder, NOS 300.19
D9-84010 Factitious disorder with physical symptoms 301.51
D9-84020 Factitious disorder with psychological symptoms 300.16

9-85 ADJUSTMENT DISORDERS

D9-85000 Adjustment disorder, NOS 309.90
D9-85010 Adjustment disorder with anxious mood 309.24
D9-85020 Adjustment disorder with depressed mood 309.00
D9-85030 Adjustment disorder with disturbance of conduct 309.30
D9-85040 Adjustment disorder with mixed disturbance of emotions and conduct 309.40
D9-85050 Adjustment disorder with mixed emotional features 309.28
D9-85060 Adjustment disorder with physical complaints 309.82
D9-85070 Adjustment disorder with withdrawal 309.83
D9-85080 Adjustment disorder with work inhibition 309.23
D9-85090 Adjustment disorder with academic inhibition 309.23

CHAPTER A — DISEASES OF THE NERVOUS SYSTEM AND SPECIAL SENSES

SECTION A-0 DISEASES OF THE CENTRAL NERVOUS SYSTEM: GENERAL TERMS

DA-00000 Disease of the central nervous system, NOS 349.9
(T-A0090) (DF-00000)

DA-00010 Disease of brain, NOS
(T-A0100) (DF-00000)

DA-00020 Intracranial mass 784.2
(T-D1400) (M-03080)
Intracranial lump 784.2
(T-D1400) (M-03080)
Intracranial swelling 784.2
(T-D1400) (M-03080)
Intracranial space-occupying lesion 784.2
(T-D1400) (M-03080)

SECTION A-1 INFLAMMATION OF THE CNS AND MISCELLANEOUS ENCEPHALOPATHIES

A-10 INFLAMMATORY DISEASES OF THE CENTRAL NERVOUS SYSTEM

DA-10000 Inflammatory disease of the central nervous system, NOS
(T-A0090) (M-40000)
Inflammation of the central nervous system, NOS
(T-A0090) (M-40000)

DA-10010 Meningitis, NOS 322.9
(T-A1110) (M-40000)

DA-10011 Nonpyogenic meningitis 322.0
(T-A1110) (M-40000)
Meningitis with clear cerebrospinal fluid 322.0
(T-A1110) (M-40000)

DA-10020 Chronic meningitis, NOS 322.2
(T-A1110) (M-43000)

DA-10021 Eosinophilic meningitis 322.1
(T-A1110) (M-40000) (T-A1000) (M-77630)

DA-10030 Leptomeningitis, NOS 322.-
(T-A1200) (M-40000)

DA-10040 Arachnoiditis, NOS 322.-
(T-A1220) (M-40000)

DA-10050 Pachymeningitis, NOS 322.-
(T-A1120) (M-40000)

DA-10080 Meningism 781.6
(T-A1110) (M-40000)
Duprés's syndrome 781.6
(T-A1110) (M-40000)
Meningismus 781.6
(T-A1110) (M-40000)

DA-10100 Encephalitis, NOS 323.9
(T-A0100) (M-40000)

DA-10110 Toxic encephalitis, NOS 327.7
(T-A0100) (M-40000) (C-.....)

DA-10111 Toxic encephalitis due to carbon tetrachloride 323.7 —982.1
(T-A0100) (M-40000) (C-20809)

DA-10112 Toxic encephalitis due to hydroxyquinoline 323.7 —961.3
(T-A0100) (M-40000) (C-21744)

DA-10113 Toxic encephalitis due to lead 323.7 —984.9
(T-A0100) (M-40000) (C-13200)

DA-10114 Toxic encephalitis due to mercury 323.7 —985.0
(T-A0100) (M-40000) (C-13300)

DA-10115 Toxic encephalitis due to thallium 323.7 —985.8
(T-A0100) (M-40000) (C-13800)

DA-10130 Encephalomyelitis, NOS 323.-
(T-A0100) (T-A7010) (M-40000)

DA-10131 Acute disseminated encephalomyelitis 323.-
(T-A0100) (T-A7010) (M-41000)

DA-10135 Meningoencephalitis 323.-
(T-A1112) (T-A0100) (M-40000)

DA-10140 Meningomyelitis 323.-
(T-A1115) (T-A7010) (M-40000)

DA-10150 Myelitis, NOS 323.-
(T-A7010) (M-40000)

DA-10151 Acute ascending myelitis 323.-
(T-A7010) (M-41000)

DA-10152 Acute transverse myelitis 323.-
(T-A7010) (M-41000)

DA-10400 Intracranial abscess, NOS 324.0
(T-D1400) (M-41610)
Intracranial embolic abscess 324.0
(T-D1400) (M-41610)

DA-10402 Cerebral abscess 324.0
(T-A0100) (M-41610)

DA-10404 Cerebellar abscess 324.0
(T-A6000) (M-41610)

DA-10405 Epidural abscess 324.0
(T-A1310) (M-41610)
Extradural abscess 324.0
(T-A1310) (M-41610)

DA-10406 Subdural abscess 324.0
(T-A1410) (M-41610)

DA-10408 Intracranial otogenic abscess 324.0
(T-D1400) (T-AB000) (M-41610)

DA-10450 Intraspinal abscess, NOS 324.1
(T-A7010) (M-41610)
Intraspinal embolic abscess 324.1
(T-A7010) (M-41610)

DA-10455 Spinal epidural abscess 324.1
(T-A1320) (M-41610)
Spinal extradural abscess 324.1
(T-A1320) (M-41610)

A-10 INFLAMMATORY DISEASES OF THE CENTRAL NERVOUS SYSTEM — Continued

DA-10456 Spinal subdural abscess 324.1
(T-A1480) (M-41610)
DA-10500V Idiopathic feline polioencephalomyelitis
DA-10510V Granulomatous meningoencephalomyelitis
Inflammatory reticulosis
DA-10520V Pyogranulomatous meningoencephalomyelitis
DA-10530V Experimental allergic encephalomyelitis

A-12 CEREBRAL SINUS THROMBOSIS, EMBOLISM AND INFLAMMATION

DA-12000 Thrombosis of intracranial venous sinus, NOS 325.-
(T-49800) (M-35100)
DA-12001 Thrombosis of cavernous venous sinus 325.-
(T-49840) (M-35100)
DA-12002 Thrombosis of lateral venous sinus 325.-
(T-49803) (M-35100)
DA-12003 Thrombosis of superior sagittal sinus 325.-
(T-49802) (M-35100)
DA-12004 Thrombosis of inferior sagittal sinus 325.-
(T-49810) (M-35100)
DA-12005 Thrombosis of basilar sinus 325.-
(T-49848) (M-35100)
DA-12006 Thrombosis of torcular Herophili 325.-
(T-49820) (M-35100)
DA-12020 Embolism of intracranial venous sinus, NOS 325.-
(T-49800) (M-35300)
DA-12021 Embolism of cavernous venous sinus 325.-
(T-49840) (M-35300)
DA-12022 Embolism of lateral venous sinus 325.-
(T-49803) (M-35300)
DA-12023 Embolism of superior sagittal sinus 325.-
(T-49802) (M-35300)
DA-12024 Embolism of inferior sagittal sinus 325.-
(T-49810) (M-35300)
DA-12025 Embolism of basilar sinus 325.-
(T-49848) (M-35300)
DA-12026 Embolism of torcular Herophili 325.-
(T-49820) (M-35300)
DA-12040 Phlebitis of intracranial venous sinus, NOS 325.-
(T-49800) (M-40000)
DA-12041 Phlebitis of cavernous venous sinus 325.-
(T-49840) (M-40000)
DA-12042 Phlebitis of lateral venous sinus 325.-
(T-49803) (M-40000)
DA-12043 Phlebitis of superior sagittal sinus 325.-
(T-49802) (M-40000)
DA-12044 Phlebitis of inferior sagittal sinus 325.-
(T-49810) (M-40000)
DA-12045 Phlebitis of basilar sinus 325.-
(T-49848) (M-40000)
DA-12046 Phlebitis of torcular Herophili 325.-
(T-49820) (M-40000)
DA-12060 Endophlebitis of intracranial venous sinus, NOS 325.-
(T-49800) (T-48031) (M-40000)
DA-12061 Endophlebitis of cavernous venous sinus 325.-
(T-49840) (T-48031) (M-40000)
DA-12062 Endophlebitis of lateral venous sinus 325.-
(T-49803) (T-48031) (M-40000)
DA-12063 Endophlebitis of superior sagittal sinus 325.-
(T-49802) (T-48031) (M-40000)
DA-12064 Endophlebitis of inferior sagittal sinus 325.-
(T-49810) (T-48031) (M-40000)
DA-12065 Endophlebitis of basilar sinus 325.-
(T-49848) (T-48031) (M-40000)
DA-12066 Endophlebitis of torcular Herophili 325.-
(T-49820) (T-48031) (M-40000)
DA-12080 Thrombophlebitis of intracranial venous sinus, NOS 325.-
(T-49800) (M-35100) (M-40000)
DA-12081 Thrombophlebitis of cavernous venous sinus 325.-
(T-48940) (M-35100) (M-40000)
DA-12082 Thrombophlebitis of lateral venous sinus 325.-
(T-49803) (M-35100) (M-40000)
DA-12083 Thrombophlebitis of superior sagittal sinus 325.-
(T-49802) (M-35100) (M-40000)
DA-12084 Thrombophlebitis of inferior sagittal sinus 325.-
(T-49810) (M-35100) (M-40000)
DA-12085 Thrombophlebitis of basilar sinus 325.-
(T-49848) (M-35100) (M-40000)
DA-12086 Thrombophlebitis of torcular Herophili 325.-
(T-49820) (M-35100) (M-40000)

A-13 ENCEPHALOPATHY AND MISCELLANEOUS CNS DISORDERS

DA-13000 Encephalopathy, NOS 348.3
DA-13005 Toxic encephalopathy 349.82
DA-13010 Cerebral cyst, NOS 348.0
DA-13012 Arachnoid cyst 348.0
DA-13020 Porencephalic cyst 348.0
DA-13021 Acquired porencephaly 348.0
Porencephaly, NOS 348.0
DA-13028 Pseudoporencephaly 348.0
DA-13030 Anoxic brain damage, NOS 348.1
DA-13040 Benign intracranial hypertension 348.2
Pseudotumor cerebri 348.2
DA-13050 Compression of brain, NOS 348.4
DA-13051 Brain stem compression 348.4
DA-13052 Brain stem herniation 348.4
DA-13055 Posterior fossa compression syndrome 348.4
DA-13070 Cerebral edema 348.5
DA-13071 Cerebral calcification 348.8
DA-13072 Cerebral fungus 348.8
DA-13075 Cerebrospinal fluid rhinorrhea 349.81

DA-13076 Pseudomeningocele 349.81
DA-13200 Disorder of meninges, NOS 349.2
DA-13210 Cyst of spinal meninges 349.2
DA-13212V Dural ossification
  Bone plaques of dura
DA-13220 Cerebral meningeal adhesions 349.2
DA-13224 Spinal meningeal adhesions 349.2
DA-13300 Nervous system complications from surgical implanted device 349.1
DA-13310 Reaction to spinal puncture 349.0
DA-13320 Reaction to lumbar puncture 349.0
DA-13324 Headache following lumbar puncture 349.0
DA-13400V Bovine progressive degenerative myeloencephalopathy
  BPDME
DA-13410V Neonatal maladjustment syndrome
  NMS
  Ischemic cerebral necrosis and hemorrhage
  Barkers
  Wanderers
  Dummies
  Convulsive foals
DA-13420V Ruminant polioencephalomalacia
  PEM
  Cerebrocortical necrosis
DA-13430V Poliomyelomalacia
DA-13440V Hepatocerebral encephalopathy
DA-13450V Hypoglycemic encephalopathy
DA-13460V Feline ischemic encephalopathy

SECTION A-2 DEGENERATIVE AND DEMYELINATING DISORDERS INCLUDING PARALYTIC SYNDROMES

A-20 HEREDITARY DEGENERATIVE DISEASES OF THE CENTRAL NERVOUS SYSTEM

DA-20000 Degenerative disease of the central nervous system, NOS
DA-20010 Cerebral degeneration, NOS 331.9
DA-20020 Alzheimer's disease 331.0
DA-20021 Pick's disease 331.1
DA-20022 Senile degeneration of brain 331.2
DA-20040 Acquired hydrocephalus, NOS 331.4
DA-20041 Acquired obstructive hydrocephalus 331.4
DA-20042 Communicating hydrocephalus 331.3
DA-20050 Reye's syndrome 331.81
    (M-27000) (F-66BF8)
  Reye's encephalopathy 331.81
    (M-27000) (F-66BF8)
  MCAD deficiency 331.81
    (M-27000) (F-66BF8)
  Medium-chain acyl-coenzyme A dehydrogenase deficiency 331.81
    (M-27000) (F-66BF8)
DA-20060 Cerebral ataxia 331.89
DA-20070V Progressive sensory ataxia of Charolais
DA-20100 Cerebral degeneration in childhood, NOS 330.9
DA-20160 Progressive sclerosing poliodystrophy 330.8
  Alpers' disease 330.8
  Gray matter degeneration 330.8
  Spongy glioneuronal dystrophy 330.8
DA-20161 Leigh's disease 330.8
  Infantile necrotizing encephalomyelopathy 330.8
  Subacute necrotizing encephalopathy 330.8
  Subacute necrotizing encephalomyelopathy 330.8
DA-20170V Dalmatian leukodystrophy
  Cavitating leukodystrophy
DA-20180 Alexander's disease
  Fibrinoid leukodystrophy
DA-20190V Leukoencephalomyelopathy of Rottweilers
  Neuroaxonal dystrophy of Rottweilers

A-21 EXTRAPYRAMIDAL DISEASES

DA-21000 Extrapyramidal disease, NOS 333.9
  Extrapyramidal disorder, NOS 333.9
DA-21010 Parkinsonism, NOS 332.0
DA-21012 Parkinson's disease, NOS 332.0
  Paralysis agitans 332.0
  Idiopathic parkinsonism 332.0
  Primary parkinsonism 332.0
  Shaking palsy 332.0
DA-21020 Secondary parkinsonism 332.1
  Symptomatic parkinsonism 332.1
DA-21021 Parkinsonism due to drug 332.1
    (C-50000)
DA-21022 Postencephalitic parkinsonism
DA-21025 MPTP-induced parkinsonism
DA-21030 Parkinson-dementia complex of Guam
DA-21050 Disease of basal ganglia, NOS 333.0
DA-21051 Olivopontocerebellar degeneration 333.0
  Olivopontocerebellar atrophy 333.0
  Déjérine-Thomas syndrome 333.0
DA-21052 Pigmentary pallidal degeneration 333.0
  Pigmentary pallidal atrophy 333.0
  Hallervorden-Spatz disease 333.0
DA-21053 Striatonigral degeneration 333.0
  Striatonigral atrophy 333.0
DA-21054 Parkinsonian syndrome associated with idiopathic orthostatic hypotension 333.0
  Parkinsonian syndrome associated with symptomatic orthostatic hypotension 333.0
DA-21055 Progressive supranuclear ophthalmoplegia 333.0
  Progressive supranuclear palsy 333.0
DA-21057 Tardive dyskinesia
DA-21058 Shy-Drager syndrome 333.0
DA-21100 Movement disorder, NOS 333.9
DA-21101 Benign essential tremor 333.1
  Familial tremor 333.1

A-21 EXTRAPYRAMIDAL DISEASES — Continued

DA-21101 (cont.) Essential tremor 333.1
Heredofamilial tremor 333.1
Hereditary essential tremor 333.1
DA-21104 Familial essential myoclonus 333.2
DA-21110 Tic of organic origin, NOS 333.3
DA-21120 Huntington's chorea 333.4
DA-21124 Hemiballism 333.5
Hemiballismus 333.5
DA-21126 Paroxysmal choreoathetosis 333.5
DA-21130 Idiopathic torsion dystonia 333.6
Dystonia deformans progressiva 333.6
Dystonia musculorum deformans 333.6
Schwalbe disease 333.6
Ziehen-Oppenheim disease 333.6
DA-21135 Symptomatic torsion dystonia 333.7
DA-21136 Athetoid cerebral palsy 333.7
Vogt's disease 333.7
DA-21138 Double athetosis 333.7
Double athetosis syndrome 333.7
DA-21140 Fragment of torsion dystonia, NOS 333.8
DA-21141 Blepharospasm 331.81
DA-21143 Orofacial dyskinesia 333.82
DA-21145 Spasmodic torticollis 333.83
DA-21147 Organic writer's cramp 333.84
DA-21151 Stiff-man syndrome 333.91
DA-21152 Restless legs 333.99

A-22 SPINOCEREBELLAR DISEASES

DA-22000 Spinocerebellar disease, NOS 334.9
DA-22010 Friedreich's ataxia 334.0
DA-22014 Hereditary spastic paraplegia 334.1
DA-22020 Primary cerebellar degeneration, NOS 334.2
DA-22021 Cerebellar ataxia, NOS 334.3
DA-22022 Marie's cerebellar ataxia 334.2
DA-22023 Sanger-Brown cerebellar ataxia 334.2
DA-22025 Dyssynergia cerebellaris myoclonica 334.2
DA-22027 Hereditary cerebellar degeneration 334.2
DA-22028 Sporadic cerebellar degeneration 334.2
DA-22034 Corticostriatal-spinal degeneration 334.8
DA-22070 Posthemiplegic athetosis
DA-22074 Posthemiplegic ataxia
DA-22090V Hereditary amblyopia with quadriplegia in the Irish Setter

A-23 MOTOR NEURON DISEASES

DA-23000 Motor neuron disease, NOS 335.2
DA-23004 Anterior horn cell disease, NOS 335.9
DA-23010 Amyotrophic lateral sclerosis 335.20
Lou Gehrig's disease 335.20
Bulbar motor neuron disease 335.20
DA-23012 Primary lateral sclerosis 335.24
DA-23020 Progressive muscular atrophy 335.21
Duchenne-Aran muscular atrophy 335.21
Pure progressive muscular atrophy 335.21
DA-23030 Progressive bulbar palsy 335.22
DA-23034 Pseudobulbar palsy 335.23
DA-23040 Lower motor neuron disease, NOS
DA-23050 Spinal muscular atrophy, NOS 335.10
DA-23052 Werdnig-Hoffmann disease 335.0
Infantile spinal muscular atrophy 335.0
Progressive muscular atrophy of infancy 335.0
DA-23054 Kugelberg-Welander disease 335.11
Familial spinal muscular atrophy 335.11
Juvenile spinal muscular atrophy 335.11
DA-23056 Adult spinal muscular atrophy 335.19
Generalized spinal muscular atrophy of late onset 335.19
DA-23060V Hereditary canine spinal muscular atrophy

A-24 MYELOPATHIES

DA-24000 Myelopathy, NOS 336.9
Disease of spinal cord, NOS 336.9
DA-24004 Cord compression, NOS 336.9
DA-24005 Radiation-induced myelopathy 336.8
DA-24010 Drug-induced myelopathy 336.8
DA-24020 Syringomyelia 336.0
DA-24022 Syringobulbia 336.0
DA-24030 Vascular myelopathy, NOS 336.1
DA-24032 Acute infarction of spinal cord 336.1
DA-24034 Arterial thrombosis of spinal cord 336.1
DA-24035V Fibrocartilagenous emboli of spinal cord
DA-24036 Edema of spinal cord 336.1
DA-24037 Hematomyelia 336.1
DA-24038 Subacute necrotic myelopathy 336.1
DA-24040 Subacute combined degeneration of spinal cord, NOS 336.2
DA-24100V Degenerative myelopathy
DA-24110V Demyelinating myelopathy of Miniature Poodles
DA-24120V Hereditary ataxia in Terriers
DA-24130V Hereditary myelopathy of Afgan Hounds

A-25 DEMYELINATING DISEASES OF THE CENTRAL NERVOUS SYSTEM

DA-25000 Demyelinating disease of central nervous system, NOS 341.9
DA-25010 Multiple sclerosis, NOS 340.-
Generalized multiple sclerosis 340.-
DA-25011 Brain stem multiple sclerosis 340.-
DA-25012 Cord multiple sclerosis 340.-
DA-25020 Neuromyelitis optica 341.0
DA-25030 Schilder's disease 341.1
Encephalitis periaxialis diffusa 341.1
DA-25032 Balo's concentric sclerosis 341.1
Encephalitis periaxialis concentrica 341.1
Balo's disease 341.1
DA-25040 Central pontine myelinosis 341.8
DA-25045 Marchiafava-Bignami disease 341.8
Central demyelination of corpus callosum 341.8
Marchiafava disease 341.8

DA-25050 Subcortical leukoencephalopathy
Binswanger's disease
Binswanger's dementia
Encephalitis subcorticalis chronica
DA-25100V Congenital tremor syndrome
Myoclonia congenita
Shaker pigs
Dancing pigs
Congenital trembles

A-26 PARALYTIC SYNDROMES

DA-26000 Paralytic syndrome, NOS 344.9
DA-26010 Hemiplegia, NOS 342.9
DA-26011 Flaccid hemiplegia 342.0
DA-26012 Spastic hemiplegia 342.1
DA-26016 Hemiparesis
DA-26020 Quadriplegia 344.0
Tetraplegia 344.0
DA-26021 Quadriparesis
Tetraparesis
DA-26030 Triplegia
DA-26031 Triparesis
DA-26040 Paraplegia 344.1
Paralysis of both lower limbs 344.1
Lower paraplegia 344.1
DA-26042 Paraparesis
DA-26050 Diplegia of upper limbs 344.2
Upper diplegia 344.2
Paralysis of both upper limbs 344.2
DA-26100 Monoplegia, NOS 344.5
DA-26110 Monoplegia of lower limb 344.3
Paralysis of lower limb 344.3
DA-26120 Monoplegia of upper limb 344.4
Paralysis of upper limb 344.4
DA-26160 Cauda equina syndrome, NOS 344.6
DA-26162 Cauda equina syndrome without neurogenic bladder 344.60
DA-26164 Cauda equina syndrome with neurogenic bladder 344.61
DA-26165 Autonomic hyperreflexia of bladder 344.61
Cord bladder 344.61
DA-26500 Spastic paralysis due to birth injury, NOS 343.-
DA-26502 Spastic paralysis due to intracranial birth injury 343.-
DA-26504 Spastic paralysis due to spinal birth injury 343.-
DA-26510 Infantile cerebral palsy, NOS 343.9
Spastic infantile paralysis 343.9
Congenital spastic paralysis 343.9
Little's disease 343.9
Cerebral palsy, NOS 343.9
DA-26520 Infantile hemiplegia 343.4
Postnatal infantile hemiplegia 343.4
DA-26530 Diplegic cerebral palsy 343.0
Congenital diplegia 343.0
Congenital paraplegia 343.0
DA-26540 Hemiplegic cerebral palsy 343.1
Congenital hemiplegia 343.1
DA-26550 Quadriplegic cerebral palsy 343.2
Tetraplegic cerebral palsy 343.2
DA-26560 Monoplegic cerebral palsy 343.3
DA-26600V Downer cow syndrome
Calving paralysis
DA-26602V Obturator nerve paralysis
DA-26604V Peroneal nerve paralysis
DA-26610V Sweeney
Suprascapular paralysis
Shoulder atrophy
Slipped shoulder
DA-26620V Inherited spastic paresis
Elso heel
DA-26630V Lethal neonatal spasticity
DA-26640V Spastic syndrome
Crampy
Krampfigkeit
Stretches

SECTION A-3 EPILEPSY AND MIGRAINE

A-30-31 CLINICAL EPILEPTIC SYNDROMES AND SEIZURES

A-30 Clinical Epilepsy Diagnoses

DA-30000 Epilepsy, NOS 345.9
Epileptic disorder, NOS 345.0
Epileptic convulsions, NOS 345.9
Epileptic fits, NOS 345.9
Epileptic seizures, NOS 345.9
DA-30010 Cursive epilepsy 345.8
(DA-31430)
Running epilepsy 345.8
(DA-31430)
DA-30020 Gelastic epilepsy 345.8
(DA-31150)
DA-30100 Generalized nonconvulsive epilepsy, NOS 345.0
(DA-31500)
DA-30110 Petit mal 345.0
(DA-31310)
DA-30120 Petit mal status 345.2
(DA-31310)
Epileptic absence status 345.2
(DA-31310)
DA-30200 Generalized convulsive epilepsy, NOS 345.1
(DA-31340)
DA-30210 Grand mal 345.1
(DA-31340)
DA-30220 Grand mal status 345.3
(DA-31340)
Status epilepticus 345.3
(DA-31340)
DA-30230 Visual epilepsy 345.5
(DA-31136)
DA-30240 Visceral epilepsy 345.5
(DA-31140)
DA-30250 Epilepsia partialis continua 345.7
(DA-31420)
Kojevnikov's epilepsy 345.7
(DA-31420)

A-30 Clinical Epilepsy Diagnoses — Continued

DA-30280 Unclassified epileptic seizures

A-31 TYPES OF SEIZURES AND EPILEPTIC SYNDROMES

A-311 Partial Seizures

DA-31100 Partial seizures, NOS 345.5
DA-31110 Simple partial seizures with consciousness preserved 345.5
DA-31120 Simple partial seizures with motor signs 345.5
  Partial motor attacks 345.5
DA-31130 Simple partial seizures with somatosensory symptoms 345.5
  Somatosensory attacks 345.5
DA-31136 Simple partial seizures with special sensory symptoms 345.5
  Special sensory attacks 345.5
DA-31140 Simple partial seizures with autonomic signs or symptoms 345.5
  Autonomic attacks 345.5
DA-31150 Simple partial seizures with psychic symptoms 345.4
DA-31160 Complex partial seizures with consciousness impaired 345.4
DA-31170 Simple partial onset seizures followed by impaired consciousness 345.4
DA-31180 Complex partial seizures with impaired consciousness at onset 345.4
DA-31190 Complex partial seizures with automatisms 345.5
DA-31200 Secondarily generalized seizures, NOS 345.4
DA-31210 Simple partial seizures evolving to generalized tonic-clonic seizures 345.4
DA-31220 Complex partial seizures evolving to generalized tonic-clonic seizures 345.4
DA-31230 Simple partial seizures evolving to complex partial seizures, then to generalized tonic-clonic seizures 345.4

A-313 Generalized-Onset Seizures

DA-31300 Generalized-onset seizures, NOS 345.0
DA-31310 Absence seizures 345.0
DA-31320 Atypical absence seizures 345.1
DA-31330 Tonic seizures 345.1
DA-31340 Tonic-clonic seizures 345.1
DA-31350 Myoclonic seizures 345.1
DA-31360 Atonic seizures 345.0

A-314 Localization-Related Epilepsies

DA-31400 Localization-related epilepsy, NOS 345.5
  Focal epilepsy, NOS 345.5
DA-31410 Benign focal epilepsy of childhood 345.5
DA-31420 Chronic progressive epilepsia partialis continua 345.7
DA-31430 Temporal lobe epilepsy 345.4
DA-31440 Extratemporal epilepsy

A-315 Generalized Epilepsies

DA-31500 Generalized epilepsy, NOS
DA-31510 Idiopathic generalized epilepsy, NOS
DA-31520 Benign neonatal convulsions
DA-31530 Childhood absence epilepsy
DA-31540 Juvenile myoclonic epilepsy
DA-31550 Symptomatic generalized epilepsy, NOS
DA-31560 West syndrome 345.6
  Infantile spasms 345.6
  Hypsarrhythmia 345.6
  Lightning spasms 345.6
  Salaam attacks 345.6
DA-31570 Early myoclonic encephalopathy
DA-31580 Lennox-Gastaut syndrome
DA-31590 Progressive myoclonic epilepsy 333.2
  Unverricht-Lundborg disease 333.2
DA-31600 Benign Rolandic epilepsy
DA-31610 Reflex epilepsy

A-38 MIGRAINES

DA-38000 Migraine, NOS 346.9
DA-38010 Classical migraine 346.0
  Migraine with aura 346.0
DA-38020 Common migraine 346.1
  Atypical migraine 346.1
  Sick headache 346.1
DA-38030 Cluster headache 346.2
  Histamine cephalgia 346.2
  Horton's neuralgia 346.2
  Ciliary neuralgia 346.2
  Migrainous neuralgia 346.2
  Horton's headache 346.2
DA-38040 Abdominal migraine 346.2
  Decapitated migraine
DA-38041 Lower half migraine 346.2
DA-38042 Basilar migraine 346.2
DA-38048 Retinal migraine 346.2
DA-38050 Hemiplegic migraine 346.8
DA-38060 Ophthalmoplegic migraine 346.8

SECTION A-4 DISORDERS OF THE PERIPHERAL NERVOUS SYSTEM

A-40 DISORDERS OF PERIPHERAL NERVOUS SYSTEM: GENERAL TERMS

DA-40000 Disorder of the peripheral nervous system, NOS
  Peripheral nerve disorder, NOS

A-41 CRANIAL NERVE DISORDERS

DA-41000 Cranial nerve disorder, NOS 352.9
DA-41010 Trigeminal nerve disorder, NOS 350.9
  Disorder of the fifth cranial nerve, NOS 350.9
DA-41012 Trigeminal neuralgia, NOS 350.1
  Tic douloureux 350.1

DA-41012 (cont.) Trifacial neuralgia 350.1
DA-41014 Atypical face pain 350.2
DA-41020 Facial nerve disorder, NOS 351.9
Disorder of of seventh cranial nerve, NOS 351.9
DA-41022 Bell's palsy 351.0
Facial palsy 351.0
DA-41024 Geniculate ganglionitis, NOS 351.1
DA-41025 Facial myokymia 351.8
DA-41026 Melkersson's syndrome 351.8
DA-41027 Supranuclear facial nerve paralysis
DA-41028 Nuclear facial nerve paralysis
DA-41029 Peripheral nerve facial nerve paralysis
DA-4102A Facial nerve motor disorder, NOS
DA-4102B Facial nerve sensory disorder, NOS
DA-41030 Disorder of olfactory nerve, NOS 352.0
Disorder of the first cranial nerve, NOS 352.0
DA-41040 Disorder of glossopharyngeal nerve 352.2
Disorder of the ninth cranial nerve 352.2
DA-41041 Glossopharyngeal neuralgia 352.1
DA-41050 Disorder of pneumogastric nerve, NOS 352.3
Disorder of the tenth cranial nerve, NOS 352.3
Disorder of vagus nerve, NOS 352.3
DA-41052 Vagus nerve laryngeal paralysis
DA-41054 Vagus nerve palate paralysis
DA-41056 Vagal hoarseness
Neurologic hoarseness
DA-41057 Vagal autonomic bradycardia
DA-41060 Disorder of accessory nerve, NOS 352.4
Disorder of the eleventh cranial nerve, NOS 352.4
DA-41070 Disorder of hypoglossal nerve, NOS 352.5
Disorder of the twelfth cranial nerve, NOS 352.5
DA-41080 Multiple cranial nerve palsy, NOS 352.6
DA-41081 Collet-Sicard syndrome 352.6
DA-41082 Polyneuritis cranialis 352.6

A-42 NERVE ROOT AND NERVE PLEXUS DISORDERS

DA-42000 Nerve root disorder, NOS 353.9
DA-42010 Nerve plexus disorder, NOS 353.9
DA-42020 Brachial plexus lesion, NOS 353.0
DA-42021 Cervical rib syndrome 353.0
Scalenus anticus syndrome 353.0
DA-42022 Costoclavicular syndrome 353.0
DA-42025 Thoracic outlet syndrome 353.0
DA-42030 Lumbosacral plexus lesion, NOS 353.1
DA-42035 Lumbosacral root lesion, NOS 353.4
DA-42040 Cervical root lesion, NOS 353.2
DA-42050 Thoracic root lesion, NOS 353.3
DA-42060 Neuralgic amyotrophy 353.5
Parsonage-Aldren-Turner syndrome 353.5
DA-42080 Phantom limb syndrome 353.6
Phantom limb pain 353.6
Phantom limb 353.6
Phantom pain 353.6

A-43-44 PERIPHERAL NERVE DISORDERS

DA-43000 Mononeuritis, NOS 355.9
DA-43003 Causalgia 354.4
DA-43005 Mononeuritis multiplex 354.5
DA-43010 Mononeuritis of upper limb, NOS 354.9
DA-43020 Carpal tunnel syndrome 354.0
Median nerve entrapment 354.0
DA-43021 Partial thenar atrophy 354.0
DA-43022 Lesion of median nerve, NOS 354.1
DA-43024 Median nerve neuritis 354.1
DA-43030 Lesion of ulnar nerve, NOS 354.2
DA-43031 Cubital tunnel syndrome 354.2
DA-43034 Tardy ulnar nerve palsy 354.2
DA-43040 Lesion of radial nerve, NOS 354.3
DA-43041 Acute radial nerve palsy 354.3
DA-43050 Mononeuritis of lower limb, NOS 355.8
DA-43060 Lesion of sciatic nerve, NOS 355.0
DA-43070 Lesion of femoral nerve, NOS 355.2
DA-43071 Meralgia paresthetica 355.1
Compression of lateral cutaneous femoral nerve of thigh 355.1
Lateral cutaneous femoral nerve of thigh syndrome 355.1
DA-43080 Lesion of lateral popliteal nerve, NOS 355.3
DA-43081 Lesion of common peroneal nerve, NOS 355.3
DA-43085 Lesion of medial popliteal nerve, NOS 355.4
DA-43090 Tarsal tunnel syndrome 355.5
DA-43095 Lesion of plantar nerve, NOS 355.6
DA-43096 Morton's metatarsalgia 355.6
Morton's neuralgia 355.6
Morton's neuroma 355.6
Morton's toe 355.6
Morton's disease 355.6
DA-44000 Hereditary peripheral neuropathy, NOS 356.9
DA-44002 Idiopathic peripheral neuropathy, NOS 356.9
DA-44010 Déjérine-Sottas disease 356.0
DA-44020 Peroneal muscular atrophy 356.1
Charcot-Marie-Tooth disease 356.1
Neuropathic muscular atrophy 356.1
DA-44030 Hereditary sensory neuropathy 356.2
DA-44050 Idiopathic progressive polyneuropathy 356.4
DA-44055 Supranuclear paralysis 356.8
DA-44100 Axonal neuropathy, NOS
DA-44200 Demyelinating neuropathy, NOS

A-45 INFLAMMATORY AND TOXIC NEUROPATHIES

DA-45000 Inflammatory neuropathy, NOS 357.9
DA-45050 Toxic neuropathy, NOS 357.9
Polyneuropathy due to toxic agents, NOS 357.7
DA-45052 Alcoholic polyneuropathy 357.5
DA-45054 Polyneuropathy due to drug, NOS 357.6

A-48 DISORDERS OF THE AUTONOMIC NERVOUS SYSTEM

DA-48000 Disorder of autonomic nervous system, NOS 337.9
  Disorder of peripheral autonomic nervous system, NOS 337.9
  Disorder of vegetative system, NOS 337.9
DA-48010 Disorder of sympathetic nervous system, NOS 337.9
DA-48020 Disorder of parasympathetic nervous system, NOS 337.9
DA-48030 Idiopathic peripheral autonomic neuropathy 337.0
DA-48032 Carotid sinus syncope 337.0
  Carotid sinus syndrome 337.0
DA-48034 Cervical sympathetic dystrophy 337.0
  Cervical sympathetic paralysis 337.0
DA-48100V Equine grass sickness

SECTION A-5 MYONEURAL DISORDERS AND MYOPATHIES

A-50 MYONEURAL DISORDERS

DA-50000 Myoneural disorder, NOS 358.9
DA-50100 Myasthenia gravis, NOS 358.0
DA-50102 Myasthenia gravis, juvenile form
DA-50104 Myasthenia gravis, adult form
DA-50110 Neonatal myasthenia
DA-50130 Eaton-Lambert syndrome 358.1
DA-50150 Toxic myoneural disorder, NOS 358.2
DA-50160 Drug-induced myasthenia
DA-50164 Antibiotic-induced neuromuscular blocking
DA-50170V Hereditary motor end-plate disease

A-51 MYOPATHIES

DA-51000 Myopathy, NOS 359.9
  Myopathic disease, NOS 359.9
  Myopathic syndrome, NOS 359.9
DA-51100 Muscular dystrophy, NOS 359.1
DA-51110 Congenital hereditary muscular dystrophy 359.0
  Benign congenital myopathy 359.0
DA-51200 Hereditary progressive muscular dystrophy, NOS 359.1
DA-51210 Gower's muscular dystrophy 359.1
  Distal muscular dystrophy 359.1
DA-51220 Duchenne muscular dystrophy 359.1
DA-51230 Erb's muscular dystrophy 359.1
DA-51240 Fascioscapulohumeral muscular dystrophy 359.1
  Landouzy-Déjérine muscular dystrophy 359.1
  Limb-girdle muscular dystrophy 359.1
DA-51250 Ocular muscular dystrophy 359.1
DA-51256 Oculopharyngeal muscular dystrophy 359.1
DA-51260 Myotonia acquisita
  Talma's disease
DA-51270 Paramyotonia congenita 359.2
  Eulenburg syndrome 359.2
DA-51280V Hereditary myopathy associated with hydrocephalus
DA-51290V Nutritional myopathy, NOS
DA-51320 Congenital myotonia, NOS
  Myotonia congenita 359.2
  Thomsen's disease 359.2
DA-51322 Congenital myotonia, autosomal dominant form
DA-51324 Congenital myotonia, autosomal recessive form
DA-51340 Isaacs syndrome
DA-51344 Myotonia levior
DA-51500 Congenital myopathy, NOS
DA-51504 Minimal change myopathy
DA-51510 Central core disease 359.0
DA-51512 Congenital fiber type disproportion
DA-51520 Myotubular myopathy 359.0
  Centronuclear myopathy 359.0
DA-51522 Myotubular myopathy with type I atrophy
DA-51528 Severe x-linked myotubular myopathy
DA-51530 Nemaline myopathy 359.0
  Nemaline body disease 359.0
  Rod myopathy 359.0
DA-51540 Megaconial myopathy
DA-51550 Mixed congenital myopathy
DA-51560 Congenital myopathy with abnormal subcellular organelles, NOS
DA-51562 Fingerprint myopathy
DA-51564 Sarcotubular myopathy
DA-51566 Zebra body myopathy
DA-51568 Reducing-body myopathy
DA-51600 Mitochondrial myopathy
  Ragged red myopathy
DA-51610 Kearns-Sayre syndrome
DA-51620 Juvenile myopathy and lactate acidosis
DA-51630 Infantile encephalopathy and lactic acidosis
DA-51640 Juvenile myopathy, encephalopathy, lactic acidosis and stroke
  MELAS
DA-51650 Juvenile cerebellar degeneration and myoclonus
DA-51660 Fukuhara syndrome
DA-51670 Myoclonus epilepsy and ragged red fibers
  MERRF
DA-51680 Oculocraniosomatic syndrome
  OCS syndrome
DA-51690 Ophthalmoplegia plus syndrome
DA-51700 Luft's hypermetabolic myopathy
DA-51710 Mitochondrial-lipid-glycogen storage myopathy
DA-51800 Toxic myopathy, NOS 359.4
DA-51810 Metabolic myopathy
DA-51820 Alcohol myopathy
  Alcoholic myopathic syndrome
DA-51830 Thyrotoxic myopathy
DA-51832 Hypothyroid myopathy
DA-51900 Secondary myopathy, NOS
DA-51910 Carcinomatous myopathic syndrome
DA-51920 Steroid-induced myopathy

SECTION A-7 DISEASES OF THE EYE
A-70 DISORDERS AFFECTING THE GLOBE

DA-70000 Disease of eye, NOS 379.90
DA-70010 Swelling of eye 379.92
  Mass of eye 379.92
DA-70020 Redness of eye 379.93
DA-70030 Discharge of eye 379.93
DA-70090 Ill-defined disorder of eye, NOS 379.99
DA-70100 Disorder of globe, NOS 360.9
DA-70110 Purulent endophthalmitis, NOS 360.00
DA-70112 Acute endophthalmitis 360.01
DA-70114 Panophthalmitis 360.02
DA-70120 Chronic endophthalmitis 360.03
DA-70130 Vitreous abscess 360.04
DA-70140 Sympathetic uveitis 360.11
DA-70150 Panuveitis 360.12
DA-70160 Parasitic endophthalmitis, NOS 360.13
DA-70170 Ophthalmia nodosa 360.14
DA-70180 Phacoanaphylactic endophthalmitis 360.19
DA-70200 Degenerative disorder of globe, NOS 360.20
DA-70210 Degenerative progressive high myopia 360.21
  Malignant myopia 360.21
DA-70220 Metallosis, NOS 360.24
DA-70230 Siderosis of eye 360.23
DA-70240 Chalcosis 360.24
DA-70300 Hypotony of eye, NOS 360.30
DA-70301 Primary hypotony 360.31
DA-70310 Ocular fistula causing hypotony 360.32
DA-70320 Hypotony associated with other ocular disorder 360.33
DA-70330 Flat anterior chamber 360.34
DA-70400 Degenerated eye, NOS 360.40
  Degenerated globe, NOS 360.40
DA-70410 Blind hypotensive eye 360.41
DA-70412 Atrophy of globe
DA-70414 Phthisis bulbi 360.41
DA-70420 Blind hypertensive eye 360.42
DA-70422 Absolute glaucoma 360.42
DA-70430 Hemophthalmos, except current injury 360.43
DA-70440 Leukocoria 360.44
DA-70500 Retained magnetic intraocular foreign body, NOS 360.50
  Old intraocular foreign body 360.50
DA-70501 Magnetic foreign body in anterior chamber 360.51
DA-70502 Retained magnetic foreign body in iris or ciliary body 560.52
DA-70503 Retained magnetic foreign body in lens 360.53
DA-70504 Retained magnetic foreign body in vitreous 360.54
DA-70505 Retained magnetic foreign body in posterior wall of eye 360.55
DA-70509 Retained magnetic foreign body in multiple sites 360.59
DA-70510 Retained nonmagnetic intraocular foreign body, NOS 360.60
DA-70511 Retained nonmagnetic foreign body in anterior chamber 360.61
DA-70512 Retained nonmagnetic foreign body in iris or ciliary body 360.62
DA-70513 Retained nonmagnetic foreign body in lens 360.63
DA-70514 Retained nonmagnetic foreign body in vitreous 360.64
DA-70515 Retained nonmagnetic foreign body in posterior wall of eye 360.65
DA-70519 Retained nonmagnetic foreign body in multiple sites 360.69
DA-70520 Luxation of globe 360.8

A-71 DISORDERS OF THE CHOROID AND RETINA

DA-71000 Chorioretinitis, NOS 363.20
DA-71010 Choroiditis, NOS 363.20
DA-71020 Retinitis, NOS 363.20
DA-71030 Posterior uveitis, NOS 363.20
DA-71040 Harada's disease 363.22
DA-71050 Pars planitis 363.21
  Posterior cyclitis 363.21
DA-71100 Focal chorioretinitis, NOS 363.00
DA-71101 Focal choroiditis, NOS 363.00
DA-71102 Focal retinitis, NOS 363.00
  Focal retinochoroiditis, NOS 363.00
DA-71103 Juxtapapillary focal choroiditis and chorioretinitis 363.01
DA-71104 Focal choroiditis and chorioretinitis of other posterior pole 363.03
DA-71105 Peripheral focal choroiditis and chorioretinitis 363.04
DA-71106 Juxtapapillary focal retinitis and retinochoroiditis 363.05
  Neuroretinitis 363.05
DA-71107 Macular focal retinitis and retinochoroiditis 363.06
  Paramacular focal retinitis and retinochoroiditis 363.06
DA-71108 Focal retinitis and retinochoroiditis of other posterior pole 363.07
DA-71109 Peripheral focal retinitis and retinochoroiditis 363.08
DA-71110 Disseminated chorioretinitis, NOS 363.10
  Disseminated retinochoroiditis 363.10
DA-71111 Disseminated choroiditis 363.10
DA-71112 Disseminated retinitis 363.10
DA-71113 Disseminated choroiditis and chorioretinitis, posterior pole 363.11
DA-71114 Peripheral disseminated choroiditis and chorioretinitis 363.12
DA-71115 Generalized disseminated choroiditis and chorioretinitis 363.13
DA-71116 Metastatic disseminated retinitis and retinochoroiditis 363.14

A-71 DISORDERS OF THE CHOROID AND RETINA — Continued

DA-71118 Pigment epitheliopathy, disseminated retinitis and retinochoroiditis 363.15
  Acute posterior multifocal placoid pigment epitheliopathy 363.15
DA-71200 Chorioretinal scar, NOS 363.30
DA-71201 Postinflammatory chorioretinal scar 363.3
DA-71202 Postsurgical chorioretinal scar 363.3
DA-71203 Posttraumatic chorioretinal scar 363.3
DA-71210 Choroid scar, NOS 363.3
DA-71211 Postinflammatory choroid scar 363.3
DA-71212 Postsurgical choroid scar 363.3
DA-71213 Posttraumatic choroid scar 363.3
DA-71220 Retinal scar, NOS 363.3
DA-71221 Postinflammatory retinal scar 363.3
DA-71222 Postsurgical retinal scar 363.3
DA-71223 Posttraumatic retinal scar 363.3
DA-71230 Solar retinopathy 363.31
DA-71231 Macular scar 363.32
DA-71232 Scar of posterior pole of eye, NOS 363.33
DA-71233 Peripheral scar of posterior pole of eye 363.34
DA-71234 Disseminated scar of retina and choroid 363.35
DA-71240 Choroidal degeneration, NOS 363.40
  Choroidal sclerosis, NOS 363.40
DA-71242 Senile atrophy of choroid 363.41
DA-71244 Diffuse secondary atrophy of choroid 363.42
DA-71246 Angioid streaks of choroid 363.43
DA-71300 Hereditary choroidal dystrophy, NOS 363.50
  Hereditary choroidal atrophy 363.50
DA-71310 Partial circumpapillary dystrophy of choroid 363.51
DA-71311 Total circumpapillary dystrophy of choroid 363.52
DA-71320 Partial central dystrophy of choroid 363.53
  Circinate choroidal dystrophy 363.53
DA-71321 Total central choroidal atrophy 363.54
  Central gyrate choroidal dystrophy 363.54
  Serpiginous choroidal dystrophy 363.54
DA-71330 Choroideremia 363.55
DA-71340 Partial generalized choroidal dystrophy 363.56
  Partial diffuse choroidal dystrophy 363.56
DA-71341 Diffuse choroidal sclerosis 363.56
DA-71350 Total generalized choroidal dystrophy 363.57
  Total diffuse choroidal dystrophy 363.57
  Generalized gyrate atrophy of choroid 363.57
DA-71400 Choroidal hemorrhage, NOS 363.61
DA-71402 Expulsive choroidal hemorrhage 363.62
DA-71404 Choroidal rupture 363.63
DA-71410 Choroidal detachment, NOS 363.70
DA-71411 Serous choroidal detachment 363.71
DA-71412 Hemorrhagic choroidal detachment 363.72
DA-71500 Retinal hemorrhage, NOS 362.81
DA-71501 Deep retinal hemorrhage 362.81
DA-71502 Superficial retinal hemorrhage 362.81
DA-71503 Preretinal hemorrhage 362.81
DA-71504 Subretinal hemorrhage 362.81
DA-71510 Retinal ischemia 362.84
DA-71520 Retinal edema, NOS 362.83
DA-71521 Localized retinal edema 362.83
DA-71522 Macular retinal edema 362.83
DA-71523 Peripheral retinal edema 362.83
DA-71524 Retinal cotton wool spots 362.83
DA-71530 Retinal nerve fiber bundle defects 362.85
DA-71600 Retinal detachment, NOS 361.9
DA-71610 Rhegmatogenous retinal detachment 361.0
DA-71620 Retinal detachment with retinal defect, NOS 361.00
DA-71621 Partial recent retinal detachment with single defect 361.01
DA-71622 Partial recent retinal detachment with multiple defects 361.02
DA-71623 Partial recent retinal detachment with giant tear 361.03
DA-71624 Partial recent retinal detachment with retinal dialysis 361.04
DA-71625 Total recent retinal detachment 361.05
DA-71626 Subtotal recent retinal detachment 361.05
DA-71627 Partial old retinal detachment 361.06
  Delimited old retinal detachment 361.06
DA-71628 Total old retinal detachment 361.07
DA-71629 Subtotal old retinal detachment 361.07
DA-71640 Retinoschisis, NOS 361.10
DA-71641 Flat retinoschisis 361.11
DA-71642 Bullous retinoschisis 361.12
DA-71648 Pseudocyst of retina 361.19
DA-71650 Primary retinal cyst 361.13
DA-71652 Secondary retinal cyst 361.14
DA-71660 Retinal detachment without retinal defect 361.2
DA-71662 Serous retinal detachment 361.2
DA-71670 Retinal defect, NOS 361.30
  Retinal break, NOS 361.30
DA-71671 Round hole of retina without detachment 361.31
DA-71672 Horseshoe tear of retina without detachment 361.32
DA-71673 Operculum of retina without mention of detachment 361.32
DA-71678 Multiple defects of retina without detachment 361.33
DA-71680 Traction detachment of retina 361.81
DA-71684 Traction detachment with vitreoretinal organization 361.81
DA-71700 Diabetic retinopathy, NOS 362.01
DA-71702 Diabetic retinal microaneurysm 362.01
DA-71712 Background diabetic retinopathy 362.01
DA-71714 Proliferative diabetic retinopathy 362.02
DA-71720 Background retinopathy, NOS 362.10
DA-71721 Hypertensive retinopathy 362.11
DA-71722 Exudative retinopathy 362.12
  Coat's syndrome 362.12

DA-71723 Changes in retinal vascular appearance 362.13
DA-71724 Vascular sheathing of retina 362.13
DA-71730 Retinal microaneurysm, NOS 362.14
DA-71732 Retinal telangiectasia 362.15
DA-71735 Retinal neovascularization, NOS 362.16
DA-71736 Choroidal retinal neovascularization 362.16
DA-71737 Subretinal neovascularization 362.16
DA-71738 Retinal varices 362.17
DA-71740 Retinal vasculitis 362.18
DA-71742 Retinal arteritis 362.18
DA-71744 Retinal endarteritis 362.18
DA-71746 Retinal perivasculitis 362.18
DA-71748 Retinal phlebitis 362.18
DA-71749 Eales's disease 362.18
DA-71751 Retrolental fibroplasia 362.21
DA-71755 Nondiabetic proliferative retinopathy, NOS 362.29
DA-71800 Retinal vascular occlusion, NOS 362.30
DA-71801 Central retinal artery occlusion 362.31
DA-71802 Arterial retinal branch occlusion 362.32
DA-71803 Partial arterial retinal occlusion 362.33
DA-71804 Transient arterial retinal occlusion 362.34
DA-71805 Central retinal vein occlusion 362.35
DA-71806 Venous retinal branch occlusion 362.36
  Venous retinal tributary occlusion 362.36
DA-71810 Hollenhorst plaque 362.33
DA-71812 Retinal microembolism 362.33
DA-71814 Amaurosis fugax 362.34
DA-71820 Venous retinal engorgement 362.37
DA-71821 Incipient occlusion of retinal vein 362.37
DA-71822 Partial occlusion of retinal vein 362.37
DA-71830 Retinal layer separation, NOS 362.40
DA-71832 Central serous retinopathy 362.41
DA-71834 Serous detachment of retinal pigment epithelium 362.42
DA-71836 Exudative detachment of retinal pigment epithelium 362.42
DA-71838 Hemorrhagic detachment of retinal pigment epithelium 362.43
DA-71840 Senile macular retinal degeneration, NOS 362.50
DA-71841 Nonexudative senile macular retinal degeneration 362.51
  Atrophic senile macular retinal degeneration 382.51
  Dry senile macular retinal degeneration 362.51
DA-71842 Exudative senile macular retinal degeneration 362.52
  Wet senile macular retinal degeneration 362.52
DA-71843 Kuhnt-Junius degeneration 362.52
  Disciform senile macular retinal degeneration 362.52
DA-71844 Cystoid macular retinal degeneration 362.53
DA-71845 Macular retinal cyst 362.54
  Hole retinal cyst 362.54
  Macular pseudohole retinal cyst 362.54
DA-71846 Toxic maculopathy 362.55
DA-71847 Macular retinal puckering 362.56
DA-71848 Preretinal fibrosis 362.56
DA-71849 Degenerative drusen 362.57
DA-71860 Peripheral retinal degeneration, NOS 362.60
DA-71861 Paving stone retinal degeneration 362.61
DA-71862 Microcystoid retinal degeneration 362.62
  Blessig's cysts 362.62
  Iwanoff's cysts 362.62
DA-71863 Retinal lattice degeneration 362.63
  Palisade degeneration of retina 362.63
DA-71864 Senile reticular retinal degeneration 362.64
DA-71865 Secondary pigmentary retinal degeneration 362.65
  Pseudoretinitis pigmentosa 362.65
DA-71868 Secondary vitreoretinal degeneration 362.66
DA-71900 Hereditary retinal dystrophy, NOS 362.70
DA-71901 Retinal dystrophy in systemic lipidosis 362.71
DA-71902 Retinal dystrophy in cerebroretinal lipidosis 362.71
DA-71903 Vitreoretinal dystrophy 362.73
DA-71904 Juvenile retinoschisis 362.73
DA-71905 Pigmentary retinal dystrophy 362.74
  Albipunctate retinal dystrophy 362.74
DA-71906 Retinitis pigmentosa 362.74
DA-71907 Progressive cone-rod dystrophy 362.75
DA-71908 Stargardt's disease 362.75
DA-71910 Fundus flavimaculatus 362.76
DA-71911 Vitelliform dystrophy 362.76
DA-71912 Hyaline dystrophy of Bruch's membrane 362.77
  Pseudoinflammatory foveal dystrophy 362.77
  Hereditary drusen 362.77

A-72 DISORDERS OF THE IRIS AND CILIARY BODY

DA-72000 Disorder of iris and ciliary body, NOS 364.8
DA-72010 Disorder of iris, NOS 364.9
DA-72020 Disorder of ciliary body, NOS 364.9
DA-72030 Prolapse of iris, NOS 364.8
DA-72100 Iridocyclitis, NOS 364.3
  Anterior uveitis, NOS 364.3
DA-72110 Primary iridocyclitis 364.01
DA-72120 Recurrent iridocyclitis 364.02
  Periodic ophthalmia
  Moon blindness
DA-72130 Infectious secondary iridocyclitis 364.03
DA-72140 Noninfectious secondary iridocyclitis 364.04
DA-72200 Acute anterior uveitis 364.00
  Acute iridocyclitis 364.00
DA-72210 Subacute anterior uveitis 364.00
  Subacute iridocyclitis 364.00
DA-72220 Acute cyclitis 364.00
DA-72230 Subacute cyclitis 364.00
DA-72240 Acute iritis 364.00
DA-72250 Subacute iritis 364.00

A-72 DISORDERS OF THE IRIS AND CILIARY BODY — Continued

DA-72280 Hypopyon 364.05
DA-72300 Chronic iridocyclitis, NOS 364.10
DA-72310 Fuchs' heterochromic cyclitis 364.21
DA-72320 Glaucomatocyclitic crisis 364.22
DA-72330 Lens-induced iridocyclitis 364.23
DA-72350 Vogt-Koyanagi syndrome 364.24
DA-72400 Vascular disorder of iris and ciliary body, NOS 364.4
DA-72410 Hemorrhage of iris or ciliary body 364.41
DA-72412 Hyphema 364.41
DA-72420 Neovascularization of iris and ciliary body 364.42
DA-72422 Rubeosis iridis 364.42
DA-72500 Degeneration of iris and ciliary body, NOS 364.5
DA-72510 Essential iris atrophy 364.51
  Progressive iris atrophy 364.51
DA-72520 Iridoschisis 364.52
DA-72530 Pigmentary iris degeneration, NOS 364.53
  Pigment dispersion syndrome of iris 364.53
DA-72532 Acquired heterochromia of iris 364.53
DA-72534 Translucency of iris 364.53
DA-72540 Degeneration of pupillary margin 364.54
  Atrophy of sphincter of iris 364.54
DA-72542 Ectropion of pigment epithelium of iris 364.54
DA-72550 Miotic cyst of pupillary margin 364.55
DA-72560 Degenerative changes of anterior chamber angle 364.56
DA-72570 Degenerative changes of ciliary body 364.57
DA-72582 Generalized iris atrophy 364.59
DA-72584 Sector shaped iris atrophy 364.59
DA-72600 Cyst of iris, NOS 364.6
DA-72601 Idiopathic cyst of iris 364.60
DA-72602 Implantation cyst of iris 364.61
DA-72603 Exudative cyst of iris 364.62
DA-72610 Cyst of ciliary body, NOS 364.6
DA-72611 Idiopathic cyst of ciliary body 364.60
DA-72612 Implantation cyst of ciliary body 364.61
DA-72613 Exudative cyst of pars plana 364.64
DA-72618 Primary cyst of pars plana 364.63
DA-72620 Cyst of anterior chamber, NOS 364.6
DA-72621 Idiopathic cyst of anterior chamber 364.60
DA-72622 Implantation cyst of anterior chamber 364.61
  Epithelial down-growth of anterior chamber 364.61
DA-72623 Exudative cyst of anterior chamber 364.62
DA-72700 Adhesions of iris, NOS 364.7
  Synechiae of iris, NOS 364.70
DA-72701 Posterior synechiae of iris 364.71
DA-72702 Anterior synechiae of iris 364.72
DA-72705 Goniosynechiae 364.73
  Peripheral anterior synechiae of iris 364.73
DA-72710 Pupillary membrane, NOS 364.74
DA-72711 Pupillary occlusion 364.74
DA-72712 Pupillary seclusion 364.74
DA-72715 Iris bombé 364.74
DA-72720 Deformed pupil 364.75
DA-72722 Ectopic pupil 364.75
DA-72724 Rupture of sphincter of pupil 364.75
DA-72730 Iridodialysis 364.76
DA-72740 Recession of anterior chamber angle 364.77
DA-72800 Abnormal pupillary function, NOS 379.40
DA-72810 Anisocoria 379.41
DA-72812 Persistent miosis 379.42
DA-72814 Persistent mydriasis 379.43
DA-72816 Atypical Argyll-Robertson pupil 379.45
  Nonsyphilitic Argyll-Robertson phenomenon 379.45
DA-72817 Tonic pupillary reaction 379.46
DA-72818 Adie's pupil 379.46
  Adie's syndrome 379.46
DA-72820 Hippus 379.49
  Pupillary athetosis 379.49
DA-72830 Pupillary paralysis 379.49

A-73 GLAUCOMAS AND DISORDERS OF THE LENS

A-730-733 Glaucomas

DA-73000 Glaucoma, NOS 365.9
DA-73010 Borderline glaucoma, NOS 365.00
  Glaucoma suspect, NOS 365.00
  Preglaucoma, NOS 365.00
DA-73020 Open angle with borderline findings, NOS 365.01
DA-73021 Open angle with borderline intraocular pressure 365.01
DA-73022 Open angle with cupping of optic discs 365.01
DA-73030 Anatomical narrow angle glaucoma 365.02
DA-73040 Steroid responders to glaucoma 365.03
DA-73050 Ocular hypertension 365.04
DA-73100 Open-angle glaucoma, NOS 365.10
  Wide-angle glaucoma, NOS 365.10
DA-73110 Primary open angle glaucoma 365.11
  Chronic simple glaucoma 365.11
DA-73120 Low tension glaucoma 365.12
DA-73130 Pigmentary glaucoma 365.13
DA-73140 Glaucoma of childhood 365.14
  Infantile glaucoma 365.14
  Juvenile glaucoma 365.14
DA-73180 Residual stage of open angle glaucoma 365.15
DA-73200 Primary angle-closure glaucoma, NOS 365.20
DA-73210 Intermittent angle-closure glaucoma 365.21
  Interval angle-closure glaucoma 365.21
  Subacute angle-closure glaucoma 365.21
DA-73220 Acute angle-closure glaucoma 365.22
DA-73230 Chronic angle-closure glaucoma 365.23
DA-73280 Residual stage angle-closure glaucoma 365.24

DA-73300 Corticosteroid-induced glaucoma, NOS 365.3
DA-73301 Glaucomatous stage of corticosteroid-induced glaucoma 365.31
DA-73302 Residual stage of corticosteroid-induced glaucoma 365.32
DA-73310 Glaucoma associated with chamber angle anomalies 365.41
DA-73311 Glaucoma associated with anomalies of iris 365.42
DA-73312 Glaucoma associated with other anterior segment anomalies 365.43
DA-73313 Glaucoma associated with systemic syndromes 365.44
DA-73320 Phacolytic glaucoma 365.51
DA-73321 Pseudoexfoliation glaucoma 365.52
DA-73322 Glaucoma associated with other lens disorders 365.59
DA-73330 Glaucoma associated with unspecified ocular disorder 365.60
DA-73331 Glaucoma associated with pupillary block 365.61
DA-73332 Glaucoma associated with ocular inflammations 365.62
DA-73333 Glaucoma associated with vascular disorders 365.63
DA-73334 Glaucoma associated with tumors or cysts 365.64
DA-73335 Glaucoma associated with ocular trauma 365.65
DA-73350 Hypersecretion glaucoma 365.81
DA-73351 Glaucoma with increased episcleral venous pressure 365.82

A-734 Disorders of The Lens

DA-73400 Disorder of lens, NOS 379.3
DA-73410 Aphakia 379.31
DA-73414 Anterior dislocation of lens 379.33
DA-73416 Posterior dislocation of lens 379.34
DA-73420 Subluxation of lens 379.32

A-735-739 Cataracts

DA-73500 Cataract, NOS 366.9
DA-73510 Nonsenile cataract, NOS 366.00
  Infantile cataract, NOS 366.00
  Juvenile cataract, NOS 366.00
  Presenile cataract, NOS 366.00
DA-73520 Anterior subcapsular polar cataract 366.01
DA-73522 Posterior subcapsular polar cataract 366.02
DA-73530 Cortical cataract 366.03
  Lamellar cataract 366.03
  Zonular cataract 366.03
DA-73540 Nuclear cataract, NOS 366.04
DA-73580 Combined form of nonsenile cataract 366.09
DA-73600 Senile cataract, NOS 366.10
DA-73610 Pseudoexfoliation of lens capsule 366.11
DA-73620 Incipient cataract 366.12
  Immature cataract 366.12
  Water clefts 366.12
DA-73621 Coronary cataract 366.12
DA-73622 Punctate cataract 366.12
DA-73630 Anterior subcapsular polar senile cataract 366.13
DA-73640 Posterior subcapsular polar senile cataract 366.14
DA-73650 Cortical senile cataract 366.15
DA-73660 Senile nuclear cataract 366.16
  Nuclear sclerosis 366.16
DA-73662 Cataracta brunescens 366.16
DA-73670 Total cataract 366.17
  Mature cataract 366.17
DA-73680 Hypermature cataract 366.18
  Morgagni cataract 366.18
DA-73690 Combined form of senile cataract 366.19
DA-73700 Traumatic cataract, NOS 366.20
DA-73710 Localized traumatic opacity 366.21
DA-73712 Vossius' ring 366.21
DA-73720 Total traumatic cataract 366.22
DA-73730 Partially resolved traumatic cataract 366.23
DA-73800 Cataract secondary to ocular disorder, NOS 366.3
  Cataracta complicata, NOS 366.30
DA-73804 Subcapsular glaucomatous flecks 366.31
DA-73810 Cataract in inflammatory disorder 366.32
DA-73820 Cataract with neovascularization 366.33
DA-73830 Cataract in degenerative disorder 366.34
DA-73840 Diabetic cataract 66.41
DA-73850 Tetanic cataract 366.42
DA-73860 Myotonic cataract 366.43
DA-73870 Toxic cataract 366.45
DA-73880 Cataract associated with radiation 366.46
DA-73900 After-cataract, NOS 366.50
  Secondary cataract 366.50
DA-73902 Soemmering's ring 366.51
DA-73904 After-cataract not obscuring vision 566.52
DA-73906 After-cataract obscuring vision 366.53
DA-73910 Calcification of lens 366.8

A-74 DISORDERS OF REFRACTION, ACCOMMODATION AND BLINDNESS

A-740-748 Disorders of Refraction and Accommodation

DA-74000 Disorder of refraction and accommodation, NOS 367.9
DA-74010 Toxic disorder of refraction and accommodation 367.89
DA-74020 Drug-induced disorder of refraction and accommodation 367.89
DA-74100 Disorder of refraction, NOS 367.-
DA-74110 Hypermetropia 367.0
  Hyperopia 367.0
  Farsightedness 367.0
DA-74120 Myopia 367.1
  Nearsightedness 367.1
DA-74122 Severe myopia 367.1
  High myopia 367.1

A-740-748 Disorders of Refraction and Accommodation — Continued

DA-74130 Astigmatism, NOS 367.20
DA-74131 Regular astigmatism 367.21
DA-74132 Irregular astigmatism 367.22
DA-74140 Anisometropia 367.31
DA-74145 Aniseikonia 367.32
DA-74150 Presbyopia 367.4
DA-74160 Transient refractive change 367.8
DA-74200 Disorder of accommodation, NOS 367.5
DA-74202 Cycloplegia 367.51
Paresis of accommodation 367.51
DA-74210 Total internal ophthalmoplegia 367.52
Complete internal ophthalmoplegia 367.52
DA-74220 Spasm of accommodation 367.53
DA-74400 Visual disturbance, NOS 368.9
DA-74410 Amblyopia, NOS 368.00
Blurred vision, NOS 368.8
DA-74411 Amblyopia ex anopsia 368.00
DA-74412 Strabismic amblyopia 368.01
Suppression amblyopia 368.01
DA-74413 Deprivation amblyopia 368.02
DA-74414 Refractive amblyopia 368.03
DA-74419 Tobacco amblyopia
DA-74420 Subjective visual disturbance, NOS 368.10
DA-74421 Sudden visual loss 368.11
DA-74422 Transient visual loss 368.12
DA-74423 Concentric fading 368.12
DA-74424 Scintillating scotoma 368.12
Flittering scotoma 368.12
Teichopsia 368.12
DA-74440 Visual distortions of shape and size 368.14
DA-74444 Metamorphopsia 368.14
DA-74450 Photopsia 368.15
DA-74452 Refractive diplopia 368.15
DA-74454 Refractive polyopia 368.15
DA-74456 Visual halos 368.15
DA-74460 Psychophysical visual disturbance, NOS 368.16
DA-74464 Visual disorientation syndrome 368.16
DA-74500 Binocular vision disorder, NOS 368.30
DA-74510 Diplopia 368.2
Double vision 368.2
DA-74514 Monocular diplopia
DA-74520 Supression of binocular vision 368.31
DA-74530 Simultaneous visual perception without fusion 368.32
DA-74540 Fusion with defective stereopsis 368.33
DA-74550 Abnormal retinal correspondence 368.34
DA-74600 Visual field defect, NOS 368.40
DA-74601 Scotoma, NOS 368.44
DA-74602 Nasal step visual field defect 368.44
DA-74603 Peripheral visual field defect 368.44
DA-74604 Relative scotoma
DA-74605 Absolute scotoma
DA-74610 Scotoma of central area 368.41
Central scotoma 368.41
DA-74611 Centrocecal scotoma 368.41
DA-74612 Paracentral scotoma 368.41
DA-74620 Scotoma of blind spot area 368.42
Enlarged angioscotoma 368.42
Enlarged blind spot 368.42
Enlarged paracecal scotoma 368.42
DA-74630 Arcuate scotoma 368.43
Arcuate defects 368.43
DA-74631 Seidel scotoma 368.43
DA-74632 Bjerrum scotoma 368.43
DA-74638 Generalized contraction of visual field 368.45
Generalized constriction of visual field 368.45
DA-74640 Hemianopsia, NOS
Hemianopia, NOS
DA-74650 Homonymous hemianopsia 368.46
Homonymous bilateral visual field defects 368.46
DA-74651 Right homonymous hemianopsia
DA-74652 Left homonymous hemianopsia
DA-74654 Altitudinal hemianopsia 368.46
DA-74656 Quadrant hemianopia 368.46
Quandrantanopia 368.46
DA-74660 Heteronymous bilateral visual field defects 368.47
DA-74662 Binasal hemianopsia 368.47
DA-74664 Bitemporal hemianopsia 368.47
DA-74700 Color vision deficiency, NOS 368.55
Color blindness, NOS 368.55
Chromatopsia 368.55
Daltonism 368.55
DA-74702 Acquired color vision deficiency, NOS 368.55
DA-74710 Protan defect 368.51
Protanomaly 368.51
Protanopia 368.51
DA-74720 Deutan defect 368.52
Deuteranomaly 368.52
Deuteranopia 368.52
DA-74730 Tritan defect 368.53
Tritanomaly 368.53
DA-74732 Tritanopia 368.53
DA-74734 Xanthopsia
DA-74735 Erythropsia
Erythropia
DA-74740 Achromatopsia 368.54
DA-74744 Cone monochromatism 368.54
Rod monochromatism 368.54
DA-74800 Night blindness, NOS 368.60
Hemeralopia 368.60
Nyctalopia 368.60
DA-74810 Congenital night blindness 368.61
Hereditary night blindness 368.61
Oguchi's disease 368.61
DA-74820 Acquired night blindness 368.62
DA-74830 Abnormal dark adaptation curve 368.63
Abnormal threshold of cones 368.63
Abnormal threshold of rods 368.63
Delayed adaptation of cones 368.63
Delayed adaptation of rods 368.63

A-749 Blindness and Vision Impairment Levels

DA-74900 Blindness, NOS 369.9
Low vision, NOS 369.9
Visual loss, NOS 369.9
Decreased vision, NOS 369.9
DA-74910 Impairment level of both eyes, NOS 369.00
DA-74911 Impairement level: total impairment of both eyes 369.01
DA-74912 Impairement level: better eye: near-total impairment; lesser-eye: not further specified 369.02
DA-74913 Impairment level: better eye: near-total impairment; lesser eye: total impairment 369.03
DA-74914 Impairment level: near-total impairment of both eyes 369.04
DA-74915 Impairment level: better eye: profound impairment; lesser eye: not further specified 369.05
DA-74916 Impairment level: better eye: profound impairment; lesser eye: total impairment 369.06
DA-74917 Impairment level: better eye: profound impairment; lesser eye: near-total impairment 369.07
DA-74918 Impairment level: profound impairment of both eyes 369.08
DA-74920 Impairment level: blindness, one eye — low vision other eye 369.10
DA-74921 Impairment level: better eye: severe impairment; lesser eye: blind, not further specified 369.11
DA-74922 Impairment level: better eye: severe impairment; lesser eye: total impairment 369.12
DA-74923 Impairment level: better eye: severe impairment; lesser eye: near-total impairment 369.13
DA-74924 Impairment level: better eye: severe impairment; lesser eye: profound impairment 369.14
DA-74925 Impairment level: better eye: moderate impairment; lesser eye: blind, not further specified 369.15
DA-74926 Impairment level: better eye: moderate impairment; lesser eye: total impairment 369.16
DA-74927 Impairment level: better eye: moderate impairment; lesser eye: near-total impairment 369.17
DA-74928 Impairment level: better eye: moderate impairment; lesser eye: profound impairment 369.18
DA-74930 Impairment level: low vision of both eyes, NOS 369.20
DA-74931 Impairment level: better eye: severe impairment; lesser eye: not further specified 369.21
DA-74932 Impairment level: severe impairment of both eyes 369.22
DA-74933 Impairment level: better eye: moderate impairment; lesser eye: not further specified 369.23
DA-74934 Impairment level: better eye: moderate impairment; lesser eye: severe impairment 369.24
DA-74935 Impairment level: moderate impairment of both eyes 369.25
DA-74938 Unqualified visual loss of both eyes 369.3
DA-74940 Blindness of one eye, NOS 369.60
DA-74941 Impairment level: one eye: total impairmen; other eye: not specified 369.61
DA-74942 Impairment level: one eye: total impairment; other eye: near-normal vision 369.62
DA-74943 Impairment level: one eye: total impairment; other eye: normal vision 369.63
DA-74944 Impairment level: one eye: near-total impairment; other eye: not specified 369.64
DA-74945 Impairment level: one eye: near-total impairment; other eye: near-normal vision 369.65
DA-74946 Impairment level: one eye: near-total impairment; other eye: normal vision 369.66
DA-74947 Impairment level: one eye: profound impairment; other eye: not specified 369.67
DA-74948 Impairment level: one eye: profound impairment; other eye: near-normal vision 369.68
DA-74949 Impairment level: one eye: profound impairment; other eye: normal vision 369.69
DA-74950 Impairment level: lovision of one eye, NOS 369.70
DA-74951 Impairment level: one eye: severe impairment; other eye: not specified 369.71
DA-74952 Impairment level: one eye: severe impairment; other eye: near-normal vision 369.72
DA-74953 Impairment level: one eye: severe impairment; other eye: normal vision 369.73
DA-74954 Impairment level: one eye: moderate impairment; other eye: not specified 369.74
DA-74955 Impairment level: one eye: moderate impairment; other eye: near-normal vision 369.75
DA-74956 Impairment level: one eye: moderate impairment; other eye: normal vision 369.76
DA-74960 Unqualified visual loss of one eye 369.8

A-75 DISEASES OF THE CORNEA AND CONJUNCTIVA

A-750-754 Diseases of The Cornea

DA-75000 Disease of cornea, NOS 370.-
DA-75010 Keratitis, NOS 370.9
DA-75100 Corneal ulcer, NOS 370.00
DA-75101 Marginal corneal ulcer 370.01
DA-75102 Ring corneal ulcer 370.02

A-750-754 Diseases of The Cornea — Continued

DA-75103 Central corneal ulcer 370.03
DA-75104 Hypopyon ulcer 370.04
DA-75105 Serpiginous ulcer 370.04
DA-75106 Mycotic corneal ulcer 370.05
DA-75107 Perforated corneal ulcer 370.06
DA-75108 Mooren's ulcer 370.07
DA-75200 Superficial keratitis, NOS 370.20
DA-75201 Punctate keratitis 370.21
Thygeson's superficial punctate keratitis 370.21
DA-75202 Macular keratitis 370.22
DA-75203 Areolar keratitis 370.22
DA-75204 Nummular keratitis 370.22
DA-75205 Stellate keratitis 370.22
DA-75206 Striate keratitis 370.22
DA-75210 Filamentary keratitis 370.23
DA-75220 Photokeratitis 370.24
DA-75221 Snow blindness 370.24
DA-75222 Welders' keratitis 370.24
DA-75230 Keratoconjunctivitis, NOS 370.40
Superficial keratitis with conjunctivitis, NOS 370.40
DA-75231 Phlyctenular keratoconjunctivitis 370.31
Phlyctenulosis 370.31
DA-75232 Keratoconjunctivitis sicca, not specified as Sjogren's 370.33
DA-75240 Limbal and corneal involvement in vernal conjunctivitis 370.32
DA-75250 Exposure keratoconjunctivitis 370.34
DA-75255 Neurotrophic keratoconjunctivitis 370.35
DA-75260 Keratitis in exanthema 370.44
Keratoconjunctivitis in exanthema 370.44
DA-75270 Interstitial keratitis, NOS 370.50
DA-75271 Diffuse interstitial keratitis 370.52
DA-75272 Cogan's syndrome 370.52
DA-75273 Sclerosing keratitis 370.54
DA-75278 Corneal abscess 370.55
DA-75280 Corneal neovascularization, NOS 370.60
DA-75281 Localized vascularization of cornea 370.61
DA-75284 Corneal pannus 370.62
DA-75286 Deep vascularization of cornea 370.63
DA-75288 Corneal ghost vessels 370.64
DA-75300 Corneal opacity, NOS 371.00
Corneal scar, NOS 371.00
DA-75301 Minor opacity of cornea 371.01
DA-75302 Corneal nebula 371.01
DA-75303 Peripheral opacity of cornea 371.02
Corneal macula not interfering with central vision 371.02
DA-75304 Central opacity of cornea, NOS 371.03
DA-75305 Corneal leukoma interfering with central vision 371.03
DA-75306 Corneal macula interfering with central vision 371.03
DA-75307 Adherent leukoma 371.04
DA-75308 Phthisical cornea 371.05
DA-75310 Corneal deposit, NOS 371.10
DA-75311 Anterior corneal pigmentation 371.11
DA-75312 Stahli's lines 371.11
DA-75313 Stromal corneal pigmentation 371.12
DA-75314 Hematocornea 371.12
DA-75315 Posterior corneal pigmentation 371.13
DA-75316 Krukenberg spindle 371.13
DA-75317 Kayser-Fleisher ring 371.14
DA-75318 Corneal deposit associated with metabolic disorder 371.15
DA-75319 Argentous corneal deposit 371.16
DA-75320 Corneal edema, NOS 371.20
DA-75321 Idiopathic corneal edema 371.21
DA-75322 Secondary corneal edema 371.22
DA-75323 Bullous keratopathy 371.23
DA-75328 Corneal edema due to wearing of contact lenses 371.24
DA-75330 Corneal membrane change, NOS 371.30
DA-75331 Folds and rupture of Bowman's membrane 371.31
DA-75332 Folds in Descemet's membrane 371.32
DA-75333 Rupture in Descemet's membrane 371.33
DA-75340 Corneal degeneration, NOS 371.40
DA-75341 Senile corneal changes 371.41
DA-75342 Arcus senilis 371.41
Gerontoxon 371.41
DA-75343 Hassall-Henle bodies 371.41
DA-75344 Recurrent erosion of cornea 371.42
DA-75345 Band-shaped keratopathy 371.43
Band keratopathy 371.43
DA-75346 Calcareous degeneration of cornea 371.44
DA-75347 Keratomalacia, NOS 371.45
DA-75348 Nodular degeneration of cornea 371.46
DA-75349 Salzmann's nodular dystrophy 371.46
DA-75350 Peripheral degeneration of cornea 371.48
DA-75351 Terrien's marginal degeneration of cornea 371.48
DA-75352 Discrete colliquative keratopathy 371.49
DA-75400 Hereditary corneal dystrophy, NOS 371.5
DA-75401 Corneal dystrophy, NOS 371.50
DA-75402 Juvenile epithelial corneal dystrophy 371.51
DA-75403 Microscopic cystic corneal dystrophy 371.52
DA-75404 Ring-like corneal dystrophy 371.52
DA-75410 Granular corneal dystrophy 371.53
DA-75412 Lattice corneal dystrophy 371.54
DA-75414 Macular corneal dystrophy 371.55
DA-75415 Crystalline corneal dystrophy 371.56
DA-75420 Endothelial corneal dystrophy 371.57
Combined corneal dystrophy 371.57
Fuchs' endothelial dystrophy 371.57
DA-75422 Cornea guttata 371.57
DA-75425 Polymorphous corneal dystrophy 371.58
DA-75430 Keratoconus, NOS 371.60
DA-75432 Stable condition keratoconus 371.61
DA-75434 Acute hydrops keratoconus 371.62
DA-75450 Corneal deformity 371.70
DA-75452 Corneal ectasia 371.71
DA-75454 Descementocele 371.72
DA-75456 Corneal staphyloma 371.73

DA-75460 Corneal anesthesia 371.81
DA-75462 Corneal hypoesthesia 371.81

A-756-759 Disorders of The Conjunctiva

DA-75600 Disorder of conjunctiva, NOS 372.9
DA-75605 Conjunctivitis, NOS 372.30
DA-75610 Acute conjunctivitis, NOS 372.00
DA-75612 Serous conjunctivitis, except viral 372.01
DA-75614 Acute follicular conjunctivitis, NOS 372.02
  Conjunctival folliculosis, NOS 372.02
DA-75617 Pseudomembranous conjunctivitis 372.04
  Membranous conjunctivitis 372.04
DA-75619 Acute atopic conjunctivitis 372.05
DA-75630 Chronic conjunctivitis, NOS 372.10
DA-75631 Simple chronic conjunctivitis 372.11
DA-75633 Chronic follicular conjunctivitis 372.12
DA-75635 Vernal conjunctivitis 372.13
DA-75637 Chronic allergic conjunctivitis, NOS 372.14
DA-75640 Blepharoconjunctivitis, NOS 372.20
DA-75642 Angular blepharoconjunctivitis, NOS 372.21
DA-75644 Contact blepharoconjunctivitis 372.22
DA-75650 Conjunctivitis in mucocutaneous disease 372.33
DA-75652 Rosacea conjunctivitis 372.31
DA-75700 Pterygium, NOS 372.40
DA-75702 Stationary peripheral pterygium 372.41
DA-75704 Progressive peripheral pterygium 372.42
DA-75706 Central pterygium 372.43
DA-75708 Double pterygium 372.44
DA-75709 Recurrent pterygium 372.45
DA-75720 Conjunctival degeneration, NOS 372.50
DA-75722 Pinguecula 372.51
  Pinguicula 372.51
DA-75724 Pseudopterygium 372.52
DA-75726 Conjunctival xerosis 372.53
DA-75730 Conjunctival concretion, NOS 372.54
DA-75740 Conjunctival pigmentation, NOS 372.55
DA-75742 Conjunctival argyrosis 372.55
DA-75744 Conjunctival deposit, NOS 372.56
DA-75800 Conjunctival scar, NOS 372.64
  Scarring of conjunctiva 372.64
DA-75810 Granuloma of conjunctiva 372.61
DA-75820 Localized adhesions and strands of conjunctiva 372.62
DA-75822 Symblepharon 372.63
DA-75830 Contraction of eye socket after enucleation 372.64
DA-75900 Conjunctival hemorrhage 373.73
DA-75902 Hyposphagma 372.72
DA-75904 Subconjunctival hemorrhage 372.72
DA-75910 Hyperemia of conjunctiva 372.71
DA-75920 Conjunctival edema 372.73
DA-75922 Chemosis of conjunctiva 372.73
DA-75924 Subconjunctival edema 372.73
DA-75930 Vascular abnormality of conjunctiva, NOS 372.74
DA-75932 Aneurysm of conjunctiva 372.74

A-76 DISORDERS OF THE EYELIDS AND LACRIMAL SYSTEM

A-760-765 Disorders of The Eyelids

DA-76000 Disorder of eyelid, NOS 374.9
DA-76010 Edema of eyelid 374.32
DA-76011 Hyperemia of eyelid 374.82
DA-76020 Hemorrhage of eyelid 374.81
DA-76030 Elephantiasis of eyelid 374.83
DA-76031 Cyst of eyelid, NOS 374.84
DA-76032 Sebaceous cyst of eyelid 374.83
DA-76040 Vascular anomaly of eyelid 374.85
DA-76050 Retained foreign body of eyelid 374.86
DA-76100 Blepharitis, NOS 373.9
  Inflammation of eyelid, NOS 373.9
DA-76102 Ulcerative blepharitis 373.01
DA-76104 Squamous blepharitis 373.02
DA-76110 Hordeolum, NOS 373.11
  Stye 373.11
DA-76112 Hordeolum externum 373.11
DA-76114 Hordeolum internum 373.12
DA-76116 Infection of meibomian gland 373.12
DA-76120 Abscess of eyelid 373.13
DA-76124 Furuncle of eyelid 373.13
DA-76130 Chalazion 373.2
  Meibomian gland cyst 373.2
DA-76200 Noninfectious dermatosis of eyelid, NOS 373.3
DA-76204 Contact dermatitis of eyelid 373.32
  Allergic dermatitis of eyelid 373.32
DA-76205 Eczematous dermatitis of eyelid 373.31
DA-76206 Xeroderma of eyelid 373.33
DA-76208 Discoid lupus erythematosus of eyelid 373.34
DA-76210 Infective dermatitis of eyelid, NOS 373.5
DA-76220 Infective dermatitis of eyelid resulting in deformity 373.4
DA-76300 Entropion, NOS 374.00
DA-76301 Senile entropion 374.01
DA-76302 Mechanical entropion 374.02
DA-76304 Spastic entropion 374.03
DA-76306 Cicatricial entropion 374.04
DA-76308 Trichiasis without entropion 374.05
DA-76310 Ectropion, NOS 374.10
DA-76312 Senile ectropion 374.11
DA-76314 Mechanical ectropion 374.12
DA-76316 Spastic ectropion 374.13
DA-76318 Cicatricial ectropion 374.14
DA-76320 Lagophthalmos, NOS 374.20
DA-76322 Paralytic lagophthalmos 374.21
DA-76324 Mechanical lagophthalmos 374.22
DA-76326 Cicatricial lagophthalmos 374.23
DA-76330 Ptosis of eyelid, NOS 374.30
DA-76332 Paralytic ptosis 374.31
DA-76334 Myogenic ptosis 374.32
DA-76336 Mechanical ptosis 374.33
DA-76337 Blepharochalasis 374.34
DA-76338 Pseudoptosis 374.34
DA-76400 Abnormal innervation syndrome 374.43

A-760-765 Disorders of The Eyelids — Continued

DA-76401 Jaw-blinking 374.43
DA-76408 Paradoxical facial movements 374.43
DA-76410 Sensory disorder of eyelid 374.44
DA-76420 Sensorimotor disorder of eyelid 374.45
DA-76430 Acquired blepharophimosis 374.46
DA-76432 Acquired ankyloblepharon 374.46
DA-76500 Degenerative disorder of eyelid, NOS 374.50
DA-76510 Xanthoma of eyelid 374.51
  Xanthelasma of eyelid 374.51
DA-76511 Xanthoma planum of eyelid
DA-76520 Hyperpigmentation of eyelid, NOS 374.52
  Dyspigmentation of eyelid 374.52
DA-76530 Hypopigmentation of eyelid 374.53
DA-76532 Vitiligo of eyelid 374.53
DA-76540 Hypertrichosis of eyelid 374.54
DA-76550 Hypotrichosis of eyelid 374.55
DA-76552 Madarosis of eyelid 374.55

A-767-769 Disorders of The Lacrimal System

DA-76700 Disorder of lacrimal system, NOS 375.9
DA-76800 Dacryoadenitis, NOS 375.00
DA-76810 Acute dacryoadenitis 375.01
DA-76820 Chronic dacryoadenitis 375.02
DA-76825 Chronic enlargement of lacrimal gland 375.03
DA-76830 Dacryops 375.11
DA-76832 Lacrimal cyst, NOS 375.12
DA-76834 Cystic degeneration of lacrimal gland 375.12
DA-76840 Primary lacrimal atrophy 375.13
DA-76842 Secondary lacrimal atrophy 375.14
DA-76844 Tear film insufficiency, NOS 375.15
  Dry eye syndrome 375.15
DA-76846 Dislocation of lacrimal gland 375.16
DA-76850 Epiphora, NOS 375.20
  Illacrimation, NOS 375.20
DA-76852 Epiphora due to excess lacrimation 375.21
DA-76854 Epiphora due to insufficient drainage 375.22
DA-76858V Chromodacryorrhea
DA-76900 Dacryocystitis, NOS 375.30
DA-76902 Acute lacrimal canaliculitis 375.31
DA-76904 Acute dacryocystitis 375.32
DA-76906 Acute peridacryocystitis 375.32
DA-76908 Phlegmonous dacryocystitis 375.33
DA-76910 Chronic dacryocystitis 375.42
DA-76912 Chronic lacrimal canaliculitis 375.41
DA-76914 Lacrimal mucocele 375.43
DA-76920 Eversion of lacrimal punctum 375.51
DA-76921 Stenosis of lacrimal punctum 375.52
DA-76922 Stenosis of lacrimal canaliculi 375.53
DA-76923 Stenosis of lacrimal sac 375.54
DA-76925 Neonatal obstruction of nasolacrimal duct 375.55
DA-76927 Acquired stenosis of nasolacrimal duct 375.56
DA-76929 Dacryolith 375.57
DA-76930 Lacrimal fistula 375.61
DA-76940 Granuloma of lacrimal passages 375.81

A-77 DISORDERS OF THE ORBIT AND VISUAL PATHWAYS

A-770-774 Disorders of The Orbit

DA-77000 Disorder of orbit, NOS 376.9
DA-77010 Retained old foreign body following penetrating wound of orbit 376.6
DA-77012 Retrobulbar foreign body 376.6
DA-77020 Orbital cyst, NOS 376.81
DA-77022 Encephalocele of orbit 376.81
DA-77030 Myopathy of extraocular muscles 376.82
DA-77100 Acute inflammation of orbit, NOS 376.00
DA-77102 Abscess of orbit 376.01
DA-77110 Orbital periostitis 376.02
DA-77112 Orbital osteomyelitis 376.03
DA-77114 Tenonitis 376.04
DA-77150 Chronic inflammation of orbit, NOS 376.10
DA-77152 Orbital granuloma 376.11
DA-77154 Inflammatory pseudotumor of orbit 376.11
DA-77160 Orbital myositis 376.12
DA-77200 Exophthalmos, NOS 376.30
DA-77202 Constant exophthalmos 376.31
DA-77204 Intermittent exophthalmos 376.34
DA-77206 Pulsating exophthalmos 376.35
DA-77207 Orbital hemorrhage 376.32
DA-77208 Orbital edema 376.33
DA-77209 Orbital congestion 376.33
DA-77210 Endocrine exophthalmos, NOS 376.2
DA-77212 Thyrotoxic exophthalmos 376.21
DA-77214 Exophthalmic ophthalmoplegia 376.22
DA-77220 Lateral displacement of globe 376.36
DA-77300 Deformity of orbit, NOS 376.40
DA-77304 Exostosis of orbit 376.42
DA-77306 Local deformities due to bone disease 376.43
DA-77308 Orbital deformity associated with craniofacial deformity 376.44
DA-77310 Atrophy of orbit 376.45
DA-77320 Enlargement of orbit 376.46
DA-77330 Orbital deformity due to trauma 376.47
DA-77332 Orbital deformity due to surgery 376.47
DA-77400 Enophthalmos, NOS 376.50
DA-77410 Enophthalmos due to atrophy of orbital tissue 376.51
DA-77420 Enophthalmos due to trauma 376.52
DA-77422 Enophthalmos due to surgery 376.52

A-775-776 Disorders of The Optic Nerve

DA-77500 Disorder of optic nerve, NOS 377.9
DA-77510 Papilledema, NOS 377.00
DA-77512 Papilledema associated with increased intracranial pressure 377.01
DA-77514 Papilledema associated with decreased ocular pressure 377.02
DA-77516 Papilledema associated with retinal disorder 377.03
DA-77518 Foster-Kennedy syndrome 377.04

DA-77520 Optic atrophy, NOS 377.10
DA-77521 Primary optic atrophy 377.11
DA-77522 Postinflammatory optic atrophy 377.12
DA-77523 Optic atrophy associated with retinal dystrophy, NOS 377.13
DA-77524 Glaucomatous atrophy of optic disc 377.14
DA-77525 Partial optic atrophy 377.15
DA-77526 Hereditary optic atrophy, NOS 376.16
DA-77527 Dominant hereditary optic atrophy 377.16
DA-77528 Leber's optic atrophy 377.16
DA-77540 Drusen of optic disc 377.2
DA-77542 Crater-like holes of optic disc 377.22
DA-77544 Coloboma of optic disc 377.23
DA-77546 Pseudopapilledema 377.24
DA-77600 Optic neuritis, NOS 377.30
DA-77604 Optic papillitis 377.31
DA-77606 Acute retrobulbar neuritis 377.32
DA-77610 Nutritional optic neuropathy 377.33
DA-77612 Toxic optic neuropathy 377.34
DA-77614 Toxic amblyopia 377.34
DA-77620 Ischemic optic neuropathy 377.41
DA-77622 Hemorrhage in optic nerve sheaths 377.42
DA-77624 Compression of optic nerve 377.49

A-778 Disorders of The Visual Pathways

DA-77800 Disorder of visual pathways, NOS 377.9
DA-77810 Disorder of optic chiasm associated with pituitary neoplasms and disorders 377.51
DA-77812 Disorder of optic chiasm associated with other neoplasm 377.52
DA-77814 Disorder of optic chiasm associated with vascular disorder 377.53
DA-77816 Disorder of optic chiasm associated with inflammatory disorder 377.54
DA-77820 Disorder of visual pathways associated with neoplasm 377.61
DA-77822 Disorder of visual pathways associated with vascular disorder 377.62
DA-77824 Disorder of visual pathways associated with inflammatory disorder 377.63
DA-77850 Disorder of visual cortex associated with neoplasm 377.71
DA-77852 Disorder of visual cortex associated with vascular disorder 377.72
DA-77854 Disorder of visual cortex associated with inflammatory disorder 377.73
DA-77856 Cortical blindness 377.75

A-78 DISORDERS OF EYE MOVEMENTS

DA-78000 Disorder of eye movements, NOS 378.9
DA-78100 Strabismus, NOS 378.9
  Heterotropia, NOS 378.9
  Squint, NOS 378.9
DA-78102 Microstrabismus 378.34
  Microtropia 378.34
DA-78110 Esotropia, NOS 378.00
  Convergent strabismus 378.0
  Cross-eye 378.0
DA-78112 Accommodative component in esotropia 378.35
DA-78120 Monocular esotropia, NOS 378.01
DA-78122 Monocular esotropia with A pattern 378.02
DA-78124 Monocular esotropia with V pattern 378.03
DA-78126 Monocular esotropia with other noncomitancies 378.04
DA-78130 Alternating esotropia, NOS 378.05
DA-78132 Alternating esotropia with A pattern 378.06
DA-78134 Alternating esotropia with V pattern 378.07
DA-78136 Alternating esotropia with other noncomitancies 378.08
DA-78138 Alternating esotropia with X or Y pattern 378.08
DA-78140 Exotropia, NOS 378.10
  Divergent concomitant strabismus 378.1
  Divergent strabismus 378.10
  External strabismus 378.10
DA-78141 Monocular exotropia, NOS 378.11
DA-78142 Monocular exotropia with A pattern 378.12
DA-78143 Monocular exotropia with V pattern 378.13
DA-78146 Monocular exotropia with other noncomitancies 378.14
DA-78148 Monocular exotropia with X or Y pattern 378.14
DA-78150 Alternating exotropia, NOS 378.15
DA-78152 Alternating exotropia with A pattern 378.16
DA-78154 Alternating exotropia with V pattern 378.17
DA-78156 Alternating exotropia with other noncomitancies 378.18
DA-78158 Alternating exotropia with X or Y pattern 378.18
DA-78160 Intermittent heterotropia, NOS 378.20
DA-78162 Intermittent esotropia, NOS 378l.20
DA-78164 Intermittent exotropia, NOS 378.20
DA-78165 Monocular intermittent esotropia 378.21
DA-78166 Alternating intermittent esotropia 378.22
DA-78167 Monocular intermittent exotropia 378.23
DA-78168 Alternating intermittent exotropia 378.24
DA-78170 Vertical heterotropia, NOS 378.30
  Vertical strabismus 378.30
DA-78172 Hypertropia 378.31
  Constant vertical heterotropia 378.31
DA-78173 Intermittent vertical heterotropia 378.31
DA-78174 Hypotropia 378.32
DA-78180 Cyclotropia, NOS 378.33
DA-78182 Incyclotropia
DA-78184 Excyclotropia
DA-78190 Monofixation syndrome 378.34
DA-78200 Heterophoria, NOS 378.40
DA-78202 Esophoria 378.41
DA-78204 Exophoria 378.42
DA-78210 Vertical heterophoria, NOS 378.43
DA-78212 Hyperphoria
DA-78213 Alternating hyperphoria 378.45
DA-78214 Hypophoria
DA-78218 Cyclophoria 378.44

A-78 DISORDERS OF EYE MOVEMENTS — Continued

DA-78220 Paralytic strabismus, NOS 378.50
DA-78221 Partial third nerve palsy 378.51
  Partial oculomotor nerve palsy 378.51
DA-78222 Total third nerve palsy 378.52
  Total oculomotor nerve palsy 378.52
DA-78230 Fourth nerve palsy 378.53
  Trochlear nerve palsy 378.53
DA-78232 Sixth nerve palsy 378.54
  Abducens nerve palsy 378.54
DA-78234 External ophthalmoplegia 378.55
DA-78236 Total ophthalmoplegia 378.56
DA-78240 Mechanical strabismus, NOS 378.60
DA-78242 Brown's tendon sheath syndrome 378.61
DA-78244 Mechanical strabismus from other musculofascial disorder 378.62
DA-78246 Limited duction associated with other condition of eye 378.63
DA-78250 Duane's syndrome 378.71
DA-78252 Progressive external ophthalmoplegia 378.72
DA-78258 Strabismus in other neuromuscular disorder 378.73
DA-78300 Palsy of conjugate gaze 378.81
DA-78302 Spasm of conjugate gaze 378.82
DA-78304 Convergence insufficiency 378.83
  Convergence palsy 378.83
DA-78306 Convergence excess 378.84
  Convergence spasm 378.84
DA-78310 Anomaly of divergence 378.85
DA-78312 Internuclear ophthalmoplegia 378.86
DA-78314 Skew deviation 378.87
DA-78500 Nystagmus, NOS 379.50
DA-78502 Congenital nystagmus 379.51
DA-78504 Latent nystagmus 379.52
DA-78510 Visual deprivation nystagmus 379.53
DA-78520 Dissociated nystagmus 379.55
DA-78524 Periodic alternating nystagmus
DA-78530 Nystagmus associated with disorders of the vestibular system 379.54
  Vestibular nystagmus 379.54
DA-78534 Deficiency of saccadic eye movements 379.57
  Abnormal optokinetic response 379.57
  Optokinetic nystagmus 379.57
DA-78536 Deficiency of smooth pursuit movements 379.58
DA-78538 Symptomatic nystagmus
DA-78540 Spontaneous ocular nystagmus
DA-78550 Horizontal nystagmus
DA-78560 Vertical nystagmus
DA-78570 Rebound nystagmus
DA-78580 Pendular nystagmus
DA-78584 Jerk nystagmus
DA-78590 End-position nystagmus

A-79 DISORDERS OF THE SCLERA AND VITREOUS BODY

A-790-791 Disorders of The Sclera

DA-79000 Disorder of sclera, NOS
DA-79100 Scleritis, NOS 379.00
DA-79102 Episcleritis, NOS 379.00
DA-79104 Episcleritis periodica fugax 379.01
DA-79106 Nodular episcleritis 379.02
DA-79108 Anterior scleritis 379.03
DA-79110 Scleromalacia perforans 379.04
DA-79112 Scleritis with corneal involvement 379.05
  Scleroperikeratitis 379.05
DA-79114 Brawny scleritis 379.06
DA-79116 Posterior scleritis 379.07
  Sclerotenonitis 379.07
DA-79118 Scleral abscess 379.09
DA-79120 Scleral staphyloma, NOS 379.11
  Scleral ectasia 379.11
DA-79122 Staphyloma posticum 379.12
DA-79124 Equatorial staphyloma 379.13
DA-79126 Localized anterior staphyloma 379.14
DA-79128 Ring staphyloma 379.15
DA-79130 Degenerative disorder of sclera, NOS 379.16

A-793 Disorders of The Vitreous Body

DA-79300 Disorder of vitreous body, NOS 379.2
DA-79310 Vitreous degeneration, NOS 379.21
DA-79312 Vitreous cavitation 379.21
DA-79314 Vitreous detachment 379.21
DA-79316 Vitreous liquifaction 379.21
DA-79320 Crystalline deposits in vitreous 379.22
DA-79322 Asteroid hyalitis 379.22
DA-79324 Synchysis scintillans 379.22
DA-79330 Vitreous hemorrhage 379.23
DA-79332 Vitreous floaters 379.24
  Muscae volitantes 379.24
  Musca volitans 379.24
DA-79334 Vitreous membranes 379.25
DA-79335 Vitreous strands 379.25
DA-79336 Vitreous prolapse 379.26

SECTION A-9 DISEASES OF THE EAR

A-90 DISEASES OF THE EAR: GENERAL TERMS

DA-90000 Disorder of ear, NOS 388.9
DA-90010 Degenerative and vascular disorder of ear, NOS 388.00
DA-90100 Otalgia, NOS 388.70
  Earache, NOS 388.70
  Pain in ear, NOS 388.70
DA-90102 Otogenic pain 388.71
DA-90104 Referred ear pain 388.72
DA-90200 Otorrhea, NOS 388.60
  Discharge of ear, NOS 388.60
DA-90210 Cerebrospinal fluid otorrhea 388.61
DA-90220 Otorrhagia 388.69

A-91 DISORDERS OF THE EXTERNAL EAR

DA-91000 Disorder of external ear, NOS 380.9
DA-91100 Disorder of pinna, NOS 380.30
DA-91102 Hematoma of pinna 380.31
  Hematoma of auricle 380.31
DA-91104 Acquired deformity of pinna 380.32
  Acquired deformity of auricle 380.32
DA-91200 Perichondritis of pinna, NOS 380.00
  Perichondritis of auricle, NOS 380.00
DA-91202 Acute perichondritis of pinna 380.01
DA-91203 Chronic perichondritis of pinna 380.02
DA-91204 Chondrodermatitis nodularis helicis 380.0
DA-91220 Infective otitis externa, NOS 380.10
DA-91222 Acute otitis externa, NOS 380.10
DA-91224 Circumscribed otitis externa 380.10
DA-91226 Diffuse otitis externa 380.10
DA-91228 Hemorrhagic otitis externa 380.10
DA-91229 Acute infection of pinna 380.11
DA-91230 Cholesteatoma of external ear 380.21
DA-91232 Keratosis obturans of external ear canal 380.21
DA-91238 Impacted cerumen 380.4
  (T-AB245)
  Excess wax in ear 380.4
  (T-AB245)
  Inspissated cerumen 380.4
  (T-AB245)
DA-91240 Acute actinic otitis externa 380.22
DA-91242 Acute chemical otitis externa 380.22
DA-91244 Acute contact otitis externa 380.22
  Acute reactive otitis externa 380.22
DA-91246 Acute eczematoid otitis externa 380.22
DA-91250 Chronic otitis externa, NOS 380.23
DA-91300 Acquired stenosis of external ear canal, NOS 380.50
DA-91302 Collapse of external ear canal 380.5
DA-91310 Acquired stenosis of external ear canal secondary to trauma 380.51
DA-91320 Acquired stenosis of external ear canal secondary to surgery 380.52
DA-91330 Acquired stenosis of external ear canal secondary to inflammation 380.53
DA-91360 Exostosis of external ear canal 380.81

A-92 DISORDERS OF THE MIDDLE EAR AND EUSTACHIAN TUBE

A-920-925 Disorders of The Middle Ear

DA-92000 Disorder of middle ear, NOS 385.9
DA-92050 Otitis media, NOS 382.9
DA-92100 Acute otitis media, NOS 382.9
DA-92101 Acute nonsuppurative otitis media, NOS 381.00
DA-92102 Acute tubotympanic catarrh 381.00
  Acute catarrhal otitis media 381.00
DA-92104 Acute exudative otitis media 381.00
DA-92106 Acute transudative otitis media 381.00
  Acute otitis media with effusion 380.00
DA-92110 Subacute nonsuppurative otitis media, NOS 381.00
DA-92112 Subacute tubotympanic catarrh 381.00
  Subacute catarrhal otitis media 381.00
DA-92114 Subacute exudative otitis media 381.00
DA-92116 Subacute transudative otitis media 381.00
  Subacute otitis media with effusion 381.00
DA-92120 Acute serous otitis media 381.01
  Acute secretory otitis media 381.01
DA-92121 Acute mucoid otitis media 381.02
  Blue drum syndrome 381.02
DA-92122 Acute seromucinous otitis media 381.02
DA-92123 Acute sanguinous otitis media 381.03
DA-92124 Acute allergic serous otitis media 381.04
DA-92125 Acute allergic mucoid otitis media 381.05
DA-92126 Acute allergic sanguinous otitis media 381.06
DA-92130 Chronic serous otitis media, NOS 381.10
  Simple chronic serous otitis media, NOS 381.10
DA-92131 Chronic tubotympanic catarrh 381.1
DA-92132 Serosanguineous chronic otitis media 381.19
DA-92140 Chronic mucoid otitis media, NOS 381.20
  Glue ear 381.2
  Simple chronic mucoid otitis media, NOS 381.20
DA-92144 Mucosanguinous chronic otitis media 381.29
DA-92150 Chronic otitis media, NOS 381.3
DA-92152 Chronic allergic otitis media 381.3
DA-92154 Chronic exudative otitis media 381.3
DA-92156 Chronic secretory otitis media 381.3
  Chronic transudative otitis media 381.3
  Chronic otitis media with effusion 381.3
DA-92158 Chronic seromucinous otitis media 381.3
DA-92170 Nonsuppurative otitis media, NOS 381.4
DA-92171 Allergic otitis media 381.4
DA-92172 Catarrhal otitis media 381.4
DA-92173 Exudative otitis media 381.4
DA-92174 Mucoid otitis media 381.4
DA-92175 Secretory otitis media 381.4
  Transudative otitis media 381.4
  Otitis media with effusion 381.4
DA-92176 Seromucinous otitis media 381.4
DA-92178 Serous otitis media 381.4
DA-92200 Acute suppurative otitis media, NOS 382.0
  Acute necrotizing otitis media 382.0
  Acute purulent otitis media 382.0
DA-92210 Acute suppurative otitis media without spontaneous rupture of ear drum 383.00
DA-92220 Acute suppurative otitis media with spontaneous rupture of ear drum 382.01
DA-92300 Purulent otitis media, NOS 382.4
DA-92310 Chronic purulent otitis media 382.3
DA-92320 Chronic tubotympanic suppurative otitis media 382.1
DA-92322 Chronic tubotympanic disease with anterior perforation of ear drum 382.1
  Benign chronic suppurative otitis media with anterior perforation of ear drum 382.1

A-920-925 Disorders of The Middle Ear — Continued

DA-92340 Chronic atticoantral suppurative otitis media 382.2
  Chronic atticoantral disease with posterior or superior marginal perforation of ear drum 382.2
  Persistent mucosal disease with posterior or superior marginal perforation of ear drum 382.2
DA-92400 Adhesive middle ear disease, NOS 385.10
  Adhesive otitis media, NOS 385.10
  Chronic adhesive otitis media 385.10
  Fibrotic adhesive otitis media 385.10
DA-92402 Adhesive middle ear disease with adhesions of drum head to incus 385.11
DA-92404 Adhesive middle ear disease with adhesions of drum head to stapes 385.12
DA-92406 Adhesive middle ear disease with adhesions of drum head to promontorium 385.13
DA-92420 Impaired mobility of malleus 385.21
DA-92422 Impaired mobility of other ear ossicles 385.22
DA-92423 Ankylosis of ear ossicles, except malleus 385.22
DA-92424 Discontinuity of ear ossicles 385.23
DA-92425 Dislocation of ear ossicles 385.23
DA-92426 Partial loss of ear ossicles 385.24
DA-92428 Partial necrosis of ear ossicles 385.24
DA-92500 Cholesteatoma of middle ear and mastoid 385.33
  Epidermosis of middle ear 385.33
DA-92502 Cholesterolosis of middle ear 385.33
DA-92504 Keratosis of middle ear 385.33
DA-92506 Polyp of middle ear 385.33
DA-92510 Cholesteatoma of attic 385.31
DA-92520 Cholesteatoma of middle ear 385.32
DA-92530 Diffuse cholesteatosis 385.35
DA-92540 Cholesterin granuloma 385.82
DA-92550 Retained foreign body of middle ear 385.83

A-928 Disorders of The Eustachian Tube

DA-92800 Eustachian tube disorder, NOS 381.9
DA-92810 Eustachian salpingitis, NOS 381.50
DA-92814 Acute eustachian salpingitis 381.51
DA-92818 Chronic eustachian salpingitis 381.52
DA-92820 Obstruction of eustachian tube, NOS 381.60
DA-92821 Stenosis of eustachian tube 381.6
  Stricture of eustachian tube 381.6
DA-92822 Osseous obstruction of eustachian tube 381.61
DA-92823 Obstruction of eustachian tube from cholesteatoma, polyp or other osseous lesion 381.62
DA-92824 Intrinsic cartilaginous obstruction of eustachian tube 381.62
DA-92825 Extrinsic cartilagenous obstruction of eustachian tube 381.63
DA-92826 Compression of eustachian tube 381.63
DA-92830 Dysfunction of eustachian tube 381.81
DA-92832 Patulous eustachian tube 381.7

A-93 DISORDERS OF THE MASTOID AND TYMPANIC MEMBRANE

A-930-934 Disorders of The Mastoid

DA-93000 Disorder of mastoid, NOS 385.9
DA-93100 Mastoiditis, NOS 383.9
DA-93200 Acute mastoiditis, NOS 383.00
  Acute mastoiditis without complications 383.00
DA-93202 Abscess of mastoid 383,00
DA-93204 Empyema of mastoid 383.00
DA-93206 Postauricular fistula 383.81
DA-93210 Subperiosteal abscess of mastoid 383.01
DA-93220 Acute mastoiditis with other complications 383.02
DA-93222 Gradenigo's syndrome 383.02
DA-93300 Chronic mastoiditis 383.1
DA-93302 Caries of mastoid 383.1
DA-93304 Fistula of mastoid 383.1
DA-93320 Petrositis, NOS 383.2
  Inflammation of petrous bone, NOS 383.2
DA-93322 Osteomyelitis of petrous bone 383.2
DA-93324 Coalescing osteitis of petrous bone 383.2
DA-93330 Acute petrositis 383.21
DA-93340 Chronic petrositis 383.22
DA-93400 Postmastoidectomy complication, NOS 383.30
DA-93402 Mucosal cyst of postmastoidectomy cavity 383.31
DA-93404 Recurrent cholesteatoma of postmastoidectomy cavity 383.32
DA-93406 Granulations of postmastoidectomy cavity 383.33
DA-93408 Chronic inflammation of postmastoidectomy cavity 383.33

A-935-936 Disorders of The Tympanic Membrane

DA-93500 Disorder of tympanic membrane, NOS 384.9
DA-93510 Acute myringitis, NOS 384.00
  Acute tympanitis, NOS 384.00
DA-93512 Bullous myringitis 384.01
  Myringitis bullosa hemorrhagica 384.01
DA-93520 Chronic tympanitis, NOS 384.1
  Chronic myringitis without mention of otitis media 384.1
DA-93530 Perforation of tympanic membrane, NOS 384.20
  Perforation of ear drum, NOS 384.20
DA-93531 Persistent posttraumatic perforation of ear drum 384.2
DA-93532 Postinflammatory perforation of ear drum 384.2

DA-93533 Central perforation of tympanic membrane 384.21

DA-93534 Attic perforation of tympanic membrane 384.22
  Pars flaccida 384.22

DA-93536 Marginal perforation of tympanic membrane, NOS 384.23

DA-93537 Multiple perforations of tympanic membrane 384.24

DA-93538 Total perforation of tympanic membrane 384.25

DA-93540 Atrophic flaccid tympanic membrane 384.81

DA-93542 Healed perforation of ear drum 384.81

DA-93550 Atrophic nonflaccid tympanic membrane 384.82

DA-93600 Tympanosclerosis, NOS 385.00

DA-93602 Tympanosclerosis involving tympanic membrane only 385.01

DA-93604 Tympanosclerosis involving tympanic membrane and ear ossicles 385.02

DA-93606 Tympanosclerosis involving tympanic membrane, ear ossicles and middle ear 385.03

DA-93608 Tympanosclerosis involving other combination of structures 385.09

A-94 VERTIGINOUS SYNDROMES AND OTHER LABYRINTHINE DISORDERS

DA-94000 Vertiginous syndrome, NOS 386.9

DA-94010 Labyrinthine disorder, NOS 386.9
  Labyrinthine vertigo 386.9

DA-94100 Ménière's disease, NOS 386.00
  Ménière's syndrome, NOS 386.00
  Ménière's vertigo, NOS 386.00
  Aural vertigo 386.00
  Auditory vertigo 386.00

DA-94101 Active Ménière's disease, NOS 386.00

DA-94102 Endolymphatic hydrops 386.0

DA-94104 Lermoyez's syndrome 386.0

DA-94110 Cochleovestibular active Ménière's disease 386.01

DA-94112 Cochlear active Ménière's disease 386.02

DA-94114 Vestibular active Ménière's disease 386.03

DA-94120 Inactive Ménière's disease 386.04
  Ménière's disease in remission 386.04

DA-94200 Peripheral vertigo, NOS 386.10
  Vestibular vertigo 386.10

DA-94210 Benign paroxysmal positional vertigo 386.11
  Benign paroxysmal positional nystagmus 386.11

DA-94220 Vestibular neuronitis 386.12
  Acute peripheral vestibulopathy 386.12

DA-94240 Vertigo of central origin 386.2
  Central positional nystagmus 386.2
  Malignant positional vertigo 386.2

DA-94300 Labyrinthitis, NOS 386.30

DA-94302 Serous labyrinthitis 386.31

DA-94304 Diffuse labyrinthitis 386.31

DA-94310 Circumscribed labyrinthitis 386.32
  Focal labyrinthitis 386.32

DA-94320 Suppurative labyrinthitis 386.33
  Purulent labyrinthitis 386.33

DA-94330 Toxic labyrinthitis 386.34

DA-94400 Labyrinthine fistula, NOS 386.40

DA-94410 Round window fistula 386.41

DA-94420 Oval window fistula 386.42

DA-94430 Semicircular canal fistula 386.43

DA-94480 Labyrinthine fistula of combined sites 386.48

DA-94500 Labyrinthine dysfunction, NOS 386.50

DA-94510 Unilateral hyperactive labyrinth 386.51

DA-94520 Bilateral hyperactive labyrinth 386.52

DA-94530 Unilateral hypoactive labyrinth 386.53

DA-94540 Bilateral hypoactive labyrinth 386.54

DA-94550 Unilateral loss of labyrinthine reactivity 386.55

DA-94560 Bilateral loss of labyrinthine reactivity 386.56

DA-94600 Otosclerosis, NOS 387.9
  Otospongiosis, NOS 387.9

DA-94610 Nonobliterative otosclerosis involving oval window 387.0

DA-94620 Obliterative otosclerosis involving oval window 387.1

DA-94630 Cochlear otosclerosis 387.2

DA-94632 Otosclerosis involving otic capsule 387.2

DA-94634 Otosclerosis involving round window 387.2

A-95 DEAFNESS AND AUDITORY PERCEPTION

A-950-955 Deafness

DA-95000 Deafness, NOS 389.9
  Hearing loss, NOS 389.9

DA-95001 Complete deafness

DA-95002 Partial deafness

DA-95007 Psychogenic deafness

DA-95008 Paradoxic hearing loss
  Paracusia willisiana

DA-95010 Presbycusis 388.01
  Senile deafness 388.01

DA-95018 Transient ischemic deafness 388.02

DA-95020 Sudden hearing loss, NOS 388.2

DA-95050 Tinnitus, NOS 388.30

DA-95052 Subjective tinnitus 388.31

DA-95054 Objective tinnitus 388.32

DA-95100 Conductive hearing loss, NOS 389.00
  Conductive deafness, NOS 389.00

DA-95102 Bone conduction deafness 389.00

DA-95104 Air conduction deafness

DA-95106 Nerve conduction deafness

DA-95110 External ear conductive hearing loss 389.01

DA-95120 Tympanic membrane conductive hearing loss 389.02

DA-95130 Middle ear conductive hearing loss 389.03

DA-95140 Inner ear conductive hearing loss 389.04

DA-95180 Conductive hearing loss of combined sites 388.08

A-950-955 Deafness — Continued

DA-95200 Sensorineural hearing loss, NOS 389.10
  Perceptive deafness, NOS 389.10
  Perceptive hearing loss, NOS 389.10
DA-95210 Sensory hearing loss 389.11
DA-95220 Neural hearing loss 389.12
DA-95222 End organ deafness
DA-95230 Central hearing loss 389.14
  Central deafness
DA-95280 Sensorineural hearing loss of combined sites 389.18
DA-95300 Mixed conductive and sensorineural hearing loss 389.2
  Mixed type deafness
DA-95400 Deaf mutism, NOS 389.7
  Nonspeaking deaf, NOS 389.7
DA-95500 Noise effects on inner ear, NOS 388.10
DA-95510 Explosive acoustic trauma to ear 388.11
  Otitic blast injury 388.11
DA-95520 Noise-induced hearing loss 388.12
DA-95580 Toxic deafness, NOS

A-956-957 Auditory Perception and Discrimination Disorders

DA-95600 Abnormal auditory perception, NOS 388.40
DA-95610 Diplacusis 388.41
  Double disharmonic hearing 388.41
DA-95612 Disharmonic diplacusis
DA-95614 Echo diplacusis
DA-95620 Hyperacusis 388.42
DA-95700 Impairment of auditory discrimination, NOS 388.43
DA-95710 Recruitment 388.44
DA-95720 Tone deafness
  Sensory amusia
DA-95721 Upper frequency deafness
DA-95722 Mid frequency deafness
DA-95723 Low frequency deafness

A-959 Disorders of The Acoustic Nerve

DA-95900 Disorder of acoustic nerve, NOS 388.5
  Disorder of eighth nerve, nOS 388.5
DA-95910 Degeneration of acoustic nerve 388.5
  Degeneration of eighth nerve 388.5
DA-95920 Acoustic neuritis 388.5

CHAPTER B — DISEASES OF THE ENDOCRINE SYSTEM

SECTION B-0 GENERAL AND POLYGLANDULAR ENDOCRINE DISORDERS

B-00 GENERAL AND GROWTH RELATED DISORDERS

DB-00000 Endocrine system disease, NOS 259.9
(T-B0000)
Endocrinopathy, NOS 259.9
(T-B0000)
Disease of endocrine glands, NOS 259.9
(T-B0000)
Disorder of endocrine glands, NEC 259.9
(T-B0000)
Endocrine disorder, NOS 259.9
(T-B0000)
Endocrine disturbance, NOS 259.9
(T-B0000)
Hormone disturbance, NOS 259.9
(T-B0000)

DB-00010 Ectopic hormone secretion, NEC 259.3
(T-B0000)

DB-00050 Carcinoid syndrome 259.2
(DF-00000) (G-C001) (M-82403)
Hormone secretion by carcinoid tumor 259.2
(DF-00000) (G-C001) (M-82403)

DB-00100 Endocrine disorder related to puberty, NOS

DB-00110 Infantilism, NOS 259.9
(T-B0000)

DB-00120 Delay in sexual development and puberty, NEC 259.0
(T-B0000) (F-96120)
Delayed puberty 259.0
(T-B0000) (F-96120)

DB-00130 Precocious sexual development and puberty, NEC 259.1
(T-B0000) (F-96400)
Sexual precocity, NOS 259.1
(T-B0000) (F-96470)
Pubertas praecox 259.1
(T-B0000) (F-96400)
Precocious true puberty 259.1
(T-B0000) (F-96400)

DB-00140 Constitutional sexual precocity 259.1
(T-B0000) (F-96470)

DB-00150 Cryptogenic sexual precocity 259.1
(T-B0000) (F-96470)
Idiopathic sexual precocity 259.1
(T-B0000) (F-96470)

DB-00160 Isosexual precocious puberty
Isosexual precocity

DB-00170 Heterosexual precocious puberty
Heterosexual precocity
Cross-sexing precocious puberty

DB-00180 Spurious sexual precocity

DB-00200 Dwarfism, NOS 259.4
(T-B0000) (M-70100)
Constitutional dwarfism 259.4
(T-B0000) (M-70100)
True dwarfism 259.4
(T-B0000) (M-70100)
Physiologic dwarfism 259.4
(T-B0000) (M-70100)
Dwarf, NOS 259.4
(T-B0000) (M-70100)

DB-00280 Dwarfism, NEC 259.4
(T-B0000) (M-70100)

DB-00300 Pineal gland dysfunction, NOS 259.8
(T-B2000) (F-25002)

DB-00350 Senile dwarfism 259.8

DB-00380 Other specified endocrine disorder, NEC 259.8
(T-B0000)

DB-00400 Gigantism, NOS
Giant, NOS

B-02 ENDOCRINE POLYGLANDULAR SYNDROMES

DB-02000 Polyglandular dysfunction and related disorders, NOS 258.9
(T-B0900) (F-25002)

DB-02100 Polyglandular activity in multiple endocrine adenomatosis 258.0
(T-B0900) (M-83601) (F-25003)
Familial polyendocrine adenomatosis 258.0
(T-B0900) (M-83601) (F-25003)
Multiple endocrine neoplasia 258.0
(T-B0900)

DB-02110 Multiple endocrine neoplasia, type 1 258.0
Wermer syndrome 258.0
(T-B0900) (M-83601) (F-25003)
MEN, type 1 258.0
Multiple endocrine adenomatosis, type 1 258.0
MEA, type 1 258.0

DB-02120 Multiple endocrine neoplasia, type 2 258.0
MEN, type 2 258.0
Sipple syndrome 258.0
Multiple endocrine adenomatosis, type 2 258.0
MEA, type 2 258.0
Familial chromaffinomatosis 258.0
PTC syndrome 258.0

DB-02130 Multiple endocrine neoplasia, type 3 258.0
MEN, type 3 258.0
Mucosal neuroma syndrome 258.0
Multiple endocrine neoplasia, type 2b 258.0

DB-02200 Other combination of endocrine dysfunction, NEC 258.1
(T-B0900) (F-25002)

B-02 ENDOCRINE POLYGLANDULAR SYNDROMES — Continued

DB-02210 Lloyd's syndrome 258.1

DB-02300 Autoimmune polyendocrinopathy, NOS 258.8
  Autoimmune polyglandular syndrome, NOS 258.8
  APS 258.8
  Polyglandular autoimmune syndrome, NOS 258.8
  PGA

DB-02310 Polyglandular autoimmune syndrome, type 1 258.8
  Polyglandular deficiency associated with mucocutaneous candidiasis 258.8
  Candidiasis-endocrinopathy syndrome 258.8
  Juvenile familial endocrinopathy 258.8
  Hypoparathyroidism, Addison's disease and moniliasis 258.8
  HAM syndrome 258.8
  Whitaker syndrome 258.8
  Autoimmune polyendocrinopathy, candidosis and ectodermal dystrophy 258.8
  APEDED 258.8
  Blizzard syndrome 258.8
  APS type 1 258.8

DB-02320 Polyglandular autoimmune syndrome, type 2 258.8
  APS type 2 258.8
  Addison's disease, toxic diffuse goiter and insulin-dependent diabetes mellitus 258.8

DB-02321 Schmidt's syndrome 258.1
  (T-B3100) (T-B6000) (F-25004)
  Primary hypothyroidism and adrenocortical insufficiency 258.1
  (T-B3100) (T-B6000) (F-25004)
  Addison's disease with struma lymphomatosa 258.1

DB-02324 Carpenter syndrome 258.1
  Addison's disease, struma lymphomatosa and insulin-dependent diabetes mellitus 258.1

DB-02390 Multiple endocrine deficiency syndrome, NEC 258.1
  (T-B3100) (T-B6000) (F-25004)

DB-02400 Other specified polyglandular dysfunction, NEC 258.8
  (T-B0900) (F-25002)

SECTION B-1 DISEASES OF THE PITUITARY GLAND

B-10 GENERAL PITUITARY DISORDERS

DB-10000 Disease of pituitary gland, NOS 253.9
  (T-B1000)
  Disorder of pituitary gland, NOS 253.9
  (T-B1000)
  Dyspituitarism, NOS 253.9
  (T-B1000)

DB-10100 Abscess of pituitary 253.8
  (T-B1100) (M-41740)

DB-10800 Other disorder of the pituitary gland, NEC 253.8
  (T-91100)

B-11-12 DISEASES OF THE ANTERIOR PITUITARY GLAND

DB-11000 Disease of anterior pituitary, NOS 253.9
  (T-B1100)
  Disorder of anterior pituitary, NOS 253.9
  (T-B1100)

DB-11100 Hyperpituitarism, NOS 253.1
  (T-B1100)
  Pituitary hyperfunction, NOS 253.1
  (T-B1100)

DB-11200 Overproduction of growth hormone, NOS 253.0
  (T-B1000) (F-25413)
  Hypersomatotropism 253.1
  (T-B1000)

DB-11220 Acromegaly 253.0
  (T-B1000)
  Growth hormone hypersecretion syndrome 253.0
  (T-B1000) (F-25413)
  Acromegalia 253.0
  (T-B1000)
  Anterior pituitary adenoma syndrome 253.0
  (T-B1000)
  Marie disease 253.0
  (T-B1000)
  STH hypersecretion syndrome 253.0
  (T-B1000)

DB-11222 Acromegaly with arthropathy 253.0 —713.0*
  (T-B1100) (T-12000) (M-01000) (F-25413)

DB-11230 Hypersomatotropic gigantism 253.0
  (T-B1100)
  Pituitary gigantism 253.0
  (T-B1100) (M-70420) (F-25413)
  Acromegalic gigantism 253.0
  (T-B1100) (M-70420) (F-25413)
  Launois syndrome 253.0
  (T-B1100)

DB-11240 Gigantism due to somatostatin deficiency 253.0

DB-11300 Thyrotropin overproduction 253.1
  Thyrotropin hypersecretion 253.1

DB-11400 Idiopathic hyperprolactinemia 253.1
  (T-B1100) (F-25453)

DB-11410 Transient hyperprolactinemia 253.1

DB-11420 Secondary hyperprolactinemia, NOS 253.1
DB-11422 Secondary hyperprolactinemia due to prolactin-secreting tumors 253.1
(T-B1100) (M-81400) (F-25453)
Forbes-Albright syndrome 253.1
(T-B1100) (M-81400) (F-25453)
DB-12000 Hypopituitarism, NOS 253.2
(T-B1100) (F-25404)
Pituitary insufficiency, NOS 253.2
(T-B1100) (F-25404)
Deficient secretion of one or more pituitary hormones 253.2
(T-B1100)
DB-12010 Panhypopituitarism, NOS 253.2
(T-B1100) (F-25404)
Primary hypopituitarism 253.2
(T-B1100) (F-25404)
Simmonds disease 253.2
(T-B1100) (F-25404)
Deficient secretion of all pituitary hormones 253.2
(T-B1100) (F-25404)
DB-12030 Pituitary cachexia 253.2
(T-B1100) (F-25404)
DB-12100 Secondary hypopituitarism 253.2
DB-12110 Necrosis of pituitary, NOS 253.2
(T-B1100) (M-54200)
DB-12120 Ischemic postpartum pituitary necrosis 253.2
(T-B1100) (M-54200) (F-31170)
Sheehan syndrome 253.2
(T-B1100) (M-54200) (F-31170)
Postpartum pituitary infarction 253.2
(T-B1100) (M-37000)
Postpartum intrapituitary hemorrhage 253.2
(T-B1100) (M-37000)
Postpartum pituitary necrosis 253.2
(T-B1100)
Reye-Sheehan syndrome 253.2
(T-B1100)
DB-12200 Hypopituitarism due to pituitary tumor 253.2
DB-12300 Lymphocytic hypopituitarism 253.2
Lymphocytic hypophysitis 253.2
DB-12500 Somatotropin deficiency, NOS 253.3
Growth hormone deficiency, NOS 253.3
GHD 253.3
STH deficiency 253.3
DB-12510 Transient somatotropin deficiency 253.3
DB-12520 Isolated somatotropin deficiency 253.3
Isolated growth hormone deficiency 253.3
DB-12530 Pituitary dwarfism 253.3
(T-B1100) (M-70120)
Isolated deficiency of growth hormone in children 253.3
(T-B1100)
Hyposomatotropic dwarfism 253.3
(T-B1100)
Pituitary nanism 253.3
(T-B1100)
Prepuberal dwarfism 253.3
(T-B1100)
Prepubertal dwarfism 253.3
(T-B1100)
Hypopituitary dwarfism 253.3
(T-B1100)
DB-12540 Ateleiotic dwarfism 253.3
Ateliotic dwarfism 253.3
Sexual ateleiotic dwarfism 253.3
Sexual ateliotic dwarfism 253.3
Sexual dwarfism 253.3
Idiopathic pituitary dwarfism 253.3
Hypopituitary dwarfism with normal sexual characteristics 253.3
DB-12550 Autosomal recessive isolated somatotropin deficiency 253.3
Isolated growth hormone deficiency type I 253.3
Pituitary dwarfism type I 253.3
DB-12560 Nonfamilial hyperinsulinemic isolated somatotropin deficiency 253.3
Ateliotic dwarfism with hyperinsulinemia 253.3
DB-12570 Autosomal dominant isolated somatotropin deficiency 253.3
Ateliotic dwarfism without insulinopenia 253.3
DB-12580 Laron-type isolated somatotropin defect 253.3
Laron-type dwarfism 253.3
Laron dwarfism 253.3
Laron-type pituitary dwarfism 253.3
DB-12590 Pituitary dwarfism with normal somatotropin level and low somatomedin 253.3
DB-12600 Asexual dwarfism 253.3
Lorain-Levi dwarfism 253.3
Hypopituitary dwarfism with failure of development of sexual characteristics 253.3
Brissaud dwarfism 253.3
Brissaud-Meige syndrome 253.3
Burnier syndrome 253.3
Frohlich dwarfism 253.3
Hypophyseal infantilism 253.3
Nebecourt syndrome 253.3
DB-12610 Nonfamilial asexual dwarfism 253.3
DB-12620 Autosomal recessive asexual dwarfism 253.3
DB-12630 X-linked asexual dwarfism 253.3
DB-12640 Pituitary dwarfism with small sella turcica 253.2
Primary empty sella syndrome 253.2
Abnormal sella turcica syndrome 253.2
Familial absence of sella turcica 253.2
Familial panhypopituitarism with abnormal sella turcica 253.2
Ferrier-Stone syndrome 253.2

B-11-12 DISEASES OF THE ANTERIOR PITUITARY GLAND — Continued

DB-12650 Pituitary dwarfism with large sella turcica 253.2
  Familial enlargement of the sella turcica 253.2
DB-12660 Immunoglobulinemia with isolated somatotropin deficiency 253.3
  Growth hormone deficiency with hypogammaglobulinemia 253.3
  Fleischer syndrome 253.3
DB-12700 Isolated gonadotropin deficiency, NOS 253.4
DB-12710 Hypogonadotropic hypogonadism 257.2
  Anosmia eunuchoidism 257.2
  Dysplasia olfactogenitalis of de Morsier 257.2
  Kallman syndrome 257.2
  Olfactogenital dysplasia 257.2
DB-12720 Isolated follitropin deficiency 253.4
DB-12730 Isolated lutropin deficiency 253.4
  Fertile eunuch 253.4
  Fertile eunuch syndrome 253.4
DB-12810 Isolated corticotropin deficiency 253.4
  Isolated ACTH deficiency 253.4
  Specific corticotropin deficiency 253.4
DB-12820 Isolated thyrotropin deficiency 253.4
  Isolated thyrotropic hormone deficiency 253.4
DB-12830 Isolated thyroliberin deficiency 253.4
  Isolated TRH deficiency 253.4
  Isolated thyroid hormone releasing hormone deficiency 253.4
DB-12840 Isolated prolactin deficiency 253.4
DB-12880 Isolated deficiency of hormone other than HGH 253.4
  Isolated deficiency of hormone other than somatotropin 253.4
DB-12990 Other anterior pituitary disorder, NEC 253.4

B-13 DISEASES OF THE POSTERIOR PITUITARY GLAND

DB-13000 Disorder of posterior pituitary, NOS 253.9
  Disorder of neurohypophysis, NOS 253.9
DB-13100 Neurohypophyseal diabetes insipidus, NOS 253.5
  Vasopressin deficiency syndrome 253.5
  Pituitary diabetes insipidus 253.5
  Neurogenic diabetes insipidus 253.5
  Cranial diabetes insipidus 253.5
  Primary central diabetes insipidus 253.5
  Diabetes insipidus, NOS 253.5
DB-13120 Idiopathic diabetes insipidus 253.5
DB-13130 Familial diabetes insipidus 253.5
DB-13140 Secondary diabetes insipidus 253.5
DB-13200 Syndrome of inappropriate vasopressin secretion 253.6
  Syndrome of inappropriate ADH production 253.6
  SIADH 253.6
  Schwarz-Bartter syndrome 253.6
DB-13210 Ectopic antidiuretic hormone secretion 259.3
  Ectopic ADH secretion
DB-13700 Adiposogenital dystrophy 253.8
  (T-B1000) (T-70200) (M-21300)
  Frohlich's syndrome 253.8
  (T-B1000) (T-70200)
DB-13740 Other syndrome of diencephalo-hypophyseal origin 253.8
  (T-B1200)
DB-13800 Other disorder of the neurohypophysis, NEC 253.6

B-14 IATROGENIC DISORDERS OF THE PITUITARY GLAND

DB-14000 Iatrogenic pituitary disorder, NOS 253.7
DB-14010 Hormone-induced hypopituitarism 253.7
  (T-91100)
DB-14020 Hypophysectomy-induced hypopituitarism 253.7
  (T-91100) (P.-.....)
DB-14030 Radiotherapy-induced hypopituitarism 253.7
  (T-91100) (P.-.....)

SECTION B-2 DISORDERS OF THE ENDOCRINE OVARIES

DB-20000 Disorder of endocrine ovary, NOS 256.9
  (T-87000) (F-25002)
  Ovarian dysfunction, NOS 256.9
  (T-87000) (F-25002)
DB-20100 Hyperestrogenism 256.0
  (T-87000) (F-26483)
DB-20200 Hypersecretion of ovarian androgens 256.1
  (T-87000) (F-26563)
DB-20300 Other ovarian hyperfunction, NEC 256.1
  (T-87000) (F-25003)
DB-20500 Iatrogenic ovarian failure, NOS 256.2
  (T-87000) (F-25004)
DB-20510 Postsurgical ovarian failure 256.2
  (T-87000)
  Postablative ovarian failure 256.2
  (T-87000)
DB-20520 Postirradiation ovarian failure 256.2
  (T-87000) (P.-.....) (F-25004)
DB-20600 Primary ovarian failure 256.3
  (T-87000) (F-25004)
DB-20800 Other ovarian failure, NEC 256.3
  (T-87000) (F-25004)
DB-21500 Polycystic ovaries 256.4
  (T-87800) (M-33830)
  Stein-Leventhal syndrome 256.4
  (T-87800) (M-33830)
  Polycystic ovarian disease
DB-21600 Isosexual virilization 256.4
DB-21700 Female hirsutism, NOS
DB-21710 Androgen-independent hirsutism
DB-21720 Androgen-dependent hirsutism

DB-21800 Other endocrine disorder of ovarian dysfunction, NEC 256.8
(T-87000)
DB-22100 Female puberty disorder, NOS
DB-22110 Precocious female puberty
DB-22120 Female pseudopuberty
DB-22130 Delayed female puberty

SECTION B-3 DISORDERS OF THE ENDOCRINE TESTES

DB-30000 Disorder of endocrine testis, NOS 257.9
(T-78000) (F-25002)
Testicular dysfunction, NOS 257.9
(T-78000) (F-25002)
Disorder of testicular function, NOS 257.9
DB-30010 Disorder of sexual differentiation, NOS
DB-30020 Disorder of testicular differentiation and development, NOS
DB-30100 Testicular hyperfunction, NOS 257.0
(T-78000) (F-25003)
Hypersecretion of testicular hormones, NOS 257.0
(T-78000) (F-25003)
DB-30600 Testicular hypogonadism, NOS 257.2
(T-78000)
DB-30610 Primary hypogonadism
Primary failure of the testes
DB-30620 Secondary hypogonadism, NOS
DB-30650 Iatrogenic testicular hypofunction 257.1
(T-78000) (F-25004)
DB-30660 Postsurgical testicular hypofunction 257.1
(T-78000) (P.-.....) (F-25004)
Postablative testicular hypofunction 257.1
(T-78000) (P.-.....) (F-25004)
DB-30670 Postirradiation testicular hypofunction 257.1
(T-78000) (P.-.....) (F-25004)
DB-30690 Other testicular hypofunction, NEC 257.2
(T-78000)
DB-30700 Deficiency of testosterone biosynthesis, NOS 257.2
Defective biosynthesis of testicular androgen, NOS 257.2
(T-78000) (F-26562)
Androgen deficiency, NOS 257.2
DB-30720 Leydig cell failure in adult 257.2
DB-30730 Seminiferous tubule failure in adult 257.2
DB-30750 Mullerian inhibiting factor deficiency
Mullerian regression factor deficiency
DB-30800 Eunuchoidism, NOS 257.2
DB-30810 Eunuchoid gigantism 257.2
DB-30980 Other specified disorder of testicular dysfunction, NEC 257.8
(T-78000)
Other testicular dysfunction, NEC 257.8

SECTION B-6 DISEASES OF THE ENDOCRINE PANCREAS INCLUDING DIABETES

DB-60000 Disease of endocrine pancreas, NOS 251.9
Disorder of endocrine pancreas, NOS 251.9
Disorder of pancreatic islets, NOS 251.9
Disorder of islets of Langerhans, NOS 251.9
DB-60020 Islet cell hyperplasia, NOS 251.9
DB-61000 Diabetes mellitus, NOS 250.0
DB-61002 Diabetes mellitus without complication 250.0
DB-61010 Insulin dependent diabetes mellitus 250.01
Diabetes mellitus type I 250.01
IDDM 250.01
DB-61020 Insulin dependent diabetes mellitus type IA 250.01
DB-61025 Insulin dependent diabetes mellitus type IB 250.01
Primary autoimmune diabetes mellitus 250.01
DB-61030 Diabetes mellitus type II 250.00
Non-insulin dependent diabetes mellitus 250.00
NCDMM 250.00
DB-61032 NIDDM in obese 250.00
DB-61034 NIDDM in nonobese 250.00
DB-61040 Maturity onset diabetes mellitus in young
MODY
Autosomal dominant diabetes mellitus
NIDDY
DB-61050 Secondary diabetes mellitus, NOS 250.-
DB-61060 Malnutrition related diabetes mellitus
MRDM
DB-61070 Fibrocalculous pancreatic diabetes
DB-61080 Protein-deficient diabetes mellitus
DB-61100 Diabetes mellitus associated with pancreatic disease
DB-61102 Diabetes mellitus associated with hormonal etiology
DB-61110 Drug-induced diabetes mellitus
DB-61120 Diabetes mellitus associated with genetic syndrome
DB-61130 Diabetes mellitus associated with receptor abnormality
DB-61140 Diabetes mellitus associated with unlisted condition
Rare form of diabetes mellitus, NOS
DB-61200 Impaired glucose tolerance, NOS
Chemical diabetes
Latent diabetes
Prediabetic nonclinical diabetes
DB-61219 Impaired glucose tolerance in obese
DB-61220 Impaired glucose tolerance in nonobese
DB-61230 Impaired glucose tolerance in MODY
DB-61240 Impaired glucose tolerance associated with pancreatic disease
DB-61242 Impaired glucose tolerance associated with hormonal etiology

SECTION B-6 DISEASES OF THE ENDOCRINE PANCREAS INCLUDING DIABETES — Continued

DB-61250 Impaired glucose tolerance associated with drugs
DB-61260 Impaired glucose tolerance associated with genetic syndrome
DB-61270 Impaired glucose tolerance associated with insulin receptor abnormality
DB-61280 Impaired glucose tolerance associated with unlisted conditions
DB-61290 Previous abnormality of glucose tolerance
  Previous AGT
DB-61292 Potential abnormality of glucose tolerance
  Potential AGT
DB-61400 Gestational diabetes mellitus, NOS
  GDM
DB-61410 Gestational diabetes mellitus, class A_1
  GDM, class A_1
DB-61414 Gestational diabetes mellitus, class A_2
  GDM, class A_2
DB-61420 Gestational diabetes mellitus, class B_1
  GDM, class B_1
DB-61460 Pregestational diabetes mellitus or impaired glucose tolerance, modified White class A
DB-61462 Pregestational diabetes mellitus or impaired glucose tolerance, modified White class B
DB-61463 Pregestational diabetes mellitus or impaired glucose tolerance, modified White class C
DB-61464 Pregestational diabetes mellitus or impaired glucose tolerance, modified White class D
DB-61465 Pregestational diabetes mellitus or impaired glucose tolerance, modified White class F
DB-61466 Pregestational diabetes mellitus or impaired glucose tolerance, modified White class R
DB-61467 Pregestational diabetes mellitus or impaired glucose tolerance, modified White class FR
DB-61500 Diabetic complication, NOS 250.9
DB-61510 Diabetic oculopathy, NOS
  Ophthalmic manifestations of diabetes
DB-61520 Diabetic neuropathy
  Diabetic neuropathy with neurologic complication
DB-61522 Symmetric diabetic proximal motor neuropathy
DB-61524 Asymmetric diabetic proximal motor neuropathy
DB-61530 Diabetic radiculopathy
DB-61532 Abdominal polyradiculopathy
DB-61538 Polyradiculopathy
DB-61540 Diabetic mononeuropathy simplex
DB-61542 Diabetic mononeuropathy multiplex
DB-61550 Diabetic polyneuropathy, NOS
DB-61552 Sensory polyneuropathy
DB-61554 Mixed sensory-motor polyneuropathy
DB-61556 Motor polyneuropathy
DB-61560 Diabetic amyotrophy
DB-61570 Diabetic autonomic neuropathy
DB-61600 Insulinopathy, NOS
  Diabetes mellitus due to abnormal insulin
DB-61610 Insulin biosynthesis defect, NOS
DB-61620 Insulin receptor defect, NOS
DB-61630 Insulin-resistant diabetes mellitus and acanthosis nigricans
DB-61632 Extreme insulin resistance with acanthosis nigricans, hirsutism and abnormal insulin receptors
  Extreme insulin resistance type A
DB-61634 Extreme insulin resistance with acanthosis nigricans, hirsutism and autoantibodies to the insulin receptors
  Extreme insulin resistance type B
DB-61700 Lipodystrophy, NOS 272.6
  Lipodystrophic diabetes, NOS 272.6
  Lipoatrophic diabetes, NOS 272.6
DB-61710 Familial generalized lipodystrophy 272.6
  Congenital lipodystrophic diabetes 272.6
  Familial lipodystrophic diabetes 272.6
  Berardinelli-Seip syndrome 272.6
  Congenital lipodystrophy 272.6
  Congenital lipoatrophic diabetes 272.6
  Lawrence-Seip syndrome 272.6
  Lipodystrophy of Berardinelli 272.6
  Total lipodystrophy and acromegaloid gigantism 272.6
DB-61720 Acquired generalized lipodystrophy 272.6
  Acquired lipodystrophic diabetes 272.6
  Lawrence syndrome 272.6
DB-61730 Familial lipodystrophy of limbs and trunk 272.6
  Kobberling-Dunnigan syndrome 272.6
DB-61740 Acquired partial lipodystrophy 272.6
  Lipodystrophic diabetes with partial lipoatrophy 272.6
  Barraquer syndrome 272.6
  Barraquer-Simons syndrome 272.6
  Hollander-Simons syndrome 272.6
  Progressive lipodystrophy 272.6
  Progressive partial lipodystrophy 272.6
DB-61780 Pineal hyperplasia and diabetes mellitus syndrome 272.6
  Mendenhall syndrome 272.6
  Rabson-Mendenhall syndrome 272.6
DB-61790 Diabetes mellitus and insipidus with optic atrophy and deafness 272.6
  DIDMOAD syndrome 272.6
  Marquardt-Loriaux syndrome 272.6
DB-61800 Hyperglycemia, NOS 790.6
DB-62010 Diabetes with ketoacidosis 250.1
  Diabetic acidosis without coma 250.1
  Diabetic ketosis without coma 250.1
DB-62020 Diabetes with hyperosmolar coma 250.2
  Hyperosmolar nonketotic coma in diabetes 250.2
DB-62030 Diabetic coma with ketoacidosis 250.3
DB-62040 Diabetes with other coma 250.3
DB-62100 Diabetes with renal manifestations 250.4 —583.8*

DB-62110 Intracapillary glomerulosclerosis 250.4 —583.81*
Diabetic nephropathy 250.4 —583.81*
Kimmelstiel-Wilson syndrome 250.4 —583.81*
Diabetic glomerulopathy 250.4 —583.81*
DB-62112 Nodular type diabetic glomerulosclerosis 250.4
DB-62114 Diffuse type diabetic glomerulosclerosis 250.4
DB-62120 Diabetes-nephrosis syndrome 250.4 —581.81*
DB-62140 Diabetes with peripheral circulatory disorders 250.7
Diabetic peripheral angiopathy 250.7 —443.8*
DB-62150 Diabetic gangrene 250.7 —785.4*
DB-62200 Diabetes mellitus due to insulin receptor antibodies 250.-
DB-63120 Hypoglycemic coma 251.0
DB-63122 Insulin coma 251.0
DB-63124 Iatrogenic hyperinsulinism 251.0
DB-63128 Factitious hypoglycemia 251.0
DB-63130 Hyperinsulinism, NOS 251.1
DB-63132 Ectopic hyperinsulinism 251.1
DB-63134 Functional hyperinsulinism 251.1
DB-63140 Hyperplasia of pancreatic islet beta cell, NOS 251.1
DB-63200 Hypoglycemia, NOS 251.2
Hypoglycemic syndrome, NOS 251.2
DB-63210 Autoimmune hypoglycemia, NOS
DB-63220 Fasting hypoglycemia 251.2
DB-63230 Idiopathic postprandial hypoglycemia 251.2
DB-63240 Reactive hypoglycemia 251.2
DB-63250 Spontaneous hypoglycemia 251.2
DB-63264 Hypoglycemia of childhood 775.6
Hypoglycemia of infancy 775.6
DB-63270 Ketotic hypoglycemia
DB-63274 Leucine-induced hypoglycemia
DB-63280 Mixed hypoglycemia
DB-63290 Postsurgical hypoinsulinemia 251.3
DB-63292 Postpancreatectomy hyperglycemia 251.3
DB-63300 Abnormality of secretion of glucagon, NOS 251.4
DB-63310 Hyperplasia of islet alpha cells with glucagon excess 251.4
DB-63320 Glucagon deficiency 251.4
DB-63330 Glucagon resistance 251.4
DB-63340 Glucagonoma syndrome, NOS 251.4
DB-63400 Abnormality of secretion of gastrin 251.5
DB-63410 Zollinger-Ellison syndrome 251.5
(T-57000) (M-38090) (F-52402) (G-C002) (M-81531)
DB-63420 Hyperplasia of islet alpha cells with gastrin excess 251.5
DB-63480 Other disorder of pancreatic internal secretion, NEC 251.8

SECTION B-7 DISEASES OF THE ADRENAL GLANDS

DB-70000 Disease of adrenal gland, NOS 255.9
Disorder of adrenal gland, NOS 255.9
DB-70100 Hypercortisolism
Cushing's syndrome III 255.0
Overproduction of cortisol 255.0
Hypercorticism
Itsenko-Cushing syndrome
Itsenko disease
Suprarenogenic syndrome
DB-70110 Hypercortisolism due to adrenal neoplasm
DB-70120 Pituitary dependent hypercortisolism 255.0
Pituitary dependent Cushing disease 255.0
Overproduction of ACTH 255.3
Cushing disease 255.0
Cushing basophilism 255.0
Pituitary Cushing syndrome 255.0
Pituitary hyperadrenal corticism 255.0
DB-70130 Hypercortisolism due to pituitary adenoma 255.0
DB-70140 Nelson syndrome 253.7
DB-70150 Hypercortisolism due to nonpituitary tumor
Ectopic ACTH syndrome 155.0
DB-70180 Iatrogenic Cushing's disease 255.0
Iatrogenic syndrome of excess cortisol 255.0
DB-70300 Aldosteronism, NOS
Hyperaldosteronism, NOS 255.1
DB-70310 Primary aldosteronism 255.1
Conn syndrome 255.1
Idiopathic aldosteronism 255.1
Aldosteronism due to neoplasm of the adrenal cortex 255.1
DB-70316 Pseudoprimary aldosteronism 255.1
Aldosteronism with hyperplasia of the adrenal cortex 255.1
Liddle's syndrome 255.1
Bartter's syndrome 255.1
Juxtaglomerular hyperplasia with secondary aldosteronism 255.1
DB-70317 Aldosteronism with nodular hyperplasia of adrenal cortex 255.1
DB-70320 Glucocorticoid-responsive primary aldosteronism 255.1
DB-70330 Secondary aldosteronism, NOS 255.1
DB-70380 Aldosterone deficiency, NOS
DB-70510 Feminizing syndrome of adrenal origin, NOS
DB-70520 Virilizing syndrome of adrenal origin, NOS
DB-70540 Achard-Thiers syndrome 255.2
Diabetic-bearded woman syndrome 255.2
DB-70550 Acquired benign adrenal androgenic overactivity 255.3
DB-70580 Other disorder of corticoadrenal overactivity, NEC 255.3
DB-70600 Adrenal cortical hypofunction, NOS 255.4
Corticoadrenal insufficiency, NOS 255.4
Adrenal insufficiency, NOS 255.4

SECTION B-7 DISEASES OF THE ADRENAL GLANDS — Continued

DB-70600 (cont.) Adrenocortical hypofunction, NOS 255.4
DB-70610 Severe adrenal insufficiency 255.4
    Addisonian crisis 255.4
    Adrenal crisis 255.4
DB-70620 Addison's disease, NOS 255.4
    Addison melanoderma 255.4
    Asthenia pigmentosa 255.4
    Bronzed disease 255.4
    Melasma addisonii 255.4
    Primary adrenal deficiency 255.4
DB-70622 Addison's disease due to tuberculosis 255.4 —017.6*
DB-70624 Addison's disease due to autoimmunity 255.4
    Autoimmune adrenal atrophy 255.4
    Autoimmune adrenalitis
DB-70630 Secondary hypocortisolism
    Adrenal supression
    Secondary adrenocortical insufficiency
DB-70640 Familial adrenocortical hypoplasia
    Familial Addison disease
    Familial cytomegalic adrenocortical hypoplasia
DB-70650 Congenital primary adrenocortical hypofunction
    Congenital Addison disease
DB-70660 Adrenoleukodystrophy
    Adrenomyeloneuropathy
    ALD
    Bronze Schilder disease
    Schilder-Addison complex
    Siemerling-Creutzfeld disease
DB-70670 Hereditary adrenal unresponsiveness to corticotropin
DB-70680 Glucocorticoid deficiency with achalasia
    Achalasia-addisonian syndrome
    Allgrove syndrome
    Triple A syndrome
    Alacrimia-achalasia-addisonianism
DB-70800 Other adrenal hypofunction, NEC 255.5
DB-70810 Adrenal medullary insufficiency 255.5
DB-70820 Hyperadrenergic postural hypotension
DB-70822 Hypoadrenergic postural hypotension
DB-70830 Epinephrine deficiency
DB-70840 Medulloadrenal hyperfunction 255.6
DB-70842 Catecholamine secretion by pheochromocytoma 255.6
DB-70850 Abnormality of cortisol-binding globulin 255.8
DB-70910 Idiopathic edema
DB-70920 Adrenal calcification 255.4
DB-70930 Adrenal hemorrhage 255.4
DB-70940 Adrenal infarction 255.4
DB-70980 Hypothalamic-adrenal dysfunction, NOS
DB-70990 Other specified adrenal disorder, NEC 255.8

SECTION B-8 DISEASES OF THE THYROID GLAND

B-80 HYPOTHYROIDISM, HYPERTHYROIDISM AND OTHER DISORDERS

DB-80000 Disease of thyroid gland, NOS 246.9
    Disorder of thyroid gland, NOS 246.9
DB-80100 Goiter, NOS 240.0
    Enlargement of thyroid 240.9
    Struma of thyroid 240.9
    Thyromegaly 240.9
DB-80110 Endemic goiter 240.9
    Simple goiter 240.0
DB-80120 Sporadic goiter 240.9
DB-80130 Substernal goiter 240.9
    Intrathoracic goiter 240.9
DB-80136 Lingual goiter 240.9
DB-80140 Colloid goiter 240.9
DB-80150 Adenomatous goiter, NOS 241.9
    Hyperplastic goiter, NOS 241.9
    Non-toxic goiter 241.9
    Non-toxic nodular goiter, NOS 241.9
DB-80160 Non-toxic uninodular goiter 241.0
    Thyroid nodule 241.0
DB-80170 Non-toxic multinodular goiter 241.1
    Multinodular non-toxic goiter 241.1
DB-80200 Hyperthyroidism, NOS 242.9
DB-80204 Thyrotoxicosis, NOS 242.9
DB-80206 Thyrotoxicosis without goiter or other cause 242.9
DB-80210 Thyrotoxic crisis 242.9
    Thyroid storm 242.9
DB-80220 Toxic diffuse goiter 242.0
    Graves' disease 242.0
    Basedow's disease 242.0
    Toxic primary thyroid hyperplasia 242.0
    Diffuse toxic goiter 242.0
DB-80230 Toxic diffuse goiter with exophthalmos 242.0
    Graves' disease with exophthalmos 242.0
DB-80240 Toxic diffuse goiter with exophthalmos and with thyrotoxic storm 242.01
    Graves' disease with exophthalmos and with thyrotoxic crisis 242.01
DB-80250 Toxic diffuse goiter with thyrotoxic crisis 242.01
    Toxic diffuse goiter with thyrotoxic storm 242.01
    Graves' disease with thyrotoxic crisis 242.01
    Graves' disease with thyrotoxic storm 242.01
DB-80260 Neonatal Graves' disease
DB-80270 Toxic uninodular goiter 242.1
    Toxic thyroid nodule 242.1
DB-80280 Toxic uninodular goiter with thyrotoxic crisis 242.11
    Toxic uninodular goiter with thyrotoxic storm 242.11

DB-80290 Toxic multinodular goiter 242.2
  Secondary thyroid hyperplasia 242.2
DB-802A0 Toxic multinodular goiter with thyrotoxic crisis 242.21
  Toxic multinodular goiter with thyrotoxic storm 242.21
DB-80300 Toxic nodular goiter, NOS 242.3
  Toxic adenomatous goiter 242.3
  Toxic struma nodosa 242.3
  Plummer's disease 242.3
DB-80310 Toxic nodular goiter with thyrotoxic storm 242.31
  Toxic nodular goiter with thyrotoxic crisis 242.31
DB-80320 Thyrotoxicosis factitia 242.8
  Factitious hyperthyroidism 242.8
  Factitious hyperthyroidism from ingestion of excessive thyroid material 242.8
DB-80322 Thyrotoxicosis factitia with thyrotoxic crisis 242.81
  Thyrotoxicosis factitia with thyrotoxic storm 242.81
DB-80324 Hyperthyroidism due to molar thyrotropin 242.8
  Hyperthyroidism due to hydatidiform mole 242.8
DB-80326 Hyperthyroidism due to hydatidiform mole with thyrotoxic crisis 242.81
  Hyperthyroidism due to hydatidiform mole with thyrotoxic storm 242.81
DB-80327 Hyperthyroidism due to struma ovarii
DB-80328 Hyperthyroidism due to ectopic thyroid nodule 242.4
DB-80340 Iodine-induced hyperthyroidism, NOS
  Iodide-induced hyperthyroidism, NOS
  Jod-Basedow phenomenon
DB-80341 Hyperthyroidism secondary to radio contrast dyes
DB-80342 Hyperthyroidism secondary to potassium iodide
DB-80343 Hyperthyroidism secondary to amiodarone
DB-80350 Hyperthyroidism with Hashimoto disease
  Hashitoxicosis
DB-80360 Toxic diffuse goiter with pretibial myxedema
  Graves' disease with pretibial myxedema
DB-80370 Graves' disease with pretibial myxedema and with thyrotoxic crisis
  Graves' disease with pretibial myxedema and with thyrotoxic storm
DB-80380 Toxic diffuse goiter with acropachy
  Graves' disease with acropachy
DB-80390 Graves' disease with acropachy and with thyrotoxic crisis
  Graves' disease with acropachy and with thyrotoxic storm
DB-80400 Hypothyroidism, NOS
DB-80410 Acquired hypothyroidism, NOS 244.9
DB-80420 Primary hypothyroidism 244.9
DB-80430 Myxedema, NOS
DB-80432 Adult myxedema
DB-80434 Juvenile myxedema
DB-80435 Hypothyroidism due to fibrous invasive thyroiditis
  Hypothyroidism due to Reidel's thyroiditis
DB-80440 Secondary hypothyroidism
DB-80442 Subclinical hypothyroidism
DB-80444 Severe hypothyroidism
DB-80446 Myxedema coma
DB-80460 Hypothyroidism following radioiodine therapy 244.1
DB-80462 Hypothyroidism following external radiotherapy 244.1
DB-80464 Post-operative hypothyroidism 244.0
  Post-surgical hypothyroidism 244.0
DB-80465 Transient hypothyroidism
DB-80470 Hypothyroidism due to infiltrative disease, NOS
DB-80471 Hypothyroidism due to cystinosis
DB-80472 Hypothyroidism due to amyloidosis
DB-80473 Hypothyroidism due to sarcoidosis
DB-80474 Hypothyroidism due to scleroderma
DB-80480 Central hypothyroidism, NOS
DB-80482 Pituitary hypothyroidism
  Hypothyrotropic hypothyroidism
DB-80484 Hypothalamic hypothyroidism
  Hypothyroidism due to TRH deficiency
DB-80553 Iatrogenic hypothyroidism 244.3
DB-80554 Hypothyroidism due to iodide excess 244.2
DB-80555 Hypothyroidism due to drugs, NOS 244.3
DB-80556 Hypothyroidism due to food stuffs 244.2
DB-80566 Intrathyroidal calcification and goiter syndrome
DB-80568 Dyshormonogenetic goiter and iodide leak
DB-80570 Transient decreased production of thyroid hormone, NOS
  Decrease thyroid hormone production associated with illness, NOS
DB-80572 Transient decreased production of T_3
DB-80574 Transient decreased production of T_4
DB-80600 Thyroiditis, NOS 245.9
DB-80602 Infectious thyroiditis, NOS
DB-80604 Viral thyroiditis
DB-80610 Acute suppurative thyroiditis 245.0
  Abscess of thyroid 245.0
  Pyogenic thyroiditis 245.0
DB-80620 Subacute thyroiditis
  de Quervain's thyroiditis
  Giant cell thyroiditis
  Granulomatous thyroiditis
  Pseudogranulomatous thyroiditis
DB-80630 Autoimmune thyroiditis, NOS
  Chronic thyroiditis, NOS 245.8
DB-80632 Hashimoto thyroiditis
  Lymphocytic thyroiditis
  Struma lymphomatosa
  Autoimmune lymphocytic chronic thyroiditis

B-80 HYPOTHYROIDISM, HYPERTHYROIDISM AND OTHER DISORDERS — Continued

DB-80634 Fibrous autoimmune thyroiditis
  Noninvasive fibrous thyroiditis
  Chronic thyroiditis, fibrous variant
  Hashimoto thyroiditis, fibrous variant
DB-80636 Idiopathic atrophic hypothyroidism
  Atrophic thyroiditis
  Gull disease
  Idiopathic atrophic myxedema
DB-80638 Self-limiting autoimmune thyroiditis with transient hyperthyroidism and/or hypothyroidism
  Atypical subacute thyroiditis
  Subacute autoimmune thyroiditis
  Subacute lymphocytic thyroiditis
  Silent thyroiditis
DB-80639 Postpartum thyroiditis
DB-80644 Focal thyroiditis
DB-80646 Reidel's thyroiditis
  Invasive fibrous thyroiditis
  Ligneous thyroiditis
  Struma fibrosa thyroid
  Woody thyroiditis
DB-80652 Chronic suppurative thyroiditis 245.8
DB-80654 Chronic nonsuppurative thyroiditis 245.8
DB-80660 Iatrogenic thyroiditis, NOS 245.4
DB-80700 Hypoplasia of thyroid 246.8
  Atrophy of thyroid 246.8
DB-80710 Cyst of thyroid 246.2
DB-80720 Hemorrhage of thyroid 246.3
DB-80730 Infarction of thyroid 246.3
DB-80900 Hypersecretion of calcitonin 246.0
  Hypersecretion of thyrocalcitonin 246.0

B-81 INHERITED DISORDERS OF THYROID METABOLISM

DB-81000 Inherited disorder of thyroid metabolism, NOS
DB-81200 Hypothyroidism due to defect in thyroid hormone synthesis, NOS 246.1
  Hypothyroidism due to defective thyroid hormonogenesis, NOS 246.1
DB-81210 Iodide transport defect 246.1
  Hypothyroidism due to iodide concentration defect 246.1
  Hypothyroidism due to iodide transport defect 246.1
  Iodine transport defect 246.1
  Iodide transport failure 246.1
  GDTH I 246.1
  Genetic defect in thyroid hormonogenesis I 246.1
  Iodine accumulation defect 246.1
DB-81220 Iodide oxidation defect 246.1
  Hypothyroidism due to iodide organification defect I 246.1
  GDTH IIA 246.1
  Genetic defect in thyroid hormonogenesis II A 246.1
  Iodide organification defect I 246.1
  Thyroid hormone organification defect II A 246.1
DB-81230 Iodide peroxidase defect 246.1 (F-670E8)
  Defective iodide peroxidase activity 246.1 (F-670E8)
DB-81250 Pendred's syndrome 246.1
  Hypothyroidism with sensorineural deafness 246.1
  GDTH IIB 246.1
  Genetic defect in thyroid hormonogenesis II B 246.1
  Goiter-deafness syndrome 246.1
  Thyroid hormone organification defect II B 246.1
DB-81260 Thyroglobulin synthesis defect 246.1
  Hypothyroidism due to thyroglobulin biosynthetic defect 246.1
  GDTH V 246.1
  Genetic defect in thyroid hormonogenesis V 246.1
DB-81270 Iodotyrosyl coupling defect 246.1 (F-670E8)
  Congenital thyroid hormone coupling defect 246.1
  GDTH III 246.1
  Genetic defect in thyroid hormonogenesis III 246.1
  Thyroid hormone coupling defect 246.1
DB-81280 Thyroglobulin proteolysis defect 246.1
DB-81290 Iodotyrosine deiodination defect 246.1
  Hypothyroidism due to iodotyrosine deiodinase defect 246.1
  Deiodinase deficiency 246.1
  GDTH IV 246.1
  Genetic defect in thyroid hormonogenesis IV 246.1
  Iodotyrosine deiodinase deficiency 246.1
  Iodotyrosine dehalogenase deficiency 246.1
DB-81300 Thyroxine transport defect, NOS 246.8
DB-81310 X-linked absence of thyroxine-binding globulin 246.8
DB-81320 X-linked reduction of thyroxine-binding globulin 246.8
DB-81330 X-linked excess of thyroxine-binding globulin 246.8
DB-81340 Autosomal dominant excess of transthyretin 246.8
  Autosomal dominant excess of thryroxine-binding prealbumin 246.8
DB-81350 X-linked variant form of thyroxine-binding globulin 246.8
DB-81360 Autosomal variant form of transthyretin 246.8

DB-81370 Autosomal dominant variant form of albumin 246.8
DB-81374 Autosomal dominant analbuminemia 246.8
DB-81380 Thyroxine plasma membrane transport defect 246.8
DB-81390 Thyroid hormone responsiveness defect 246.8
  Hypothyroidism due to thyroid insensitivity to TSH 246.8
  Congenital unresponsiveness to thyrotropin 246.8
  General resistance to thyrotropin 246.8
  Thyroid hormone resistance syndrome 246.8
  Unresponsiveness of thyroid gland to thyrotropin 246.8
  Resistance to thyrotropin 246.8
  Resistance to thyroid stimulating hormone 246.8
  TSH resistance 246.8
  Thyroid hormone resistance 246.8
  Thyroid hormone unresponsiveness 246.8
DB-813A0 Refetoff syndrome 246.8

SECTION B-9 DISEASES OF THE PARATHYROID GLANDS

DB-90000 Disease of parathyroid glands, NOS 252.9
  Disorder of parathyroid glands, NOS 252.9
DB-90100 Hyperparathyroidism, NOS 252.0
DB-90110 Primary hyperparathyroidism 252.0
DB-90120 Parathyroid hyperplasia 252.0
DB-90130 Familial hyperparathyroidism 252.0
  Familial hypocalciuric hypercalcemia 252.0
  FFH 252.0
  Familial benign hypercalcemia 252.0
DB-90140 Secondary hyperparathyroidism, NOS 252.0
DB-90150 Hyperparathyroidism due to renal insufficiency 588.8
DB-90160 Hyperparathyroidism due to vitamin D deficiency
  Hyperparathyroidism due to $1,25(OH)_2D_3$
DB-90170 Hyperparathyroidism due to lithium therapy
  Hypercalcemia due to lithium
DB-90180 Vitamin D intoxication
DB-90200 Hypercalcemia due to granulomatous disease, NOS
DB-90210 Hypercalcemia due to sarcoidosis
DB-90230 Hypercalcemia due to hyperthyroidism
DB-90240 Hypercalcemia due to immobilization
DB-90250 Hypercalcemia due to a drug, NOS
DB-90260 Hypercalcemia due to thiazide and vitamin A
DB-90270 Hyperparathyroidism due to intestinal malabsorption 252.0
DB-90280 Hypercalcemia associated with chronic dialysis
DB-90300 Tertiary hyperparathyroidism 252.0
DB-90310 Ectopic hyperparathyroidism, NOS 259.3
DB-90320 Humoral hypercalcemia of malignancy 259.3
  HHM 259.3
  Malignancy associated hypercalcemia 259.3
  MAHC 259.3
DB-90340 Osteitis fibrosa cystica generalisata 252.0
  Fibro-osteoclasia 252.0
  Von Recklinghausen's disease of bone 252.0
  Fibrous osteodystrophy 252.0
  Osteitis fibrosa cystica 252.0
  Osteodystrophia fibrosa 252.0
  Bran disease
  Big head
DB-90500 Hypoparathyroidism, NOS 252.1
  Deficiency of parathyroid hormone 252.1
  Deficiency of PTH 252.1
  Deficiency of parathyrin
DB-90510 Parathyroid hypocalcemic tetany 252.1
  Parathyroidal tetany 252.1
DB-90520 Postablative hypoparathyroidism 252.1
  Transient hypoparathyroidism 252.1
DB-90530 Idiopathic parathyroidism 252.1
  Absence of parathyroid hormone 252.1
  Absence of PTH
DB-90540 Transitory neonatal hypoparathyroidism 775.4
DB-90550 Senile osteopenia
  Osteopenia of the elderly
DB-90800 Autoimmune hypoparathyroidism
DB-90840 Isolated persistent neonatal hypoparathyroidism
DB-90842 Isolated late onset hypoparathyroidism
DB-90850 Pseudohypoparathyroidism, NOS 275.4
  Constitutional chronic hypocalcemia 275.4
  Familial pseudohypoparathyroidism 275.4
  Parathyroid hormone resistant hypoparathyroidism 275.4
DB-90851 Albright hereditary osteodystrophy, NOS 275.4
DB-90852 Pseudohypoparathyroidism type I A 275.4
  Albright hereditary osteodystrophy, classical type 275.4
DB-90854 Pseudohypoparathyroidism type I B 275.4
DB-90856 Pseudohypoparathyroidism type II 275.4
DB-90858 Normocalcemic pseudohypoparathyroidism 275.4
  Pseudopseudohypoparathyroidism 275.4
  Albright hereditary osteodystrophy type 2 275.4
DB-90860 Rickets, NOS 275.3
DB-90862 Calcipenic type rickets 275.3
DB-90864 Phosphopenic type rickets 275.3
DB-90870 Hereditary vitamin D dependency syndrome, NOS
DB-90872 Hereditary vitamin D dependency syndrome, type I
  Hereditary selective and simple deficiency of 1 alpha, $25(OH)_2$ D
  ARUDD-I

SECTION B-9 DISEASES OF THE PARATHYROID GLANDS — Continued

DB-90880 Hereditary vitamin D dependency syndrome type, II
ARUDD-II
Hereditary generalized resistance to 1 alpha, $25(OH)_2$ D

DB-90894 Anticonvulsant drug-induced osteomalacia, NOS

DB-90896 Steroid-induced oesteopenia

SECTION B-A FUNCTIONAL DISEASES OF THE CENTRAL NERVOUS SYSTEM WITH NEUROENDOCRINE DISTURBANCES

DB-A0000 Functional disease of the CNS with neuroendocrine disturbance, NOS

DB-A0100 Central nervous system disorder of water regulation, NOS

DB-A0110 Cerebral hyponatremia

DB-A0120 Cerebral hypernatremia

DB-A0200 Disorder of neurometabolic regulation, NOS

DB-A0210 Hypothalamic obesity

CHAPTER C — DISEASES OF THE HEMATOPOIETIC AND IMMUNE SYSTEMS

SECTION C-0 HEMATOPOIETIC SYSTEM DISEASES: GENERAL TERMS

DC-00000 Disease of hematopoietic system, NOS 289.9
  Disorder of hematopoietic system, NOS 289.9
  Hematopoietic system syndrome, NOS 289.9
  Hematologic disease, NOS 289.9
  Blood dyscrasia, NOS 289.9
  Disease of blood and blood forming organ, NOS 289.9
DC-00010 Cytopenia, NOS 285.9
DC-00020 Acquired pancytopenia 285.8

SECTIONS C-1-3 RED BLOOD CELL DISORDERS
C-10 RED BLOOD CELL DISORDERS: GENERAL TERMS

DC-10000 Red blood cell disorder, NOS
DC-10002 Erythropenia
  Erythrocytopenia
DC-10010 Anemia, NOS 285.9
  Oligocythemia of red blood cells 285.9
  Absolute anemia
  Oligocytosis of red blood cells 285.9
DC-10014 Relative anemia
DC-10020 Normocytic normochromic anemia 285.9
DC-10022 Normocytic hypochromic anemia 280.9
  Idiopathic hypochromic anemia 280.9
DC-10030 Microcytic hypochromic anemia 280.-
  Hypochromic microcytic anemia 280.-
DC-10032 Microcytic normochromic anemia
DC-10040 Macrocytic anemia 285.9
DC-10050 Blood loss anemia 285.1
  Acute blood loss anemia 285.1
  Acute post-hemorrhagic anemia 285.1
DC-10060 Nutritional anemia, NOS 281.9
DC-10100 Hemolytic anemia, NOS 283.1
DC-10101 Hemolysis, NOS
  Hemolytic
DC-10102 Extravascular hemolysis, NOS
DC-10103 Intravascular hemolysis, NOS 283.2
DC-10106 Acquired hemolytic anemia, NOS 283.9
DC-10107 Congenital hemolytic anemia, NOS 282.9
DC-10108 Hereditary hemolytic anemia, NOS 282.9
DC-10109 Chronic idiopathic hemolytic anemia 283.9
DC-10110 Hypoplastic anemia 284.9
  Medullary hypoplasia of bone marrow 284.9
DC-10120 Refractory anemia
DC-10130 Aregenerative anemia
  Non regenerative anemia
DC-10160 Hemoglobinuria, NOS 791.2
DC-10170 Methemoglobinemia, NOS 289.7
DC-10180 Acquired methemoglobinuria 289.7
  Toxic methemoglobinuria 289.7

C-11 ANEMIAS DUE TO DECREASED RED CELL PRODUCTION

DC-11000 Anemia due to decreased red cell production, NOS
DC-11010 Aplastic anemia, NOS 294.9
DC-11020 Constitutional aplastic anemia, NOS
DC-11040 Estren-Dameshek anemia
DC-11050 Acquired aplastic anemia, NOS 284.9
  Idiopathic acquired aplastic anemia, NOS 284.9
DC-11060 Secondary aplastic anemia, NOS 284.8
DC-11070 Aplastic anemia secondary to drugs 284.8
DC-11080 Aplastic anemia secondary to radiation 284.8
DC-11090 Aplastic anemia secondary to chemicals 284.8
  Toxic aplastic anemia 284.8
DC-11100 Aplastic anemia secondary to infection 284.8
DC-11110 Aplastic anemia secondary to metabolic alteration, NOS
DC-11120 Aplastic anemia secondary to pancreatitis
DC-11130 Aplastic anemia secondary to pregnancy 284.8
DC-11140 Aplastic anemia secondary to chronic systemic disease, NOS 284.8
DC-11300 Immunologic aplastic anemia, NOS
DC-11302 Humoral immunologic aplastic anemia
DC-11304 Cellular immunologic aplastic anemia
DC-11400 Anemia due to disturbance of proliferation and differentiation of hematopoietic stem cells, NOS
DC-11410 Anemia due to disturbance of proliferation and differentiation of erythroid precursor cells, NOS
DC-11420 Pure red cell aplasia, NOS 284.0
  Pure red cell anemia, NOS 284.0
  Primary red cell aplasia 284.0
DC-11430 Acute pure red cell aplasia
  Acute pure red cell anemia
DC-11440 Chronic constitutional pure red cell aplasia 284.0
  Diamond-Blackfan anemia 284.0
  Chronic constitutional pure red cell anemia 284.0
  Congenital erythroid hypoplasia 284.0
  Congenital hypoplastic anemia 284.0
  Familial hypoplastic anemia 284.0
DC-11450 Chronic acquired pure red cell aplasia
  Chronic acquired pure red cell anemia
DC-11600 Anemia of endocrine disorder, NOS
DC-11610 Anemia of pituitary deficiency
DC-11620 Anemia of thyroid dysfunction
DC-11630 Anemia of adrenal dysfunction

C-11 ANEMIAS DUE TO DECREASED RED CELL PRODUCTION — Continued

DC-11640 Anemia of gonadal dysfunction
DC-11650 Anemia of parathyroid dysfunction
DC-11660 Anemia of pregnancy
DC-11670 Anemia of diabetes
DC-11680 Anemia of chronic renal failure
DC-11900 Congenital dyserythropoietic anemia, NOS 285.8
  CDA, NOS
DC-11910 Congenital dyserythropoietic anemia, type I 285.8
DC-11920 Congenital dyserythropoietic anemia, type II 285.8
  HEMPAS 285.8
DC-11930 Congenital dyserythropoietic anemia, type III 285.8

C-12 ANEMIAS RELATED TO DISTURBED DNA SYNTHESIS

DC-12010 Megaloblastic anemia, NOS 281.9
DC-12020 Megaloblastic anemia due to folate deficiency, NOS 281.2
  Folate deficiency anemia 281.2
  Folic acid deficiency anemia 281.2
DC-12022 Drug-induced folate deficiency anemia 281.2
DC-12024 Megaloblastic anemia due to poor nutrition 281.2
  Dietary folate deficiency anemia 281.2
DC-12040 Megaloblastic anemia due to alcoholism
DC-12050 Megaloblastic anemia due to hyperalimentation
DC-12060 Megaloblastic anemia due to hemodialysis 281.2
DC-12070 Megaloblastic anemia of premature infant 281.2
  Nutritional megaloblastic anemia of infancy 281.2
DC-12080 Goats' milk anemia 281.2
DC-12200 Megaloblastic anemia due to impaired absorption of folate, NOS 281.2
  Congenital folate malabsorption 281.2
DC-12210 Megaloblastic anemia due to tropical sprue
DC-12220 Megaloblastic anemia due to nontropical sprue
DC-12230 Megaloblastic anemia due to disease of small intestine
  Megaloblastic anemia due to ileal disease
DC-12240 Megaloblastic anemia due to increased requirements, NOS
DC-12250 Megaloblastic anemia due to pregnancy
DC-12260 Megaloblastic anemia due to chronic hemolytic anemia
DC-12270 Megaloblastic anemia due to exfoliative dermatitis
DC-12300 Pernicious anemia, NOS 280.0
  Megaloblastic anemia due to impaired absorption of cobalamin 280.0
  Addison's anemia 281.0
  Biermer's anemia 281.0
DC-12310 Megaloblastic anemia due to vitamin B_{12} deficiency 281.1
  Megaloblastic anemia due to cobalamin deficiency 281.1
  Vitamin B_{12} deficiency anemia 281.1
DC-12320 Megaloblastic anemia due to decreased intake of vitamin B_{12}, NOS 281.1
  Dietary vitamin B_{12} deficiency anemia 281.1
DC-12400 Megaloblastic anemia due to gastrectomy
DC-12410 Megaloblastic anemia due to Zollinger-Ellison syndrome
DC-12422 Megaloblastic anemia due to vitamin B_{12} malabsorption with proteinuria 281.1
DC-12430 Megaloblastic anemia due to blind loop syndrome
DC-12440 Megaloblastic anemia due to fish tapeworm
DC-12450 Megaloblastic anemia due to pancreatic insufficiency
DC-12470 Megaloblastic anemia due to vegetarianism 281.1
  Vegans' anemia 281.1
DC-12600 Acute megaloblastic anemia, NOS
DC-12610 Acute megaloblastic anemia due to nitrous oxide
DC-12620 Acute megaloblastic anemia due to severe illness
DC-12630 Acute megaloblastic anemia due to dialysis
DC-12640 Acute megaloblastic anemia secondary to total parenteral nutrition
DC-12650 Megaloblastic anemia due to drugs, NOS
DC-12800 Megaloblastic anemia due to inborn errors of metabolism, NOS 281.0
  Congenital pernicious anemia, NOS 281.0
DC-12810 Juvenile type megaloblastic anemia, NOS
DC-12820 Familial megaloblastic anemia 281.1
  Imerslund-Grasbeck disease 281.1
  Imerslund's syndrome 281.1
DC-12830 Megaloblastic anemia due to congenital deficiency of intrinsic factor 281.0
  Congenital intrinsic factor deficiency anemia 281.0
DC-12850 Megaloblastic anemia due to error of folate metabolism
DC-12860 Megaloblastic anemia due to error of cobalamin metabolism
DC-12870 Thiamine-responsive megaloblastic anemia
DC-12872 Combined B_{12} and folate deficiency anemia 281.3
DC-12880 Refractory megaloblastic anemia, NOS 281.3

C-13 ANEMIAS DUE TO DISTURBANCE OF HEMOGLOBIN SYNTHESIS AND THALASSEMIAS

C-130 Anemias Due to Disturbance of Hemoglobin Synthesis

DC-13000 Anemia due to disturbance of hemoglobin synthesis, NOS
DC-13010 Iron deficiency anemia, NOS 280.9
Asiderotic anemia 280.9
Chlorotic anemia 280.9
Sideropenic anemia 280.9
DC-13012 Iron deficiency anemia secondary to chronic blood loss 280.0
Chronic blood loss anemia 280.0
DC-13014 Iron deficiency anemia secondary to inadequate dietary iron intake 280.1
DC-13016 Plummer-Vinson syndrome 280.8 (T-56000) (F-51702) (G-C001) (M-34200)
Paterson-Kelly syndrome 280.8 (T-56000) (F-51702) (G-C001) (M-34200)
Sideropenic dysphagia 280.8 (T-56000) (F-51702) (G-C001) (M-34200)
DC-13018 Achlorhydric anemia 280.9
Achylic anemia 280.9
Faber syndrome 280.9
DC-13020 Congenital atransferinemia

C-132-136 Thalassemias

DC-13200 Thalassemia, NOS 282.4
DC-13210 Thalassemia syndrome, NOS
DC-13230 Thalassemia major, NOS
Homozygous thalassemia, NOS
DC-13250 Thalassemia intermedia, NOS
DC-13260 Thalassemia minor, NOS
DC-13270 Heterozygous thalassemia, NOS
Thalassemia trait, NOS
DC-13500 beta Thalassemia, NOS
DC-13510 Homozygous beta thalassemia 282.4
Cooley's anemia 282.4
Mediterranean anemia 282.4
DC-13520 $beta^0$ Thalassemia, NOS
DC-13530 $beta^0$ Thalassemia, deletion type
DC-13540 $beta^0$ Thalassemia, nondeletion type
DC-13550 $beta^+$ Thalassemia, NOS
DC-13560 $beta^+$ Thalassemia, normal Hb A_2, type 1, silent
DC-13570 $beta^+$ Thalassemia, normal Hb A_2, type 2
DC-13580 delta beta Thalassemia, NOS
DC-13590 delta $beta^0$ Thalassemia
DC-13600 A_{gamma} delta $beta^0$ Thalassemia
DC-13610 Hb Lepore thalassemia
DC-13620 A_{gamma} $beta^+$ HPFH and $beta^0$ thalassemia in cis
DC-13630 delta Thalassemia, NOS
DC-13640 $delta^0$ Thalassemia
DC-13650 epsilon gamma delta beta Thalassemia
DC-13660 epsilon gamma delta $beta^0$ Thalassemia
DC-13700 Hereditary persistence of fetal hemoglobin thalassemia, NOS 282.7
HPFH, NOS 282.7
DC-13710 HPFH deletion type, NOS 282.7
DC-13720 HPFH delta $beta^0$ thalassemia 282.7
DC-13730 HPFH nondeletion type, NOS 282.7
DC-13740 HPFH linked to beta-globulin gene cluster, NOS 282.7
DC-13750 HPFH G gamma $beta^+$ thalassemia 282.7
DC-13760 HPFH A gamma $beta^+$ thalassemia 282.7
DC-13770 HPFH unlinked to beta-globulin gene cluster, NOS 282.7
DC-13800 alpha Thalassemia, NOS 282.7
DC-13810 $alpha^0$ Thalassemia 282.7
alpha Thalassemia 1 282.7
DC-13820 $alpha^+$ Thalassemia, NOS 282.7
alpha Thalassemia 2 282.7
DC-13830 $alpha^+$ Thalassemia, deletion type 282.7
DC-13840 $alpha^+$ Thalassemia, nondeletion type 282.7
DC-13850 Hemoglobin Bart's hydrops syndrome 282.7
Hemoglobin Bart's disease 282.7
DC-13860 Hemoglobin H disease
DC-13880 Unstable hemoglobin disease, NOS 282.7
Congenital Heinz body anemia 282.7

C-14 ANEMIAS DUE TO UNKNOWN OR MULTIPLE MECHANISMS

DC-14010 Anemia due to unknown mechanism, NOS
DC-14020 Anemia due to multiple mechanisms, NOS
DC-14030 Anemia of chronic disorder, NOS 281.9
Sideropenic anemia with reticuloendothelial siderosis 281.9
Chronic simple anemia 281.9
Anemia of infection, NOS 281.9
Simple chronic anemia 281.9
DC-14040 Myelophthisic anemia
Anemia associated with marrow infiltration
DC-14050 Non megaloblastic anemia associated with nutritional deficiency, NOS 281.9
Non megaloblastic nutritional anemia, NOS 281.9
DC-14060 Anemia due to vitamin A deficiency
DC-14070 Anemia due to vitamin B_6 deficiency
DC-14080 Anemia due to riboflavin deficiency
DC-14090 Anemia due to pantothenic deficiency
DC-14100 Anemia due to niacin deficiency
DC-14110 Anemia due to vitamin C deficiency 281.8
Anemia due to ascorbic acid deficiency 281.8
Scorbutic anemia 281.8
DC-14120 Anemia due to vitamin E deficiency
DC-14130 Anemia due to copper deficiency
DC-14140 Anemia due to zinc deficiency
DC-14150 Anemia due to starvation

C-14 ANEMIAS DUE TO UNKNOWN OR MULTIPLE MECHANISMS — Continued

DC-14152 Anemia due to protein deficiency 281.3
  Anemia related to kwashiorkor 281.3
  Protein deficiency anemia 281.3
DC-14154 Amino acid deficiency anemia 281.4
DC-14170 Non megaloblastic anemia due to alcoholism
DC-14180 Sideroblastic anemia, NOS 285.0
    (M-99821)
  Primary sideroblastic anemia, NOS 285.0
    (M-99821)
  Refractory sideroblastic anemia, NOS 285.0
    (M-99821)
  Sideroachrestic anemia, NOS 285.0
    (M-99821)
DC-14300 Secondary acquired sideroblastic anemia, NOS 285.0
  Secondary sideroblastic anemia, NOS 285.0
  Acquired sideroblastic anemia, NOS 285.0
DC-14302 Drug-induced sideroblastic anemia, NOS 285.0
DC-14310 Hereditary sideroblastic anemia, NOS 281.9
  Dimorphic anemia 281.9
  Congenital sideroblastic anemia 285.9
DC-14320 X chromosome-linked sideroblastic anemia, NOS
DC-14330 X chromosome-linked pyridoxine responsive sideroblastic anemia 285.0
  Pyridoxine responsive sideroblastic anemia 285.0
DC-14340 X chromosome-linked pyridoxine refractory sideroblastic anemia
DC-14350 Autosomal-linked pyridoxine refractory sideroblastic anemia

C-15 ANEMIAS DUE TO INTRINSIC RED CELL ABNORMALITY

DC-15000 Anemia due to intrinsic red cell abnormality, NOS
DC-15020 Anemia due to membrane defect, NOS
DC-15100 Hereditary spherocytosis, NOS 282.0
  Familial spherocytosis 282.0
  Minkowsky-Chauffard syndrome 282.0
  Congenital spherocytosis 282.0
  Familial acholuric jaundice 282.0
  Congenital spherocytic hemolytic anemia 282.0
DC-15110 Hereditary spherocytosis due to spectrin deficiency, NOS
DC-15112 Mild hereditary spherocytosis due to spectrin deficiency
DC-15114 Severe hereditary spherocytosis due to spectrin deficiency
DC-15130 Hereditary spherocytosis due to combined deficiency of spectrin and ankyrin, NOS
DC-15132 Mild hereditary spherocytosis due to combined deficiency of spectrin and ankyrin
DC-15134 Severe hereditary spherocytosis due to combined deficiency of spectrin and ankyrin
DC-15170 Hereditary spherocytosis due to deficiency of protein 4.2
DC-15180 Hereditary spherocytosis due to beta spectrin defect
DC-15300 Hereditary elliptocytosis, NOS 282.1
  Hereditary ovalocytosis, NOS 282.1
  Congenital elliptocytosis, NOS 282.1
  Congenital ovalocytosis, NOS 282.1
  Hereditary pyropoikilocytosis
  HPP
DC-15310 Hereditary elliptocytosis due to alpha spectrin defect
DC-15320 Hereditary elliptocytosis due to beta spectrin defect in self-association
DC-15330 Hereditary elliptocytosis due to beta spectrin-ankyrin interaction
DC-15340 Hereditary elliptocytosis due to deficiency of protein 4.1
DC-15350 Hereditary elliptocytosis due to abnormal protein 4.1
DC-15360 Hereditary elliptocytosis due to glycophorin C deficiency
DC-15500 Hereditary acanthocytosis, NOS
DC-15510 Chorea acanthocytosis syndrome
DC-15520 Stomatocytosis, NOS 282.8
DC-15530 Hereditary stomatocytosis
  Hereditary hydrocytosis
DC-15540 Acquired stomatocytosis
DC-15570 Hereditary xerocytosis
  Xerocytosis
  Dessicocytosis
DC-15580 Rh deficiency syndrome
DC-15600 Paroxysmal noctural hemoglobinuria 283.2
  Marchiafava-Micheli syndrome 283.2
  PNH 283.2

C-17 ANEMIAS DUE TO ENZYME DEFICIENCIES

DC-17000 Anemia due to enzyme deficiency, NOS 282.3
DC-17002 Drug-induced enzyme deficiency anemia, NOS 282.2
DC-17010 Glucose-6-phosphate deficiency anemia, NOS 282.2
  G-6-PD deficiency anemia, NOS 282.2
DC-17020 G-6-PD variant enzyme deficiency anemia, NOS 282.2
DC-17021 G-6-PD class I variant anemia 282.2
DC-17022 G-6-PD class II variant anemia 282.2
DC-17023 G-6-PD class III variant anemia 282.2
DC-17024 G-6-PD class IV variant anemia 282.2
DC-17025 G-6-PD class V variant anemia 282.2
DC-17090 Anemia due to pentose phosphate pathway defect, NOS 282.2

DC-17100 Congenital nonspherocytic hemolytic anemia, NOS 282.9
Hereditary nonspherocytic hemolytic anemia, NOS 282.9
HNSHA 282.9
DC-17130 HNSHA due to pyruvate kinase deficiency 282.3
Pyruvate kinase deficiency anemia 282.3
PK deficiency anemia 282.3
DC-17140 HNSHA due to hexokinase deficiency 282.3
Hexokinase deficiency anemia 282.3
DC-17150 HNSHA due to glucose phosphate isomerase deficiency 282.3
DC-17160 HNSHA due to phosphofructokinase deficiency 282.3
DC-17170 HNSHA due to aldolase deficiency 282.3
DC-17180 HNSHA due to triosephosphate isomerase deficiency 282.3
Triosephosphate deficiency anemia 282.3
DC-17190 HNSHA due to phophoglycerate kinase deficiency
DC-17200 HNSHA due to diphosphoglycerate mutase deficiency
DC-17210 HNSHA due to glutathione reductase deficiency 282.2
Erythrocytic glutathione deficiency anemia 282.2
DC-17220 HNSHA due to gamma glutamyl cysteine synthetase deficiency
DC-17240 HNSHA due to glutathione synthetase deficiency
DC-17250 HNSHA due to pyrimidine-5'-nucleotidase deficiency
DC-17260 HNSHA due to increased adenosine deaminase activity
DC-17262 HNSHA due to decreased adenosine deaminase activity
DC-17270 HNSHA due to NADH diaphorase deficiency
DC-17280 HNSHA due to NADH-methemoglobin reductase deficiency 289.7

C-20 HEMOGLOBINOPATHIES

DC-20000 Hemoglobinopathy, NOS 282.7
Globin abnormality, NOS 282.7
Hemoglobin disease, NOS 282.7
Hemoglobin disorder, NOS 282.7
DC-20020 Hemoglobin S disease 282.60
Hemoglobin S-S disease 282.60
Sickle cell anemia 282.60
Sickle cell disease 282.60
DC-20022 Hemoglobin S disease without crisis 282.61
Sickle cell disease without crisis 282.61
DC-20024 Hemoglobin S disease with crisis 282.62
Sickle cell crisis 282.62
DC-20028 Sickle cell trait 282.5
Hemoglobin S-A disorder 282.5
Hemoglobin A-S genotype 282.5
Hemoglobin S trait 282.5
Heterozygous hemoglobin S 282.5
DC-20100 Hemoglobin C disease 282.7
Hemoglobin C-C disease 282.7
DC-20110 Hemoglobin C trait
Hemoglobin C-A disorder
DC-20200 Hemoglobin D disease 282.7
Hemoglobin D-D disease 282.7
DC-20210 Hemoglobin D trait
Hemoglobin D-A disorder
DC-20300 Hemoglobin E disease 282.7
Hemoglobin E-E disease 282.7
DC-20310 Hemoglobin E trait
Hemoglobin E-A disorder
DC-20400 Mixed hemoglobin disorder, NOS
Mixed hemoglobinopathy, NOS
DC-20410 Sickle cell-hemoglobin C disease 282.63
Hemoglobin S-C disease 282.63
HbS-HbC disease 282.63
DC-20420 Sickle cell-hemoglobin D disease 282.69
Hemoglobin S-D disease 282.69
HbS-HbD disease 282.69
DC-20430 Sickle cell-hemoglobin E disease 282.69
Hemoglobin S-E disease 282.69
HbS-HbE disease 282.69
DC-20440 Hemoglobin S-F disease 282.4
Thalassemia-hemoglobin S disease 282.4
Sickle cell-thalassemia disease 282.4
Microdrepanocytic disease 282.4
Microdrepanocytosis 282.4
DC-20450 Hemoglobin C-F disease
Thalassemia-hemoglobin C disease
DC-20458 Thalassemia with other hemoglobinopathy, NOS 282.4
DC-20460 Hemoglobin M disease 289.7
Hereditary M hemoglobinopathy 289.7
Hereditary methemoglobinuria 289.7
DC-20500 Hemoglobinopathy with cyanosis, NOS
DC-20510 Hemoglobinopathy with erythrocytosis, NOS
DC-20520 Sulfhemoglobinemia 289.7

C-30 ANEMIAS DUE TO EXTRINSIC RED CELL ABNORMALITIES

DC-30000 Anemia due to extrinsic red cell abnormality, NOS
DC-30010 Anemia due to mechanical damage
DC-30020 March hemoglobinuria 283.2
Sports anemia 283.2
Hemoglobinuria from exertion 283.2
DC-30030 Traumatic cardiac hemolytic anemia 283.1
Hemolytic anemia due to vascular prosthesis 283.1
Mechanical hemolytic anemia 283.1
DC-30040 Microangiopathic hemolytic anemia 283.1

C-32 ANEMIAS DUE TO CHEMICAL OR PHYSICAL AGENTS

DC-32200 Anemia due to chemical agent, NOS 283.1
Toxic hemolytic anemia 283.1

C-32 ANEMIAS DUE TO CHEMICAL OR PHYSICAL AGENTS — Continued

DC-32210 Anemia due to arsenic hydride
DC-32220 Anemia due to lead
DC-32230 Anemia due to copper
DC-32240 Anemia due to chlorates
DC-32250 Anemia due to oxygen
DC-32260 Anemia due to insect venoms
DC-32300 Anemia due to physical agent, NOS
DC-32310 Anemia due to heat
DC-32320 Anemia due to radiation
DC-32402 Stokvis' disease 289.7

C-35 ANEMIAS DUE TO INFECTIONS

DC-35000 Hemolytic anemia due to infection, NOS
DC-35010 Hemolytic anemia due to malaria
DC-35020 Hemolytic anemia due to Bartonella
DC-35030 Hemolytic anemia due to Clostridium welchii
DC-35040 Hemolytic anemia due to babesiosis

C-36 ANTIBODY-MEDIATED ANEMIAS

DC-36000 Antibody-mediated anemia, NOS
DC-36120 Autoimmune hemolytic anemia, NOS 283.0
  Hemolytic anemia due to antibody, NOS 283.0
  Neonatal isoerythrolysis
DC-36130 Hemolytic anemia due to warm antibody, NOS 283.0
DC-36140 Hemolytic anemia associated with lymphoproliferative disorder
DC-36145 Hemolytic anemia associated with rheumatic disorder
DC-36150 Hemolytic anemia associated with systemic lupus erythematosus
DC-36160 Hemolytic anemia associated with infection
DC-36170 Hemolytic anemia due to nonlymphoid neoplasm
DC-36180 Hemolytic anemia associated with chronic inflammatory disease, NOS
DC-36190 Hemolytic anemia associated with ulcerative colitis
DC-36200 Evans syndrome
DC-36400 Hemolytic anemia due to cold antibody, NOS 283.0
  Cryopathic hemolytic anemia 283.0
  Cold antibody hemolytic anemia 283.0
  Cold agglutinin disease 283.0
  Cold agglutinin hemoglobinuria 283.0
  Cold hemolytic disease
DC-36410 Cold agglutinin disease due to Mycoplasma pneumonia
DC-36420 Idiopathic chronic cold agglutinin disease
DC-36450 Idiopathic paroxysmal cold hemoglobinuria 283.2
  Donath-Landsteiner hemolytic anemia 283.2
DC-36452 Transient paroxysmal cold hemoglobinuria
DC-36454 Secondary paroxysmal cold hemoglobinuria
DC-36600 Hemolytic anemia due to drugs, NOS 283.0
  Drug-induced hemolytic anemia, NOS 283.0
DC-36610 Hapten type high affinity hemolytic anemia
DC-36620 Hapten type low affinity hemolytic anemia
DC-36630 Drug-induced autoantibody type hemolytic anemia 283.0
DC-36640 Innocent bystander type hemolytic anemia
DC-36800 Autoerythrocyte sensitivity disorder, NOS
DC-36810 Erythroblastosis fetalis
  Alloimmune hemolytic disease of newborn
DC-36820 Polyagglutinable erythrocyte syndrome
  TN syndrome
DC-36840 Hemolytic uremic syndrome 283.1
DC-36860 Erythroblastosis, NOS
  Erythroblastemia, NOS
  Erythroleukosis, NOS

C-38 SECONDARY POLYCYTHEMIAS

DC-38000 Secondary polycythemia, NOS
  Secondary erythrocytosis, NOS
  Acquired polycythemia, NOS
  Polycythemia, NOS
DC-38010 Erythrocytosis due to low atmospheric pressure 289.0
  High altitude polycythemia 289.0
DC-38020 Stress polycythemia 289.0
  Emotional polycythemia 289.0
DC-38040 Erythrocytosis due to pulmonary disease, NOS
DC-38050 Erythrocytosis due to cardiovascular disease, NOS
DC-38060 Erythrocytosis due to alveolar hypoventilation
DC-38200 Erythrocytosis due to defective oxygen transport
DC-38210 Erythrocytosis due to tissue hypoxemia
DC-38220 Inappropriate secondary erythrocytosis
DC-38230 Erythrocytosis due to renal cyst
DC-38240 Erythrocytosis due to hydronephrosis
DC-38250 Erythrocytosis due to renal tumor 289.0
  Nephrogenous polycythemia 289.0
DC-38260 Erythrocytosis due to uterine myoma
DC-38270 Erythrocytosis due to cerebellar hemangioma
DC-38280 Erythrocytosis due to hepatoma
DC-38290 Erythrocytosis due to endocrine disorders
DC-38400 Neonatal polycythemia
DC-38410 Hereditary pure erythrocytosis 289.0
  Congenital erythrocytosis 289.0
  Essential hypererythropoietinemia 289.0
  Familial polycythemia 289.0
  Erythropoietin polycythemia 289.0
  Familial erythrocytosis 289.0
DC-38420 Erythrocytosis due to autotransfusion
  Blood doping
DC-38450 Relative erythrocytosis 289.0
  Relative polycythemia 289.0

DC-38450 (cont.) Benign polycythemia 289.0
Spurious polycythemia 289.0
Benign polycythemia due to fall in plasma volume 289.0

DC-38490 High oxygen affinity hemoglobin polycythemia 289.0

SECTION C-4 WHITE BLOOD CELL DISORDERS
C-40 WHITE BLOOD CELL DISORDERS: GENERAL TERMS

DC-40000 White blood cell disorder, NOS 288.9

C-41 DISORDERS OF NEUTROPHILS
C-410 Quantitative Disorders of Neutrophils

DC-41000 Leukocytosis, NOS 288.8
DC-41010 Neutrophilia, NOS
Neutrophilic leukocytosis
Granulocytosis
DC-41012 Acute neutrophilia
DC-41014 Chronic neutrophilia
DC-41040 Leukemoid reaction, NOS 288.8
DC-41042 Neutrophilic leukemoid reaction 288.8
Granulocytic leukemoid reaction 288.8
Myelocytic leukemoid reaction 288.8
DC-41050 Pseudoneutrophilia
DC-41052 Drug-induced neutrophilia
DC-41060 Leukoerythroblastotic reaction 285.8

C-412-416 Quantitative Abnormalities of Granulocytes

DC-41200 Leukopenia, NOS
DC-41210 Neutropenia, NOS 288.0
Granulocytopenia 288.0
DC-41220 Agranulocytosis 288.0
DC-41230 Agranulocytic angina
DC-41240 Congenital neutropenia 288.0
Kostmann's syndrome 288.0
Severe infantile genetic neutropenia 288.0
Severe infantile genetic agranulocytosis 288.0
DC-41250 Reticular dysgenesis
DC-41260 Reticular dysgenesis with congenital aleukocytosis
DC-41270 Neutropenia with dysgranulopoiesis
DC-41280 Schwachmann-Diamond syndrome
DC-41290 Cyclic neutropenia 288.0
Periodic neutropenia 288.0
DC-41292V Cyclic neutropenia in Gray Collie dogs
Gray Collie syndrome
DC-41400 Chronic idiopathic neutropenia
Familial neutropenia
Familial benign neutropenia
Chronic benign neutropenia
DC-41410 Myelokathexis
DC-41420 Lazy leukocyte syndrome
DC-41600 Immune neutropenia, NOS 288.0
DC-41610 Alloimmune neonatal neutropenia
Isoimmune neonatal neutropenia
DC-41620 Neutropenia associated with autoimmune disease
DC-41630 Drug-induced neutropenia, NOS 288.0
Idiosyncratic neutropenia, NOS 288.0
DC-41632 Dose-related drug-induced neutropenia
DC-41634 Non dose-related drug-induced neutropenia
Immunologic drug-induced neutropenia
Allergic drug-induced neutropenia
DC-41640 Neutropenia associated with infectious disease
DC-41650 Toxic neutropenia, NOS 288.0

C-418 Qualitative Abnormalities of Granulocytes

DC-41800 Qualitative abnormality of granulocyte, NOS 288.2
Neutrophil dysfunction, NOS 288.2
Granulocyte anomaly 288.2
DC-41810 Chediak-Higashi syndrome
DC-41820 Granulocyte abnormality due to immune defect
DC-41830 Granulocyte granule deficiency, NOS 288.2
Granulation anomaly 288.2
DC-41840 Congenital leukocyte adherence deficiency
DC-41844 Pelger-Huët anomaly 288.2
DC-41850 Neutrophil motility disorder, NOS
DC-41860 Congenital neutrophil actin dysfunction
DC-41870 Neutrophil cytomatrix disorder, NOS
DC-41880 Genetic anomaly of leukocyte, NOS 288.2
DC-41890 Job's syndrome 288.1
Recurring cold staphylococcal abscesses 288.1

C-45 EOSINOPHILIAS

DC-45000 Eosinophilic syndrome, NOS
DC-45010 Eosinophilia, NOS 288.3
Idiopathic eosinophilia 288.3
Eosinophilic leukocytosis 288.3
DC-45030 Familial eosinophilia 288.3
Hereditary eosinophilia 288.3
DC-45040 Allergic eosinophilia 288.3
DC-45050 Secondary eosinophilia 288.3
DC-45100 Eosinopenia
Eosinophilic cytopenia

C-46 MONOCYTOSES

DC-46000 Monocytosis, NOS
DC-46001 Reactive monocytosis
DC-46004 Chronic idiopathic monocytosis
DC-46010 Monocytic leukemoid reaction
DC-46030 Familial hemophagocytic histiocytosis
DC-46040 Infection-induced hemophagocytic histiocytosis

C-47 MAST CELL DISEASES

DC-47000 Mast cell disease, NOS
DC-47020 Localized extracutaneous mastocytosis
DC-47040 Systemic mastocytosis, NOS
DC-47050 Indolent systemic mastocytosis
DC-47060 Progressive systemic mastocytosis
DC-47070 Malignant mastocytosis
DC-47080 Reactive mastocytosis
DC-47090 Basophilia

C-48 NON MALIGNANT LYMPHOCYTE AND PLASMA CELL DISORDERS

DC-48100 Lymphocyte disorder, NOS
DC-48110 B lymphocyte disorder, NOS
DC-48120 T lymphocyte disorder, NOS
DC-48200 Mononucleosis syndrome, NOS
DC-48202 Heterophil-positive mononucleosis syndrome
Epstein Barr virus positive mononucleosis syndrome
DC-48204 Heterophil-negative mononucleosis syndrome
DC-48400 Lymphocytosis, NOS 288.8
DC-48402 Acute infectious lymphocytosis
DC-48404 Persistent lymphocytosis
DC-48410 Lymphocytic leukemoid reaction 288.8
DC-48430 Lymphocytopenia, NOS 288.8
Lymphopenia 288.8
DC-48440 Episodic lymphocytopenia, NOS
DC-48450 Plasmacytosis, NOS 288.8

C-49 CHRONIC GRANULOMATOUS DISEASES

DC-49010 Chronic granulomatous disease, NOS 288.1
DC-49020 Chronic granulomatous disease, type I 288.1
DC-49030 Chronic granulomatous disease, type IA 288.1
DC-49040 Chronic granulomatous disease, type II 288.1
DC-49050 Chronic granulomatous disease, type IIA 288.1
DC-49060 Chronic granulomatous disease, type III 288.1
DC-49070 Chronic granulomatous disease, type IV 288.1
DC-49080 Chronic granulomatous disease, type IVA 288.1

SECTION C-5 DISEASES OF THE IMMUNE SYSTEM

C-50 DISEASES OF THE IMMUNE SYSTEM: GENERAL TERMS

DC-50000 Disease of immune system, NOS
Disorder of immune system, NOS

C-51 CONGENITAL IMMUNODEFICIENCY DISEASES

DC-51000 Congenital immunodeficiency disease, NOS 279.2
DC-51010 Severe combined immunodeficiency disease, NOS 279.2
SCID, NOS 279.2
DC-51020 SCID due to absent lymphoid stem cells 279.2
Swiss type agammaglobulinemia 279.2
DC-51030 SCID due to absent adenosine deaminase 279.2
SCID due to absent ADA 279.2
DC-51040 SCID due to absent T cell receptor 279.2
DC-51050 SCID due to absent IL-2 production 279.2
DC-51060 SCID due to absent IL-2 receptor 279.2
DC-51070 SCID due to absent class II HLA antigens 279.2
Bare lymphocyte syndrome 279.2
DC-51080 SCID due to absent peripheral T cell maturation 279.2
DC-51090V Combined immunodeficiency disease in Arab foals
DC-51210 Wiskott-Aldrich syndrome 279.2
Immunodeficiency with thrombocytopenia and eczema 279.2
DC-51220 X-linked agammaglobulinemia 279.2
Bruton's type agammaglobulinemia 279.2
Congenital agammaglobulinemia 279.2
DC-51400 Hyperimmunoglobulin M syndrome
DC-51410 Immunoglobulin A deficiency
IgA deficiency
DC-51420 Common variable agammaglobulinemia
CVAG
DC-51430 Nezelof's syndrome
Congenital thymic dysplasia syndrome
DC-51440 Transient hypogammaglobulinemia of infancy
DC-51450 Immunodeficiency with thymoma
DC-51460 Hyperimmunoglobulin E syndrome
HIE syndrome
DC-51470 Hypergammaglobulinemia, NOS 289.8

C-53 DISORDERS OF COMPLEMENT

DC-53000 Disorder of complement, NOS
DC-53010 Complement abnormality, NOS
DC-53020 Complement deficiency disease, NOS
DC-53050 Hereditary angioneurotic edema 995.1
C-1 esterase inhibitor deficiency 995.1
Quincke's edema 995.1
Hereditary angioedema 995.1
DC-53070 Familial C3B inhibitor deficiency syndrome 995.1

C-55 CLONAL PROTEIN DISEASES

DC-55000 Clonal protein disease, NOS
DC-55100 Monoclonal gammopathy
Paraproteinemia
DC-55102 Benign monoclonal gammopathy
Asymptomatic monoclonal gammopathy
DC-55104 Secondary monoclonal gammopathy
DC-55130 Biclonal gammopathy, NOS

DC-55140 Triclonal gammopathy, NOS
DC-55150 Polyclonal gammopathy, NOS
DC-55160 Light chain disease, NOS
DC-55162 Kappa light chain disease
DC-55164 Lambda light chain disease
DC-55300 Heavy chain disease, NOS
DC-55310 Gamma heavy chain disease
  Franklin's disease
  IgG heavy chain disease
DC-55320 Alpha heavy chain disease, NOS
  IgA heavy chain disease, NOS
DC-55330 Alpha heavy chain disease, enteric form
  Immunoproliferative small intestinal disease
  Mediterranean lymphoma
DC-55340 Alpha heavy chain disease, respiratory form
DC-55350 Mu heavy chain disease
  IgM heavy chain disease
DC-55360 Delta heavy chain disease
  IgD heavy chain disease
DC-55370 Epsilon heavy chain disease
  IgE heavy chain disease
DC-55380 Hyperviscosity syndrome
  Reimann's syndrome

C-56 CRYOPATHIES

DC-56000 Cryopathy, NOS
DC-56010 Cryoglobulinemia, NOS
  Cryoimmunoglobulinemia, NOS
DC-56012 Primary cryoglobulinemia
DC-56014 Secondary cryoglobulinemia
DC-56020 Monoclonal cryoimmunoglobulinemia
DC-56022 Mixed cryoimmunoglobulinemia with monoclonal component
DC-56024 Mixed polyclonal cryoimmunoglobulinemia
DC-56030 Cryofibrinogenemia, NOS
DC-56032 Primary cryofibrinogenemia
DC-56034 Secondary cryofibrinogenemia
DC-56040 Mixed cryofibrinogenemia

SECTION C-6 DISORDERS OF BLOOD COAGULATION

C-60 DISORDERS OF BLOOD COAGULATION: GENERAL CONDITIONS

DC-60000 Blood coagulation disorder, NOS 286.9
  Coagulopathy, NOS 286.9
  Disorder of hemostasis, NOS 286.9
  Coagulation disorder, NOS 286.9
DC-60010 Blood coagulation disorder due to liver disease 286.7
DC-60020 Disseminated intravascular coagulation 286.6
  Consumptive thrombohemorrhagic disorder, NOS 286.6
  Consumptive coagulopathy 286.6
  DIC syndrome 286.6
  Defibrination syndrome 286.6
  Hemorrhagic fibrinogenolysis 286.6
DC-60026 Purpura fulminans 286.6
  Fibrinolytic purpura 286.6
DC-60030 Systemic fibrinogenolysis 286.6
DC-60040 Hyperheparinemia
DC-60050 Familial hemorrhagic diathesis, NOS 287.9
DC-60060 White clot syndrome

C-61 PLATELET DISORDERS

DC-61000 Platelet disorder, NOS 287.5
DC-61010 Thrombocytopenia, NOS 287.8
DC-61020 Thrombocytopenia due to diminished platelet production
DC-61030 Thrombocytopenia due to defective platelet production
DC-61040 Congenital thrombocytopenia 287.3
  Hereditary thrombocytopenia 287.3
DC-61050 Amegakaryocytic thrombocytopenia with congenital malformation 287.3
  Megakaryocytic hypoplasia 287.3
DC-61060 Sex-linked thrombocytopenia
DC-61070 Mediterranean macrothrombocytopenia
DC-61080 Neonatal thrombocytopenia
DC-61090 Acquired thrombocytopenia 287.4
  Secondary thrombocytopenia 287.4
DC-61100 Cyclic thrombocytopenia 287.3
  Tidal platelet dysgenesis 287.3
DC-61110 Thrombocytopenia due to non-immune destruction, NOS
DC-61120 Kasabach-Merritt syndrome
  Thrombocytopenia-hemangioma syndrome
DC-61130 Thrombotic thrombocytopenic purpura 446.6
  Moschowitz's syndrome 446.6
  TTP 446.6
  Thrombotic microangiopathy 446.6
DC-61136 Dilutional thrombocytopenia 287.4
DC-61140 Heparin-induced thrombocytopenia
DC-61300 Thrombocytopenia due to immune destruction, NOS
  Thrombocytopenia due to platelet alloimmunization
DC-61310 Neonatal alloimmune thrombocytopenia
  Neonatal isoimmune thrombocytopenia
  NATP
DC-61320 Neonatal thrombocytopenia associated with maternal idiopathic thrombocytopenic purpura
DC-61340 T activation syndrome
DC-61500 Idiopathic thrombocytopenic purpura, NOS 287.3
  ITP, NOS
DC-61510 Drug-induced thrombocytopenic purpura 287.4
  Drug-induced ITP 287.4
DC-61520 Post infectious thrombocytopenic purpura
  ITP secondary to infection
DC-61530 Acute idiopathic thrombocytopenic purpura
DC-61600 Chronic idiopathic thrombocytopenic purpura, NOS
  Chronic thrombocytopenic purpura, NOS

C-61 PLATELET DISORDERS — Continued

DC-61600 (cont.) Werlhof's disease
  Purpura hemorrhagica
  Autoimmune thrombocytopenia
DC-61610 Posttransfusion purpura, NOS 287.4
DC-61630 Purpura rheumatica 287.0
  Peliosis rheumatica 287.0
DC-61800 Thrombocytopenia due to sequestration, NOS
DC-61810 Thrombocytopenia due to hypersplenism
DC-61820 Thrombocytopenia due to hypothermia
  Thrombocytopenia due to cold
DC-61830 Thrombocytopenia due to blood loss 287.4
DC-61840 Thrombocytopenia due to extracorporal circulation 287.4
DC-61850 Thrombocytosis
  Increased platelets
DC-61900 Qualitative platelet disorder, NOS 287.1
  Thromboasthenia, NOS 287.1
DC-61910 Bernard Soulier syndrome 287.1
DC-61920 Hereditary thromboasthenia, NOS 287.1
  Glanzmann thromboasthenia
DC-61930 Platelet secretory disorder, NOS
DC-61940 Gray platelet syndrome
  Deficient alpha granule syndrome
DC-61950 Hermansky-Pudlack syndrome
  Alpha storage pool disease
DC-61960 Nucleotide storage pool disorder
  Platelet dense granule deficiency
  Delta storage pool disease
DC-61970 Platelet procoagulant activity deficiency
DC-61980 Platelet dysfunction due to drugs, NOS
DC-61990 Platelet dysfunction due to aspirin

C-62 PURPURAS

DC-62010 Non allergic purpura, NOS
DC-62020 Purpura simplex 287.2
  Simple bruising 287.2
DC-62030 Mechanical purpura
DC-62040 Senile purpura 287.2
DC-62050 Factitious purpura
DC-62060 Steroid purpura
DC-62070 Infection-associated purpura
DC-62200 Allergic purpura 287.0
DC-62204 Autoimmune purpura 287.0
  Henoch-Schonlein purpura 287.0
  Anaphylactoid purpura 287.0
  Henoch's purpura 287.0
DC-62220 Vascular hemostatic disease, NOS 287.0
  Vascular purpura 287.0
DC-62230 Capillary fragility abnormality, NOS 287.8

C-63 COAGULATION FACTOR DEFICIENCY SYNDROMES

DC-63000 Coagulation factor deficiency syndrome, NOS 286,9
  Coagulation factor disorder, NOS 286.9
DC-63002 Hereditary coagulation factor deficiency, NOS 286.9
DC-63004 Acquired coagulation factor deficiency, NOS 286.9
DC-63010 Hereditary factor I deficiency disease, NOS
  Hereditary hypofibrinogenemia
  Congenital hypofibrinogenemia
  Congenital afibrinogenemia
DC-63014 Acquired hypofibrinogenemia 286.3
  Fibrinogen deficiency 286.3
DC-63020 Factor II deficiency, NOS 286.3
  Prothrombin deficiency, NOS 286.3
DC-63030 Hereditary factor II deficiency disease 286.3
  Hereditary hypoprothrombinemia 286.3
DC-63040 Hemorrhagic disease of the newborn due to factor II deficiency 286.3
  Acquired neonatal factor II deficiency disease 286.3
DC-63042 Acquired hypoprothrombinemia, NOS 286.3
DC-63050 Factor V deficiency, NOS 286.3
DC-63060 Hereditary factor V deficiency disease 286.3
  Parahemophilia 286.3
  Hereditary hypoproaccelerinemia 286.3
  Owren's disease 286.3
  Labile factor deficiency 286.3
  AC globulin deficiency 286.3
DC-63070 Acquired factor V deficiency disease 286.3
  Acquired hypoproaccelerinemia 286.3
DC-63080 Factor VII deficiency, NOS 286.3
  Stable factor deficiency, NOS 286.3
DC-63082 Hereditary factor VII deficiency syndrome 286.3
  Hereditary hypoproconvertinemia 286.3
DC-63090 Acquired factor VII deficiency disease 286.3
  Acquired hypoproconvertinemia 286.3
DC-63100 Hemophilia, NOS
DC-63120 Hemophilia A, NOS 286.0
  Hereditary factor VIII deficiency disease 286.0
  Classical hemophilia 286.0
  AHG deficiency disease 286.0
  Sex-linked factor VIII deficiency 286.0
  Congenital factor VIII deficiency disease 286.0
DC-63121 Severe hemophilia A
  Less than 1% of normal factor VIII
DC-63122 Moderate hemophilia A
  1-5% of normal factor VIII
DC-63123 Mild hemophilia A
  6-60% of normal factor VIII
DC-63130 Acquired factor VIII deficiency disease
DC-63160 Hemophilia B, NOS 286.1
  Hereditary factor IX deficiency disease 286.1
  Christmas disease
  Sex-linked factor IX deficiency disease
  PTC deficiency disease 286.1
DC-63170 Acquired factor IX deficiency disease
DC-63200 Factor X deficiency, NOS 286.3
DC-63210 Hereditary factor X deficiency disease 286.3
  Hereditary Stuart factor deficiency disease 286.3

DC-63210 (cont.) Hereditary Stuart-Prower deficiency disease 286.3
DC-63220 Acquired factor X deficiency disease
  Acquired Stuart factor deficiency disease
DC-63240 Hereditary factor XI deficiency disease 286.2
  Hemophilia C 286.2
  Congenital factor XI deficiency disease 286.2
  Plasma thromboplastin antecedent deficiency 286.2
  PTA deficiency 286.2
  Rosenthal's disease 286.2
DC-63241 Factor XI deficiency, type I
DC-63242 Factor XI deficiency, type II
DC-63243 Factor XI deficiency, type III
DC-63250 Acquired factor XI deficiency disease
DC-63300 Factor XII deficiency disease, NOS
DC-63304 Hereditary factor XII deficiency disease 286.3
  Hereditary Hageman factor deficiency disease 286.3
DC-63308 Acquired factor XII deficiency disease 286.3
  Acquired Hageman factor deficiency disease 286.3
DC-63320 Factor XIII deficiency disease, NOS 286.3
  Fibrin stabilizing factor deficiency 286.3
DC-63330 Hereditary factor XIII deficiency disease 286.3
  Laki-Lorand factor deficiency disease 286.3
DC-63340 Acquired factor XIII deficiency disease
DC-63400 Prekallikrein deficiency
  Fletcher factor deficiency
DC-63410 High molecular weight kininogen deficiency
  Fitzgerald factor deficiency
DC-63500 Familial multiple factor deficiency syndrome, NOS
  FMFD syndrome
DC-63510 Familial multiple factor deficiency syndrome, type I
  FMFD syndrome, type I
  Factor V and factor VIII deficiency
DC-63520 Familial multiple factor deficiency syndrome, type II
  FMFD syndrome, type II
  Factor VIII and factor IX deficiency
DC-63530 Familial multiple factor deficiency syndrome, type III
  Factors II, VII, IX and X deficiency
  FMFD syndrome, type III
DC-63540 Familial multiple factor deficiency syndrome, type IV
  FMFD syndrome, type IV
  Factors VII and VIII deficiency
DC-63550 Familial multiple factor deficiency syndrome, type V
  FMFD syndrome, type V
  Factors VIII, IX and XI deficiency
DC-63560 Familial multiple factor deficiency syndrome, type VI
  FMFD syndrome, type VI
  Factor IX and factor XI deficiency
DC-63580 Vitamin K deficiency coagulation disorder, NOS 286.7
  Bleeding diathesis due to vitamin K deficiency 286.7

C-64 DYSFIBRINOGENEMIAS

DC-64000 Dysfibrinogenemia, NOS 286.3
DC-64010 Congenital dysfibrinogenemia, NOS 286.3
DC-64100 von Willebrand disease, NOS 286.4
  Angiohemophilia 286.4
  Factor VIII deficiency with vascular defect 286.4
  Pseudohemophilia type B 286.4
  Vascular hemophilia 286.4
  von Willebrand-Jürgens disease 286.4
  Constitutional thrombopathy 286.4
DC-64110 von Willebrand disease, type 1[a] 286.4
DC-64120 von Willebrand disease, type IS/III 286.4
DC-64130 von Willebrand disease, type IIA 286.4
DC-64140 von Willebrand disease, type IIB 286.4
DC-64150 von Willebrand disease, type IIC 286.4
DC-64160 von Willebrand disease, type IID 286.4
DC-64170 von Willebrand disease, type IIE 286.4
DC-64180 von Willebrand disease, type IIF 286.4
DC-64190 von Willebrand disease, type IIG 286.4
DC-64200 von Willebrand disease, type IIH 286.4
DC-64210 von Willebrand disease, platelet type 286.4
  von Willebrand disease, pseudo type 286.4
DC-64280 Acquired von Willebrand disease 286.4

C-65 ANTICOAGULANT DISORDERS

DC-65100 Circulating anticoagulant disorder, NOS 286.5
  Acquired anticoagulants, NOS 286.5
  Acquired inhibitor of coagulation, NOS 286.5
DC-65110 Factor VIII inhibitor disorder, NOS 286.5
DC-65120 Factor IX inhibitor disorder 286.5
DC-65130 Factor X inhibitor disorder
DC-65140 Factor XI inhibitor disorder 286.5
DC-65150 Factor XIII inhibitor disorder 286.5
DC-65160 Factor I inhibitor disorder 286.5
  Fibrinogen-fibrin inhibitor disorder 286.5
DC-65170 von Willebrand factor inhibitor disorder 286.5
DC-65180 Factor V inhibitor disorder 286.5
DC-65190 Drug-induced coagulation inhibitor, NOS 286.5
DC-65200 Lupus anticoagulant disorder 286.5
  Antiphospholipid syndrome 286.5
  Lupus anticoagulant inhibitor syndrome 286.5
  SLE inhibitor syndrome 286.5
DC-65220 Non-immune anticoagulant disorder, NOS
DC-65250 Anticoagulant overdosage, NOS
DC-65260 Warfarin overdosage

C-71 DISEASES OF THE TONSILS AND ADENOIDS — Continued

SECTION C-7 DISEASES OF THE LYMPHOID TISSUES

C-71 DISEASES OF THE TONSILS AND ADENOIDS

DC-71100 Disease of tonsils and adenoids, NOS 463.-
DC-71110 Disease of tonsils, NOS 463.-
DC-71200 Tonsillitis, NOS 463.-
(T-C5100) (M-40000)
DC-71210 Acute tonsillitis 463.-
(T-C5100) (M-41000)
Infective tonsillitis 463.-
(T-C5100) (M-41000)
DC-71220 Follicular tonsillitis 463.-
(T-C5100) (M-43020)
DC-71230 Gangrenous tonsillitis 463.-
(T-C5100) (M-40700)
DC-71240 Suppurative tonsillitis 463.-
(T-C5100) (M-40600)
Septic tonsillitis 463.-
(T-C5100) (M-40600)
DC-71250 Ulcerative tonsillitis 463.-
(T-C5100) (M-40750)
DC-71400 Chronic disease of tonsils and adenoids, NOS 474.9
(M-40700)
DC-71410 Chronic tonsillitis
(T-C5100) (M-43000)
DC-71420 Hypertrophy of tonsils and adenoids 474.10
(T-C5100) (T-C5300) (M-71000)
Enlargement of tonsils and adenoids 474.10
(T-C5100) (T-C5300) (M-71000)
DC-71430 Hyperplasia of tonsils and adenoids 474.10
(T-C5100) (T-C5300) (M-72000)
DC-71440 Hypertrophy of tonsils 474.11
(T-C5100) (M-71000)
Enlargement of tonsils 474.11
(T-C5100) (M-71000)
DC-71450 Hyperplasia of tonsils 474.11
(T-C5100) (M-72000)
DC-71460 Amygdalolith 474.8
(T-C5100) (M-30000)
Calculus of tonsil 474.8
(T-C5100) (M-30000)
DC-71470 Cicatrix of tonsil 474.8
(T-C5100) (M-78060)
DC-71480 Cicatrix of adenoid 474.8
(T-C5300) (M-78060)
DC-71490 Tonsillar tag 474.8
(T-C5100) (M-76822)
DC-7149A Ulcer of tonsil 474.8
(T-C5100) (M-38000)
DC-71600 Peritonsillar abscess 475.-
(T-C5230) (M-41610)
Peritonsillar cellulitis 475.-
(T-C5230) (M-41650)
Quinsy 475.-
(T-C5230) (M-41650)
DC-71610 Abscess of tonsil 475.-
(T-C5100) (M-41610)
DC-71700 Disease of adenoids, NOS
(T-C5300)
DC-71710 Hypertrophy of adenoids 474.12
(T-C5300) (M-71000)
Enlargement of adenoids 474.12
(T-C5300) (M-71000)
DC-71720 Hyperplasia of adenoids 474.12
(T-C5300) (M-72000)
Adenoid vegetations 474.2
(T-C5300) (M-72000)

C-72 DISEASES OF THE LYMPH NODES

DC-72000 Disease of lymph node, NOS
DC-72010 Lymphadenitis, NOS 289.3
(T-C4000) (M-40000)
Adenitis, NOS 289.3
(T-C4000) (M-40000)
DC-72020 Acute lymphadenitis except mesenteric 683.-
DC-72100 Chronic lymphadenitis, NOS 289.1
(T-C4000) (M-43000)
Chronic adenitis, NOS 289.1
(T-C4000) (M-43000)
DC-72110 Mesenteric lymphadenitis, NOS 289.2
(T-C4510) (M-40000)
DC-72120 Lymph node abscess 683.-
DC-72130 Enlargement of lymph nodes, NOS 785.6
Unspecified lymphadenopathy 785.6
Swelling of lymph nodes, NOS 785.6
DC-72200 Dermatopathic lymphadenitis
Dermatopathic lymphadenopathy
Lipomelanotic reticuloendothelial cell hyperplasia
DC-72210 Angiolymphoid hyperplasia
Pseudopyogenic granuloma
Benign angiofollicular hyperplasia
Angiomatous lymphoid hamartoma
Castleman's disease
Kimura's disease
DC-72250 Piringer-Kuchinka's syndrome
Piringer's lymphadenitis

SECTION C-8 DISEASES OF THE SPLEEN

DC-80000 Splenic disorder, NOS 289.50
Splenic syndrome, NOS 289.50
Disease of spleen, NOS 289.50
DC-80050 Unspecified splenomegaly 789.2
Enlargement of spleen, NOS 789.2
DC-80100 Hypersplenism, NOS 289.4
Big spleen syndrome 289.4
Dyssplenism 289.4
Hypersplenia 289.4
(T-C3000) (M-71000)

DC-80110 Doan-Wright syndrome 288.0
Splenic pancytopenia syndrome 288.0
DC-80120 Doan-Wiseman syndrome 288.0
Primary splenic neutropenia syndrome 288.0
Neutropenic splenomegaly 288.0
DC-80130 Hyposplenism
DC-80140 Congenital asplenia
DC-80150 Congestive splenomegaly 289.51
Banti syndrome
DC-80160 Splenic infarction 289.59
(T-C3000) (M-54700)
DC-80162 Splenic atrophy 289.59
(T-C3000) (M-58000)
DC-80170 Splenic cyst 289.59
(T-C3000) (M-33400)
DC-80172 Splenic fibrosis 289.59
(T-C3000) (M-78000)
DC-80180 Nontraumatic splenic rupture 289.59
(T-C3000) (M-14400)
DC-80200 Splenitis 289.59
(T-C3000) (M-40000)
DC-80204 Splenic abscess 289.59
(T-C3000) (M-41610)
DC-80210 Perisplenitis 289.59
(T-C3010) (M-40000)
DC-80250 Lien migrans 289.59
(T-C3000)
Wandering spleen 289.59
(T-C3000)
DC-80260 Splenosis
DC-80300 Splenic vein thrombosis
(T-48890) (M-35100)

SECTION C-9 DISEASES OF THE THYMUS GLAND

DC-90000 Disease of thymus gland, NOS 254.9
(T-C8000)
Disorder of thymus, NOS 254.9
(T-C8000)
DC-90100 Aplasia of thymus gland with immunodeficiency 279.2
(T-C8000) (M-75400) (F-C0450)
DC-90200 Dysplasia of thymus gland with immunodeficiency 279.2
(T-C8000) (M-74000) (F-C0450)
DC-90300 Hypertrophy of thymus 254.0
(T-C8000) (M-71000)
Persistent hyperplasia of thymus 254.0
(T-C8000) (M-72000)
DC-90500 Abscess of thymus 254.1
(T-C8000) (M-41610)
DC-90600 Atrophy of thymus gland 254.8
(T-C8000) (M-58000)
DC-90700 Cyst of thymus gland 254.8
(T-C8000) (M-33400)
DC-90790 Disease of thymus gland, NEC 254.9
(T-C8000)

CHAPTER D — INJURIES AND POISONINGS

SECTION D-0 INJURIES: GENERAL TERMS

DD-00100 Injury of face and neck, NOS 959.0
(T-D1200) (T-D1600) (M-10000)

DD-00101 Injury of neck 959.0
(T-D1600) (M-10000)

DD-00102 Injury of ear 959.0
(T-AB100) (M-10000)

DD-00103 Injury of eyebrow 959.0
(T-01520) (M-10000)

DD-00104 Injury of lip 959.0
(T-52000) (M-10000)

DD-00105 Injury of mouth 959.0
(T-51000) (M-10000)

DD-00106 Injury of nose 959.0
(T-21000) (M-10000)

DD-00107 Injury of throat 959.0
(T-D1602) (M-10000)
Injury of anterior neck 959.0
(T-D1602) (M-10000)

DD-00200 Injury of trunk, NOS 959.1
(T-D2000) (M-10000)

DD-00201 Injury of abdominal wall 959.1
(T-D4300) (M-10000)

DD-00202 Injury of back 959.1
(T-D2100) (M-10000)

DD-00203 Injury of buttock 959.1
(T-D2600) (M-10000)

DD-00204 Injury of interscapular region 959.1
(T-D2210) (M-10000)

DD-00210 Injury of breast 959.1
(T-04000) (M-10000)

DD-00212 Injury of chest wall 959.1
(T-D3050) (M-10000)

DD-00220 Injury of female external genital organs, NOS 959.1
(T-80010) (M-10000)

DD-00230 Injury of male external genital organs, NOS 959.1
(T-90010) (M-10000)

DD-00250 Injury of flank 959.1
(T-D2310) (M-10000)

DD-00252 Injury of groin 959.1
(T-D7000) (M-10000)

DD-00260 Injury of perineum 959.1
(T-D2700) (M-10000)

DD-00300 Injury of shoulder and upper arm, NOS 959.2
(T-D2220) (T-D8200) (M-10000)

DD-00310 Injury of axilla 959.2
(T-D8100) (M-10000)

DD-00320 Injury of scapular region 959.2
(T-D2200) (M-10000)

DD-00400 Injury of elbow, forearm and wrist 959.3
(T-D8300) (T-D8500) (T-D8600)
(M-10000)

DD-00410 Injury of hand, except finger 959.4
(T-D8700) (M-10000) (G-C030)
(T-D8800)

DD-00420 Injury of finger 959.5
(T-D8800) (M-10000)

DD-00500 Injury of hip and thigh 959.6
(T-D2500) (T-D9100) (M-10000)

DD-00510 Injury of upper leg 959.6
(T-D9100) (M-10000)
Injury to thigh 959.6
(T-D9100) (M-10000)

DD-00600 Injury of knee, leg, ankle and foot 959.7
(T-D9200) (T-D9400) (T-D9500)
(T-D9700) (M-10000)

SECTION D-1 INJURIES OF THE MUSCULOSKELETAL SYSTEM
D-10 FRACTURES OF THE SKULL

DD-10000 Fracture of skull, NOS 803.-
(T-11100) (M-12000)

DD-10008 Multiple fractures of skull, NOS 803.-
(T-11100) (M-12800)

DD-10010 Fracture of vault of skull, NOS 800.-
(T-11195) (M-12000)

DD-10012 Fracture of frontal bone 800.-
(T-11110) (M-12000)

DD-10014 Fracture of parietal bone 800.-
(T-11120) (M-12000)

DD-10020 Closed fracture of vault of skull without intracranial injury 800.0
(T-11195) (M-12100) (G-C009)
(T-D1400) (M-10060)

DD-10030 Closed fracture of vault of skull with cerebral laceration and contusion 800.1
(T-11195) (T-12100) (G-C008)
(T-A0100) (M-14400) (M-14200)

DD-10040 Closed fracture of vault of skull with subarachnoid, subdural and extradural hemorrhage 800.2
(T-11195) (M-12100) (G-C008)
(T-A1502) (T-A1410) (T-A1310)
(M-37000)

DD-10050 Closed fracture of vault of skull with other and unspecified intracranial hemorrhage 800.3
(T-11195) (M-12100) (G-C008)
(T-D1400) (M-37000)

DD-10060 Closed fracture of vault of skull with intracranial injury of other and unspecified nature 800.4
(T-11195) (M-12100) (G-C008)
(T-D1400) (M-10060)

DD-10070 Open fracture of vault of skull without intracranial injury 800.5
(T-11195) (M-12200) (G-C009)
(T-D1400) (M-10060)

DD-10080 Open fracture of vault of skull with cerebral laceration and contusion 800.6
(T-11195) (M-12200) (G-C008) (T-A0100) (M-14400) (M-14200)

DD-10090 Open fracture of vault of skull with subarachnoid, subdural and extradural hemorrhage 800.7
(T-11195) (M-12200) (G-C008) (T-A1502) (T-A1410) (T-A1310) (M-37000)

DD-100A0 Open fracture of vault of skull with other and unspecified intracranial hemorrhage 800.8
(T-11195) (M-12200) (G-C008) (T-D1400) (M-37000)

DD-100B0 Open fracture of vault of skull with intracranial injury of other and unspecified nature 800.9
(T-11195) (M-12200) (G-C008) (T-D1400) (M-10060)

DD-10100 Fracture of base of skull, NOS 801.-
(T-11000) (T-D1451) (M-12000)

DD-10101 Fracture of anterior fossa 801.-
(T-11000) (T-D1420) (M-12000)

DD-10102 Fracture of middle fossa 801.-
(T-11000) (T-D1430) (M-12000)

DD-10103 Fracture of posterior fossa 801.-
(T-11000) (T-D1450) (M-12000)

DD-10104 Fracture of occipital bone 801.-
(T-11140) (M-12000)

DD-10105 Fracture of orbital roof 801.-
(T-D1484) (M-12000)

DD-10106 Fracture of ethmoid sinus 801.-
(T-22300) (M-12000)

DD-10107 Fracture of frontal sinus 801.-
(T-22200) (M-12000)

DD-10108 Fracture of temporal bone 801.-
(T-11130) (M-12000)

DD-10109 Fracture of sphenoid bone 801.-
(T-11131) (M-12000)

DD-10110 Closed fracture of base of skull without mention of intracranial injury 801.0
(T-11000) (T-D1451) (M-12100) (G-C009) (T-D1400) (M-10060)

DD-10120 Closed fracture of base of skull with cerebral laceration and contusion 801.1
(T-11000) (T-D1451) (M-12100) (G-C008) (T-A0100) (M-14400) (M-14200)

DD-10130 Closed fracture of base of skull with subarachnoid, subdural and extradural hemorrhage 801.2
(T-11000) (T-D1451) (M-12100) (G-C008) (T-A1502) (T-A1410) (T-A1310) (M-37000)

DD-10140 Closed fracture of base of skull with other and unspecified intracranial hemorrhage 801.3
(T-11000) (T-D1451) (M-12100) (G-C008) (T-D1400) (M-37000)

DD-10150 Closed fracture of base of skull with intracranial injury of other and unspecified nature 801.4
(T-11000) (T-D1451) (M-12100) (G-C008) (T-D1400) (M-10060)

DD-10160 Open fracture of base of skull without intracranial injury 801.5
(T-11000) (T-D1451) (M-12200) (G-C009) (T-D1400) (M-10060)

DD-10170 Open fracture of base of skull with cerebral laceration and contusion 801.6
(T-11000) (T-D1451) (M-12200) (G-C008) (T-A0100) (M-14400) (M-14200)

DD-10180 Open fracture of base of skull with subarachnoid, subdural and extradural hemorrhage 801.7
(T-11000) (T-D1451) (M-12200) (G-C008) (T-A1502) (T-A1410) (T-A1310) (M-37000)

DD-10190 Open fracture of base of skull with other and unspecified intracranial hemorrhage 801.8
(T-11000) (T-D1451) (M-12200) (G-C008) (T-D1400) (M-37000)

DD-101A0 Open fracture of base of skull with intracranial injury of other and unspecified nature 801.9
(T-11000) (T-D1451) (M-12200) (G-C008) (T-D1400) (M-10060)

DD-10200 Fracture of face bones, NOS 802.-
(T-11000) (T-D1200) (M-12000)

DD-10210 Closed fracture of nasal bones 802.0
(T-11149) (M-12100)

DD-10215 Open fracture of nasal bones 802.1
(T-11149) (M-12200)

DD-10220 Closed fracture of mandible, NOS 802.20
(T-11180) (M-12100)
Closed fracture of inferior maxilla 802.20
(T-11180) (M-12100)
Closed fracture of lower jaw bone 802.20
(T-11180) (M-12100)

DD-10221 Closed fracture of condylar process of mandible 802.21
(T-11185) (M-12100)

DD-10222 Closed subcondylar fracture of mandible 802.22
(T-11187) (M-12100)

DD-10223 Closed fracture of coronoid process of mandible 802.23
(T-11188) (M-12100)

DD-10224 Closed fracture of ramus of mandible 802.24
(T-11184) (M-12100)

DD-10225 Closed fracture of angle of jaw 802.25
(T-11189) (M-12100)

DD-10226 Closed fracture of symphysis of body of mandible 802.26
(T-11181) (M-12100)

D-10 FRACTURES OF THE SKULL — Continued

DD-10227 Closed fracture of alveolar border of body of mandible 802.27
(T-1118B) (M-12100)

DD-10228 Closed fracture of body of mandible, NOS 802.28
(T-11181) (M-12100)

DD-10229 Closed fracture of multiple sites of mandible 802.29
(T-11180) (M-12810)

DD-10230 Open fracture of mandible, NOS 802.30
(T-11180) (M-12200)

DD-10231 Open fracture of condylar process of mandible 802.31
(T-11185) (M-12200)

DD-10232 Open subcondylar fracture of mandible 802.32
(T-11187) (M-12200)

DD-10233 Open fracture of coronoid process of mandible 802.33
(T-11188) (M-12200)

DD-10234 Open fracture of ramus of mandible 802.34
(T-11184) (M-12200)

DD-10235 Open fracture of angle of jaw 802.35
(T-11189) (M-12200)

DD-10236 Open fracture of symphysis of body of mandible 802.36
(T-11181) (M-12200)

DD-10237 Open fracture of alveolar border of body of mandible 802.37
(T-1118B) (M-12200)

DD-10238 Open fracture of body of mandible, NOS 802.38
(T-11181) (M-12200)

DD-10239 Open fracture of multiple sites of mandible 802.39
(T-11180) (M-12820)

DD-10240 Closed fracture of malar and maxillary bones, NOS 802.4
(T-11166) (T-11170) (M-12100)

DD-10241 Closed fracture of superior maxilla 802.4
(T-11170) (M-12100)
Closed fracture of upper jaw bone 802.4
(T-11170) (M-12100)

DD-10242 Closed fracture of zygoma 802.4
(T-11168) (M-12100)

DD-10243 Closed fracture of zygomatic arch 802.4
(T-11167) (M-12100)

DD-10245 Open fracture of malar and maxillary bones 802.5
(T-11166) (T-11170) (M-12200)

DD-10246 Open fracture of superior maxilla 802.4
(T-11170) (M-12200)
Open fracture of upper jaw bone 802.4
(T-11170) (M-12200)

DD-10247 Open fracture of zygoma 802.4
(T-11168) (M-12200)

DD-10248 Open fracture of zygomatic arch 802.4
(T-11167) (M-12200)

DD-10250 Closed fracture of orbital floor (blow-out) 802.6
(T-D1485) (M-12100)

DD-10255 Open fracture of orbital floor (blow-out) 802.7
(T-D1485) (M-12200)

DD-10257 Closed fracture of alveolus 802.8
(T-11177) (M-12100)

DD-10258 Closed fracture of orbit 802.8
(T-D1480) (M-12100)

DD-10259 Closed fracture of palate 802.8
(T-11160) (M-12100)

DD-1025A Open fracture of other facial bones 802.9
(T-11000) (T-D1200) (M-12200)

DD-10400 Closed skull fracture without intracranial injury 803.0
(T-11100) (M-12100) (G-C009)
(T-D1400) (M-10060)

DD-10410 Closed skull fracture with cerebral laceration and contusion 803.1
(T-11100) (M-12100) (G-C008)
(T-A0100) (M-14400) (M-14200)

DD-10420 Closed skull fracture with subarachnoid, subdural and extradural hemorrhage 803.2
(T-11100) (M-12100) (G-C008)
(T-A1502) (T-A1410) (T-A1310)
(M-37000)

DD-10430 Closed skull fracture with other and unspecified intracranial hemorrhage 803.3
(T-11100) (M-12100) (G-C008)
(T-D1400) (M-37000)

DD-10440 Closed skull fracture with intracranial injury of other and unspecified nature 803.4
(T-11100) (M-12100) (G-C008)
(T-D1400) (M-10060)

DD-10450 Open skull fracture without intracranial injury 803.5
(T-11100) (M-12200) (G-C009)
(T-D1400) (M-10060)

DD-10460 Open skull fracture with cerebral laceration and contusion 803.6
(T-11100) (M-12200) (G-C008)
(T-A0100) (M-14400) (M-14200)

DD-10470 Open skull fracture with subarachnoid, subdural and extradural hemorrhage 803.7
(T-11100) (M-12200) (G-C008)
(T-A1502) (T-A1410) (T-A1310)
(M-37000)

DD-10480 Open skull fracture with other and unspecified intracranial hemorrhage 803.8
(T-11100) (M-12200) (G-C008)
(T-D1400) (M-37000)

DD-10490 Open skull fracture with intracranial injury of other and unspecified nature 803.9
(T-11100) (M-12200) (G-C008)
(T-D1400) (M-10060)

DD-10500 Multiple closed fractures of skull and face without intracranial injury, NOS 804.0
(T-11100) (T-11000) (T-D1200)
(M-12810) (G-C009) (T-D1400)
(M-10060)

DD-10510 Multiple closed fractures of skull and face with cerebral laceration and contusion 804.1
(T-11100) (T-11000) (T-D1200)
(M-12810) (G-C008) (T-A0100)
(M-14400) (M-14200)

DD-10520 Multiple closed fractures of skull and face with subarachnoid, subdural and extradural hemorrhage 804.2
(T-11100) (T-11000) (T-D1200)
(M-12810) (G-C008) (T-A1502)
(T-A1410) (T-A1310) (M-37000)

DD-10530 Multiple closed fractures of skull and face with other and unspecified intracranial hemorrhage 804.3
(T-11100) (T-11000) (T-D1200)
(M-12810) (G-C008) (T-D1400)
(M-37000)

DD-10540 Multiple closed fractures of skull and face with intracranial injury of other and unspecified nature 804.4
(T-11100) (T-11000) (T-D1200)
(M-12810) (G-C008) (T-D1400)
(M-10060)

DD-10550 Multiple open fractures of skull and face without intracranial injury 804.5
(T-11100) (T-11000) (T-D1200)
(M-12820) (G-C009) (T-D1400)
(M-10060)

DD-10560 Multiple open fractures of skull and face with cerebral laceration and contusion 804.6
(T-11100) (T-11000) (T-D1200)
(M-12820) (G-C008) (T-A0100)
(M-14400) (M-14200)

DD-10570 Multiple open fractures of skull and face with subarachnoid, subdural and extradural hemorrhage 804.7
(T-11100) (T-11000) (T-D1200)
(M-12820) (G-C008) (T-A1502)
(T-A1410) (T-A1310) (M-37000)

DD-10580 Multiple open fractures of skull and face with other and unspecified intracranial hemorrhage 804.8
(T-11100) (T-11000) (T-D1200)
(M-12820) (G-C008) (T-D1400)
(M-37000)

DD-10590 Multiple open fractures of skull and face with intracranial injury of other and unspecified nature 804.9
(T-11100) (T-11000) (T-D1200)
(M-12820) (G-C008) (T-D1400)
(M-10060)

D-11 FRACTURES OF THE NECK, TRUNK AND VERTEBRAL COLUMN

DD-11000 Fracture of neck and trunk, NOS
(T-D1600) (T-D2000) (M-12000)

DD-11002 Fracture of bones of trunk, NOS 809.-
(T-11000) (T-D2000) (M-12000)

DD-11004 Closed fracture of bones of trunk 809.0
(T-11000) (T-D2000) (M-12100)

DD-11006 Open fracture of bones of trunk 809.1
(T-11000) (T-D2000) (M-12200)

DD-11010 Fracture of vertebral column, NOS 805.-
(T-11500) (M-12000)
Fracture of spine 805.-
(T-11500) (M-12000)

DD-11020 Closed fracture of vertebral column, NOS 805.8
(T-11500) (M-12100)

DD-11030 Open fracture of vertebral column, NOS 805.9
(T-11500) (M-12200)

DD-11100 Fracture of vertebral column without spinal cord injury, NOS 805.-
(T-11500) (M-12000) (G-C009)
(T-A7010) (M-10000)

DD-11110 Closed fracture of vertebral column without spinal cord injury 805.8
(T-11500) (M-12100) (G-C009)
(T-A7010) (M-10000)

DD-11120 Open fracture of vertebral column without spinal cord injury 805.9
(T-11500) (M-12200) (G-C009)
(T-A7010) (M-10000)

DD-11130 Fracture of neural arch 805.-
(T-11511) (M-12000)

DD-11134 Fracture of spinous process of vertebra 805.-
(T-11512) (M-12000)

DD-11136 Fracture of transverse process of vertebra 805.-
(T-11513) (M-12000)

DD-11140 Closed fracture of cervical vertebra without spinal cord injury, NOS 805.00
(T-11600) (M-12100) (G-C009)
(T-A7600) (M-10000)

DD-11141 Closed fracture of first cervical vertebra without spinal cord injury 805.01
(T-11610) (M-12100) (G-C009)
(T-A7600) (M-10000)
Closed fracture of atlas without spinal cord injury 805.01
(T-11610) (M-12100) (G-C009)
(T-A7600) (M-10000)

DD-11142 Closed fracture of second cervical vertebra without spinal cord injury 805.02
(T-11620) (M-12100) (G-C009)
(T-A7600) (M-10000)
Closed fracture of axis without spinal cord injury 805.02
(T-11620) (M-12100) (G-C009)
(T-A7600) (M-10000)

D-11 FRACTURES OF THE NECK, TRUNK AND VERTEBRAL COLUMN — Continued

DD-11143 Closed fracture of third cervical vertebra without spinal cord injury 805.03
(T-11630) (M-12100) (G-C009) (T-A7600) (M-10000)

DD-11144 Closed fracture of fourth cervical vertebra without spinal cord injury 805.04
(T-11640) (M-12100) (G-C009) (T-A7600) (M-10000)

DD-11145 Closed fracture of fifth cervical vertebra without spinal cord injury 805.05
(T-11650) (M-12100) (G-C009) (T-A7600) (M-10000)

DD-11146 Closed fracture of sixth cervical vertebra without spinal cord injury 805.06
(T-11660) (M-12100) (G-C009) (T-A7600) (M-10000)

DD-11147 Closed fracture of seventh cervical vertebra without spinal cord injury 805.07
(T-11670) (M-12100) (G-C009) (T-A7600) (M-10000)

DD-11148 Closed fracture of multiple cervical vertebrae without spinal cord injury 805.08
(T-11600) (M-12810) (G-C009) (T-A7600) (M-10000)

DD-11150 Open fracture of cervical vertebra without spinal cord injury, NOS 805.10
(T-11600) (M-12200) (G-C009) (T-A7600) (M-10000)

DD-11151 Open fracture of first cervical vertebra without spinal cord injury 805.11
(T-11610) (M-12200) (G-C009) (T-A7600) (M-10000)
Open fracture of atlas without spinal cord injury 805.11
(T-11610) (M-12200) (G-C009) (T-A7600) (M-10000)

DD-11152 Open fracture of second cervical vertebra without spinal cord injury 805.12
(T-11620) (M-12200) (G-C009) (T-A7600) (M-10000)
Open fracture of axis without spinal cord injury 805.12
(T-11620) (M-12200) (G-C009) (T-A7600) (M-10000)

DD-11153 Open fracture of third cervical vertebra without spinal cord injury 805.13
(T-11630) (M-12200) (G-C009) (T-A7600) (M-10000)

DD-11154 Open fracture of fourth cervical vertebra without spinal cord injury 805.14
(T-11640) (M-12200) (G-C009) (T-A7600) (M-10000)

DD-11155 Open fracture of fifth cervical vertebra without spinal cord injury 805.15
(T-11650) (M-12200) (G-C009) (T-A7600) (M-10000)

DD-11156 Open fracture of sixth cervical vertebra without spinal cord injury 805.16
(T-11660) (M-12200) (G-C009) (T-A7600) (M-10000)

DD-11157 Open fracture of seventh cervical vertebra without spinal cord injury 805.17
(T-11670) (M-12200) (G-C009) (T-A7600) (M-10000)

DD-11158 Open fracture of multiple cervical vertebrae without spinal cord injury 805.18
(T-11600) (M-12820) (G-C009) (T-A7600) (M-10000)

DD-11160 Closed fracture of dorsal vertebra without spinal cord injury 805.2
(T-11700) (M-12100) (G-C009) (T-A7700) (M-10000)
Closed fracture of thoracic vertebra without spinal cord injury 805.2
(T-11700) (M-12100) (G-C009) (T-A7700) (M-10000)

DD-11170 Open fracture of dorsal vertebra without spinal cord injury 805.3
(T-11700) (M-12200) (G-CC09) (T-A7700) (M-10000)
Open fracture of thoracic vertebra without spinal cord injury 805.3
(T-11700) (M-12200) (G-C009) (T-A7700) (M-10000)

DD-11180 Closed fracture of lumbar vertebra without spinal cord injury 805.4
(T-11900) (M-12100) (G-C009) (T-A7801) (M-10000)

DD-11185 Open fracture of lumbar vertebra without spinal cord injury 805.5
(T-11900) (M-12200) (G-C009) (T-A7801) (M-10000)

DD-11190 Closed fracture of sacrum and coccyx without spinal cord injury 805.6
(T-11AD0) (T-11BF0) (M-12100) (G-C009) (T-A7802) (M-10000)

DD-11195 Open fracture of sacrum and coccyx without spinal cord injury 805.7
(T-11AD0) (T-11BF0) (M-12200) (G-C009) (T-A7802) (M-10000)

DD-11300 Fracture of vertebral column with spinal cord injury, NOS 806.-
(T-11500) (M-12000) (G-C008) (T-A7010) (M-10000)

DD-11310 Closed fracture of vertebral column with spinal cord injury 806.8
(T-11500) (M-12100) (G-C008) (T-A7010) (M-10000)

DD-11320 Open fracture of vertebral column with spinal cord injury 806.9
(T-11500) (M-12200) (G-C008) (T-A7010) (M-10000)

DD-11330 Closed fracture of cervical region with spinal cord injury, NOS 806.00
(T-11600) (M-12100) (G-C008) (T-A7600) (M-10000)

DD-11331 Closed fracture of C1-C4 level with unspecified spinal cord injury 806.00
(T-11610) (T-11640) (M-12100)
(G-C008) (T-A7602) (M-10000)

DD-11332 Closed fracture of C1-C4 level with complete lesion of cord 806.01
(T-11610) (T-11640) (M-12100)
(G-C008) (T-A7602) (M-17110)

DD-11333 Closed fracture of C1-C4 level with anterior cord syndrome 806.02
(T-11610) (T-11640) (M-12100)
(G-C008) (T-A7640) (M-10000)

DD-11334 Closed fracture of C1-C4 level with central cord syndrome 806.03
(T-11610) (T-11640) (M-12100)
(G-C008) (T-A7681) (M-10000)

DD-11335 Closed fracture of C1-C4 level with posterior cord syndrome 806.04
(T-11610) (T-11640) (M-12100)
(G-C008) (T-A7620) (M-10000)

DD-11336 Closed fracture of C1-C4 level with incomplete cord lesion, NOS 806.04
(T-11610) (T-11640) (M-12100)
(G-C008) (T-A7600) (M-10000)

DD-11337 Closed fracture of C1-C4 level with other specified spinal cord injury 806.04
(T-11610) (T-11640) (M-12100)
(G-C008) (T-A7600) (M-10000)

DD-11338 Closed fracture of C5-C7 level with unspecified spinal cord injury 806.05
(T-11650) (T-11670) (M-12100)
(G-C008) (T-A7604) (M-10000)

DD-11339 Closed fracture of C5-C7 level with complete lesion of cord 806.06
(T-11650) (T-11670) (M-12100)
(G-C008) (T-A7600) (M-17110)

DD-1133A Closed fracture of C5-C7 level with anterior cord syndrome 806.07
(T-11650) (T-11670) (M-12100)
(G-C008) (T-A7640) (M-10000)

DD-1133B Closed fracture of C5-C7 level with central cord syndrome 806.08
(T-11650) (T-11670) (M-12100)
(G-C008) (T-A7681) (M-10000)

DD-1133C Closed fracture of C5-C7 level with posterior cord syndrome 806.09
(T-11650) (T-11670) (M-12100)
(G-C008) (T-A7620) (M-10000)

DD-1133D Closed fracture of C5-C7 level with incomplete spinal cord lesion, NOS 806.09
(T-11650) (T-11670) (M-12100)
(G-C008) (T-A7600) (M-10000)

DD-1133E Closed fracture of C5-C7 level with other specified spinal cord injury 806.09
(T-11650) (T-11670) (M-12100)
(G-C008) (T-A7600) (M-10000)

DD-11340 Open fracture of C1-C4 level with unspecified spinal cord injury 806.10
(T-11610) (T-11640) (M-12200)
(G-C008) (T-A7602) (T-10000)

DD-11341 Open fracture of C1-C4 level with complete lesion of cord 806.11
(T-11610) (T-11640) (M-12200)
(G-C008) (T-A7600) (M-17110)

DD-11342 Open fracture of C1-C4 level with anterior cord syndrome 806.12
(T-11610) (T-11640) (M-12200)
(G-C008) (T-A7640) (M-10000)

DD-11343 Open fracture of C1-C4 level with central cord syndrome 806.13
(T-11610) (T-11640) (M-12200)
(G-C008) (T-A7681) (M-10000)

DD-11344 Open fracture of C1-C4 level with posterior cord syndrome 806.14
(T-11610) (T-11640) (M-12200)
(G-C008) (T-A7620) (M-10000)

DD-11345 Open fracture of C1-C4 level with incomplete spinal cord lesion, NOS 806.14
(T-11610) (T-11640) (M-12200)
(G-C008) (T-A7600) (M-10000)

DD-11346 Open fracture of C1-C4 level with other specified spinal cord injury 806.14
(T-11610) (T-11640) (M-12200)
(G-C008) (T-A7600) (M-10000)

DD-11348 Open fracture of C5-C7 level with unspecified spinal cord injury 806.15
(T-11650) (T-11670) (M-12200)
(G-C008) (T-A7604) (M-10000)

DD-11349 Open fracture of C5-C7 level with complete lesion of cord 806.16
(T-11650) (T-11670) (M-12200)
(G-C008) (T-A7600) (M-17110)

DD-1134A Open fracture of C5-C7 level with anterior cord syndrome 806.17
(T-11650) (T-11670) (M-12200)
(G-C008) (T-A7600) (M-10000)

DD-1134B Open fracture of C5-C7 level with central cord syndrome 806.18
(T-11650) (T-11670) (M-12200)
(G-C008) (T-A7681) (M-10000)

DD-1134C Open fracture of C5-C7 level with posterior cord syndrome 806.19
(T-11650) (T-11670) (M-12200)
(G-C008) (T-A7620) (M-10000)

DD-1134D Open fracture of C5-C7 level with incomplete spinal cord lesion, NOS 806.19
(T-11650) (T-11670) (M-12200)
(G-C008) (T-A7604) (M-10000)

DD-1134E Open fracture of C5-C7 level with other specified spinal cord injury 806.19
(T-11650) (T-11670) (M-12200)
(G-C008) (T-A7600) (M-10000)

DD-11350 Closed fracture of thoracic region with spinal cord injury, NOS 806.20
(T-11700) (M-12100) (G-C008)
(T-A7700) (M-10000)

DD-11351 Closed fracture of T1-T6 level with unspecified spinal cord injury 806.20
(T-11710) (T-11760) (M-12100)
(G-C008) (T-A7700) (M-10000)

D-11 FRACTURES OF THE NECK, TRUNK AND VERTEBRAL COLUMN — Continued

DD-11352 Closed fracture of T1-T6 level with complete lesion of cord 806.21
(T-11710) (T-11760) (M-12100) (G-C008) (T-A7700) (M-17110)

DD-11353 Closed fracture of T1-T6 level with anterior cord syndrome 806.22
(T-11710) (T-11760) (M-12100) (G-C008) (T-A7740) (M-10000)

DD-11354 Closed fracture of T1-T6 level with central cord syndrome 806.23
(T-11710) (T-11760) (M-12100) (G-C008) (T-A7781) (M-10000)

DD-11355 Closed fracture of T1-T6 level with posterior cord syndrome 806.24
(T-11710) (T-11760) (M-12100) (G-C008) (T-A7720) (M-10000)

DD-11356 Closed fracture of T1-T6 level with incomplete spinal cord lesion, NOS 806.24
(T-11710) (T-11760) (M-12100) (G-C008) (T-A7700) (M-10000)

DD-11357 Closed fracture of T1-T6 level with other specified spinal cord injury 806.24
(T-11710) (T-11760) (M-12100) (G-C008) (T-A7700) (M-10000)

DD-11358 Closed fracture of T7-T12 level with unspecified spinal cord injury 806.25
(T-11770) (T-117C0) (M-12100) (G-C008) (T-A7700) (M-10000)

DD-11359 Closed fracture of T7-T12 level with complete lesion of cord 806.26
(T-11770) (T-117C0) (M-12100) (G-C008) (T-A7700) (M-17110)

DD-1135A Closed fracture of T7-T12 level with anterior cord syndrome 806.27
(T-11770) (T-117C0) (M-12100) (G-C008) (T-A7740) (M-10000)

DD-1135B Closed fracture of T7-T12 level with central cord syndrome 806.28
(T-11770) (T-117C0) (M-12100) (G-C008) (T-A7781) (M-10000)

DD-1135C Closed fracture of T7-T12 level with posterior cord syndrome 806.29
(T-11770) (T-117C0) (M-12100) (G-C008) (T-A7720) (M-10000)

DD-1135D Closed fracture of T7-T12 level with incomplete spinal cord lesion, NOS 806.29
(T-11770) (T-117C0) (M-12100) (G-C008) (T-A7700) (M-10000)

DD-1135E Closed fracture of T7-T12 level with other specified spinal cord injury 806.29
(T-11770) (T-117C0) (M-12100) (G-C008) (T-A7700) (M-10000)

DD-11360 Open fracture of thoracic region with spinal cord injury, NOS 806.30
(T-11700) (M-12200) (G-C008) (T-A7700) (M-10000)

DD-11361 Open fracture of T1-T6 level with unspecified spinal cord injury 806.30
(T-11710) (T-11760) (M-12200) (G-C008) (T-A7700) (M-10000)

DD-11362 Open fracture of T1-T6 level with complete lesion of cord 806.31
(T-11710) (T-11760) (M-12200) (G-C008) (T-A7700) (M-17110)

DD-11363 Open fracture of T1-T6 level with anterior cord syndrome 806.32
(T-11710) (T-11760) (M-12200) (G-C008) (T-A7740) (M-10000)

DD-11364 Open fracture of T1-T6 level with central cord syndrome 806.33
(T-11710) (T-11760) (M-12200) (G-C008) (T-A7781) (M-10000)

DD-11365 Open fracture of T1-T6 level with posterior cord syndrome 806.34
(T-11710) (T-11760) (M-12200) (G-C008) (T-A7720) (M-10000)

DD-11366 Open fracture of T1-T6 level with incomplete spinal cord lesion, NOS 806.34
(T-11710) (T-11760) (M-12200) (G-C008) (T-A7700) (M-10000)

DD-11367 Open fracture of T1-T6 level with other specified spinal cord injury 806.34
(T-11710) (T-11760) (M-12200) (G-C008) (T-A7700) (M-10000)

DD-11368 Open fracture of T7-T12 level with unspecified spinal cord injury 806.35
(T-11770) (T-117C0) (M-12200) (G-C008) (T-A7700) (M-10000)

DD-11369 Open fracture of T7-T12 level with complete lesion of cord 806.36
(T-11770) (T-117C0) (M-12200) (G-C008) (T-A7700) (M-17110)

DD-1136A Open fracture of T7-T12 level with anterior cord syndrome 806.37
(T-11770) (T-117C0) (M-12200) (G-C008) (T-A7740) (M-10000)

DD-1136B Open fracture of T7-T12 level with central cord syndrome 806.38
(T-11770) (T-117C0) (M-12200) (G-C008) (T-A7781) (M-10000)

DD-1136C Open fracture of T7-T12 level with posterior cord syndrome 806.39
(T-11770) (T-117C0) (M-12200) (G-C008) (T-A7720) (M-10000)

DD-1136D Open fracture of T7-T12 level with incomplete spinal cord lesion, NOS 806.39
(T-11770) (T-117C0) (M-12200) (G-C008) (T-A7700) (M-10000)

DD-1136E Open fracture of T7-T12 level with other specified spinal cord injury 806.39
(T-11770) (T-117C0) (M-12200) (G-C008) (T-A7700) (M-10000)

DD-11370 Closed fracture of lumbar vertebra with spinal cord injury 806.4
(T-11900) (M-12100) (G-C008) (T-A7801) (M-10000)

DD-11375 Open fracture of lumbar vertebra with spinal cord injury 806.5
(T-11900) (M-12200) (G-C008)
(T-A7801) (M-10000)

DD-11380 Closed fracture of sacrum and coccyx with unspecified spinal cord injury 806.60
(T-11AD0) (T-11BF0) (M-12100)
(G-C008) (T-A7802) (M-10000)

DD-11381 Closed fracture of sacrum and coccyx with complete cauda equina lesion 806.61
(T-11AD0) (T-11BF0) (M-12100)
(G-CC08) (T-A7900) (M-17110)

DD-11382 Closed fracture of sacrum and coccyx with other cauda equina injury 806.62
(T-11AD0) (T-11BF0) (M-12100)
(G-C008) (T-A7900) (M-10000)

DD-11383 Closed fracture of sacrum and coccyx with other spinal cord injury 806.69
(T-11AD0) (T-11BF0) (M-12100)
(G-C008) (T-A7802) (M-10000)

DD-11390 Open fracture of sacrum and coccyx with unspecified spinal cord injury 806.70
(T-11AD0) (T-11BF0) (M-12200)
(G-C008) (T-A7802) (M-10000)

DD-11391 Open fracture of sacrum and coccyx with complete cauda equina lesion 806.71
(T-11AD0) (T-11BF0) (M-12200)
(G-C008) (T-A7900) (M-17110)

DD-11392 Open fracture of sacrum and coccyx with other cauda equina injury 806.72
(T-11AD0) (T-11BF0) (M-12200)
(G-C008) (T-A7900) (M-10000)

DD-11393 Open fracture of sacrum and coccyx with other spinal cord injury 806.79
(T-11AD0) (T-11BF0) (M-12200)
(G-C008) (T-A7802) (M-10000)

DD-11400 Fracture of rib, NOS 807.-0
(T-11300) (M-12000)

DD-11401 Fracture of one rib 807.-1
(T-11300) (G-A721) (T-12000)

DD-11402 Fracture of two ribs 807.-2
(T-11300) (G-A722) (M-12000)

DD-11403 Fracture of three ribs 807.-3
(T-11300) (G-A723) (M-12000)

DD-11404 Fracture of four ribs 807.-4
(T-11300) (G-A724) (M-12000)

DD-11405 Fracture of five ribs 807.-5
(T-11300) (G-A725) (M-12000)

DD-11406 Fracture of six ribs 807.-6
(T-11300) (G-A726) (M-12000)

DD-11407 Fracture of seven ribs 807.-7
(T-11300) (G-A727) (M-12000)

DD-11408 Fracture of eight or more ribs 807.-8
(T-11300) (G-A728) (M-12000)

DD-11409 Fracture of multiple ribs, NOS 807.-9
(T-11300) (G-A445) (M-12800)

DD-11410 Closed fracture of rib, NOS 807.00
(T-11300) (M-12100)

DD-11411 Closed fracture of one rib 807.01
(T-11300) (G-A721) (M-12100)

DD-11412 Closed fracture of two ribs 807.02
(T-11300) (G-A722) (M-12100)

DD-11413 Closed fracture of three ribs 807.03
(T-11300) (G-A723) (M-12100)

DD-11414 Closed fracture of four ribs 807.04
(T-11300) (G-A724) (M-12100)

DD-11415 Closed fracture of five ribs 807.05
(T-11300) (G-A725) (M-12100)

DD-11416 Closed fracture of six ribs 807.06
(T-11300) (G-A726) (M-12100)

DD-11417 Closed fracture of seven ribs 807.07
(T-11300) (G-A727) (M-12100)

DD-11418 Closed fracture of eight or more ribs 807.08
(T-11300) (G-A728) (M-12100)

DD-11419 Closed fracture of multiple ribs, NOS 807.09
(T-11300) (G-A445) (M-12810)

DD-11420 Open fracture of rib, NOS 807.10
(T-11300) (M-12200)

DD-11421 Open fracture of one rib 807.11
(T-11300) (G-A721) (M-12200)

DD-11422 Open fracture of two ribs 807.12
(T-11300) (G-A722) (M-12200)

DD-11423 Open fracture of three ribs 807.13
(T-11300) (G-A723) (M-12200)

DD-11424 Open fracture of four ribs 807.14
(T-11300) (G-A724) (M-12200)

DD-11425 Open fracture of five ribs 807.15
(T-11300) (G-A725) (M-12200)

DD-11426 Open fracture of six ribs 807.16
(T-11300) (G-A726) (M-12200)

DD-11427 Open fracture of seven ribs 807.17
(T-11300) (G-A727) (M-12200)

DD-11428 Open fracture of eight or more ribs 807.18
(T-11300) (G-A728) (M-12200)

DD-11429 Open fracture of multiple ribs, NOS 807.19
(T-11300) (G-A445) (M-12820)

DD-11430 Fracture of sternum, NOS 807.-
(T-11210) (M-12000)

DD-11432 Closed fracture of sternum 807.2
(T-11210) (M-12100)

DD-11434 Open fracture of sternum 807.3
(T-11210) (M-12200)

DD-11438 Flail chest 807.4
(T-11200) (M-12000)

DD-11450 Fracture of larynx, NOS 807.-
(T-24100) (M-12000)

DD-11451 Closed fracture of larynx, NOS 807.5
(T-24100) (M-12100)

DD-11452 Closed fracture of trachea 807.5
(T-25000) (M-12100)

DD-11454 Closed fracture of hyoid bone 807.5
(T-11190) (M-12100)

DD-11456 Closed fracture of thyroid cartilage 807.5
(T-24160) (M-12100)

DD-11460 Open fracture of larynx 807.6
(T-24100) (M-12200)

D-11 FRACTURES OF THE NECK, TRUNK AND VERTEBRAL COLUMN — Continued

DD-11462 Open fracture of trachea 807.6
(T-25000) (M-12200)

DD-11500 Fracture of pelvis, NOS 808.-
(T-12380) (M-12000)

DD-11502 Closed fracture of pelvis, NOS 808.8
(T-12380) (M-12100)

DD-11504 Open fracture of pelvis, NOS 808.9
(T-12380) (M-12200)

DD-11510 Closed fracture of acetabulum 808.0
(T-12390) (M-12100)

DD-11512 Open fracture of acetabulum 808.1
(T-12390) (M-12200)

DD-11514 Closed fracture of pubis 808.2
(T-12360) (M-12100)

DD-11516 Open fracture of pubis 808.3
(T-12360) (M-12200)

DD-11520 Closed fracture of ilium 808.41
(T-12340) (M-12100)

DD-11522 Closed fracture of ischium 808.42
(T-12350) (M-12100)

DD-11524 Closed fracture of innominate bone 808.49
(T-12370) (M-12100)
Closed fracture of pelvic rim 808.49
(T-12370) (M-12100)

DD-11528 Multiple closed fractures of pelvis with disruption of pelvic circle 808.43
(T-12380) (M-12810) (G-C008) (M-31000)

DD-11530 Open fracture of ilium 808.51
(T-12340) (M-12200)

DD-11532 Open fracture of ischium 808.52
(T-12350) (M-12200)

DD-11534 Open fracture of innominate bone 808.59
(T-12370) (M-12200)
Open fracture of pelvic rim 808.59
(T-12370) (M-12200)

DD-11538 Multiple open fractures of pelvis with disruption of pelvic circle 808.53
(T-12380) (M-12820) (G-C008) (M-31000)

D-12 FRACTURES OF THE UPPER LIMB

DD-12000 Fracture of upper limb, NOS 818.-
(T-11000) (T-D8000) (M-12000)
Fracture of arm, NOS 818.-
(T-11000) (T-D8000) (M-12000)

DD-12010 Fracture of multiple bones of upper limb, NOS 818.-
(T-11000) (T-D8000) (M-12800)

DD-12011 Multiple fractures of both upper limbs, NOS 819.-
(T-11000) (T-D8000) (G-A102) (M-12800)
Multiple fractures of both arms, NOS 819.-
(T-11000) (T-D8000) (G-A102) (M-12800)

DD-12012 Multiple fractures of upper limb with ribs 819.-
(T-11000) (T-D8000) (T-11300) (M-12800)

DD-12013 Multiple fractures of upper limb with sternum 819.-
(T-11000) (T-D8000) (T-11210) (M-12800)

DD-12014 Multiple fractures of upper limb with sternum and ribs 819.-
(T-11000) (T-D8000) (T-11210) (T-11300) (M-12800)

DD-12020 Closed fracture of upper limb, NOS 818.0
(T-11000) (T-D8000) (M-12100)
Closed fracture of arm, NOS 818.0
(T-11000) (T-D8000) (M-12100)

DD-12030 Closed fracture of multiple bones of upper limb, NOS 818.0
(T-11000) (T-D8000) (M-12810)

DD-12031 Closed multiple fractures of both upper limbs, NOS 819.0
(T-11000) (T-D8000) (G-A102) (M-12810)
Closed multiple fractures of both arms, NOS 819.0
(T-11000) (T-D8000) (G-A102) (M-12810)

DD-12032 Closed multiple fractures of upper limb with ribs 819.0
(T-11000) (T-D8000) (T-11300) (M-12810)

DD-12033 Closed multiple fractures of upper limb with sternum 819.0
(T-11000) (T-D8000) (T-11210) (M-12810)

DD-12034 Closed multiple fractures of upper limb with sternum and ribs 819.0
(T-11000) (T-D8000) (T-11210) (T-11300) (M-12810)

DD-12040 Open fracture of upper limb, NOS 818.1
(T-11000) (T-D8000) (M-12200)
Open fracture of arm, NOS 818.1
(T-11000) (T-D8000) (M-12200)

DD-12050 Open fracture of multiple bones of upper limbs, NOS 818.1
(T-11000) (T-D8000) (M-12820)

DD-12051 Open multiple fractures of both upper limbs, NOS 819.1
(T-11000) (T-D8000) (G-A102) (M-12820)
Open multiple fractures of both arms, NOS 819.1
(T-11000) (T-D8000) (G-A102) (M-12820)

DD-12052 Open multiple fractures of upper limb with ribs 819.1
(T-11000) (T-D8000) (T-11300) (M-12820)

DD-12053 Open multiple fractures of upper limb with sternum 819.1
(T-11000) (T-D8000) (T-11210) (M-12820)

DD-12054 Open multiple fractures of upper limb with sternum and ribs 819.1
(T-11000) (T-D8000) (T-11210) (T-11300) (M-12820)

DD-12100 Fracture of clavicle, NOS 810.-0
(T-12310) (M-12000)
Fracture of collar bone 810.-0
(T-12310) (M-12000)

DD-12101 Fracture of sternal end of clavicle 810.-1
(T-12315) (M-12000)

DD-12102 Fracture of shaft of clavicle 810.-2
(T-12316) (M-12000)

DD-12103 Fracture of acromial end of clavicle 810.-3
(T-12317) (M-12000)

DD-12109 Fracture of interligamentous part of clavicle 810.-0
(T-12310) (M-12000)

DD-12110 Closed fracture of clavicle, NOS 810.00
(T-12310) (M-12100)

DD-12111 Closed fracture of sternal end of clavicle 810.01
(T-12315) (M-12100)

DD-12112 Closed fracture of shaft of clavicle 810.02
(T-12316) (M-12100)

DD-12113 Closed fracture of acromial end of clavicle 810.03
(T-12317) (M-12100)

DD-12120 Open fracture of clavicle, NOS 810.10
(T-12310) (M-12200)

DD-12121 Open fracture of sternal end of clavicle 810.11
(T-12315) (M-12200)

DD-12122 Open fracture of shaft of clavicle 810.12
(T-12316) (M-12200)

DD-12123 Open fracture of acromial end of clavicle 810.13
(T-12317) (M-12200)

DD-12140 Fracture of scapula, NOS 811.-0
(T-12280) (M-12000)
Fracture of shoulder blade, NOS 811.-0
(T-12280) (M-12000)

DD-12141 Fracture of acromial process of scapula 811.-1
(T-12281) (M-12000)
Fracture of acromion of scapula 811.-1
(T-12281) (M-12000)

DD-12142 Fracture of coracoid process of scapula 811.-2
(T-12282) (M-12000)

DD-12143 Fracture of glenoid cavity and neck of scapula 811.-3
(T-1228A) (T-12288) (M-12000)

DD-12144 Fracture of scapular body 811.-9
(T-1228D) (M-12000)

DD-12150 Closed fracture of scapula, NOS 811.00
(T-12280) (M-12100)
Closed fracture of shoulder blade, NOS 811.00
(T-12280) (M-12100)

DD-12151 Closed fracture of acromial process of scapula 811.01
(T-12281) (M-12100)
Closed fracture of acromion of scapula 811.01
(T-12281) (M-12100)

DD-12152 Closed fracture of coracoid process of scapula 811.02
(T-12282) (M-12100)

DD-12153 Closed fracture of glenoid cavity and neck of scapula 811.03
(T-1228A) (T-12288) (M-12100)

DD-12160 Open fracture of scapula, NOS 811.10
(T-12280) (M-12200)
Open fracture of shoulder blade 811.10
(T-12280) (M-12200)

DD-12161 Open fracture of acromial process of scapula 811.11
(T-12281) (M-12200)
Open fracture of acromion of scapula 811.11
(T-12281) (M-12200)

DD-12162 Open fracture of coracoid process of scapula 811.12
(T-12282) (M-12200)

DD-12163 Open fracture of glenoid cavity and neck of scapula 811.13
(T-1228A) (T-12288) (M-12200)

DD-12200 Fracture of humerus, NOS 812.-
(T-12410) (M-12000)
Fracture of upper arm, NOS 812.-
(T-12410) (M-12000)

DD-12202 Closed fracture of humerus, NOS 812.20
(T-12410) (M-12100)
Closed fracture of upper arm, NOS 812.20
(T-12410) (M-12100)

DD-12204 Open fracture of humerus, NOS 812.30
(T-12410) (M-12200)
Open fracture of upper arm, NOS 812.30
(T-12410) (M-12200)

DD-12210 Closed fracture of upper end of humerus, NOS 812.00
(T-1241C) (M-12100)
Closed fracture of proximal end of humerus 812.00
(T-1241C) (M-12100)

DD-12212 Closed fracture of surgical neck of humerus 812.01
(T-12413) (M-12100)
Closed fracture of neck of humerus, NOS 812.01
(T-12413) (M-12100)

D-12 FRACTURES OF THE UPPER LIMB — Continued

DD-12214 Closed fracture of anatomical neck of humerus 812.02
(T-12413) (M-12100)

DD-12216 Closed fracture of greater tuberosity of humerus 812.03
(T-12414) (M-12100)

DD-12218 Closed fracture of head of humerus 812.09
(T-12411) (M-12100)
Closed fracture of upper epiphysis of humerus 812.09
(T-12411) (M-12100)

DD-12220 Open fracture of upper end of humerus, NOS 812.10
(T-1241C) (M-12200)
Open fracture of proximal end of humerus 812.10
(T-1241C) (M-12200)

DD-12222 Open fracture of surgical neck of humerus 812.11
(T-12413) (M-12200)
Open fracture of neck of humerus, NOS 812.11
(T-12413) (M-12200)

DD-12224 Open fracture of anatomical neck of humerus 812.12
(T-12413) (M-12200)

DD-12226 Open fracture of greater tuberosity of humerus 812.13
(T-12414) (M-12200)

DD-12230 Fracture of shaft of humerus 812.21
(T-12412) (M-12000)

DD-12232 Closed fracture of shaft of humerus 812.2
(T-12412) (M-12100)

DD-12234 Open fracture of shaft of humerus 812.31
(T-12412) (M-12200)

DD-12240 Fracture of lower end of humerus, NOS 814.4
(T-1241E) (M-12000)
Fracture of distal end of humerus, NOS 814.4
(T-1241E) (M-12000)
Fracture of elbow, NOS 814.4
(T-1241E) (M-12000)

DD-12250 Closed fracture of lower end of humerus 812.40
(T-1241E) (M-12100)
Closed fracture of distal end of humerus 812.40
(T-1241E) (M-12100)
Closed fracture of elbow 812.40
(T-1241E) (M-12100)

DD-12251 Closed supracondylar fracture of humerus 812.41
(T-1241A) (M-12100)

DD-12252 Closed fracture of condyle of humerus, NOS 812.44
(T-12418) (T-12419) (M-12100)
Closed fracture of articular process of humerus, NOS 812.44
(T-12418) (M-12419) (M-12100)
Closed fracture of lower epiphysis of humerus, NOS 812.44
(T-12418) (T-12419) (M-12100)

DD-12253 Closed fracture of lateral condyle of humerus 812.42
(T-12419) (M-12100)
Closed fracture of external condyle of humerus 812.42
(T-12419) (M-12100)

DD-12254 Closed fracture of medial condyle of humerus 812.43
(T-12418) (M-12100)
Closed fracture of internal epicondyle of humerus 812.43
(T-12418) (M-12100)

DD-12256 Closed fracture of trochlea of humerus 812.49
(T-12417) (M-12100)

DD-12258 Closed multiple fractures of lower end of humerus 812.49
(T-1241E) (M-12810)

DD-12260 Open fracture of lower end of humerus 812.50
(T-1241E) (M-12200)
Open fracture of distal end of humerus 812.50
(T-1241E) (M-12000)
Open fracture of elbow 812.50
(T-1241E) (M-12200)

DD-12261 Open supracondylar fracture of humerus 812.51
(T-1241A) (M-12200)

DD-12262 Open fracture of condyle of humerus, NOS 812.54
(T-12418) (T-12419) (M-12200)
Open fracture of articular process of humerus 812.54
(T-12418) (T-12419) (M-12200)
Open fracture of lower epiphysis of humerus 812.54
(T-12418) (T-12419) (M-12200)

DD-12263 Open fracture of lateral condyle of humerus 812.52
(T-12419) (M-12200)
Open fracture of external condyle of humerus 812.52
(T-12419) (M-12200)

DD-12264 Open fracture of medial condyle of humerus 812.53
(T-12418) (M-12200)
Open fracture of internal epicondyle of humerus 812.53
(T-12418) (M-12200)

DD-12300 Fracture of forearm, NOS 813.-
(T-11000) (T-D8500) (M-12000)

DD-12302 Fracture of radius, NOS 813.-
(T-12420) (M-12000)

DD-12304 Fracture of ulna, NOS 813.-
(T-12430) (M-12000)

DD-12306 Fracture of radius and ulna, NOS 813.-
(T-12420) (T-12430) (M-12000)

DD-12310 Closed fracture of forearm, NOS 813.80
(T-11000) (T-D8500) (M-12100)

DD-12312 Closed fracture of radius 813.81
(T-12420) (M-12100)

DD-12314 Closed fracture of ulna 813.82
(T-12430) (M-12100)

DD-12316 Closed fracture of radius and ulna 813.83
(T-12420) (T-12430) (M-12100)

DD-12320 Open fracture of forearm, NOS 813.90
(T-11000) (T-D8500) (M-12200)

DD-12322 Open fracture of radius 813.91
(T-12420) (M-12200)

DD-12324 Open fracture of ulna 813.92
(T-12430) (M-12200)

DD-12326 Open fracture of radius and ulna 813.93
(T-12420) (T-12430) (M-12200)

DD-12330 Closed fracture of upper end of forearm, NOS 813.00
(T-1242A) (T-1243A) (M-12100)
Closed fracture of proximal end of forearm, NOS 813.00
(T-1242A) (T-1243A) (M-12100)

DD-12331 Closed fracture of olecranon process of ulna 813.01
(T-12431) (M-12100)

DD-12332 Closed fracture of coronoid process of ulna 813.02
(T-12432) (M-12100)

DD-12333 Closed Monteggia's fracture 813.03
(T-1243A) (M-12100) (G-C008)
(T-12421) (M-13000)

DD-12334 Closed fracture of proximal end of ulna 813.04
(T-1243A) (m-12100)

DD-12335 Closed multiple fractures of upper end of ulna 813.04
(T-1243A) (M-12810)

DD-12336 Closed fracture of head of radius 813.05
(T-12421) (M-12100)

DD-12337 Closed fracture of neck of radius 813.06
(T-12422) (M-12100)

DD-12338 Closed fracture of proximal end of radius 813.07
(T-1242A) (M-12100)

DD-12339 Closed multiple fractures of upper end of radius 813.07
(T-1242A) (M-12810)

DD-1233A Closed fracture of upper end of radius and ulna 813.08
(T-1242A) (T-1243A) (M-12100)

DD-12340 Open fracture of upper end of forearm, NOS 813.10
(T-1242A) (T-1243A) (M-12200)
Open fracture of proximal end of forearm, NOS 813.10
(T-1242A) (T-1243A) (M-12200)

DD-12341 Open fracture of olecranon process of ulna 813.11
(T-12431) (M-12200)

DD-12342 Open fracture of coronoid process of ulna 813.12
(T-12432) (M-12200)

DD-12343 Open Monteggia's fracture 813.13
(T-1243A) (M-12200) (G-C008)
(T-12421) (M-13000)

DD-12344 Open fracture of proximal end of ulna 813.14
(T-1243A) (M-12200)

DD-12345 Open multiple fractures of upper end of ulna 813.14
(T-1243A) (M-12820)

DD-12346 Open fracture of head of radius 813.15
(T-12421) (M-12200)

DD-12347 Open fracture of neck of radius 813.16
(T-12422) (M-12200)

DD-12348 Open fracture of proximal end of radius 813.17
(T-1242A) (M-12200)

DD-12349 Open multiple fractures of upper end of radius 813.17
(T-1242A) (M-12820)

DD-1234A Open fracture of upper end of radius and ulna 813.18
(T-1242A) (T-1243A) (M-12200)

DD-12350 Closed fracture of shaft of bone of forearm, NOS 813.20
(T-11050) (T-D8500) (M-12100)

DD-12351 Closed fracture of shaft of radius 813.21
(T-12423) (M-12100)

DD-12352 Closed fracture of shaft of ulna 813.22
(T-12435) (M-12100)

DD-12353 Closed fracture of shaft of radius and ulna 813.23
(T-12423) (T-12435) (M-12100)

DD-12360 Open fracture of shaft of bone of forearm, NOS 813.30
(T-11050) (T-D8500) (M-12200)

DD-12361 Open fracture of shaft of radius 813.31
(T-12423) (M-12200)

DD-12362 Open fracture of shaft of ulna 813.32
(T-12435) (M-12200)

DD-12363 Open fracture of shaft of radius and ulna 813.33
(T-12423) (T-12435) (M-12200)

DD-12370 Closed fracture of lower end of forearm, NOS 813.40
(T-1242E) (T-1243E) (M-12100)
Closed fracture of distal end of forearm, NOS 813.40
(T-1242E) (T-1243E) (M-12100)

DD-12371 Closed Colles' fracture 813.41
(T-1242B) (M-12100) (G-C008)
(M-31040)
Closed Smith's fracture 813.41
(T-1242B) (M-12100) (G-C008)
(M-31040)

D-12 FRACTURES OF THE UPPER LIMB — Continued

DD-12372 Closed fracture of distal end of radius, NOS 813.42
(T-1242B) (M-12100)
Closed fracture of lower end of radius, NOS 813.42
(T-1242B) (M-12100)

DD-12373 Dupuytren's fracture of radius 813.42
(T-1242B) (M-12100) (G-C008) (T-1243B) (M-13000)
Galeazzi's fracture of radius 813.42
(T-1242B) (M-12100) (G-C008) (T-1243B) (M-13000)

DD-12375 Closed fracture of distal end of ulna 813.43
(T-1243B) (M-12100)
Closed fracture of lower end of ulna 813.43
(T-1243B) (M-12100)
Closed fracture of lower epiphysis 813.43
(T-1243B) (M-12100)

DD-12376 Closed fracture of head of ulna 813.43
(T-12437) (M-12100)

DD-12377 Closed fracture of styloid process of ulna 813.43
(T-12438) (M-12100)

DD-12378 Closed fracture of lower end of radius and ulna 813.44
(T-1242B) (T-1243B) (M-12100)

DD-12380 Open fracture of lower end of forearm, NOS 813.50
(T-1242E) (T-1243E) (M-12200)
Open fracture of distal end of forearm, NOS 813.50
(T-1242E) (T-1243E) (M-12200)

DD-12381 Open Colles' fracture 813.51
(T-1242B) (M-12200) (G-C008) (M-31040)
Open Smith's fracture 813.51
(T-1242B) (M-12200) (G-C008) (M-31040)

DD-12382 Open fracture of distal end of radius, NOS 813.52
(T-1242B) (M-12200)

DD-12383 Open fracture of distal end of ulna 813.53
(T-1243B) (M-12200)

DD-12388 Open fracture of lower end of radius and ulna 813.54
(T-1242B) (T-1243B) (M-12200)

DD-12400 Fracture of carpal bone, NOS 814.-0
(T-12440) (M-12000)
Fracture of wrist, NOS 814.-0
(T-12440) (M-12000)

DD-12401 Fracture of navicular bone of wrist 814.-1
(T-12450) (M-12000)
Fracture of scaphoid bone of wrist 814.-1
(T-12450) (M-12000)

DD-12402 Fracture of lunate bone of wrist 814.-2
(T-12470) (M-12000)
Fracture of seminular bone of wrist 814.-2
(T-12470) (M-12000)

DD-12403 Fracture of triquetal bone of wrist 814.-3
(T-12510) (M-12000)
Fracture of cuneiform bone of wrist 814.-3
(T-12510) (M-12000)

DD-12404 Fracture of pisiform bone of wrist 814.-4
(T-12460) (M-12000)

DD-12405 Fracture of trapezium of wrist 814.-5
(T-12490) (M-12000)
Fracture of larger multangular bone of wrist 814.-5
(T-12490) (M-12000)

DD-12406 Fracture of trapezoidal bone of wrist 814.-6
(T-12520) (M-12000)
Fracture of small multangular bone of wrist 814.-6
(T-12520) (M-12000)

DD-12407 Fracture of capitate bone of wrist 814.-7
(T-12480) (M-12000)
Fracture of os magnum of wrist 814.-7
(T-12480) (M-12000)

DD-12408 Fracture of hamate bone of wrist 814.-8
(T-12530) (M-12000)
Fracture of unciform bone of wrist 814.-8
(T-12530) (M-12000)

DD-12410 Closed fracture carpal bone, NOS 814.00
(T-12440) (M-12100)
Closed fracture of wrist, NOS 814.00
(T-12440) (M-12100)

DD-12411 Closed fracture of of navicular bone of wrist 814.01
(T-12450) (M-12100)
Closed fracture of scaphoid bone of wrist 814.01
(T-12450) (M-12100)

DD-12412 Closed fracture of lunate bone of wrist 814.02
(T-12470) (M-12100)
Closed fracture of semilunar bone of wrist 814.02
(T-12470) (M-12100)

DD-12413 Closed fracture of triquetal bone of wrist 814.03
(T-12510) (M-12100)
Closed fracture of cuneiform bone of wrist 814.03
(T-12510) (M-12100)

DD-12414 Closed fracture of pisiform bone of wrist 814.04
(T-12460) (M-12100)

DD-12415 Closed fracture of trapezium bone of wrist 814.05
(T-12490) (M-12100)
Closed fracture of larger multangular bone of wrist 814.05
(T-12490) (M-12100)

DD-12416 Closed fracture of trapezoidal bone of wrist 814.06
(T-12520) (M-12100)
Closed fracture of small multangular bone of wrist 814.06
(T-12520) (M-12100)

DD-12417 Closed fracture of capitate bone of wrist 814.07
(T-12480) (M-12100)
Closed fracture of os magnum of wrist 814.07
(T-12480) (M-12100)

DD-12418 Closed fracture of hamate bone of wrist 814.08
(T-12530) (M-12100)
Closed fracture of uniciform bone of wrist 814.08
(T-12530) (M-12100)

DD-12420 Open fracture of carpal bone, NOS 814.10
(T-12440) (M-12200)
Open fracture of wrist, NOS 814.10
(T-12440) (M-12200)

DD-12421 Open fracture of navicular bone of wrist 814.11
(T-12450) (M-12200)
Open fracture of scaphoid bone of wrist 814.11
(T-12450) (M-12200)

DD-12422 Open fracture of lunate bone of wrist 814.12
(T-12470) (M-12200)
Open fracture of semilunar bone of wrist 814.12
(T-12470) (M-12200)

DD-12423 Open fracture of triquetal bone of wrist 814.13
(T-12510) (M-12200)
Open fracture of cuneiform bone of wrist 814.13
(T-12510) (M-12200)

DD-12424 Open fracture of pisiform bone of wrist 814.14
(T-12460) (M-12200)

DD-12425 Open fracture of trapezium of wrist 814.15
(T-12490) (M-12200)
Open fracture of larger multangular bone of wrist 814.15
(T-12490) (M-12200)

DD-12426 Open fracture of trapezoidal bone of wrist 814.16
(T-12520) (M-12200)
Open fracture of small multangular bone of wrist 814.16
(T-12520) (M-12200)

DD-12427 Open fracture of capitate bone of wrist 814.17
(T-12480) (M-12200)
Open fracture of os magnum of wrist 814.17
(T-12480) (M-12200)

DD-12428 Open fracture of hamate bone of wrist 814.18
(T-12530) (M-12200)
Open fracture of unciform bone of wrist 814.18
(T-12530) (M-12200)

DD-12430 Fracture of metacarpal bone, NOS 815.-0
(T-12540) (M-12000)
Fracture of hand except finger, NOS 815.-0
(T-12540) (M-12000)
Fracture of metacarpus, NOS 815.-0
(T-12540) (M-12000)

DD-12431 Fracture of base of thumb 815.-1
(T-12551) (M-12200)
Fracture of first metacarpal 815.-
(T-12551) (M-12000)

DD-12432 Bennett's fracture 815.-1
(T-12551) (M-12000) (G-C008)
(T-15522) (M-13020)

DD-12433 Fracture of base of other metacarpal bone 815.-2
(T-12541) (M-12000)

DD-12434 Fracture of shaft of metacarpal bone 815.-3
(T-12542) (M-12000)

DD-12435 Fracture of neck of metacarpal bone 815.-4
(T-12543) (M-12000)

DD-12439 Fracture of multiple sites of metacarpus 815.-9
(T-12540) (M-12800)

DD-12440 Closed fracture of metacarpal bone, NOS 815.00
(T-12540) (M-12100)

DD-12441 Closed fracture of base of thumb 815.01
(T-12551) (M-12100)
Closed fracture of first metacarpal 815.01
(T-12551) (M-12100)

DD-12442 Closed Bennett's fracture 815.01
(T-12551) (M-12100) (G-C008)
(T-15522) (M-13020)

DD-12443 Closed fracture of base of other metacarpal bone 815.02
(T-12541) (M-12100)

DD-12444 Closed fracture of shaft of metacarpal bone 815.03
(T-12542) (M-12100)

DD-12445 Closed fracture of neck of metacarpal bone 815.04
(T-12543) (M-12100)

DD-12449 Closed fracture of multiple sites of metacarpus 815.09
(T-12540) (M-12810)

DD-12450 Open fracture of metacarpal bone, NOS 815.10
(T-12540) (M-12200)

DD-12451 Open fracture of base of thumb 815.11
(T-12551) (M-12200)
Open fracture of first metacarpal 815.11
(T-12551) (M-12200)

D-12 FRACTURES OF THE UPPER LIMB — Continued

DD-12452 Open Bennett's fracture 815.11
(T-12551) (M-12200) (G-C008)
(T-15522) (M-13020)

DD-12453 Open fracture of base of other metacarpal bone 815.12
(T-12541) (M-12200)

DD-12454 Open fracture of shaft of metacarpal bone 815.13
(T-12542) (M-12200)

DD-12455 Open fracture of neck of metacarpal bone 815.14
(T-12543) (M-12200)

DD-12459 Open fracture of multiple sites of metacarpus 815.19
(T-12540) (M-12820)

DD-12460 Fracture of phalanx of finger, NOS 816.-0
(T-12610) (M-12000)
Fracture of finger, NOS 816.-0
(T-12610) (M-12000)

DD-12461 Fracture of middle or proximal phalanx of finger 816.-1
(T-12611) (T-12612) (M-12000)

DD-12462 Fracture of distal phalanx of finger 816.-2
(T-12613) (M-12000)

DD-12463 Fracture of multiple sites of phalanges of hand 816.-3
(T-12610) (M-12800)

DD-12470 Closed fracture of phalanx of finger, NOS 816.00
(T-12610) (M-12100)
Closed fracture of finger, NOS 816.00
(T-12610) (M-12100)

DD-12471 Closed fracture of middle or proximal phalanx of finger 816.01
(T-12611) (T-12612) (M-12100)

DD-12472 Closed fracture of distal phalanx of finger 816.02
(T-12613) (M-12100)

DD-12473 Closed fracture of multiple sites of phalanges of hand 816.03
(T-12610) (M-12810)

DD-12480 Open fracture of phalanx of finger, NOS 816.10
(T-12610) (M-12200)
Open fracture of finger, NOS 816.10
(T-12610) (M-12200)

DD-12481 Open fracture of middle or proximal phalanx of finger 816.11
(T-12611) (T-12612) (M-12200)

DD-12482 Open fracture of distal phalanx of finger 816.12
(T-12613) (M-12200)

DD-12483 Open fracture of multiple sites of phalanges of hand 816.13
(T-12610) (M-12820)

DD-12490 Multiple fractures of hand bones, NOS 817.-
(T-11000) (T-D8700) (M-12800)

DD-12494 Multiple closed fractures of hand bones 817.0
(T-11000) (T-D8700) (M-12810)

DD-12498 Multiple open fractures of hand bones 817.1
(T-11000) (T-D8700) (M-12820)

D-13 FRACTURES OF THE LOWER LIMB

DD-13000 Fracture of lower limb, NOS 829.-
(T-11000) (T-D9000) (M-12000)
Fracture of leg, NOS 829.-
(T-11000) (T-D9000) (M-12000)

DD-13002 Fracture of unspecified bone of lower limb 829.-
(T-11000) (T-D9000) (M-12000)

DD-13004 Closed fracture of unspecified bone of lower limb 829.0
(T-11000) (T-D9000) (M-12100)

DD-13006 Open fracture of unspecified bone of lower limb 829.1
(T-11000) (T-D9000) (M-12200)

DD-13010 Fractures of multiple bones of lower limb, NOS 827.-
(T-11000) (T-D9000) (M-12800)

DD-13011 Multiple fractures of both lower limbs, NOS 828.-
(T-11000) (T-D9000) (M-12800)
(G-A102)
Multiple fractures of both legs, NOS 828.-
(T-11000) (T-D9000) (M-12800)
(G-A102)

DD-13012 Multiple fractures of upper and lower limbs 828.-
(T-11000) (T-D8000) (T-D9000)
(M-12800)

DD-13013 Multiple fractures of lower limb and ribs 828.-
(T-11000) (T-D9000) (T-11300)
(M-12800)

DD-13014 Multiple fractures of lower limb and sternum 828.-
(T-11000) (T-D9000) (T-11210)
(M-12800)

DD-13015 Multiple fractures of lower limb with ribs and sternum 828.-
(T-11000) (T-D9000) (T-11300)
(T-11210) (M-12800)

DD-13020 Closed fracture of lower limb, NOS 827.0
(T-11000) (T-D9000) (M-12100)
Closed fracture of leg, NOS 728.0
(T-11000) (T-D9000) (M-12100)

DD-13030 Closed fractures of multiple bones of lower limb, NOS 827.0
(T-11000) (T-D9000) (T-12810)

DD-13031 Closed multiple fractures of both lower limbs, NOS 828.0
(T-11000) (T-D9000) (M-12810)
(G-A102)
Closed multiple fractures of both legs, NOS 828.0
(T-11000) (T-D9000) (M-12810)
(G-A102)

DD-13032 Closed multiple fractures of upper and lower limbs 828.0
(T-11000) (T-D8000) (T-D9000) (M-12810)

DD-13033 Closed multiple fractures of lower limb and ribs 828.0
(T-11000) (T-D9000) (T-11300) (M-12810)

DD-13034 Closed multiple fractures of lower limb and sternum 828.0
(T-11000) (T-D9000) (T-11210) (M-12810)

DD-13035 Closed multiple fractures of lower limb with ribs and sternum 828.0
(T-11000) (T-D9000) (T-11300) (T-11210) (M-12810)

DD-13040 Open fracture of lower limb, NOS 827.1
(T-11000) (T-D9000) (M-12200)
Open fracture of leg, NOS 827.1
(T-11000) (T-D9000) (T-12200)

DD-13050 Open fracture of multiple bones of lower limb, NOS 827.1
(T-11000) (T-D9000) (T-12820)

DD-13051 Open multiple fractures of both lower limbs, NOS 828.1
(T-11000) (T-D9000) (M-12820) (G-A102)
Open multiple fractures of both legs, NOS 828.1
(T-11000) (T-D9000) (M-12820) (G-A102)

DD-13052 Open multiple fractures of upper and lower limbs 828.1
(T-11000) (T-D8000) (T-D9000) (M-12820)

DD-13053 Open multiple fractures of lower limb and ribs 828.1
(T-11000) (T-D9000) (T-11300) (M-12820)

DD-13054 Open multiple fractures of lower limb and sternum 828.1
(T-11000) (T-D9000) (T-11210) (M-12820)

DD-13055 Open multiple fractures of lower limb with ribs and sternum 828.1
(T-11000) (T-D9000) (T-11300) (T-11210) (M-12820)

DD-13100 Fracture of femur, NOS 821.00
(T-12710) (M-12000)
Fracture of thigh, NOS 821.00
(T-12710) (M-12000)
Fracture of upper leg, NOS 821.00
(T-12710) (M-12000)

DD-13102 Closed fracture of femur, NOS 821.00
(T-12710) (M-12100)
Closed fracture of thigh 821.00
(T-12710) (M-12100)
Closed fracture of upper leg 821.00
(T-12710) (M-12100)

DD-13104 Open fracture of femur, NOS 821.10
(T-12710) (M-12200)
Open fracture of thigh 821.10
(T-12710) (M-12200)
Open fracture of upper leg 821.10
(T-12710) (M-12200)

DD-13110 Fracture of neck of femur 820.8
(T-12712) (M-12000)
Fracture of hip, NOS 820.8
(T-12712) (M-12000)

DD-13111 Closed transcervical fracture of femur, NOS 820.02
(T-12712) (M-12100)

DD-13112 Closed fracture of intracapsular section of femur, NOS 820.00
(T-12726) (M-12100)

DD-13113 Closed fracture of epiphysis of femur 820.01
(T-12724) (M-12100)
Closed transepiphyseal fracture of femur 820.01
(T-12724) (M-12100)

DD-13115 Closed fracture of midcervical section of femur 820.02
(T-12727) (M-12100)

DD-13116 Closed fracture of base of neck of femur 820.03
(T-12728) (M-12100)
Closed fracture of cervicotrochanteric section of femur 820.03
(T-12728) (M-12100)

DD-13117 Closed fracture of head of femur 820.09
(T-12711) (M-12100)

DD-13118 Closed subcapital fracture of femur 820.09
(T-12729) (M-12100)

DD-13120 Open transcervical fracture of femur, NOS 820.12
(T-12712) (M-12200)

DD-13121 Open fracture of intracapsular section of femur, NOS 820.10
(T-12726) (M-12200)

DD-13122 Open fracture of epiphysis of femur 820.11
(T-12724) (M-12200)
Open transepiphyseal fracture of femur 820.11
(T-12724) (M-12200)

DD-13123 Open fracture of midcervical section of femur 820.12
(T-12727) (M-12200)

DD-13124 Open fracture of base of neck of femur 820.13
(T-12728) (M-12200)
Open fracture of cervicotrochanteric section of femur 820.13
(T-12728) (M-12200)

DD-13126 Open fracture of head of femur 820.19
(T-12711) (M-12200)

D-13 FRACTURES OF THE LOWER LIMB — Continued

DD-13127 Open subcapital fracture of femur 820.19
(T-12729) (M-12200)

DD-13130 Closed pertrochanteric fracture, NOS 820.20
(T-12713) (T-12714) (M-12100)

DD-13131 Closed fracture of greater trochanter of femur 820.20
(T-12713) (M-12100)

DD-13132 Closed fracture of lesser trochanter of femur 820.20
(T-12714) (M-12100)

DD-13133 Closed intertrochanteric fracture 820.21
(T-12715) (M-12100)

DD-13134 Closed subtrochanteric fracture 820.22
(T-1272A) (M-12100)

DD-13135 Open pertrochanteric fracture, NOS 820.30
(T-12713) (T-12714) (M-12200)

DD-13136 Open fracture of greater trochanter of femur 820.30
(T-12713) (M-12200)

DD-13137 Open fracture of lesser trochanter of femur 820.30
(T-12714) (M-12200)

DD-13138 Open intertrochanteric fracture 820.31
(T-12715) (M-12200)

DD-13139 Open subtrochanteric fracture 820.32
(T-1272A) (M-12200)

DD-13140 Closed fracture of neck of femur, NOS 820.8
(T-12712) (M-12100)
Closed fracture of hip, NOS 820.8
(T-12712) (M-12100)

DD-13144 Open fracture of neck of femur, NOS 820.9
(T-12712) (M-12200)
Open fracture of hip, NOS 820.9
(T-12712) (M-12200)

DD-13150 Fracture of shaft of femur 821.01
(T-12717) (M-12000)

DD-13152 Closed fracture of shaft of femur 821.01
(T-12717) (M-12100)

DD-13154 Open fracture of shaft of femur 821.11
(T-12717) (M-12200)

DD-13170 Closed fracture of lower end of femur 821.20
(T-12723) (M-12100)
Closed fracture of distal end of femur 821.20
(T-12723) (M-12100)

DD-13172 Closed fracture of femoral condyle of femur 821.21
(T-12718) (T-12719) (M-12100)

DD-13174 Closed fracture of lower epiphysis of femur 821.22
(T-12725) (M-12100)

DD-13176 Closed supracondylar fracture of femur 821.23
(T-1271B) (M-12100)

DD-13178 Multiple closed fractures of lower end of femur 821.29
(T-12723) (M-12810)

DD-13180 Open fracture of lower end of femur 821.30
(T-12723) (M-12200)
Open fracture of distal end of femur 821.30
(T-12723) (M-12200)

DD-13182 Open fracture of femoral condyle of femur 821.31
(T-12718) (T-12719) (M-12200)

DD-13184 Open fracture of lower epiphysis of femur 821.32
(T-12725) (M-12200)

DD-13186 Open supracondylar fracture of femur 821.33
(T-1271B) (M-12200)

DD-13188 Multiple open fractures of lower end of femur 821.39
(T-12723) (M-12820)

DD-13300 Fracture of patella, NOS 822.-
(T-12730) (M-12000)

DD-13302 Closed fracture of patella 822.0
(T-12730) (M-12100)

DD-13304 Open fracture of patella 822.1
(T-12730) (M-12200)

DD-13400 Fracture of lower leg, NOS 823.82
(T-12740) (T-12750) (M-12000)
Fracture of tibia and fibula, NOS 823.82
(T-12740) (T-12750) (M-12000)

DD-13402 Closed fracture of lower leg 823.82
(T-12740) (T-12750) (M-12100)
Closed fracture of tibia and fibula 823.82
(T-12740) (T-12750) (M-12100)

DD-13404 Open fracture of lower leg 823.92
(T-12740) (T-12750) (M-12200)
Open fracture of tibia and fibula 823.92
(T-12740) (T-12750) (M-12200)

DD-13410 Fracture of upper end of lower leg, NOS 823.02
(T-1274A) (T-1275C) (M-12000)
Fracture of upper end of tibia and fibula, NOS 823.02
(T-1274A) (T-1275C) (M-12000)

DD-13412 Closed fracture of upper end of lower leg 823.02
(T-1274A) (T-1275C) (M-12100)
Closed fracture of upper end of tibia and fibula 823.02
(T-1274A) (T-1275C) (M-12100)

DD-13414 Open fracture of upper end of lower leg 823.12
(T-1274A) (T-1275C) (M-12200)
Open fracture of upper end of tibia and fibula 823.12
(T-1274A) (T-1275C) (M-12200)

DD-13417 Closed fracture of head of fibula 823.01
(T-12751) (M-12100)

DD-13418 Closed fracture of condyle of tibia 823.00
(T-1274F) (M-12100)

DD-13419 Closed fracture of tuberosity of tibia 823.00
(T-12745) (M-12100)

DD-13420 Fracture of upper end of tibia 823.00
(T-1274A) (M-12000)

DD-13421 Fracture of upper end of fibula 823.01
(T-1275C) (M-12000)

DD-13422 Closed fracture of upper end of tibia 823.00
(T-1274A) (M-12100)

DD-13423 Closed fracture of upper end of fibula 823.01
(T-1275C) (M-12100)

DD-13424 Open fracture of upper end of tibia 823.10
(T-1274A) (M-12200)

DD-13425 Open fracture of upper end of fibula 823.11
(T-1275C) (M-12200)

DD-13440 Fracture of shaft of tibia 823.20
(T-12746) (M-12000)

DD-13441 Fracture of shaft of fibula 823.21
(T-12754) (M-12000)

DD-13442 Closed fracture of shaft of tibia 823.20
(T-12746) (M-12100)

DD-13443 Closed fracture of shaft of fibula 823.21
(T-12754) (M-12100)

DD-13446 Open fracture of shaft of tibia 823.30
(T-12746) (M-12200)

DD-13447 Open fracture of shaft of fibula 823.31
(T-12754) (M-12200)

DD-13500 Fracture of ankle, NOS 824.8
(T-11000) (T-D9500) (M-12000)

DD-13502 Closed fracture of ankle 824.8
(T-11000) (T-D9500) (M-12100)

DD-13504 Open fracture of ankle 824.9
(T-11000) (T-D9500) (M-12200)

DD-13510 Closed fracture of medial malleolus 824.0
(T-12744) (M-12100)

DD-13512 Open fracture of medial malleolus 824.1
(T-12744) (M-12200)

DD-13514 Closed fracture of lateral malleolus 824.2
(T-12755) (M-12100)

DD-13516 Open fracture of lateral malleolus 824.3
(T-12755) (M-12200)

DD-13520 Closed bimalleolar fracture 824.4
(T-12744) (T-12755) (M-12100)

DD-13522 Pott's fracture 824.4
(T-1275D) (T-12744) (M-12000)
Dupuytren's fracture of fibula 824.4
(T-1275D) (T-12744) (M-12000)

DD-13530 Open bimalleolar fracture 824.5
(T-12744) (T-12755) (M-12200)

DD-13540 Closed trimalleolar fracture 824.6
(T-12744) (T-12755) (T-12757)
(M-12100)

DD-13550 Open trimalleolar fracture 824.7
(T-12744) (T-12755) (T-12757)
(M-12200)

DD-13600 Fracture of foot, NOS 825.-
(T-11000) (T-D9700) (M-12000)

DD-13602 Closed fracture of foot, NOS 825.-
(T-11000) (T-D9700) (M-12100)
Closed fracture of unspecified bone of foot, except toes 825.20
(T-11000) (T-D9700) (M-12100)

DD-13604 Open fracture of foot, NOS 825.-
(T-11000) (T-D9700) (M-12200)
Open fracture of unspecified bone of foot except toes 825.30
(T-11000) (T-D9700) (M-12200)

DD-13610 Closed fracture of calcaneus 825.0
(T-12770) (M-12100)
Closed fracture of heel bone 825.0
(T-12770) (M-12100)
Closed fracture of os calcis 825.0
(T-12770) (M-12100)

DD-13612 Open fracture of calcaneus 825.1
(T-12770) (M-12200)
Open fracture of heel bone 825.1
(T-12770) (M-12200)
Open fracture of os calcis 825.1
(T-12270) (M-12200)

DD-13620 Closed fracture of astragalus 825.21
(T-12780) (M-12100)
Closed fracture of talus 825.21
(T-12780) (M-12100)

DD-13621 Closed fracture of navicular bone of foot 825.22
(T-12800) (M-12100)
Closed fracture of scaphoid bone of foot 825.22
(T-12800) (M-12100)

DD-13622 Closed fracture of cuboid bone of foot 825.23
(T-12790) (M-12100)

DD-13623 Closed fracture of cuneiform bone of foot, NOS 825.24
(T-12810) (T-12820) (T-12830)
(M-12100)

DD-13624 Closed fracture of lateral cuneiform bone of foot 824.24
(T-12810) (M-12100)

DD-13625 Closed fracture of intermediate cuneiform bone of foot 824.24
(T-12830) (M-12100)

DD-13626 Closed fracture of medial cuneiform bone of foot 824.24
(T-12820) (M-12100)

DD-13630 Closed fracture of metatarsal bone, NOS 825.25
(T-12840) (M-12100)

DD-13631 Closed fracture of first metatarsal bone 825.25
(T-12850) (M-12100)

DD-13632 Closed fracture of second metatarsal bone 825.25
(T-12860) (M-12100)

DD-13633 Closed fracture of third metatarsal bone 825.25
(T-12870) (M-12100)

DD-13634 Closed fracture of fourth metatarsal bone 825.25
(T-12880) (M-12100)

D-13 FRACTURES OF THE LOWER LIMB — Continued

DD-13635 Closed fracture of fifth metatarsal bone 825.25
(T-12890) (M-12100)

DD-13638 Closed fractures of tarsal and metatarsal bones 825.29
(T-11000) (T-D9500) (T-12840) (M-12100)

DD-13640 Open fracture of astragalus 825.31
(T-12780) (M-12200)
Open fracture of talus 825.31
(T-12780) (M-12200)

DD-13641 Open fracture of navicular bone of foot 825.32
(T-12800) (M-12200)
Open fracture of scaphoid bone of foot 825.32
(T-12800) (M-12200)

DD-13642 Open fracture of cuboid bone of foot 825.33
(T-12790) (M-12200)

DD-13643 Open fracture of cuneiform bone of foot, NOS 825.34
(T-12810) (T-12820) (T-12830) (M-12200)

DD-13644 Open fracture of lateral cuneiform bone of foot 825.34
(T-12810) (M-12200)

DD-13645 Open fracture of intermediate cuneiform bone of foot 824.34
(T-12830) (M-12200)

DD-13646 Open fracture of medial cuneiform bone of foot 825.34
(T-12820) (M-12200)

DD-13650 Open fracture of metatarsal bone, NOS 825.35
(T-12840) (M-12200)

DD-13651 Open fracture of first metatarsal bone 825.35
(T-12850) (M-12200)

DD-13652 Open fracture of second metatarsal bone 825.35
(T-12860) (M-12200)

DD-13653 Open fracture of third metatarsal bone 825.35
(T-12870) (M-12200)

DD-13654 Open fracture of fourth metatarsal bone 825.35
(T-12880) (M-12200)

DD-13655 Open fracture of fifth metatarsal bone 825.35
(T-12890) (M-12200)

DD-13658 Open fracture of tarsal and metatarsal bones 835.39
(T-11000) (T-D9500) (T-12840) (M-12200)

DD-13660 Fracture of phalanx of foot, NOS 826.-
(T-12910) (M-12000)
Fracture of toe, NOS 826.-
(T-12910) (M-12000)

DD-13662 Closed fracture of phalanx of foot 826.0
(T-12910) (M-12100)
Closed fracture of toe 826.0
(T-12910) (M-12100)

DD-13664 Open fracture of phalanx of foot 826.1
(T-12910) (M-12200)
Open fracture of toe 826.1
(T-12910) (M-12200)

D-14 DISLOCATIONS

DD-14100 Dislocation of jaw, NOS 830.-
(T-15290) (M-13000)
Dislocation of mandible 830.-
(T-15290) (M-13000)
Dislocation of inferior maxilla 830.-
(T-15290) (M-13000)
Dislocation of temporomandibular joint 830.-
(T-15290) (M-13000)

DD-14110 Closed dislocation of jaw 830.0
(T-15290) (M-13100)
Closed dislocation of mandible 830.0
(T-15290) (M-13100)
Closed dislocation of inferior maxilla 830.0
(T-15290) (M-13100)
Closed dislocation of temporomandibular joint 830.0
(T-15290) (M-13100)

DD-14120 Open dislocation of jaw 830.1
(T-15290) (M-13200)
Open dislocation of mandible 830.1
(T-15290) (M-13200)
Open dislocation of inferior maxilla 830.1
(T-15290) (M-13200)
Open dislocation of temporomandibular joint 830.1
(T-15290) (M-13200)

DD-14300 Dislocation of cervical vertebra, NOS 839.00
(T-11600) (T-15320) (M-13000)

DD-14310 Closed dislocation of cervical vertebra, NOS 839.00
(T-11600) (T-15320) (M-13100)

DD-14311 Closed dislocation of first cervical vertebra 839.01
(T-11610) (M-13100)

DD-14312 Closed dislocation of second cervical vertebra 838.02
(T-11620) (M-13100)

DD-14313 Closed dislocation of third cervical vertebra 839.03
(T-11630) (M-13100)

DD-14314 Closed dislocation of fourth cervical vertebra 839.04
(T-11640) (M-13100)

DD-14315 Closed dislocation of fifth cervical vertebra 839.05
(T-11650) (M-13100)

DD-14316 Closed dislocation of sixth cervical vertebra 838.06
(T-11660) (M-13100)

DD-14317 Closed dislocation of seventh cervical vertebra 839.07
(T-11670) (M-13100)

DD-14318 Closed dislocations of multiple cervical vertebrae 838.08
(T-11600) (M-13810)

DD-14320 Open dislocation of cervical vertebra, NOS 839.10
(T-11600) (T-15320) (M-13200)

DD-14321 Open dislocation of first cervical vertebra 839.11
(T-11610) (M-13200)

DD-14322 Open dislocation of second cervical vertebra 839.12
(T-11620) (M-13200)

DD-14323 Open dislocation of third cervical vertebra 839.13
(T-11630) (M-13200)

DD-14324 Open dislocation of fourth cervical vertebra 839.14
(T-11640) (M-13200)

DD-14325 Open dislocation of fifth cervical vertebra 839.15
(T-11650) (M-13200)

DD-14326 Open dislocation of sixth cervical vertebra 839.16
(T-11660) (M-13200)

DD-14327 Open dislocation of seventh cervical vertebra 839.17
(T-11670) (M-13200)

DD-14328 Open dislocations of multiple cervical vertebrae 839.18
(T-11600) (M-13820)

DD-14330 Closed dislocation of thoracic vertebra 839.21
(T-11700) (M-13100)
Closed dislocation of dorsal vertebra 839.21
(T-11700) (M-13100)

DD-14340 Closed dislocation of lumbar vertebra 839.20
(T-11900) (M-13100)

DD-14350 Open dislocation of thoracic vertebra 839.31
(T-11700) (M-13200)
Open dislocation of dorsal vertebra 839.31
(T-11700) (M-13200)

DD-14360 Open dislocation of lumbar vertebra 839.30
(T-11900) (M-13200)

DD-14370 Closed dislocation of sacrum 839.42
(T-11AD0) (T-15680) (M-13100)
Closed dislocation of sacroiliac joint 839.42
(T-11AD0) (T-15680) (M-13100)

DD-14372 Open dislocation of sacrum 839.52
(T-11AD0) (T-15680) (M-13200)
Open dislocation of sacroiliac joint 839.52
(T-11AD0) (T-15680) (M-13200)

DD-14380 Closed dislocation of coccyx 839.41
(T-11BF0) (M-13100)

DD-14382 Open dislocation of coccyx 839.51
(T-11BF0) (M-13200)

DD-14390 Closed dislocation of vertebra, NOS 839.40
(T-11500) (M-13100)
Closed dislocation of spine, NOS 839.40
(T-11500) (M-13100)

DD-14392 Open dislocation of vertebra, NOS 839.50
(T-11500) (M-13200)
Open dislocation of spine, NOS 839.50
(T-11500) (M-13200)

DD-14400 Closed dislocation of sternum 839.61
(T-11210) (M-13100)

DD-14402 Closed dislocation of sternocalvicular joint 839.61
(T-15610) (M-13100)

DD-14410 Open dislocation of sternum 839.71
(T-11210) (M-13200)

DD-14412 Open dislocation of sternoclavicular joint 839.71
(T-15610) (M-13200)

DD-14420 Closed dislocation of pelvis 839.69
(T-12380) (M-13100)

DD-14422 Open dislocation of pelvis 839.79
(T-12380) (M-13200)

DD-14500 Closed dislocation of shoulder, NOS 831.00
(T-12410) (M-13100)
Closed dislocation of humerus, NOS 831.00
(T-12410) (M-13100)

DD-14501 Closed anterior dislocation of humerus 831.01
(T-12410) (M-13101)

DD-14502 Closed posterior dislocation of humerus 831.02
(T-12410) (M-13102)

DD-14503 Closed inferior dislocation of humerus 831.03
(T-12410) (M-13105)

DD-14504 Closed dislocation of acromioclavicular joint 831.04
(T-15420) (M-13100)

DD-14505 Closed dislocation of clavicle 831.04
(T-12310) (M-13100)

DD-14506 Closed dislocation of scapula 831.09
(T-12280) (M-13100)

DD-14510 Open dislocation of shoulder, NOS 831.10
(T-12410) (M-13200)
Open dislocation of humerus, NOS 831.10
(T-12410) (M-13200)

DD-14511 Open anterior dislocation of humerus 831.11
(T-12410) (M-13201)

DD-14512 Open posterior dislocation of humerus 831.12
(T-12410) (M-13202)

DD-14513 Open inferior dislocation of humerus 831.13
(T-12410) (M-13205)

D-14 DISLOCATIONS — Continued

DD-14514 Open dislocation of acromioclavicular joint 831.14
(T-15420) (M-13200)

DD-14515 Open dislocation of clavicle 831.14
(T-12310) (M-13200)

DD-14516 Open dislocation of scapula 831.19
(T-12280) (M-13200)

DD-14520 Closed dislocation of elbow, NOS 832.00
(T-15000) (T-D8300) (M-13100)

DD-14521 Closed anterior dislocation of elbow 832.01
(T-15000) (T-D8300) (M-13101)

DD-14522 Closed posterior dislocation of elbow 832.02
(T-15000) (T-D8300) (M-13102)

DD-14523 Closed medial dislocation of elbow 832.03
(T-15000) (T-D8300) (M-13103)

DD-14524 Closed lateral dislocation of elbow 832.04
(T-15000) (T-D8300) (M-13104)

DD-14530 Open dislocation of elbow, NOS 832.10
(T-15000) (T-D8300) (M-13200)

DD-14531 Open anterior dislocation of elbow 832.11
(T-15000) (T-D8300) (M-13201)

DD-14532 Open posterior dislocation of elbow 832.12
(T-15000) (T-D8300) (M-13202)

DD-14533 Open medial dislocation of elbow 832.13
(T-15000) (T-D8300) (M-13203)

DD-14534 Open lateral dislocation of elbow 832.14
(T-15000) (T-D8300) (M-13204)

DD-14550 Closed dislocation of wrist, NOS 833.00
(T-15000) (T-D8600) (M-13100)

DD-14551 Closed dislocation of distal radioulnar joint of wrist 833.01
(T-15470) (M-13100)

DD-14552 Closed dislocation of radiocarpal joint of wrist 833.02
(T-15480) (M-13100)

DD-14553 Closed dislocation of midcarpal joint of wrist 833.03
(T-15510) (M-13100)

DD-14554 Closed dislocation of carpometacarpal joint of wrist 833.04
(T-15520) (M-13100)

DD-14555 Closed dislocation of proximal end of metacarpal bone of wrist 833.05
(T-12541) (M-13100)

DD-14556 Closed dislocation of distal end of ulna 833.09
(T-1243B) (M-13100)

DD-14560 Open dislocation of wrist, NOS 833.10
(T-15000) (T-D8600) (M-13200)

DD-14561 Open dislocation of distal radioulnar joint of wrist 833.11
(T-15470) (M-13200)

DD-14562 Open dislocation of radiocarpal joint of wrist 833.12
(T-15480) (M-13200)

DD-14563 Open dislocation of midcarpal joint of wrist 833.13
(T-15510) (M-13200)

DD-14564 Open dislocation of carpometacarpal joint of wrist 833.14
(T-15520) (M-13200)

DD-14565 Open dislocation of proximal end of metacarpal bone of wrist 833.15
(T-12541) (M-13200)

DD-14566 Open dislocation of distal end of ulna 833.19
(T-1243B) (M-13200)

DD-14570 Closed dislocation of finger, NOS 834.00
(T-15000) (T-12610) (M-13100)
Closed dislocation of phalanx of hand, NOS 834.00
(T-15000) (M-12610) (M-13100)

DD-14571 Closed dislocation of metacarpophalangeal joint of finger 834.01
(T-15530) (M-13100)

DD-14572 Closed dislocation of interphalangeal joint of hand 834.02
(T-15590) (T-15592) (M-13100)

DD-14574 Closed dislocation of thumb, NOS 834.00
(T-15000) (T-12620) (M-13100)

DD-14575 Closed dislocation of metacarpophalangeal joint of thumb 834.01
(T-15540) (M-13100)

DD-14576 Closed dislocation of interphalangeal joint of thumb 834.02
(T-15594) (M-13100)

DD-14580 Open dislocation of finger, NOS 834.10
(T-15000) (T-12610) (M-13200)
Open dislocation of phalanx of hand, NOS 834.10
(T-15000) (T-12610) (M-13200)

DD-14581 Open dislocation of metacarpophalangeal joint of finger 834.11
(T-15530) (M-13200)

DD-14582 Open dislocation of interphalangeal joint of hand 834.12
(T-15590) (T-15592) (M-13200)

DD-14584 Open dislocation of thumb, NOS 834.10
(T-15000) (T-12620) (M-13200)

DD-14585 Open dislocation of metacarpophalangeal joint of thumb 834.11
(T-15540) (M-13200)

DD-14586 Open dislocation of interphalangeal joint of thumb 834.12
(T-15594) (M-13200)

DD-14600 Closed dislocation of hip, NOS 835.00
(T-15000) (T-D2500) (M-13100)

DD-14601 Closed posterior dislocation of hip 835.01
(T-15000) (T-D2500) (M-13102)

DD-14602 Closed obturator dislocation of hip 835.02
(T-15000) (T-D2500) (M-13101)

DD-14604 Other closed anterior dislocation of hip, NEC 835.03
(T-15000) (T-D2500) (M-13101)

DD-14610 Open dislocation of hip, NOS 835.10
(T-15000) (T-D2500) (M-13200)

DD-14611 Open posterior dislocation of hip 835.11
(T-15000) (T-D2500) (M-13202)
DD-14613 Open obturator dislocation of hip 835.12
(T-15000) (T-D2500) (M-13201)
DD-14614 Other open anterior dislocation of hip, NEC 835.13
(T-15000) (T-D2500) (M-13201)
DD-14620 Dislocation of knee, NOS 836.-
(T-15000) (T-D9200) (M-13000)
DD-14622 Current tear of semilunar cartilage, NOS 836.2
(T-15722) (M-14400)
Current tear of meniscus of knee, NOS 836.2
(T-15722) (M-14400)
DD-14623 Current tear of medial cartilage or meniscus of knee 836.0
(T-15724) (M-14400)
DD-14624 Current tear of lateral cartilage or meniscus of knee 836.1
(T-15723) (M-14400)
DD-14626 Closed dislocation of patella 836.3
(T-12730) (M-13100)
DD-14628 Open dislocation of patella 836.4
(T-12730) (M-13200)
DD-14630 Closed dislocation of knee, NOS 836.50
(T-15000) (T-D9200) (M-13100)
DD-14631 Closed anterior dislocation of proximal end of tibia 836.51
(T-1274A) (M-13101)
DD-14632 Closed posterior dislocation of distal end of femur 836.51
(T-12725) (M-13102)
DD-14633 Closed posterior dislocation of proximal end of tibia 836.52
(T-1274A) (M-13102)
DD-14634 Closed anterior dislocation of distal end of femur 836.52
(T-12725) (M-13101)
DD-14635 Closed medial dislocation of proximal end of tibia 836.53
(T-1274A) (M-13103)
DD-14636 Closed lateral dislocation of proximal end of tibia 836.54
(T-1274A) (M-13104)
DD-14640 Open dislocation of knee, NOS 836.60
(T-15000) (T-D9200) (M-13200)
DD-14641 Open anterior dislocation of proximal end of tibia 836.61
(T-1274A) (M-13201)
DD-14642 Open posterior dislocation of distal end of femur 836.61
(T-12725) (M-13202)
DD-14643 Open posterior dislocation of proximal end of tibia 836.62
(T-1274A) (M-13202)
DD-14644 Open anterior dislocation of distal end of femur 836.62
(T-12725) (M-13203)
DD-14645 Open medial dislocation of proximal end of tibia 836.63
(T-1274A) (M-13203)
DD-14646 Open lateral dislocation of proximal end of tibia 836.64
(T-1274A) (M-13204)
DD-14650 Closed dislocation of ankle, NOS 837.0
(T-15000) (T-D9500) (M-13100)
DD-14651 Closed dislocation of astragalus 837.0
(T-12780) (M-13100)
DD-14652 Closed dislocation of distal end of fibula 837.0
(T-1275D) (M-13100)
DD-14653 Closed dislocation of navicular bone of foot 837.0
(T-12800) (M-13100)
Closed dislocation of scaphoid bone of foot 837.00
(T-12800) (M-13100)
DD-14655 Closed dislocation of distal end of tibia 837.0
(T-1274B) (M-13100)
DD-14660 Open dislocation of ankle, NOS 837.1
(T-15000) (T-D9500) (M-13200)
DD-14661 Open dislocation of astragalus 837.1
(T-12780) (M-13200)
DD-14662 Open dislocation of distal end of fibula 837.1
(T-1275D) (M-13200)
DD-14663 Open dislocation of navicular bone of foot 837.1
(T-12800) (M-13200)
Open dislocation of scaphoid bone of foot 837.1
(T-12800) (M-13200)
DD-14665 Open dislocation of distal end of tibia 837.1
(T-1274B) (M-13200)
DD-14670 Closed dislocation of foot, NOS 838.00
(T-15000) (T-D9700) (M-13100)
DD-14671 Closed dislocation of tarsal joint, NOS 838.01
(T-15770) (M-13100)
DD-14672 Closed dislocation of midtarsal joint, NOS 838.02
(T-15771) (M-13100)
DD-14673 Closed dislocation of tarsometatarsal joint, NOS 838.03
(T-15780) (M-13100)
DD-14674 Closed dislocation of metatarsal joint, NOS 838.04
(T-15810) (M-13100)
DD-14675 Closed dislocation of metatarsophalangeal joint, NOS 838.05
(T-15810) (M-13100)
DD-14676 Closed dislocation of phalanx of foot, NOS 838.09
(T-15000) (T-12910) (M-13100)
Closed dislocation of toe, NOS 838.09
(T-15000) (T-12910) (M-13100)
DD-14678 Closed dislocation of interphalangeal joint of foot 838.06
(T-15870) (T-15872) (M-13100)

D-14 DISLOCATIONS — Continued

DD-14680 Open dislocation of foot, NOS 838.10
(T-15000) (T-D9700) (M-13200)

DD-14681 Open dislocation of tarsal joint, NOS 838.11
(T-15770) (M-13200)

DD-14682 Open dislocation of midtarsal joint, NOS 838.12
(T-15771) (M-13200)

DD-14683 Open dislocation of tarsometatarsal joint, NOS 838.13
(T-15780) (M-13200)

DD-14684 Open dislocation of metatarsal joint, NOS 838.14
(T-15810) (M-13200)

DD-14685 Open dislocation of metatarsophalangeal joint, NOS 838.15
(T-15810) (M-13200)

DD-14686 Open dislocation of phalanx of foot, NOS 838.19
(T-15000) (T-12910) (M-13200)
Open dislocation of toe, NOS 838.19
(T-15000) (T-12910) (M-13200)

DD-14688 Open dislocation of interphalangeal joint of foot, NOS 838.16
(T-15870) (T-15872) (M-13200)

DD-14802 Multiple closed dislocations of arm 839.8
(T-D8200) (M-13810)

DD-14804 Multiple closed dislocations of back 839.8
(T-D2100) (M-13810)

DD-14806 Multiple closed dislocations of hand 839.8
(T-D8700) (M-13810)

DD-14822 Multiple open dislocations of arm 839.9
(T-D8200) (M-13820)

DD-14824 Multiple open dislocations of back 839.9
(T-D2100) (M-13820)

DD-14826 Multiple open dislocations of hand 839.9
(T-D8700) (M-13820)

D-15 SPRAINS AND STRAINS

D-150 Sprains and Strains: General Terms

DD-15020 Repetitive strain injury, NOS
(T-D0003) (F-11350)
RSI
(T-D0003) (F-11350)

D-151 Sprains and Strains of The Upper Extremities

DD-15100 Sprain of shoulder, NOS 840.9
(T-15000) (T-D2220) (M-13400)

DD-15110 Sprain of acromioclavicular joint or ligament 840.0
(T-15420) (T-18230) (M-13400)

DD-15111 Sprain of coracoclavicular ligament 840.1
(T-18232) (M-13400)

DD-15112 Sprain of coracohumeral ligament 840.2
(T-18312) (M-13400)

DD-15113 Strain of infraspinatus muscle or tendon 840.3
(T-13620) (T-17212) (F-11350)

DD-15114 Strain of rotator cuff capsule 840.4
(T-13601) (F-11350)

DD-15115 Strain of subscapularis muscle 840.5
(T-13650) (F-11350)

DD-15116 Strain of supraspinatus muscle or tendon 840.6
(T-13610) (T-17211) (F-11350)

DD-15118 Sprain of other site of shoulder and upper arm 840.8
(T-15000) (T-D2220) (T-D8200) (M-13400)

DD-15119 Sprain of arm, NOS 840.9
(T-15000) (T-D8000) (M-13400)

DD-15130 Sprain of elbow, NOS 841.9
(T-15000) (T-D8300) (M-13400)

DD-15131 Strain of radial collateral ligament 840.0
(T-18322) (F-11350)

DD-15132 Strain of ulnar collateral ligament 841.1
(T-18321) (F-11350)

DD-15133 Sprain of radiohumeral joint 841.2
(T-15440) (M-13400)

DD-15134 Sprain of ulnohumeral joint 841.3
(T-15445) (M-13400)

DD-15135 Sprain of other specified site of elbow and forearm 841.8
(T-15000) (T-D8300) (T-D8500) (M-13400)

DD-15150 Sprain of wrist, NOS 842.00
(T-15000) (T-D8600) (M-13400)

DD-15151 Sprain of carpal joint 842.01
(T-15000) (T-D8600) (M-13400)

DD-15152 Sprain of radiocarpal joint or ligament 842.02
(T-15480) (T-18340) (M-13400)

DD-15158 Sprain of distal radioulnar joint 842.09
(T-15470) (M-13400)

DD-15170 Sprain of hand, NOS 842.10
(T-15000) (T-D8700) (M-13400)

DD-15171 Sprain of carpometacarpal joint 842.11
(T-15520) (M-13400)

DD-15172 Sprain of metacarpophalangeal joint 842.12
(T-15530) (M-13400)

DD-15173 Sprain of interphalangeal joint of finger 842.13
(T-15590) (T-15592) (M-13400)

DD-15174 Sprain of midcarpal joint 842.19
(T-15510) (M-13400)

D-152 Sprains and Strains of The Lower Extremities

DD-15200 Sprain of lower extremity, NOS 843.-
(T-15000) (T-D9000) (M-13400)

DD-15210 Sprain of hip, NOS 843.9
(T-15000) (T-D2500) (M-13400)

DD-15212 Sprain of iliofemoral ligament 843.0
(T-18402) (M-13400)

DD-15214 Sprain of ischiocapsular ligament 843.1
(T-18403) (M-13400)

DD-15216 Sprain of other specified site of hip and thigh 843.8
(T-15000) (T-D2500) (T-D9100) (M-13400)

DD-15218 Sprain of thigh, NOS 843.9
(T-15000) (T-D9100) (M-13400)

DD-15230 Sprain of knee, NOS 844.9
(T-15000) (T-D9200) (M-13400)

DD-15231 Sprain of lateral collateral ligament of knee 844.0
(T-18440) (M-13400)

DD-15232 Sprain of medial collateral ligament of knee 844.1
(T-18430) (M-13400)

DD-15233 Sprain of cruciate ligament of knee 844.2
(T-18422) (M-13400)

DD-15234 Sprain of superior tibiofibular joint or ligament 844.3
(T-15730) (T-18460) (M-13400)

DD-15237 Sprain of other specified site of knee and leg 844.8
(T-15000) (T-D9400) (M-13400)

DD-15238 Sprain of leg, NOS 844.9
(T-15000) (T-D9400) (M-13400)

DD-15250 Sprain of ankle, NOS 845.00
(T-15000) (T-D9500) (M-13400)

DD-15251 Sprain of deltoid ligament of ankle 845.01
(T-18521) (M-13400)
Sprain of internal collateral ligament of ankle 845.01
(T-18521) (M-13400)
Sprain of medial ligament of talocrural joint 845.01
(T-18521) (M-13400)

DD-15253 Sprain of calcaneofibular ligament 845.2
(T-18528) (M-13400)

DD-15254 Sprain of distal tibiofibular ligament 845.03
(T-18480) (M-13400)

DD-15255 Strain of Achilles tendon 845.09
(T-17860) (F-11350)

DD-15270 Sprain of foot, NOS 845.1
(T-15000) (T-D9700) (M-13400)

DD-15271 Sprain of tarsometatarsal joint or ligament 845.11
(T-15780) (T-18550) (M-13400)

DD-15272 Sprain of metatarsophalangeal joint 845.12
(T-15810) (T-18580) (M-13400)

DD-15273 Sprain of interphalangeal joint of toe 845.13
(T-15870) (T-15872) (M-13400)

D-154 Sprains and Strains of The Neck and Vertebral Column

DD-15410 Sprain of neck, NOS 847.0
(T-15320) (M-13400)

DD-15412 Whiplash injury to neck 847.0
(T-15320) (T-18111) (T-13000) (T-D1600) (M-13400) (F-11350)
Acute cervical sprain 847.0
(T-15320) (T-18111) (T-13000) (T-D1600) (M-13400) (F-11350)

DD-15414 Sprain of atlanto-axial joint 847.0
(T-15317) (M-13400)

DD-15416 Sprain of atlanto-occipital joint 847.0
(T-15311) (M-13400)

DD-15420 Strain of back, NOS 847.9
(T-D2100) (T-D1409) (F-11350)

DD-15430 Strain of thoracic region, NOS 847.1
(T-D2110) (F-11350)

DD-15440 Strain of lumbar region, NOS 847.2
(T-D2120) (F-11350)

DD-15442 Sprain of sacrum 847.3
(T-15000) (T-11AD0) (M-13400)

DD-15444 Sprain of sacrococcygeal ligament 847.3
(T-15370) (T-18150) (M-13400)

DD-15448 Sprain of coccyx 847.4
(T-15372) (M-13400)

DD-15460 Sprain or strain of sacroiliac region, NOS 846.9
(T-D2330) (M-13400) (F-11350)

DD-15461 Sprain of lumbosacral joint or ligament 846.0
(T-15360) (T-18140) (M-13400)

DD-15462 Sprain of sacroiliac ligament 846.1
(T-18293) (T-18295) (M-13400)

DD-15463 Sprain of sacrospinatus ligament 846.2
(T-18292) (M-13400)

DD-15464 Sprain of sacrotuberous ligament 846.3
(T-18291) (M-13400)

DD-15468 Sprain of other specified site of sacroiliac region 846.8
(T-D2330) (M-13400)

D-155 Sprains of Other Joints

DD-15510 Sprain of septal cartilage of nose 848.0
(T-21230) (M-13400)

DD-15512 Sprain of jaw, NOS 848.1
(T-15290) (M-13400)
Sprain of temporomandibular joint or ligament 848.1
(T-15290) (M-13400)

DD-15520 Sprain of cricoarytenoid joint or ligament 848.2
(T-2418C) (M-13400)

DD-15522 Sprain of cricothyroid joint or ligament 848.2
(T-24175) (M-13400)

DD-15524 Sprain of thyroid cartilage 848.2
(T-24160) (M-13400)

DD-15530 Sprain of chondrocostal joint without injury to sternum 848.3
(T-15652) (M-13400) (G-C009) (T-11210) (M-10000)
Sprain of costal cartilage without injury to sternum 848.3
(T-15652) (M-13400) (G-C009) (T-11210) (M-10000)

DD-15550 Sprain of sternum, NOS 848.40
(T-15000) (T-11210) (M-13400)

DD-15552 Sprain of sternoclavicular joint or ligament 848.41
(T-15610) (M-13400)

D-155 Sprains of Other Joints — Continued

DD-15554 Sprain of chondrosternal joint 848.42
(T-15650) (M-13400)

DD-15556 Sprain of xiphoid cartilage 848.49
(T-15622) (M-13400)

DD-15570 Sprain of symphysis pubis 848.5
(T-15690) (M-13400)

SECTION D-2 INJURIES OF THE INTERNAL ORGANS
D-21 INTRACRANIAL INJURIES WITHOUT SKULL FRACTURE

DD-21000 Intracranial injury, NOS, without skull fracture 854.-
(T-D1400) (M-10060)
Head injury, NOS, without skull fracture 854.-
(T-D1400) (M-10060)

DD-21010 Brain injury, NOS, without skull fracture 854.-
(T-A0100) (T-D1400) (M-10060)

DD-21040 Brain injury without open intracranial wound, NOS 854.0
(T-A0100) (M-10060) (G-C009)
(T-D1400) (M-14010)

DD-21041 Brain injury without open intracranial wound and with unspecified state of consciousness 854.00
(T-A0100) (M-10060) (G-C009)
(T-D1400) (M-14010) (G-C008)
(F-A5500)

DD-21042 Brain injury without open intracranial wound and with no loss of consciousness 854.01
(T-A0100) (M-10060) (G-C009)
(T-D1400) (M-14010) (G-C009)
(F-A5570)

DD-21043 Brain injury without open intracranial wound and with brief loss of consciousness (less than one hour) 854.02
(T-A0100) (M-10060) (G-C009)
(T-D1400) (M-14010) (G-C008)
(F-A5574)

DD-21044 Brain injury without open intracranial wound and with moderate loss of consciousness (1-24 hours) 854.03
(T-A0100) (M-10060) (G-C009)
(T-D1400) (M-14010) (G-C008)
(F-A5575)

DD-21045 Brain injury without open intracranial wound and with prolonged loss of consciousness (more than 24 hours) with return to pre-existing conscious level 854.04
(T-A0100) (M-10060) (G-C009)
(T-D1400) (M-14010) (G-C008)
(G-4010) (G-4003) (F-A5500)

DD-21046 Brain injury without open intracranial wound and with prolonged loss of consciousness (more than 24 hours) without return to pre-existing conscious level 854.05
(T-A0100) (M-10060) (G-C009)
(T-D1400) (M-14010) (G-C008)
(F-A5576) (G-C009) (G-4010) (G-4003)
(F-A5500)

DD-21047 Brain injury without open intracranial wound and with loss of consciousness of unspecified duration 854.06
(T-A0100) (M-10060) (G-C009)
(T-D1400) (M-14010) (G-C008)
(F-A5570)

DD-21048 Brain injury without open intracranial wound and with unspecified concussion 854.09
(T-A0100) (M-10060) (G-C009)
(T-D1400) (M-14010) (G-C008)
(F-A5680)

DD-21060 Brain injury with open intracranial wound, NOS 854.1
(T-A0100) (M-10060) (G-C008)
(T-D1400) (M-14010)

DD-21061 Brain injury with open intracranial wound and unspecified state of consciousness 854.10
(T-A0100) (M-10060) (G-C008)
(T-D1400) (M-14010) (G-C008)
(F-A5500)

DD-21062 Brain injury with open intracranial wound and no loss of consciousness 854.11
(T-A0100) (M-10060) (G-C008)
(T-D1400) (M-14010) (G-C009)
(F-A5570)

DD-21063 Brain injury with open intracranial wound and brief loss of consciousness (less than one hour) 854.12
(T-A0100) (M-10060) (G-C008)
(T-D1400) (M-14010) (G-C008)
(F-A5574)

DD-21064 Brain injury with open intracranial wound and moderate loss of consciousness (1-24 hours) 854.13
(T-A0100) (M-10060) (G-C008)
(T-D1400) (M-14010) (G-C008)
(F-A5575)

DD-21065 Brain injury with open intracranial wound and prolonged loss of consciousness (more than 24 hours) and return to pre-existing conscious level 854.14
(T-A0100) (M-10060) (G-C008)
(T-D1400) (M-14010) (G-C008)
(G-4010) (G-4003) (F-A5500)

DD-21066 Brain injury with open intracranial wound and prolonged loss of consciousness (more than 24 hours) without return to pre-existing conscious level 854.15
(T-A0100) (M-10060) (G-C008)
(T-D1400) (M-14010) (G-C009)
(G-4010) (G-4003) (F-A5500)

DD-21067 Brain injury with open intracranial wound and loss of consciousness of unspecified duration 854.16
(T-A0100) (M-10060) (G-C008)
(T-D1400) (M-14010) (G-C008)
(F-A5570)

DD-21068 Brain injury with open intracranial wound and unspecified concussion 854.19
(T-A0100) (M-10060) (G-C008)
(T-D1400) (M-14010) (G-C008)
(F-A5680)

DD-21101 Concussion with no loss of consciousness 850.0
(T-A0100) (F-A5680) (G-C009)
(F-A5570)
Concussion with mental confusion or disorientation without loss of consciousness 850.0
(T-A0100) (F-A5680) (G-C008)
(F-A5562) (G-C009) (F-A5570)

DD-21102 Concussion with brief loss of consciousness 850.1
(T-A0100) (F-A5680) (G-C008)
(F-A5574)
Concussion with loss of consciousness for less than one hour 850.1
(T-A0100) (F-A5680) (G-C008)
(F-A5574)

DD-21103 Concussion with moderate loss of consciousness 850.2
(T-A0100) (F-A5680) (G-C008)
(F-A5575)
Concussion with loss of consciousness for 1-24 hours 850.2
(T-A0100) (F-A5680) (G-C008)
(F-A5575)

DD-21104 Concussion with prolonged loss of consciousness and return to pre-existing conscious level 850.3
(T-A0100) (F-A5680) (G-C008)
(F-A5576) (G-C008) (G-4010) (G-4003)
(F-A5500)
Concussion with loss of consciousness for more than 24 hours with complete recovery 850.3
(T-A0100) (F-A5680) (G-C008)
(F-A5576) (G-C008) (G-4010) (G-4003)
(F-A5500)

DD-21105 Concussion with prolonged loss of consciousness without return to pre-existing conscious level 850.4
(T-A0100) (F-A5680) (G-C008)
(F-A5576) (G-C009) (G-4010) (G-4003)
(F-A5500)

DD-21106 Concussion with loss of consciousness of unspecified duration 850.5
(T-A0100) (F-A5680) (G-C008)
(F-A5570)

DD-21200 Contusion of brain, NOS 851.8
(T-A0100) (M-14200)
Cerebral contusion, NOS 851.8
(T-A0100) (M-14200)

DD-21201 Laceration of brain, NOS 851.8
(T-A0100) (M-14400)
Cerebral laceration, NOS 851.8
(T-A0100) (M-14400)

DD-21202 Contusion of brain without open intracranial wound 851.8
(T-A0100) (M-14200) (G-C009)
(T-D1400) (M-14010)

DD-21203 Laceration of brain without open intracranial wound 851.8
(T-A0100) (M-14400) (G-C009)
(T-D1400) (M-14010)

DD-21205 Contusion of brain with open intracranial wound 851.9
(T-A0100) (M-14200) (G-C008)
(T-D1400) (M-14010)

DD-21206 Laceration of brain with open intracranial wound 851.9
(T-A0100) (M-14400) (G-C008)
(T-D1400) (M-14010)

DD-21210 Contusion of cerebral cortex, NOS 851.0
(T-A2020) (M-14200)

DD-21211 Cortex contusion without open intracranial wound 851.0
(T-A2020) (M-14200) (G-C009)
(M-14010)

DD-21212 Cortex contusion without open intracranial wound and with unspecified state of consciousness 851.00
(T-A2020) (M-14200) (G-C009)
(T-D1400) (M-14010) (G-C008)
(F-A5500)

DD-21213 Cortex contusion without open intracranial wound and with no loss of consciousness 851.01
(T-A2020) (M-14200) (G-C009)
(T-D1400) (M-14010) (G-C009)
(F-A5570)

DD-21214 Cortex contusion without open intracranial wound and with brief loss of consciousness (less than one hour) 851.02
(T-A2020) (M-14200) (G-C009)
(T-D1400) (M-14010) (G-C008)
(F-A5574)

DD-21215 Cortex contusion without open intracranial wound and with moderate loss of consciousness (1-24 hours) 851.03
(T-A2020) (M-14200) (G-C009)
(T-D1400) (M-14010) (G-C008)
(F-A5575)

DD-21216 Cortex contusion without open intracranial wound and with prolonged loss of consciousness (more than 24 hours) and return to pre-existing conscious level 851.04
(T-A2020) (M-14200) (G-C009)
(T-D1400) (M-14010) (G-C008)
(G-4010) (G-4003) (F-A5500)

DD-21217 Cortex contusion without open intracranial wound and with prolonged loss of consciousness (more than 24 hours) without return to pre-existing conscious level 851.05
(T-A2020) (M-14200) (G-C009)
(T-D1400) (M-14010) (G-C008)
(F-A5576) (G-C009) (G-4010) (G-4003)
(F-A5500)

D-21 INTRACRANIAL INJURIES WITHOUT SKULL FRACTURE — Continued

DD-21218 Cortex contusion without open intracranial wound and with loss of consciousness of unspecified duration 851.06
(T-A2020) (M-14200) (G-C009)
(T-D1400) (M-14010) (G-C008)
(F-A5570)

DD-21219 Cortex contusion without open intracranial wound and with unspecified concussion 851.09
(T-A2020) (M-14200) (G-C009)
(T-D1400) (M-14010) (G-C008)
(F-A5680)

DD-21221 Cortex contusion with open intracranial wound 851.1
(T-A2020) (M-14200) (G-C008)
(T-D1400) (M-14010)
Contusion of cerebral cortex with open intracranial wound 851.1
(T-A2020) (M-14200) (G-C008)
(T-D1400) (M-14010)

DD-21222 Cortex contusion with open intracranial wound and unspecified state of consciousness 851.10
(T-A2020) (M-14200) (G-C008)
(T-D1400) (M-14010) (G-C008)
(F-A5500)

DD-21223 Cortex contusion with open intracranial wound and no loss of consciousness 851.11
(T-A2020) (M-14200) (G-C008)
(T-D1400) (M-14010) (G-C009)
(F-A5570)

DD-21224 Cortex contusion with open intracranial wound and brief loss of consciousness (less than one hour) 851.12
(T-A2020) (M-14200) (G-C008)
(T-D1400) (M-14010) (G-C008)
(F-A5574)

DD-21225 Cortex contusion with open intracranial wound and moderate loss of consciousness (1-24 hours) 851.13
(T-A2020) (M-14200) (G-C008)
(T-D1400) (M-14010) (G-C008)
(F-A5575)

DD-21226 Cortex contusion with open intracranial wound and prolonged loss of consciousness (more than 24 hours) and return to pre-existing conscious level 851.14
(T-A2020) (M-14200) (G-C008)
(T-D1400) (M-14010) (G-C008)
(F-A5576) (G-C008) (G-4010) (G-4003)
(F-A5500)

DD-21227 Cortex contusion with open intracranial and prolonged loss of consciousness (more than 24 hours) without return to pre-existing conscious level 851.15
(T-A2020) (M-14200) (G-C008)
(T-D1400) (M-14010) (G-C009)
(G-4010) (G-4003) (F-A5500)

DD-21228 Cortex contusion with open intracranial wound and loss of consciousness of unspecified duration 851.16
(T-A2020) (M-14200) (G-C008)
(T-D1400) (M-14010) (G-C008)
(F-A5570)

DD-21229 Cortex contusion with open intracranial wound and unspecified concussion 821.19
(T-A2020) (M-14200) (G-C008)
(T-D1400) (M-14010) (G-C008)
(F-A5680)

DD-21230 Cortex laceration without open intracranial wound 851.2
(T-A2020) (M-14400) (G-C009)
(T-D1400) (M-14010)

DD-21231 Cortex laceration without open intracranial wound and with unspecified state of consciousness 851.20
(T-A2020) (M-14400) (G-C009)
(T-D1400) (M-14010) (G-C008)
(F-A5500)

DD-21232 Cortex laceration without open intracranial wound and with no loss of consciousness 851.21
(T-A2020) (M-14400) (G-C009)
(T-D1400) (M-14010) (G-C008)
(F-A5570)

DD-21233 Cortex laceration without open intracranial wound and with brief loss of consciousness (less than one hour) 851.22
(T-A2020) (M-14400) (G-C009)
(T-D1400) (M-14010) (G-C008)
(F-A5574)

DD-21234 Cortex laceration without open intracranial wound and with moderate loss of consciousness (1-24 hours) 851.23
(T-A2020) (M-14400) (G-C009)
(T-D1400) (M-14010) (G-C008)
(F-A5575)

DD-21235 Cortex laceration without open intracranial wound and with prolonged loss of consciousness (more than 24 hours) and return to pre-existing conscious level 851.24
(T-A2020) (M-14400) (G-C009)
(T-D1400) (M-14010) (G-C008)
(F-A5576) (G-C008) (G-4010) (G-4003)
(F-A5500)

DD-21236 Cortex laceration without open intracranial wound and with prolonged loss of consciousness (more than 24 hours) without return to pre-existing conscious level 851.25
(T-A2020) (M-14400) (G-C009)
(T-D1400) (M-14010) (G-C009)
(G-4010) (G-4003) (F-A5500)

DD-21237 Cortex laceration without open intracranial wound and with loss of consciousness of unspecified duration 851.26
(T-A2020) (M-14400) (G-C009)
(T-D1400) (M-14010) (G-C008)
(F-A5570)

DD-21238 Cortex laceration without open intracranial wound and with unspecified concussion 851.29
(T-A2020) (M-14400) (G-C009)
(T-D1400) (M-14010) (G-C008)
(F-A5680)

DD-21240 Cortex laceration with open intracranial wound 851.3
(T-A2020) (M-14400) (G-C008)
(T-D1400) (M-14010)

DD-21241 Cortex laceration with open intracranial wound and unspecified state of consciousness 851.30
(T-A2020) (M-14010) (G-C008)
(T-D1400) (M-14010) (G-C008)
(F-A5500)

DD-21242 Cortex laceration with open intracranial wound and no loss of consciousness 851.31
(T-A2020) (M-14400) (G-C008)
(T-D1400) (M-14010) (G-C009)
(F-A5570)

DD-21243 Cortex laceration with open intracranial wound and brief loss of consciousness (less than one hour) 851.32
(T-A2020) (M-14400) (G-C008)
(T-D1400) (M-14010) (G-C008)
(F-A5574)

DD-21244 Cortex laceration with open intracranial wound and moderate loss of consciousness (1-24 hours) 851.33
(T-A2020) (M-14400) (G-C008)
(T-D1400) (M-14010) (G-C008)
(F-A5575)

DD-21245 Cortex laceration with open intracranial wound and prolonged loss of consciousness (more than 24 hours) and return to pre-existing conscious level 851.34
(T-A2020) (M-14400) (G-C008)
(T-D1400) (M-14010) (G-C008)
(F-A5576) (G-C008) (G-4010) (G-4003)
(F-A5500)

DD-21246 Cortex laceration with open intracranial wound and prolonged loss of consciousness (more than 24 hours) without return to pre-existing conscious level 851.35
(T-A2020) (M-14400) (G-C008)
(T-D1400) (M-14010) (G-C008)
(F-A5576) (G-C009) (G-4010) (G-4003)
(F-A5500)

DD-21247 Cortex laceration with open intracranial wound and loss of consciousness of unspecified duration 851.36
(T-A2020) (M-14400) (G-C008)
(T-D1400) (M-14010) (G-C008)
(F-A5570)

DD-21248 Cortex laceration with open intracranial wound and unspecified concussion 851.39
(T-A2020) (M-14400) (G-C008)
(T-D1400) (M-14010) (G-C008)
(F-A5680)

DD-21250 Cerebellar contusion without open intracranial wound 851.4
(T-A6000) (M-14200) (G-C009)
(T-D1400) (M-14010)

DD-21251 Cerebellar contusion without open intracranial wound and with unspecified state of consciousness 851.40
(T-A6000) (M-14200) (G-C009)
(T-D1400) (M-14010) (G-C008)
(F-A5500)

DD-21252 Cerebellar contusion without open intracranial wound and with no loss of consciousness 851.41
(T-A6000) (M-14200) (G-C009)
(T-D1400) (M-14010) (G-C009)
(F-A5570)

DD-21253 Cerebellar contusion without open intracranial wound and with brief loss of consciousness (less than one hour) 851.42
(T-A6000) (M-14200) (G-C009)
(T-D1400) (M-14010) (G-C008)
(F-A5574)

DD-21254 Cerebellar contusion without open intracranial wound and with moderate loss of consciousness (1-24 hours) 851.43
(T-A6000) (M-14200) (G-C009)
(T-D1400) (M-14010) (G-C008)
(F-A5575)

DD-21255 Cerebellar contusion without open intracranial wound and with prolonged loss of consciousness (more than 24 hours) and return to pre-existing conscious level 851.44
(T-A6000) (M-14200) (G-C009)
(T-D1400) (M-14010) (G-C008)
(F-A5576) (G-C008) (G-4010) (G-4003)
(F-A5500)

DD-21256 Cerebellar contusion without open intracranial wound and with prolonged loss of consciousness (more than 24 hours) without return to pre-existing conscious level 851.45
(T-A6000) (M-14200) (G-C009)
(T-D1400) (M-14010) (G-C008)
(F-A5576) (G-C009) (G-4010) (G-4003)
(F-A5500)

DD-21257 Cerebellar contusion without open intracranial wound and with loss of consciousness of unspecified duration 851.46
(T-A6000) (M-14200) (G-C009)
(T-D1400) (M-14010) (G-C008)
(F-A5570)

DD-21258 Cerebellar contusion without open intracranial wound and with unspecified concussion 851.49
(T-A6000) (M-14200) (G-C009)
(T-D1400) (M-14010) (G-C008)
(F-A5680)

DD-21260 Brain stem contusion without open intracranial wound 851.4
(T-A2050) (M-14200) (G-C009)
(T-D1400) (M-14010)

D-21 INTRACRANIAL INJURIES WITHOUT SKULL FRACTURE — Continued

DD-21261 Brain stem contusion without open intracranial wound and with unspecified state of consciousness 851.40
(T-A2050) (M-14200) (G-C009)
(T-D1400) (M-14010) (G-C008)
(F-A5500)

DD-21262 Brain stem contusion without open intracranial wound and with no loss of consciousness 851.41
(T-A2050) (M-14200) (G-C009)
(T-D1400) (M-14010) (G-C009)
(F-A5570)

DD-21263 Brain stem contusion without open intracranial wound and with brief loss of consciousness (less than one hour) 851.42
(T-A2050) (M-14200) (G-C009)
(T-D1400) (M-14010) (G-C008)
(F-A5574)

DD-21264 Brain stem contusion without open intracranial wound and with moderate loss of consciousness (1-24 hours) 851.43
(T-A2050) (M-14200) (G-C009)
(T-D1400) (M-14010) (G-C008)
(F-A5575)

DD-21265 Brain stem contusion without open intracranial wound and with prolonged loss of consciousness (more than 24 hours) and return to pre-existing conscious level 851.44
(T-A2050) (M-14200) (G-C009)
(T-D1400) (M-14010) (G-C008)
(F-A5576) (G-C008) (G-4010) (G-4003)
(F-A5500)

DD-21266 Brain stem contusion without open intracranial wound and with prolonged loss of consciousness (more than 24 hours) without return to pre-existing conscious level 851.45
(T-A2050) (M-14200) (G-C009)
(T-D1400) (M-14010) (G-C008)
(F-A5576) (G-C009) (G-4010) (G-4003)
(F-A5500)

DD-21267 Brain stem contusion without open intracranial wound and with loss of consciousness of unspecified duration 851.46
(T-A2050) (M-14200) (G-C009)
(T-D1400) (M-14010) (G-C008)
(F-A5570)

DD-21268 Brain stem contusion without open intracranial wound and with unspecified concussion 851.49
(T-A2050) (M-14200) (G-C009)
(T-D1400) (M-14010) (G-C008)
(F-A5680)

DD-21270 Cerebellar contusion with open intracranial wound 851.5
(T-A6000) (M-14200) (G-C008)
(T-D1400) (M-14010)

DD-21271 Cerebellar contusion with open intracranial wound and unspecified state of consciousness 851.50
(T-A6000) (M-14200) (G-C008)
(T-D1400) (M-14010) (G-C008)
(F-A5500)

DD-21272 Cerebellar contusion with open intracranial wound and no loss of consciousness 851.51
(T-A6000) (M-14200) (G-C008)
(T-D1400) (M-14010) (G-C009)
(F-A5570)

DD-21273 Cerebellar contusion with open intracranial wound and brief loss of consciousness (less than one hour) 851.52
(T-A6000) (M-14200) (G-C008)
(T-D1400) (M-14010) (G-C008)
(F-A5574)

DD-21274 Cerebellar contusion with open intracranial wound and moderate loss of consciousness (1-24 hours) 851.53
(T-A6000) (M-14200) (G-C008)
(T-D1400) (M-14010) (G-C008)
(F-A5575)

DD-21275 Cerebellar contusion with open intracranial wound and prolonged loss of consciousness (more than 24 hours) and return to pre-existing conscious level 851.54
(T-A6000) (M-14200) (G-C008)
(T-D1400) (M-14010) (G-C008)
(F-A5576) (G-C008) (G-4010) (G-4003)
(F-A5500)

DD-21276 Cerebellar contusion with open intracranial wound and prolonged loss of consciousness (more than 24 hours) without return to pre-existing conscious level 851.55
(T-A6000) (M-14200) (G-C008)
(T-D1400) (M-14010) (G-C008)
(F-A5576) (G-C009) (G-4010) (G-4003)
(F-A5500)

DD-21277 Cerebellar contusion with open intracranial wound and loss of consciousness of unspecified duration 851.56
(T-A6000) (M-14200) (G-C008)
(T-D1400) (M-14010) (G-C008)
(F-A5570)

DD-21278 Cerebellar contusion with open intracranial wound and unspecified concussion 851.59
(T-A6000) (M-14200) (G-C008)
(T-D1400) (M-14010) (G-C008)
(F-A5680)

DD-21280 Brain stem contusion with open intracranial wound 851.5
(T-A2050) (M-14200) (G-C008)
(T-D1400) (M-14010)

DD-21281 Brain stem contusion with open intracranial wound and unspecified state of consciousness 851.50
(T-A2050) (M-14200) (G-C008)
(T-D1400) (M-14010) (G-C008)
(F-A5500)

DD-21282 Brain stem contusion with open intracranial wound and no loss of consciousness 851.51
(T-A2050) (M-14200) (G-C008)
(T-D1400) (M-14010) (G-C009)
(F-A5570)

DD-21283 Brain stem contusion with open intracranial wound and brief loss of consciousness (less than one hour) 851.52
(T-A2050) (M-14200) (G-C008)
(T-D1400) (M-14010) (G-C008)
(F-A5574)

DD-21284 Brain stem contusion with open intracranial wound and moderate loss of consciousness (1-24 hours) 851.53
(T-A2050) (M-14200) (G-C008)
(T-D1400) (M-14010) (G-C008)
(F-A5575)

DD-21285 Brain stem contusion with open intracranial wound and prolonged loss of consciousness (more than 24 hours) and return to pre-existing conscious level 851.54
(T-A2050) (M-14200) (G-C008)
(T-D1400) (M-14010) (G-C008)
(F-A5576) (G-C008) (G-4010) (G-4003)
(F-A5500)

DD-21286 Brain stem contusion with open intracranial wound and prolonged loss of consciousness (more than 24 hours) without return to pre-existing conscious level 851.55
(T-A2050) (M-14200) (G-C008)
(T-D1400) (M-14010) (G-C008)
(F-A5576) (G-C009) (G-4010) (G-4003)
(F-A5500)

DD-21287 Brain stem contusion with open intracranial wound and loss of consciousness of unspecified duration 851.56
(T-A2050) (M-14200) (G-C008)
(T-D1400) (M-14010) (G-C008)
(F-A5570)

DD-21288 Brain stem contusion with open intracranial wound and unspecified concussion 851.59
(T-A2050) (M-14200) (G-C008)
(T-D1400) (M-14010) (G-C008)
(F-A5680)

DD-21290 Cerebellar laceration without open intracranial wound 851.6
(T-A6000) (M-14400) (G-C009)
(T-D1400) (M-14010)

DD-21291 Cerebellar laceration without open intracranial wound and with unspecified state of consciousness 851.60
(T-A6000) (M-14400) (G-C009)
(T-D1400) (M-14010) (G-C008)
(F-A5500)

DD-21292 Cerebellar laceration without open intracranial wound and with no loss of consciousness 851.61
(T-A6000) (M-14400) (G-C009)
(T-D1400) (M-14010) (G-C009)
(F-A5570)

DD-21293 Cerebellar laceration without open intracranial wound and with brief loss of consciousness (less than one hour) 851.62
(T-A6000) (M-14400) (G-C009)
(T-D1400) (M-14010) (G-C008)
(F-A5574)

DD-21294 Cerebellar laceration without open intracranial wound and with moderate loss of consciousness (1-24 hours) 851.63
(T-A6000) (M-14400) (G-C009)
(T-D1400) (M-14010) (G-C008)
(F-A5575)

DD-21295 Cerebellar laceration without open intracranial wound and with prolonged loss of consciousness (more than 24 hours) and return to pre-existing conscious level 851.64
(T-A6000) (M-14400) (G-C009)
(T-D1400) (M-14010) (G-C008)
(F-A5576) (G-C008) (G-4010) (G-4003)
(F-A5500)

DD-21296 Cerebellar laceration without open intracranial wound and with prolonged loss of consciousness (more than 24 hours) without return to pre-existing conscious level 851.65
(T-A6000) (M-14400) (G-C009)
(T-D1400) (M-14010) (G-C008)
(F-A5576) (G-C009) (G-4010) (G-4003)
(F-A5500)

DD-21297 Cerebellar laceration without open intracranial wound and with loss of consciousness of unspecified duration 851.66
(T-A6000) (M-14400) (G-C009)
(T-D1400) (M-14010) (G-C008)
(F-A5570)

DD-21298 Cerebellar laceration without open intracranial wound and with unspecified concussion 851.69
(T-A6000) (M-14400) (G-C009)
(T-D1400) (M-14010) (G-C008)
(F-A5680)

DD-212A0 Brain stem laceration without open intracranial wound 851.6
(T-A2050) (M-14400) (G-C009)
(T-D1400) (M-14010)

DD-212A1 Brain stem laceration without open intracranial wound and with unspecified state of consciousness 851.60
(T-A2050) (M-14400) (G-C009)
(T-D1400) (M-14010) (G-C008)
(F-A5500)

DD-212A2 Brain stem laceration without open intracranial wound and with no loss of consciousness 851.61
(T-A2050) (M-14400) (G-C009)
(T-D1400) (M-14010) (G-C009)
(F-A5570)

DD-212A3 Brain stem laceration without open intracranial wound and with brief loss of consciousness (less than one hour) 851.62
(T-A2050) (M-14400) (G-C009)
(T-D1400) (M-14010) (G-C008)
(F-A5574)

D-21 INTRACRANIAL INJURIES WITHOUT SKULL FRACTURE — Continued

DD-212A4 Brain stem laceration without open intracranial wound and with moderate loss of consciousness (1-24 hours) 851.63
(T-A2050) (M-14400) (G-C009)
(T-D1400) (M-14010) (G-C008)
(F-A5575)

DD-212A5 Brain stem laceration without open intracranial wound and with prolonged loss of consciousness (more than 24 hours) and return to pre-existing conscious level 851.64
(T-A2050) (M-14400) (G-C009)
(T-D1400) (M-14010) (G-C008)
(F-A5576) (G-C008) (G-4010) (G-4003)
(F-A5500)

DD-212A6 Brain stem laceration without open intracranial wound and with prolonged loss of consciousness (more than 24 hours) without return to pre-existing conscious level 851.65
(T-A2050) (M-14400) (G-C009)
(T-D1400) (M-14010) (G-C008)
(F-A5576) (G-C009) (G-4010) (G-4003)
(F-A5500)

DD-212A7 Brain stem laceration without open intracranial wound and with loss of consciousness of unspecified duration 851.66
(T-A2050) (M-14400) (G-C009)
(T-D1400) (M-14010) (G-C008)
(F-A5570)

DD-212A8 Brain stem laceration without open intracranial wound and with unspecified concussion 851.69
(T-A2050) (M-14400) (G-C009)
(T-D1400) (M-14010) (G-C008)
(F-A5680)

DD-212B0 Cerebellar laceration with open intracranial wound 851.7
(T-A6000) (M-14400) (G-C008)
(T-D1400) (M-14010)

DD-212B1 Cerebellar laceration with open intracranial wound and unspecified state of consciousness 851.70
(T-A6000) (M-14400) (G-C008)
(T-D1400) (M-14010) (G-C008)
(F-A5500)

DD-212B2 Cerebellar laceration with open intracranial wound and no loss of consciousness 851.71
(T-A6000) (M-14400) (G-C008)
(T-D1400) (M-14010) (G-C009)
(F-A5570)

DD-212B3 Cerebellar laceration with open intracranial wound and brief loss of consciousness (less than one hour) 851.72
(T-A6000) (M-14400) (G-C008)
(T-D1400) (M-14010) (G-C008)
(F-A5574)

DD-212B4 Cerebellar laceration with open intracranial wound and moderate loss of consciousness (1-24 hours) 851.73
(T-A6000) (M-14400) (G-C008)
(T-D1400) (M-14010) (G-C008)
(F-A5575)

DD-212B5 Cerebellar laceration with open intracranial wound and prolonged loss of consciousness (more than 24 hours) and return to pre-existing conscious level 851.74
(T-A6000) (M-14400) (G-C008)
(T-D1400) (M-14010) (G-C008)
(F-A5576) (G-C008) (G-4010) (G-4003)
(F-A5500)

DD-212B6 Cerebellar laceration with open intracranial wound and prolonged loss of consciousness (more than 24 hours) without return to pre-existing conscious level 851.75
(T-A6000) (M-14400) (G-C008)
(T-D1400) (M-14010) (G-C008)
(F-A5576) (G-C009) (G-4010) (G-4003)
(F-A5500)

DD-212B7 Cerebellar laceration with open intracranial wound and loss of consciousness of unspecified duration 851.76
(T-A6000) (M-14400) (G-C008)
(T-D1400) (M-14010) (G-C008)
(F-A5570)

DD-212B8 Cerebellar laceration with open intracranial wound and unspecified concussion 851.79
(T-A6000) (M-14400) (G-C008)
(T-D1400) (M-14010) (G-C008)
(F-A5680)

DD-212C0 Brain stem laceration with open intracranial wound 851.7
(T-A2050) (M-14400) (G-C008)
(T-D1400) (M-14010)

DD-212C1 Brain stem laceration with open intracranial wound and unspecified state of consciousness 851.70
(T-A2050) (M-14400) (G-C008)
(T-D1400) (M-14010) (G-C008)
(F-A5500)

DD-212C2 Brain stem laceration with open intracranial wound and no loss of consciousness 851.71
(T-A2050) (M-14400) (G-C008)
(T-D1400) (M-14010) (G-C008)
(F-A5570)

DD-212C3 Brain stem laceration with open intracranial wound and brief loss of consciousness (less than one hour) 851.72
(T-A2050) (M-14400) (G-C008)
(T-D1400) (M-14010) (G-C008)
(F-A5574)

DD-212C4 Brain stem laceration with open intracranial wound and moderate loss of consciousness (1-24 hours) 851.73
(T-A2050) (M-14400) (G-C008)
(T-D1400) (M-14010) (G-C008)
(F-A5575)

DD-212C5 Brain stem laceration with open intracranial wound and prolonged loss of consciousness (more than 24 hours) and return to pre-existing conscious level 851.74
(T-A2050) (M-14400) (G-C008)
(T-D1400) (M-14010) (G-C008)
(F-A5576) (G-C008) (G-4010) (G-4003)
(F-A5500)

DD-212C6 Brain stem laceration with open intracranial wound and prolonged loss of consciousness (more than 24 hours) without return to pre-existing conscious level 851.75
(T-A2050) (M-14400) (G-C008)
(T-D1400) (M-14010) (G-C008)
(F-A5576) (G-C009) (G-4010) (G-4003)
(F-A5500)

DD-212C7 Brain stem laceration with open intracranial wound and loss of consciousness of unspecified duration 851.76
(T-A2050) (M-14400) (G-C008)
(T-D1400) (M-14010) (G-C008)
(F-A5570)

DD-212C8 Brain stem laceration with open intracranial wound and unspecified concussion 851.79
(T-A2050) (M-14400) (G-C008)
(T-D1400) (M-14010) (G-C008)
(F-A5680)

DD-21400 Intracranial hemorrhage following injury, NOS 853.-
(T-D1400) (M-37000) (G-C001)
(M-10060)
Traumatic cerebral hemorrhage, NOS 853.0
(T-D1400) (M-37000) (G-C001)
(M-10060)

DD-21402 Intracranial hematoma following injury 853.0
(T-D1400) (M-35060) (G-C001)
(M-10060)

DD-21404 Cerebral compression due to injury 853.0
(T-A0100) (M-01460) (G-C001)
(M-10060)

DD-21420 Intracranial hemorrhage following injury without open intracranial wound 853.0
(T-D1400) (M-37000) (G-C001)
(M-10060) (G-C009) (T-D1400)
(M-14010)

DD-21421 Intracranial hemorrhage following injury without open intracranial wound and unspecified state of consciousness 853.00
(T-D1400) (M-37000) (G-C001)
(M-10060) (G-C009) (T-D1400)
(M-14010) (G-C008) (F-A5500)

DD-21422 Intracranial hemorrhage following injury without open intracranial wound and with no loss of consciousness 853.01
(T-D1400) (M-37000) (G-C001)
(M-10060) (G-C009) (T-D1400)
(M-14010) (G-C009) (F-A5570)

DD-21423 Intracranial hemorrhage following injury without open intracranial wound and with brief loss of consciousness (less than one hour) 853.02
(T-D1400) (M-37000) (G-C001)
(M-10060) (G-C009) (T-D1400)
(M-14010) (G-C008) (F-A5574)

DD-21424 Intracranial hemorrhage following injury without intracranial wound and with moderate loss of consciousness (1-24 hours) 853.03
(T-D1400) (M-37000) (G-C001)
(M-10060) (G-C009) (T-D1400)
(M-14010) (G-C008) (F-A5575)

DD-21425 Intracranial hemorrhage following injury without open intracranial wound and with prolonged loss of consciousness (more than 24 hours) and return to pre-existing conscious level 853.04
(T-D1400) (M-37000) (G-C001)
(M-10060) (G-C009) (T-D1400)
(M-14010) (G-C008) (F-A5576)
(G-C008) (G-4010) (G-4003) (F-A5500)

DD-21426 Intracranial hemorrhage following injury without open intracranial wound and with prolonged loss of consciousness (more than 24 hours) without return to pre-existing level 853.05
(T-D1400) (M-37000) (G-C001)
(M-10060) (G-C009) (T-D1400)
(M-14010) (G-C008) (F-A5576)
(G-C009) (G-4010) (G-4003) (F-A5500)

DD-21427 Intracranial hemorrhage following injury without open intracranial wound and with loss of consciousness of unspecified duration 852.06
(T-D1400) (M-37000) (G-C001)
(M-10060) (G-C009) (T-D1400)
(M-14010) (G-C008) (F-A5570)

DD-21428 Intracranial hemorrhage following injury without open intracranial wound and with unspecified concussion 853.09
(T-D1400) (M-37000) (G-C001)
(M-10060) (G-C009) (T-D1400)
(M-14010) (G-C008) (F-A5680)

DD-21440 Intracranial hemorrhage following injury with open intracranial wound 853.1
(T-D1400) (M-37000) (G-C001)
(M-10060) (G-C008) (T-D1400)
(M-14010)

DD-21441 Intracranial hemorrhage following injury with open intracranial wound and unspecified state of consciousness 853.10
(T-D1400) (M-37000) (G-C001)
(M-10060) (G-C008) (T-D1400)
(M-14010) (G-C008) (F-A5500)

DD-21442 Intracranial hemorrhage following injury with open intracranial wound and no loss of consciousness 853.11
(T-D1400) (M-37000) (G-C001)
(M-10060) (G-C008) (T-D1400)
(M-14010) (G-C009) (F-A5570)

D-21 INTRACRANIAL INJURIES WITHOUT SKULL FRACTURE — Continued

DD-21443 Intracranial hemorrhage following injury with open intracranial wound and brief loss of consciousness (less than one hour) 853.12
(T-D1400) (M-37000) (G-C001) (M-10060) (G-C008) (T-D1400) (M-14010) (G-C008) (F-A5574)

DD-21444 Intracranial hemorrhage following injury with intracranial wound and moderate loss of consciousness (1-24 hours) 853.13
(T-D1400) (M-37000) (G-C001) (M-10060) (G-C008) (T-D1400) (M-14010) (G-C008) (F-A5575)

DD-21445 Intracranial hemorrhage following injury with open intracranial wound and prolonged loss of consciousness (more than 24 hours) and return to pre-existing conscious level 853.14
(T-D1400) (M-37000) (G-C001) (M-10060) (G-C008) (T-D1400) (M-14010) (G-C008) (F-A5576) (G-C008) (G-4010) (G-4003) (F-A5500)

DD-21446 Intracranial hemorrhage following injury with open intracranial wound and prolonged loss of consciousness (more than 24 hours) without return to pre-existing level 853.15
(T-D1400) (M-37000) (G-C001) (M-10060) (G-C008) (T-D1400) (M-14010) (G-C008) (F-A5576) (G-C009) (G-4010) (G-4003) (F-A5500)

DD-21447 Intracranial hemorrhage following injury with open intracranial wound and loss of consciousness of unspecified duration 853.16
(T-D1400) (M-37000) (G-C001) (M-10060) (G-C008) (T-D1400) (M-14010) (G-C008) (F-A5570)

DD-21448 Intracranial hemorrhage following injury with open intracranial wound and unspecified concussion 853.19
(T-D1400) (M-37000) (G-C001) (M-10060) (G-C008) (T-D1400) (M-14010) (G-C008) (F-A5680)

DD-21500 Subarachnoid hemorrhage following injury without open intracranial wound 852.0
(T-A1502) (M-37000) (G-C001) (M-10060) (G-C009) (T-D1400) (M-14010)

DD-21501 Subarachnoid hemorrhage following injury without open intracranial wound and unspecified state of consciousness 852.00
(T-A1502) (M-37000) (G-C001) (M-10060) (G-C009) (T-D1400) (M-14010) (G-C008) (F-A5500)

DD-21502 Subarachnoid hemorrhage following injury without open intracranial wound and with no loss of consciousness 852.01
(T-A1502) (M-37000) (G-C001) (M-10060) (G-C009) (T-D1400) (M-14010) (G-C009) (F-A5570)

DD-21503 Subarachnoid hemorrhage following injury without open intracranial wound and with brief loss of consciousness (less than one hour) 852.02
(T-A1502) (M-37000) (G-C001) (M-10060) (G-C009) (T-D1400) (M-14010) (G-C008) (F-A5574)

DD-21504 Subarachnoid hemorrhage following injury without open intracranial wound and with moderate loss of consciousness (1-24 hours) 852.03
(T-A1502) (M-37000) (G-C001) (M-10060) (G-C009) (T-D1400) (M-14010) (G-C008) (F-A5575)

DD-21505 Subarachnoid hemorrhage following injury without open intracranial wound and with prolonged loss of consciousness (more than 24 hours) and return to pre-existing conscious level 852.04
(T-A1502) (M-37000) (G-C001) (M-10060) (G-C009) (T-D1400) (M-14010) (G-C008) (F-A5576) (G-C008) (G-4010) (G-4003) (F-A5500)

DD-21506 Subarachnoid hemorrhage following injury without open intracranial wound and with prolonged loss of consciousness (more than 24 hours) and without return to pre-existing conscious level 852.05
(T-A1502) (M-37000) (G-C001) (M-10060) (G-C009) (T-D1400) (M-14010) (G-C008) (F-A5576) (G-C009) (G-4010) (G-4003) (F-A5500)

DD-21507 Subarachnoid hemorrhage following injury without open intracranial wound and with loss of consciousnes of unspecified duration 852.06
(T-A1502) (M-37000) (G-C001) (M-10060) (G-C009) (T-D1400) (M-14010) (G-C008) (F-A5570)

DD-21508 Subarachnoid hemorrhage following injury without open intracranial wound and with unspecified concussion 852.09
(T-A1502) (M-37000) (G-C001) (M-10060) (G-C009) (T-D1400) (M-14010) (G-C008) (F-A5680)

DD-21509 Middle meningeal hemorrhage following injury 852.0
(T-45290) (M-37000) (G-C001) (M-10000)

DD-21510 Subarachnoid hemorrhage following injury with open intracranial wound 852.1
(T-A1502) (M-37000) (G-C001) (M-10060) (G-C008) (T-D1400) (M-14010)

DD-21511 Subarachnoid hemorrhage following injury with open intracranial wound and unspecified state of consciousness 852.00
(T-A1502) (M-37000) (G-C001) (M-10060) (G-C008) (T-D1400) (M-14010) (G-C008) (F-A5500)

DD-21512 Subarachnoid hemorrhage following injury with open intracranial wound and no loss of consciousness 852.11
(T-A1502) (M-37000) (G-C001)
(M-10060) (G-C008) (T-D1400)
(M-14010) (G-C009) (F-A5570)

DD-21513 Subarachnoid hemorrhage following injury with open intracranial wound and brief loss of consciousness (less than one hour) 852.12
(T-A1502) (M-37000) (G-C001)
(M-10060) (G-C008) (T-D1400)
(M-14010) (G-C008) (F-A5574)

DD-21514 Subarachnoid hemorrhage following injury with open intracranial wound and moderate loss of consciousness (1-24 hours) 852.13
(T-A1502) (M-37000) (G-C001)
(M-10060) (G-C008) (T-D1400)
(M-14010) (G-C008) (F-A5575)

DD-21515 Subarachnoid hemorrhage following injury with open intracranial wound and prolonged loss of consciousness (more than 24 hours) and return to pre-existing conscious level 851.14
(T-A1502) (M-37000) (G-C001)
(M-10060) (G-C008) (T-D1400)
(M-14010) (G-C008) (F-A5576)
(G-C008) (G-4010) (G-4003) (F-A5500)

DD-21516 Subarachnoid hemorrhage following injury with open intracranial wound and prolonged loss of consciousness (more than 24 hours) without return to pre-existing conscious level 852.15
(T-A1502) (M-37000) (G-C001)
(M-10060) (G-C008) (T-D1400)
(M-14010) (G-C008) (F-A5576)
(G-C009) (G-4010) (G-4003) (F-A5500)

DD-21517 Subarachnoid hemorrhage following injury with open intracranial wound and loss of consciousness of unspecified duration 851.16
(T-A1502) (M-37000) (G-C001)
(M-10060) (G-C008) (T-D1400)
(M-14010) (G-C008) (F-A5570)

DD-21518 Subarachnoid hemorrhage following injury with open intracranial wound and unspecified concussion 852.19
(T-A1502) (M-37000) (G-C001)
(M-10060) (G-C008) (T-D1400)
(M-14010) (G-C008) (F-A5680)

DD-21520 Subdural hemorrhage following injury without open intracranial wound 852.2
(T-A1400) (M-37000) (G-C001)
(M-10000) (G-C009) (T-D1400)
(M-14010)

DD-21521 Subdural hemorrhage following injury without open intracranial wound with unspecified state of consciousness 852.20
(T-A1400) (M-37000) (G-C001)
(M-10000) (G-C009) (T-D1400)
(M-14010) (G-C008) (F-A5500)

DD-21522 Subdural hemorrhage following injury without open intracranial wound and with no loss of consciousness 852.21
(T-A1400) (M-37000) (G-C001)
(M-10000) (G-C009) (T-D1400)
(M-14010) (G-C009) (F-A5570)

DD-21523 Subdural hemorrhage following injury without open intracranial wound and with brief loss of consciousness (less than one hour) 852.22
(T-A1400) (M-37000) (G-C001)
(M-10000) (G-C009) (T-D1400)
(M-14010) (G-C008) (F-A5574)

DD-21524 Subdural hemorrhage following injury without open intracranial wound and with moderate loss of consciousness (1-24 hours) 852.23
(T-A1400) (M-37000) (G-C001)
(M-10000) (G-C009) (T-D1400)
(M-14010) (G-C008) (F-A5575)

DD-21525 Subdural hemorrhage following injury without open intracranial wound and with prolonged loss of consciousness (more than 24 hours) and return to pre-existing conscious level 852.24
(T-A1400) (M-37000) (G-C001)
(M-10000) (G-C009) (T-D1400)
(M-14010) (G-C008) (F-A5576)
(G-C008) (G-4010) (G-4003) (F-A5500)

DD-21526 Subdural hemorrhage following injury without open intracranial wound and with prolonged loss of consciousness (more than 24 hours) without return to pre-existing conscious level 852.25
(T-A1400) (M-37000) (G-C001)
(M-10000) (G-C009) (T-D1400)
(M-14010) (G-C008) (F-A5576)
(G-C009) (G-4010) (G-4003) (F-A5500)

DD-21527 Subdural hemorrhage following injury without open intracranial wound and with loss of consciousness of unspecified duration 852.26
(T-A1400) (M-37000) (G-C001)
(M-10000) (G-C009) (T-D1400)
(M-14010) (G-C008) (F-A5570)

DD-21528 Subdural hemorrhage following injury without open intracranial wound and with unspecified concussion 852.29
(T-A1400) (M-37000) (G-C001)
(M-10000) (G-C009) (T-D1400)
(M-14010) (G-C008) (F-A5680)

DD-21530 Subdural hemorrhage following injury with open intracranial wound 852.3
(T-A1400) (M-37000) (G-C001)
(M-10000) (G-C008) (T-D1400)
(M-14010)

DD-21531 Subdural hemorrhage following injury with open intracranial wound and unspecified state of consciousness 852.30
(T-A1400) (M-37000) (G-C001)
(M-10000) (G-C008) (T-D1400)
(M-14010) (G-C008) (F-A5500)

D-21 INTRACRANIAL INJURIES WITHOUT SKULL FRACTURE — Continued

DD-21532 Subdural hemorrhage following injury with open intracranial wound and no loss of consciousness 852.31
(T-A1400) (M-37000) (G-C001) (M-10000) (G-C008) (T-D1400) (M-14010) (G-C009) (F-A5570)

DD-21533 Subdural hemorrhage following injury with open intracranial wound and brief loss of consciousness (less than one hour) 852.32
(T-A1400) (M-37000) (G-C001) (M-10000) (G-C008) (T-D1400) (M-14010) (G-C008) (F-A5574)

DD-21534 Subdural hemorrhage following injury with open intracranial wound and moderate loss of consciousness (1-24 hours) 852.33
(T-A1400) (M-37000) (G-C001) (M-10000) (G-C008) (T-D1400) (M-14010) (G-C008) (F-A5575)

DD-21535 Subdural hemorrhage following injury with open intracranial wound and prolonged loss of consciousness (more than 24 hours) and return to pre-existing conscious level 852.34
(T-A1400) (M-37000) (G-C001) (M-10000) (G-C008) (T-D1400) (M-14010) (G-C008) (F-A5576) (G-C008) (G-4010) (G-4003) (F-A5500)

DD-21536 Subdural hemorrhage following injury with open intracranial wound and prolonged loss of consciousness (more than 24 hours) and without return to pre-existing conscious level 852.35
(T-A1400) (M-37000) (G-C001) (M-10000) (G-C008) (T-D1400) (M-14010) (G-C008) (F-A5576) (G-C009) (G-4010) (G-4003) (F-A5500)

DD-21537 Subdural hemorrhage following injury with open intracranial wound and loss of consciousness of unspecified duration 852.36
(T-A1400) (M-37000) (G-C001) (M-10000) (G-C008) (T-D1400) (M-14010) (G-C008) (F-A5570)

DD-21538 Subdural hemorrhage following injury with open intracranial wound and unspecified concussion 852.39
(T-A1400) (M-37000) (G-C001) (M-10000) (G-C008) (T-D1400) (M-14010) (G-C008) (F-A5680)

DD-21540 Extradural hemorrhage following injury without open intracranial wound 852.4
(T-A1310) (M-37000) (G-C001) (M-10000) (G-C009) (T-D1400) (M-14010)

DD-21541 Extradural hemorrhage following injury without open intracranial wound and with unspecified state of consciousness 852.40
(T-A1310) (M-37000) (G-C001) (M-10000) (G-C009) (T-D1400) (M-14010) (G-C008) (F-A5500)

DD-21542 Extradural hemorrhage following injury without open intracranial wound and with no loss of consciousness 852.41
(T-A1310) (M-37000) (G-C001) (M-10000) (G-C009) (T-D1400) (M-14010) (G-C009) (F-A5570)

DD-21543 Extradural hemorrhage following injury without open intracranial wound and with brief loss of consciousness (less than one hour) 852.42
(T-A1310) (M-37000) (G-C001) (M-10000) (G-C009) (T-D1400) (M-14010) (G-C008) (F-A5574)

DD-21544 Extradural hemorrhage following injury without open intracranial wound and with moderate loss of consciousness (1-24 hours) 852.43
(T-A1310) (M-37000) (G-C001) (M-10000) (G-C009) (T-D1400) (M-14010) (G-C008) (F-A5575)

DD-21545 Extradural hemorrhage following injury without open intracranial wound and with prolonged loss of consciousness (more than 24 hours) and return to pre-existing conscious level 852.44
(T-A1310) (M-37000) (G-C001) (M-10000) (G-C009) (T-D1400) (M-14010) (G-C008) (F-A5576) (G-C008) (G-4010) (G-4003) (F-A5500)

DD-21546 Extradural hemorrhage following injury without open intracranial wound and with prolonged loss of consciousness (more than 24 hours) without return to pre-existing conscious level 852.45
(T-A1310) (M-37000) (G-C001) (M-10000) (G-C009) (T-D1400) (M-14010) (G-C008) (F-A5576) (G-C009) (G-4010) (G-4003) (F-A5500)

DD-21547 Extradural hemorrhage following injury without open intracranial wound and with loss of consciousness of unspecified duration 852.46
(T-A1310) (M-37000) (G-C001) (M-10000) (G-C009) (T-D1400) (M-14010) (G-C008) (F-A5570)

DD-21548 Extradural hemorrhage following injury without open intracranial wound and with unspecified concussion 852.49
(T-A1310) (M-37000) (G-C001) (M-10000) (G-C009) (T-D1400) (M-14010) (G-C008) (F-A5680)

DD-21550 Extradural hemorrhage following injury with open intracranial wound 852.5
(T-A1310) (M-37000) (G-C001) (M-10000) (G-C008) (T-D1400) (M-14010)

DD-21551 Extradural hemorrhage following injury with open intracranial wound and unspecified state of consciousness 852.50
(T-A1310) (M-37000) (G-C001) (M-10000) (G-C008) (T-D1400) (M-14010) (G-C008) (F-A5500)

DD-21552 Extradural hemorrhage following injury with open intracranial wound and no loss of consciousness 852.51
(T-A1310) (M-37000) (G-C001) (M-10000) (G-C008) (T-D1400) (M-14010) (G-C009) (F-A5570)

DD-21553 Extradural hemorrhage following injury with open intracranial wound and brief loss of consciousness (less than one hour) 852.52
(T-A1310) (M-37000) (G-C001) (M-10000) (G-C008) (T-D1400) (M-14010) (G-C008) (F-A5574)

DD-21554 Extradural hemorrhage following injury with open intracranial wound and moderate loss of consciousness (1-24 hours) 852.53
(T-A1310) (M-37000) (G-C001) (M-10000) (G-C008) (T-D1400) (M-14010) (G-C008) (F-A5575)

DD-21555 Extradural hemorrhage following injury with open intracranial wound and prolonged loss of consciousness (more than 24 hours) and return to pre-existing conscious level 852.54
(T-A1310) (M-37000) (G-C001) (M-10000) (G-C009) (T-D1400) (M-14010) (G-C008) (F-A5576) (G-C008) (G-4010) (G-4003) (F-A5500)

DD-21556 Extradural hemorrhage following injury with open intracranial wound and prolonged loss of consciousness (more than 24 hours) without return to pre-existing conscious level 852.55
(T-A1310) (M-37000) (G-C001) (M-10000) (G-C008) (T-D1400) (M-14010) (G-C008) (F-A5576) (G-C009) (G-4010) (G-4003) (F-A5500)

DD-21557 Extradural hemorrhage following injury with open intracranial wound and loss of consciousness of unspecified duration 852.56
(T-A1310) (M-37000) (G-C001) (M-10000) (G-C008) (T-D1400) (M-14010) (G-C008) (F-A5570)

DD-21558 Extradural hemorrhage following injury with open intracranial wound and unspecified concussion 852.59
(T-A1310) (M-37000) (G-C001) (M-10000) (G-C008) (T-D1400) (M-14010) (G-C008) (F-A5680)

D-22 INTERNAL INJURIES OF THE CHEST

DD-22100 Internal injury of chest, NOS
(T-D3000) (M-10060)

DD-22110 Traumatic pneumothorax without open wound into thorax 860.0
(D2-80300) (G-C001) (M-10000) (G-C009) (T-D3200) (M-14010)

DD-22112 Traumatic pneumothorax with open wound into thorax 860.1
(D2-80300) (G-C001) (M-10000) (G-C008) (T-D3200) (M-14010)

DD-22113 Traumatic hemothorax without open wound into thorax 860.2
(D2-80120) (G-C001) (M-10000) (G-C009) (T-D3200) (M-14010)

DD-22114 Traumatic hemothorax with open wound into thorax 860.3
(D2-80120) (G-C001) (M-10000) (G-C008) (T-D3200) (M-14010)

DD-22116 Traumatic pneumohemothorax without open wound into thorax 860.4
(D2-80110) (G-C001) (M-10000) (G-C009) (T-D3200) (M-14010)

DD-22118 Traumatic pneumohemothorax with open wound into thorax 860.5
(D2-80110) (G-C001) (M-10000) (G-C008) (T-D3200) (M-14010)

DD-22200 Injury of heart, NOS 861.00
(T-32000) (M-10000)

DD-22210 Injury of heart without open wound into thorax 861.0
(T-32000) (M-10000) (G-C009) (T-D3200) (M-14010)

DD-22212 Contusion to heart 861.01
(T-32000) (M-14200)
Cardiac contusion 861.01
(T-32000) (M-14200)
Myocardial contusion 861.01
(T-32000) (M-14200)

DD-22214 Laceration of heart without penetration of heart chambers 861.02
(T-32000) (M-14400) (G-C009) (T-32080) (M-14100)

DD-22216 Laceration of heart with penetration of heart chambers 861.03
(T-32000) (M-14400) (G-C008) (T-32080) (M-14100)

DD-22220 Unspecified injury to heart with open wound into thorax 861.10
(T-32000) (M-10000) (G-C008) (M-14010) (G-C007) (T-D3200)

DD-22222 Contusion to heart with open wound into thorax 861.11
(T-32000) (M-14200) (G-C008) (M-14010) (G-C007) (T-D3200)

DD-22224 Laceration of heart with open wound into thorax and without penetration of heart chambers 861.12
(T-32000) (M-14400) (G-C008) (M-14010) (G-C007) (T-D3200) (G-C009) (M-14100) (T-32080)

DD-22226 Laceration of heart with open wound into thorax and with penetration of heart chambers 861.13
(T-32000) (M-14400) (G-C008) (M-14010) (T-D3200) (G-C008) (M-14100) (T-32080)

DD-22300 Unspecified injury of lung, NOS 861.20
(T-28000) (M-10000)

D-22 INTERNAL INJURIES OF THE CHEST — Continued

DD-22310 Injury of lung without open wound into thorax 861.2
(T-28000) (M-10000) (G-C009)
(M-14010) (G-C007) (T-D3200)

DD-22312 Contusion of lung without open wound into thorax 861.21
(T-28000) (M-14200) (G-C009)
(M-14010) (G-C007) (T-D3200)

DD-22314 Laceration of lung without open wound into thorax 861.22
(T-28000) (M-14400) (G-C009)
(M-14010) (G-C007) (T-D3200)

DD-22320 Unspecified injury of lung with open wound into thorax 861.30
(T-28000) (M-14400) (G-C008)
(M-14010) (G-C007) (T-D3200)

DD-22322 Contusion of lung with open wound into thorax 861.31
(T-28000) (M-14200) (G-C008)
(M-14010) (G-C007) (T-D3200)

DD-22324 Laceration of lung with open wound into thorax 861.32
(T-28000) (M-14400) (G-C008)
(M-14010) (G-C007) (T-D3200)

DD-22330 Injury of pleura 862.29
(T-29000) (M-10000)

DD-22340 Injury of bronchus without open wound into thoracic cavity 862.21
(T-26000) (M-10000) (G-C009)
(M-14010) (G-C007) (T-D3200)

DD-22345 Injury of bronchus with open wound into thoracic cavity 862.31
(T-26000) (M-10000) (G-C008)
(M-14010) (G-C007) (T-D3200)

DD-22410 Injury of diaphragm without open wound into cavity 862.0
(T-D3400) (M-10000) (G-C009)
(M-14010) (G-C007) (T-D3200)

DD-22420 Injury of diaphragm with open wound into cavity 862.1
(T-D3400) (M-10000) (G-C008)
(M-14010) (G-C007) (T-D3200)

DD-22430 Injury of esophagus without open wound into thoracic cavity 862.22
(T-56000) (M-10000) (G-C009)
(M-14010) (G-C007) (T-D3200)

DD-22435 Injury of esophagus with open wound into thoracic cavity 862.32
(T-56000) (M-10000) (G-C008)
(M-14010) (G-C007) (T-D3200)

DD-22440 Injury of thymus gland 862.29
(T-C8000) (M-10000)

DD-22500 Injury of multiple intrathoracic organs without open wound into cavity 862.8
(T-D3030) (M-10000) (G-C009)
(G-C009) (M-14010) (G-C007)
(T-D3200)

DD-22510 Crushed chest without open wound into thoracic cavity 862.8
(T-D3000) (M-10400) (G-C009)
(M-14010) (G-C007) (T-D3200)

DD-22520 Crushed chest with open wound into thoracic cavity 862.9
(T-D3000) (M-10400) (G-C008)
(M-14010) (G-C007) (T-D3200)

DD-22530 Injury of multiple intrathoracic organs with open wound into cavity 862.9
(T-D3030) (M-10000) (G-C008)
(M-14010) (G-C007) (T-D3200)

D-23 INTERNAL INJURIES OF THE ABDOMEN

DD-23000 Internal injury of abdominal organs, NOS 869.-
(T-D4030) (M-10060)
Internal injury of abdomen, NOS
(T-D4030) (M-10060)

DD-23002 Internal injury of abdominal organs without open wound into cavity 869.0
(T-D4030) (M-10060) (G-C009)
(M-14010) (G-C007) (T-D4010)

DD-23004 Internal injury of abdominal organs with open wound into cavity 869.1
(T-D4030) (M-10060) (G-C008)
(M-14010) (G-C007) (T-D4010)

DD-23010 Multiple extreme injuries of abdominal organs, NOS 869.-
(T-D4030) (M-10062)

DD-23012 Multiple extreme injuries of abdominal organs without open wound into cavity 869.0
(T-D4030) (M-10062) (G-C009)
(M-14010) (G-C007) (T-D4010)

DD-23014 Multiple extreme injuries of abdominal organs with open wound into cavity 869.1
(T-D4030) (M-10062) (G-C008)
(M-14010) (G-C007) (T-D4010)

DD-23020 Severe crushing injury of abdominal organs, NOS 869.-
(T-D4030) (M-10400)

DD-23022 Severe crushing injury of abdominal organs without open wound into cavity 869.0
(T-D4030) (M-10400) (G-C009)
(M-14010) (G-C007) (T-D4010)

DD-23024 Severe crushing injury of abdominal organs with open wound into cavity 869.1
(T-D4030) (M-10400) (G-C008)
(M-14010) (G-C007) (T-D4010)

DD-23100 Injury of gastrointestinal tract, NOS 863.-
(T-50100) (M-10060)

DD-23102 Injury of gastrointestinal tract without open wound into abdominal cavity 863.80
(T-50100) (M-10060) (G-C009)
(M-14010) (G-C007) (T-D4010)

DD-23104 Injury of gastrointestinal tract with open wound into abdominal cavity 863.90
(T-50100) (M-10060) (G-C008)
(M-14010) (G-C007) (T-D4010)

DD-23110 Injury of intestine without open wound into abdominal cavity 863.89
(T-50100) (M-10060) (G-C009) (M-14010) (G-C007) (T-D4010)

DD-23120 Injury of intestine with open wound into abdominal cavity 863.99
(T-50100) (M-10060) (G-C008) (M-14010) (G-C007) (T-D4010)

DD-23200 Injury of stomach without open wound into abdominal cavity 863.0
(T-57000) (M-10060) (G-C009) (M-14010) (G-C007) (T-D4010)

DD-23210 Injury of stomach with open wound into abdominal cavity 863.1
(T-57000) (M-10060) (G-C008) (M-14010) (G-C007) (T-D4010)

DD-23220 Injury of small intestine without open wound into abdominal cavity 823.20
(T-58000) (M-10060) (G-C009) (M-14010) (G-C007) (T-D4010)

DD-23222 Injury of duodenum without open wound into abdominal cavity 863.21
(T-58200) (M-10060) (G-C009) (M-14010) (G-C007) (T-D4010)

DD-23230 Injury of small intestine with open wound into abdominal cavity 863.3
(T-58000) (M-10060) (G-C008) (M-14010) (G-C007) (T-D4010)

DD-23232 Injury of duodenum with open wound into abdominal cavity 863.31
(T-58200) (M-10060) (G-C008) (M-14010) (G-C007) (T-D4010)

DD-23300 Injury of colon without open wound into abdominal cavity 863.40
(T-59300) (M-10060) (G-C009) (M-14010) (G-C007) (T-D4010)

DD-23301 Injury of appendix without open wound into abdominal cavity 863.85
(T-59200) (M-10060) (G-C009) (M-14010) (G-C007) (T-D4010)

DD-23302 Injury of ascending right colon without open wound into abdominal cavity 863.41
(T-59420) (M-10060) (G-C009) (M-14010) (G-C007) (T-D4010)

DD-23304 Injury of transverse colon without open wound into abdominal cavity 863.42
(T-59440) (M-10060) (G-C009) (M-14010) (G-C007) (T-D4010)

DD-23305 Injury of descending left colon without open wound into abdominal cavity 863.43
(T-59460) (M-10060) (G-C009) (M-14010) (G-C007) (T-D4010)

DD-23306 Injury of sigmoid colon without open wound into abdominal cavity 863.44
(T-59470) (M-10060) (G-C009) (M-14010) (G-C007) (T-D4010)

DD-23307 Injury of rectum without open wound into abdominal cavity 863.45
(T-59300) (M-10062) (G-C009) (M-14010) (G-C007) (T-D4010)

DD-23308 Injury of multiple sites in colon and rectum without open wound into abdominal cavity 863.46
(T-59300) (T-59600) (M-10062) (G-C009) (M-14010) (G-C007) (T-D4010)

DD-23310 Injury of colon with open wound into abdominal cavity 863.50
(T-59300) (M-10060) (G-C008) (M-14010) (G-C007) (T-D4010)

DD-23311 Injury of appendix with open wound into abdominal cavity 863.95
(T-59200) (M-10060) (G-C008) (M-14010) (G-C007) (T-D4010)

DD-23312 Injury of ascending right colon with open wound into abdominal cavity 863.51
(T-59420) (M-10060) (G-C008) (M-14010) (G-C007) (T-D4010)

DD-23314 Injury of transverse colon with open wound into abdominal cavity 863.52
(T-59440) (M-10060) (G-C008) (M-14010) (G-C007) (T-D4010)

DD-23315 Injury of descending left colon with open wound into abdominal cavity 863.53
(T-59460) (M-10060) (G-C008) (M-14010) (G-C007) (T-D4010)

DD-23316 Injury of sigmoid colon with open wound into abdominal cavity 863.54
(T-59470) (M-10060) (G-C008) (M-14010) (G-C007) (T-D4010)

DD-23317 Injury of rectum with open wound into abdominal cavity 863.55
(T-59600) (M-10060) (G-C008) (M-14010) (G-C007) (T-D4010)

DD-23318 Injury of multiple sites in colon and rectum with open wound into abdominal cavity 863.56
(T-59300) (T-59600) (M-10062) (G-C009) (M-14010) (G-C007) (T-D4010)

DD-23400 Injury of pancreas, NOS 863.84
(T-65000) (M-10060)

DD-23402 Injury of head of pancreas without open wound into cavity 863.81
(T-65100) (M-10060) (G-C009) (M-14010) (G-C007) (T-D4010)

DD-23404 Injury of body of pancreas without open wound into abdominal cavity 863.82
(T-65200) (M-10060) (G-C009) (M-14010) (G-C007) (T-D4010)

DD-23406 Injury of tail of pancreas without open wound into abdominal cavity 863.83
(T-65300) (M-10060) (G-C009) (M-14010) (G-C007) (T-D4010)

DD-23408 Injury of multiple sites of pancreas without open wound into abdominal cavity 863.84
(T-65000) (M-10062) (G-C009) (M-14010) (G-C007) (T-D4010)

D-23 INTERNAL INJURIES OF THE ABDOMEN — Continued

DD-23410 Injury of head of pancreas with open wound into abdominal cavity 863.91
(T-65100) (M-10060) (G-C008) (M-14010) (G-C007) (T-D4010)

DD-23412 Injury of body of pancreas with open wound into abdominal cavity 863.92
(T-65200) (M-10060) (G-C008) (M-14010) (G-C007) (T-D4010)

DD-23414 Injury of tail of pancreas with open wound into abdominal cavity 863.93
(T-65300) (M-10060) (G-C008) (M-14010) (G-C007) (T-D4010)

DD-23418 Injury of multiple sites of pancreas with open wound into abdominal cavity 863.94
(T-65000) (M-10062) (G-C008) (M-14010) (G-C007) (T-D4010)

DD-23510 Unspecified injury of liver without open wound into abdominal cavity 864.00
(T-62000) (M-10060) (G-C009) (M-14010) (G-C007) (T-D4010)

DD-23511 Hematoma and contusion of liver without open wound into abdominal cavity 864.01
(T-62000) (M-35060) (M-14200) (G-C009) (M-14010) (G-C007) (T-D4010)

DD-23512 Minor laceration of liver without open wound into abdominal cavity 864.02
(T-62000) (M-14401) (G-C009) (M-14010) (G-C007) (T-D4010)

DD-23513 Moderate laceration of liver without open wound into abdominal cavity 864.03
(T-62000) (M-14402) (G-C009) (M-14010) (G-C007) (T-D4010)

DD-23514 Major laceration of liver without open wound into abdominal cavity 864.04
(T-62000) (M-14403) (G-C009) (M-14010) (G-C007) (T-D4010)

DD-23515 Stellate laceration of liver without open wound into abdominal cavity 864.04
(T-62000) (M-14410) (G-C009) (M-14010) (G-C007) (T-D4010)

DD-23520 Unspecified injury of liver with open wound into abdominal cavity 864.10
(T-62000) (M-10060) (G-C008) (M-14010) (G-C007) (T-D4010)

DD-23521 Hematoma and contusion of liver with open wound into abdominal cavity 864.11
(T-62000) (M-35060) (M-14200) (G-C008) (M-14010) (G-C007) (T-D4010)

DD-23522 Minor laceration of liver with open wound into abdominal cavity 864.12
(T-62000) (M-14401) (G-C008) (M-14010) (G-C007) (T-D4010)

DD-23523 Moderate laceration of liver with open wound into abdominal cavity 864.13
(T-62000) (M-14402) (G-C008) (M-14010) (G-C007) (T-D4010)

DD-23524 Major laceration of liver with open wound into abdominal cavity 864.14
(T-62000) (M-14403) (G-C008) (M-14010) (G-C007) (T-D4010)

DD-23525 Stellate laceration of liver with open wound into abdominal cavity 864.14
(T-62000) (M-14410) (G-C008) (M-14010) (G-C007) (T-D4010)

DD-23600 Injury of spleen, NOS 865.-
(T-C3000) (M-10060)

DD-23610 Injury of spleen without open wound into abdominal cavity 865.0
(T-C3000) (M-10060) (G-C009) (M-14010) (G-C007) (T-D4010)

DD-23611 Hematoma of spleen without rupture of capsule and without open wound into abdominal cavity 865.01
(T-C3000) (M-35060) (G-C009) (M-14400) (G-C009) (M-14010) (G-C007) (T-D4010)

DD-23612 Capsular tear without major disruption of parenchyma of spleen and without open wound into abdominal cavity 865.02
(T-C3010) (M-14400) (G-C009) (M-01442) (T-C3080) (G-C009) (M-14010) (G-C007) (T-D4010)

DD-23614 Laceration extending into parenchyma of spleen without open wound into abdominal cavity 865.03
(T-C3080) (M-14400) (G-C009) (M-14010) (G-C007) (T-D4010)

DD-23616 Massive parenchymal disruption of spleen without open wound into abdominal cavity 865.04
(T-C3080) (M-01442) (G-C009) (M-14010) (G-C007) (T-D4010)

DD-23620 Injury of spleen with open wound into abdominal cavity 865.1
(T-C3000) (M-10060) (G-C008) (M-14010) (G-C007) (T-D4010)

DD-23621 Hematoma of spleen without rupture of capsule and with open wound into abdominal cavity 865.11
(T-C3000) (M-35060) (G-C009) (M-14400) (T-C3010) (G-C008) (M-14010) (G-C007) (T-D4010)

DD-23622 Capsular tear without major disruption of parenchyma of spleen and with open wound in abdominal cavity 865.12
(T-C3010) (M-14400) (G-C009) (M-01442) (T-C3080) (G-C008) (M-14010) (G-C007) (T-D4010)

DD-23624 Laceration extending into parenchyma of spleen with open wound into abdominal cavity 865.13
(T-C3080) (M-14400) (G-C008) (M-14010) (G-C007) (T-D4010)

DD-23626 Massive parenchymal disruption of spleen with open wound into abdominal cavity 865.14
(T-C3080) (M-01442) (G-C008)
(M-14010) (G-C007) (T-D4010)

DD-23700 Injury of kidney, NOS 866.-
(T-71000) (M-10060)

DD-23710 Injury of kidney without open wound into abdominal cavity 866.0
(T-71000) (M-10060) (G-C009)
(M-14010) (G-C007) (T-D4010)

DD-23711 Hematoma of kidney without rupture of capsule and without open wound into abdominal cavity 866.01
(T-71000) (M-35060) (G-C009)
(T-71030) (M-14400) (G-C009)
(M-14010) (G-C007) (T-D4010)

DD-23712 Laceration of kidney without open wound into abdominal cavity 866.02
(T-71000) (M-14400) (G-C009)
(M-14010) (G-C007) (T-D4010)

DD-23713 Complete disruption of kidney parenchyma without open wound into cavity 866.03
(T-71040) (M-01443) (G-C009)
(M-14010) (G-C007) (T-D4010)

DD-23720 Injury of kidney with open wound into abdominal cavity 866.1
(T-71000) (M-10060) (G-C008)
(M-14010) (G-C007) (T-D4010)

DD-23721 Hematoma of kidney without rupture of capsule and with open wound into abdominal cavity 866.11
(T-71000) (M-35060) (G-C009)
(T-71030) (M-14400) (G-C008)
(M-14010) (G-C007) (T-D4010)

DD-23722 Laceration of kidney with open wound into abdominal cavity 866.12
(T-71000) (M-14400) (G-C008)
(M-14010) (G-C007) (T-D4010)

DD-23723 Complete disruption of kidney parenchyma with open wound into cavity 866.13
(T-71040) (M-01443) (G-C008)
(M-14010) (G-C007) (T-D4010)

DD-23800 Injury of adrenal gland without open wound into abdominal cavity 868.01
(T-B3000) (M-10060) (G-C009)
(M-14010) (G-C007) (T-D4010)

DD-23802 Injury of adrenal gland with open wound into abdominal cavity 868.11
(T-B3000) (M-10060) (G-C008)
(M-14010) (G-C007) (T-D4010)

DD-23810 Injury of bile duct without open wound into abdominal cavity 868.02
(T-60610) (M-10060) (G-C009)
(M-14010) (G-C007) (T-D4010)

DD-23812 Injury of gallbladder without open wound into abdominal cavity 868.02
(T-63000) (M-10060) (G-C009)
(M-14010) (G-C007) (T-D4010)

DD-23814 Injury of bile duct with open wound into abdominal cavity 868.12
(T-60610) (M-10060) (G-C008)
(M-14010) (G-C007) (T-D4010)

DD-23816 Injury of gallbladder with open wound into abdominal cavity 868.12
(T-63000) (M-10060) (G-C008)
(M-14010) (G-C007) (T-D4010)

DD-23820 Injury of peritoneum without open wound into abdominal cavity 868.03
(T-D4400) (M-10060) (G-C009)
(M-14010) (G-C007) (T-D4010)

DD-23822 Injury of peritoneum with open wound into abdominal cavity 868.13
(T-D4400) (M-10060) (G-C008)
(M-14010) (G-C007) (T-D4010)

DD-23830 Injury of retroperitoneum without open wound into abdominal cavity 868.04
(T-D4900) (M-10060) (G-C009)
(M-14010) (G-C007) (T-D4010)

DD-23832 Injury of retroperitoneum with open wound into abdominal cavity 868.14
(T-D4900) (M-10060) (G-C008)
(M-14010) (G-C007) (T-D4010)

DD-23850 Injury of multiple intra-abdominal organs without open wound into abdominal cavity 868.09
(T-D4030) (M-10080) (G-C009)
(M-14010) (G-C007) (T-D4010)

DD-23852 Injury of multiple intra-abdominal organs with open wound into abdominal cavity 868.19
(T-D4030) (M-10080) (G-C008)
(M-14010) (G-C007) (T-D4010)

D-24 INTERNAL INJURIES OF THE PELVIC ORGANS

DD-24000 Internal injury of pelvic organs, NOS 867.8
(T-D6100) (M-10060)

DD-24010 Unspecified pelvic organ injury without open wound into abdominal cavity 867.8
(T-D6100) (M-10060) (G-C009)
(M-14010) (G-C007) (T-D4010)

DD-24020 Unspecified pelvic organ injury with open wound into abdominal cavity 867.9
(T-D6100) (M-10060) (G-C008)
(M-14010) (G-C007) (T-D4010)

DD-24110 Injury of bladder and urethra without open wound into abdominal cavity 867.0
(T-74000) (T-75000) (M-10060)
(G-C009) (M-14010) (G-C007)
(T-D4010)

DD-24120 Injury of bladder and urethra with open wound into abdominal cavity 867.1
(T-74000) (T-75000) (M-10060)
(G-C008) (M-14010) (G-C007)
(T-D4010)

DD-24130 Injury of ureter without open wound into abdominal cavity 867.2
(T-73000) (M-10060) (G-C009)
(M-14010) (G-C007) (T-D4010)

D-24 INTERNAL INJURIES OF THE PELVIC ORGANS — Continued

DD-24134 Injury of ureter with open wound into abdominal cavity 867.3
(T-73000) (M-10060) (G-C008)
(M-14010) (G-C007) (T-D4010)

DD-24140 Injury of uterus without open wound into abdominal cavity 867.4
(T-83000) (M-10060) (G-C009)
(M-14010) (G-C007) (T-D4010)

DD-24144 Injury of uterus with open wound into abdominal cavity 867.5
(T-83000) (M-10060) (G-C008)
(M-14010) (G-C007) (T-D4010)

DD-24150 Injury of Fallopian tube without open wound into abdominal cavity 867.6
(T-88000) (M-10060) (G-C009)
(M-14010) (G-C007) (T-D4010)

DD-24152 Injury of Fallopian tube with open wound into abdominal cavity 867.7
(T-88000) (M-10060) (G-C008)
(M-14010) (G-C007) (T-D4010)

DD-24156 Injury of ovary without open wound into abdominal cavity 867.6
(T-87000) (M-10060) (G-C009)
(M-14010) (G-C007) (T-D4010)

DD-24157 Injury of ovary with open wound into abdominal cavity 867.7
(T-87000) (M-10060) (G-C008)
(M-14010) (G-C007) (T-D4010)

DD-24160 Injury of prostate without open wound into abdominal cavity 867.6
(T-92000) (M-10060) (G-C009)
(M-14010) (G-C007) (T-D4010)

DD-24162 Injury of prostate with open wound into abdominal cavity 867.7
(T-92000) (M-10060) (G-C008)
(M-14010) (G-C007) (T-D4010)

DD-24164 Injury of seminal vesicle without open wound into abdominal cavity 867.6
(T-93000) (M-10060) (G-C009)
(M-14010) (G-C007) (T-D4010)

DD-24165 Injury of seminal vesicle with open wound into abdominal cavity 867.7
(T-93000) (M-10060) (G-C008)
(M-14010) (G-C007) (T-D4010)

DD-24166 Injury of vas deferens without open injury to abdominal cavity 867.6
(T-96000) (M-10060) (G-C009)
(M-14010) (G-C007) (T-D4010)

DD-24167 Injury of vas deferens with open wound into abdominal cavity 867.7
(T-96000) (M-10060) (G-C008)
(M-14010) (G-C007) (T-D4010)

SECTION D-3 OPEN WOUNDS AND CRUSHING INJURIES

D-30 OPEN WOUNDS: GENERAL TERMS

DD-30010 Open wound of unspecified site without complication 879.8
(T-D0003) (M-14010) (G-C009)
(F-01450)

DD-30020 Open wound of unspecified site with complication 879.9
(T-D0003) (M-14010) (G-C008)
(F-01450)

DD-30040 Multiple open wounds without complication 879.8
(T-D0003) (M-14018) (G-C009)
(F-01450)

DD-30050 Multiple open wounds with complication 879.9
(T-D0003) (M-14018) (G-C008)
(F-01450)

D-31 OPEN WOUNDS OF THE HEAD AND NECK

DD-31000 Open wound of head, NOS 873.8
(T-D1100) (M-14010)

DD-31010 Open wound of head without complication 873.8
(T-D1100) (M-14010) (G-C009)
(F-01450)

DD-31020 Open wound of head with complication 873.9
(T-D1100) (M-14010) (G-C008)
(F-01450)

DD-31100 Open wound of eyeball, NOS 871.9
(T-AA000) (M-14010)

DD-31101 Ocular laceration without prolapse of intraocular tissue 871.0
(T-AA000) (M-14400) (G-C009)
(M-31050) (T-AA770)

DD-31102 Ocular laceration with prolapse or exposure of intraocular tissue 871.1
(T-AA000) (M-14400) (G-C008)
(M-31050) (T-AA770)

DD-31103 Rupture of eye with partial loss of intraocular tissue 871.2
(T-AA000) (M-14400) (G-C008)
(M-16010) (T-AA770)

DD-31104 Avulsion of eye 871.3
(T-AA000) (M-14120)

DD-31105 Traumatic enucleation of eye 871.3
(T-AA000) (M-17010)

DD-31106 Unspecified laceration of eye 871.4
(T-AA000) (M-14400)

DD-31110 Ocular penetration, NOS 871.7
(T-AA000) (M-14100)
Penetrating wound of eyeball, NOS 871.7
(T-AA000) (M-14100)

DD-31112 Penetration of eyeball with magnetic foreign body 871.5
(T-AA000) (M-14100) (G-C001)
(M-30410)

DD-31114 Penetration of eyeball with nonmagnetic foreign body 871.6
(T-AA000) (M-14100) (G-C001) (M-30400)

DD-31200 Open wound of ocular adnexa, NOS 870.9
(T-AA800) (M-14010)

DD-31201 Laceration of skin of eyelid and periocular area 870.0
(T-01000) (T-AA810) (T-AA006) (M-14400)

DD-31202 Laceration of eyelid, full-thickness, not involving lacrimal passages 870.1
(T-AA810) (M-14400) (G-C009) (T-AA900)

DD-31203 Laceration of eyelid involving lacrimal passages 870.2
(T-AA810) (M-14400) (G-C008) (T-AA900)

DD-31204 Penetrating wound of orbit without foreign body 870.3
(T-D1480) (M-14100) (G-C009) (M-30400)

DD-31205 Penetrating wound of orbit with foreign body 870.4
(T-D1480) (M-14100) (G-C008) (M-30400)

DD-31208 Other specified wound of ocular adnexa, NEC 870.8
(T-AA800) (M-14000)

DD-31300 Open wound of ear, NOS 872.8
(T-AB000) (M-14010)

DD-31302 Open wound of ear without complication, NOS 872.8
(T-AB000) (M-14010) (G-C009) (F-01450)

DD-31303 Open wound of external ear without complication 872.00
(T-AB100) (M-14010) (G-C009) (F-01450)

DD-31304 Open wound of auricle of ear without complication 872.01
(T-AB105) (M-14010) (G-C009) (F-01450)
Open wound of pinna of ear without complication 872.01
(T-AB105) (M-14010) (G-C009) (F-01450)

DD-31306 Open wound of auditory canal without complication 872.02
(T-AB200) (M-14010) (G-C009) (F-01450)

DD-31310 Open wound of ear with complication, NOS 872.9
(T-AB000) (M-14010) (G-C008) (F-01450)

DD-31313 Open wound of external ear with complication 872.10
(T-AB100) (M-14010) (G-C008) (F-01450)

DD-31314 Open wound of auricle of ear with complication 872.11
(T-AB105) (M-14010) (G-C008) (F-01450)
Open wound of pinna of ear with complication 872.11
(T-AB105) (M-14010) (G-C008) (F-01450)

DD-31316 Open wound of auditory canal with complication 872.12
(T-AB200) (M-14010) (G-C008) (F-01450)

DD-31320 Open wound of ear drum without complication 872.61
(T-AB320) (M-14010) (G-C009) (F-01450)
Open wound of drumhead without complication 872.61
(T-AB320) (M-14010) (G-C009) (F-01450)
Open wound of tympanic membrane without complication 872.61
(T-AB320) (M-14010) (G-C009) (F-01450)

DD-31323 Open wound of ossicles without complication 872.62
(T-AB400) (M-14010) (G-C009) (F-01450)

DD-31324 Open wound of Eustachian tube without complication 872.63
(T-AB600) (M-14010) (G-C009) (F-01450)

DD-31325 Open wound of cochlea without complication 872.64
(T-AB800) (M-14010) (G-C009) (F-01450)

DD-31328 Open wound of multiple sites of ear without complication 872.69
(T-AB000) (M-14018) (G-C009) (F-01450)

DD-31330 Open wound of ear drum with complication 872.71
(T-AB320) (M-14010) (G-C008) (F-01450)
Open wound of tympanic membrane with complication 872.71
(T-AB320) (M-14010) (G-C008) (F-01450)
Open wound of drumhead with complication 872.71
(T-AB320) (M-14010) (G-C008) (F-01450)

DD-31333 Open wound of ossicles with complication 872.72
(T-AB400) (M-14010) (G-C008) (F-01450)

DD-31334 Open wound of Eustachian tube with complication 872.73
(T-AB600) (M-14010) (G-C008) (F-01450)

D-31 OPEN WOUNDS OF THE HEAD AND NECK — Continued

DD-31335 Open wound of cochlea with complication 872.74
(T-AB800) (M-14010) (G-C008) (F-01450)

DD-31338 Open wound of multiple sites of ear with complication 872.79
(T-AB000) (M-14018) (G-C008) (F-01450)

DD-31350 Open wound of scalp without complication 873.0
(T-D1160) (M-14010) (G-C009) (F-01450)

DD-31352 Open wound of scalp with complication 873.1
(T-D1160) (M-14010) (G-C008) (F-01450)

DD-31360 Open wound of nose without complication, NOS 873.20
(T-21000) (M-14010) (G-C009) (F-01450)

DD-31362 Open wound of nasal septum without complication 873.21
(T-21340) (M-14010) (G-C009) (F-01450)

DD-31363 Open wound of nasal cavity without complication 873.22
(T-21300) (M-14010) (G-C009) (F-01450)

DD-31364 Open wound of nasal sinus without complication 873.23
(T-22000) (M-14010) (G-C009) (F-01450)

DD-31368 Open wound of multiple sites of nose without complication 873.29
(T-21000) (M-14018) (G-C009) (F-01450)

DD-31370 Open wound of nose with complication, NOS 873.30
(T-21000) (M-14010) (G-C008) (F-01450)

DD-31371 Open wound of nasal septum with complication 873.31
(T-21340) (M-14010) (G-C008) (F-01450)

DD-31372 Open wound of nasal cavity with complication 873.32
(T-21300) (M-14010) (G-C008) (F-01450)

DD-31373 Open wound of nasal sinus with complication 873.33
(T-22000) (M-14010) (G-C008) (F-01450)

DD-31378 Open wound of multiple sites of nose with complication 873.39
(T-21000) (M-14018) (G-C008) (F-01450)

DD-31380 Open wound of face without complication, NOS 873.40
(T-D1200) (M-14010) (G-C009) (F-01450)

DD-31381 Open wound of cheek without complication 873.41
(T-D1206) (M-14010) (G-C009) (F-01450)

DD-31382 Open wound of forehead without complication 873.42
(T-D1110) (M-14010) (G-C009) (F-01450)

DD-31383 Open wound of eyebrow without complication 873.42
(T-01520) (M-14010) (G-C009) (F-01450)

DD-31384 Open wound of lip without complication 873.43
(T-52000) (M-14010) (G-C009) (F-01450)

DD-31385 Open wound of jaw without complication 873.44
(T-D1213) (M-14010) (G-C009) (F-01450)

DD-31388 Open wound of multiple sites of face without complication 873.49
(T-D1200) (M-14018) (G-C009) (F-01450)

DD-31390 Open wound of face with complication, NOS 873.50
(T-D1200) (M-14010) (G-C008) (F-01450)

DD-31391 Open wound of cheek with complication 873.51
(T-D1206) (M-14010) (G-C008) (F-01450)

DD-31392 Open wound of forehead with complication 873.52
(T-D1110) (M-14010) (G-C008) (F-01450)

DD-31393 Open wound of eyebrow with complication 873.52
(T-01520) (M-14010) (G-C008) (F-01450)

DD-31394 Open wound of lip with complication 873.53
(T-52000) (M-14010) (G-C008) (F-01450)

DD-31395 Open wound of jaw with complication 873.54
(T-D1213) (M-14010) (G-C008) (F-01450)

DD-31398 Open wound of multiple sites of face with complication 873.59
(T-D1200) (M-14010) (G-C008) (F-01450)

DD-31400 Open wound of mouth without complication, NOS 873.60
(T-51000) (M-14010) (G-C009) (F-01450)

DD-31401 Open wound of buccal mucosa without complication 873.61
(T-51300) (M-14010) (G-C009) (F-01450)

DD-31402 Open wound of gum without complication 873.62
(T-54910) (M-14010) (G-C009) (F-01450)

DD-31403 Open wound of alveolar process without complication 873.62
(T-11177) (T-1118B) (M-14010) (G-C009) (F-01450)

DD-31404 Broken tooth without complication 873.63
(T-54010) (M-12000) (G-C009) (F-01450)

DD-31405 Open wound of tongue without complication 873.64
(T-53000) (M-14010) (G-C009) (F-01450)

DD-31406 Open wound of floor of mouth without complication 873.64
(T-51200) (M-14010) (G-C009) (F-01450)

DD-31407 Open wound of palate without complication 873.65
(T-51100) (M-14010) (G-C009) (F-01450)

DD-31408 Open wound of multiple sites of mouth without complication 873.69
(T-51000) (M-14018) (G-C009) (F-01450)

DD-31410 Open wound of mouth with complication, NOS 873.70
(T-51000) (M-14010) (G-C008) (F-01450)

DD-31411 Open wound of buccal mucosa with complication 873.71
(T-51300) (M-14010) (G-C008) (F-01450)

DD-31412 Open wound of gum with complication 873.72
(T-54910) (M-14010) (G-C008) (F-01450)

DD-31413 Open wound of alveolar process with complication 873.72
(T-11177) (T-1118B) (M-14010) (G-C008) (F-01450)

DD-31414 Broken tooth with complication 873.73
(T-54010) (M-12000) (G-C008) (F-01450)

DD-31415 Open wound of tongue with complication 873.74
(T-53000) (M-14010) (G-C008) (F-01450)

DD-31416 Open wound of floor of mouth with complication 873.74
(T-51200) (M-14010) (G-C008) (F-01450)

DD-31417 Open wound of palate with complication 873.75
(T-51100) (M-14010) (G-C008) (F-01450)

DD-31418 Open wound of multiple sites of mouth with complication 873.79
(T-51000) (M-14018) (G-C008) (F-01450)

DD-31610 Open wound of neck without complication 874.8
(T-D1600) (M-14010) (G-C009) (F-01450)

DD-31612 Open wound of throat without complication 874.8
(T-55000) (M-14010) (G-C009) (F-01450)

DD-31614 Open wound of supraclavicular region without complication 874.8
(T-D1620) (M-14010) (G-C009) (F-01450)

DD-31616 Open wound of nape of neck without complication 874.8
(T-D1610) (M-14010) (G-C009) (F-01450)

DD-31620 Open wound of neck with complication 874.9
(T-D1600) (M-14010) (G-C008) (F-01450)

DD-31622 Open wound of throat with complication 874.9
(T-55000) (M-14010) (G-C008) (F-01450)

DD-31624 Open wound of supraclavicular region with complication 874.9
(T-D1620) (M-14010) (G-C008) (F-01450)

DD-31626 Open wound of nape of neck with complication 874.9
(T-D1610) (M-14010) (G-C008) (F-01450)

DD-31640 Open wound of larynx with trachea without complication 874.00
(T-24100) (T-25000) (M-14010) (G-C009) (F-01450)

DD-31642 Open wound of larynx without complication 874.01
(T-24100) (M-14010) (G-C009) (F-01450)

DD-31644 Open wound of trachea without complication 874.02
(T-25000) (M-14010) (G-C009) (F-01450)

DD-31650 Open wound of larynx with trachea and with complication 874.10
(T-24100) (T-25000) (M-14010) (G-C008) (F-01450)

DD-31652 Open wound of larynx with complication 874.11
(T-24100) (M-14010) (G-C008) (F-01450)

D-31 OPEN WOUNDS OF THE HEAD AND NECK — Continued

DD-31654 Open wound of trachea with complication 874.12
(T-25000) (M-14010) (G-C008) (F-01450)

DD-31660 Open wound of thyroid gland without complication 874.2
(T-B6000) (M-14010) (G-C009) (F-01450)

DD-31664 Open wound of thyroid gland with complication 874.3
(T-B6000) (M-14010) (G-C008) (F-01450)

DD-31670 Open wound of pharynx without complication 874.4
(T-55000) (M-14010) (G-C009) (F-01450)

DD-31672 Open wound of cervical esophagus without complication 874.4
(T-56100) (M-14010) (G-C009) (F-01450)

DD-31674 Open wound of pharynx with complication 874.5
(T-55000) (M-14010) (G-C008) (F-01450)

DD-31676 Open wound of cervical esophagus with complication 874.5
(T-56100) (M-14010) (G-C008) (F-01450)

D-32 OPEN WOUNDS OF THE TRUNK

DD-32000 Open wound of trunk without complication, NOS 879.6
(T-D2000) (M-14010) (G-C009) (F-01450)

DD-32010 Open wound of pelvic region without complication 879.6
(T-D6000) (M-14010) (G-C009) (F-01450)

DD-32020 Open wound of perineum without complication 879.6
(T-D2700) (M-14010) (G-C009) (F-01450)

DD-32040 Open wound of trunk with complication, NOS 879.7
(T-D2000) (M-14010) (G-C008) (F-01450)

DD-32050 Open wound of pelvic region with complication 879.7
(T-D6000) (M-14010) (G-C008) (F-01450)

DD-32060 Open wound of perineum with complication 879.7
(T-D2700) (M-14010) (G-C008) (F-01450)

DD-32100 Open wound of chest wall without complication 875.0
(T-D3050) (M-14010) (G-C009) (F-01450)

DD-32120 Open wound of chest wall with complication 875.1
(T-D3050) (M-14010) (G-C008) (F-01450)

DD-32200 Open wound of back without complication 876.0
(T-D2100) (M-14010) (G-C009) (F-01450)

DD-32202 Open wound of loin without complication 876.0
(T-D2300) (M-14010) (G-C009) (F-01450)
Open wound of lumbar region without complication 876.0
(T-D2300) (M-14010) (G-C009) (F-01450)

DD-32210 Open wound of back with complication 876.1
(T-D2100) (M-14010) (G-C008) (F-01450)

DD-32212 Open wound of loin with complication 876.1
(T-D2300) (M-14010) (G-C008) (F-01450)
Open wound of lumbar region with complication 876.1
(T-D2300) (M-14010) (G-C008) (F-01450)

DD-32230 Open wound of buttock without complication 877.0
(T-D2600) (M-14010) (G-C009) (F-01450)

DD-32232 Open wound of sacroiliac region without complication 877.0
(T-D2330) (M-14010) (G-C009) (F-01450)

DD-32236 Open wound of buttock with complication 877.1
(T-D2600) (M-14010) (G-C008) (F-01450)

DD-32238 Open wound of sacroiliac region with complication 877.1
(T-D2330) (M-14010) (G-C008) (F-01450)

DD-32300 Open wound of external genital organs, NOS 878.-
(T-70260) (M-14010)

DD-32302 Open wound of external genital organs without complication 878.8
(T-70260) (M-14010) (G-C009) (F-01450)

DD-32303 Open wound of external genital organs with complication 878.9
(T-70260) (M-14010) (G-C008) (F-01450)

DD-32310 Open wound of penis without complication 878.0
(T-91000) (M-14010) (G-C009) (F-01450)

DD-32312 Open wound of penis with complication 878.1
(T-91000) (M-14010) (G-C008) (F-01450)

DD-32314 Open wound of scrotum without complication 878.2
(T-98000) (M-14010) (G-C009) (F-01450)

DD-32315 Open wound of testis without complication 878.2
(T-94000) (M-14010) (G-C009) (F-01450)

DD-32316 Open wound of scrotum with complication 878.3
(T-98000) (M-14010) (G-C008) (F-01450)

DD-32317 Open wound of testis with complication 878.3
(T-94000) (M-14010) (G-C008) (F-01450)

DD-32340 Open wound of vulva without complication 878.4
(T-81000) (M-14010) (G-C009) (F-01450)
Open wound of labium majus and minus without complication 878.4
(T-81000) (M-14010) (G-C009) (F-01450)

DD-32342 Open wound of vulva with complication 878.5
(T-81000) (M-14010) (G-C008) (F-01450)
Open wound of labium majus and minus with complication 878.5
(T-81000) (M-14010) (G-C008) (F-01450)

DD-32346 Open wound of vagina without complication 878.6
(T-82000) (M-14010) (G-C009) (F-01450)

DD-32348 Open wound of vagina with complication 878.7
(T-82000) (M-14010) (G-C008) (F-01450)

DD-32400 Open wound of breast without complication 879.0
(T-04000) (M-14010) (G-C009) (F-01450)

DD-32410 Open wound of breast with complication 879.1
(T-04000) (M-14010) (G-C008) (F-01450)

DD-32500 Open wound of abdominal wall without complication, NOS 879.2
(T-D4300) (M-14010) (G-C009) (F-01450)

DD-32505 Open wound of abdominal wall with complication, NOS 879.3
(T-D4300) (M-14010) (G-C008) (F-01450)

DD-32510 Open wound of anterior abdominal wall without complication 879.2
(T-D4310) (M-14010) (G-C009) (F-01450)

DD-32511 Open wound of epigastric region without complication 879.2
(T-D4200) (M-14010) (G-C009) (F-01450)

DD-32512 Open wound of hypogastric region without complication 879.2
(T-D4240) (M-14010) (G-C009) (F-01450)
Open wound of pubic region without complication 879.2
(T-D4240) (M-14010) (G-C009) (F-01450)

DD-32516 Open wound of umbilical region without complication 879.2
(T-D4230) (M-14010) (G-C009) (F-01450)

DD-32520 Open wound of anterior abdominal wall with complication 879.3
(T-D4310) (M-14010) (G-C008) (F-01450)

DD-32521 Open wound of epigastric region with complication 879.3
(T-D4200) (M-14010) (G-C008) (F-01450)

DD-32522 Open wound of hypogastric region with complication 879.3
(T-D4240) (M-14010) (G-C008) (F-01450)
Open wound of pubic region with complication 879.3
(T-D4240) (M-14010) (G-C008) (F-01450)

DD-32526 Open wound of umbilical region with complication 879.3
(T-D4230) (M-14010) (G-C008) (F-01450)

DD-32540 Open wound of lateral abdominal wall without complication 879.4
(T-D2310) (M-14010) (G-C009) (F-01450)
Open wound of flank without complication 879.4
(T-D2310) (M-14010) (G-C009) (F-01450)

DD-32542 Open wound of groin without complication 879.4
(T-D7000) (M-14010) (G-C009) (F-01450)
Open wound of iliac region without complication 879.4
(T-D7000) (M-14010) (G-C009) (F-01450)

D-32 OPEN WOUNDS OF THE TRUNK — Continued

DD-32542 (cont.) Open wound of inguinal region without complication 879.4
(T-D7000) (M-14010) (G-C009) (F-01450)

DD-32544 Open wound of hypochondrium without complication 879.4
(T-D4210) (M-14010) (G-C009) (F-01450)

DD-32550 Open wound of lateral abdominal wall with complication 879.5
(T-D2310) (M-14010) (G-C008) (F-01450)
Open wound of flank with complication 879.5
(T-D2310) (M-14010) (G-C008) (F-01450)

DD-32552 Open wound of groin with complication 879.5
(T-D7000) (M-14010) (G-C008) (F-01450)
Open wound of iliac region with complication 879.5
(T-D7000) (M-14010) (G-C008) (F-01450)
Open wound of inguinal region with complication 879.5
(T-D7000) (M-14010) (G-C008) (F-01450)

DD-32554 Open wound of hypochondrium with complication 879.5
(T-D4210) (M-14010) (G-C008) (F-01450)

D-33 OPEN WOUNDS OF THE LIMBS

DD-33000 Open wound of upper limb, NOS 884.0
(T-D8000) (M-14010)
Open wound of arm, NOS 884.0
(T-D8000) (M-14010)

DD-33001 Open wound of upper limb without complication 884.0
(T-D8000) (M-14010) (G-C009) (F-01450)
Open wound of arm without complication 884.0
(T-D8000) (M-14010) (G-C009) (F-01450)

DD-33002 Open wound of upper limb with complication 884.1
(T-D8000) (M-14010) (G-C008) (F-01450)
Open wound of arm with complication 884.1
(T-D8000) (M-14010) (G-C008) (F-01450)

DD-33003 Open wound of upper limb with tendon involvement 884.2
(T-D8000) (M-14010) (G-C008) (T-17010) (M-10000)
Open wound of arm with tendon involvement 884.2
(T-D8000) (M-14010) (G-C008) (T-17010) (M-10000)

DD-33005 Open wound of multiple sites of one upper limb, NOS 884.0
(T-D8000) (M-14018)

DD-33006 Open wound of multiple sites of one upper limb without complication 884.0
(T-D8000) (M-14018) (G-C009) (F-01450)

DD-33007 Open wound of multiple sites of one upper limb with complication 884.1
(T-D8000) (M-14018) (G-C008) (F-01450)

DD-33008 Open wound of multiple sites of one upper limb with tendon involvement 884.2
(T-D8000) (M-14018) (G-C008) (T-17010) (M-10000)

DD-33100 Open wound of shoulder region without complication 880.00
(T-D2220) (M-14010) (G-C009) (F-01450)

DD-33102 Open wound of scapular region without complication 880.01
(T-D2200) (M-14010) (G-C009) (F-01450)

DD-33104 Open wound of axillary region without complication 880.02
(T-D8104) (M-14010) (G-C009) (F-01450)

DD-33106 Open wound of upper arm without complication 880.03
(T-D8200) (M-14010) (G-C009) (F-01450)

DD-33108 Open wound of multiple sites of shoulder and upper arm without complication 880.09
(T-D2220) (T-D8200) (M-14018) (G-C009) (F-01450)

DD-33110 Open wound of shoulder region with complication 880.10
(T-D2220) (M-14010) (G-C008) (F-01450)

DD-33112 Open wound of scapular region with complication 880.11
(T-D2200) (M-14010) (G-C008) (F-01450)

DD-33114 Open wound of axillary region with complication 880.12
(T-D8104) (M-14010) (G-C008) (F-01450)

DD-33116 Open wound of upper arm with complication 880.13
(T-D8200) (M-14010) (G-C008) (F-01450)

DD-33118 Open wound of multiple sites of shoulder and upper arm with complication 880.19
(T-D2220) (T-D8200) (M-14018) (G-C008) (F-01450)

DD-33120 Open wound of shoulder region with tendon involvement 880.20
(T-D2220) (M-14010) (G-C008) (T-17010) (M-10000)

DD-33122 Open wound of scapular region with tendon involvement 880.21
(T-D2200) (M-14010) (G-C008) (F-01450)

DD-33124 Open wound of axillary region with tendon involvement 880.22
(T-D8104) (M-14010) (G-C008) (F-01450)

DD-33126 Open wound of upper arm with tendon involvement 880.23
(T-D8200) (M-14010) (G-C008) (F-01450)

DD-33128 Open wound of multiple sites of shoulder and upper arm with tendon involvement 880.29
(T-D2220) (T-D8200) (M-14018) (G-C008) (T-17010) (M-10000)

DD-33130 Open wound of forearm without complication 881.00
(T-D8500) (M-14010) (G-C009) (F-01450)

DD-33132 Open wound of elbow without complication 881.01
(T-D8300) (M-14010) (G-C009) (F-01450)

DD-33134 Open wound of wrist without complication 881.02
(T-D8600) (M-14010) (G-C009) (F-01450)

DD-33140 Open wound of forearm with complication 881.10
(T-D8500) (M-14010) (G-C008) (F-01450)

DD-33142 Open wound of elbow with complication 881.11
(T-D8300) (M-14010) (G-C008) (F-01450)

DD-33144 Open wound of wrist with complication 881.12
(T-D8600) (M-14010) (G-C008) (F-01450)

DD-33150 Open wound of forearm with tendon involvement 881.20
(T-D8500) (M-14010) (G-C008) (T-17010) (M-10000)

DD-33152 Open wound of elbow with tendon involvement 881.21
(T-D8300) (M-14010) (G-C008) (T-17010) (M-10000)

DD-33154 Open wound of wrist with tendon involvement 881.22
(T-D8600) (M-14010) (G-C008) (T-17010) (M-10000)

DD-33160 Open wound of hand except fingers without complication 882.0
(T-D8700) (G-C030) (T-D8800) (M-14010) (G-C009) (F-01450)

DD-33162 Open wound of hand except fingers with complication 882.1
(T-D8700) (G-C030) (T-D8800) (M-14010) (G-C008) (F-01450)

DD-33164 Open wound of hand except fingers with tendon involvement 882.2
(T-D8700) (G-C030) (T-D8800) (M-14010) (G-C008) (T-17010) (M-10000)

DD-33170 Open wound of finger without complication 883.0
(T-D8800) (M-14010) (G-C009) (F-01450)

DD-33171 Open wound of finger with complication 883.1
(T-D8800) (M-14010) (G-C008) (F-01450)

DD-33172 Open wound of finger with tendon involvement 883.2
(T-D8800) (M-14010) (G-C008) (T-17010) (M-10000)

DD-33174 Open wound of thumb without complication 883.0
(T-D8810) (M-14010) (G-C009) (F-01450)

DD-33175 Open wound of thumb with complication 883.1
(T-D8810) (M-14010) (G-C008) (F-01450)

DD-33176 Open wound of thumb with tendon involvement 883.2
(T-D8810) (M-14010) (G-C008) (T-17010) (M-10000)

DD-33180 Open wound of fingernail without complication 883.0
(T-01600) (T-D8800) (M-14010) (G-C009) (F-01450)

DD-33181 Open wound of fingernail with complication 883.1
(T-01600) (T-D8800) (M-14010) (G-C008) (F-01450)

DD-33182 Open wound of fingernail with tendon involvement 883.2
(T-01600) (T-D8800) (M-14010) (G-C008) (F-01450)

DD-33184 Open wound of thumbnail without complication 883.0
(T-01600) (T-D8810) (M-14010) (G-C009) (F-01450)

DD-33185 Open wound of thumbnail with complication 883.1
(T-01600) (T-D8810) (M-14010) (G-C008) (F-01450)

DD-33186 Open wound of thumbnail with tendon involvement 883.2
(T-01600) (T-D8810) (M-14010) (G-C008) (T-17010) (M-10000)

DD-33200 Traumatic amputation of thumb with fingers of either hand, NOS 885.0
(T-D8800) (T-D8810) (M-17010)

DD-33202 Traumatic amputation of thumb with fingers of either hand without complication 885.0
(T-D8800) (T-D8810) (M-17010) (G-C009) (F-01450)

D-33 OPEN WOUNDS OF THE LIMBS — Continued

DD-33204 Traumatic amputation of thumb with fingers of either hand with complication 885.1
(T-D8800) (T-D8810) (M-17010) (G-C008) (F-01450)

DD-33206 Traumatic amputation of thumb and fingers of one hand without complication 885.0
(T-D8800) (T-D8810) (M-17011) (G-C009) (F-01450)

DD-33208 Traumatic amputation of thumb and fingers of one hand with complication 885.1
(T-D8800) (T-D8810) (M-17011) (G-C008) (F-01450)

DD-33220 Traumatic amputation of finger without complication 886.0
(T-D8800) (M-17010) (G-C009) (F-01450)

DD-33222 Traumatic amputation of finger with complication 886.1
(T-D8800) (M-17010) (G-C008) (F-01450)

DD-33300 Unilateral traumatic amputation of arm level not specified without complication 887.4
(T-D8000) (M-17011) (G-C009) (F-01450)

DD-33302 Unilateral traumatic amputation of arm level not specified with complication 887.5
(T-D8000) (M-17011) (G-C008) (F-01450)

DD-33310 Bilateral traumatic amputation of arms at any level without complication 887.6
(T-D8000) (M-17012) (G-C009) (F-01450)

DD-33312 Bilateral traumatic amputation of arms at any level with complication 887.7
(T-D8000) (M-17012) (G-C008) (F-01450)

DD-33320 Unilateral traumatic amputation at or above elbow without complication 887.2
(T-D8300) (M-17011) (G-C009) (F-01450)

DD-33322 Unilateral traumatic amputation at or above elbow with complication 887.3
(T-D8300) (M-17011) (G-C008) (F-01450)

DD-33330 Unilateral traumatic amputation below elbow without complication 887.0
(T-D8300) (G-A115) (M-17011) (G-C009) (F-01450)

DD-33332 Unilateral traumatic amputation below elbow with complication 887.1
(T-D8300) (G-A115) (M-17011) (G-C008) (F-01450)

DD-33500 Open wound of lower limb, NOS 894.0
(T-D9000) (M-14010)

DD-33501 Open wound of lower limb without complication 894.0
(T-D9000) (M-14010) (G-C009) (F-01450)

DD-33502 Open wound of lower limb with complication 894.1
(T-D9000) (M-14010) (G-C008) (F-01450)

DD-33503 Open wound of lower limb with tendon involvement 894.2
(T-D9000) (M-14010) (G-C008) (T-17010) (M-10000)

DD-33505 Open wound of multiple sites of one lower limb and thigh, NOS 894.0
(T-D9000) (T-D9100) (M-14018)

DD-33506 Open wound of multiple sites of one lower limb and thigh without complication 894.0
(T-D9000) (T-D9100) (M-14018) (G-C009) (F-01450)

DD-33507 Open wound of multiple sites of one lower limb and thigh with complication 894.1
(T-D9000) (T-D9100) (M-14018) (G-C008) (F-01450)

DD-33508 Open wound of multiple sites of one lower limb and thigh with tendon involvement 894.2
(T-D9000) (T-D9100) (M-14018) (G-C008) (T-17010) (M-10000)

DD-33600 Open wound of hip and thigh without complication 890.0
(T-D2500) (T-D9100) (M-14010) (G-C009) (F-01450)

DD-33602 Open wound of hip and thigh with complication 890.1
(T-D2500) (T-D9100) (M-14010) (G-C008) (F-01450)

DD-33604 Open wound of hip and thigh with tendon involvement 890.2
(T-D2500) (T-D9100) (M-14010) (G-C008) (T-17010) (M-10000)

DD-33620 Open wound of knee without complication 891.0
(T-D9200) (M-14010) (G-C009) (F-01450)

DD-33621 Open wound of knee with complication 891.1
(T-D9200) (M-14010) (G-C008) (F-01450)

DD-33622 Open wound of knee with tendon involvement 891.2
(T-D9200) (M-14010) (G-C008) (T-17010) (M-10000)

DD-33631 Open wound of leg without complication 891.0
(T-D9400) (M-14010) (G-C009) (F-01450)

DD-33632 Open wound of leg with complication 891.1
(T-D9400) (M-14010) (G-C008) (F-01450)

DD-33633 Open wound of leg with tendon involvement 891.2
(T-D9400) (M-14010) (G-C008) (T-17010) (M-10000)

DD-33641 Open wound of ankle without complication 891.0
(T-D9500) (M-14010) (G-C009) (F-01450)

DD-33642 Open wound of ankle with complication 891.1
(T-D9500) (M-14010) (G-C008) (F-01450)

DD-33643 Open wound of ankle with tendon involvement 891.2
(T-D9500) (M-14010) (G-C008) (T-17010) (M-10000)

DD-33650 Open wound of foot except toes without complication 892.0
(T-D9700) (G-C030) (T-D9800) (M-14010) (G-C009) (F-01450)

DD-33651 Open wound of foot except toes with complication 892.1
(T-D9700) (G-C030) (T-D9800) (M-14010) (G-C008) (F-01450)

DD-33652 Open wound of foot except toes with tendon involvement 892.2
(T-D9700) (G-C030) (T-D9800) (M-14010) (G-C008) (T-17010) (M-10000)

DD-33658V Puncture wound of foot
Pricked foot
Nail bind

DD-33660 Open wound of toe without complication 893.0
(T-D9800) (M-14010) (G-C009) (F-01450)

DD-33661 Open wound of toe with complication 893.1
(T-D9800) (M-14010) (G-C008) (F-01450)

DD-33662 Open wound of toe with tendon involvement 893.2
(T-D9800) (M-14010) (G-C008) (T-17010) (M-10000)

DD-33700 Traumatic amputation of toe or toes without complication 895.0
(T-D9800) (M-17010) (G-C009) (F-01450)

DD-33702 Traumatic amputation of toe or toes with complication 895.1
(T-D9800) (M-17010) (G-C008) (F-01450)

DD-33710 Unilateral traumatic amputation of foot without complication 896.0
(T-D9700) (M-17011) (G-C009) (F-01450)

DD-33712 Unilateral traumatic amputation of foot with complication 896.1
(T-D9700) (M-17011) (G-C008) (F-01450)

DD-33714 Bilateral traumatic amputation of feet without complication 896.2
(T-D9700) (M-17012) (G-C009) (F-01450)

DD-33716 Bilateral traumatic amputation of feet with complication 896.3
(T-D9700) (M-17012) (G-C008) (F-01450)

DD-33730 Unilateral traumatic amputation of leg level not specified without complication 897.4
(T-D9000) (M-17011) (G-C009) (F-01450)

DD-33731 Unilateral traumatic amputation of leg level not specified with complication 897.5
(T-D9000) (M-17011) (G-C008) (F-01450)

DD-33732 Unilateral traumatic amputation of leg below knee without complication 897.0
(T-D9240) (M-17011) (G-C009) (F-01450)

DD-33733 Unilateral traumatic amputation of leg below knee with complication 897.1
(T-D9240) (M-17011) (G-C008) (F-01450)

DD-33734 Unilateral traumatic amputation of leg at or above knee without complication 897.2
(T-D9160) (M-17011) (G-C009) (F-01450)

DD-33735 Unilateral traumatic amputation of leg at or above knee with complication 897.3
(T-D9160) (M-17011) (G-C008) (F-01450)

DD-33738 Bilateral traumatic amputation of legs at any level without complication 897.6
(T-D9000) (M-17012) (G-C009) (F-01450)

DD-33739 Bilateral traumatic amputation of legs at any level with complication 897.7
(T-D9000) (M-17012) (G-C008) (F-01450)

D-35 CRUSHING INJURIES

DD-35010 Crushing injury of multiple sites, NEC 929.0
(T-D0020) (M-10400)

DD-35100 Crushing injury of face 925.-
(T-D1200) (M-10400)

DD-35102 Crushing injury of cheek 925.-
(T-D1206) (M-10400)

DD-35104 Crushing injury of ear 925.-
(T-AB000) (M-10400)

DD-35110 Crushing injury of scalp 925.-
(T-D1160) (M-10400)

DD-35120 Crushing injury of neck 925.-
(T-D1600) (M-10400)

DD-35122 Crushing injury of throat 925.-
(T-55000) (M-10400)
Crushing injury of pharynx 925.-
(T-55000) (M-10400)

DD-35124 Crushing injury of larynx 925.-
(T-24100) (M-10400)

DD-35200 Crushing injury of trunk, NOS 926.9
(T-D2000) (M-10400)

D-35 CRUSHING INJURIES — Continued

DD-35210 Crushing injury of back 926.11
(T-D2100) (M-10400)

DD-35220 Crushing injury of buttock 926.12
(T-D2600) (M-10400)

DD-35228 Crushing injury of multiple sites of trunk 926.8
(T-D2000) (T-D0020) (M-10400)

DD-35400 Crushing injury of external genitalia, NOS 926.0
(T-70260) (M-10400)

DD-35410 Crushing injury of female external genitalia, NOS 926.0
(T-80010) (M-10400)

DD-35412 Crushing injury of vulva 926.0
(T-81000) (M-10400)
Crushing injury of labium majus and minus 926.0
(T-81000) (M-10400)

DD-35430 Crushing injury of male external genitalia, NOS 926.0
(T-90010) (M-10400)

DD-35432 Crushing injury of penis 926.0
(T-91000) (M-10400)

DD-35434 Crushing injury of scrotum 926.0
(T-98000) (M-10400)

DD-35436 Crushing injury of testis 926.0
(T-94000) (M-10400)

DD-35500 Crushing injury of upper limb, NOS 927.9
(T-D8000) (M-10400)
Crushing injury of arm, NOS 927.9
(T-D8000) (M-10400)

DD-35508 Crushing injury of multiple sites of upper limb 927.8
(T-D8000) (T-D0020) (M-10400)

DD-35510 Crushing injury of shoulder and upper arm 927.0
(T-D2220) (T-D8200) (M-10400)

DD-35512 Crushing injury of shoulder region 927.00
(T-D2220) (M-10400)

DD-35513 Crushing injury of scapular region 927.01
(T-D2200) (M-10400)

DD-35514 Crushing injury of axillary region 927.02
(T-D8104) (M-10400)

DD-35516 Crushing injury of upper arm 927.03
(T-D8200) (M-10400)

DD-35518 Crushing injury of multiple sites of shoulder and upper arm 927.09
(T-D2220) (T-D8200) (T-D0020) (M-10400)

DD-35530 Crushing injury of elbow and forearm 927.1
(T-D8300) (T-D8500) (M-10400)

DD-35532 Crushing injury of forearm 927.10
(T-D8500) (M-10400)

DD-35534 Crushing injury of elbow 927.11
(T-D8300) (M-10400)

DD-35540 Crushing injury of wrist and hand except fingers 927.2
(T-D8600) (T-D8700) (G-C030) (T-D8800) (M-10400)

DD-35542 Crushing injury of hand 927.20
(T-D8700) (M-10400)

DD-35544 Crushing injury of wrist 927.21
(T-D8600) (M-10400)

DD-35550 Crushing injury of finger 927.3
(T-D8800) (M-10400)

DD-35600 Crushing injury of lower limb, NOS 928.9
(T-D9000) (M-10400)
Crushing injury of leg, NOS 928.9
(T-D9000) (M-10400)

DD-35608 Crushing injury of multiple sites of lower limb 928.8
(T-D9000) (T-D0020) (M-10400)

DD-35610 Crushing injury of hip and thigh 928.0
(T-D2500) (T-D9100) (M-10400)

DD-35612 Crushing injury of thigh 928.00
(T-D9100) (M-10400)

DD-35614 Crushing injury of hip 928.01
(T-D2500) (M-10400)

DD-35630 Crushing injury of knee and lower leg 928.1
(T-D9200) (T-D9400) (M-10400)

DD-35632 Crushing injury of lower leg 928.10
(T-D9400) (M-10400)

DD-35634 Crushing injury of knee 928.11
(T-D9200) (M-10400)

DD-35640 Crushing injury of ankle and foot excluding toes 928.2
(T-D9500) (T-D9700) (M-10400)

DD-35642 Crushing injury of foot 928.20
(T-D9500) (M-10400)

DD-35643 Crushing injury of heel 928.20
(T-D9600) (M-10400)

DD-35644 Crushing injury of ankle 928.21
(T-D9700) (M-10400)

DD-35650 Crushing injury of toe 928.3
(T-D9800) (M-10400)

SECTION D-4 INJURIES OF THE BLOOD VESSELS, NERVES AND SPINAL CORD

D-40 INJURIES OF THE BLOOD VESSELS

DD-40000 Injury of blood vessel, NOS 904.9
(T-40000) (M-10000)

DD-40100 Injury of blood vessels of head and neck, NOS 900.90
(T-40000) (T-D1100) (T-D1600) (M-10000)

DD-40108 Injury of multiple blood vessels of head and neck 900.82
(T-40000) (T-D1100) (T-D1600) (M-10080)

DD-40110 Injury of carotid artery, NOS 900.00
(T-45010) (M-10000)

DD-40112 Injury of common carotid artery 900.01
(T-45100) (M-10000)

DD-40114 Injury of external carotid artery 900.02
(T-45200) (M-10000)

DD-40116 Injury of internal carotid artery 900.03
(T-45300) (M-10000)

DD-40120 Injury of internal jugular vein 900.1
(T-48170) (M-10000)

DD-40122 Injury of external jugular vein 900.81
(T-48160) (M-10000)

DD-40200 Injury of blood vessels of thorax, NOS 901.9
(T-40000) (T-D3000) (M-10000)

DD-40210 Injury of thoracic aorta 901.0
(T-42070) (M-10000)

DD-40212 Injury of innominate artery 901.1
(T-46010) (M-10000)

DD-40214 Injury of subclavian artery 901.1
(T-46100) (M-10000)

DD-40220 Injury of superior vena cava 901.2
(T-48610) (M-10000)

DD-40222 Injury of innominate vein 901.3
(T-48620) (M-10000)

DD-40224 Injury of subclavian vein 901.3
(T-48330) (M-10000)

DD-40230 Injury of pulmonary vessels, NOS 901.40
(T-30200) (M-10000)

DD-40232 Injury of pulmonary artery 901.41
(T-44000) (M-10000)

DD-40234 Injury of pulmonary vein 901.42
(T-48500) (M-10000)

DD-40240 Injury of intercostal artery 901.81
(T-46207) (M-10000)

DD-40242 Injury of internal mammary artery 901.82
(T-46200) (M-10000)

DD-40250 Injury of intercostal vein 901.81
(T-48349) (M-10000)

DD-40252 Injury of internal mammary vein 901.82
(T-48321) (M-10000)

DD-40254 Injury of azygos vein 901.89
(T-48340) (M-10000)

DD-40256 Injury of hemiazygos vein 901.89
(T-48351) (M-10000)

DD-40280 Injury of multiple blood vessels of thorax 901.83
(T-40000) (T-D3000) (M-10080)

DD-40400 Injury of blood vessels of abdomen and pelvis, NOS 902.9
(T-40000) (T-D4000) (T-D6000) (M-10000)

DD-40402 Injury of mutiple blood vessels of abdomen and pelvis, NOS 902.87
(T-40000) (T-D4000) (T-D6000) (M-10080)

DD-40410 Injury of abdominal aorta 902.0
(T-42500) (M-10000)

DD-40420 Injury of inferior vena cava, NOS 902.10
(T-48710) (M-10000)

DD-40422 Injury of hepatic vein 902.11
(T-48720) (M-10000)

DD-40430 Injury of celiac and mesenteric arteries, NOS 902.20
(T-46400) (T-46500) (M-10000)

DD-40431 Injury of gastric artery 902.21
(T-46410) (M-10000)

DD-40432 Injury of hepatic artery 902.22
(T-46420) (M-10000)

DD-40433 Injury of splenic artery 902.23
(T-46460) (M-10000)

DD-40434 Injury of other specified branch of celiac axis, NEC 902.24
(T-46400) (M-10000)

DD-40435 Injury of superior mesenteric artery 902.25
(T-46510) (M-10000)

DD-40437 Injury of primary branches of superior mesenteric artery 902.26
(T-46510) (M-10000)

DD-40438 Injury of ileocolic artery 902.26
(T-46560) (M-10000)

DD-40439 Injury of inferior mesenteric artery 902.27
(T-46520) (M-10000)

DD-40440 Injury of portal and splenic veins 902.3
(T-48810) (T-48890) (M-10000)

DD-40441 Injury of superior mesenteric vein and primary subdivisions 902.31
(T-48840) (M-10000)

DD-40442 Injury of ileocolic vein 902.31
(T-48842) (M-10000)

DD-40443 Injury of inferior mesenteric vein 902.32
(T-48910) (M-10000)

DD-40444 Injury of portal vein 902.33
(T-48810) (M-10000)

DD-40445 Injury of splenic vein 902.34
(T-48890) (M-10000)

DD-40446 Injury of cystic vein 902.39
(T-48830) (M-10000)

DD-40447 Injury of gastric veins 902.35
(T-48821) (T-48822) (M-10000)

DD-40450 Injury of renal vessels, NOS 902.40
(T-40000) (T-71000) (M-10000)

DD-40452 Injury of renal artery 902.41
(T-46600) (M-10000)

DD-40454 Injury of renal vein 902.42
(T-48740) (M-10000)

DD-40456 Injury of suprarenal arteries 902.49
(T-46950) (M-10000)

DD-40460 Injury of iliac blood vessels, NOS 902.50
(T-46700) (T-48920) (M-10000)

DD-40461 Injury of hypogastric artery 902.51
(T-46740) (M-10000)

DD-40462 Injury of hypogastric vein 902.52
(T-48940) (M-10000)

DD-40463 Injury of iliac artery 902.53
(T-46700) (M-10000)

DD-40464 Injury of iliac vein 902.54
(T-48920) (M-10000)

DD-40465 Injury of uterine artery 902.55
(T-46820) (M-10000)

DD-40466 Injury of uterine vein 902.56
(T-49010) (M-10000)

D-40 INJURIES OF THE BLOOD VESSELS — Continued

DD-40470 Injury of ovarian artery 902.81
(T-46980) (M-10000)
DD-40472 Injury of ovarian vein 902.82
(T-48780) (M-10000)
DD-40600 Injury of blood vessels of upper extremity, NOS 903.9
(T-40000) (T-D8000) (M-10000)
DD-40602 Injury of multiple blood vessels of upper extremity, NOS 903.8
(T-40000) (T-D8000) (M-10080)
DD-40610 Injury of axillary vessel, NOS 903.00
(T-40000) (T-D8100) (M-10000)
DD-40612 Injury of axillary artery 903.01
(T-47100) (M-10000)
DD-40614 Injury of axillary vein 903.02
(T-49100) (M-10000)
DD-40620 Injury of brachial blood vessels, NOS 903.1
(T-47160) (T-49350) (M-10000)
DD-40622 Injury of brachial artery 903.1
(T-47160) (M-10000)
DD-40624 Injury of brachial vein 903.1
(T-49350) (M-10000)
DD-40630 Injury of radial blood vessels, NOS 903.2
(T-47300) (T-49340) (M-10000)
DD-40632 Injury of radial artery 903.2
(T-47300) (M-10000)
DD-40634 Injury of radial vein 903.2
(T-49340) (M-10000)
DD-40640 Injury of ulnar blood vessels, NOS 903.3
(T-47200) (T-49330) (M-10000)
DD-40642 Injury of ulnar artery 903.3
(T-47200) (M-10000)
DD-40644 Injury of ulnar vein 903.3
(T-49330) (M-10000)
DD-40650 Injury of palmar artery 903.4
(T-47350) (M-10000)
DD-40652 Injury of digital blood vessels, NOS 903.5
(T-40000) (T-D8800) (M-10000)
DD-40800 Injury of blood vessels of lower extremity, NOS 904.8
(T-40000) (T-D9000) (M-10000)
DD-40802 Injury of multiple blood vessels of lower extremity, NOS 904.7
(T-40000) (T-D9000) (M-10080)
DD-40810 Injury of common femoral artery 904.0
(T-47400) (M-10000)
DD-40812 Injury of superficial femoral artery 904.1
(T-47400) (T-D9101) (M-10000)
DD-40813 Injury of femoral vein 904.2
(T-49410) (M-10000)
DD-40814 Injury of saphenous vein 904.3
(T-49530) (M-10000)
DD-40820 Injury of popliteal vessels, NOS 904.40
(T-47500) (T-49650) (M-10000)
DD-40822 Injury of popliteal artery 904.41
(T-47500) (M-10000)
DD-40824 Injury of popliteal vein 904.42
(T-49650) (M-10000)
DD-40830 Injury of tibial blood vessels, NOS 904.50
(T-47700) (T-49630) (T-47600)
(T-49620) (M-10000)
DD-40832 Injury of anterior tibial artery 904.51
(T-47700) (M-10000)
DD-40834 Injury of anterior tibial vein 904.52
(T-49630) (M-10000)
DD-40836 Injury of posterior tibial artery 904.53
(T-47600) (M-10000)
DD-40838 Injury of posterior tibial vein 904.54
(T-49620) (M-10000)
DD-40840 Injury of deep plantar blood vessels 904.6
(T-47770) (T-49643) (M-10000)

D-42 INJURIES OF THE NERVES AND SPINAL CORD

DD-42000 Nerve injury, NOS 957.9
(T-A9001) (M-10000)
DD-42002 Multiple nerve injury, NOS 957.8
(T-A9001) (M-10080)
DD-42100 Injury of cranial nerve, NOS 951.9
(T-A8000) (M-10000)
DD-42110 Optic nerve injury, NOS 950.9
(T-A8040) (M-10000)
Second cranial nerve injury, NOS 950.9
(T-A8040) (M-10000)
DD-42112 Injury of optic chiasm 950.1
(T-A8050) (M-10000)
DD-42114 Injury of optic pathways 950.2
(T-A2880) (M-10000)
DD-42116 Injury of visual cortex 950.3
(T-A2430) (M-10000)
DD-42118 Traumatic blindness, NOS 950.9
(DA-54900) (G-C001) (M-10000)
DD-42120 Injury of oculomotor nerve 951.0
(T-A8070) (M-10000)
Injury of third cranial nerve 951.0
(T-A8070) (M-10000)
DD-42122 Injury of trochlear nerve 951.1
(T-A8110) (M-10000)
Injury of fourth cranial nerve 951.1
(T-A8110) (M-10000)
DD-42124 Injury of trigeminal nerve 951.2
(T-A8150) (M-10000)
Injury of fifth cranial nerve 951.2
(T-A8150) (M-10000)
DD-42126 Injury of abducens nerve 951.3
(T-A8130) (M-10000)
Injury of sixth cranial nerve 951.3
(T-A8130) (M-10000)
DD-42128 Injury of facial nerve 951.4
(T-A8410) (M-10000)
Injury of seventh cranial nerve 951.4
(T-A8410) (M-10000)
DD-42130 Injury of accessory nerve 951.6
(T-A8780) (M-10000)
Injury of eleventh cranial nerve 951.6
(T-A8780) (M-10000)

DD-42132 Injury of hypoglossal nerve 951.7
(T-A8820) (M-10000)
Injury of twelfth cranial nerve 951.7
(T-A8820) (M-10000)

DD-42134 Injury of glossopharyngeal nerve 951.8
(T-A8570) (M-10000)
Injury to ninth cranial nerve 951.8
(T-A8570) (M-10000)

DD-42136 Injury of pneumogastric nerve 951.8
(T-A8640) (M-10000)
Injury of vagus nerve 951.8
(T-A8640) (M-10000)
Injury of tenth cranial nerve 951.8
(T-A8640) (M-10000)

DD-42140 Injury of olfactory nerve 951.8
(T-A8020) (M-10000)
Injury of first cranial nerve 951.8
(T-A8020) (M-10000)

DD-42142 Traumatic anosmia, NOS 951.8
(F-A3025) (G-C001) (M-10000)

DD-42144 Injury of acoustic nerve 951.5
(T-A8500) (M-10000)
Injury of auditory nerve 951.5
(T-A8500) (M-10000)
Injury of eighth cranial nerve 951.5
(T-A8500) (M-10000)

DD-42146 Traumatic deafness, NOS 951.5
(F-F6000) (G-C001) (M-10000)

DD-42300 Spinal cord injury, NOS 952.9
(T-A7010) (M-10000)

DD-42301 Spinal cord injury without spinal bone injury, NOS 952.9
(T-A7010) (M-10000) (G-C009)
(T-11500) (M-10000)

DD-42302 Multiple spinal cord injuries without spinal bone injury, NOS 952.8
(T-A7010) (M-10080) (G-C009)
(T-11500) (M-10000)

DD-42310 Spinal cord injury to cervical region without bone injury, NOS 952.00
(T-A7600) (M-10000) (G-C009)
(T-11600) (M-10000)

DD-42311 Injury at C1-C4 level with unspecified spinal cord injury and without bone injury 952.00
(T-A7602) (M-10000) (G-C009)
(T-11600) (M-10000)

DD-42312 Injury at C1-C4 level with complete lesion of spinal cord and without bone injury 952.01
(T-A7602) (M-17110) (G-C009)
(T-11600) (M-10000)

DD-42313 Injury at C1-C4 level with anterior cord syndrome and without bone injury 952.02
(T-A7602) (T-A7640) (M-10000)
(G-C009) (T-11600) (M-10000)

DD-42314 Injury at C1-C4 level with central cord syndrome and without bone injury 952.03
(T-A7602) (T-A7681) (M-10000)
(G-C009) (T-11600) (M-10000)

DD-42315 Injury at C1-C4 level with posterior cord syndrome and without bone injury 952.04
(T-A7602) (T-A7620) (M-10000)
(G-C009) (T-11600) (M-10000)

DD-42316 Injury at C1-C4 level with other specified spinal cord injury and without bone injury 952.04
(T-A7602) (M-10000) (G-C009)
(T-11600) (M-10000)

DD-42317 Incomplete spinal cord lesion at C1-C4 level without bone injury, NOS 952.04
(T-A7602) (M-10000) (G-C009)
(T-11600) (M-10000)

DD-42321 Injury at C5-C7 level with unspecified spinal cord injury and without bone injury 952.05
(T-A7604) (M-10000) (G-C009)
(T-11600) (M-10000)

DD-42322 Injury at C5-C7 level with complete lesion of spinal cord and without bone injury 952.06
(T-A7604) (M-17110) (G-C009)
(T-11600) (M-10000)

DD-42323 Injury at C5-C7 level with anterior cord syndrome and without bone injury 952.07
(T-A7604) (T-A7640) (M-10000)
(G-C009) (T-11600) (M-10000)

DD-42324 Injury at C5-C7 level with central cord syndrome and without bone injury 952.08
(T-A7604) (T-A7681) (M-10000)
(G-C009) (T-11600) (M-10000)

DD-42325 Injury at C5-C7 level with posterior cord syndrome and without bone injury 952.09
(T-A7604) (T-A7620) (M-10000)
(G-C009) (T-11600) (M-10000)

DD-42326 Injury at C5-C7 level with other specified spinal cord injury and without bone injury 952.09
(T-A7604) (M-10000) (G-C009)
(T-11600) (M-10000)

DD-42327 Incomplete spinal cord lesion at C5-C7 level without bone injury, NOS 952.09
(T-A7604) (M-10000) (G-C009)
(T-11600) (M-10000)

DD-42340 Spinal cord injury of thoracic region without bone injury, NOS 952.10
(T-A7700) (M-10000) (G-C009)
(T-11700) (M-10000)
Spinal cord injury of dorsal region without bone injury, NOS 952.10
(T-A7700) (M-10000) (G-C009)
(T-11700) (M-10000)

DD-42342 Injury at T1-T6 level with unspecified spinal cord injury and without bone injury 952.10
(T-A7702) (M-10000) (G-C009)
(T-11700) (M-10000)

DD-42343 Injury at T1-T6 level with complete lesion of spinal cord and without bone injury 952.11
(T-A7702) (M-17110) (G-C009)
(T-11700) (M-10000)

D-42 INJURIES OF THE NERVES AND SPINAL CORD — Continued

DD-42344 Injury at T1-T6 level with anterior cord syndrome and without bone injury 952.12
(T-A7702) (T-A7740) (M-10000) (G-C009) (T-11700) (M-10000)

DD-42345 Injury at T1-T6 level with central cord syndrome and without bone injury 952.13
(T-A7702) (M-10000) (G-C009) (T-11700) (M-10000)

DD-42346 Injury at T1-T6 level with posterior cord syndrome and without bone injury 952.14
(T-A7702) (M-10000) (G-C009) (T-11700) (M-10000)

DD-42347 Incomplete spinal cord lesion at T1-T6 level without bone injury, NOS 952.14
(T-A7702) (M-10000) (G-C009) (T-11700) (M-10000)

DD-42352 Injury at T7-T12 level with unspecified spinal cord injury and without bone injury 952.15
(T-A7704) (M-10000) (G-C009) (T-11700) (M-10000)

DD-42353 Injury at T7-T12 level with complete lesion of spinal cord and without bone injury 952.16
(T-A7704) (M-17110) (G-C009) (T-11700) (M-10000)

DD-42354 Injury at T7-T12 level with anterior cord syndrome and without bone injury 952.17
(T-A7704) (T-A7740) (M-10000) (G-C009) (T-11700) (M-10000)

DD-42355 Injury at T7-T12 level with central cord syndrome and without bone injury 952.18
(T-A7704) (T-A7781) (M-10000) (G-C009) (T-11700) (M-10000)

DD-42356 Injury at T7-T12 level with posterior cord syndrome and without bone injury 952.19
(T-A7704) (T-A7720) (M-10000) (G-C009) (T-11700) (M-10000)

DD-42357 Incomplete spinal cord lesion at T7-T12 level without bone injury, NOS 952.19
(T-A7704) (M-10000) (G-C009) (T-11700) (M-10000)

DD-42360 Lumbar spinal cord injury without bone injury 952.2
(T-A7801) (M-10000) (G-C009) (T-11900) (M-10000)

DD-42370 Sacral spinal cord injury without bone injury 952.3
(T-A7802) (M-10000) (G-C009) (T-11A00) (M-10000)

DD-42380 Cauda equina injury without bone injury 952.4
(T-A7900) (M-10000) (G-C009) (T-11A70) (M-10000)

DD-42400 Injury of nerve roots and spinal plexus, NOS 953.9
(T-A7160) (T-A7170) (M-10000)

DD-42402 Injury of nerve roots and spinal plexus of multiple sites 953.8
(T-A7160) (T-A7170) (M-10080)

DD-42410 Injury of cervical nerve roots 953.0
(T-A7690) (M-10000)

DD-42411 Injury of dorsal nerve roots 953.1
(T-A7790) (M-10000)

DD-42412 Injury of lumbar nerve roots 953.2
(T-A7890) (M-10000)

DD-42413 Injury of sacral nerve roots 953.3
(T-A7890) (M-10000)

DD-42416 Injury of brachial plexus 953.4
(T-A9090) (M-10000)

DD-42417 Injury of lumbosacral plexus 953.5
(T-A9330) (M-10000)

DD-42500 Injury of nerve of trunk, NOS 954.9
(T-A9000) (T-D2000) (M-10000)

DD-42510 Injury of cervical sympathetic nerves 954.0
(T-A9710) (M-10000)

DD-42512 Injury of celiac ganglion or plexus 954.1
(T-A9810) (T-A9821) (M-10000)

DD-42514 Injury of inferior mesenteric plexus 954.1
(T-A9830) (M-10000)

DD-42516 Injury of splanchnic nerve 954.1
(T-A9780) (T-A9782) (M-10000)

DD-42518 Injury of stellate ganglion 954.1
(T-A9740) (M-10000)

DD-42700 Injury of peripheral nerve of shoulder girdle and upper limb, NOS 955.9
(T-A0500) (T-12200) (T-D8000) (M-10000)

DD-42702 Injury of multiple nerves of shoulder girdle and upper limb, NOS 955.8
(T-A0500) (T-12200) (T-D8000) (M-10080)

DD-42710 Injury of axillary nerve 955.0
(T-A9210) (M-10000)

DD-42712 Injury of median nerve 955.1
(T-A9180) (M-10000)

DD-42714 Injury of ulnar nerve 955.2
(T-A9170) (M-10000)

DD-42716 Injury of radial nerve 955.3
(T-A9190) (M-10000)

DD-42718 Injury of musculocutaneous nerve 955.4
(T-A9140) (M-10000)

DD-42720 Injury of cutaneous sensory nerve of upper limb 955.5
(T-A9012) (T-01000) (T-D8000) (M-10000)

DD-42722 Injury of digital nerve 955.6
(T-A9485) (M-10000)

DD-42800 Injury of peripheral nerve of pelvic girdle and lower limb, NOS 956.9
(T-A0500) (T-D6000) (T-D9000) (M-10000)

DD-42802 Injury of multiple nerves of pelvic girdle and lower limb 956.8
(T-A0500) (T-D6000) (T-D9000) (M-10080)

DD-42810 Injury of sciatic nerve 956.0
(T-A9440) (M-10000)

DD-42812 Injury of femoral nerve 956.1
(T-A9380) (M-10000)

DD-42814 Injury of tibial nerve 956.2
(T-A9450) (M-10000)

DD-42816 Injury of peroneal nerve 956.3
(T-A9490) (M-10000)

DD-42820 Injury of cutaneous sensory nerve of lower limb 956.4
(T-A9012) (T-01000) (T-D9000) (M-10000)

DD-42830 Injury of other specified nerve of pelvic girdle and lower limb 956.5
(T-A9001) (T-D6000) (T-D9000) (M-10000)

DD-42900 Injury of superficial nerves of head and neck 957.0
(T-A9001) (T-01000) (T-D1100) (T-D1600) (M-10000)

SECTION D-5 SUPERFICIAL INJURIES, BURNS AND CONTUSIONS

D-50 SUPERFICIAL INJURIES

DD-50002 Unspecified superficial injury without infection 919.8
(T-D0003) (M-10050) (G-C009) (DE-00050)

DD-50004 Unspecified superficial injury with infection 919.9
(T-D0003) (M-10050) (G-C008) (DE-00050)

DD-50010 Abrasion or friction burn of unspecified site without infection 919.0
(T-D0003) (M-14700) (M-14710) (G-C009) (DE-00050)

DD-50012 Abrasion or friction burn of unspecified site with infection 919.1
(T-D0003) (M-14700) (M-14710) (G-C008) (DE-00050)

DD-50020 Friction blister of unspecified site without infection 919.2
(T-D0003) (M-14720) (G-C009) (DE-00050)

DD-50022 Friction blister of unspecified site with infection 919.3
(T-D0003) (M-14720) (G-C008) (DE-00050)

DD-50030 Nonvenomous insect bite of unspecified site without infection 919.4
(T-D0003) (M-14368) (G-C009) (DE-00050)

DD-50032 Nonvenomous insect bite of unspecified site with infection 919.5
(T-D0003) (M-14368) (G-C008) (DE-00050)

DD-50040 Superficial foreign body of unspecified site without major open wound and without infection 919.6
(T-D0003) (M-30408) (G-C009) (M-14014) (DE-00050)

DD-50042 Superficial foreign body of unspecified site without major open wound but with infection 919.7
(T-D0003) (M-30408) (G-C008) (M-14014) (DE-00050)

DD-50100 Superficial injury of eye and adnexa, NOS 918.-
(T-AA000) (T-AA800) (M-10050)

DD-50102 Superficial injury of eye, NOS 918.9
(T-AA000) (M-10050)

DD-50110 Superficial injury of eyelid and periocular area 918.0
(T-AA810) (T-AA006) (M-10050)

DD-50120 Superficial injury of cornea 918.1
(T-AA200) (M-10050)

DD-50122 Corneal abrasion 918.1
(T-AA200) (M-14700)

DD-50124 Superficial laceration of cornea 918.1
(T-AA200) (M-14401)

DD-50130 Superficial injury of conjunctiva 918.2
(T-AA860) (M-10050)

DD-50200 Superficial injury of face without infection 910.8
(T-D1200) (M-10050) (G-C009) (DE-00050)

DD-50201 Superficial injury of face with infection 910.9
(T-D1200) (M-10050) (G-C008) (DE-00050)

DD-50202 Abrasion or friction burn of face without infection 910.0
(T-D1200) (M-14700) (M-14710) (G-C009) (DE-00050)

DD-50203 Abrasion or friction burn of face with infection 910.1
(T-D1200) (M-14700) (M-14710) (G-C008) (DE-00050)

DD-50204 Blister of face without infection 910.2
(T-D1200) (M-14720) (G-C009) (DE-00050)

DD-50205 Blister of face with infection 910.3
(T-D1200) (M-14720) (G-C008) (DE-00050)

DD-50206 Nonvenomous insect bite of face without infection 910.4
(T-D1200) (M-14368) (G-C009) (DE-00050)

DD-50207 Nonvenomous insect bite of face with infection 910.5
(T-D1200) (M-14368) (G-C009) (DE-00050)

DD-50208 Superficial foreign body of face without major open wound and without infection 910.6
(T-D1200) (M-30408) (M-14014) (G-C009) (DE-00050)

D-50 SUPERFICIAL INJURIES — Continued

DD-50209 Superficial foreign body of face without major open wound but with infection 910.7
(T-D1200) (M-30408) (G-C009) (M-14014) (G-C008) (DE-00050)

DD-50210 Superficial injury of cheek without infection 910.8
(T-D1206) (M-10050) (G-C009) (DE-00050)

DD-50211 Superficial injury of cheek with infection 910.9
(T-D1206) (M-10050) (G-C008) (DE-00050)

DD-50212 Abrasion or friction burn of cheek without infection 910.0
(T-D1206) (M-14700) (M-14710) (G-C009) (DE-00050)

DD-50213 Abrasion or friction burn of cheek with infection 910.1
(T-D1206) (M-14700) (M-14720) (G-C008) (DE-00050)

DD-50214 Blister of cheek without infection 910.2
(T-D1206) (M-14720) (G-C009) (DE-00050)

DD-50215 Blister of cheek with infection 910.3
(T-D1206) (M-14720) (G-C008) (DE-00050)

DD-50216 Nonvenomous insect bite of cheek without infection 910.4
(T-D1206) (M-14368) (G-C009) (DE-00050)

DD-50217 Nonvenomous insect bite of cheek with infection 910.5
(T-D1206) (M-14368) (G-C008) (DE-00050)

DD-50218 Superficial foreign body of cheek without major open wound and without infection 910.6
(T-D1206) (M-30408) (G-C009) (M-14014) (DE-00050)

DD-50219 Superficial foreign body of cheek without major open wound but with infection 910.7
(T-D1206) (M-30408) (G-C009) (M-14014) (G-C008) (DE-00050)

DD-50220 Superficial injury of ear without infection 910.8
(T-AB100) (M-10050) (G-C009) (DE-00050)

DD-50221 Superficial injury of ear with infection 910.9
(T-AB100) (M-10050) (G-C008) (DE-00050)

DD-50222 Abrasion or friction burn of ear without infection 910.0
(T-AB100) (M-14700) (M-14710) (G-C009) (DE-00050)

DD-50223 Abrasion or friction burn of ear with infection 910.1
(T-AB100) (M-14700) (M-14710) (G-C008) (DE-00050)

DD-50224 Blister of ear without infection 910.2
(T-AB100) (M-14720) (G-C009) (DE-00050)

DD-50225 Blister of ear with infection 910.3
(T-AB100) (M-14720) (G-C008) (DE-00050)

DD-50226 Nonvenomous insect bite of ear without infection 910.4
(T-AB100) (M-14368) (G-C009) (DE-00050)

DD-50227 Nonvenomous insect bite of ear with infection 910.5
(T-AB100) (M-14368) (G-C008) (DE-00050)

DD-50228 Superficial foreign body of ear without major open wound and without infection 910.6
(T-AB100) (M-30408) (G-C009) (M-14014) (DE-00050)

DD-50229 Superficial foreign body of ear without major open wound but with infection 910.7
(T-AB100) (M-30408) (G-C009) (M-14014) (G-C008) (DE-00050)

DD-50230 Superficial injury of gum without infection 910.8
(T-54910) (M-10050) (G-C009) (DE-00050)

DD-50231 Superficial injury of gum with infection 910.9
(T-54910) (M-10050) (G-C008) (DE-00050)

DD-50232 Abrasion or friction burn of gum without infection 910.0
(T-54910) (M-14700) (M-14710) (G-C009) (DE-00050)

DD-50233 Abrasion or friction burn of gum with infection 910.1
(T-54910) (M-14700) (M-14710) (G-C008) (DE-00050)

DD-50234 Blister of gum without infection 910.2
(T-54910) (M-14720) (G-C009) (DE-00050)

DD-50235 Blister of gum with infection 910.3
(T-54910) (M-14720) (G-C008) (DE-00050)

DD-50236 Nonvenomous insect bite of gum without infection 910.4
(T-54910) (M-14368) (G-C009) (DE-00050)

DD-50237 Nonvenomous insect bite of gum with infection 910.5
(T-54910) (M-14368) (G-C008) (DE-00050)

DD-50238 Superficial foreign body of gum without major open wound and without infection 910.6
(T-54910) (M-30408) (G-C009) (M-14014) (DE-00050)

DD-50239 Superficial foreign body of gum without major open wound but with infection 910.7
(T-54910) (M-30408) (G-C009) (M-14014) (G-C008) (DE-00050)

DD-50240 Superficial injury of lip without infection 910.8
(T-52000) (M-10050) (G-C009) (DE-00050)

DD-50241 Superficial injury of lip with infection 910.9
(T-52000) (M-10050) (G-C008) (DE-00050)

DD-50242 Abrasion or friction burn of lip without infection 910.0
(T-52000) (M-14700) (M-14710) (G-C009) (DE-00050)

DD-50243 Abrasion or friction burn of lip with infection 910.1
(T-52000) (M-14700) (M-14710) (G-C008) (DE-00050)

DD-50244 Blister of lip without infection 910.2
(T-52000) (M-14720) (G-C009) (DE-00050)

DD-50245 Blister of lip with infection 910.3
(T-52000) (M-14720) (G-C008) (DE-00050)

DD-50246 Nonvenomous insect bite of lip without infection 910.4
(T-52000) (M-14368) (G-C009) (DE-00050)

DD-50247 Nonvenomous insect bite of lip with infection 910.5
(T-52000) (M-14368) (G-C008) (DE-00050)

DD-50248 Superficial foreign body of lip without major open wound and without infection 910.6
(T-52000) (M-30408) (G-C009) (M-14014) (DE-00050)

DD-50249 Superficial foreign body of lip without major open wound but with infection 910.7
(T-52000) (M-30408) (G-C009) (M-14014) (G-C008) (DE-00050)

DD-50250 Superficial injury of nose without infection 910.8
(T-21000) (M-10050) (G-C009) (DE-00050)

DD-50251 Superficial injury of nose with infection 910.9
(T-21000) (M-10050) (G-C008) (DE-00050)

DD-50252 Abrasion or friction burn of nose without infection 910.0
(T-21000) (M-14700) (M-14710) (G-C009) (DE-00050)

DD-50253 Abrasion or friction burn of nose with infection 910.1
(T-21000) (M-14700) (M-14710) (G-C008) (DE-00050)

DD-50254 Blister of nose without infection 910.2
(T-21000) (M-14720) (G-C009) (DE-00050)

DD-50255 Blister of nose with infection 910.3
(T-21000) (M-14720) (G-C008) (DE-00050)

DD-50256 Nonvenomous insect bite of nose without infection 910.4
(T-21000) (M-14368) (G-C009) (DE-00050)

DD-50257 Nonvenomous insect bite of nose with infection 910.5
(T-21000) (M-14368) (G-C008) (DE-00050)

DD-50258 Superficial foreign body of nose without major open wound and without infection 910.6
(T-21000) (M-30408) (G-C009) (M-14014) (DE-00050)

DD-50259 Superficial foreign body of nose without major open wound but with infection 910.7
(T-21000) (M-30408) (G-C009) (M-14014) (G-C008) (DE-00050)

DD-50260 Superficial injury of neck without infection 910.8
(T-D1600) (M-10050) (G-C009) (DE-00050)

DD-50261 Superficial injury of neck with infection 910.9
(T-D1600) (M-10050) (G-C008) (DE-00050)

DD-50262 Abrasion or friction burn of neck without infection 910.0
(T-D1600) (M-14700) (M-14710) (G-C009) (DE-00050)

DD-50263 Abrasion or friction burn of neck with infection 910.1
(T-D1600) (M-14700) (M-14710) (G-C008) (DE-00050)

DD-50264 Blister of neck without infection 910.2
(T-D1600) (M-14720) (G-C009) (DE-00050)

DD-50265 Blister of neck with infection 910.3
(T-D1600) (M-14720) (G-C008) (DE-00050)

DD-50266 Nonvenomous insect bite of neck without infection 910.4
(T-D1600) (M-14368) (G-C009) (DE-00050)

DD-50267 Nonvenomous insect bite of neck with infection 910.5
(T-D1600) (M-14368) (G-C008) (DE-00050)

DD-50268 Superficial foreign body of neck without major open wound and without infection 910.6
(T-D1600) (M-30408) (G-C009) (M-14014) (DE-00050)

DD-50269 Superficial foreign body of neck without major open wound but with infection 910.7
(T-D1600) (M-30408) (G-C009) (M-14014) (G-C008) (DE-00050)

DD-50280 Superficial injury of scalp without infection 910.8
(T-D1160) (M-10050) (G-C009) (DE-00050)

D-50 SUPERFICIAL INJURIES — Continued

DD-50281 Superficial injury of scalp with infection 910.9
(T-D1160) (M-10050) (G-C008) (DE-00050)

DD-50282 Abrasion or friction burn of scalp without infection 910.0
(T-D1160) (M-14700) (M-14710) (G-C009) (DE-00050)

DD-50283 Abrasion or friction burn of scalp with infection 910.1
(T-D1160) (M-14700) (M-14710) (G-C008) (DE-00050)

DD-50284 Blister of scalp without infection 910.2
(T-D1160) (M-14720) (G-C009) (DE-00050)

DD-50285 Blister of scalp with infection 910.3
(T-D1160) (M-14720) (G-C008) (DE-00050)

DD-50286 Nonvenomous insect bite of scalp without infection 910.4
(T-D1160) (M-14368) (G-C009) (DE-00050)

DD-50287 Nonvenomous insect bite of scalp with infection 910.5
(T-D1160) (M-14368) (G-C008) (DE-00050)

DD-50288 Superficial foreign body of scalp without major open wound and without infection 910.6
(T-D1160) (M-30408) (G-C009) (M-14014) (DE-00050)

DD-50289 Superficial foreign body of scalp without major open wound but with infection 910.7
(T-D1160) (M-30408) (G-C009) (M-14014) (G-C008) (DE-00050)

DD-50300 Superficial injury of trunk without infection 911.8
(T-D2000) (M-10050) (G-C009) (DE-00050)

DD-50301 Superficial injury of trunk with infection 911.9
(T-D2000) (M-10050) (G-C008) (DE-00050)

DD-50302 Abrasion or friction burn of trunk without infection 911.0
(T-D2000) (M-14700) (M-14700) (G-C009) (DE-00050)

DD-50303 Abrasion or friction burn of trunk with infection 911.1
(T-D2000) (M-14700) (M-14710) (G-C008) (DE-00050)

DD-50304 Blister of trunk without infection 911.2
(T-D2000) (M-14720) (G-C009) (DE-00050)

DD-50305 Blister of trunk with infection 911.3
(T-D2000) (M-14720) (G-C008) (DE-00050)

DD-50306 Nonvenomous insect bite of trunk without infection 911.4
(T-D2000) (M-14368) (G-C009) (DE-00050)

DD-50307 Nonvenomous insect bite of trunk with infection 911.5
(T-D2000) (M-14368) (G-C008) (DE-00050)

DD-50308 Superficial foreign body of trunk without major open wound and without infection 911.6
(T-D2000) (M-30408) (G-C009) (M-14014) (DE-00050)

DD-50309 Superficial foreign body of trunk without major open wound but with infection 911.7
(T-D2000) (M-30408) (G-C009) (M-14014) (G-C008) (DE-00050)

DD-50310 Superficial injury of abdominal wall without infection 911.8
(T-D4300) (M-10050) (G-C009) (DE-00050)

DD-50311 Superficial injury of abdominal wall with infection 911.9
(T-D4300) (M-10050) (G-C008) (DE-00050)

DD-50312 Abrasion or friction burn of abdominal wall without infection 911.0
(T-D4300) (M-14700) (M-14710) (G-C009) (DE-00050)

DD-50313 Abrasion or friction burn of abdominal wall with infection 911.1
(T-D4300) (M-14700) (M-14710) (G-C008) (DE-00050)

DD-50314 Blister of abdominal wall without infection 911.2
(T-D4300) (M-14720) (G-C009) (DE-00050)

DD-50315 Blister of abdominal wall with infection 911.3
(T-D4300) (M-14720) (G-C008) (DE-00050)

DD-50316 Nonvenomous insect bite of abdominal wall without infection 911.4
(T-D4300) (M-14368) (G-C009) (DE-00050)

DD-50317 Nonvenomous insect bite of abdominal wall with infection 911.5
(T-D4300) (M-14368) (G-C008) (DE-00050)

DD-50318 Superficial foreign body of abdominal wall without major open wound and without infection 911.6
(T-D4300) (M-30408) (G-C009) (M-14014) (DE-00050)

DD-50319 Superficial foreign body of abdominal wall without major open wound but with infection 911.7
(T-D4300) (M-30408) (G-C009) (M-14014) (G-C008) (DE-00050)

DD-50320 Superficial injury of back without infection 911.8
(T-D2100) (M-10050) (G-C009) (DE-00050)

DD-50321 Superficial injury of back with infection 911.9
(T-D2100) (M-10050) (G-C008) (DE-00050)

DD-50322 Abrasion or friction burn of back without infection 911.0
(T-D2100) (M-14700) (M-14710) (G-C009) (DE-00050)

DD-50323 Abrasion or friction burn of back with infection 911.1
(T-D2100) (M-14700) (M-14710) (G-C008) (DE-00050)

DD-50324 Blister of back without infection 911.2
(T-D2100) (M-14720) (G-C009) (DE-00050)

DD-50325 Blister of back with infection 911.3
(T-D2100) (M-14720) (G-C008) (DE-00050)

DD-50326 Nonvenomous insect bite of back without infection 911.4
(T-D2100) (M-14368) (G-C009) (DE-00050)

DD-50327 Nonvenomous insect bite of back with infection 911.5
(T-D2100) (M-14368) (G-C008) (DE-00050)

DD-50328 Superficial foreign body of back without major open wound and without infection 911.6
(T-D2100) (M-30408) (G-C009) (M-14014) (DE-00050)

DD-50329 Superficial foreign body of back without major open wound but with infection 911.7
(T-D2100) (M-30408) (G-C009) (M-14014) (G-C008) (DE-00050)

DD-50330 Superficial injury of breast without infection 911.8
(T-04000) (M-10050) (G-C009) (DE-00050)

DD-50331 Superficial injury of breast with infection 911.9
(T-04000) (M-10050) (G-C008) (DE-00050)

DD-50332 Abrasion or friction burn of breast without infection 911.0
(T-04000) (M-14700) (M-14710) (G-C009) (DE-00050)

DD-50333 Abrasion or friction burn of breast with infection 911.1
(T-04000) (M-14700) (M-14710) (G-C008) (DE-00050)

DD-50334 Blister of breast without infection 911.2
(T-04000) (M-14720) (G-C009) (DE-00050)

DD-50335 Blister of breast with infection 911.3
(T-04000) (M-14720) (G-C008) (DE-00050)

DD-50336 Nonvenomous insect bite of breast without infection 911.4
(T-04000) (M-14368) (G-C009) (DE-00050)

DD-50337 Nonvenomous insect bite of breast with infection 911.5
(T-04000) (M-14368) (G-C008) (DE-00050)

DD-50338 Superficial foreign body of breast without major open wound and without infection 911.6
(T-04000) (M-30408) (G-C009) (M-14014) (DE-00050)

DD-50339 Superficial foreign body of breast without major open wound but with infection 911.7
(T-04000) (M-30408) (G-C009) (M-14014) (G-C008) (DE-00050)

DD-50340 Superficial injury of buttock without infection 911.8
(T-D2600) (M-10050) (G-C009) (DE-00050)

DD-50341 Superficial injury of buttock with infection 911.9
(T-D2600) (M-10050) (G-C008) (DE-00050)

DD-50342 Abrasion or friction burn of buttock without infection 911.0
(T-D2600) (M-14700) (M-14710) (G-C009) (DE-00050)

DD-50343 Abrasion or friction burn of buttock with infection 911.1
(T-D2600) (M-14700) (M-14710) (G-C008) (DE-00050)

DD-50344 Blister of buttock without infection 911.2
(T-D2600) (M-14720) (G-C009) (DE-00050)

DD-50345 Blister of buttock with infection 911.3
(T-D2600) (M-14720) (G-C008) (DE-00050)

DD-50346 Nonvenomous insect bite of buttock without infection 911.4
(T-D2600) (M-14368) (G-C009) (DE-00050)

DD-50347 Nonvenomous insect bite of buttock with infection 911.5
(T-D2600) (M-14368) (G-C008) (DE-00050)

DD-50348 Superficial foreign body of buttock without major open wound and without infection 911.6
(T-D2600) (M-30408) (G-C009) (M-14014) (DE-00050)

DD-50349 Superficial foreign body of buttock without major open wound but with infection 911.7
(T-D2600) (M-30408) (G-C009) (M-14014) (G-C008) (DE-00050)

D-50 SUPERFICIAL INJURIES — Continued

DD-50350 Superficial injury of anus without infection 911.8
(T-59900) (M-10050) (G-C009) (DE-00050)

DD-50351 Superficial injury of anus with infection 911.9
(T-59900) (M-10050) (G-C008) (DE-00050)

DD-50352 Abrasion or friction burn of anus without infection 911.0
(T-59900) (M-14700) (M-14710) (G-C009) (DE-00050)

DD-50353 Abrasion or friction burn of anus with infection 911.1
(T-59900) (M-14700) (M-14710) (G-C008) (DE-00050)

DD-50354 Blister of anus without infection 911.2
(T-59900) (M-14720) (G-C009) (DE-00050)

DD-50355 Blister of anus with infection 911.3
(T-59900) (M-14720) (G-C008) (DE-00050)

DD-50356 Nonvenomous insect bite of anus without infection 911.4
(T-59900) (M-14368) (G-C009) (DE-00050)

DD-50357 Nonvenomous insect bite of anus with infection 911.5
(T-59900) (M-14368) (G-C008) (DE-00050)

DD-50358 Superficial foreign body of anus without major open wound and without infection 911.6
(T-59900) (M-30408) (G-C009) (M-14014) (DE-00050)

DD-50359 Superficial foreign body of anus without major open wound but with infection 911.7
(T-59900) (M-30408) (G-C009) (M-14014) (G-C008) (DE-00050)

DD-50360 Superficial injury of chest wall without infection 911.8
(T-D3050) (M-10050) (G-C009) (DE-00050)

DD-50361 Superficial injury of chest wall with infection 911.9
(T-D3050) (M-10050) (G-C008) (DE-00050)

DD-50362 Abrasion or friction burn of chest wall without infection 911.0
(T-D3050) (M-14700) (M-14710) (G-C009) (DE-00050)

DD-50363 Abrasion or friction burn of chest wall with infection 911.1
(T-D3050) (M-14700) (M-14710) (G-C008) (DE-00050)

DD-50364 Blister of chest wall without infection 911.2
(T-D3050) (M-14720) (G-C009) (DE-00050)

DD-50365 Blister of chest wall with infection 911.3
(T-D3050) (M-14720) (G-C008) (DE-00050)

DD-50366 Nonvenomous insect bite of chest wall without infection 911.4
(T-D3050) (M-14368) (G-C009) (DE-00050)

DD-50367 Nonvenomous insect bite of chest wall with infection 911.5
(T-D3050) (M-14368) (G-C008) (DE-00050)

DD-50368 Superficial foreign body of chest wall without major open wound and without infection 911.6
(T-D3050) (M-30408) (G-C009) (M-14014) (DE-00050)

DD-50369 Superficial foreign body of chest wall without major open wound but with infection 911.7
(T-D3050) (M-30408) (G-C009) (M-14014) (G-C009) (DE-00050)

DD-50370 Superficial injury of flank without infection 911.8
(T-D2310) (M-10050) (G-C009) (DE-00050)

DD-50371 Superficial injury of flank with infection 911.9
(T-D2310) (M-10050) (G-C008) (DE-00050)

DD-50372 Abrasion or friction burn of flank without infection 911.0
(T-D2310) (M-14700) (M-14710) (G-C009) (DE-00050)

DD-50373 Abrasion or friction burn of flank with infection 911.1
(T-D2310) (M-14700) (M-14710) (G-C008) (DE-00050)

DD-50374 Blister of flank without infection 911.2
(T-D2310) (M-14720) (G-C009) (DE-00050)

DD-50375 Blister of flank with infection 911.3
(T-D2310) (M-14720) (G-C008) (DE-00050)

DD-50376 Nonvenomous insect bite of flank without infection 911.4
(T-D2310) (M-14368) (G-C009) (DE-00050)

DD-50377 Nonvenomous insect bite of flank with infection 911.5
(T-D2310) (M-14368) (G-C008) (DE-00050)

DD-50378 Superficial foreign body of flank without major open wound and without infection 911.6
(T-D2310) (M-30408) (G-C009) (M-14014) (DE-00050)

DD-50379 Superficial foreign body of flank without major open wound but with infection 911.7
(T-D2310) (M-30408) (G-C009) (T-14014) (G-C008) (DE-00050)

DD-50380 Superficial injury of groin without infection 911.8
(T-D7000) (M-10050) (G-C009) (DE-00050)

DD-50381 Superficial injury of groin with infection 911.9
(T-D7000) (M-10050) (G-C008) (DE-00050)

DD-50382 Abrasion or friction burn of groin without infection 911.0
(T-D7000) (M-14700) (M-14710) (G-C009) (DE-00050)

DD-50383 Abrasion or friction burn of groin with infection 911.1
(T-D7000) (M-14700) (M-14710) (G-C008) (DE-00050)

DD-50384 Blister of groin without infection 911.2
(T-D7000) (M-14720) (G-C009) (DE-00050)

DD-50385 Blister of groin with infection 911.3
(T-D7000) (M-14720) (G-C008) (DE-00050)

DD-50386 Nonvenomous insect bite of groin without infection 911.4
(T-D7000) (M-14368) (G-C009) (DE-00050)

DD-50387 Nonvenomous insect bite of groin with infection 911.5
(T-D7000) (M-14368) (G-C008) (DE-00050)

DD-50388 Superficial foreign body of groin without major open wound and without infection 911.6
(T-D7000) (M-30408) (G-C009) (M-14014) (DE-00050)

DD-50389 Superficial foreign body of groin without major open wound but with infection 911.7
(T-D7000) (M-30408) (G-C009) (M-14014) (G-C008) (DE-00050)

DD-50390 Superficial injury of interscapular region without infection 911.8
(T-D2210) (M-10050) (G-C009) (DE-00050)

DD-50391 Superficial injury of interscapular region with infection 911.9
(T-D2210) (M-10050) (G-C008) (DE-00050)

DD-50392 Abrasion or friction burn of interscapular region without infection 911.0
(T-D2210) (M-14700) (M-14710) (G-C009) (DE-00050)

DD-50393 Abrasion or friction burn of interscapular region with infection 911.1
(T-D2210) (M-14700) (M-14710) (G-C008) (DE-00050)

DD-50394 Blister of interscapular region without infection 911.2
(T-D2210) (M-14720) (G-C009) (DE-00050)

DD-50395 Blister of interscapular region with infection 911.3
(T-D2210) (M-14720) (G-C008) (DE-00050)

DD-50396 Nonvenomous insect bite of interscapular region without infection 911.4
(T-D2210) (M-14368) (G-C009) (DE-00050)

DD-50397 Nonvenomous insect bite of interscapular region with infection 911.5
(T-D2210) (M-14368) (G-C008) (DE-00050)

DD-50398 Superficial foreign body of interscapular region without major open wound and without infection 911.6
(T-D2210) (M-30408) (G-C009) (M-14014) (DE-00050)

DD-50399 Superficial foreign body of interscapular region without major open wound but with infection 911.7
(T-D2210) (M-30408) (G-C009) (M-14014) (G-C008) (DE-00050)

DD-50400 Superficial injury of penis without infection 911.8
(T-91000) (M-10050) (G-C009) (DE-00050)

DD-50401 Superficial injury of penis with infection 911.9
(T-91000) (M-10050) (G-C008) (DE-00050)

DD-50402 Abrasion or friction burn of penis without infection 911.0
(T-91000) (M-14700) (M-14710) (G-C009) (DE-00050)

DD-50403 Abrasion or friction burn of penis with infection 911.1
(T-91000) (M-14700) (M-14710) (G-C008) (DE-00050)

DD-50404 Blister of penis without infection 911.2
(T-91000) (M-14720) (G-C009) (DE-00050)

DD-50405 Blister of penis with infection 911.3
(T-91000) (M-14720) (G-C008) (DE-00050)

DD-50406 Nonvenomous insect bite of penis without infection 911.4
(T-91000) (M-14368) (G-C009) (DE-00050)

DD-50407 Nonvenomous insect bite of penis with infection 911.5
(T-91000) (M-14368) (G-C008) (DE-00050)

DD-50408 Superficial foreign body of penis without major open wound and without infection 911.6
(T-91000) (M-30408) (G-C009) (M-14014) (DE-00050)

D-50 SUPERFICIAL INJURIES — Continued

DD-50409 Superficial foreign body of penis without major open wound but with infection 911.7
(T-91000) (M-30408) (G-C009) (M-14014) (G-C008) (DE-00050)

DD-50410 Superficial injury of scrotum without infection 911.8
(T-98000) (M-10050) (G-C009) (DE-00050)

DD-50411 Superficial injury of scrotum with infection 911.9
(T-98000) (M-10050) (G-C008) (DE-00050)

DD-50412 Abrasion or friction burn of scrotum without infection 911.0
(T-98000) (M-14700) (M-14710) (G-C009) (DE-00050)

DD-50413 Abrasion or friction burn of scrotum with infection 911.1
(T-98000) (M-14700) (M-14710) (G-C008) (DE-00050)

DD-50414 Blister of scrotum without infection 911.2
(T-98000) (M-14720) (G-C009) (DE-00050)

DD-50415 Blister of scrotum with infection 911.3
(T-98000) (M-14720) (G-C008) (DE-00050)

DD-50416 Nonvenomous insect bite of scrotum without infection 911.4
(T-98000) (M-14368) (G-C009) (DE-00050)

DD-50417 Nonvenomous insect bite of scrotum with infection 911.5
(T-98000) (M-14368) (G-C008) (DE-00050)

DD-50418 Superficial foreign body of scrotum without major open wound and without infection 911.6
(T-98000) (M-30408) (G-C009) (M-14014) (DE-00050)

DD-50419 Superficial foreign body of scrotum without major open wound but with infection 911.7
(T-98000) (M-30408) (G-C009) (M-14014) (G-C008) (DE-00050)

DD-50420 Superficial injury of testis without infection 911.8
(T-94000) (M-10050) (G-C009) (DE-00050)

DD-50421 Superficial injury of testis with infection 911.9
(T-94000) (M-10050) (G-C008) (DE-00050)

DD-50422 Abrasion or friction burn of testis without infection 911.0
(T-94000) (M-14700) (M-14710) (G-C009) (DE-00050)

DD-50423 Abrasion or friction burn of testis with infection 911.1
(T-94000) (M-14700) (M-14710) (G-C008) (DE-00050)

DD-50424 Blister of testis without infection 911.2
(T-94000) (M-14720) (G-C009) (DE-00050)

DD-50425 Blister of testis with infection 911.3
(T-94000) (M-14720) (G-C008) (DE-00050)

DD-50426 Nonvenomous insect bite of testis without infection 911.4
(T-94000) (M-14368) (G-C009) (DE-00050)

DD-50427 Nonvenomous insect bite of testis with infection 911.5
(T-94000) (M-14368) (G-C008) (DE-00050)

DD-50428 Superficial foreign body of testis without major open wound and without infection 911.6
(T-94000) (M-30408) (G-C009) (M-14014) (DE-00050)

DD-50429 Superficial foreign body of testis without major open wound but with infection 911.7
(T-94000) (M-30408) (G-C009) (M-14014) (G-C008) (DE-00050)

DD-50430 Superficial injury of vulva without infection 911.8
(T-81000) (M-10050) (G-C009) (DE-00050)

DD-50431 Superficial injury of vulva with infection 911.9
(T-81000) (M-10050) (G-C008) (DE-00050)

DD-50432 Abrasion or friction burn of vulva without infection 911.0
(T-81000) (M-14700) (M-14710) (G-C009) (DE-00050)

DD-50433 Abrasion or friction burn of vulva with infection 911.1
(T-81000) (M-14700) (M-14710) (G-C008) (DE-00050)

DD-50434 Blister of vulva without infection 911.2
(T-81000) (M-14720) (G-C009) (DE-00050)

DD-50435 Blister of vulva with infection 911.3
(T-81000) (M-14720) (G-C008) (DE-00050)

DD-50436 Nonvenomous insect bite of vulva without infection 911.4
(T-81000) (M-14368) (G-C009) (DE-00050)

DD-50437 Nonvenomous insect bite of vulva with infection 911.5
(T-81000) (M-14368) (G-C008) (DE-00050)

DD-50438 Superficial foreign body of vulva without major open wound and without infection 911.6
(T-81000) (M-30408) (G-C009) (M-14014) (DE-00050)

DD-50439 Superficial foreign body of vulva without major open wound but with infection 911.7
(T-81000) (M-30408) (G-C009) (M-14014) (G-C008) (DE-00050)

DD-50440 Superficial injury of vagina without infection 911.8
(T-82000) (M-10050) (G-C009) (DE-00050)

DD-50441 Superficial injury of vagina with infection 911.9
(T-82000) (M-10050) (G-C008) (DE-00050)

DD-50442 Abrasion or friction burn of vagina without infection 911.0
(T-82000) (M-14700) (M-14710) (G-C009) (DE-00050)

DD-50443 Abrasion or friction burn of vagina with infection 911.1
(T-82000) (M-14700) (M-14710) (G-C008) (DE-00050)

DD-50444 Blister of vagina without infection 911.2
(T-82000) (M-14720) (G-C009) (DE-00050)

DD-50445 Blister of vagina with infection 911.3
(T-82000) (M-14720) (G-C008) (DE-00050)

DD-50446 Nonvenomous insect bite of vagina without infection 911.4
(T-82000) (M-14368) (G-C009) (DE-00050)

DD-50447 Nonvenomous insect bite of vagina with infection 911.5
(T-82000) (M-14368) (G-C008) (DE-00050)

DD-50448 Superficial foreign body of vagina without major open wound and without infection 911.6
(T-82000) (M-30408) (G-C009) (M-14014) (DE-00050)

DD-50449 Superficial foreign body of vagina without major open wound but with infection 911.7
(T-82000) (M-30408) (G-C009) (M-14014) (G-C008) (DE-00050)

DD-50450 Superficial injury of perineum without infection 911.8
(T-D2700) (M-10050) (G-C009) (DE-00050)

DD-50451 Superficial injury of perineum with infection 911.9
(T-D2700) (M-10050) (G-C008) (DE-00050)

DD-50452 Abrasion or friction burn of perineum without infection 911.0
(T-D2700) (M-14700) (M-14710) (G-C009) (DE-00050)

DD-50453 Abrasion or friction burn of perineum with infection 911.1
(T-D2700) (M-14700) (M-14710) (G-C008) (DE-00050)

DD-50454 Blister of perineum without infection 911.2
(T-D2700) (M-14720) (G-C009) (DE-00050)

DD-50455 Blister of perineum with infection 911.3
(T-D2700) (M-14720) (G-C008) (DE-00050)

DD-50456 Nonvenomous insect bite of perineum without infection 911.4
(T-D2700) (M-14368) (G-C009) (DE-00050)

DD-50457 Nonvenomous insect bite of perineum with infection 911.5
(T-D2700) (M-14368) (G-C008) (DE-00050)

DD-50458 Superficial foreign body of perineum without major open wound and without infection 911.6
(T-D2700) (M-30408) (G-C009) (M-14014) (DE-00050)

DD-50459 Superficial foreign body of perineum without major open wound but with infection 911.7
(T-D2700) (M-30408) (G-C009) (M-14014) (G-C008) (DE-00050)

DD-50500 Superficial injury of shoulder without infection 912.8
(T-D2220) (M-10050) (G-C009) (DE-00050)

DD-50501 Superficial injury of shoulder with infection 912.9
(T-D2220) (M-10050) (G-C008) (DE-00050)

DD-50502 Abrasion or friction burn of shoulder without infection 912.0
(T-D2220) (M-14700) (M-14710) (G-C009) (DE-00050)

DD-50503 Abrasion or friction burn of shoulder with infection 912.1
(T-D2220) (M-14700) (M-14710) (G-C008) (DE-00050)

DD-50504 Blister of shoulder without infection 912.2
(T-D2220) (M-14720) (G-C009) (DE-00050)

DD-50505 Blister of shoulder with infection 912.3
(T-D2220) (M-14720) (G-C008) (DE-00050)

DD-50506 Nonvenomous insect bite of shoulder without infection 912.4
(T-D2220) (M-14368) (G-C009) (DE-00050)

DD-50507 Nonvenomous insect bite of shoulder with infection 912.5
(T-D2220) (M-14368) (G-C008) (DE-00050)

DD-50508 Superficial foreign body of shoulder without major open wound and without infection 912.6
(T-D2220) (M-30408) (G-C009) (M-14014) (DE-00050)

D-50 SUPERFICIAL INJURIES — Continued

DD-50509 Superficial foreign body of shoulder without major open wound but with infection 912.7
(T-D2220) (M-30408) (G-C009) (M-14014) (G-C008) (DE-00050)

DD-50510 Superficial injury of axilla without infection 912.8
(T-D8100) (M-10050) (G-C009) (DE-00050)

DD-50511 Superficial injury of axilla with infection 912.9
(T-D8100) (M-10050) (G-C008) (DE-00050)

DD-50512 Abrasion or friction burn of axilla without infection 912.0
(T-D8100) (M-14700) (M-14710) (G-C009) (DE-00050)

DD-50513 Abrasion or friction burn of axilla with infection 912.1
(T-D8100) (M-14700) (M-14710) (G-C008) (DE-00050)

DD-50514 Blister of axilla without infection 912.2
(T-D8100) (M-14720) (G-C009) (DE-00050)

DD-50515 Blister of axilla with infection 912.3
(T-D8100) (M-14720) (G-C008) (DE-00050)

DD-50516 Nonvenomous insect bite of axilla without infection 912.4
(T-D8100) (M-14368) (G-C009) (DE-00050)

DD-50517 Nonvenomous insect bite of axilla with infection 912.5
(T-D8100) (M-14368) (G-C008) (DE-00050)

DD-50518 Superficial foreign body of axilla without major open wound and without infection 912.6
(T-D8100) (M-30408) (G-C009) (M-14014) (DE-00050)

DD-50519 Superficial foreign body of axilla without major open wound but with infection 912.7
(T-D8100) (M-30408) (G-C009) (M-14014) (G-C008) (DE-00050)

DD-50520 Superficial injury of scapular region without infection 912.8
(T-D2200) (M-10050) (G-C009) (DE-00050)

DD-50521 Superficial injury of scapular region with infection 912.9
(T-D2200) (M-10050) (G-C008) (DE-00050)

DD-50522 Abrasion or friction burn of scapular region without infection 912.0
(T-D2200) (M-14700) (M-14710) (G-C009) (DE-00050)

DD-50523 Abrasion or friction burn of scapular region with infection 912.1
(T-D2200) (M-14700) (M-14710) (G-C008) (DE-00050)

DD-50524 Blister of scapular region without infection 912.2
(T-D2200) (M-14720) (G-C009) (DE-00050)

DD-50525 Blister of scapular region with infection 912.3
(T-D2200) (M-14720) (G-C008) (DE-00050)

DD-50526 Nonvenomous insect bite of scapular region without infection 912.4
(T-D2200) (M-14368) (G-C009) (DE-00050)

DD-50527 Nonvenomous insect bite of scapular region with infection 912.5
(T-D2200) (M-14368) (G-C008) (DE-00050)

DD-50528 Superficial foreign body of scapular region without major open wound and without infection 912.6
(T-D2200) (M-30408) (G-C009) (M-14014) (DE-00050)

DD-50529 Superficial foreign body of scapular region without major open wound but with infection 912.7
(T-D2200) (M-30408) (G-C009) (M-14014) (G-C008) (DE-00050)

DD-50530 Superficial injury of upper arm without infection 912.8
(T-D8200) (M-10050) (G-C009) (DE-00050)

DD-50531 Superficial injury of upper arm with infection 912.9
(T-D8200) (M-10050) (G-C008) (DE-00050)

DD-50532 Abrasion or friction burn of upper arm without infection 912.0
(T-D8200) (M-14700) (M-14710) (G-C009) (DE-00050)

DD-50533 Abrasion or friction burn of upper arm with infection 912.1
(T-D8200) (M-14700) (M-14710) (G-C008) (DE-00050)

DD-50534 Blister of upper arm without infection 912.2
(T-D8200) (M-14720) (G-C009) (DE-00050)

DD-50535 Blister of upper arm with infection 912.3
(T-D8200) (M-14720) (G-C008) (DE-00050)

DD-50536 Nonvenomous insect bite of upper arm without infection 912.4
(T-D8200) (M-14368) (G-C009) (DE-00050)

DD-50537 Nonvenomous insect bite of upper arm with infection 912.5
(T-D8200) (M-14368) (G-C008) (DE-00050)

DD-50538 Superficial foreign body of upper arm without major open wound and without infection 912.6
(T-D8200) (M-30408) (G-C009) (M-14014) (DE-00050)

DD-50539 Superficial foreign body of upper arm without major open wound but with infection 912.7
(T-D8200) (M-30408) (G-C009) (M-14014) (G-C008) (DE-00050)

DD-50540 Superficial injury of elbow without infection 913.8
(T-D8300) (M-10050) (G-C009) (DE-00050)

DD-50541 Superficial injury of elbow with infection 913.9
(T-D8300) (M-10050) (G-C008) (DE-00050)

DD-50542 Abrasion or friction burn of elbow without infection 913.0
(T-D8300) (M-14700) (M-14710) (G-C009) (DE-00050)

DD-50543 Abrasion or friction burn of elbow with infection 913.1
(T-D8300) (M-14700) (M-14710) (G-C008) (DE-00050)

DD-50544 Blister of elbow without infection 913.2
(T-D8300) (M-14720) (G-C009) (DE-00050)

DD-50545 Blister of elbow with infection 913.3
(T-D8300) (M-14720) (G-C008) (DE-00050)

DD-50546 Nonvenomous insect bite of elbow without infection 913.4
(T-D8300) (M-14368) (G-C009) (DE-00050)

DD-50547 Nonvenomous insect bite of elbow with infection 913.5
(T-D8300) (M-14368) (G-C008) (DE-00050)

DD-50548 Superficial foreign body of elbow without major open wound and without infection 913.6
(T-D8300) (M-30408) (G-C009) (M-14014) (DE-00050)

DD-50549 Superficial foreign body of elbow without major open wound but infection 913.7
(T-D8300) (M-30408) (G-C009) (M-14014) (G-C008) (DE-00050)

DD-50550 Superficial injury of forearm without infection 913.8
(T-D8500) (M-10050) (G-C009) (DE-00050)

DD-50551 Superficial injury of forearm with infection 913.9
(T-D8500) (M-10050) (G-C008) (DE-00050)

DD-50552 Abrasion or friction burn of forearm without infection 913.0
(T-D8500) (M-14700) (M-14710) (G-C009) (DE-00050)

DD-50553 Abrasion or friction burn of forearm with infection 913.1
(T-D8500) (M-14700) (M-14710) (G-C008) (DE-00050)

DD-50554 Blister of forearm without infection 913.2
(T-D8500) (M-14720) (G-C009) (DE-00050)

DD-50555 Blister of forearm with infection 913.3
(T-D8500) (M-14720) (G-C008) (DE-00050)

DD-50556 Nonvenomous insect bite of forearm without infection 913.4
(T-D8500) (M-14368) (G-C009) (DE-00050)

DD-50557 Nonvenomous insect bite of forearm with infection 913.5
(T-D8500) (M-14368) (G-C008) (DE-00050)

DD-50558 Superficial foreign body of forearm without major open wound and without infection 913.6
(T-D8500) (M-30408) (G-C009) (M-14014) (DE-00050)

DD-50559 Superficial foreign body of forearm without major open wound but with infection 913.7
(T-D8500) (M-30408) (G-C009) (M-14014) (G-C008) (DE-00050)

DD-50560 Superficial injury of wrist without infection 913.8
(T-D8600) (M-10050) (G-C009) (DE-00050)

DD-50561 Superficial injury of wrist with infection 913.9
(T-D8600) (M-10050) (G-C008) (DE-00050)

DD-50562 Abrasion or friction burn of wrist without infection 913.0
(T-D8600) (M-14700) (M-14710) (G-C009) (DE-00050)

DD-50563 Abrasion or friction burn of wrist with infection 913.1
(T-D8600) (M-14700) (M-14710) (G-C008) (DE-00050)

DD-50564 Blister of wrist without infection 913.2
(T-D8600) (M-14720) (G-C009) (DE-00050)

DD-50565 Blister of wrist with infection 913.3
(T-D8600) (M-14720) (G-C008) (DE-00050)

DD-50566 Nonvenomous insect bite of wrist without infection 913.4
(T-D8600) (M-14368) (G-C009) (DE-00050)

DD-50567 Nonvenomous insect bite of wrist with infection 913.5
(T-D8600) (M-14368) (G-C008) (DE-00050)

DD-50568 Superficial foreign body of wrist without major open wound and without infection 913.6
(T-D8600) (M-30408) (G-C009) (M-14014) (DE-00050)

D-50 SUPERFICIAL INJURIES — Continued

DD-50569 Superficial foreign body of wrist without major open wound but with infection 913.7
(T-D8600) (M-30408) (G-C009) (M-14014) (G-C008) (DE-00050)

DD-50570 Superficial injury of hand without infection 914.8
(T-D8700) (M-10050) (G-C009) (DE-00050)

DD-50571 Superficial injury of hand with infection 913.9
(T-D8700) (M-10050) (G-C008) (DE-00050)

DD-50572 Abrasion or friction burn of hand without infection 914.0
(T-D8700) (M-14700) (M-14710) (G-C009) (DE-00050)

DD-50573 Abrasion or friction burn of hand with infection 914.1
(T-D8700) (M-14700) (M-14710) (G-C008) (DE-00050)

DD-50574 Blister of hand without infection 914.2
(T-D8700) (M-14720) (G-C009) (DE-00050)

DD-50575 Blister of hand with infection 914.3
(T-D8700) (M-14720) (G-C008) (DE-00050)

DD-50576 Nonvenomous insect bite of hand without infection 914.4
(T-D8700) (M-14368) (G-C009) (DE-00050)

DD-50577 Nonvenomous insect bite of hand with infection 914.5
(T-D8700) (M-14368) (G-C008) (DE-00050)

DD-50578 Superficial foreign body of hand without major open wound and without infection 914.6
(T-D8700) (M-30408) (G-C009) (M-14014) (DE-00050)

DD-50579 Superficial foreign body of hand without major open wound but with infection 914.7
(T-D8700) (M-30408) (G-C009) (M-14014) (G-C008) (DE-00050)

DD-50580 Superficial injury of finger without infection 915.8
(T-D8800) (M-10050) (G-C009) (DE-00050)

DD-50581 Superficial injury of finger with infection 915.9
(T-D8800) (M-10050) (G-C008) (DE-00050)

DD-50582 Abrasion or friction burn of finger without infection 915.0
(T-D8800) (M-14700) (M-14710) (G-C009) (DE-00050)

DD-50583 Abrasion or friction burn of finger with infection 915.1
(T-D8800) (M-14700) (M-14710) (G-C008) (DE-00050)

DD-50584 Blister of finger without infection 915.2
(T-D8800) (M-14720) (G-C009) (DE-00050)

DD-50585 Blister of finger with infection 915.3
(T-D8800) (M-14720) (G-C008) (DE-00050)

DD-50586 Nonvenomous insect bite of finger without infection 915.4
(T-D8800) (M-14368) (G-C009) (DE-00050)

DD-50587 Nonvenomous insect bite of finger with infection 915.5
(T-D8800) (M-14368) (G-C008) (DE-00050)

DD-50588 Superficial foreign body of finger without major open wound and without infection 915.6
(T-D8800) (M-30408) (G-C009) (M-14014) (DE-00050)

DD-50589 Superficial foreign body of finger without major open wound but with infection 915.7
(T-D8800) (M-30408) (G-C009) (M-14014) (G-C008) (DE-00050)

DD-50600 Superficial injury of hip without infection 916.8
(T-D2500) (M-10050) (G-C009) (DE-00050)

DD-50601 Superficial injury of hip with infection 916.9
(T-D2500) (M-10050) (G-C008) (DE-00050)

DD-50602 Abrasion or friction burn of hip without infection 916.0
(T-D2500) (M-14700) (M-14710) (G-C009) (DE-00050)

DD-50603 Abrasion or friction burn of hip with infection 916.1
(T-D2500) (M-14700) (M-14710) (G-C008) (DE-00050)

DD-50604 Blister of hip without infection 916.2
(T-D2500) (M-14720) (G-C009) (DE-00050)

DD-50605 Blister of hip with infection 916.3
(T-D2500) (M-14720) (G-C008) (DE-00050)

DD-50606 Nonvenomous insect bite of hip without infection 916.4
(T-D2500) (M-14368) (G-C009) (DE-00050)

DD-50607 Nonvenomous insect bite of hip with infection 916.5
(T-D2500) (M-14368) (G-C008) (DE-00050)

DD-50608 Superficial foreign body of hip without major open wound and without infection 916.6
(T-D2500) (M-30408) (G-C009) (M-14014) (DE-00050)

DD-50609 Superficial foreign body of hip without major open wound but with infection 916.7
(T-D2500) (M-30408) (G-C009) (M-14010) (G-C008) (DE-00050)

DD-50610 Superficial injury of thigh without infection 916.8
(T-D9100) (M-10050) (G-C009) (DE-00050)

DD-50611 Superficial injury of thigh with infection 916.9
(T-D9100) (M-10050) (G-C008) (DE-00050)

DD-50612 Abrasion or friction burn of thigh without infection 916.0
(T-D9100) (M-14700) (M-14710) (G-C009) (DE-00050)

DD-50613 Abrasion or friction burn of thigh with infection 916.1
(T-D9100) (M-14700) (M-14710) (G-C008) (DE-00050)

DD-50614 Blister of thigh without infection 916.2
(T-D9100) (M-14720) (G-C009) (DE-00050)

DD-50615 Blister of thigh with infection 916.3
(T-D9100) (M-14720) (G-C008) (DE-00050)

DD-50616 Nonvenomous insect bite of thigh without infection 916.4
(T-D9100) (M-14368) (G-C009) (DE-00050)

DD-50617 Nonvenomous insect bite of thigh with infection 916.5
(T-D9100) (M-14368) (G-C008) (DE-00050)

DD-50618 Superficial foreign body of thigh without major open wound and without infection 916.7
(T-D9100) (M-30408) (G-C009) (M-14014) (DE-00050)

DD-50619 Superficial foreign body of thigh without major open wound but with infection 916.7
(T-D9100) (M-40308) (G-C009) (M-14014) (G-C008) (DE-00050)

DD-50620 Superficial injury of leg without infection 916.8
(T-D9400) (M-10050) (G-C009) (DE-00050)

DD-50621 Superficial injury of leg with infection 916.9
(T-D9400) (M-10050) (G-C008) (DE-00050)

DD-50622 Abrasion or friction burn of leg without infection 916.0
(T-D9400) (M-14700) (M-14710) (G-C009) (DE-00050)

DD-50623 Abrasion or friction burn of leg with infection 916.1
(T-D9400) (M-14700) (M-14710) (G-C008) (DE-00050)

DD-50624 Blister of leg without infection 916.2
(T-D9400) (M-14720) (G-C009) (DE-00050)

DD-50625 Blister of leg with infection 916.3
(T-D9400) (M-14720) (G-C008) (DE-00050)

DD-50626 Nonvenomous insect bite of leg without infection 916.4
(T-D9400) (M-14368) (G-C009) (DE-00050)

DD-50627 Nonvenomous insect bite of leg with infection 916.5
(T-D9400) (M-14368) (G-C008) (DE-00050)

DD-50628 Superficial foreign body of leg without major open wound and without infection 916.6
(T-D9400) (M-30408) (G-C009) (M-14014) (DE-00050)

DD-50629 Superficial foreign body of leg without major open wound but with infection 916.7
(T-D9400) (M-30408) (G-C009) (M-14014) (G-C008) (DE-00050)

DD-50630 Superficial injury of ankle without infection 916.8
(T-D9500) (M-10050) (G-C009) (DE-00050)

DD-50631 Superficial injury of ankle with infection 916.9
(T-D9500) (M-10050) (G-C008) (DE-00050)

DD-50632 Abrasion or friction burn of ankle without infection 916.0
(T-D9500) (M-14700) (M-14710) (G-C009) (DE-00050)

DD-50633 Abrasion or friction burn of ankle with infection 916.1
(T-D9500) (M-14700) (M-14710) (G-C008) (DE-00050)

DD-50634 Blister of ankle without infection 916.2
(T-D9500) (M-14720) (G-C009) (DE-00050)

DD-50635 Blister of ankle with infection 916.3
(T-D9500) (M-14720) (G-C008) (DE-00050)

DD-50636 Nonvenomous insect bite of ankle without infection 916.4
(T-D9500) (M-14368) (G-C009) (DE-00050)

DD-50637 Nonvenomous insect bite of ankle with infection 916.5
(T-D9500) (M-14368) (G-C008) (DE-00050)

DD-50638 Superficial foreign body of ankle without major open wound and without infection 916.6
(T-D9500) (M-30408) (G-C009) (M-14014) (DE-00050)

DD-50639 Superficial foreign body of ankle without major open wound but with infection 916.7
(T-D9500) (M-30408) (G-C009) (M-14014) (G-C008) (DE-00050)

D-50 SUPERFICIAL INJURIES — Continued

DD-50640 Superficial injury of foot without infection 917.8
(T-D9700) (M-10050) (G-C009) (DE-00050)

DD-50641 Superficial injury of foot with infection 917.9
(T-D9700) (M-10050) (G-C008) (DE-00050)

DD-50642 Abrasion or friction burn of foot without infection 917.0
(T-D9700) (M-14700) (M-14710) (G-C009) (DE-00050)

DD-50643 Abrasion or friction burn of foot with infection 917.1
(T-D9700) (M-14700) (M-14710) (G-C009) (DE-00050)

DD-50644 Blister of foot without infection 917.2
(T-D9700) (M-14720) (G-C009) (DE-00050)

DD-50645 Blister of foot with infection 917.3
(T-D9700) (M-14720) (G-C008) (DE-00050)

DD-50646 Nonvenomous insect bite of foot without infection 917.4
(T-D9700) (M-14368) (G-C009) (DE-00050)

DD-50647 Nonvenomous insect bite of foot with infection 917.5
(T-D9700) (M-14368) (G-C008) (DE-00050)

DD-50648 Superficial foreign body of foot without major open wound and without infection 917.6
(T-D9700) (M-30408) (G-C009) (M-14014) (DE-00050)

DD-50649 Superficial foreign body of foot without major open wound but with infection 917.7
(T-D9700) (M-30408) (G-C009) (M-14014) (G-C008) (DE-00050)

DD-50650 Superficial injury of toe without infection 917.8
(T-D9800) (M-10050) (G-C009) (DE-00050)

DD-50651 Superficial injury of toe with infection 917.9
(T-D9800) (M-10050) (G-C008) (DE-00050)

DD-50652 Abrasion or friction burn of toe without injury 917.0
(T-D9800) (M-14700) (M-14710) (G-C009) (DE-00050)

DD-50653 Abrasion or friction burn of toe with infection 917.1
(T-D9800) (M-14700) (M-14710) (G-C008) (DE-00050)

DD-50654 Blister of toe without infection 917.2
(T-D9800) (M-14720) (G-C009) (DE-00050)

DD-50655 Blister of toe with infection 917.3
(T-D9800) (M-14720) (G-C008) (DE-00050)

DD-50656 Nonvenomous insect bite of toe without infection 917.4
(T-D9700) (M-14368) (G-C009) (DE-00050)

DD-50657 Nonvenomous insect bite of toe with infection 917.5
(T-D9800) (M-14368) (G-C008) (DE-00050)

DD-50658 Superficial foreign body of toe without major open wound and without infection 917.6
(T-D9800) (M-30408) (G-C009) (M-14014) (DE-00050)

DD-50659 Superficial foreign body of toe without major open wound but with infection 917.7
(T-D9800) (M-30408) (G-C009) (M-14014) (G-C008) (DE-00050)

D-52 BURNS

DD-52005 Burn with deep necrosis of underlying tissues without loss of body part of unspecified site 949.4
(T-D0003) (M-11104) (G-C009) (M-16010) (T-D0011)
Deep third degree burn without loss of body part of unspecified site 949.4
(T-D0003) (M-11104) (G-C009) (M-16010) (T-D0011)

DD-52006 Burn with deep necrosis of underlying tissues with loss of body part of unspecified site 949.5
(T-D0003) (M-11104) (G-C008) (M-16010) (T-D0011)
Deep third degree burn with loss of body part of unspecified site 949.5
(T-D0003) (M-11104) (G-C008) (M-16010) (T-D0011)

DD-52020 Burn any degree involving less than 10 percent of body surface 948.0
(T-D0022) (M-11100)

DD-52021 Burn any degree involving 10-19 percent of body surface 948.1
(T-D0022) (M-11100)

DD-52022 Burn any degree involving 20-29 percent of body surface 948.2
(T-D0023) (M-11100)

DD-52023 Burn any degree involving 30-39 percent of body surface 948.3
(T-D0024) (M-11100)

DD-52024 Burn any degree involving 40-49 percent of body surface 948.4
(T-D0025) (M-11100)

DD-52025 Burn any degree involving 50-59 percent of body surface 948.5
(T-D0026) (M-11100)

DD-52026 Burn any degree involving 60-69 percent of body surface 948.6
(T-D0027) (M-11100)

DD-52027 Burn any degree involving 70-79 percent of body surface 948.7
(T-D0028) (M-11100)

DD-52028 Burn any degree involving 80-89 percent of body surface 948.8
(T-D0029) (M-11100)

DD-52029 Burn any degree involving 90 percent or more of body surface 948.9
(T-D0030) (M-11100)

DD-52100 Burn of eye and adnexa, NOS 940.9
(T-AA000) (T-AA800) (M-11100)

DD-52101 Chemical burn of eyelid and periocular area 940.0
(T-AA810) (T-AA006) (M-11100) (G-C001) (C-10030)

DD-52102 Other burns of eyelid and periocular area 940.1
(T-AA810) (T-AA006) (M-11100)

DD-52103 Alkaline chemical burn of cornea and conjunctival sac 940.2
(T-AA200) (T-AA865) (M-11100) (G-C001) (C-10055)

DD-52104 Acid chemical burn of cornea and conjunctival sac 940.3
(T-AA200) (T-AA865) (M-11100) (G-C001) (C-10040)

DD-52105 Other burns of cornea and conjunctival sac 940.4
(T-AA200) (T-AA865) (M-11100)

DD-52108 Burn with resulting rupture and destruction of eyeball 940.5
(T-AA000) (M-11100) (G-C008) (M-14400)

DD-52200 Burn of face, head and neck, NOS 941.09
(T-D1200) (T-D1100) (T-D1600) (M-11100)

DD-52201 Erythema of face, head and neck 941.19
(T-D1200) (T-D1100) (T-D1600) (M-11101)
First degree burn of face, head and neck 941.19
(T-D1200) (T-D1100) (T-D1600) (M-11101)

DD-52202 Second degree burn of face, head and neck 941.29
(T-D1200) (T-D1100) (T-D1600) (M-11102)

DD-52203 Third degree burn of face, head and neck 941.39
(T-D1200) (T-D1100) (T-D1600) (M-11102)

DD-52204 Deep third degree burn of face, head and neck 941.49
(T-D1200) (T-D1100) (T-D1600) (M-11103)

DD-52205 Deep third degree burn of face, head and neck with loss of body part 941.59
(T-D1200) (T-D1100) (T-D1600) (M-11104) (G-C008) (M-16010) (T-D0011)

DD-52210 Burn of face and head, NOS 941.00
(T-D1200) (T-D1100) (M-11100)

DD-52211 Erythema of face and head 941.10
(T-D1200) (T-D1100) (M-11101)
First degree burn of face and head 941.10
(T-D1200) (T-D1100) (M-11101)

DD-52212 Second degree burn of face and head 941.20
(T-D1200) (T-D1100) (M-11102)

DD-52213 Third degree burn of face and head 941.30
(T-D1200) (T-D1100) (M-11103)

DD-52214 Deep third degree burn of face and head 941.40
(T-D1200) (T-D1100) (M-11104)

DD-52215 Deep third degree burn of face and head with loss of body part 941.50
(T-D1200) (T-D1100) (M-11104) (G-C008) (M-16010) (T-D0011)

DD-52220 Burn of ear, NOS 941.01
(T-Ab100) (M-11100)

DD-52221 Erythema of ear 941.11
(T-AB100) (M-11101)
First degree burn of ear 941.11
(T-AB100) (M-11101)

DD-52222 Second degree burn of ear 941.21
(T-AB100) (M-11102)

DD-52223 Third degree burn of ear 941.31
(T-AB100) (M-11103)

DD-52224 Deep third degree burn of ear 914.41
(T-AB100) (M-11104)

DD-52225 Deep third degree burn of ear with loss of body part 941.51
(T-AB100) (M-11104) (G-C008) (M-16010) (T-D0011)

DD-52230 Burn of lip, NOS 941.03
(T-52000) (M-11100)

DD-52231 Erythema of lip 941.13
(T-52000) (M-11101)
First degree burn of lip 941.13
(T-52000) (M-11101)

DD-52232 Second degree burn of lip 941.23
(T-52000) (M-11102)

DD-52233 Third degree burn of lip 941.33
(T-52000) (M-11103)

DD-52234 Deep third degree burn of lip 941.43
(T-52000) (M-11104)

DD-52235 Deep third degree burn of lip with loss of body part 941.53
(T-52000) (M-11104) (G-C008) (M-16010) (T-D0011)

DD-52240 Burn of chin, NOS 941.04
(T-D1210) (M-11100)

DD-52241 Erythema of chin 941.14
(T-D1210) (M-11101)
First degree burn of chin 941.14
(T-D1210) (M-11101)

DD-52242 Second degree burn of chin 941.24
(T-D1210) (M-11102)

D-52 BURNS — Continued

DD-52243 Third degree burn of chin 941.34
(T-D1210) (M-11103)

DD-52244 Deep third degree burn of chin 941.44
(T-D1210) (M-11104)

DD-52245 Deep third degree burn of chin with loss of body part 941.54
(T-D1210) (M-11104) (G-C008)
(M-16010) (T-D0011)

DD-52250 Burn of nose, NOS 941.05
(T-21000) (M-11100)

DD-52251 Erythema of nose 941.15
(T-21000) (M-11101)
First degree burn of nose 941.15
(T-21000) (M-11101)

DD-52252 Second degree burn of nose 941.25
(T-21000) (M-11100)

DD-52253 Third degree burn of nose 941.35
(T-21000) (M-11103)

DD-52254 Deep third degree burn of nose 941.45
(T-21000) (M-11104)

DD-52255 Deep third degree burn of nose with loss of body part 941.55
(T-21000) (M-11104) (G-C008)
(M-16010) (T-D0011)

DD-52260 Burn of scalp, NOS 941.06
(T-D1160) (M-11100)

DD-52261 Erythema of scalp 941.16
(T-D1160) (M-11101)
First degree burn of scalp 941.16
(T-D1160) (M-11101)

DD-52262 Second degree burn of scalp 941.26
(T-D1160) (M-11102)

DD-52263 Third degree burn of scalp 941.36
(T-D1160) (M-11103)

DD-52264 Deep third degree burn of scalp 941.46
(T-D1160) (M-11104)

DD-52265 Deep third degree burn of scalp with loss of body part 941.56
(T-D1160) (M-11104) (G-C008)
(M-16010) (T-D0011)

DD-52270 Burn of forehead and cheek, NOS 941.07
(T-D1110) (T-D1206) (M-11100)

DD-52271 Erythema of forehead and cheek 941.17
(T-D1110) (T-D1206) (M-11101)
First degree burn of forehead and cheek 941.17
(T-D1110) (T-D1206) (M-11101)

DD-52272 Second degree burn of forehead and cheek 941.27
(T-D1110) (T-D1206) (M-11102)

DD-52273 Third degree burn of forehead and cheek 941.37
(T-D1110) (T-D1206) (M-11103)

DD-52274 Deep third degree burn of forehead and cheek 941.47
(T-D1110) (T-D1206) (M-11104)

DD-52275 Deep third degree burn of forehead and cheek with loss of body part 941.57
(T-D1110) (T-D1206) (M-11104)
(G-C008) (M-16010) (T-D0011)

DD-52280 Burn of neck, NOS 941.08
(T-D1600) (M-11100)

DD-52281 Erythema of neck 941.18
(T-D1600) (M-11101)
First degree burn of neck 941.18
(T-D1600) (M-11101)

DD-52282 Second degree burn of neck 941.28
(T-D1600) (M-11102)

DD-52283 Third degree burn of neck 941.38
(T-D1600) (M-11103)

DD-52284 Deep third degree burn of neck 941.48
(T-D1600) (M-11104)

DD-52285 Deep third degree burn of neck with loss of body part 941.58
(T-D1600) (M-11104) (G-C008)
(M-16010) (T-D0011)

DD-52300 Burn of trunk, NOS 942.00
(T-D2000) (M-11100)

DD-52301 Erythema of trunk 942.10
(T-D2000) (M-11101)
First degree burn of trunk 942.10
(T-D2000) (M-11101)

DD-52302 Second degree burn of trunk 942.20
(T-D2000) (M-11102)

DD-52303 Third degree burn of trunk 942.30
(T-D2000) (M-11103)

DD-52304 Deep third degree burn of trunk 942.40
(T-D2000) (M-11104)

DD-52305 Deep third degree burn of trunk with loss of body part 942.50
(T-D2000) (M-11104) (G-C008)
(M-16010) (T-D0011)

DD-52310 Burn of breast, NOS 942.01
(T-04000) (M-11100)

DD-52311 Erythema of breast 942.11
(T-04000) (M-11101)
First degree burn of breast 942.11
(T-04000) (M-11101)

DD-52312 Second degree burn of breast 942.21
(T-04000) (M-11102)

DD-52313 Third degree burn of breast 942.31
(T-04000) (M-11103)

DD-52314 Deep third degree burn of breast 942.41
(T-04000) (M-11104)

DD-52315 Deep third degree burn of breast with loss of body part 942.51
(T-04000) (M-11104) (G-C008)
(M-16010) (T-D0011)

DD-52320 Burn of chest wall, NOS 942.02
(T-D3050) (M-11100)

DD-52321 Erythema of chest wall 941.12
(T-D3050) (M-11101)
First degree burn of chest wall 942.12
(T-D3050) (M-11101)

DD-52322 Second degree burn of chest wall 942.22
(T-D3050) (M-11102)
DD-52323 Third degree burn of chest wall 942.32
(T-D3050) (M-11103)
DD-52324 Deep third degree burn of chest wall 942.42
(T-D3050) (M-11104)
DD-52325 Deep third degree burn of chest wall with loss of body part 942.52
(T-D3050) (M-11104) (G-C008)
(M-16010) (T-D0011)
DD-52330 Burn of abdominal wall, NOS 942.03
(T-D4300) (M-11100)
DD-52331 Erythema of abdominal wall 942.13
(T-D4300) (M-11101)
First degree burn of abdominal wall 942.13
(T-D4300) (M-11101)
DD-52332 Second degree burn of abdominal wall 942.23
(T-D4300) (M-11102)
DD-52333 Third degree burn of abdominal wall 942.33
(T-D4300) (M-11103)
DD-52334 Deep third degree burn of abdominal wall 942.43
(T-D4300) (M-11104)
DD-52335 Deep third degree burn of abdominal wall with loss of body part 942.53
(T-D4300) (M-11104) (G-C008)
(M-16010) (T-D0011)
DD-52340 Burn of back, NOS 942.04
(T-D2100) (M-11100)
DD-52341 Erythema of back 942.14
(T-D2100) (M-11101)
First degree burn of back 942.14
(T-D2100) (M-11101)
DD-52342 Second degree burn of back 942.24
(T-D2100) (M-11102)
DD-52343 Third degree burn of back 942.34
(T-D2100) (M-11103)
DD-52344 Deep third degree burn of back 942.44
(T-D2100) (M-11104)
DD-52345 Deep third degree burn of back with loss of body part 942.54
(T-D2100) (M-11104) (G-C008)
(M-16010) (T-D0011)
DD-52350 Burn of male genitalia, NOS 942.05
(T-90010) (M-11100)
DD-52351 Erythema of male genitalia 942.15
(T-90010) (M-11101)
First degree burn of male genitalia 942.15
(T-90010) (M-11101)
DD-52352 Second degree burn of male genitalia 942.25
(T-90010) (M-11102)
DD-52353 Third degree burn of male genitalia 942.35
(T-90010) (M-11103)
DD-52354 Deep third degree burn of male genitalia 942.45
(T-90010) (M-11104)
DD-52355 Deep third degree burn of male genitalia with loss of body part 942.55
(T-90010) (M-11104) (G-C008)
(M-16010) (T-D0011)
DD-52360 Burn of female genitalia, NOS 942.05
(T-80010) (M-11100)
DD-52361 Erythema of female genitalia 942.15
(T-80010) (M-11101)
First degree burn of female genitalia 942.15
(T-80010) (M-11101)
DD-52362 Second degree burn of female genitalia 942.25
(T-80010) (M-11102)
DD-52363 Third degree burn of female genitalia 942.35
(T-80010) (M-11103)
DD-52364 Deep third degree burn of female genitalia 942.45
(T-80010) (M-11104)
DD-52365 Deep third degree burn of female genitalia with loss of body part 942.55
(T-80010) (M-11104) (G-C008)
(M-16010) (T-D0011)
DD-52380 Burn of multiple sites of trunk, NOS 942.09
(T-D2000) (M-11100) (M-11180)
DD-52381 Erythema of multiple sites of trunk 942.19
(T-D2000) (M-11101) (M-11180)
First degree burn of multiple sites of trunk 942.19
(T-D2000) (M-11101) (M-11180)
DD-52382 Second degree burn of multiple sites of trunk 942.29
(T-D2000) (M-11102) (M-11180)
DD-52383 Third degree burn of multiple sites of trunk 942.39
(T-D2000) (M-11103) (M-11180)
DD-52384 Deep third degree burn of multiple sites of trunk 942.49
(T-D2000) (M-11104) (M-11180)
DD-52385 Deep third degree burn of multiple sites of trunk with loss of body part 942.59
(T-D2000) (M-11104) (M-11180)
(G-C008) (M-16010) (T-D0011)
DD-52400 Burn of upper limb, NOS 943.00
(T-D8000) (M-11100)
DD-52401 Erythema of upper limb 943.10
(T-D8000) (M-11101)
First degree burn of upper limb 943.10
(T-D8000) (M-11101)
DD-52402 Second degree burn of upper limb 943.20
(T-D8000) (M-11102)
DD-52403 Third degree burn of upper limb 943.30
(T-D8000) (M-11103)
DD-52404 Deep third degree burn of upper limb 943.40
(T-D8000) (M-11104)
DD-52405 Deep third degree burn of upper limb with loss of body part 943.50
(T-D8000) (M-11104) (G-C008)
(M-16010) (T-D0011)

D-52 BURNS — Continued

DD-52410 Burn of shoulder, NOS 943.05
(T-D2220) (M-11100)

DD-52411 Erythema of shoulder 943.15
(T-D2220) (M-11101)
First degree burn of shoulder 943.15
(T-D2220) (M-11101)

DD-52412 Second degree burn of shoulder 943.25
(T-D2220) (M-11102)

DD-52413 Third degree burn of shoulder 943.35
(T-D2220) (M-11103)

DD-52414 Deep third degree burn of shoulder 943.45
(T-D2220) (M-11104)

DD-52415 Deep third degree burn of shoulder with loss of body part 943.55
(T-D2220) (M-11104) (G-C008)
(M-16010) (T-D0011)

DD-52420 Burn of scapular region, NOS 943.06
(T-D2200) (M-11100)

DD-52421 Erythema of scapular region 943.16
(T-D2200) (M-11101)
First degree burn of scapular region 943.16
(T-D2200) (M-11101)

DD-52422 Second degree burn of scapular region 943.26
(T-D2200) (M-11102)

DD-52423 Third degree burn of scapula region 943.36
(T-D2200) (M-11103)

DD-52424 Deep third degree burn of scapular region 943.46
(T-D2200) (M-11104)

DD-52425 Deep third degree burn of scapular region with loss of body part 943.56
(T-D2200) (M-11104) (G-C008)
(M-16010) (T-D0011)

DD-52430 Burn of axilla, NOS 943.04
(T-D8100) (M-11100)

DD-52431 Erythema of axilla 943.14
(T-D8100) (M-11101)
First degree burn of axilla 943.14
(T-D8100) (M-11101)

DD-52432 Second degree burn of axilla 943.24
(T-D8100) (M-11102)

DD-52433 Third degree burn of axilla 943.34
(T-D8100) (M-11103)

DD-52434 Deep third degree burn of axilla 943.44
(T-D8100) (M-11104)

DD-52435 Deep third degree burn of axilla with loss of body part 943.54
(T-D8100) (M-11104) (G-C008)
(M-16010) (T-D0011)

DD-52440 Burn of upper arm, NOS 943.03
(T-D8200) (M-11100)

DD-52441 Erythema of upper arm 943.13
(T-D8200) (M-11101)
First degree burn of upper arm 943.13
(T-D8200) (M-11101)

DD-52442 Second degree burn of upper arm 943.23
(T-D8200) (M-11102)

DD-52443 Third degree burn of upper arm 943.33
(T-D8200) (M-11103)

DD-52444 Deep third degree burn of upper arm 943.43
(T-D8200) (M-11104)

DD-52445 Deep third degree burn of upper arm with loss of body part 943.53
(T-D8200) (M-11104) (G-C008)
(M-16010) (T-D0011)

DD-52450 Burn of elbow, NOS 943.02
(T-D8300) (M-11100)

DD-52451 Erythema of elbow 943.12
(T-D8300) (M-11101)
First degree burn of elbow 943.12
(T-D8300) (M-11101)

DD-52452 Second degree burn of elbow 943.22
(T-D8300) (M-11102)

DD-52453 Third degree burn of elbow 943.32
(T-D8300) (M-11103)

DD-52454 Deep third degree burn of elbow 943.42
(T-D8300) (M-11104)

DD-52455 Deep third degree burn of elbow with loss of body part 943.52
(T-D8300) (M-11104) (G-C008)
(M-16010) (T-D0011)

DD-52460 Burn of forearm, NOS 943.01
(T-D8500) (M-11100)

DD-52461 Erythema of forearm 943.11
(T-D8500) (M-11101)
First degree burn of forearm 943.11
(T-D8500) (M-11101)

DD-52462 Second degree burn of forearm 943.21
(T-D8500) (M-11102)

DD-52463 Third degree burn of forearm 943.31
(T-D8500) (M-11103)

DD-52464 Deep third degree burn of forearm 943.41
(T-D8500) (M-11104)

DD-52465 Deep third degree burn of forearm with loss of body part 943.51
(T-D8500) (M-11104) (G-C001)
(M-16010) (T-D0011)

DD-52480 Burn of multiple sites of upper limb, NOS 943.09
(T-D8000) (M-11100) (M-11180)

DD-52481 Erythema of multiple sites of upper limb 943.19
(T-D8000) (M-11101) (M-11180)
First degree burn of multiple sites of upper arm 943.19
(T-D8000) (M-11101) (M-11180)

DD-52482 Second degree burn of multiple sites of upper arm 943.29
(T-D8000) (M-11102) (M-11180)

DD-52483 Third degree burn of multiple sites of upper limb 943.39
(T-D8000) (M-11103) (M-11180)

DD-52484 Deep third degree burn of multiple sites of upper limb 943.49
(T-D8000) (M-11104) (M-11180)

DD-52485 Deep third degree burn of multiple sites of upper limb with loss of body part 943.59
(T-D8000) (M-11104) (M-11180) (G-C008) (M-16010) (T-D0011)

DD-52500 Burn of wrist, NOS 944.07
(T-D8600) (M-11100)

DD-52501 Erythema of wrist 944.17
(T-D8600) (M-11101)
First degree burn of wrist 944.17
(T-D8600) (M-11101)

DD-52502 Second degree burn of wrist 944.27
(T-D8600) (M-11102)

DD-52503 Third degree burn of wrist 944.37
(T-D8600) (M-11103)

DD-52504 Deep third degree burn of wrist 944.47
(T-D8600) (M-11104)

DD-52505 Deep third degree burn of wrist with loss of body part 944.57
(T-D8600) (M-11104) (G-C008) (M-16010) (T-D0011)

DD-52510 Burn of hand, NOS 944.00
(T-D8700) (M-11100)

DD-52511 Erythema of hand 944.10
(T-D8700) (M-11101)
First degree burn of hand 944.10
(T-D8700) (M-11101)

DD-52512 Second degree burn of hand 944.20
(T-D8700) (M-11102)

DD-52513 Third degree burn of hand 944.30
(T-D8700) (M-11103)

DD-52514 Deep third degree burn of hand 944.40
(T-D8700) (M-11104)

DD-52515 Deep third degree burn of hand with loss of body part 944.50
(T-D8700) (M-11104) (G-C008) (M-16010) (T-D0011)

DD-52520 Burn of palm, NOS 944.05
(T-D8740) (M-11100)

DD-52521 Erythema of palm 944.15
(T-D8740) (M-11101)
First degree burn of palm 944.15
(T-D8740) (M-11101)

DD-52522 Second degree burn of palm 944.25
(T-D8740) (M-11102)

DD-52523 Third degree burn of palm 944.35
(T-D8740) (M-11103)

DD-52524 Deep third degree burn of palm 944.45
(T-D8740) (M-11104)

DD-52525 Deep third degree burn of palm with loss of body part 944.55
(T-D8740) (M-11104) (G-C008) (M-16010) (T-D0011)

DD-52530 Burn of back of hand, NOS 944.06
(T-D8730) (M-11100)

DD-52531 Erythema of back of hand 944.16
(T-D8730) (M-11101)
First degree burn of back of hand 944.16
(T-D8730) (M-11101)

DD-52532 Second degree burn of back of hand 944.26
(T-D8730) (M-11102)

DD-52533 Third degree burn of back of hand 944.36
(T-D8730) (M-11103)

DD-52534 Deep third degree burn of back of hand 944.46
(T-D8730) (M-11104)

DD-52535 Deep third degree burn of back of hand with loss of body part 944.56
(T-D8730) (M-11104) (G-C008) (M-16010) (T-D0011)

DD-52540 Burn of single finger, not thumb, NOS 944.01
(T-D8800) (M-11100) (G-C030) (T-D8810)

DD-52541 Erythema of single finger, not thumb 944.11
(T-D8800) (M-11101) (G-C030) (T-D8810)
First degree burn of single finger, not thumb 944.11
(T-D8800) (M-11101) (G-C030) (T-D8810)

DD-52542 Second degree burn of single finger, not thumb 944.21
(T-D8800) (M-11102) (G-C030) (T-D8810)

DD-52543 Third degree burn of single finger, not thumb 944.31
(T-D8800) (M-11103) (G-C030) (T-D8810)

DD-52544 Deep third degree burn of finger, not thumb 944.41
(T-D8800) (M-11104) (G-C030) (T-D8810)

DD-52545 Deep third degree burn of finger, not thumb with loss of body part 944.51
(T-D8800) (M-11104) (G-C030) (T-D8810) (G-C008) (M-16010) (T-D0011)

DD-52550 Burn of two or more fingers not including thumb, NOS 944.03
(T-D8800) (G-A722) (M-11100) (G-C030) (T-D8810)

DD-52551 Erythema of two or more fingers not including thumb 944.13
(T-D8800) (G-A722) (M-11101) (G-C030) (T-D8810)
First degree burn or two or more fingers not including thumb 944.13
(T-D8800) (G-A722) (M-11101) (G-C030) (T-D8810)

DD-52552 Second degree burn of two or more fingers not including thumb 944.23
(T-D8800) (G-A722) (M-11102) (G-C030) (T-D8810)

D-52 BURNS — Continued

DD-52553 Third degree burn of two or more fingers not including thumb 944.33
(T-D8800) (G-A722) (M-11103) (G-C030) (T-D8810)

DD-52554 Deep third degree burn of two or more fingers not including thumb 944.43
(T-D8800) (G-A722) (M-11104) (G-C030) (T-D8810)

DD-52555 Deep third degree burn of two or more fingers not including thumb with loss of body part 944.53
(T-D8800) (G-A722) (M-11104) (G-C030) (T-D8810) (G-C008) (M-16010) (T-D0011)

DD-52560 Burn of two or more fingers including thumb 944.04
(T-D8800) (G-A722) (M-11100) (G-A656) (T-D8810)

DD-52561 Erythema of two or more fingers including thumb 944.14
(T-D8800) (G-A722) (M-11101) (G-A656) (T-D8810)
First degree burn of two or more fingers including thumb 944.14
(T-D8800) (G-A722) (M-11101) (G-A656) (T-D8810)

DD-52562 Second degree burn of two or more fingers including thumb 944.24
(T-D8800) (G-A722) (M-11102) (G-A656) (T-D8810)

DD-52563 Third degree burn of two or more fingers including thumb 944.34
(T-D8800) (G-A722) (M-11103) (G-A656) (T-D8810)

DD-52564 Deep third degree burn of two or more fingers including thumb 944.44
(T-D8800) (G-A722) (M-11104) (G-A656) (T-D8810)

DD-52565 Deep third degree burn of two or more fingers including thumb with loss of body part 944.55
(T-D8800) (G-A722) (M-11104) (G-A656) (T-D8810) (G-C008) (M-16010) (T-D0011)

DD-52570 Burn of thumb, NOS 944.02
(T-D8810) (M-11100)

DD-52571 Erythema of thumb 944.12
(T-D8810) (M-11101)
First degree burn of thumb 944.12
(T-D8810) (M-11101)

DD-52572 Second degree burn of thumb 944.22
(T-D8810) (M-11102)

DD-52573 Third degree burn of thumb 944.32
(T-D8810) (M-11103)

DD-52574 Deep third degree burn of thumb 944.42
(T-D8810) (M-11104)

DD-52575 Deep third degree burn of thumb with loss of body part 944.52
(T-D8810) (M-11104) (G-C008) (M-16010) (T-D0011)

DD-52580 Burn of multiple sites of wrist and hand, NOS 944.08
(T-D8600) (T-D8700) (M-11100) (M-11180)

DD-52581 Erythema of multiple sites of wrist and hand 944.18
(T-D8600) (T-D8700) (M-11101) (M-11180)
First degree burn of wrist and hand 944.18
(T-D8600) (T-D8700) (M-11101) (M-11180)

DD-52582 Second degree burn of wrist and hand 944.28
(T-D8600) (T-D8700) (M-11102) (M-11180)

DD-52583 Third degree burn of wrist and hand 944.38
(T-D8600) (T-D8700) (M-11103) (M-11180)

DD-52584 Deep third degree burn of wrist and hand 944.48
(T-D8600) (T-D8700) (M-11104) (M-11180)

DD-52585 Deep third degree burn of wrist and hand with loss of body part 944.58
(T-D8600) (T-D8700) (M-11104) (M-11180) (G-C008) (M-16010) (T-D0011)

DD-52600 Burn of lower limb, NOS 945.00
(T-D9000) (M-11100)

DD-52601 Erythema of lower limb 945.10
(T-D9000) (M-11101)
First degree burn of lower limb 945.10
(T-D9000) (M-11101)

DD-52602 Second degree burn of lower limb 945.20
(T-D9000) (M-11102)

DD-52603 Third degree burn of lower limb 945.30
(T-D9000) (M-11103)

DD-52604 Deep third degree burn of lower limb 945.40
(T-D9000) (M-11104)

DD-52605 Deep third degree burn of lower limb with loss of body part 945.50
(T-D9000) (M-11104) (G-C008) (M-16010) (T-D0011)

DD-52610 Burn of thigh, NOS 945.06
(T-D9100) (M-11100)

DD-52611 Erythema of thigh 945.16
(T-D9100) (M-11101)
First degree burn of thigh 945.16
(T-D9100) (M-11101)

DD-52612 Second degree burn of thigh 945.26
(T-D9100) (M-11102)

DD-52613 Third degree burn of thigh 945.36
(T-D9100) (M-11103)

DD-52614 Deep third degree burn of thigh 945.46
(T-D9100) (M-11104)

DD-52615 Deep third degree burn of thigh with loss of body part 945.56
(T-D9100) (M-11104) (G-C008) (M-16010) (T-D0011)

DD-52620 Burn of knee, NOS 945.05
(T-D9200) (M-11100)

DD-52621 Erythema of knee 945.15
(T-D9200) (M-11101)
First degree burn of knee 945.15
(T-D9200) (M-11101)

DD-52622 Second degree burn of knee 945.25
(T-D9200) (M-11102)

DD-52623 Third degree burn of knee 945.35
(T-D9200) (M-11103)

DD-52624 Deep third degree burn of knee 945.45
(T-D9200) (M-11104)

DD-52625 Deep third degree burn of knee with loss of body part 945.55
(T-D9200) (M-11104) (G-C008) (M-16010) (T-D0011)

DD-52630 Burn of lower leg, NOS 945.04
(T-D9400) (M-11100)

DD-52631 Erythema of lower leg 945.14
(T-D9400) (M-11101)
First degree burn of lower leg 945.14
(T-D9400) (M-11101)

DD-52632 Second degree burn of lower leg 945.24
(T-D9400) (M-11102)

DD-52633 Third degree burn of lower leg 945.34
(T-D9400) (M-11103)

DD-52634 Deep third degree burn of lower leg 945.44
(T-D9400) (M-11104)

DD-52635 Deep third degree burn of lower leg with loss of body part 945.54
(T-D9400) (M-11104) (G-C008) (M-16010) (T-D0011)

DD-52640 Burn of ankle, NOS 945.03
(T-D9500) (M-11100)

DD-52641 Erythema of ankle 945.13
(T-D9500) (M-11101)
First degree burn of ankle 945.13
(T-D9500) (M-11101)

DD-52642 Second degree burn of ankle 945.23
(T-D9500) (M-11102)

DD-52643 Third degree burn of ankle 945.33
(T-D9500) (M-11103)

DD-52644 Deep third degree burn of ankle 945.43
(T-D9500) (M-11104)

DD-52645 Deep third degree burn of ankle with loss of body part 945.53
(T-D9500) (M-11104) (G-C008) (M-16010) (T-D0011)

DD-52650 Burn of foot, NOS 945.02
(T-D9700) (M-11100)

DD-52651 Erythema of foot 945.12
(T-D9700) (M-11101)
First degree burn of foot 945.12
(T-D9700) (M-11101)

DD-52652 Second degree burn of foot 945.22
(T-D9700) (M-11102)

DD-52653 Third degree burn of foot 945.32
(T-D9700) (M-11103)

DD-52654 Deep third degree burn of foot 945.42
(T-D9700) (M-11104)

DD-52655 Deep third degree burn of foot with loss of body part 945.52
(T-D9700) (M-11104) (G-C008) (M-16010) (T-D0011)

DD-52660 Burn of toe, NOS 945.01
(T-D9800) (M-11100)

DD-52661 Erythema of toe 945.11
(T-D9800) (M-11101)
First degree burn of toe 945.11
(T-D9800) (M-11101)

DD-52662 Second degree burn of toe 945.21
(T-D9800) (M-11102)

DD-52663 Third degree burn of toe 945.31
(T-D9800) (M-11103)

DD-52664 Deep third degree burn of toe 945.41
(T-D9800) (M-11104)

DD-52665 Deep third degree burn of toe with loss of body part 945.51
(T-D9800) (M-11104) (G-C008) (M-16010) (T-D0011)

DD-52680 Burn of multiple sites of lower limb 945.09
(T-D9000) (M-11100) (M-11180)

DD-52681 Erythema of multiple sites of lower limb 945.19
(T-D9000) (M-11101) (M-11180)
First degree burn of multiple sites of lower limb 945.19
(T-D9000) (M-11101) (M-11180)

DD-52682 Second degree burn of multiple sites of lower limb 945.29
(T-D9000) (M-11102) (M-11180)

DD-52683 Third degree burn of multiple sites of lower limb 945.39
(T-D9000) (M-11103) (M-11180)

DD-52684 Deep third degree burn of multiple sites of lower limb 945.49
(T-D9000) (M-11104) (M-11180)

DD-52685 Deep third degree burn of multiple sites of lower limb with loss of body part 945.59
(T-D9000) (M-11104) (M-11180) (G-C008) (M-16010) (T-D0011)

DD-52700 Burns of multiple specified sites 946.0
(T-D0020) (M-11100) (M-11180)

DD-52701 Erythema of multiple specified sites 946.1
(T-D0020) (M-11101) (M-11180)
First degree burns of multiple specified sites 946.1
(T-D0020) (M-11101) (M-11180)

DD-52702 Second degree burns of multiple specified sites 946.2
(T-D0020) (M-11102) (M-11180)

D-52 BURNS — Continued

DD-52703 Third degree burns of multiple specified sites 946.3
(T-D0020) (M-11103) (M-11180)

DD-52704 Deep third degree burns of multiple specified sites 946.4
(T-D0020) (M-11104) (M-11180)

DD-52705 Deep third degree burns of multiple specified sites with loss of body part 946.5
(T-D0020) (M-11104) (M-11180) (G-C008) (M-16010) (T-D0011)

DD-52800 Burn of internal organs, NOS 947.9
(T-D0060) (M-11100)

DD-52802 Chemical burn of internal organs 947.9
(T-D0060) (M-11100) (G-C008) (C-00000)

DD-52810 Burn of mouth and pharynx 947.0
(T-51000) (T-55000) (M-11100)

DD-52812 Burn of mouth 947.0
(T-51000) (M-11100)

DD-52814 Burn of pharynx 947.0
(T-55000) (M-11100)

DD-52816 Burn of gum 947.0
(T-54910) (M-11100)

DD-52818 Burn of tongue 947.0
(T-53000) (M-11100)

DD-52820 Burn of larynx, trachea and lung 947.1
(T-24100) (T-25000) (T-28000) (M-11100)

DD-52822 Burn of larynx 947.1
(T-24100) (M-11100)

DD-52824 Burn of trachea 947.1
(T-25000) (M-11100)

DD-52826 Burn of lung 947.1
(T-28000) (M-11100)

DD-52830 Burn of esophagus 947.2
(T-56000) (M-11100)

DD-52840 Burn of gastrointestinal tract, NOS 947.3
(T-50100) (M-11100)

DD-52842 Burn of stomach 947.3
(T-57000) (M-11100)

DD-52844 Burn of small intestine 947.3
(T-58000) (M-11100)

DD-52846 Burn of colon 947.3
(T-59300) (M-11100)

DD-52848 Burn of rectum 947.3
(T-59600) (M-11100)

DD-52850 Burn of vagina and uterus 947.4
(T-82000) (T-83000) (M-11100)

DD-52852 Burn of vagina 947.4
(T-82000) (M-11100)

DD-52854 Burn of cervix 947.4
(T-83200) (M-11100)

DD-52856 Burn of uterus 947.4
(T-83000) (M-11100)

DD-52880 Burn of other internal organ, NEC 947.8
(T-D0060) (M-11100)

D-53 CONTUSIONS WITH INTACT SKIN

DD-53002 Contusion of multiple sites, NEC 924.8
(T-D0020) (M-14200)

DD-53100 Contusion of face, except eye 920.-
(T-D1200) (M-14200) (G-C030) (T-AA000)

DD-53101 Contusion of cheek 920.-
(T-D1206) (M-14200)

DD-53102 Contusion of ear 920.-
(T-AB100) (M-14200)

DD-53103 Contusion of nose 920.-
(T-21000) (M-14200)

DD-53104 Contusion of lip 920.-
(T-52000) (M-14200)

DD-53105 Contusion of gum 920.-
(T-54910) (M-14200)

DD-53106 Contusion of mandibular joint area 920.-
(T-D1216) (M-14200)

DD-53110 Contusion of scalp 920.-
(T-D1160) (M-14200)

DD-53120 Contusion of neck 920.-
(T-D1600) (M-14200)

DD-53122 Contusion of throat 920.-
(T-D1602) (M-14200)

DD-53200 Contusion of eye and adnexa, NOS 921.-
(T-AA000) (T-AA800) (M-14200)

DD-53210 Contusion of eye, NOS 921.9
(T-AA000) (M-14200)
Black eye, NOS 921.0
(T-AA000) (M-14200)
Contusion of eyeball 921.3
(T-AA000) (M-14200)
Injury of eye, NOS 921.9
(T-AA000) (M-14200)

DD-53220 Contusion of eyelids and periocular area 921.1
(T-AA810) (T-AA006) (M-14200)

DD-53230 Contusion of orbital tissues 921.2
(T-AA006) (M-14200)

DD-53300 Contusion of trunk, NOS 922.9
(T-D2000) (M-14200)

DD-53310 Contusion of chest 922.1
(T-D3000) (M-14200)

DD-53312 Contusion of breast 922.0
(T-04000) (M-14200)

DD-53320 Contusion of abdominal wall 922.2
(T-D4300) (M-14200)

DD-53322 Contusion of flank 922.2
(T-D2310) (M-14200)

DD-53324 Contusion of groin 922.2
(T-D7000) (M-14200)

DD-53330 Contusion of back 922.3
(T-D2100) (M-14200)

DD-53332 Contusion of buttock 922.3
(T-D2600) (M-14200)

DD-53334 Contusion of interscapular region 922.3
(T-D2210) (M-14200)

DD-53340 Contusion of male genital organs, NOS 922.4
(T-90010) (M-14200)

DD-53342 Contusion of penis 922.4
(T-91000) (M-14200)

DD-53344 Contusion of scrotum 922.4
(T-98000) (M-14200)

DD-53346 Contusion of testis 922.4
(T-94000) (M-14200)

DD-53350 Contusion of female genital organs, NOS 922.4
(T-80010) (M-14200)

DD-53352 Contusion of labium 922.4
(T-81210) (M-14200)

DD-53354 Contusion of vulva 922.4
(T-81000) (M-14200)

DD-53356 Contusion of vagina 922.4
(T-82000) (M-14200)

DD-53360 Contusion of perineum 922.4
(T-D2700) (M-14200)

DD-53380 Contusion of multiple sites of trunk 922.8
(T-D2000) (T-D0020) (M-14200)

DD-53400 Contusion of upper limb, NOS 923.9
(T-D8000) (M-14200)
Contusion of arm, NOS 923.9
(T-D8000) (M-14200)

DD-53410 Contusion of shoulder and upper arm 923.0
(T-D2220) (T-D8200) (M-14200)

DD-53412 Contusion of shoulder region 923.00
(T-D2220) (M-14200)

DD-53413 Contusion of scapular region 923.01
(T-D2200) (M-14200)

DD-53414 Contusion of axillary region 923.02
(T-D8104) (M-14200)

DD-53416 Contusion of upper arm 923.-3
(T-D8200) (M-14200)

DD-53420 Contusion of elbow and forearm 923.1
(T-D8300) (T-D8500) (M-14200)

DD-53422 Contusion of forearm 923.10
(T-D8500) (M-14200)

DD-53424 Contusion of elbow 923.11
(T-D8300) (M-14200)

DD-53440 Contusion of wrist and hand, except fingers 923.2
(T-D8700) (T-D8700) (M-14200)
(G-C030) (T-D8800)

DD-53442 Contusion of hand 923.20
(T-D8700) (M-14200)

DD-53444 Contusion of wrist 923.21
(T-D8600) (M-14200)

DD-53450 Contusion of finger 923.3
(T-D8800) (M-14200)

DD-53452 Contusion of fingernail 923.3
(T-01600) (T-D8800) (M-14200)

DD-53454 Contusion of thumb 923.3
(T-D8810) (M-14200)

DD-53456 Contusion of thumb nail 923.3
(T-01600) (T-D8810) (M-14200)

DD-53480 Contusion of multiple sites of upper limb 923.8
(T-D8000) (T-D0020) (M-14200)

DD-53600 Contusion of lower limb, NOS 924.5
(T-D9000) (M-14200)
Contusion of leg, NOS 924.5
(T-D9000) (M-14200)

DD-53610 Contusion of hip and thigh 924.0
(T-D2500) (T-D9100) (M-14200)

DD-53612 Contusion of thigh 924.00
(T-D9100) (M-14200)

DD-53614 Contusion of hip 924.01
(T-D2500) (M-14200)

DD-53620 Contusion of knee and lower leg 924.10
(T-D9200) (T-D9400) (M-14200)

DD-53622 Contusion of lower leg 924.10
(T-D9400) (M-14200)

DD-53624 Contusion of knee 924.11
(T-D9200) (M-14200)

DD-53630 Contusion of ankle and foot, excluding toes 924.2
(T-D9500) (T-D9700) (M-14200)
(G-C030) (T-D9800)

DD-53632 Contusion of foot 924.20
(T-D9700) (M-14200)

DD-53634 Contusion of heel 924.20
(T-D9600) (M-14200)

DD-53638 Contusion of ankle 924.21
(T-D9500) (M-14200)

DD-53640 Contusion of toe 924.3
(T-D9800) (M-14200)

DD-53642 Contusion of toenail 924.3
(T-01600) (T-D9800) (M-14200)

DD-53680 Contusion of multiple sites of lower limb 924.4
(T-D9000) (T-D0020) (M-14200)

SECTION D-6 EFFECTS AND COMPLICATIONS OF INJURY, EXPOSURE AND CARE

D-61 EFFECTS OF FOREIGN BODIES

DD-61100 Foreign body on external eye 930.9
(T-AA880) (M-30400)

DD-61110 Corneal foreign body 930.0
(T-AA200) (M-30400)

DD-61120 Foreign body in conjuntival sac 930.1
(T-AA865) (M-30400)

DD-61130 Foreign body in lacrimal punctum 930.2
(T-AA931) (M-30400)

DD-61200 Foreign body in ear 931.-
(T-AB100) (M-30400)

DD-61210 Foreign body in auditory canal 931.-
(T-AB200) (M-30400)

DD-61220 Foreign body in auricle 931.-
(T-AB105) (M-30400)

DD-61300 Foreign body in nose 932.-
(T-21300) (M-30400)

D-61 EFFECTS OF FOREIGN BODIES — Continued

DD-61310 Foreign body in nostril 932.-
(T-21310) (M-30400)

DD-61320 Foreign body in nasal sinus 932.-
(T-22000) (M-30400)

DD-61330 Foreign body in hypopharynx
(T-55300) (M-30400)

DD-61400 Foreign body in pharynx and larynx 933.-
(T-55000) (T-24100) (M-30400)

DD-61410 Foreign body in pharynx 930.0
(T-55000) (M-30400)
Foreign body in throat, NOS 933.0
(T-55000) (M-30400)

DD-61412 Foreign body in nasopharynx 933.0
(T-23000) (M-30400)

DD-61420 Foreign body in larynx 933.1
(T-24100) (M-30400)

DD-61422 Asphyxia due to foreign body in larynx 933.1
(F-20150) (G-C001) (M-30400)
(T-24100)

DD-61424 Choking due to food in larynx 933.1
(F-20110) (G-C001) (M-30400)
(C-F0000) (T-24100)

DD-61426 Choking due to phlegm in larynx 933.1
(F-20110) (G-C001) (T-20141)
(G-C006) (T-24100)

DD-61500 Foreign body in respiratory tree, NOS 943.9
(T-20000) (M-30400)
Foreign body in trachea, bronchus and lung 934.9
(T-25000) (T-26000) (T-28000)
(M-30400)

DD-61510 Foreign body in trachea 934.0
(T-25000) (M-30400)

DD-61520 Foreign body in main bronchus 934.1
(T-26000) (M-30400)

DD-61530 Foreign body in bronchioles 934.8
(T-27000) (M-30400)

DD-61540 Foreign body in lung 934.8
(T-28000) (M-30400)

DD-61550 Inhalation of liquid in lower respiratory tract 934.9
(T-20010) (C-00300) (T-20200)

DD-61552 Inhalation of vomitus in lower respiratory tract 934.9
(F-20010) (T-50270) (T-20200)

DD-61600 Foreign body in digestive system, NOS 938.-
(T-50100) (M-30400)
Foreign body in alimentary tract, NOS 938.-
(T-50100) (M-30400)
Swallowed foreign body 938.-
(T-50100) (M-30400)

DD-61610 Foreign body in mouth 935.0
(T-51000) (M-30400)

DD-61620 Foreign body in esophagus 935.1
(T-56000) (M-30400)

DD-61630 Foreign body in stomach 935.2
(T-57000) (M-30400)

DD-61640 Foreign body in intestine 936.-
(T-50500) (M-30400)
Foreign body in intestinal tract 936.-
(T-50500) (M-30400)

DD-61650 Foreign body in colon 936.-
(T-59300) (M-30400)

DD-61660 Foreign body in rectum 937.-
(T-59600) (M-30400)

DD-61666 Foreign body in rectosigmoid junction 937.-
(T-59670) (M-30400)

DD-61670 Foreign body in anus 937.-
(T-59900) (M-30400)

DD-61700 Foreign body in genitourinary tract, NOS 939.-
(T-70200) (M-30400)

DD-61710 Foreign body in bladder and urethra 939.0
(T-74000) (T-75000) (M-30400)

DD-61720 Foreign body in uterus, any part 939.1
(T-83000) (M-30400)

DD-61730 Foreign body in vulva 939.2
(T-81000) (M-30400)

DD-61740 Foreign body in vagina 939.2
(T-82000) (M-30400)

DD-61750 Foreign body in penis 939.3
(T-91000) (M-30400)

D-62 EARLY TRAUMATIC COMPLICATIONS OF INJURY

DD-62000 Traumatic complication of injury of unspecified site, NOS 759.9
(T-D0003) (M-10000) (F-01452)

DD-62100 Early complication of trauma of unspecified site, NOS 958.-
(T-D0003) (M-10000) (F-01452)

DD-62110 Air embolism as early complication of trauma 958.0
(T-D0003) (M-10000) (F-01452)
(M-35320)
Pneumathemia as early complication of trauma 958.0
(T-D0003) (M-10000) (F-01452)
(M-35320)

DD-62120 Fat embolism as early complication of trauma 958.1
(T-D0003) (M-10000) (F-01452)
(M-35450)

DD-62130 Secondary and recurrent hemorrhage as early complication of trauma 958.2
(T-D0003) (M-10000) (F-01452)
(M-37000)

DD-62140 Posttraumatic wound infection, NEC 958.3
(T-D0003) (M-10000) (F-01452)
(DE-00050)

DD-62150 Traumatic shock, NOS 958.4
Shock following injury, NOS 958.4

DD-62160 Traumatic anuria 958.5

DD-62164 Crush syndrome 958.5
Renal failure following crushing injury 958.5

DD-62200 Volkmann's ischemic contracture following injury 958.6
Posttraumatic muscle contracture following injury 958.6

DD-62300 Traumatic subcutaneous emphysema 958.7
(T-03000) (M-33900) (F-01452) (M-10000)

DD-62400 Other early complication of trauma, NEC 958.8

D-63 LATE EFFECTS OF INJURY

DD-63000 Late effect of injury, NOS 908.9
(T-D0003) (M-10000) (F-01460)

DD-63100 Late effect of musculoskeletal and connective tissue injuries 905.-
(T-10000) (T-1A200) (M-10000) (F-01460)

DD-63110 Late effect of fracture of skull and face bones 905.0
(T-11100) (T-11000) (T-D1200) (M-12000) (F-01460)

DD-63120 Late effect of fracture of spine and trunk without spinal cord lesion 905.1
(T-11500) (T-11000) (T-D2000) (M-12000) (G-C009) (T-A7600) (M-10000) (F-01460)

DD-63130 Late effect of fracture of upper extremities 905.2
(T-11000) (T-D8000) (M-12000) (F-01460)

DD-63140 Late effect of fracture of neck of femur 905.3
(T-12712) (M-12000) (F-01460)

DD-63150 Late effect of fracture of lower extremities 905.4
(T-11000) (T-D9000) (M-12000) (F-01460)

DD-63160 Late effect of fracture of multiple and unspecified bones 905.5
(T-11000) (G-A445) (M-12000) (F-01460)

DD-63170 Late effect of dislocation 905.6
(T-15000) (M-13000) (F-01460)

DD-63180 Late effect of sprain and strain without tendon injury 905.7
(T-15000) (M-13400) (G-C008) (T-17010) (M-10000) (F-01460)

DD-63190 Late effect of tendon injury 905.8
(T-17010) (M-10000) (F-01460)

DD-631A0 Late effect of traumatic amputation 905.9
(T-D2800) (M-17010) (F-01460)

DD-63300 Late effect of injuries to skin and subcutaneous tissues 906.-
(T-01000) (T-03000) (M-10000) (F-01460)

DD-63310 Late effect of open wound of head, neck and trunk 906.0
(T-D1100) (T-D1600) (T-D2000) (M-14010) (F-01460)

DD-63320 Late effect of open wound of extremities without tendon injury 906.1
(T-D8000) (T-D9000) (M-14010) (G-C009) (T-17010) (M-10000) (F-01460)

DD-63330 Late effect of superficial injury 906.2
(T-D0003) (M-10050) (F-01460)

DD-63340 Late effect of contusion 906.3
(T-D0003) (M-14200) (F-01460)

DD-63350 Late effect of crushing injury 906.4
(T-D0003) (M-10400) (F-01460)

DD-63360 Late effect of burns of eye, face, head and neck 906.5
(T-AA000) (T-D1200) (T-D1100) (T-D1600) (M-11100) (F-01460)

DD-63370 Late effect of burn of wrist and hand 906.6
(T-D8600) (T-D8700) (M-11100) (F-01460)

DD-63380 Late effect of burn of other extremities 906.7
(T-D8000) (T-D9000) (M-11100) (F-01460)

DD-63390 Late effect of burns of other specified sites, NEC 906.8
(T-D0000) (M-11180) (F-01460)

DD-633A0 Late effect of burn of unspecified site 906.9
(T-D0003) (M-11100) (F-01460)

DD-63500 Late effect of injuries to the nervous system 907.-
(T-A0000) (M-10000) (F-01460)

DD-63510 Late effect of intracranial injury without skull fracture 907.0
(T-D1400) (M-10060) (G-C009) (M-11100) (F-01460)

DD-63520 Late effect of injury to cranial nerve 907.1
(T-A8000) (M-10000) (F-01460)

DD-63530 Late effect of spinal cord injury 907.2
(T-A7010) (M-10000) (F-01460)

DD-63540 Late effect of injury to nerve roots, spinal plexus and other nerves of trunk 907.3
(T-A7160) (T-A7170) (T-A9000) (T-D2000) (M-10000) (F-01460)

DD-63550 Late effect of injury to peripheral nerve of shoulder girdle and upper limb 907.4
(T-A0500) (T-D2220) (T-D8000) (M-10000) (F-01460)

DD-63560 Late effect of injury to peripheral nerve of pelvic girdle and lower limb 907.5
(T-A0500) (T-D6000) (T-D9000) (M-10000) (F-01460)

DD-63570 Late effect of injury to other and unspecified nerve 907.9
(T-A0500) (M-10000) (F-01460)

DD-63710 Late effect of internal injury to chest 908.0
(T-D3000) (M-10060) (F-01460)

D-63 LATE EFFECTS OF INJURY — Continued

DD-63720 Late effect of internal injury to intra-abdominal organs 908.1
(T-D4030) (M-10060) (F-01460)

DD-63730 Late effect of internal injury to other internal organs 908.2
(T-D0060) (M-10060) (F-01460)

DD-63740 Late effect of injury to blood vessels of head, neck and extremities 908.3
(T-40000) (T-D1100) (T-D1600) (M-10000) (F-01460)

DD-63750 Late effect of injury to blood vessels of thorax, abdomen and pelvis 908.4
(T-40000) (T-D3000) (T-D4000) (T-D6000) (M-10000) (F-01460)

DD-63760 Late effect of foreign body in orifice 908.5
(T-D0090) (M-30400) (F-01460)

DD-63770 Late effect of certain complications of trauma 908.6
(T-D0003) (M-10000) (F-01450) (F-01460)

DD-63900 Late effect of other and unspecified external causes 909.9

DD-63910 Late effect of poisoning due to drug, medicinal or biological substance 909.0

DD-63920 Late effect of toxic effects of nonmedical substances 909.1

DD-63930 Late effect of radiation 909.2

DD-63940 Late effect of complications of surgical and medical care 909.3

DD-63980 Late effect of certain other external causes, NEC 909.4

D-64 EFFECTS OF EXPOSURE TO EXTERNAL CAUSES

DD-64000 Effects of exposure to external cause, NOS

DD-64100 Effects of radiation, NOS 990.-

DD-64110 Effects of radiation therapy 990.-
Radiation sickness 990.-

DD-64112 Complication of phototherapy 990.-

DD-64200 Effects of reduced temperature, NOS 991.9
Effects of freezing or excessive cold, NOS 991.9

DD-64210 Frostbite of face 991.0

DD-64220 Frostbite of hand 991.1

DD-64230 Frostbite of foot 991.2

DD-64240 Frostbite of other site, NEC 991.3

DD-64250 Immersion foot 991.4
Trench foot 991.4

DD-64260 Chilblains 991.5
Erythema pernio 991.5
Perniosis 991.5

DD-64270 Hypothermia due to cold environment 991.6

DD-64280 Effects of reduced temperature, NEC 991.8

DD-64300 Effects of heat or light, NOS 992.9

DD-64310 Heat stroke, NOS 992.0
Heat apoplexy 992.0
Thermoplegia 992.0
Heat exhaustion, NOS 992.5
Heat prostration, NOS 992.5

DD-64312 Heat pyrexia 992.0

DD-64313 Heat syncope 992.1
Heat collapse 992.1

DD-64314 Heat cramps 992.2

DD-64315 Transient heat fatigue 992.6

DD-64318 Heat edema 992.7

DD-64320 Sunstroke, NOS 992.0
Ictus solaris 992.0
Siriasis 992.0

DD-64330 Anhidrotic heat exhaustion 992.3
Heat prostration due to water depletion 992.3

DD-64340 Heat exhaustion due to salt depletion 992.4

DD-64380 Other heat effect, NEC 992.8

DD-64500 Effects of air pressure, NOS 993.9

DD-64510 Otitic barotrauma 993.0
Aero-otitis media 993.0

DD-64512 Effects of high altitude on ears, NOS 993.0

DD-64520 Sinus barotrauma 993.1
Aerosinusitis 993.1

DD-64522 Effects of high altitude on sinuses, NOS 993.1

DD-64540 Effects of high altitude, NOS 993.2
Hypobaropathy 993.2

DD-64541 Anoxia due to high altitude 993.2
(T-28000) (F-60294) (DF-00001) (G-C001) (A-80263)
Alpine sickness 993.2
(T-28000) (F-60294) (DF-00001) (G-C001) (A-80263)
Mountain sickness 993.2
(T-28000) (F-60294) (DF-00001) (G-C001) (A-80263)

DD-64542 Acute mountain sickness 993.2
(T-28000) (F-60294) (DF-00001) (G-C001) (A-80263)
Acosta's disease 993.2
(T-28000) (F-60294) (DF-00001) (G-C001) (A-80263)
Soroche 993.2
(T-28000) (F-60294) (DF-00001) (G-C001) (A-80263)

DD-64543 Subacute mountain sickness 993.2
(T-28000) (F-60294) (DF-00002) (G-C001) (A-80263)

DD-64544 Chronic mountain sickness 993.2
(T-28000) (F-60294) (DF-00003) (G-C001) (A-80263)
Andes disease 993.2
(T-28000) (F-60294) (DF-00003) (G-C001)
Monge's disease 993.2
(T-28000) (F-60294) (DF-00003) (G-C001) (A-80263)

DD-64548V Brisket disease 993.2
(T-28000) (F-60294) (DF-00003) (G-C001) (A-80263)

DD-64560 Caisson disease 993.3
Compressed-air disease 993.3
Decompression sickness 993.3
DD-64562 Bends 993.3
Divers' palsy 993.3
Divers' paralysis 993.3
DD-64570 Effects of air pressure caused by explosion 993.4
DD-64580 Other effect of air pressure, NOS 993.8
DD-64600 Effects of lightning, NOS 994.0
Struck by lightning, NOS 994.0
DD-64602 Shock from lightning, NOS 994.0
DD-64612 Nonfatal submersion, NOS 994.1
Near drowning 994.1
DD-64614 Bathing cramp 994.1
DD-64616 Immersion, NOS 994.1
DD-64640 Exhaustion due to exposure 994.4
DD-64644 Exhaustion due to excessive exertion 994.5
Overexertion 994.5
DD-64650 Motion sickness, NOS 994.6
Travel sickness 994.6
DD-64651 Air sickness 994.6
(T-D0010) (F-52760) (F-51700) (F-42220) (G-C001) (A-80254) (A-52000)
DD-64652 Sea sickness 994.6
(T-D0010) (F-52760) (F-52770) (G-C001) (A-51000) (A-80450)
DD-64653 Car sickness
(T-D0010) (F-52760) (F-52770) (G-C001) (A-80450) (A-50100)
DD-64660 Outerspace sickness
(T-D0010) (F-52760) (G-C001) (A-80450) (A-80500) (A-52500)
DD-64730 Nonfatal effect of electric current, NOS 994.8
DD-64732 Shock from electric current 994.8
DD-64740 Effects of abnormal gravitational (G) forces or states 994.9
Weightlessness 994.9
DD-64800 Adverse effect, NOS, due to correct medicinal substance properly administered 995.2
DD-64810 Allergic reaction, NOS, due to correct medicinal substance properly administered 995.2
Hypersensitivity reaction, NOS, due to correct medicinal substance properly administered 995.2
Drug hypersensitivity, NOS, due to correct medicinal substance properly administered 995.2
Drug reaction, NOS, due to correct medicinal substance properly administered 995.2
DD-64820 Idiosyncrasy, NOS, due to correct medicinal substance properly administered 995.2
DD-64840 Anaphylactic shock, NOS, due to adverse effect of correct medicinal substance properly administered 995.0
Allergic shock, NOS, due to adverse effect of correct medicinal substance properly administered 995.0
Anaphylactic reaction, NOS, due to adverse effect of correct medicinal substance properly administered 995.0
Anaphylaxis, NOS, due to adverse effect of correct medicinal substance properly administered 995.0
DD-64860 Shock due to anesthesia 995.4
DD-64B00 Malignant hyperpyrexia due to anesthesia 995.89
DD-64B10 Malignant hypothermia due to anesthesia 995.89

D-66-67 COMPLICATIONS OF SURGICAL AND MEDICAL CARE

D-660 Complications of Surgical and Medical Care: General Terms

DD-66000 Complication of surgical procedure, NOS 998.9
Misadventure of surgical procedure, NOS 998.9
DD-66010 Complication of transplant 996.-
Complication of graft 996.-
DD-66012 Complication of bypass graft, NOS 996.-
DD-66014 Complication of implant 996.-
DD-66016 Complication of reimplant 996.-
DD-66020 Complication of internal anastomosis 996.-
DD-66030 Complication of internal device, NOS 996.-
DD-66031 Complication of catheter 996.-
DD-66032 Complication of electronic internal device 996.-
DD-66034 Complication of internal fixation device 996.-
DD-66035 Complication of internal prosthetic device 996.-
DD-66080 Complication peculiar to a certain specified procedure, NEC 996.-

D-661 Mechanical Complications of Cardiovascular Devices

DD-66110 Mechanical complication of cardiac device, implant or graft, NOS 996.00
DD-66111 Mechanical breakdown of cardiac device, NOS 996.00
DD-66112 Displacement of cardiac device 996.00
DD-66113 Leakage of cardiac device 996.00
DD-66114 Mechanical obstruction of cardiac device 996.00
DD-66115 Perforation of cardiac device 996.00
DD-66116 Protrusion of cardiac device 996.00
DD-66120 Mechanical complication due to cardiac pacemaker (electrode) 996.01
DD-66130 Mechanical complication due to heart valve prosthesis 996.02
DD-66140 Mechanical complication due to coronary bypass graft 996.03
DD-66142 Mechanical complication of other vascular device, implant or graft, NOS 996.1
DD-66161 Mechanical complication of aortic graft 996.1
DD-66162 Mechanical complication of arteriovenous fistula surgically created 996.1
Mechanical complication of arteriovenous shunt surgically created 996.1

D-661 Mechanical Complications of Cardiovascular Devices — Continued

DD-66164 Mechanical complication of intra-aortic balloon device 996.1

DD-66165 Mechanical complication of carotid artery bypass graft 996.1

DD-66166 Mechanical complication of dialysis catheter 996.1

DD-66167 Mechanical complication of umbrella device of vena cava 996.1

D-662 Mechanical Complications of Nervous System Devices

DD-66200 Mechanical complication of nervous system device, implant or graft, NOS 996.2

DD-66202 Mechanical complication of dorsal column stimulator 996.2

DD-66203 Mechanical complication of electrodes implanted in brain 996.2

DD-66204 Mechanical complication of peripheral nerve graft 996.2

DD-66207 Mechanical complication of ventricular communicating shunt 996.2

D-663 Mechanical Complications of Genitourinary Devices

DD-66300 Mechanical complication of genitourinary device, implant or graft, NOS 996.30

DD-66310 Mechanical complication due to urethral indwelling catheter 996.31

DD-66320 Mechanical complication due to intrauterine contraceptive device 996.32

DD-66330 Mechanical complication due to cystostomy catheter 996.39

DD-66340 Mechanical complication due to prosthetic reconstruction of vas deferens 996.39

DD-66350 Mechanical complication due to repair of ureter without resection 996.39

D-664 Mechanical Complications of Internal Orthopedic Devices

DD-66400 Mechanical complication of internal orthopedic device, implant or graft, NOS 996.4

DD-66410 Mechanical complication of graft of bone, cartilage, muscle or tendon 996.4

DD-66420 Mechanical complication of internal fixation device such as nail, plate or rod 996.4

D-665 Mechanical Complications of Other Devices

DD-66500 Mechanical complication of other specified device, implant or graft, NOS 996.5

DD-66510 Mechanical complication due to corneal graft 996.51

DD-66520 Mechanical complication due to skin graft failure or rejection 996.52

DD-66530 Mechanical complication due to ocular lens prosthesis, NOS 996.53

DD-66540 Mechanical complication due to breast prosthesis, NOS 996.54
  Mechanical complication due to breast implant 996.54

DD-66550 Mechanical complication due to other implant or internal device, NOS 996.59

DD-66560 Mechanical complication of prosthetic implant in bile duct 996.59

DD-66570 Mechanical complication of prosthetic implant in chin 996.59

DD-66580 Mechanical complication of prosthetic implant in orbit of eye 996.59

D-666 Infections and Inflammatory Reactions Due to Internal Devices

DD-66600 Infection or inflammatory reaction due to internal prosthetic device, implant or graft, NOS 996.6

DD-66620 Thrombus due to any device, implant or graft 996.7

DD-66622 Embolism due to any device, implant or graft 996.7

DD-66630 Stenosis due to any device, implant or graft 996.7

DD-66632 Fibrosis due to any device, implant or graft 996.7

DD-66640 Hemorrhage due to any device, implant or graft 996.7

DD-66650 Pain due to any device, implant or graft 996.7

D-667 Complications of Transplanted Organs

DD-66700 Complication of transplanted organ, NOS 996.80
  Transplant rejection 996.80
  Transplant failure due to rejection 996.80

DD-66710 Complication of transplanted kidney 996.81

DD-66720 Complication of transplanted liver 996.82

DD-66730 Complication of transplanted heart 996.83

DD-66740 Complication of transplanted lung 996.84

DD-66750 Complication of transplanted pancreas 996.86

DD-66760 Complication of transplanted intestines 996.89

DD-66780 Complication of other specified transplanted organ, NEC 996.89

D-668 Complications of Reattached Extremity or Body Part

DD-66800 Complication of reattached extremity or body part, NOS 996.9

DD-66810 Complication of reattached forearm 996.91

DD-66820 Complication of reattached hand 996.92

DD-66830 Complication of reattached finger 996.93

DD-66840 Complication of reattached upper extremity, NOS 996.94

DD-66859 Complication of reattached foot and toe 996.95

DD-66860 Complication of reattached lower extremity, NOS 996.96

DD-66880 Complication of other attached specified body part 996.99

D-669 Other Complications of Specified Body Systems

DD-66900 Complication affecting specified body system, NEC 997.-

DD-66910 Central nervous system complication, NOS 997.0

DD-66912 Anoxic brain damage during or resulting from a procedure 997.0
  Cerebral hypoxia during or resulting from a procedure 997.0

DD-66920 Cardiac complication, NOS 997.1

DD-66922 Cardiac arrest during or resulting from a procedure 997.1

DD-66923 Cardiac insufficiency during or resulting from a procedure 997.1
  Heart failure during or resulting from a procedure 997.1

DD-66928 Cardiorespiratory failure during or resulting from a procedure 997.1

DD-66930 Peripheral vascular complication, NOS 997.2

DD-66932 Phlebitis or thrombophlebitis during or resulting from a procedure 997.2

DD-66940 Respiratory complication, NOS 997.3

DD-66942 Mendelson's syndrome resulting from a procedure 997.3

DD-66944 Aspiration pneumonia resulting from a procedure 997.3

DD-66950 Gastrointestinal complication, NOS 997.4

DD-66952 Complication of external stoma of gastrointestinal tract, NEC 997.4

DD-66954 Complication of internal intestinal anastomosis and bypass, NEC 997.4

DD-66955 Hepatic failure specified as due to a procedure 997.4

DD-66956 Hepatorenal syndrome specified as due to a procedure 997.4

DD-66958 Intestinal obstruction, NOS, specified as due to a procedure 997.4

DD-66960 Urinary complication, NOS 997.5

DD-66962 Complication of external stoma of urinary tract 997.5

DD-66963 Complication of internal anastomosis and bypass of urinary tract including that involving intestinal tract 997.5

DD-66964 Oliguria or anuria specified as due to procedure 997.5

DD-66966 Acute renal failure specified as due to procedure 997.5
  Acute renal insufficiency specified as due to procedure 997.5
  Acute tubular necrosis specified as due to procedure 997.5

DD-66970 Late amputation stump complication, NOS 997.60

DD-66972 Neuroma of amputation stump 997.61
  Amputation neuroma 997.61

DD-66974 Chronic infection as complication of amputation 997.62

DD-66980 Vitreous touch syndrome 997.9

D-66A Complications of Procedures, NEC

DD-66A00 Complication of procedure, NEC 998.-

DD-66A05 Complication of administrative procedure, NOS

DD-66A10 Postoperative shock, NOS 998.0
  Shock, NOS, during or resulting from a surgical procedure 998.0

DD-66A20 Hemorrhage or hematoma complicating procedure 998.1

DD-66A30 Accidental puncture or laceration during a procedure, NOS 998.2

DD-66A32 Accidental puncture or laceration during a procedure on a blood vessel 998.2

DD-66A34 Accidental puncture or laceration during a procedure on a nerve 998.2

DD-66A36 Accidental puncture or laceration during a procedure on an organ 998.2

DD-66A40 Disruption of operation wound 998.3
  Dehiscence of operation wound 998.3
  Rupture of operation wound 998.3

DD-66A50 Foreign body accidentally left during a procedure, NOS 998.4

DD-66A52 Adhesions due to foreign body accidentally left in operative wound or body cavity during a procedure 998.4

DD-66A54 Obstruction due to foreign body accidentally left in operative wound or body cavity during a procedure 998.4

DD-66A56 Perforation due to foreign body accidentally left in operative wound or body cavity during a procedure 998.4

DD-66A60 Postoperative infection 998.5

DD-66A61 Postoperative intra-abdominal abscess 998.5

DD-66A62 Postoperative stitch abscess 998.5

DD-66A63 Postoperative subphrenic abscess 998.5

DD-66A64 Postoperative wound abscess 998.5

DD-66A68 Postoperative septicemia 998.5

DD-66A70 Persistent postoperative fistula 998.6

DD-66A80 Acute reaction to foreign substance accidentally left during a procedure 998.7

DD-66A82 Aseptic peritonitis following a procedure 998.7

DD-66A84 Chemical peritonitis following a procedure 998.7

DD-66A90 Subcutaneous emphysema resulting from a procedure 998.8

DD-66A99 Postoperative complication, NOS 998.9

D-67 COMPLICATIONS OF MEDICAL CARE

DD-67000 Complication of medical care, NOS 999.-

D-67 COMPLICATIONS OF MEDICAL CARE — Continued

DD-67010 Complication of electroshock therapy 999.9
DD-67020 Complication of inhalation therapy 999.9
DD-67030 Complication of ultrasound therapy 999.9
DD-67050 Complication of ventilation therapy 999.9
DD-67100 Complication of dialysis 999.-
DD-67101 Complication of hemodialysis 999.-
DD-67102 Complication of peritoneal dialysis 999.-
DD-67103 Complication of renal dialysis 999.-
DD-67110 Complication of extracorporeal circulation 999.-
DD-67200 Vascular complication of medical care, NOS 999.2
DD-67210 Phlebitis following infusion, perfusion or transfusion 999.2
DD-67220 Thrombophlebitis following infusion, perfusion or transfusion 999.2
DD-67230 Thromboembolism following infusion, perfusion or transfusion 999.2
DD-67300 Complication of injection, NOS 999.-
DD-67310 Complication of infusion, NOS 999.-
DD-67320 Complication of perfusion, NOS 999.-
DD-67330 Air embolism complicating injection 999.1
DD-67400 Complication due to immunization, NOS 999.-
DD-67410 Complication due to vaccination, NOS 999.-
  Complication due to inoculation, NOS 999.-
DD-67480 Complication of preventive medicine procedure, NOS
DD-67700 Infection as complication of medical care, NOS 999.3
DD-67710 Sepsis following infusion, injection, transfusion or vaccination 999.3
  Septicemia following infusion, injection, transfusion or vaccination 999.3
DD-67712 Infection following infusion, injection, transfusion or vaccination 999.3

D-68-69 BLOOD TRANSFUSION REACTIONS

DD-68000 Blood transfusion reaction, NOS 999.8
  Complication of blood transfusion, NOS 999.8
  Transfusion reaction, NOS 999.8
DD-68010 Hemolytic transfusion reaction, NOS
DD-68012 Immediate hemolytic transfusion reaction
DD-68014 Delayed hemolytic transfusion reaction
DD-68020 Febrile transfusion reaction
  Transfusion reaction chill fever type
DD-68030 Transfusion reaction due to leukagglutinins
  Transfusion reaction mediated by HLA antibody
DD-68040 Transfusion reaction due to platelet antibody
DD-68050 Urticarial transfusion reaction
  Allergic transfusion reaction
  Transfusion reaction due to allergens in blood
DD-68054 Anaphylactic transfusion reaction, NOS
  Anaphylactic shock due to serum 999.4
DD-68060 Transfusion reaction due to serum protein reaction, NOS
  Serum reaction 999.5
  Intoxication by serum 999.5
  Protein sickness 999.5
  Serum rash 999.5
  Serum sickness 999.5
  Urticaria due to serum 999.5
DD-68064 Transfusion reaction due to IgA
DD-68070 Transfusion reaction due to excess volume
DD-68072 Transfusion reaction due to toxic effect of anticoagulants
DD-68074 Transfusion reaction due to products of cell metabolism
DD-68076 Transfusion reaction due to air embolism
DD-68080 Transfusion reaction due to faulty storage of blood
DD-68082 Transfusion reaction due to toxic substance in blood
  Transfusion reaction due to contaminant in blood
DD-68086 Septic shock due to transfusion 999.8
DD-68090 Transfusion reaction due to clerical error
DD-69000 Transfusion reaction due to isoantibody, NOS
DD-69010 Transfusion reaction due to specific isoantibody
DD-69012 Transfusion reaction due to minor incompatibility
DD-69020 ABO incompatibility reaction 999.6
  Incompatible blood transfusion 999.6
  Reaction to blood group incompatibility in transfusion 999.6
DD-69022 Transfusion reaction due to anti A
    (F-51610)
DD-69024 Transfusion reaction due to anti B
    (F-51630)
DD-69050 Rh incompatibility reaction 999.7
  Reaction due to Rh factor in infusion or transfusion 999.7

SECTION D-8 POISONINGS

D-80 POISONINGS: GENERAL TYPES

DD-80000 Poisoning, NOS
  Poisoning syndrome, NOS
  Poisoning by
  Toxicosis, NOS
DD-80010 Accidental poisoning
DD-80012 Self-administered accidental poisoning
DD-80020 Suicidal deliberate poisoning
DD-80030 Homocidal deliberate poisoning
DD-80050 Toxic effect
  Toxicity
  Toxic effect of

D-81-82 POISONING BY DRUGS AND BIOLOGICALS

D-811 Poisoning by Nonantibiotic Anti-Infectives

DD-81100 Poisoning by nonantibiotic anti-infective, NOS 961.9
(DD-80000) (C-52000)

DD-81110 Poisoning by sulfonamide, NOS 961.0
(DD-80000) (C-55900)

DD-81112 Poisoning by sulfadiazine 961.0
(DD-80000) (C-55920)

DD-81114 Poisoning by sulfafurazole 961.0
(DD-80000) (C-55970)
Poisoning by sulfisoxazole 961.0
(DD-80000) (C-55970)

DD-81116 Poisoning by sulfamethoxazole 961.0
(DD-80000) (C-55940)

DD-81130 Poisoning by heavy metal anti-infective, NOS 961.2
(DD-80000) (C-52000) (C-11820)

DD-81140 Poisoning by arsenical anti-infective, NOS 961.1
(DD-80000) (C-52000) (C-11500)

DD-81142 Poisoning by anti-infective compound of antimony 961.2
(DD-80000) (C-52000) (C-12100)

DD-81144 Poisoning by anti-infective compound of bismuth 961.2
(DD-80000) (C-52000) (C-12500)

DD-81146 Poisoning by anti-infective compound of lead 961.2
(DD-80000) (C-52000) (C-13200)

DD-81148 Poisoning by anti-infective compound of mercury 961.2
(DD-80000) (C-52000) (C-13300)

DD-81150 Poisoning by quinoline and hydroxyquinoline derivative 961.3
(DD-80000) (C-21743) (C-21740)

DD-81154 Poisoning by chiniofon 961.3
(DD-80000) (C-56320)

DD-81156 Poisoning by diiodohydroxyquin 961.3
(DD-80000) (C-56120)

DD-81160 Poisoning by antiprotozoal drug, NOS 961.4
(DD-80000) (C-56010)

DD-81161 Poisoning by antimalarial drug, NOS 961.4
(DD-80000) (C-56500)

DD-81162 Poisoning by chloroquine 961.4
(DD-80000) (C-56510)

DD-81163 Poisoning by cycloguanil 961.4
(DD-80000) (C-56574)

DD-81164 Poisoning by primaquine 961.4
(DD-80000) (C-56530)

DD-81165 Poisoning by proguanil 961.4
(DD-80000) (C-56570)
Poisoning by chlorguanide 961.4
(DD-80000) (C-56570)

DD-81166 Poisoning by quinine 961.4
(DD-80000) (C-56550)

DD-81167 Poisoning by pyrimethamine 961.4
(DD-80000) (C-56540)

DD-81168 Poisoning by emetine 961.5
(DD-80000) (C-56110)

DD-81180 Poisoning by anthelmintic, NOS 961.6
(DD-80000) (C-56A00)

DD-81181 Poisoning by hexylresorcinol 961.6
(DD-80000) (C-56A93)

DD-81182 Poisoning by piperazine 961.6
(DD-80000) (C-51800)

DD-81183 Poisoning by thiabendazole 961.6
(DD-80000) (C-56A80)

DD-81190 Poisoning by antiviral drug, NOS 961.7
(DD-80000) (C-55B00)

DD-81191 Poisoning by methisazone 961.7
(DD-80000) (C-55B70)

DD-811A0 Poisoning by antimycobacterial drug, NOS 961.8
(DD-80000) (C-55200)

DD-811A1 Poisoning by ethambutol 961.8
(DD-80000) (C-55240)

DD-811A2 Poisoning by ethionamide 961.8
(DD-80000) (C-55250)

DD-811A3 Poisoning by isoniazid 961.8
(DD-80000) (C-55260)

DD-811A4 Poisoning by para-aminosalicyclic acid derivative 961.8
(DD-80000) (C-55210)

DD-811A5 Poisoning by sulfone 961.8
(DD-80000) (C-55D00)

DD-811C0 Poisoning by flucytosine 961.9
(DD-80000) (C-52B30)

DD-811C1 Poisoning by nitrofuran derivatives 961.9
(DD-80000) (C-55620)

DD-811C2 Poisoning by unspecified anti-infective, NOS 961.9
(DD-80000) (C-52000)

D-812 Poisoning by Antibiotics

DD-81200 Poisoning by antibiotic, NOS 960.9
(DD-80000) (C-52200)

DD-81210 Poisoning by penicillin, NOS 960.0
(DD-80000) (C-54000)

DD-81211 Poisoning by ampicillin 960.0
(DD-80000) (C-54640)

DD-81212 Poisoning by carbenicillin 960.0
(DD-80000) (C-54910)

DD-81213 Poisoning by cloxacillin 960.0
(DD-80000) (C-54420)

DD-81214 Poisoning by penicillin G 960.0
(DD-80000) (C-54220)

DD-81220 Poisoning by antifungal antibiotic, NOS 960.1
(DD-80000) (C-52B00)

DD-81221 Poisoning by amphotericin B 960.1
(DD-80000) (C-52B20)

DD-81222 Poisoning by griseofulvin 960.1
(DD-80000) (C-52B40)

D-812 Poisoning by Antibiotics — Continued

DD-81223 Poisoning by nystatin 960.1
(DD-80000) (C-52B70)

DD-81224 Poisoning by trichomycin 960.1
(DD-80000) (C-52BB0)

DD-81230 Poisoning by chloramphenicol group antibiotic, NOS 960.2
(DD-80000) (C-52800)

DD-81231 Poisoning by chloramphenicol 960.2
(DD-80000) (C-52800)

DD-81232 Poisoning by thiamphenicol 960.2
(DD-80000) (C-52810)

DD-81240 Poisoning by erythromycin or other macrolide, NOS 960.3
(DD-80000) (C-52A00)

DD-81241 Poisoning by oleandomycin 960.3
(DD-80000) (C-522B9)

DD-81242 Poisoning by spiramycin 960.3
(DD-80000) (C-522B5)

DD-81250 Poisoning by tetracycline group antibiotic, NOS 960.4
(DD-80000) (C-55000)

DD-81251 Poisoning by doxycycline 960.4
(DD-80000) (C-55020)

DD-81252 Poisoning by minocycline 960.4
(DD-80000) (C-55040)

DD-81253 Poisoning by oxytetracycline 960.4
(DD-80000) (C-55050)

DD-81260 Poisoning by cephalosporin group antiobiotic, NOS 960.5
(DD-80000) (C-53000)

DD-81261 Poisoning by cephalexin 960.5
(DD-80000) (C-53130)

DD-81262 Poisoning by cephaloglycin 960.5
(DD-80000) (C-53020)

DD-81263 Poisoning by cephaloridine 960.5
(DD-80000) (C-53010)

DD-81264 Poisoning by cephalothin 960.5
(DD-80000) (C-53140)

DD-81270 Poisoning by antimycobacterial antibiotic, NOS 960.6
(DD-80000) (C-55200)

DD-81271 Poisoning by cycloserine 960.6
(DD-80000) (C-55230)

DD-81272 Poisoning by kanamycin 960.6
(DD-80000) (C-52540)

DD-81273 Poisoning by rifampin 960.6
(DD-80000) (C-55280)

DD-81274 Poisoning by streptomycin 960.6
(DD-80000) (C-52570)

DD-81280 Poisoning by antineoplastic antibiotic, NOS 960.7
(DD-80000) (C-78003)

DD-81281 Poisoning by actinomycin, NOS 960.7
(DD-80000) (C-780A0)
Poisoning by dactinomycin 960.7
(DD-80000) (C-780A0)

DD-81282 Poisoning by cactinomycin 960.7
(DD-80000) (C-780A1)

DD-81284 Poisoning by bleomycin 960.7
(DD-80000) (C-78020)

DD-81285 Poisoning by daunorubicin 960.7
(DD-80000) (C-780B0)

DD-81286 Poisoning by mitomycin 960.7
(DD-80000) (C-78190)

DD-81290 Poisoning by other antibiotic, NEC 960.8
(DD-80000) (C-52200)

D-813 Poisoning by Hormones and Synthetic Substitutes

DD-81300 Poisoning by hormone or synthetic substitute, NOS 962.9
(DD-80000)

DD-81310 Poisoning by adrenal cortical steroid 962.0
(DD-80000)

DD-81311 Poisoning by cortisone derivative 962.0
(DD-80000)

DD-81312 Poisoning by desoxycorticosterone derivative 962.0
(DD-80000)

DD-81313 Poisoning by fluorinated corticosteroid 962.0
(DD-80000)

DD-81320 Poisoning by androgen or anabolic congener, NOS 962.1
(DD-80000)

DD-81321 Poisoning by methandriol 962.1
(DD-80000)

DD-81322 Poisoning by nandrolone 962.1
(DD-80000)

DD-81323 Poisoning by oxymetholone 962.1
(DD-80000)

DD-81324 Poisoning by testosterone 962.1
(DD-80000)

DD-81340 Poisoning by ovarian hormone or synthetic substitute, NOS 962.2
(DD-80000)

DD-81341 Poisoning by oral contraceptive 962.2
(DD-80000)

DD-81342 Poisoning by estrogen 962.2
(DD-80000) (C-A0900)
Estrogen toxicity
(DD-80000) (C-A0900)

DD-81343 Poisoning by progestogen 962.2
(DD-80000)

DD-81344 Poisoning by combined estrogen and progestogen 962.2
(DD-80000)

DD-81345 Diethylstilbestrol poisoning 962.2
(DD-80000) (C-A0930)

DD-81350 Poisoning by insulin or antidiabetic agent, NOS 926.3
(DD-80000)

DD-81351 Poisoning by acetohexamide 962.3
(DD-80000)

DD-81352 Poisoning by oral biguanide derivative 962.3
(DD-80000)

DD-81353 Poisoning by chlorpropamide 962.3
(DD-80000)

DD-81354 Poisoning by glucagon 962.3
(DD-80000)

DD-81355 Poisoning by insulin 962.3
(DD-80000)

DD-81356 Poisoning by phenformin 962.3
(DD-80000)

DD-81357 Poisoning by oral sulfonylurea derivative 962.3
(DD-80000)

DD-81358 Poisoning by tolbutamide 962.3
(DD-80000)

DD-81370 Poisoning by pituitary hormone, NOS 962.4
(DD-80000)

DD-81371 Poisoning by anterior pituitary hormone, NOS 962.4
(DD-80000)

DD-81372 Poisoning by corticotropin 962.4
(DD-80000)

DD-81373 Poisoning by gonadotropin 962.4
(DD-80000)

DD-81374 Poisoning by somatotropin 962.4
(DD-80000)
Poisoning by growth hormone 962.4
(DD-80000)

DD-81376 Poisoning by posterior pituitary hormone, NOS 962.5
(DD-80000)

DD-81377 Poisoning by vasopressin 962.5
(DD-80000)

DD-81380 Poisoning by parathyroid hormone or parathyroid derivative, NOS 962.6
(DD-80000)

DD-81390 Poisoning by thyroid hormone or thyroid derivative, NOS 962.7
(DD-80000)

DD-81391 Poisoning by dextrothyroxin 962.7
(DD-80000)

DD-81392 Poisoning by levothyroxine sodium 962.7
(DD-80000)

DD-81393 Poisoning by liothyronine 962.7
(DD-80000)

DD-81394 Poisoning by thyroglobulin 962.7
(DD-80000)

DD-813A0 Poisoning by antithyroid agent, NOS 962.8
(DD-80000)

DD-813A1 Poisoning by iodide 962.8
(DD-80000)

DD-813A2 Poisoning by thiouracil 962.8
(DD-80000)

DD-813A3 Poisoning by thiourea 962.8
(DD-80000)

D-814 Poisoning by Systemic Agents

DD-81400 Poisoning by primarily systemic agent, NOS 963.9
(DD-80000)
Poisoning by unspecified systemic agent, NOS 963.9
(DD-80000)

DD-81410 Poisoning by antiallergic and antiemetic drug, NOS 963.0
(DD-80000)

DD-81412 Poisoning by antihistamine 963.0
(DD-80000)

DD-81413 Poisoning by chlorpheniramine 963.0
(DD-80000)

DD-81414 Poisoning by diphenhydramine 963.0
(DD-80000)

DD-81415 Poisoning by diphenylpyraline 963.0
(DD-80000)

DD-81416 Poisoning by thonzylamine 963.0
(DD-80000)

DD-81417 Poisoning by tripelennamine 963.0
(DD-80000)

DD-81430 Poisoning by antineoplastic and immunosuppressive drug, NOS 963.1
(DD-80000)

DD-81431 Poisoning by azathioprine 963.1
(DD-80000)

DD-81432 Poisoning by busulfan 963.1
(DD-80000)

DD-81433 Poisoning by chlorambucil 963.1
(DD-80000)

DD-81434 Poisoning by cyclophosphamide 963.1
(DD-80000)

DD-81435 Poisoning by cytarabine 963.1
(DD-80000)

DD-81436 Poisoning by fluorouracil 963.1
(DD-80000)

DD-81437 Poisoning by mercaptopurine 963.1
(DD-80000)

DD-81438 Poisoning by thio-TEPA 963.1
(DD-80000)

DD-81450 Poisoning by acidifying agent, NOS 963.2
(DD-80000)

DD-81455 Poisoning by alkalinizing agent, NOS 963.3
(DD-80000)

DD-81460 Poisoning by enzyme, NEC 963.4
(DD-80000)

DD-81461 Poisoning by penicillinase 963.4
(DD-80000)

DD-81470 Poisoning by vitamin, NEC 963.5
(DD-80000)

DD-81471 Poisoning by vitamin A 963.5
(DD-80000) (C-BB010)
Vitamin A toxicity 963.5
(DD-80000) (C-BB010)

DD-81472 Poisoning by vitamin D 963.5
(DD-80000) (C-BB070)
Vitamin D toxicity 963.5
(DD-80000) (C-BB070)

D-814 Poisoning by Systemic Agents — Continued

DD-81480 Poisoning by heavy metal antagonist, NOS 963.8
(DD-80000)

D-815 Poisoning by Agents Affecting Blood Constituents

DD-81500 Poisoning by agent primarily affecting blood constituent, NOS 964.9
(DD-80000)

DD-81510 Poisoning by iron and its compounds, NOS 964.0
(DD-80000)

DD-81511 Poisoning by ferric salt, NOS 964.0
(DD-80000)

DD-81512 Poisoning by ferrous salt, NOS 964.0
(DD-80000)

DD-81513 Poisoning by ferrous sulfate, NOS 964.0
(DD-80000)

DD-81520 Poisoning by liver preparation or other antianemic agent, NOS 964.1
(DD-80000)

DD-81522 Poisoning by folic acid 964.1
(DD-80000)

DD-81530 Poisoning by anticoagulant, NOS 964.2
(DD-80000)

DD-81531 Poisoning by coumarin 964.2
(DD-80000)

DD-81532 Poisoning by heparin 964.2
(DD-80000)

DD-81533 Poisoning by phenindione 964.2
(DD-80000)

DD-81534 Poisoning by warfarin sodium 964.2
(DD-80000)
Warfarin toxicity 964.2

DD-81540 Poisoning by vitamin K 964.3
(DD-80000) (C-BB180)
Poisoning by phytonadione 964.3
(DD-80000) (C-BB180)
Vitamin K toxicity 964.3
(DD-80000) (C-BB180)
Hypervitaminosis K 964.3
(DD-80000) (C-BB180)

DD-81550 Poisoning by fibrinolysis-affecting drug, NOS 964.4
(DD-80000)

DD-81551 Poisoning by aminocaproic acid 964.4
(DD-80000)

DD-81552 Poisoning by streptodornase 964.4
(DD-80000)

DD-81553 Poisoning by streptokinase 964.4
(DD-80000)

DD-81554 Poisoning by urokinase 964.4
(DD-80000)

DD-81560 Poisoning by anticoagulant antagonist, NOS 964.5
(DD-80000)

DD-81561 Poisoning by hexadimethrine 964.5
(DD-80000)

DD-81562 Poisoning by protamine sulfate 964.5
(DD-80000)

DD-81570 Poisoning by natural blood or blood product, NOS 964.7
(DD-80000)

DD-81571 Poisoning by blood plasma 964.7
(DD-80000)

DD-81572 Poisoning by human fibrinogen 964.7
(DD-80000)

DD-81573 Poisoning by packed red cells 964.7
(DD-80000)

DD-81574 Poisoning by whole blood 964.7
(DD-80000)

DD-81580 Poisoning by gamma globulin 964.6
(DD-80000)

DD-81584 Poisoning by macromolecular blood substitute 964.8
(DD-80000)

DD-81586 Poisoning by plasma expander 964.8
(DD-80000)

D-816 Poisoning by Analgesics, Antipyretics and Antirheumatics

DD-81600 Poisoning by analgesic or antipyretic, NOS 965.9
(DD-80000)

DD-81610 Poisoning by opiate or related narcotic, NOS 965.0
(DD-80000)
Opiate poisoning 965.0

DD-81611 Poisoning by opium alkakoid, NOS 965.00
(DD-80000)

DD-81612 Poisoning by heroin 965.01
(DD-80000)
Poisoning by diacetylmorphine 965.01
(DD-80000)

DD-81614 Poisoning by methadone 965.02
(DD-80000)

DD-81615 Poisoning by codeine 965.09
(DD-80000)
Poisoning by methylmorphine 965.09
(DD-80000)

DD-81616 Poisoning by meperidine 965.09
(DD-80000)
Poisoning by pethidine 965.09
(DD-80000)

DD-81617 Poisoning by morphine 965.09
(DD-80000)

DD-81630 Poisoning by salicylate, NOS 965.1
(DD-80000)

DD-81631 Poisoning by acetylsalicylic acid 965.1
(DD-80000)
Poisoning by aspirin 965.1
(DD-80000)

DD-81632 Poisoning by salicylic acid salt, NOS 965.1
(DD-80000)

DD-81640 Poisoning by aromatic analgesic, NEC 965.4
(DD-80000)

DD-81641 Poisoning by acetanilid 965.4
(DD-80000)

DD-81642 Poisoning by paracetamol 965.4
(DD-80000)
Poisoning by acetaminophen 965.4
(DD-80000)

DD-81643 Poisoning by phenacetin 965.4
(DD-80000)
Poisoning by acetophenetidin 965.4
(DD-80000)

DD-81650 Poisoning by pyrazole derivative, NOS 965.5
(DD-80000)

DD-81651 Poisoning by aminophenazone 965.5
(DD-80000)
Poisoning by aminopyrine 965.5
(DD-80000)

DD-81652 Poisoning by phenylbutazone 965.5
(DD-80000)

DD-81660 Poisoning by antirheumatic, NEC 965.6
(DD-80000)
Poisoning by antiphlogistic, NEC 965.6
(DD-80000)

DD-81662 Poisoning by gold salt, NOS 965.6
(DD-80000)

DD-81664 Poisoning by indomethacin 965.6
(DD-80000)

DD-81680 Poisoning by other analgesic or antipyretic, NEC 965.8
(DD-80000)

DD-81681 Poisoning by pentazocine 965.8
(DD-80000)

D-817 Poisoning by Anticonvulsants and Anti-Parkinsonism Drugs

DD-81700 Poisoning by anticonvulsant, NOS 966.3
(DD-80000)

DD-81710 Poisoning by oxazolidine derivative, NOS 966.0
(DD-80000)

DD-81711 Poisoning by paramethadione 966.0
(DD-80000)

DD-81712 Poisoning by trimethadione 966.0
(DD-80000)

DD-81720 Poisoning by hydantoin derivative, NOS 966.1
(DD-80000)

DD-81721 Poisoning by phenytoin 966.1
(DD-80000)

DD-81730 Poisoning by succinimide, NOS 966.2
(DD-80000)

DD-81731 Poisoning by ethosuximide 966.2
(DD-80000)

DD-81732 Poisoning by phensuximide 966.2
(DD-80000)

DD-81740 Poisoning by other anticonvulsant, NEC 966.3
(DD-80000)

DD-81741 Poisoning by primidone 966.3
(DD-80000)

DD-81760 Poisoning by anti-parkinsonism drug, NOS 966.4
(DD-80000)

DD-81761 Poisoning by amantadine 966.4
(DD-80000)

DD-81762 Poisoning by ethopropazine 966.4
(DD-80000)
Poisoning by profenamine 966.4
(DD-80000)

DD-81763 Poisoning by levodopa 966.4
(DD-80000)
Poisoning by L-dopa 966.4
(DD-80000)

D-818 Poisoning by Sedatives and Hypnotics

DD-81800 Poisoning by sedative or hypnotic, NOS 967.9
(DD-80000)
Poisoning by sleeping drug, NOS 967.9
(DD-80000)
Poisoning by sleeping pill, NOS 967.9
(DD-80000)
Poisoning by sleeping tablet, NOS 967.9
(DD-80000)

DD-81810 Poisoning by barbiturate, NOS 967.0
(DD-80000)

DD-81811 Poisoning by amobarbital 967.0
(DD-80000)
Poisoning by amylobarbitone 967.0
(DD-80000)

DD-81812 Poisoning by barbital 967.0
(DD-80000)
Poisoning by barbitone 967.0
(DD-80000)

DD-81813 Poisoning by butabarbital 967.0
(DD-80000)
Poisoning by butabarbitone 967.0
(DD-80000)

DD-81814 Poisoning by pentobarbital 967.0
(DD-80000)
Poisoning by pentobarbitone 967.0
(DD-80000)

DD-81815 Poisoning by phenobarbital 967.0
(DD-80000)
Poisoning by phenobarbitone 967.0
(DD-80000)

DD-81816 Poisoning by secobarbital 967.0
(DD-80000)
Poisoning by quinalbarbitone 967.0
(DD-80000)

DD-81830 Poisoning by chloral hydrate group, NOS 967.1
(DD-80000)

D-818 Poisoning by Sedatives and Hypnotics — Continued

DD-81840 Poisoning by paraldehyde 967.2
(DD-80000)

DD-81850 Poisoning by bromine compound, NOS 967.3
(DD-80000)

DD-81851 Poisoning by bromide, NOS 967.3
(DD-80000)

DD-81852 Poisoning by carbromal derivative, NOS 967.3
(DD-80000)

DD-81860 Poisoning by methaqualone compound, NOS 967.4
(DD-80000)

DD-81870 Poisoning by glutethimide group, NOS 967.5
(DD-80000)

DD-81880 Poisoning by mixed sedative, NEC 967.6
(DD-80000)

DD-81890 Poisoning by other sedative or hypnotic, NEC 967.8
(DD-80000)

D-819 Poisoning by Anesthetics and Muscle-Tone Depressants

DD-81900 Poisoning by anesthetic or muscle-tone depressant, NOS 968.-
(DD-80000)

DD-81910 Poisoning by gaseous anesthetic, NOS 968.2
(DD-80000)

DD-81911 Poisoning by ether 968.2
(DD-80000)

DD-81912 Poisoning by halogenated hydrocarbon derivative, NOS 968.2
(DD-80000)

DD-81913 Poisoning by nitrous oxide, NOS 968.2
(DD-80000)

DD-81914 Poisoning by halothane 968.1
(DD-80000)

DD-81920 Poisoning by intravenous anesthetic, NOS 968.3
(DD-80000)

DD-81921 Poisoning by ketamine 968.3
(DD-80000)

DD-81922 Poisoning by methohexital 968.3
(DD-80000)
Poisoning by methohexitone 968.3
(DD-80000)

DD-81925 Poisoning by thiobarbiturate, NOS 968.3
(DD-80000)

DD-81926 Poisoning by thiopental sodium 968.3
(DD-80000)

DD-81930 Poisoning by surface (topical) or infiltration anesthetic, NOS 968.5
(DD-80000)

DD-81941 Poisoning by cocaine 968.5
(DD-80000)

DD-81942 Poisoning by lidocaine 968.5
(DD-80000)
Poisoning by lignocaine 968.5
(DD-80000)

DD-81943 Poisoning by procaine 968.5
(DD-80000)

DD-81944 Poisoning by tetracaine 968,5
(DD-80000)

DD-81950 Poisoning by peripheral nerve and plexus-blocking anesthetic, NOS 968.6
(DD-80000)

DD-81960 Poisoning by spinal anesthetic, NOS 968.7
(DD-80000)

DD-81970 Poisoning by local anesthetic, NEC 968.9
(DD-80000)

DD-81980 Poisoning by central nervous system muscle tone depressant, NOS 968.0
(DD-80000)

DD-81981 Poisoning by chlorphenesin carbamate 968.0
(DD-80000)

DD-81982 Poisoning by mephenesin 968.0
(DD-80000)

DD-81983 Poisoning by methocarbamol 968.0
(DD-80000)

D-81A Poisoning by Psychotropic Agents

DD-81A00 Poisoning by psychotropic agent, NOS 969.9
(DD-80000)

DD-81A10 Poisoning by antidepressant, NOS 969.0
(DD-80000)

DD-81A11 Poisoning by amitriptyline 969.0
(DD-80000)

DD-81A12 Poisoning by imipramine 969.0
(DD-80000)

DD-81A13 Poisoning by monoamine oxidase inhibitor, NOS 969.0
(DD-80000)
Poisoning by MAO inhibitor, NOS 969.0
(DD-80000)

DD-81A20 Poisoning by phenothiazine-based tranquilizer, NOS 969.1
(DD-80000)

DD-81A21 Poisoning by chlorpromazine 969.1
(DD-80000)

DD-81A22 Poisoning by fluphenazine 969.1
(DD-80000)

DD-81A23 Poisoning by prochlorperazine 969.1
(DD-80000)

DD-81A24 Poisoning by promazine 969.1
(DD-80000)

DD-81A30 Poisoning by butyrophenone-based tranquilizer, NOS 969.2
(DD-80000)

DD-81A31 Poisoning by haloperidol 969.1
(DD-80000)

DD-81A32 Poisoning by spiperone 969.2
(DD-80000)

DD-81A33 Poisoning by trifluperidol 969.2
(DD-80000)

DD-81A40 Poisoning by benzodiazepine-based tranquilizer 969.4
(DD-80000)

DD-81A41 Poisoning by chlordiazepoxide 969.4
(DD-80000)
DD-81A42 Poisoning by diazepam 969.4
(DD-80000)
DD-81A43 Poisoning by flurazepam 969.4
(DD-80000)
DD-81A44 Poisoning by lorazepam 969.4
(DD-80000)
DD-81A45 Poisoning by medazepam 969.4
(DD-80000)
DD-81A46 Poisoning by nitrazepam 969.4
(DD-80000)
DD-81A50 Poisoning by tranquilizer, NEC 969.5
(DD-80000)
DD-81A51 Poisoning by hydroxyzine 969.5
(DD-80000)
DD-81A52 Poisoning by meprobamate 969.5
(DD-80000)
DD-81A60 Poisoning by psychodysleptic, NOS 969.6
(DD-80000)
Poisoning by hallucinogen, NOS 969.6
(DD-80000)
DD-81A61 Poisoning by cannabis derivative, NOS 969.6
(DD-80000)
Poisoning by marihuana derivative, NOS 969.6
(DD-80000)
DD-81A62 Poisoning by lysergide 969.6
(DD-80000)
Poisoning by LSD 969.6
(DD-80000)
DD-81A66 Poisoning by mescaline 969.6
(DD-80000)
DD-81A67 Poisoning by psilocin 969.6
(DD-80000)
DD-81A68 Poisoning by psilocybin 969.6
(DD-80000)
DD-81A70 Poisoning by psychostimulant, NOS 969.7
(DD-80000)
DD-81A71 Poisoning by amphetamine 969.7
(DD-80000)
DD-81A72 Poisoning by caffeine 969.7
(DD-80000)
DD-81A80 Poisoning by other psychotropic agent, NEC 969.8
(DD-80000)

D-81B Poisoning by Central Nervous System Stimulants

DD-81B00 Poisoning by central nervous system stimulant, NOS 970.9
(DD-80000)
DD-81B10 Poisoning by analeptic, NOS 970.0
(DD-80000)
DD-81B11 Poisoning by lobeline 970.0
(DD-80000)
DD-81B12 Poisoning by nikethamide 970.0
(DD-80000)
DD-81B30 Poisoning by opiate antagonist, NOS 970.1
(DD-80000)
DD-81B31 Poisoning by levallorphan 970.1
(DD-80000)
DD-81B32 Poisoning by nalorphine 970.1
(DD-80000)
DD-81B33 Poisoning by naloxone 970.1
(DD-80000)
DD-81B80 Poisoning by central nervous system stimulant, NEC 970.8
(DD-80000)

D-821 Poisoning by Autonomous Nervous System Drugs

DD-82100 Poisoning by autonomous nervous system drug, NOS 971.9
(DD-80000)
DD-82110 Poisoning by parasympathomimetic drug, NOS 971.0
(DD-80000)
Poisoning by cholinergic drug, NOS 971.0
(DD-80000)
DD-82111 Poisoning by acetylcholine 971.0
(DD-80000)
DD-82112 Poisoning by anticholinesterase, NOS 971.0
(DD-80000)
DD-82113 Poisoning by organophosphorus anticholinesterase 971.0
(DD-80000)
DD-82114 Poisoning by reversible anticholinesterase 971.0
(DD-80000)
DD-82118 Poisoning by pilocarpine 971.0
(DD-80000)
DD-82130 Poisoning by parasympatholytic drug, NOS 971.1
(DD-80000)
Poisoning by anticholinergic drug, NOS 971.1
(DD-80000)
DD-82131 Poisoning by antimuscarinic drug, NOS 971.1
(DD-80000)
DD-82132 Poisoning by spasmolytic drug, NOS 971.1
(DD-80000)
DD-82133 Poisoning by atropine 971.1
(DD-80000)
DD-82134 Poisoning by homatropine 971.1
(DD-80000)
DD-82135 Poisoning by hyoscine 971.1
(DD-80000)
Poisoning by scopolamine 971.1
(DD-80000)
DD-82138 Poisoning by quaternary ammonium derivative, NOS 971.1
(DD-80000)
DD-82150 Poisoning by sympathomimetic drug, NOS 971.2
(DD-80000)
Poisoning by adrenergic drug, NOS 971.2
(DD-80000)

D-821 Poisoning by Autonomous Nervous System Drugs — Continued

DD-82151 Poisoning by epinephrine 971.2
(DD-80000)
Poisoning by adrenaline 971.2
(DD-80000)

DD-82152 Poisoning by levarterenol 971.2
(DD-80000)
Poisoning by noradrenaline 971.2
(DD-80000)

DD-82160 Poisoning by antiadrenergic drug, NOS 971.3
(DD-80000)
Poisoning by sympatholytic drug, NOS 971.3
(DD-80000)

DD-82171 Poisoning by phenoxybenzamine 971.3
(DD-80000)

DD-82172 Poisoning by tolazoline hydrochloride 971.3
(DD-80000)

D-822 Poisoning by Cardiovascular System Drugs

DD-82200 Poisoning by cardiovascular system drug, NOS 972.9
(DD-80000)

DD-82210 Poisoning by cardiac rhythm regulator, NOS 972.0
(DD-80000)

DD-82211 Poisoning by practolol 972.0
(DD-80000)

DD-82212 Poisoning by procainamide 972.0
(DD-80000)

DD-82213 Poisoning by propranolol 972.0
(DD-80000)

DD-82214 Poisoning by quinidine 972.0
(DD-80000)

DD-82220 Poisoning by cardiotonic glycoside, NOS 972.1
(DD-80000)

DD-82221 Poisoning by digitalis glycoside, NOS 972.1
(DD-80000)
Digitalis poisoning 972.1

DD-82222 Poisoning by digoxin 972.1
(DD-80000)

DD-82226 Poisoning by strophantin, NOS 972.1
(DD-80000)

DD-82230 Poisoning by antilipemic or antiarteriosclerotic drug, NOS 972.2
(DD-80000)

DD-82231 Poisoning by clofibrate 972.2
(DD-80000)

DD-82232 Poisoning by nicotinic acid derivative 972.2
(DD-80000)

DD-82240 Poisoning by ganglion-blocking agent, NOS 972.3
(DD-80000)

DD-82241 Poisoning by pentamethonium bromide 972.3
(DD-80000)

DD-82250 Poisoning by coronary vasodilator, NOS 972.4
(DD-80000)

DD-82251 Poisoning by dipyridamole 972.4
(DD-80000)

DD-82252 Poisoning by nitrate, NOS 972.4
(DD-80000)

DD-82253 Poisoning by nitroglycerin 972.4
(DD-80000)

DD-82256 Poisoning by nitrite, NOS 972.4
(DD-80000)

DD-82260 Poisoning by vasodilator, NEC 972.5
(DD-80000)

DD-82261 Poisoning by cyclandelate 972.5
(DD-80000)

DD-82262 Poisoning by diazoxide 972.5
(DD-80000)

DD-82263 Poisoning by papaverine 972.5
(DD-80000)

DD-82270 Poisoning by antihypertensive agent, NEC 972.6
(DD-80000)

DD-82271 Poisoning by clonidine 972.6
(DD-80000)

DD-82272 Poisoning by guanethidine 972.6
(DD-80000)

DD-82273 Poisoning by rauwolfia alkaloid, NOS 972.6
(DD-80000)

DD-82274 Poisoning by reserpine 972.6
(DD-80000)

DD-82280 Poisoning by antivaricose drug or sclerosing agent, NOS 972.7
(DD-80000)

DD-82281 Poisoning by sodium morrhuate 972.7
(DD-80000)

DD-82284 Poisoning by zinc salt, NOS 972.7
(DD-80000)

DD-82290 Poisoning by capillary-active drug, NOS 972.8
(DD-80000)

DD-82291 Poisoning by adrenochrome derivative, NOS 972.8
(DD-80000)

DD-82292 Poisoning by metaraminol 972.8
(DD-80000)

D-823 Poisoning by Gastrointestinal System Drugs

DD-82300 Poisoning by gastrointestinal system drug, NOS 973.9
(DD-80000)

DD-82310 Poisoning by antacid or antigastric secretion drug, NOS 973.0
(DD-80000)

DD-82311 Poisoning by aluminum hydroxide 973.0
(DD-80000)

DD-82312 Poisoning by magnesium trisilicate 973.0
(DD-80000)

DD-82330 Poisoning by irritant cathartic, NOS 973.1 (DD-80000)

DD-82331 Poisoning by bisacodyl 973.1 (DD-80000)

DD-82332 Poisoning by castor oil 973.1 (DD-80000)

DD-82335 Poisoning by phenolphthalein 973.1 (DD-80000)

DD-82340 Poisoning by emollient cathartic, NOS 973.2 (DD-80000)

DD-82341 Poisoning by dioctyl sulfosuccinate, NOS 973.2 (DD-80000)

DD-82348 Poisoning by magnesium sulfate 973.3 (DD-80000)

DD-82350 Poisoning by digestant, NOS 973.4 (DD-80000)

DD-82351 Poisoning by pancreatin 973.4 (DD-80000)

DD-82352 Poisoning by papain 973.4 (DD-80000)

DD-82355 Poisoning by pepsin 973.4 (DD-80000)

DD-82360 Poisoning by antidiarrheal drug, NOS 973.5 (DD-80000)

DD-82361 Poisoning by kaolin 973.5 (DD-80000)

DD-82362 Poisoning by pectin 973.5 (DD-80000)

DD-82370 Poisoning by emetic, NOS 973.6 (DD-80000)

DD-82380 Poisoning by other gastrointestinal system drug, NEC 973.8 (DD-80000)

D-824 Poisoning by Water and Mineral Metabolism Drugs

DD-82400 Poisoning by water and mineral metabolism drug, NOS 974.- (DD-80000)

DD-82410 Poisoning by mercurial diuretic, NOS 974.0 (DD-80000)

DD-82411 Poisoning by chlormerodrin 974.0 (DD-80000)

DD-82412 Poisoning by mercaptomerin 974.0 (DD-80000)

DD-82414 Poisoning by mersalyl 974.0 (DD-80000)

DD-82420 Poisoning by purine derivative diuretic, NOS 974.1 (DD-80000)

DD-82421 Poisoning by theobromine 974.1 (DD-80000)

DD-82422 Poisoning by theophylline 974.1 (DD-80000)

DD-82430 Poisoning by carbonic acid anhydrase inhibitor, NOS 974.2 (DD-80000)

DD-82431 Poisoning by acetazolamide 974.2 (DD-80000)

DD-82440 Poisoning by saluretic, NOS 974.3 (DD-80000)

DD-82441 Poisoning by benzothiadiazide, NOS 974.3 (DD-80000)

DD-82442 Poisoning by chlorothiazide group, NOS 974.3 (DD-80000)

DD-82450 Poisoning by diuretic, NEC 974.4 (DD-80000)

DD-82451 Poisoning by ethacrynic acid 974.4 (DD-80000)

DD-82452 Poisoning by furosemide 974.4 (DD-80000)

DD-82460 Poisoning by electrolytic, caloric and water-balanced agent, NEC 974.5 (DD-80000)

D-825 Poisoning by Uric Acid Metabolism Drugs

DD-82500 Poisoning by uric acid metabolism drug, NOS 974.7 (DD-80000)

DD-82501 Poisoning by allopurinol 974.7 (DD-80000)

DD-82502 Poisoning by colchicine 974.7 (DD-80000)

DD-82503 Poisoning by probenecid 974.7 (DD-80000)

D-826 Poisoning by Smooth and Skeletal Muscle Agents

DD-82600 Poisoning by drug acting on smooth or skeletal muscle, NOS 975.3 (DD-80000)

DD-82610 Poisoning by oxytocic agent, NOS 975.0 (DD-80000)

DD-82611 Poisoning by ergot alkaloid, NOS 975.0 (DD-80000)

DD-82615 Poisoning by oxytocin 975.0 (DD-80000)

DD-82617 Poisoning by prostaglandin, NOS 975.0 (DD-80000)

DD-82620 Poisoning by smooth muscle relaxant, NOS 975.1 (DD-80000)

DD-82621 Poisoning by adiphenine 975.1 (DD-80000)

DD-82622 Poisoning by metaproterenol 975.1 (DD-80000)
Poisoning by orciprenaline 975.1 (DD-80000)

DD-82640 Poisoning by skeletal muscle relaxant, NOS 975.2 (DD-80000)

D-827 Poisoning by Drugs Acting on The Respiratory System

DD-82700 Poisoning by drug acting on the respiratory system, NOS 975.8
(DD-80000)

DD-82710 Poisoning by antitussive, NOS 975.4
(DD-80000)

DD-82711 Poisoning by dextromethorphan 975.4
(DD-80000)

DD-82712 Poisoning by pipazethate 975.4
(DD-80000)

DD-82720 Poisoning by expectorant, NOS 975.5
(DD-80000)

DD-82721 Poisoning by acetylcysteine 975.5
(DD-80000)

DD-82726 Poisoning by terpin hydrate 975.5
(DD-80000)

DD-82730 Poisoning by anti-common cold drug, NOS 976.5
(DD-80000)

DD-82750 Poisoning by antiasthmatic, NOS 975.7
(DD-80000)

DD-82752 Poisoning by aminophylline 975.7
(DD-80000)
Poisoning by theophylline ethylenediamine 975.7
(DD-80000)

D-828 Poisoning by Agents Affecting Skin and Mucous Membranes

DD-82800 Poisoning by skin or mucous membrane drug, NOS 976.9
(DD-80000)

DD-82810 Poisoning by local anti-infective, NOS 976.0
(DD-80000)

DD-82812 Poisoning by local anti-inflammatory drug, NOS 976.0
(DD-80000)

DD-82814 Poisoning by local antipruritic, NOS 976.1
(DD-80000)

DD-82820 Poisoning by local astringent, NOS 976.2
(DD-80000)

DD-82824 Poisoning by local detergent, NOS 976.2
(DD-80000)

DD-82830 Poisoning by emollient, NOS 976.3
(DD-80000)

DD-82832 Poisoning by demulcent, NOS 976.3
(DD-80000)

DD-82834 Poisoning by protectant, NOS 976.3
(DD-80000)

DD-82840 Poisoning by keratolytic agent, NOS 976.4
(DD-80000)

DD-82842 Poisoning by keratoplastic drug, NOS 976.4
(DD-80000)

DD-82848 Poisoning by hair treatment drug or preparation, NOS 976.4
(DD-80000)

DD-82850 Poisoning by ear anti-infective, NOS 976.6
(DD-80000)

DD-82852 Poisoning by nose anti-infective, NOS 976.6
(DD-80000)

DD-82854 Poisoning by throat anti-infective, NOS 976.6
(DD-80000)

DD-82860 Poisoning by topical dental drug, NOS 976.7
(DD-80000)

DD-82870 Poisoning by eye anti-infective, NOS 976.5
(DD-80000)

DD-82872 Poisoning by idoxuridine 976.5
(DD-80000)

DD-82880 Poisoning by other agent affecting skin and mucous membrane, NEC 976.8
(DD-80000)

DD-82882 Poisoning by vaginal contraceptive, NOS 976.8
(DD-80000)

DD-82884 Poisoning by spermicide, NOS 976.8
(DD-80000)

D-829 Poisoning by Unclassified Drugs and Medicinal Substances

DD-82900 Poisoning by drug or medicinal substance, NEC 977.9
(DD-80000)

DD-82910 Poisoning by dietetic drug, NOS 977.0
(DD-80000)

DD-82912 Poisoning by central appetite depressant, NOS 977.0
(DD-80000)

DD-82920 Poisoning by lipotropic drug, NOS 977.1
(DD-80000)

DD-82930 Poisoning by antidote or chelating agent, NEC 977.2
(DD-80000)

DD-82940 Poisoning by alcohol deterrent, NOS 977.3
(DD-80000)

DD-82950 Poisoning by pharmaceutical excipient, NOS 977.4
(DD-80000)

DD-82952 Poisoning by pharmaceutical adjunct, NOS 977.4
(DD-80000)

DD-82960 Poisoning by contrast media used for diagnostic x-ray procedure, NOS 977.8
(DD-80000)

DD-82970 Poisoning by diagnostic agent or kit, NOS 977.8
(DD-80000)

D-82A Poisoning by Vaccines and Biological Substances

DD-82A00 Poisoning by vaccine or biological substance, NOS 979.9
(DD-80000)

DD-82A10 Poisoning by smallpox vaccine 979.0
(DD-80000)

DD-82A20 Poisoning by rabies vaccine 979.1
(DD-80000)

DD-82A30 Poisoning by typhus vaccine 979.2
(DD-80000)

DD-82A40 Poisoning by yellow fever vaccine 979.3
(DD-80000)

DD-82A50 Poisoning by measles vaccine 979.4
(DD-80000)

DD-82A60 Poisoning by poliomyelitis vaccine 979.5
(DD-80000)

DD-82A70 Poisoning by mumps vaccine 979.6
(DD-80000)

DD-82A80 Poisoning by viral and rickettsial vaccine, NOS 979.6
(DD-80000)

DD-82A90 Poisoning by mixed viral-rickettsial and bacterial vaccine, NOS 979.7
(DD-80000)

D-82B Poisoning by Bacterial Vaccines

DD-82B00 Poisoning by bacterial vaccine, NOS 978.8
(DD-80000)

DD-82B02 Poisoning by BCG vaccine 978.0
(DD-80000)

DD-82B10 Poisoning by typhoid and paratyphoid vaccine 978.1
(DD-80000)

DD-82B20 Poisoning by cholera vaccine 978.2
(DD-80000)

DD-82B30 Poisoning by plague vaccine 978.3
(DD-80000)

DD-82B40 Poisoning by tetanus vaccine 978.4
(DD-80000)

DD-82B50 Poisoning by diphtheria vaccine 978.5
(DD-80000)

DD-82B60 Poisoning by pertussis vaccine including combinations with a pertussis component 978.6
(DD-80000)

DD-82B80 Poisoning by mixed bacterial vaccine except combinations with a pertussis component 978.9
(DD-80000)

D-84 TOXIC EFFECTS OF NONMEDICINAL SUBSTANCES

DD-84000 Toxic effect of chiefly nonmedicinal substance, NOS 989.9

DD-84010 Toxic effect of chiefly nonmedicinal substance, NEC 989.8

DD-84100 Toxic effect of alcohol, NOS 980.9

DD-84110 Toxic effect of ethyl alcohol 980.0
Toxic effect of ethanol 980.0
Toxic effect of grain alcohol 980.0
Ethyl alcohol poisoning 980.0
(C-21005)
Ethanol poisoning 980.0

DD-84112 Toxic effect of denatured alcohol 980.0

DD-84120 Toxic effect of methyl alcohol 980.1
Toxic effect of methanol 980.1
Toxic effect of wood alcohol 980.1
Methyl alcohol poisoning 980.1
(C-21002)
Methanol poisoning 980.1
(C-21002)

DD-84130 Toxic effect of isopropyl alcohol 980.2
Toxic effect of dimethyl carbinol 980.2
Toxic effect of isopropanol 980.2
Toxic effect of rubbing alcohol 980.2
Isopropyl alcohol poisoning 980.2

DD-84140 Toxic effect of fusel oil, NOS 980.3

DD-84141 Toxic effect of amyl alcohol 980.3

DD-84142 Toxic effect of butyl alcohol 980.3

DD-84143 Toxic effect of propyl alcohol 980.3

DD-84180 Toxic effect of other alcohol, NEC 980.8

DD-84190 Ethylene glycol poisoning 980.8
Anti-freeze poisoning 980.8

DD-84200 Toxic effect of petroleum product, NOS 981.-

DD-84201 Toxic effect of benzine 981.-

DD-84210 Toxic effect of gasoline 981.-

DD-84220 Toxic effect of kerosine 981.-

DD-84230 Toxic effect of paraffin wax 981.-

DD-84240 Toxic effect of petroleum ether 981.-
Toxic effect of petroleum naphtha 981.-
Toxic effect of petroleum spirit 981.-

DD-84250 Toxic effect of naphthaline
(C-20212)
Naphthalene poisoning
(C-20212)
Mothball poisoning
(C-20212)

DD-84300 Toxic effect of non-petroleum-based solvent, NOS 982.-

DD-84310 Toxic effect of benzene or homologue, NOS 982.0

DD-84320 Toxic effect of carbon tetrachloride 982.1
Carbon tetrachloride poisoning
(C-20809)

DD-84330 Toxic effect of carbon disulfide 982.2
Toxic effect of carbon bisulfide 982.2
Carbon disulfide poisoning
(C-10515)

DD-84340 Toxic effect of other chlorinated hydrocarbon solvent, NOS 982.3

DD-84342 Toxic effect of tetrachloroethylene 982.3

DD-84344 Toxic effect of trichloroethylene 982.3

DD-84350 Toxic effect of nitroglycol 982.4

DD-84360 Toxic effect of other nonpetroleum-based solvent, NEC 982.8

DD-84362 Toxic effect of acetone 982.8
Acetone poisoning

DD-84400 Toxic effect of caustic substance, NOS 983.9

DD-84410 Toxic effect of corrosive aromatic, NOS 983.0

DD-84411 Toxic effect of carbolic acid 983.0
Toxic effect of phenol 983.0

D-84 TOXIC EFFECTS OF NONMEDICINAL SUBSTANCES — Continued

DD-84412 Toxic effect of cresol 983.0
DD-84420 Toxic effect of acid, NOS 983.1
DD-84422 Toxic effect of hydrochloric acid 983.1
DD-84424 Toxic effect of nitric acid 983.1
DD-84426 Toxic effect of sulfuric acid 983.1
DD-84430 Toxic effect of caustic alkali, NOS 983.2
  Toxic effect of lye 983.2
DD-84431 Toxic effect of sodium hydroxide 983.2
DD-84432 Toxic effect of potassium hydroxide 983.2
DD-84500 Toxic effect of lead compound, NOS 984.8
  Lead poisoning 984.8
    (C-13200)
  Plumbism 984.8
    (C-13200)
  Saturnine poisoning 984.8
    (C-13200)
DD-84510 Toxic effect of inorganic lead compound, NOS 984.0
DD-84512 Toxic effect of lead dioxide 984.0
DD-84514 Toxic effect of lead salt, NOS 984.0
DD-84540 Toxic effect of organic lead compound, NOS 984.1
DD-84542 Toxic effect of lead acetate 984.1
DD-84544 Toxic effect of tetraethyl lead 984.1
DD-84600 Toxic effect of other metal, NOS 985.9
DD-84610 Toxic effect of mercury and its compounds, NOS 985.0
    (C-13300)
  Mercury poisoning 985.0
    (C-13300)
  Mercurialism 985.0
    (C-13300)
  Hydrargyria 985.0
    (C-13300)
  Hydrargyrism 985.0
    (C-13300)
  Hydrargyrosis 985.0
    (C-13300)
DD-84611 Inorganic mercury poisoning
DD-84615 Organic mercury poisoning
DD-84616 Minamata disease 985.0
  Toxic effect of alkyl mercury compounds 985.0
DD-84620 Toxic effect of arsenic and its compounds, NOS 985.1
  Arsenic poisoning 985.1
    (C-11500)
  Arsenical toxicity
DD-84622 Inorganic arsenic poisoning
    (C-11500)
DD-84624 Organic arsenic poisoning
    (C-11500)
DD-84625 Arsanilic acid poisoning
DD-84630 Toxic effect of manganese and its compounds, NOS 985.2
DD-84640 Toxic effect of beryllium and its compounds, NOS 985.3
DD-84650 Toxic effect of antimony and its compounds, NOS 985.4
    (T-28000) (M-55700) (C-12100)
  Antimony poisoning 985.4
    (T-28000) (M-55700) (C-12100)
  Antimoniosis 985.4
  Stibialism 985.4
DD-84660 Toxic effect of cadmium and its compounds, NOS 985.5
DD-84670 Toxic effect of chromium, NOS 985.6
DD-84681 Toxic effect of brass fumes 985.8
DD-84682 Toxic effect of copper salt, NOS 985.8
DD-84683 Toxic effect of iron compound, NOS 985.8
DD-84684 Toxic effect of nickel compound, NOS 985.8
DD-84685 Toxic effect of selenium compound, NOS 985.8
DD-84700 Toxic effect of gas, fumes or vapors, NOS 987.9
DD-84710 Toxic effect of liquefied petroleum gas, NOS 987.0
DD-84711 Toxic effect of butane 987.0
DD-84712 Toxic effect of propane 987.0
DD-84720 Toxic effect of hydrocarbon gas, NEC 987.1
DD-84730 Toxic effect of nitrogen oxide, NOS 987.2
DD-84731 Toxic effect of nitrogen dioxide 987.2
DD-84732 Toxic effect of nitrous fumes 987.2
DD-84740 Toxic effect of sulfur dioxide 987.3
DD-84750 Toxic effect of freon 987.4
  Toxic effect of dichloromonofluoromethane 987.4
DD-84760 Toxic effect of lacrimogenic gas 987.5
DD-84761 Toxic effect of bromobenzyl cyanide 987.5
DD-84762 Toxic effect of chloroacetophenone 987.5
DD-84763 Toxic effect of ethyliodoacetate 987.5
DD-84770 Toxic effect of chlorine gas 987.6
DD-84780 Toxic effect of hydrocyanic acid gas 987.7
DD-84790 Toxic effect of other gas, fumes or vapors, NEC 987.8
DD-84791 Toxic effect of phosgene 987.8
DD-84794 Toxic effect of polyester fumes 987.8
DD-847A0 Toxic effect of carbon monoxide 986.-
  Carbon monoxide poisoning
    (C-10526)
DD-84800 Toxic effect of noxious substance eaten as food, NOS 988.9
DD-84810 Toxic effect from eating fish 988.0
DD-84814 Toxic effect from eating shellfish, NOS 988.0
  Shellfish poisoning, NOS 988.0
  Poisoning by eating contaminated shellfish, NOS 988.0
DD-84820 Toxic effect from eating mushrooms 988.1
    (L-42200)
  Mushroom poisoning 988.1
    (L-42200)
DD-84821 Amanita species poisoning
    (L-42220)
DD-84822 Amanita phalloides poisoning
    (L-42221)

DD-84830 Toxic effect from eating berries and other plants 988.2
DD-84880 Toxic effect from noxious substance eaten as food, NEC 988.8
DD-84890 Jamaican vomiting sickness 988.8
(T-57000) (F-52772) (L-D7C01)
(C-30212) (C-30211)
Akee poisoning 988.8
(T-57000) (F-52772) (L-D7C01)
(C-30212) (C-30211)
DD-84900 Toxic effect of hydrocyanic acid, NOS 989.0
DD-84901 Toxic effect of cyanide, NOS 989.0
Cyanide poisoning
(C-10550)
DD-84902 Toxic effect of potassium cyanide 989.0
DD-84903 Toxic effect of sodium cyanide 989.0
DD-84910 Toxic effect of strychnine, NOS 989.1
Strychnine poisoning 989.1
(C-30364)
Strychnine toxicity 989.1
DD-84920 Toxic effect of chlorinated hydrocarbon pesticide, NOS 989.2
DD-84921 Toxic effect of aldrin 989.2
Aldrin poisoning 989.2
DD-84922 Toxic effect of chlordane 989.2
Chlordane poisoning
DD-84923 Toxic effect of DDT 989.2
Dichlorodiphenyltrichloroethane poisoning 989.2
DDT toxicity 989.2
(C-23114)
DD-84924 Toxic effect of dieldrin 989.2
Dieldrin poisoning 989.2
DD-84930 Toxic effect of organophosphate or carbamate pesticide, NOS 989.3
Carbamate insecticide toxicity 989.3
Organophosphate toxicity 989.3
(C-22100)
DD-84931 Toxic effect of carbaryl 989.3
Carbaryl poisoning 989.3
DD-84932 Toxic effect of dichlorvos 989.3
Dichlorvos poisoning 989.3
DD-84933 Toxic effect of malathion 989.3
Malathion poisoning 989.3
DD-84934 Toxic effect of parathion 989.3
Parathion poisoning 989.3
DD-84935 Toxic effect of phorate 989.3
Phorate poisoning 989.3
DD-84936 Toxic effect of phosdrin 989.3
DD-84940 Toxic effect of mixtures of insecticides 989.4
DD-84A00 Toxic effect of venom, NOS 989.5
DD-84A10 Toxic effect of bite of venomous snake, NOS 989.5
DD-84A20 Toxic effect of bite of venomous lizard, NOS 989.5
DD-84A30 Toxic effect of bite of venomous spider, NOS 989.5
DD-84B00 Toxic effect of soap or detergent, NOS 989.6
DD-84C00 Toxic effect of food contaminant, NOS 989.7
DD-84C10 Toxic effect of mycotoxin, NOS 989.7
DD-84C12 Toxic effect of aflatoxin 989.7

SECTION D-9 POISONING SYNDROMES MAINLY IN ANIMALS

D-90 POISONING SYNDROMES MAINLY IN ANIMALS: GENERAL TERMS

DD-90000V Poisoning syndrome in animal, NOS
(DD-80000)
Poisoning in animal, NOS
(DD-80000)
Poisoning of animal, NOS
(DD-80000)
Toxic syndrome in animal, NOS
(DD-80000)
DD-90010V Organic poisoning syndrome of animal, NOS
(DD-80000)
DD-90020V Inorganic poisoning syndrome of animal, NOS
(DD-80000)

D-91 POISONING OF ANIMALS BY CHEMICALS AND DRUGS

DD-91000V Chemical or drug poisoning of animal, NOS
(DD-80000)
DD-91010V 1,3 Indandion poisoning
(DD-80000)
DD-91012V 4-aminopyridine poisoning
(DD-80000)
Avitrol poisoning
(DD-80000)
DD-91018V Benzoic and salicylic acid poisoning
(DD-80000) (C-72620)
DD-91070V Bismuth poisoning
(DD-80000)
DD-91074V Cadmium poisoning
(DD-80000) (C-12600)
DD-91090V Chlorate poisoning
(DD-80000) (C-10481)
DD-91092V Chlorinated naphthalene poisoning
(DD-80000)
Bovine hyperkeratosis
(DD-80000)
DD-91094V Chloroform poisoning
(DD-80000) (C-20821)
DD-91100V Cacao poisoning
(DD-80000)
Chocolate poisoning
(DD-80000)
Theobromine poisoning
(DD-80000)
DD-91110V Coal-tar-pitch poisoning
(DD-80000)
Clay pigeon poisoning
(DD-80000) (C-20202)

D-91 POISONING OF ANIMALS BY CHEMICALS AND DRUGS — Continued

DD-91120V Cobalt poisoning
(DD-80000) (C-14400)

DD-91140V Copper poisoning
(DD-80000) (C-12700)

DD-91142V Acute copper poisoning
(DD-80000)

DD-91144V Chronic copper poisoning
(DD-80000)

DD-91145V Phytogenous chronic copper poisoning
(DD-80000) (L-D6414)

DD-91146 Hepatogenous chronic copper poisoning
(DD-80000) (L-D9C31)

DD-91150V Cresol poisoning
(DD-80000)

DD-91152V Creosote poisoning
(DD-80000)

DD-91160V Comafuryl poisoning
(DD-80000)

DD-91184V Diamidine poisoning
(DD-80000)

DD-91214V Dioxin poisoning
(DD-80000)

DD-91220V Diphacinone/diphenadione poisoning
(DD-80000)

DD-91230V Dynamite poisoning
(DD-80000)

DD-91245V Oxalate poisoning
(DD-80000) (C-21618)

DD-91250V Fleet-like enema poisoning
(DD-80000)

DD-91260V Flumixin poisoning
(DD-80000)

DD-91270 Chronic fluoride poisoning
(DD-80000) (C-11100)
Fluorosis
(DD-80000)

DD-91280V Garbage poisoning
(DD-80000)

DD-91290V Gold poisoning
(DD-80000)

DD-91294V Gossypol poisoning
(DD-80000) (C-30632)

DD-91300V Hexachlorophene poisoning
(DD-80000) (C-72130)

DD-91306V Hydrogen sulfide poisoning
(DD-80000) (C-10812)

DD-91310V Iodine poisoning
(DD-80000)

DD-91314V Ionophor poisoning
(DD-80000)

DD-91320V Iron dextran toxicity
(DD-80000)

DD-91340V Lewisite poisoning
(DD-80000) (C-27220)

DD-91370V Metaldehyde poisoning
(DD-80000)

DD-91372V Methane/propane poisoning
(DD-80000)

DD-91380V Molybdenum poisoning
(DD-80000) (C-15000)

DD-91410V Mustard gas poisoning
(DD-80000) (C-27201)

DD-91430V Nicotine poisoning
(DD-80000)
Nicotinism
(DD-80000)

DD-91432V Nicotine sulfate poisoning
(DD-80000)
Blackleaf 40 poisoning
(DD-80000)

DD-91450V Nitrogen dioxide poisoning
(DD-80000) (C-10713)

DD-91454V Nitrogen trichloride poisoning
(DD-80000) (C-10717)
Agene poisoning
(DD-80000) (C-10717)
Fright disease
(DD-80000) (C-10717)

DD-91470V Ortho-tricresyl phosphate poisoning
(DD-80000) (C-22103)

DD-91480V Phenanthrene poisoning
(DD-80000) (C-20731)

DD-91482V Phenanthrene derivative poisoning
(DD-80000) (C-58620)

DD-91486V Phencyclidine poisoning
(DD-80000)
PCP poisoning
(DD-80000)

DD-91490V Pindone poisoning
(DD-80000)

DD-91500V Polybrominated biphenyl poisoning
(DD-80000)
PBB poisoning
(DD-80000)

DD-91504V Polychlorinated biphenyl poisoning
(DD-80000)
PCB poisoning
(DD-80000)
Yusko
(DD-80000)

DD-91510V Petroleum poisoning
(DD-80000) (C-20220)
Petroleum product toxicity
(DD-80000)

DD-91520V Phenol poisoning
(DD-80000) (C-21100)
Carbolic acid poisoning
(DD-80000)
Phenolic disinfectant poisoning
(DD-80000)
Phenolic product poisoning
(DD-80000)

DD-91530V Phenothiazine poisoning
(DD-80000) (C-5A600)

DD-91540V Phosphate salt poisoning
(DD-80000) (C-10630)
Organic phosphate poisoning
(DD-80000) (C-22100)

DD-91550V Phosphorus poisoning
(DD-80000) (C-10600)
Phosphorus toxicity
(DD-80000)

DD-91560V Polyurethane poisoning
(DD-80000)

DD-91570V Red squill poisoning
(DD-80000) (C-30048)

DD-91580V Reserpine poisoning
(DD-80000) (C-57530)

DD-91600V Salt poisoning
(DD-80000) (C-63470)
Sodium chloride poisoning
(DD-80000)
Saline poisoning
(DD-80000)

DD-91610V Selenium poisoning
(DD-80000) (C-11600)
Alkali disease
(DD-80000)
Blind staggers
(DD-80000)

DD-91611V Acute selenium poisoning
(DD-80000)

DD-91613V Chronic selenium poisoning
(DD-80000)

DD-91620V Silver poisoning
(DD-80000)

DD-91650V Tannic acid poisoning
(DD-80000)

DD-91660V Teflon poisoning
(DD-80000)

DD-91670V Tetrachlorodibenzodioxin poisoning
(DD-80000)
TCDD poisoning
(DD-80000)

DD-91676V Tetrachloroethylene poisoning
(DD-80000) (C-20841)

DD-91680V Thallium poisoning
(DD-80000) (C-13800)

DD-91690V Thalidomide poisoning
(DD-80000)

DD-91700V Tricyclic antidepressant poisoning
(DD-80000)

DD-91710V Turpentine poisoning
(DD-80000) (C-31170)

DD-91720V Urea poisoning
(DD-80000) (C-63A60)

DD-91760V Zinc poisoning
(DD-80000) (C-14100)

DD-91764V Zinc phosphide poisoning
(DD-80000) (C-23813)
Zinc phosphide toxicity
(DD-80000)

D-92 POISONING OF ANIMALS BY HERBICIDES

DD-92000V Herbicide poisoning, NOS
(DD-80000)
Herbicide toxicity, NOS
(DD-80000)
Poisoning of animal by herbicide, NOS
(DD-80000)

DD-92010V Amide compound toxicity
(DD-80000)

DD-92012V Ammonium sulfamate toxicity
(DD-80000)

DD-92020V Borax toxicity
(DD-80000)

DD-92030V Chlorobenzoic acid toxicty
(DD-80000)

DD-92040V Dinitro compound toxicity
(DD-80000)

DD-92050V Dipyridyl compound toxicity
(DD-80000)

DD-92060V Glyphosate toxicity
(DD-80000)

DD-92070V Methyluracil compound toxicity
(DD-80000)

DD-92080V Paraquat toxicity
(DD-80000) (C-23512)

DD-92090V Pentachlorophenol toxicity
(DD-80000)

DD-92100V Phenoxyacetate herbicide toxicity
(DD-80000)

DD-92110V 2,4-Dichlorophenoxyacetic acid poisoning
(DD-80000)
2,4-D poisoning
(DD-80000)

DD-92112V MCPP poisoning
(DD-80000)

DD-92114V Monochloromethylphenoxyacetic acid poisoning
(DD-80000)
MCPA poisoning
(DD-80000)

DD-92120V Phenylurea compound toxicity
(DD-80000)

DD-92130V Plant hormone herbicide toxicity
(DD-80000)

DD-92140V Sodium chlorate toxicity
(DD-80000)

DD-92150V Thiocarbamate compound toxicity
(DD-80000)

DD-92160V Triazine compound toxicity
(DD-80000)

D-93 POISONING OF ANIMALS BY PESTICIDES

DD-93000V Pesticide poisoning, NOS
(DD-80000)
Pesticide toxicity, NOS
(DD-80000)

D-93 POISONING OF ANIMALS BY PESTICIDES — Continued

DD-93010V Insecticide poisoning, NOS (DD-80000)
Insecticide toxicity, NOS (DD-80000)

DD-93020V Acaricide poisoning, NOS (DD-80000)
Acaricide toxicity, NOS (DD-80000)

DD-93100V Borate toxicity (DD-80000)

DD-93114V Carbofuran poisoning (DD-80000)

DD-93116V Methomyl poisoning (DD-80000)

DD-93118V Propoxur poisoning (DD-80000)

DD-93120V Chlorinated hydrocarbon toxicity (DD-80000) (C-20801)
Organochlorine toxicity (DD-80000)

DD-93130V Benzene hexachloride poisoning (DD-80000)
BHC poisoning (DD-80000)

DD-93142V Endrin poisoning (DD-80000)

DD-93150V Heptachlor poisoning (DD-80000)

DD-93152V Methoxychlor poisoning (DD-80000)

DD-93160V Lindane poisoning (DD-80000) (C-23112)

DD-93164V Strobane poisoning (DD-80000) (C-31420)

DD-93170V Toxaphene poisoning (DD-80000)

DD-93200V Pyrethrin toxicity (DD-80000)

DD-93204V Pyrethroid toxicity (DD-80000)

DD-93212V Azinphos-methyl poisoning (DD-80000)

DD-93214V Azinphos-ethyl poisoning (DD-80000)

DD-93216V Carbophenothion poisoning (DD-80000)

DD-93220V Chlorfenvinphos poisoning (DD-80000)

DD-93222V Chlorpyrifos poisoning (DD-80000)

DD-93224V Coumaphos poisoning (DD-80000)

DD-93226V Crotoxyphos poisoning (DD-80000)

DD-93230V Demeton poisoning (DD-80000)

DD-93232V Diazinon poisoning (DD-80000)

DD-93240V Dimethoate poisoning (DD-80000)

DD-93242V Dioxathion poisoning (DD-80000)

DD-93244V Disulfoton poisoning (DD-80000)

DD-93250V EPN poisoning (DD-80000)

DD-93252V Famphur poisoning (DD-80000)

DD-93260V Fenthion poisoning (DD-80000)

DD-93264V Methyl parathion poisoning (DD-80000)

DD-93270V Mevinphos poisoning (DD-80000)

DD-93274V Naled poisoning (DD-80000)

DD-93280V Oxydemeton-methyl poisoning (DD-80000)

DD-93288V Phosmet poisoning (DD-80000)

DD-93290V Ronnel poisoning (DD-80000)

DD-93300V Ruelene poisoning (DD-80000)

DD-93310V Temephos poisoning (DD-80000)

DD-93320V Terbufos poisoning (DD-80000)

DD-93324V Tetrachlorvinphos poisoning (DD-80000)

DD-93330V Tetraethyl pyrophosphate poisoning (DD-80000)
TEPP poisoning (DD-80000)

DD-93340V Trichlorfon poisoning (DD-80000)

DD-93410V Solvent and emulsifier toxicity (DD-80000)

DD-93420V Sulfur and lime-sulfur toxicity (DD-80000)

DD-93700V Rodenticide poisoning, NOS (DD-80000)

DD-93710V Alpha chloralose toxicity (DD-80000)

DD-93720V Alphanaphthylthiourea toxicity (DD-80000)
ANTU toxicity (DD-80000)

DD-93730V Anticoagulant rodenticide toxicity (DD-80000)

DD-93740V Cholecalciferol toxicity (DD-80000)

DD-93750V Congener toxicity (DD-80000)

DD-93760V Crimidine toxicity
(DD-80000)
DD-93770V Fluoroacetate toxicity
(DD-80000)
DD-93780V Norbromide toxicity
(DD-80000)
DD-93800V Pyriminil toxicity
(DD-80000)
DD-93820V Sodium fluoroacetate toxicity
(DD-80000)
1080 toxicity
(DD-80000)
DD-93824V Sodium fluoroacetamide toxicity
(DD-80000)
1081 toxicity
(DD-80000)
DD-93840V Thallium sulfate toxicity
(DD-80000)
DD-93850V Vacor toxicity
(DD-80000)

D-94 ANIMAL MYCOTOXICOSES

DD-94000V Animal mycotoxicosis, NOS
(DD-80000)
Poisoning caused by fungal or bacterial toxin, NOS
(DD-80000)
Poisoning caused by ingestion of fungi, NOS
(DD-80000)
DD-94100V Aflatoxicosis poisoning
(DD-80000) (C-30810) (L-44135)
Aspergillus flavus toxicosis
(DD-80000) (C-30810) (L-44135)
DD-94110V Alimentary toxic aleukia
(DD-80000) (L-45912) (L-45918)
DD-94112V Aspergillus versicolor toxicosis
(DD-80000) (L-44146)
DD-94114V Aspergillus clavatus tremors
(DD-80000) (L-44133)
DD-94120V Atypical interstitial pneumonia of cattle
(DD-80000) (C-30822) (L-45903)
DD-94130V Cardiac beriberi
(DD-80000) (C-30823) (L-44331)
Shoskin-Kakke
(DD-80000) (C-30823) (L-44331)
DD-94140V Cephalosporium toxicosis
(DD-80000) (L-44100)
DD-94150V Dikoor
(DD-80000) (L-DB920) (L-45731)
DD-94160V Diplodiosis
(DD-80000) (L-DB941) (L-46102)
Diplodia zea toxicity
(DD-80000) (L-DB941) (L-46102)
Diplodia toxicosis
(DD-80000) (L-DB941) (L-46102)
DD-94170V Drechslera toxicosis
(DD-80000) (L-45170)
DD-94180V Equine leukoencephalomalacia
(DD-80000) (L-45901)
Moldy corn poisoning
(DD-80000) (L-45901)
DD-94190V Ergotism, NOS
(DD-80000) (L-41171)
DD-94192V Gangrenous ergotism
(DD-80000) (C-55870) (L-41171)
DD-94194V Spasmodic ergotism
(DD-80000) (L-41174)
DD-94200V Estrogenic mycotoxicosis
(DD-80000)
DD-94210V Facial eczema
(DD-80000) (C-30865) (L-45731)
Pithomycotoxicosis
(DD-80000) (L-45731)
DD-94220V Fusariotoxicosis
(DD-80000) (L-45900) (L-45904)
(C-45915)
DD-94222V Vomiting and feed refusal in swine
(DD-80000) (L-45904)
Fusariotoxicosis due to Fusarium graminearum
(DD-80000) (L-45904)
DD-94230V Fescue poisoning
(DD-80000) (L-DB750)
Fescue foot
(DD-80000) (L-DB750)
Summer fescue toxicosis
(DD-80000) (L-DB750) (L-44109)
DD-94232V Festuca arundinacea poisoning
(DD-80000) (L-DB750)
Tall fescue toxicosis
(DD-80000) (L-DB750)
Tall fescue poisoning
(DD-80000) (L-DB750)
DD-94240V Fusarium estrogenism and vulvovaginitis
(DD-80000)
Porcine vulvovaginitis
(DD-80000) (L-45904)
DD-94250V Hepatic necrosis in animals
(DD-80000) (C-30821) (L-44328)
DD-94270V Maroek poisoning
(DD-80000) (L-44133)
DD-94280V Mold nephropathy of swine
(DD-80000) (C-30820) (L-44321)
(L-44141)
DD-94290V Moldy walnut poisoning
(DD-80000)
DD-94410V Myrotheciotoxicosis
(DD-80000) (L-44671)
DD-94420V Neurotoxicosis in animals
(DD-80000) (C-30827) (L-44329)
DD-94430V Ochratoxicosis
(DD-80000) (L-44141) (L-44321)
Porcine nephropathy
(DD-80000) (L-44141) (L-44321)

D-94 ANIMAL MYCOTOXICOSES — Continued

DD-94440V Penicillium cyclopium toxicosis
(DD-80000) (L-44372)

DD-94442V Penicillium rubrum toxicosis
(DD-80000) (C-30862) (L-44319)

DD-94460V Poultry hemorrhagic syndrome
(DD-80000) (L-44135)

DD-94470V Slaframine toxicosis
(DD-80000) (T-61083) (F-57102)
(G-C001) (F-50440) (L-D6410)
(G-C008) (L-45561) (C-30864)
Slobbers
(DD-80000) (T-61083) (F-57102)
(G-C001) (F-50440) (L-D6410)
(G-C008) (L-45561) (C-30864)

DD-94480V Stachybotryotoxicosis
(DD-80000) (C-30863) (L-45721)

DD-94520V Tremorgenataxia syndrome
(DD-80000) (L-44333)

DD-94530V Tricothecium toxicosis
(DD-80000) (L-44240)

D-95 POISONING BY ARTHROPODS AND OTHER ANIMALS

D-950 Poisoning by Arthropods: General Terms

DD-95000V Poisoning by arthropod, NOS
(DD-80000)

D-951 Insect-Related Poisonings

DD-95100V Insect-related poisoning, NOS
(DD-80000)
Insect poisoning, NOS
(DD-80000)

DD-95110V Poisoning by ingestion of insect-infested food, NOS
(DD-80000)

DD-95120V Blister beetle poisoning
(DD-80000) (C-60202)
Cantharidin poisoning
(DD-80000)

DD-95121V Poisoning by Epicauta, NOS
(DD-80000)

DD-95122V Poisoning by Epicauta vittata
(DD-80000)

DD-95130V Poisoning by caterpillar, NOS
(DD-80000)

DD-95132V Poisoning by puss caterpillar
(DD-80000)

DD-95140V Poisoning by sawfly larvae
(DD-80000)
Sawfly larvae toxicity
(DD-80000)

DD-95142V Poisoning by Lophyrotoma interrupta
(DD-80000)

DD-95200V Poisoning by insect bite, NOS
(DD-80000)
Poisoning by insect sting, NOS
(DD-80000)

DD-95210V Poisoning by bee sting, NOS
(DD-80000)

DD-95212V Poisoning by honey bee sting, NOS
(DD-80000)
Poisoning by Apis mellifera
(DD-80000)

DD-95214V Poisoning by African honey bee sting
(DD-80000)
Poisoning by Apis mellifera scutellata
(DD-80000)

DD-95216V Poisoning by bumble bee sting, NOS
(DD-80000)
Poisoning by Bombus, NOS
(DD-80000)

DD-95230V Poisoning by wasp sting, NOS
(DD-80000)

DD-95240V Poisoning by hornet sting, NOS
(DD-80000)
Poisoning by yellow jacket, NOS
(DD-80000)

DD-95250V Poisoning by sting or bite of fire ant, NOS
(DD-80000)
Poisoning by sting or bite of Solenopis, NOS
(DD-80000)

DD-95254V Poisoning by sting of harvester ant, NOS
(DD-80000)
Poisoning by sting of Pogomyrmex, NOS
(DD-80000)

DD-95300V Poisoning by venomous spider bite, NOS
(DD-80000)

DD-95304V Poisoning by black widow spider bite
(DD-80000)
Poisoning by Lactrodectus mactans bite
(DD-80000)

DD-95305V Poisoning by brown recluse spider bite
(DD-80000)
Poisoning by Loxosceles bite
(DD-80000)

DD-95330V Poisoning by scorpion sting, NOS
(DD-80000)

DD-95340V Poisoning by Centruroides sculpturatus
(DD-80000)

DD-95400V Toad poisoning
(DD-80000) (C-34210)
Poisoning by ingesting toad
(DD-80000) (C-34210)

DD-95402V Poisoning by Colorado river toad
(DD-80000) (C-34210) (L-B1502)
Poisoning by Bufo alvarius
(DD-80000) (C-34210) (L-B1502)

DD-95404V Poisoning by marine toad
(DD-80000) (C-34210) (L-B1503)
Poisoning by Bufo marinus
(DD-80000) (C-34210) (L-B1503)

DD-95406V Poisoning by giant toad
(DD-80000) (C-34210) (L-B1511)

DD-95500V Poisoning by venomous reptile bite, NOS
(DD-80000)

DD-95510V Poisoning by venomous lizard bite, NOS
(DD-80000)

DD-95512V Poisoning by Gila monster bite
(DD-80000)
Poisoning by Heloderma suspectum bite
(DD-80000)

DD-95514V Poisoning by Mexican beaded lizard bite
(DD-80000)
Poisoning by Heloderma horridum bite
(DD-80000)

DD-95520V Poisoning by venomous snake, NOS
(DD-80000)
Snake venom poisoning, NOS
(DD-80000)
Snake bite poisoning, NOS
(DD-80000)

DD-95700V Poisoning by marine animal, NOS
(DD-80000)

DD-95710V Jellyfish poisoning
(DD-80000)

DD-95720V Poisoning by Portuguese man-of-war
(DD-80000)

DD-95730V Stingray poisoning
(DD-80000)

DD-95800V Fish poisoning, NOS
(DD-80000)
Ichthyosarcotoxism, NOS
(DD-80000)
Poisoning by eating contaminated fish
(DD-80000)
Ciguatera
(DD-80000)

DD-95810V Fugu poisoning
(DD-80000)
Puffer fish poisoning
(DD-80000)
Tetrodotoxism
(DD-80000)

DD-95820V Scombroid fish poisoning
(DD-80000)

DD-95910V Paralytic shellfish poisoning
(DD-80000)
Poisoning due to red tide of dinoflagellates
(DD-80000)

DD-95912V Shellfish poisoning due to Gonyaulax catenalla
(DD-80000)

DD-95914V Shellfish poisoning due to Gonyaulax tamarensis
(DD-80000)

DD-95920V Neurotoxic shellfish poisoning
(DD-80000)
Poisoning due to shellfish contaminated with Gymnodinium
(DD-80000)

D-97-98 POISONING OF ANIMALS BY PLANTS

DD-97000V Poisoning of animal by plant, NOS
(DD-80000) (L-D0000)
Plant poisoning
(DD-80000) (L-D0000)

DD-97100V Abrus precatorius poisoning
(DD-80000) (L-D6201)
Precatory bean poisoning
(DD-80000) (L-D6201)
Rosary pea poisoning
(DD-80000) (L-D6201)

DD-97110V Acacia species poisoning
(DD-80000) (L-D6210)

DD-97111V Acacia berlandieri poisoning
(DD-80000) (L-D6211)
Guajillo poisoning
(DD-80000) (L-D6211)

DD-97112V Acacia georginae poisoning
(DD-80000) (L-D6212)
Gidgee tree poisoning
(DD-80000) (L-D6212)
Gorgina river poisoning
(DD-80000) (L-D6212)

DD-97114V Acacia nilotica poisoning
(DD-80000) (L-D6213)

DD-97120V Acer rubrum poisoning
(DD-80000) (L-D8201)
Red maple poisoning
(DD-80000) (L-D8201)

DD-97130V Acokanthera species poisoning
(DD-80000) (L-D9100)
Arrow poison poisoning
(DD-80000) (L-D9100)

DD-97140V Aconitum species poisoning
(DD-80000) (L-D2800)
Aconite poisoning
(DD-80000) (L-D2800)
Monkshood poisoning
(DD-80000) (L-D2800)

DD-97150V Adenia species poisoning
(DD-80000) (L-D4200)

DD-97160V Adenium species poisoning
(DD-80000) (L-D9110)

DD-97162V Adenium multiflorum poisoning
(DD-80000) (L-D9112)
Impala lily poisoning
(DD-80000) (L-D9112)

DD-97170V Aesculus species poisoning
(DD-80000) (L-D8300)
Buckeye poisoning
(DD-80000) (L-D8300)

DD-97172V Aesculus hippocastanum poisoning
(DD-80000) (L-D8301)
Horsechestnut poisoning
(DD-80000) (L-D8301)

DD-97180V Agave species poisoning
(DD-80000) (L-DC100)
Sisal plant poisoning
(DD-80000) (L-DC100)

D-97-98 POISONING OF ANIMALS BY PLANTS — Continued

DD-97182V Agave lecheguilla poisoning (DD-80000) (L-DC101)
Lechuguilla poisoning (DD-80000) (L-DC101)
DD-97190V Agrostemma species poisoning (DD-80000) (L-D3600)
DD-97192V Agrostemma githago poisoning (DD-80000) (L-D3601)
Corn cockle poisoning (DD-80000) (L-D3601)
DD-971A0V Albizia species poisoning (DD-80000) (L-D6300)
Paper bark poisoning (DD-80000) (L-D6300)
Poison pod poisoning (DD-80000) (L-D6300)
DD-971B0V Aleurites fordii poisoning (DD-80000) (L-D5471)
Tung-oil tree poisoning (DD-80000) (L-D5471)
DD-97200V Algae poisoning (DD-80000) (L-DD100)
DD-97202V Microcystis species poisoning (DD-80000) (L-DD130)
DD-97204V Microcystis flos-aquae poisoning (DD-80000) (L-DD131)
Blue green algae poisoning (DD-80000) (L-DD131)
DD-97220V Allium species poisoning (DD-80000) (L-DC110)
DD-97222V Allium cepa poisoning (DD-80000) (L-DC112)
Onion poisoning (DD-80000) (L-DC112)
DD-97240V Amaranthus species poisoning (DD-80000) (L-D3500)
DD-97242V Amaranthus retroflexus poisoning (DD-80000) (L-D3502)
Pigweed poisoning (DD-80000) (L-D3502)
Perirenal edema disease (DD-80000) (L-D3502)
DD-97250V Amianthium muscaetoxicum poisoning (DD-80000) (L-DC121)
Fly poison poisoning (DD-80000) (L-DC121)
Staggergrass poisoning (DD-80000) (L-DC121)
Crow poison poisoning (DD-80000) (L-DC121)
DD-97260V Ammi species poisoning (DD-80000) (L-D8A90)
DD-97262V Ammi majus poisoning (DD-80000) (L-D8A91)
Bishop's weed poisoning (DD-80000) (L-D8A91)
DD-97270V Amsinckia species poisoning (DD-80000) (L-D9C00)
DD-97272V Amsinckia intermedia poisoning (DD-80000) (L-D9C01)
Tarweed poisoning (DD-80000) (L-D9C01)
DD-97280V Anagallis arvensis poisoning (DD-80000) (L-D3D01)
Scarlet pimpernel poisoning (DD-80000) (L-D3D01)
DD-97290V Anemone species poisoning (DD-80000) (L-D2830)
DD-972A0V Anthoxanthum odoratum poisoning (DD-80000) (L-DB7A1)
Sweet vernal grass poisoning (DD-80000) (L-DB7A1)
DD-97300V Apocynum species poisoning (DD-80000) (L-D9121)
Dogbane poisoning (DD-80000) (L-D9121)
DD-97310V Argemone species poisoning (DD-80000) (L-D2B00)
Mexican poppy poisoning (DD-80000) (L-D2B01)
DD-97320V Arisaema species poisoning (DD-80000) (L-DB010)
DD-97322V Arisaema triphyllum poisoning (DD-80000) (L-DB011)
Jack-in-the-pulpit poisoning (DD-80000) (L-DB011)
DD-97330V Arum maculatum poisoning (DD-80000) (L-DB001)
Arum lily poisoning (DD-80000) (L-DB001)
DD-97340V Asaemia axillaris poisoning (DD-80000) (L-DA953)
Vuursiekte (DD-80000) (L-DA953)
DD-97350V Asclepias species poisoning (DD-80000) (L-D9300)
DD-97352V Asclepias fructicosa poisoning (DD-80000) (L-D9301)
Milkweed poisoning (DD-80000) (L-D9301)
DD-97360V Astragalus species poisoning (DD-80000) (L-D6660)
Locoweed astragalus poisoning (DD-80000) (L-D6660)
Locoism (DD-80000) (L-D6660)
DD-97370V Athanasia trifurcata poisoning (DD-80000) (L-DA957)
DD-97380V Atropa belladonna poisoning (DD-80000) (L-D9801)
Deadly nightshade poisoning (DD-80000) (L-D9801)
DD-97390V Avena sativa poisoning (DD-80000) (L-DB701)
Oats poisoning (DD-80000) (L-DB701)

DD-973A0V Baccharis species poisoning
(DD-80000) (L-DA430)
Silverling poisoning
(DD-80000) (L-DA430)

DD-973B0V Baileya multiradiata poisoning
(DD-80000) (L-DA451)

DD-97400V Beta species poisoning
(DD-80000) (L-D3730)

DD-97402V Beta vulgaris poisoning
(DD-80000) (L-D3731)
Sugar beet poisoning
(DD-80000) (L-D3731)

DD-97410V Bowiea species poisoning
(DD-80000) (L-DC310)

DD-97420V Brachiaria species poisoning
(DD-80000) (L-DB760)

DD-97430V Brassica species poisoning
(DD-80000) (L-D4800)

DD-97432V Brassica rapa poisoning
(DD-80000) (L-D4804)
Turnip poisoning
(DD-80000) (L-D4804)

DD-97433V Brassica napus poisoning
(DD-80000) (L-D4802)
Rape poisoning
(DD-80000) (L-D4802)

DD-97434V Brassica oleracea poisoning
(DD-80000) (L-D4801)
Kale poisoning
(DD-80000) (L-D4801)

DD-97435V Brassica sinapis poisoning
(DD-80000) (L-D4807)
Mustard seed poisoning
(DD-80000) (L-D4807)

DD-97440V Bulnesia sarmientii poisoning
(DD-80000)
Palo Santo tree poisoning
(DD-80000)

DD-97450V Buxus sempervirens poisoning
(DD-80000) (L-D5900)
Common box poisoning
(DD-80000) (L-D5900)

DD-97460V Cannabis sativa poisoning
(DD-80000) (L-D5101)
Marihuana poisoning
(DD-80000) (L-D5101)

DD-97470V Cassia species poisoning
(DD-80000) (L-D6240)
Coffee senna poisoning
(DD-80000) (L-D6240)

DD-97480V Castalis species poisoning
(DD-80000) (L-DA950)

DD-97490V Centaurea species poisoning
(DD-80000) (L-DA460)

DD-97492V Centaurea solstitialis poisoning
(DD-80000) (L-DA461)
Yellow star thistle poisoning
(DD-80000) (L-DA461)
Nigropallidal encephalomalacia
(DD-80000) (L-DA461)
Chewing disease
(DD-80000) (L-DA461)

DD-97500V Cestrum species poisoning
(DD-80000) (L-D9810)
Chase valley disease
(DD-80000) (L-D9810)

DD-97502V Cestrum diurnum poisoning
(DD-80000) (L-D9812)
Wild jasmine poisoning
(DD-80000) (L-D9812)
Cestrum enzootic calcinosis
(DD-80000) (L-D9812)

DD-97504V Cestrum laevigatum poisoning
(DD-80000) (L-D9813)
Ink-berry poisoning
(DD-80000) (L-D9813)

DD-97506V Cestrum parqui poisoning
(DD-80000) (L-D9814)

DD-97510V Cheilanthes sieberi poisoning
(DD-80000) (L-DD443)
Mulga poisoning
(DD-80000) (L-DD443)
Rock fern poisoning
(DD-80000) (L-DD443)
Hepatic lipofuscinosis
(DD-80000) (L-DD443)

DD-97514V Cheilanthes sinnata poisoning
(DD-80000) (L-DD442)
Jimmy fern poisoning
(DD-80000) (L-DD442)

DD-97520V Chelidonium majus poisoning
(DD-80000) (L-D2B11)
Celandine poisoning
(DD-80000) (L-D2B11)

DD-97530V Chenopodium album species poisoning
(DD-80000) (L-D3411)
Lambsquarters poisoning
(DD-80000) (L-D3411)

DD-97540V Christmas tree poisoning
(DD-80000)

DD-97550V Chrysocoma tenuifolia poisoning
(DD-80000) (L-DA541)
Bitterbush poisoning
(DD-80000) (L-DA541)
Kaalsiekte in lambs
(DD-80000) (L-DA541)
Lakseersiekte
(DD-80000) (L-DA541)
Purging disease
(DD-80000) (L-DA541)
Valsiekte
(DD-80000) (L-DA541)
Falling disease
(DD-80000) (L-DA541)

DD-97560V Cicuta species poisoning
(DD-80000) (L-D8A20)

D-97-98 POISONING OF ANIMALS BY PLANTS — Continued

DD-97562V Cicuta maculata poisoning
(DD-80000) (L-D8A22)
Water hemlock poisoning
(DD-80000) (L-D8A22)
DD-97564V Cicuta virosa poisoning
(DD-80000) (L-D8A23)
Cowbane poisoning
(DD-80000) (L-D8A23)
DD-97570V Colchicum autumnale poisoning
(DD-80000) (L-DC131)
Autumn crocus poisoning
(DD-80000) (L-DC131)
DD-97580V Colocasia antiquorum poisoning
(DD-80000) (L-DB091)
Elephant's ear poisoning
(DD-80000) (L-DB091)
DD-97590V Conium maculatum poisoning
(DD-80000) (L-D8A31)
Poison hemlock poisoning
(DD-80000) (L-D8A31)
DD-975A0V Convallaria majalis poisoning
(DD-80000) (L-DC141)
Lily of the valley poisoning
(DD-80000) (L-DC141)
DD-975B0V Cotyledon species poisoning
(DD-80000) (L-D5C20)
Krimpsiekte
(DD-80000) (L-D5C20)
DD-97600V Crotalaria species poisoning
(DD-80000) (L-D6220)
DD-97602V Crotalaria burkeana poisoning
(DD-80000) (L-D6221)
Rattlebox poisoning
(DD-80000) (L-D6221)
DD-97604V Crotalaria dura poisoning
(DD-80000) (L-D6222)
Wild lucerne poisoning
(DD-80000) (L-D6222)
DD-97605V Crotalaria globifera poisoning
(DD-80000) (L-D6223)
DD-97606V Crotalaria juncea poisoning
(DD-80000) (L-D6224)
DD-97607V Crotalaria spartioides poisoning
(DD-80000) (L-D6225)
DD-97608V Crotalaria spectabilis poisoning
(DD-80000) (L-D6229)
DD-97620V Croton species poisoning
(DD-80000) (L-D5320)
DD-97630V Cryptostegia grandiflora poisoning
(DD-80000) (L-DB931)
Rubber vine poisoning
(DD-80000) (L-DB931)
DD-97640V Cucumis species poisoning
(DD-80000) (L-D4450)
DD-97650V Cupressus species poisoning
(DD-80000) (L-D1100)
Cypress poisoning
(DD-80000) (L-D1100)
DD-97660V Cycas species poisoning
(DD-80000) (L-D1200)
Cycada poisoning
(DD-80000) (L-D1200)
Zamia staggers
(DD-80000) (L-D1200)
DD-97670V Cymopterus watsonii poisoning
(DD-80000) (L-D8A70)
Spring parsley poisoning
(DD-80000) (L-D8A70)
DD-97680V Cynanchum species poisoning
(DD-80000) (L-D9360)
DD-97690V Cynodon species poisoning
(DD-80000) (L-DB710)
DD-97692V Cynodon dactylon poisoning
(DD-80000) (L-DB711)
Bermuda grass tremors
(DD-80000) (L-DB711)
Kweek tremors
(DD-80000) (L-DB711)
Couch grass poisoning
(DD-80000) (L-DB711)
DD-976A0V Cynoglossum officinale poisoning
(DD-80000) (L-D9C10)
Hound's tongue poisoning
(DD-80000) (L-D9C10)
DD-976B0V Daphne species poisoning
(DD-80000) (L-D5700)
DD-97700V Datura species poisoning
(DD-80000) (L-D9820)
DD-97702V Datura stramonium poisoning
(DD-80000) (L-D9821)
Thornapple poisoning
(DD-80000) (L-D9821)
Jimsonweed poisoning
(DD-80000) (L-D9821)
Stinkweed poisoning
(DD-80000) (L-D9821)
DD-97710V Delphinium species poisoning
(DD-80000) (L-D2850)
Larkspur poisoning
(DD-80000) (L-D2850)
DD-97720V Descurainia pinnata poisoning
(DD-80000) (L-D4831)
Tansy mustard poisoning
(DD-80000) (L-D4831)
DD-97730V Dicentra species poisoning
(DD-80000) (L-D2B30)
DD-97732V Dicentra spectabilis poisoning
(DD-80000) (L-D2B31)
Bleeding heart poisoning
(DD-80000) (L-D2B31)
DD-97734V Dicentra canadensis poisoning
(DD-80000) (L-D2B33)
Squirrel corn poisoning
(DD-80000) (L-D2B33)
DD-97736V Dicentra cucullaria poisoning
(DD-80000) (L-D2B32)
Dutchman's breeches poisoning
(DD-80000) (L-D2B32)

DD-97740V Dichapetalum species poisoning
(DD-80000) (L-D5600)

DD-97742V Dichapetalum cymosum poisoning
(DD-80000) (L-D5601)
Gifblaar poisoning
(DD-80000) (L-D5601)

DD-97750V Dieffenbachia species poisoning
(DD-80000) (L-DB050)
Dumbcane poisoning
(DD-80000) (L-DB050)

DD-97760V Digitalis species poisoning
(DD-80000) (L-D9700)

DD-97762V Digitalis purpurea poisoning
(DD-80000) (L-D9701)
Foxglove poisoning
(DD-80000) (L-D9701)

DD-97770V Dipcadi glaucum poisoning
(DD-80000) (L-DC221)
Wild onion poisoning
(DD-80000) (L-DC221)

DD-97780V Drymaria pachyphylla poisoning
(DD-80000) (L-D3612)
Inkweed poisoning
(DD-80000) (L-D3612)
Drymary poisoning
(DD-80000) (L-D3612)

DD-97790V Dryopteris species poisoning
(DD-80000) (L-DD450)
Male fern poisoning
(DD-80000) (L-DD450)
Retrobulbar neuropathy
(DD-80000) (L-DD450)

DD-977A0V Echinopogon ovatus poisoning
(DD-80000) (L-DB841)
Rough-bearded grass poisoning
(DD-80000) (L-DB841)

DD-977B0V Echium species poisoning
(DD-80000) (L-D9C20)

DD-97800V Echium lycopis poisoning
(DD-80000) (L-D9C22)
Paterson's curse
(DD-80000) (L-D9C22)

DD-97810V Encephalartos species poisoning
(DD-80000) (L-D1330)

DD-97820V Equisetum species poisoning
(DD-80000) (L-DD500)

DD-97822V Equisetum arvense poisoning
(DD-80000) (L-DD501)

DD-97824V Equisetum palustre poisoning
(DD-80000) (L-DD502)
Horsetails poisoning
(DD-80000) (L-DD502)

DD-97830V Erodium species poisoning
(DD-80000) (L-D7120)

DD-97840V Erythrophloeum species poisoning
(DD-80000) (L-D6370)

DD-97842V Erythrophloeum chlorostachys poisoning
(DD-80000) (L-D6372)
Ironwood tree poisoning
(DD-80000) (L-D6372)

DD-97850V Eucalyptus species poisoning
(DD-80000) (L-D6B00)

DD-97852V Eucalyptus cladocalyx poisoning
(DD-80000) (L-D6B01)
Gum tree poisoning
(DD-80000) (L-D6B01)

DD-97860V Eupatorium adenophorum poisoning
(DD-80000) (L-DA502)
Crofton weed poisoning
(DD-80000) (L-DA502)

DD-97862V Eupatorium rugosum poisoning
(DD-80000) (L-DA501)
White snakeroot poisoning
(DD-80000) (L-DA501)

DD-97870V Euphorbia species poisoning
(DD-80000) (L-D5300)
Caustic creeper poisoning
(DD-80000) (L-D5300)

DD-97872V Euphorbia mauritanica poisoning
(DD-80000) (L-D5311)
Yellow milkbush poisoning
(DD-80000) (L-D5311)

DD-97880V Fadogia homblei poisoning
(DD-80000) (L-D9431)
Wild date poisoning
(DD-80000) (L-D9431)

DD-97890V Fagopyrum species poisoning
(DD-80000) (L-D3740)
Fagopyrism
(DD-80000) (L-D3740)

DD-97892V Fagopyrum esculentum poisoning
(DD-80000) (L-D3742)
Buckwheat poisoning
(DD-80000) (L-D3742)

DD-978A0V Fagus sylvatica poisoning
(DD-80000) (L-D2D01)
Beech nut poisoning
(DD-80000) (L-D2D01)

DD-97910V Galega species poisoning
(DD-80000) (L-D6540)
Goat's rue poisoning
(DD-80000) (L-D6540)

DD-97920V Galenia africana poisoning
(DD-80000) (L-D3351)
Kraalbos poisoning
(DD-80000) (L-D3351)
Waterpens
(DD-80000) (L-D3351)

DD-97930V Gastrolobium species poisoning
(DD-80000) (L-D6390)

DD-97940V Geigeria species poisoning
(DD-80000) (L-DA730)
Vermeersiekte
(DD-80000) (L-DA730)

DD-97950V Gelsemium sempervirens poisoning
(DD-80000) (L-D9001)
Yellow jessamine poisoning
(DD-80000) (L-D9001)

D-97-98 POISONING OF ANIMALS BY PLANTS — Continued

DD-97960V Glycine max poisoning
(DD-80000) (L-D6331)
Trichloroethylene-extracted soybean meal poisoning
(DD-80000) (L-D6331)
DD-97970V Gnidia species poisoning
(DD-80000) (L-D5720)
DD-97980V Gomphrena celosiodes poisoning
(DD-80000) (L-D3521)
Soft khaki weed poisoning
(DD-80000) (L-D3521)
DD-97990V Gossypium species poisoning
(DD-80000) (L-D4D00)
Cottonseed cake poisoning
(DD-80000) (L-D4D00)
DD-979A0V Gutierrezia species poisoning
(DD-80000) (L-DA630)
DD-979A2V Gutierrezia microcephala poisoning
(DD-80000) (L-DA631)
Perennial broomweed poisoning
(DD-80000) (L-DA631)
DD-97A00V Halogeton species poisoning
(DD-80000) (L-D3750)
DD-97A02V Halogeton glomeratus poisoning
(DD-80000) (L-D3751)
DD-97A10V Haplopappus heterophyllus poisoning
(DD-80000) (L-DA641)
Rayless goldenrod poisoning
(DD-80000) (L-DA641)
Burroweed poisoning
(DD-80000) (L-DA641)
DD-97A20V Hedera helix poisoning
(DD-80000) (L-D8911)
Common ivy poisoning
(DD-80000) (L-D8911)
DD-97A30V Helenium species poisoning
(DD-80000) (L-DA650)
Sneezeweed poisoning
(DD-80000) (L-DA650)
DD-97A32V Helenium hoopesii poisoning
(DD-80000) (L-DA651)
Orange sneezeweed poisoning
(DD-80000) (L-DA651)
DD-97A34V Helenium microcephalum poisoning
(DD-80000) (L-DA652)
Small head sneezeweed poisoning
(DD-80000) (L-DA652)
DD-97A40V Helichrysum species poisoning
(DD-80000) (L-DA740)
DD-97A42V Helichrysum argyosphaerum
(DD-80000) (L-DA741)
Wild everlasting poisoning
(DD-80000) (L-DA741)
DD-97A50V Heliotropium europaeum poisoning
(DD-80000) (L-D9C31)
Heliotrope poisoning
(DD-80000) (L-D9C31)
DD-97A60V Hertia pallens poisoning
(DD-80000) (L-DA941)
Springbokbush poisoning
(DD-80000) (L-DA941)
DD-97A70V Homeria species poisoning
(DD-80000) (L-DC910)
Cape tulip poisoning
(DD-80000) (L-DC910)
Homeria tulp poisoning
(DD-80000) (L-DC910)
DD-97A72V Homeria pallida poisoning
(DD-80000) (L-DC911)
DD-97A80V Hordeum vulgare poisoning
(DD-80000) (L-DB900)
DD-97A90V Hymenoxys species poisoning
(DD-80000) (L-DA660)
DD-97A92V Hymenoxys oderata poisoning
(DD-80000) (L-DA661)
Bitterweed poisoning
(DD-80000) (L-DA661)
Rubberweed poisoning
(DD-80000) (L-DA661)
DD-97A94V Hymenoxys richardsonii poisoning
(DD-80000) (L-DA662)
Pingue poisoning
(DD-80000) (L-DA662)
Colorado rubberweed poisoning
(DD-80000) (L-DA662)
DD-97AA0V Hyoscyamus niger poisoning
(DD-80000) (L-D9831)
Black henbane poisoning
(DD-80000) (L-D9831)
DD-97B00V Hypericum species poisoning
(DD-80000) (L-D3900)
DD-97B02V Hypericum perforatum poisoning
(DD-80000) (L-D3901)
St.John's wort poisoning
(DD-80000) (L-D3901)
Goatweed poisoning
(DD-80000) (L-D3901)
DD-98010V Indigofera dominii poisoning
(DD-80000) (L-D6352)
Birdsville indigo poisoning
(DD-80000) (L-D6352)
Birdsville horse disease
(DD-80000) (L-D6352)
DD-98020V Inula conyza poisoning
(DD-80000) (L-DA971)
Fly-bane poisoning
(DD-80000) (L-DA971)
DD-98022V Inula graveolens poisoning
(DD-80000) (L-DA972)
Cape khakiweed poisoning
(DD-80000) (L-DA972)
DD-98030V Ipomoea species poisoning
(DD-80000) (L-D9B10)
DD-98032V Ipomoea batatas poisoning
(DD-80000) (L-D9B12)
Moldy sweet potato poisoning
(DD-80000) (L-D9B12)

DD-98034V Ipomoea muelleri poisoning
(DD-80000) (L-D9B14)
Morning glory poisoning
(DD-80000) (L-D9B14)

DD-98040V Isotropis species poisoning
(DD-80000) (L-D6328)

DD-98050V Jatropha curcas poisoning
(DD-80000) (L-D5361)
Purge nut poisoning
(DD-80000) (L-D5361)

DD-98060V Juglans nigra poisoning
(DD-80000) (L-D7B11)
Black walnut poisoning
(DD-80000) (L-D7B11)

DD-98070V Kalanchoe species poisoning
(DD-80000) (L-D5C10)

DD-98080V Kallstroemia hirsutissima poisoning
(DD-80000) (L-D7331)
Carpet weed poisoning
(DD-80000) (L-D7331)

DD-98090V Kalmia species poisoning
(DD-80000) (L-D3A10)
Laurel poisoning
(DD-80000) (L-D3A10)

DD-98091V Mountain laurel poisoning
(DD-80000) (L-D3A11)

DD-98092V Kalmia angustifolia poisoning
(DD-80000) (L-D3A12)
Lambkill poisoning
(DD-80000) (L-D3A12)

DD-980A0V Karwinskia humboldtiana poisoning
(DD-80000) (L-D5A11)
Coyotillo poisoning
(DD-80000) (L-D5A11)
Limberleg
(DD-80000) (L-D5A11)

DD-980B0V Kochia scoparia poisoning
(DD-80000) (L-D3421)
Mexican fireweed poisoning
(DD-80000) (L-D3421)

DD-98100V Laburnum anagyroides poisoning
(DD-80000) (L-D6318)
Golden rain poisoning
(DD-80000) (L-D6318)

DD-98110V Lantana species poisoning
(DD-80000) (L-DA020)

DD-98112V Lantana camara poisoning
(DD-80000) (L-DA021)

DD-98120V Lasiospermum bipinnatum poisoning
(DD-80000) (L-DA954)
Ganskweek poisoning
(DD-80000) (L-DA954)

DD-98130V Lathyrus species poisoning
(DD-80000) (L-D6260)
Vetchling poisoning
(DD-80000) (L-D6260)
Lathyrism
(DD-80000) (L-D6260)

DD-98132V Lathyrus sylvestris poisoning
(DD-80000) (L-D6265)
Everlasting pea poisoning
(DD-80000) (L-D6265)

DD-98140V Leucaena species poisoning
(DD-80000) (L-D6630)
Jumbey
(DD-80000) (L-D6630)

DD-98150V Lidneria species poisoning
(DD-80000) (L-DC240)
Slangkop poisoning
(DD-80000) (L-DC240)

DD-98160V Linum species poisoning
(DD-80000) (L-D7000)

DD-98162V Linum usitatissium poisoning
(DD-80000) (L-D7001)
Flax poisoning
(DD-80000) (L-D7001)

DD-98170V Lippia species poisoning
(DD-80000) (L-DA030)

DD-98180V Lobelia species poisoning
(DD-80000) (L-DA240)

DD-98182V Lobelia cardinalis poisoning
(DD-80000) (L-DA241)
Cardinal flower poisoning
(DD-80000) (L-DA241)

DD-98184V Lobelia inflata poisoning
(DD-80000) (L-DA242)
Indian tobacco poisoning
(DD-80000) (L-DA242)

DD-98190V Lolium species poisoning
(DD-80000) (L-DB910)
Ryegrass toxicity
(DD-80000) (L-DB910)

DD-98192V Lolium temulentum poisoning
(DD-80000) (L-DB911)

DD-98194V Lolium perenne poisoning
(DD-80000) (L-DB913)
Perennial ryegrass staggers
(DD-80000) (L-44111) (L-DB913)

DD-98196V Lolium rigidum poisoning
(DD-80000) (L-DB914)
Annual ryegrass staggers
(DD-80000) (C-30874) (L-55210)
(L-DB914)

DD-981A0V Lupinus species poisoning
(DD-80000) (L-D6500) (L-46022)
Mycotoxic lupinosis
(DD-80000) (L-D6500) (L-46022)
Lupinosis
(DD-80000) (L-D6500) (L-46022)

DD-981A2V Lupinus sericeus poisoning
(DD-80000) (L-D6504) (L-46022)
Crooked calf disease
(DD-80000) (L-D6504) (L-46022)

DD-981A4V Lupinus digitatus poisoning
(DD-80000) (L-D6503) (L-46022)
Lupine poisoning
(DD-80000) (L-D6503) (L-46022)

D-97-98 POISONING OF ANIMALS BY PLANTS — Continued

DD-98200V Macrozamia species poisoning
(DD-80000) (L-D1300)
DD-98210V Malva species poisoning
(DD-80000) (L-D4D20)
DD-98212V Mallow poisoning
(DD-80000) (L-D4D20)
DD-98220V Manihot species poisoning
(DD-80000) (L-D5370)
DD-98230V Marsilea drummondii poisoning
(DD-80000) (L-DD431)
Nardoo fern poisoning
(DD-80000) (L-DD431)
DD-98240V Matricaria nigellifolia poisoning
(DD-80000) (L-DA751)
Staggerweed poisoning
(DD-80000) (L-DA751)
Stootsiekte
(DD-80000) (L-DA751)
Pushing disease
(DD-80000) (L-DA751)
DD-98250V Medicago species poisoning
(DD-80000) (L-D6380)
DD-98252V Medicago sativa poisoning
(DD-80000) (L-D6381)
Alfalfa poisoning
(DD-80000) (L-D6381)
DD-98254V Medicago denticulatum poisoning
(DD-80000) (L-D6383)
Burr trefoil poisoning
(DD-80000) (L-D6383)
DD-98260V Melia azedarach poisoning
(DD-80000) (L-D7901)
Chinaberry tree poisoning
(DD-80000) (L-D7901)
DD-98270V Melianthus species poisoning
(DD-80000) (L-D8110)
DD-98280V Melica species poisoning
(DD-80000) (L-DB830)
DD-98282V Melica decumbens poisoning
(DD-80000) (L-DB831)
Dronkgras poisoning
(DD-80000) (L-DB831)
DD-98290V Melilotus species poisoning
(DD-80000) (L-D6530)
DD-98292V Melilotus alba poisoning
(DD-80000) (L-D6531) (L-44310)
Sweet clover poisoning
(DD-80000) (L-D6531) (L-44310)
DD-982A0V Mercurialis species poisoning
(DD-80000) (L-D5380)
DD-982A2V Mercurialis annua poisoning
(DD-80000) (L-D5381)
Annual mercury poisoning
(DD-80000) (L-D5381)
DD-98300V Mesembryanthemum species poisoning
(DD-80000) (L-D3360)
DD-98320V Mimosa pudica poisoning
(DD-80000) (L-D6561)
Sensitive plant poisoning
(DD-80000) (L-D6561)
DD-98330V Moraea species poisoning
(DD-80000) (L-DC920)
Moraea tulp poisoning
(DD-80000) (L-DC920)
DD-98340V Myoporum species poisoning
(DD-80000) (L-D9550)
Ngaio tree poisoning
(DD-80000) (L-D9550)
DD-98350V Narthecium ossifragum poisoning
(DD-80000) (L-DC261)
Bog asphodel poisoning
(DD-80000) (L-DC261)
DD-98360V Nerium oleander poisoning
(DD-80000) (L-D9142)
Oleander poisoning
(DD-80000) (L-D9142)
DD-98370V Nicotiana species poisoning
(DD-80000) (L-D9870)
DD-98372V Nicotiana glauca poisoning
(DD-80000) (L-D9878)
Tree tobacco poisoning
(DD-80000) (L-D9878)
DD-98374V Nicotiana tabacum poisoning
(DD-80000) (L-D9871)
Cigarette poisoning
(DD-80000)
Tobacco poisoning
(DD-80000) (L-D9871)
DD-98380V Nidorella species poisoning
(DD-80000) (L-DA920)
DD-98390V Nolina texana poisoning
(DD-80000) (L-DC521)
Sacahuiste poisoning
(DD-80000) (L-DC521)
Beargrass poisoning
(DD-80000) (L-DC521)
DD-983A0V Oenanthe species poisoning
(DD-80000) (L-D8A50)
Water dropwort poisoning
(DD-80000) (L-D8A50)
DD-983B0V Onoclea sensibilis poisoning
(DD-80000) (L-DD421)
Sensitive fern poisoning
(DD-80000) (L-DD421)
DD-98400V Opuntia species poisoning
(DD-80000) (L-D3220)
Prickly pear poisoning
(DD-80000) (L-D3220)
DD-98410V Ornithogalum species poisoning
(DD-80000) (L-DC160)
DD-98412V Ornithogalum thyrosides poisoning
(DD-80000) (L-DC163)
Chinkerinchee poisoning
(DD-80000) (L-DC163)

DD-98420V Ornithoglossum viride poisoning
(DD-80000) (L-DC233)
DD-98430V Osteospermum species poisoning
(DD-80000) (L-DA930)
DD-98440V Osteospermum ecklonis poisoning
(DD-80000) (L-DA932)
Dimorphotheca eckloni poisoning
(DD-80000) (L-DA932)
South African daisy poisoning
(DD-80000) (L-DA932)
DD-98450V Oxalis species poisoning
(DD-80000) (L-D7400)
Wood sorrel poisoning
(DD-80000) (L-D7400)
Soursob poisoning
(DD-80000) (L-D7400)
DD-98460V Oxylobium species poisoning
(DD-80000) (L-D63C0)
DD-98470V Oxytenia acerosa poisoning
(DD-80000) (L-DA690)
Prickly copperweed poisoning
(DD-80000) (L-DA691)
DD-98480V Oxytropis species poisoning
(DD-80000) (L-D6650)
Locoweed oxtropis poisoning
(DD-80000) (L-D6650)
DD-98490V Pachystigma species poisoning
(DD-80000) (L-D9440)
Gousiekte bush poisoning
(DD-80000) (L-D9440)
DD-984A0V Panicum species poisoning
(DD-80000) (L-DB920)
Dikkor
(DD-80000) (L-DB920)
DD-984A2V Panicum coloratum poisoning
(DD-80000) (L-DB924)
Kleingrass poisoning
(DD-80000) (L-DB924)
DD-984A4V Panicum effusum poisoning
(DD-80000) (L-DB926)
Hairy millet poisoning
(DD-80000) (L-DB926)
DD-98500V Papaver species poisoning
(DD-80000) (L-D2B40)
Poppy poisoning
(DD-80000) (L-D2B40)
DD-98510V Paspalum species poisoning
(DD-80000) (L-DB780)
DD-98512V Paspalum commersonii poisoning
(DD-80000) (L-DB786)
DD-98514V Paspalum dilatatum poisoning
(DD-80000) (L-DB781)
Dallas grass poisoning
(DD-80000) (L-DB781)
Paspalum staggers
(DD-80000) (L-41174) (L-DB781)
DD-98520V Pavetta species poisoning
(DD-80000) (L-D9450)
Gousiekte tree poisoning
(DD-80000) (L-D9450)
DD-98530V Peganum harmala poisoning
(DD-80000) (L-D7321)
African rue poisoning
(DD-80000) (L-D7321)
DD-98540V Pennisetum clandestinum poisoning
(DD-80000) (C-30830) (L-DB862)
(L-44671)
Kikuyu poisoning
(DD-80000) (C-30830) (L-DB862)
(L-44671)
Kikuyu grass poisoning
(DD-80000) (C-30830) (L-DB862)
(L-44671)
DD-98550V Perilla frutescens poisoning
(DD-80000) (L-DA261)
Purple mint poisoning
(DD-80000) (L-DA261)
Beefsteak plant poisoning
(DD-80000) (L-DA261)
DD-98560V Phalaris species poisoning
(DD-80000) (L-DB960)
DD-98562V Phalaris minor poisoning
(DD-80000) (L-DB962)
Canary grass poisoning
(DD-80000) (L-DB962)
Phalaris staggers
(DD-80000) (L-DB962)
DD-98564V Phalaris tuberosa poisoning
(DD-80000) (L-DB961)
Phalaris grass poisoning
(DD-80000) (L-DB961)
DD-98570V Phaseolus species poisoning
(DD-80000) (L-D6620)
DD-98580V Philodendron species poisoning
(DD-80000) (L-DB060)
DD-98590V Phyllanthus abnormis poisoning
(DD-80000) (L-D5401)
Spurge poisoning
(DD-80000) (L-D5401)
DD-985A0V Phytolacca species poisoning
(DD-80000) (L-D3000)
DD-985A2V Phytolacca americana poisoning
(DD-80000) (L-D3001)
Pokeweed poisoning
(DD-80000) (L-D3001)
DD-98600V Pieris japonica poisoning
(DD-80000) (L-D3A51)
Japanese pieris poisoning
(DD-80000) (L-D3A51)
DD-98610V Pimelea species poisoning
(DD-80000) (L-D5740)
DD-98612V Pimelea trichostachya poisoning
(DD-80000) (L-D5743)
Desert riceflower poisoning
(DD-80000) (L-D5743)
St.George disease
(DD-80000) (L-D5743)

D-97-98 POISONING OF ANIMALS BY PLANTS — Continued

DD-98620V Pinus species poisoning
(DD-80000) (L-D1500)

DD-98622V Pinus ponderosa poisoning
(DD-80000) (L-D1501)
Western yellow pine poisoning
(DD-80000) (L-D1501)

DD-98626V Pine needle abortion
(DD-80000) (L-D1501)

DD-98630V Pithecellobium jiringa poisoning
(DD-80000) (L-D66A1)
Djenkol bean poisoning
(DD-80000) (L-D66A1)

DD-98640V Podophyllum peltatum poisoning
(DD-80000) (L-D2A11)
Mandrake poisoning
(DD-80000) (L-D2A11)
Mayapple poisoning
(DD-80000) (L-D2A11)

DD-98650V Polygonum species poisoning
(DD-80000) (L-D3700)
Smartweed poisoning
(DD-80000) (L-D3700)

DD-98660V Portulacca species poisoning
(DD-80000) (L-D3300)

DD-98662V Portulacca oleracea poisoning
(DD-80000) (L-D3301)
Purslane poisoning
(DD-80000) (L-D3301)

DD-98670V Prosopis glandulosa poisoning
(DD-80000) (L-D6461)
Mesquite poisoning
(DD-80000) (L-D6461)

DD-98680V Prunus species poisoning
(DD-80000) (L-D5B40)

DD-98682V Prunus virginiana poisoning
(DD-80000) (L-D5B48)
Choke cherry poisoning
(DD-80000) (L-D5B48)

DD-98684V Prunus serotina poisoning
(DD-80000) (L-D5B41)
Wild cherry poisoning
(DD-80000) (L-D5B41)

DD-98686V Prunus caroliniana poisoning
(DD-80000) (L-D5B45)
Cherry laurel poisoning
(DD-80000) (L-D5B45)

DD-98690V Psilocaulon species poisoning
(DD-80000) (L-D3380)

DD-986A0V Psilostrophe species poisoning
(DD-80000) (L-DA700)
Paper-flowers poisoning
(DD-80000) (L-DA700)

DD-986B0V Pteridium aquilinum poisoning
(DD-80000) (L-DD411)
Bracken fern poisoning
(DD-80000) (L-DD411)
Enzootic hematuria
(DD-80000) (L-DD411)
Bright blindness
(DD-80000) (L-DD411)

DD-98700V Pteronia pallens poisoning
(DD-80000) (L-DA531)
Scholtz bush poisoning
(DD-80000) (L-DA531)

DD-98710V Quercus species poisoning
(DD-80000) (L-D2D10)
Oak bud poisoning
(DD-80000) (L-D2D10)
Acorn poisoning
(DD-80000) (L-D2D10)

DD-98712V Quercus havardi poisoning
(DD-80000) (L-D2D14)
Shin oak poisoning
(DD-80000) (L-D2D14)

DD-98720V Ranunculus species poisoning
(DD-80000) (L-D2870)
Buttercup poisoning
(DD-80000) (L-D2870)
Crowfoot poisoning
(DD-80000) (L-D2870)

DD-98730V Raphanus raphanistrum poisoning
(DD-80000) (L-D4851)
Wild radish poisoning
(DD-80000) (L-D4851)

DD-98740V Rheum rhaponicum poisoning
(DD-80000) (L-D3711)
Rhubarb poisoning
(DD-80000) (L-D3711)

DD-98750V Rhododendron species poisoning
(DD-80000) (L-D3A60)

DD-98752V Rhododendron indicum poisoning
(DD-80000) (L-D3A63)
Azealea poisoning
(DD-80000) (L-D3A63)

DD-98760V Ricinus communis poisoning
(DD-80000) (L-D5421)
Castor bean poisoning
(DD-80000) (L-D5421)
Castor oil plant poisoning
(DD-80000) (L-D5421)

DD-98770V Robinia pseudoacacia poisoning
(DD-80000) (L-D6451)
Black locust poisoning
(DD-80000) (L-D6451)

DD-98772V Robinia viscosa poisoning
(DD-80000) (L-D6452)
Clammy locust poisoning
(DD-80000) (L-D6452)

DD-98780V Romulea species poisoning
(DD-80000) (L-DC930)
Onion grass poisoning
(DD-80000) (L-DC930)

DD-98790V Rumex species poisoning
(DD-80000) (L-D3720)
Dock poisoning
(DD-80000) (L-D3720)

DD-98790V (cont.) Tongblaar poisoning
(DD-80000) (L-D3720)

DD-987A0V Salsola species poisoning
(DD-80000) (L-D3430)

DD-987A2V Salsola tuberculatiformis poisoning
(DD-80000) (L-D3432)
Saltwort poisoning
(DD-80000) (L-D3432)
Blomkoolganna poisoning
(DD-80000) (L-D3432)
Grootlamsiekte
(DD-80000) (L-D3432)
Big-lamb disease
(DD-80000) (L-D3432)

DD-98800V Sapium sebiferum poisoning
(DD-80000) (L-D5430)
Chinese tallow tree poisoning
(DD-80000) (L-D5430)

DD-98810V Saponaria species poisoning
(DD-80000) (L-D3620)

DD-98812V Saponaria officinalis poisoning
(DD-80000) (L-D3621)
Soapwort poisoning
(DD-80000) (L-D3621)

DD-98820 Sarcobatus vermiculatus poisoning
(DD-80000) (L-D3451)
Greasewood poisoning
(DD-80000) (L-D3451)

DD-98830V Sarcostemma species poisoning
(DD-80000) (L-D9340)
Melktou poisoning
(DD-80000) (L-D9340)

DD-98840V Scilla species poisoning
(DD-80000) (L-DC180)
Squill poisoning
(DD-80000) (L-DC180)

DD-98850V Secale cereale poisoning
(DD-80000) (L-DB971)
Rye poisoning
(DD-80000) (L-DB971)

DD-98860V Senecio species poisoning
(DD-80000) (L-DA810)
Seneciosis
(DD-80000) (L-DA810)
Dunsiekte
(DD-80000) (L-DA810)
Molteno straining disease
(DD-80000) (L-DA810)

DD-98862V Senecio jacobaea poisoning
(DD-80000) (L-DA811)
Tansy ragwort poisoning
(DD-80000) (L-DA811)

DD-98870V Sesbania species poisoning
(DD-80000) (L-D6290)
Sesbane poisoning
(DD-80000) (L-D6290)
Coffee bean poisoning
(DD-80000) (L-D6290)

DD-98872V Sesbania vesicaria poisoning
(DD-80000) (L-D6292)
Bladder pod poisoning
(DD-80000) (L-D6292)

DD-98874V Sesbania punicea poisoning
(DD-80000) (L-D6293)
Red sesbania poisoning
(DD-80000) (L-D6293)

DD-98880V Setaria species poisoning
(DD-80000) (L-DB950)

DD-98882V Setaria lutescens poisoning
(DD-80000) (L-DB951)
Foxtail grass
(DD-80000) (L-DB951)

DD-98890V Solanum species poisoning
(DD-80000) (L-D9900)

DD-98892V Solanum incanum poisoning
(DD-80000) (L-D9915)
Bitter apple poisoning
(DD-80000) (L-D9915)

DD-98893V Solanum kwebense poisoning
(DD-80000) (L-D9922)
Maldronksiekte
(DD-80000) (L-D9922)
Mad-drunk-disease
(DD-80000) (L-D9922)

DD-98894V Solanum malacoxylon poisoning
(DD-80000) (L-D9914)
Solanum enzootic calcinosis
(DD-80000) (L-D9914)
Enteque seco
(DD-80000) (L-D9914)
Manchester wasting disease
(DD-80000) (L-D9914)

DD-98895V Solanum nigrum poisoning
(DD-80000) (L-D9904)
Black nightshade poisoning
(DD-80000) (L-D9904)

DD-98896V Solanum tuberosum poisoning
(DD-80000) (L-D9909)
Potato poisoning
(DD-80000) (L-D9909)

DD-98900V Sophora secundiflora poisoning
(DD-80000) (L-D6441)
Mescal bean poisoning
(DD-80000) (L-D6441)

DD-98920V Sorghum species poisoning
(DD-80000) (L-DB930)
Prussic acid poisoning
(DD-80000) (L-DB930)
HCN poisoning
(DD-80000) (L-DB930)
Geilsiekte
(DD-80000) (L-DB930)

DD-98922V Sorghum almum poisoning
(DD-80000) (L-DB933)

DD-98923V Sorghum vulgare poisoning
(DD-80000) (L-DB931)
Milo poisoning
(DD-80000) (L-DB931)

D-97-98 POISONING OF ANIMALS BY PLANTS — Continued

DD-98924V Sorghum bicolor poisoning
(DD-80000) (L-DB934)
Sudan grass poisoning
(DD-80000) (L-DB934)

DD-98925V Sorghum halepense poisoning
(DD-80000) (L-DB932)
Johnson grass poisoning
(DD-80000) (L-DB932)

DD-98930V Sphenosciadium capitellatum poisoning
(DD-80000)
Whiteheads poisoning
(DD-80000)

DD-98940V Stipa species poisoning
(DD-80000) (L-DB790)
Spear grass poisoning
(DD-80000) (L-DB790)

DD-98950V Strophanthus species poisoning
(DD-80000) (L-D9190)
Poison rope poisoning
(DD-80000) (L-D9190)

DD-98960V Stypandra species poisoning
(DD-80000) (L-DC230)
Blind grass poisoning
(DD-80000) (L-DC230)

DD-98970V Swainsona species poisoning
(DD-80000) (L-D6670)
Darling pea poisoning
(DD-80000) (L-D6670)
Pea struck
(DD-80000) (L-D6670)

DD-98980V Taxus species poisoning
(DD-80000) (L-D1600)
Yew poisoning
(DD-80000) (L-D1600)

DD-98982V Taxus baccata poisoning
(DD-80000) (L-D1601)
English yew poisoning
(DD-80000) (L-D1601)

DD-98984V Taxus cuspidata poisoning
(DD-80000) (L-D1602)
Japanese yew poisoning
(DD-80000) (L-D1602)

DD-98990V Terminalia oblongata poisoning
(DD-80000) (L-D6A02)
Mackenzie river disease
(DD-80000) (L-D6A02)

DD-989A0V Tetradymia glabrata poisoning
(DD-80000) (L-DA841)
Horsebrush poisoning
(DD-80000) (L-DA841)

DD-989B0V Thamnosma texana poisoning
(DD-80000) (L-D7751)
Dutchmans breeches texana poisoning
(DD-80000) (L-D7751)

DD-98A00V Thesium species poisoning
(DD-80000) (L-D33A0)

DD-98A10V Thevetia peruviana poisoning
(DD-80000) (L-D9231)
Yellow oleander poisoning
(DD-80000) (L-D9231)

DD-98A20V Threlkeldia proceriflora poisoning
(DD-80000) (L-D3441)

DD-98A30V Toxicodendron diversilobum poisoning
(DD-80000) (L-D7A26)
Western poison oak poisoning
(DD-80000) (L-D7A26)

DD-98A32V Toxicodendron radicans poisoning
(DD-80000) (L-D7A30)
Poison ivy poisoning
(DD-80000) (L-D7A30)

DD-98A34V Toxicodendron vernix poisoning
(DD-80000) (L-D7A28)
Poison sumac poisoning
(DD-80000) (L-D7A28)

DD-98A40V Trachyandra species poisoning
(DD-80000) (L-DC250)

DD-98A50V Trachymene species poisoning
(DD-80000) (L-D8A81)
Bowie
(DD-80000) (L-D8A81)

DD-98A60V Trema aspera poisoning
(DD-80000) (L-D4E01)
Poison peach poisoning
(DD-80000) (L-D4E01)

DD-98A70V Trianthema species poisoning
(DD-80000) (L-D3370)
Hogweed poisoning
(DD-80000) (L-D3370)

DD-98A80V Tribulus terrestris poisoning
(DD-80000) (L-D7312)
Devil's thorn poisoning
(DD-80000) (L-D7312)
Puncture vine poisoning
(DD-80000) (L-D7312)
Geeldikkop
(DD-80000) (L-D7312)
Tribulosis ovis
(DD-80000) (L-D7312)

DD-98A90V Trifolium species poisoning
(DD-80000) (L-D6410)
Clover poisoning
(DD-80000) (L-D6410)

DD-98A92V Trifolium hybridum poisoning
(DD-80000) (L-D6412)
Alsike clover poisoning
(DD-80000) (L-D6412)

DD-98A94V Trifolium pratense poisoning
(DD-80000) (L-D6413)
Red clover poisoning
(DD-80000) (L-D6413)

DD-98A95V Trifolium repens poisoning
(DD-80000) (L-D6411)
White clover poisoning
(DD-80000) (L-D6411)

DD-98A96V Trifolium subterraneum poisoning
(DD-80000) (L-D6414)
Subterranean clover poisoning
(DD-80000) (L-D6414)
DD-98B00V Triglochin species poisoning
(DD-80000) (L-DAB00)
Arrowgrass poisoning
(DD-80000) (L-DAB00)
DD-98B10V Trisetum flavescens poisoning
(DD-80000) (L-DB851)
Yellow oat grass poisoning
(DD-80000) (L-DB851)
Trisetum enzootic calcinosis
(DD-80000) (L-DB851)
DD-98B20V Tylecodon species poisoning
(DD-80000) (L-D5C30)
DD-98B30V Urginea species poisoning
(DD-80000) (L-DC170)
DD-98B32V Urginea maritima poisoning
(DD-80000) (L-DC171) (C-30048)
Red squill toxicity
(DD-80000) (L-DC171) (C-30048)
Sea onion poisoning
(DD-80000) (L-DC171) (C-30048)
White squill poisoning
(DD-80000) (L-DC171) (C-30048)
Scilla maritima poisoning
(DD-80000) (L-DC171) (C-30048)
DD-98B40V Urtica incisa poisoning
(DD-80000) (L-D5201)
Stinging nettle poisoning
(DD-80000) (L-D5201)
DD-98B50V Veratrum species poisoning
(DD-80000) (L-DC200)
DD-98B52V Veratrum californicum poisoning
(DD-80000) (L-DC202)
False hellebore poisoning
(DD-80000) (L-DC202)
Skunk cabbage poisoning
(DD-80000) (L-DC202)
DD-98B60V Vicia species poisoning
(DD-80000) (L-D6420)
Vetch poisoning
(DD-80000) (L-D6420)
DD-98B62 Vicia faba poisoning 282.2
(DD-80000) (L-D6421)
Broad bean poisoning 282.2
(DD-80000) (L-D6421)
Favism 282.2
(DD-80000) (L-D6421)
DD-98B64V Vicia villosa poisoning
(DD-80000) (L-D6425)
Hairy vetch poisoning
(DD-80000) (L-D6425)
DD-98B70V Vinca species poisoning
(DD-80000) (L-D9240)
Periwinkle poisoning
(DD-80000) (L-D9240)
DD-98B80V Wedelia asperrima poisoning
(DD-80000) (L-DA980)
Yellow daisy poisoning
(DD-80000) (L-DA980)
DD-98B90V Xanthium species poisoning
(DD-80000) (L-DA850)
Cocklebur poisoning
(DD-80000) (L-DA850)
DD-98BA0V Xanthorrhoea species poisoning
(DD-80000) (L-DD600)
Grass tree poisoning
(DD-80000) (L-DD600)
DD-98BB0V Zamia species poisoning
(DD-80000) (L-D1320)
Burrawang palm poisoning
(DD-80000) (L-D1320)
DD-98BC0V Zieria arborescens poisoning
(DD-80000) (L-D7741)
Stinkwood poisoning
(DD-80000) (L-D7741)
DD-98BD0V Zygadenus species poisoning
(DD-80000) (L-DC190)
Death cama poisoning
(DD-80000) (L-DC190)

CHAPTER E — INFECTIOUS AND PARASITIC DISEASES

SECTION E-0 INFECTIOUS AND PARASITIC DISEASES: GENERAL TERMS

DE-00000 Infectious disease, NOS 136.9
  Infection, NOS 136.9
DE-00001 Acute infectious disease
  Acute infection
DE-00002 Subacute infectious disease
  Subacute infection
DE-00003 Chronic infectious disease
  Chronic infection
DE-00010 Communicable disease, NOS 136.9
  Transmissible disease, NOS 136.9
  Contagious disease, NOS 136.9
DE-00018 Infectious disease in mother complicating pregnancy, childbirth or puerperium, NOS 647.8
DE-00020 Systemic infection, NOS 038.9
  (T-C2000)
  Sepsis, NOS 038.9
  (T-C2000)
  Septicemia, NOS 038.9
  (T-C2000)
DE-00030 Clinical infection 136.9
DE-00040 Subclinical infection 136.9
DE-00050 Localized infection 136.9
DE-00060 Mixed infectious disease, NOS 136.9
  Mixed infection, NOS 136.9
DE-00070 Exanthematous infectious disease, NOS 136.9
  (T-01000) (M-01710)
  Exanthematous infection, NOS 136.9
  (T-01000) (M-01710)
DE-00080 Enanthematous infectious disease, NOS 136.9
  (T-00400) (M-01800)
  Enanthematous infection, NOS 136.9
  (T-00400) (M-01800)
DE-01100 Opportunistic infectious disease, NOS
DE-01200 Nosocomial infectious disease, NOS
DE-01300 Fomite transmitted disease, NOS
DE-01320 Dust-borne infectious disease, NOS
  (C-20060)
DE-01400 Immunosuppression-related infectious disease, NOS
DE-01500 Human transmitted disease, NOS
  (L-85B00)
DE-01600 Sexually transmitted disease, NOS 099.9
  (F-9B900)
  Venereal disease, NOS 099.9
  (F-9B900)
DE-01608 Venereal disease in mother complicating pregnancy, childbirth or puerperium, NOS 647.2
DE-01700 Animal transmitted disease, NOS
  (L-80010)
DE-01750 Zoonosis, NOS
  (L-80010) (L-85B00)
DE-01752 Anthropozoonosis
DE-01753 Amphixenosis
DE-01754 Zooanthroponosis
DE-01761 Cyclozoonosis
DE-01762 Metazoonosis
DE-01763 Saprozoonosis
DE-01800 Arthropod-borne disease, NOS 088.9
  (L-60000)
DE-01810 Insect-transmitted disease, NOS 088.9
  (L-60001)
DE-01820 Mosquito-borne disease, NOS 088.9
  (L-60008)
DE-01830 Louse-borne disease, NOS 088.9
  (L-60007)
DE-01900 Congenital infectious disease, NOS 771.-
  (D4-00000)

SECTION E-1 BACTERIAL INFECTIOUS DISEASES

E-100 Bacterial Infectious Diseases: General Terms

DE-10000 Bacterial infectious disease, NOS 041.9
  (L-10000)
  Disease caused by bacteria, NOS 041.9
  (L-10000)
  Bacterial infection, NOS 041.9
  (L-10000)
DE-10010 Zoonotic bacterial disease, NOS 027.9
  (L-10000) (DE-01750)
  Bacterial zoonosis, NOS 027.9
  (L-10000) (DE-01750)
DE-10020 Spirochetal infection, NOS 104.9
  (L-10016)
DE-10021 Spirochetal infection, NEC 104.8
  (L-10016)
DE-10100 Bacterial pneumonia, NOS 482.9
  (T-28000) (M-40000) (L-10000)
DE-10101 Bacterial pleurisy, NOS 511.0
  (T-29000) (M-40000) (L-10000)
DE-10102 Bacterial pleurisy with effusion 511.1
  (T-29000) (M-40000) (L-10000)
  (M-36700)
DE-10105 Acute bacterial peritonitis
  (T-D4400) (M-41000) (L-10000)
DE-10106 Primary bacterial peritonitis
  (T-D4400) (M-40000) (L-10000)
  Spontaneous bacterial peritonitis
  (T-D4400) (M-40000) (L-10000)
DE-10108 Bacterial myocarditis, NOS 422.92
  (T-32020) (M-40000) (L-10000)
  Septic myocarditis, NOS 422.92
  (T-32020) (M-40000) (L-10000)

DE-10110 Acute bacterial inflammation of external ear, NOS 380.12
(T-AB100) (M-41000) (L-10000)
Acute swimmers' ear 380.12
(T-AB100) (M-41000) (L-10000)
Beach ear 380.12
(T-AB100) (M-41000) (L-10000)
Tank ear 380.12
(T-AB100) (M-41000) (L-10000)

DE-10115 Chronic bacterial otitis externa 380.16
(T-AB100) (M-43000) (L-10000)
Chronic infective otitis externa 380.16
(T-AB100) (M-43000) (L-10000)

DE-10120 Bacterial cholangitis
(T-60610) (M-40000) (L-10000)

E-110 Actinomycotic Infections

DE-11000 Actinomycotic infection, NOS 039.9
(L-10800)

DE-11010 Actinomycosis, NOS 039.9
(L-10800)
Actinomycosis due to Actinomyces israelii 039.9
(L-10803)
Actinomycosis due to Actinomyces naeslundii 039.9
(L-10804)
Actinomycosis due to Actinomyces viscosus 039.9
(L-10805)
Actinomycosis due to Actinomyces odontolyticus 039.9
(L-10802)
Actinomycosis due to Actinomyces meyeri 039.9
(L-10808)
Actinomycosis due to Actinomyces suis
(L-10807)
Actinomycosis due to Actinomyces eriksonii
(L-10814)

DE-11011 Disseminated actinomycosis 039.8
(T-D0010) (L-10800)

DE-11012 Cervicofacial actinomycosis 039.3
(T-C4100) (T-C4200) (L-10800)
Lumpy jaw 039.3
(T-C4100) (T-C4200) (L-10800)

DE-11013 Abdominal actinomycosis 039.2
(T-D4010) (L-10800)
Ray fungus disease of the intestines 039.2
(T-D4010) (L-10800)

DE-11014 Pulmonary actinomycosis 039.1
(T-28000) (L-10800)
Thoracic actinomycosis 039.1
(T-28000) (L-10800)

DE-11015 Cutaneous actinomycosis 039.0
(T-01000) (L-10800)

DE-11020V Bovine actinomycosis
(L-10801)
Actinomycosis due to Actinomyces bovis
(L-10801)
Bovine lumpy jaw
(L-10801)

DE-11024V Poll evil
(T-16115) (L-10801) (L-13202)

DE-11026V Fistulous withers
(T-16192) (L-10801) (L-13202)

DE-11030V Dermatophilus infection, NOS
(T-01000) (L-14500)
Dermatophilosis, NOS
(T-01000) (L-14500)

DE-11032V Dermatophilosis due to Dermatophilus congolensis
(T-01000) (L-14501)
Cutaneous dermatophilosis
(T-01000) (L-14501)
Cutaneous streptotrichosis
(T-01000) (L-14501)
Lumpy wool disease
(T-01000) (L-14501)
Strawberry foot rot
(T-01000) (L-14501)
Proliferative dermatitis
(T-01000) (L-14501)

DE-11050 Actinomycotic madura foot 039.4
(T-D9700) (L-10800)
Actinomycotic maduromycosis 039.4
(T-D9700) (L-10800)
Actinomycotic mycetoma 039.4
(T-D9700) (L-10800)
Actinomycotic schizomycetoma 039.9
(T-D9700) (L-10800)

DE-11052 Madura foot due to Streptomyces, NOS 039.4
(T-D9700) (L-25300)

DE-11053 Madura foot due to Streptomyces somaliensis 039.4
(T-D9700) (L-25301)

DE-11055 Madura foot due to Actinomadura, NOS 039.4
(T-D9700) (L-10700)

DE-11056 Madura foot due to Actinomadura pelletieri 039.4
(T-D9700) (L-10702)

DE-11060 Nocardiosis, NOS 039.9
(L-22300)
Nocardiosis due to Nocardia caviae 039.9
(L-22303)
Nocardiosis due to Nocardia asteroides 039.9
(L-22301)
Nocardiosis due to Nocardia farcinica 039.9
(L-22306)
Nocardiosis due to Nocardia brasiliensis 039.9
(L-22302)

DE-11062V Bovine farcy
(L-21833) (L-22306)

E-110 Actinomycotic Infections — Continued

DE-11063V Bovine granulomatous mastitis
(T-04000) (L-22301)

DE-11064V Pulmonary nocardiosis
(T-28000) (L-22303)

DE-11066V Cutaneous nocardiosis
(T-01000) (L-22301)
Pyogranulomatous dermatitis
(T-01000) (L-22301)

DE-11070 Trichomycosis axillaris 039.0
(T-01400) (T-D8104) (L-14427)
Trichonocardiasis axillaris 039.0
(T-01400) (T-D8104) (L-14427)
Axillary trichomycosis due to Corynebacterium tenuis 039.0
(T-01400) (T-D8104) (L-14427)

DE-11080 Erythrasma 039.0
(T-01000) (M-43000) (L-14420)
Infection due to Corynebacterium minutissimum 039.0
(T-01000) (M-43000) (L-14420)

DE-11090 Botryomycosis 041.1
(T-01000) (M-44000) (L-24801)
Chronic granulomatous infection due mostly to Staphylococcus aureus 041.1
(T-01000) (M-44000) (L-24801)
Staphylococcal granuloma
(T-01000) (M-44000) (L-24801)

E-111 Angular Conjunctivitis

DE-11100 Angular conjunctivitis 372.0
(T-AA860) (L-21601)
Morax-Axenfeld conjunctivitis 372.0
(T-AA860) (L-21601)
Infection due to Moraxella lacunata 372.0
(T-AA860) (L-21601)
Infection due to Morax-Axenfeld bacillus 372.0
(T-AA860) (L-21601)

DE-11120V Bovine infectious keratoconjunctivitis
(T-AA860) (L-21602)
Bovine infectious ophthalmia
(T-AA860) (L-21602)
Pinkeye in animals
(T-AA860) (L-21602)
New Forest disease
(T-AA860) (L-21602)
Blight
(T-AA860) (L-21602)
Infection due to Moraxella bovis
(T-AA860) (L-21602)

DE-11130V Contagious ovine ophthalmitis
(T-AA860) (L-21609)
Infection due to Moraxella ovis
(T-AA860) (L-21609)

E-112 Anthrax

DE-11200 Anthrax, NOS 022.9
(L-12202)
Infection due to Bacillus anthracis 022.9
(L-12202)
Splenic fever
(T-12202)
Charbon
(L-12202)
Milzbrand
(L-12202)

DE-11201 Cutaneous anthrax 022.0
(T-01000) (L-12202)
Malignant pustule 022.0
(T-01000) (L-12202)

DE-11204 Pulmonary anthrax 022.1
(T-28000) (L-12202)
Woolsorters' disease 022.1
(T-28000) (L-12202)
Respiratory anthrax 022.1
(T-28000) (L-12202)

DE-11205 Pneumonia in anthrax 484.5
(T-28000) (M-40000)

DE-11206 Gastrointestinal anthrax 022.2
(T-50100) (L-12202)

DE-11207 Anthrax septicemia 022.3
(T-C2000) (L-12202)

DE-11208 Other specified anthrax manifestations 022.8
(T-.....) (L-12202)

E-113 Bacterial Food Poisoning

DE-11300 Bacterial food poisoning, NOS 005.9
(T-50100) (L-10000)
Food poisoning due to bacteria, NOS 005.8
(T-50100) (L-10000)

DE-11310 Botulism 005.1
(L-10038) (L-14118)
Food poisoning due to Clostridium botulinum toxin 005.1
(L-10038) (L-14118)
Lamziekte
(L-10038) (L-14121)
Lame sickness
(L-10038) (L-14121)
Loin disease
(L-10038) (L-14121)
Limberneck
(L-10038) (L-14118)
Western duck sickness
(L-10038) (L-14118)

DE-11312V Toxicoinfectious botulism
(L-10038) (L-14120)
Shaker foal syndrome
(L-14120)

DE-11320 Food poisoning due to Bacillus cereus 005.8
(T-50100) (L-12205)

DE-11330 Food poisoning due to Clostridium perfringens 005.2
(T-50100) (L-14210)

DE-11332 Food poisoning due to other Clostridia 005.3
(T-50100) (L-14100)

DE-11340 Food poisoning due to staphylococcus 005.0
(T-50100) (L-24800)
Staphylococcal toxemia specified as due to food 005.0
(T-50100) (L-24800)

DE-11350 Food poisoning due to streptococcus 005.8
(T-50100) (L-25100)

DE-11360 Food poisoning due to Vibrio parahaemolyticus 005.4
(T-50100) (L-26209)

E-114 Brucellosis

DE-11400 Brucellosis, NOS 023.9
(L-13200)
Malta fever 023.9
(L-13200)
Mediterranean fever 023.9
(L-13200)
Undulant fever 023.9
(L-13200)

DE-11410V Bovine brucellosis
(L-13202)
Infection due to Brucella abortus 023.1
(L-13202)
Bang's disease
(L-13202)
Contagious abortion
(L-13202)

DE-11420V Ovine brucellosis
(L-13205)
Epididymitis of rams
(L-13205)
Infection due to Brucella ovis
(L-13205)

DE-11430V Porcine brucellosis
(L-13203)
Infection due to Brucella suis 023.2
(L-13203)

DE-11440V Caprine brucellosis
(L-13201)
Infection due to Brucella melitensis 023.0
(L-13201)

DE-11450V Canine brucellosis
(L-13206)
Infection due to Brucella canis 023.3
(L-13206)

DE-11480 Brucellosis due to other Brucella sp. 023.8
(L-132..)

E-115 Chancroid

DE-11500 Chancroid 099.0
(T-70260) (T-C4810) (M-38000)
(L-1F710) (DE-01600)
Soft chancre 099.0
(T-70260) (T-C4810) (M-38000)
(L-1F710) (DE-01600)
Ulcus molle 099.0
(T-70260) (T-C4810) (M-38000)
(L-1F710) (DE-01600)
Ducrey's disease 099.0
(T-70260) (T-C4810) (M-38000)
(L-1F710) (DE-01600)
Ducrey's chancre 099.0
(T-70260) (T-C4810) (M-38000)
(L-1F710) (DE-01600)
Inguinal bubo 099.0
(T-70260) (T-C4810) (M-38000)
(L-1F710) (DE-01600)
Chancroidal bubo 099.0
(T-70260) (T-C4810) (M-38000)
(L-1F710) (DE-01600)
Bubo due to Haemophilus ducreyi 099.0
(T-70260) (T-C4810) (M-38000)
(L-1F710) (DE-01600)
Simple chancre 099.0
(T-70260) (T-C4810) (M-38000)
(L-1F710) (DE-01600)

E-116 Cholera

DE-11600 Cholera, NOS 001.9
(L-26200)

DE-11601 Cholera due to Vibrio cholerae 001.0
(L-26201)

DE-11602 Cholera due to Vibrio cholerae El Tor 001.1
(L-26205)

E-117 Diphteria

DE-11700 Diphtheria, NOS 032.9
(L-14401)
Infection due to Corynebacterium diphtheriae 032.9
(L-14401)

DE-11710 Anterior nasal diphtheria 032.2
(T-21000) (L-14401)

DE-11720 Faucial diphtheria 032.0
(T-55200) (L-14401)
Diphtheritic membranous angina 032.0
(T-55200) (L-14401)

DE-11730 Laryngeal diphtheria 032.3
(T-24100) (L-14401)
Diphtheritic laryngotracheitis 032.3
(T-24100) (L-14401)

DE-11740 Nasopharyngeal diphtheria 032.1
(T-23000) (L-14401)

DE-11750 Cutaneous diphtheria 032.85
(T-01000) (L-14401)

DE-11760 Diphtheritic myocarditis 032.82
(T-32020) (L-14401)

DE-11770 Diphtheritic cystitis 032.84
(T-74000) (L-14401)

DE-11780 Diphtheritic peritonitis 032.83
(T-D4400) (L-14401)

DE-11790 Conjunctival diphtheria 032.81
(T-AA860) (L-14401)
Pseudomembranous diphtheritic conjunctivitis 032.81
(T-AA860) (L-14401)

E-119 Erysipelothrix

DE-11900 Erysipelothrix 027.1
(T-01000) (L-1E701)
Erysipelothrix infection 027.1
(T-01000) (L-1E701)
Erysipeloid of Rosenbach 027.1
(T-01000) (L-1E701)
Infection due to Erysipelothrix insidiosa 027.1
(T-01000) (L-1E701)
Infection due to Erysipelothrix rhusiopathiae 027.1
(T-01000) (L-1E701)
Erysipeloid 027.1
(T-01000) (L-1E701)
Swine erysipelas
(T-01000) (L-1E701)
Diamond skin disease
(T-01000) (L-1E701)
Fish handlers' disease
(T-01000) (L-1E701)

DE-11910 Septicemia due to Erysipelothrix insidiosa 027.1
(T-C2000) (L-1E701)

DE-11912V Septicemia due to Erysipelothrix rhusiopathiae
(T-C2000) (L-1E701)

DE-11920V Nonsuppurative polyarthritis in lambs
(L-1E701)

DE-11922V Post-dipping lameness in sheep
(L-1E701)

E-11A Clostridial Infections

DE-11A00V Clostridial infection, NOS
(L-14100)

DE-11A10 Gas gangrene, NOS 040.0
(T-13000) (T-03000) (M-54600) (L-14100)
Gas bacillus infection 040.0
(T-13000) (T-03000) (M-54600) (L-14100)
Gas gangrene due to Clostridia, NOS 040.0
(T-13000) (T-03000) (M-54600) (L-14100)
Malignant edema 040.0
(T-13000) (T-03000) (M-54600) (L-14100)
Clostridial myositis 040.0
(T-13000) (T-03000) (M-54600) (L-14100)
Clostridial myonecrosis 040.0
(T-13000) (T-03000) (M-54600) (L-14100)
Gas gangrene due to Clostridium perfringens 040.0
(T-13000) (T-03000) (M-54600) (L-14210)
Gas gangrene due to Clostridium welchii 040.0
(T-13000) (T-03000) (M-54600) (L-14210)
Gas gangrene due to Clostridium histolyticum 040.0
(T-13000) (T-03000) (M-54600) (L-14127)
Gas gangrene due to Clostridium oedematiens 040.0
(T-13000) (T-03000) (M-54600) (L-14129)
Gas gangrene due to Clostridium septicum 040.0
(T-13000) (T-03000) (M-54600) (L-14136)
Gas gangrene due to Clostridium sordellii 040.0
(T-13000) (T-03000) (M-54600) (L-14112)

DE-11A12 Gas gangrene septicemia 040.0
(T-C2000) (T-13000) (T-03000) (M-54600) (L-14100)

DE-11A15V Clostridial wound infection in animal, NOS
(L-14100)

DE-11A20V Avian gangrenous dermatitis due to Clostridium, NOS
(T-01000) (L-14136) (L-14210)
Avian gangrenous cellulitis
(T-01000) (L-14136) (L-14210)

DE-11A21V Infection due to Clostridium novyi
(L-14131)
Infectious necrotic hepatitis
(L-14131)
Black disease
(L-14131)

DE-11A22V Ovine bighead
(L-14129)

DE-11A24V Infection due to Clostridium haemolyticum
(L-14133)
Bovine bacillary hemoglobinuria
(L-14133)
Red water disease
(L-14133)

DE-11A26V Infection due to Clostridium chauvoei
(L-14135)
Blackleg
(L-14135)
Clostridial myositis/myonecrosis
(L-14135)

DE-11A28V Infection due to Clostridium septicum
(L-14136)
Malignant edema of animals
(L-14136)
Vibrion septique
(L-14136)
Pseudo-blackleg
(L-14136)

DE-11A29V Braxy
(T-57A40) (L-14136)
Bradsot
(T-57A40) (L-14136)

DE-11A30V Infection due to Clostridium perfringens, NOS
(L-14210)

DE-11A31V Infection due to Clostridium perfringens type A
(L-10038) (L-14211)
Clostridium perfringens type A enterotoxemia
(L-10038) (L-14211)

DE-11A32V Infection due to Clostridium perfringens type B
(L-14212) (L-10038)
Clostridium perfringens type B enterotoxemia
(L-14212) (L-10038)

DE-11A33V Lamb dysentery
(L-14212)

DE-11A34V Calf enterotoxemia
(L-14212)

DE-11A35V Foal enterotoxemia
(L-14212)

DE-11A40V Infection due to Clostridium perfringens type C
(L-14213) (L-10038)
Clostridium perfringens type C enterotoxemia
(L-14213) (L-10038)

DE-11A42V Struck
(L-14213)
Romney Marsh disease
(L-14213)
Enterotoxemia of sheep due to Clostridium perfringens type C
(L-14213)

DE-11A44V Goat enterotoxemia
(L-14213)

DE-11A46V Pig enterotoxemia
(L-14213)

DE-11A48V Enterotoxic hemorrhagic enteritis of calves and lambs
(L-14213)

DE-11A50V Infection due to Clostridium perfringens type D
(L-14214) (L-10038)
Clostridium perfringens type D enterotoxemia
(L-14214) (L-10038)

DE-11A52V Pulpy kidney disease
(L-14214)

DE-11A54V Overeating disease
(L-14214)

DE-11A60 Enteritis necroticans 005.2
(T-50500) (M-41000) (L-14210)
Pigbel 005.2
(T-50500) (M-41000) (L-14210)
Enteritis necroticans due to Clostridium perfringens 005.2
(T-50500) (M-41000) (L-14210)

DE-11A70V Avian necrotic enteritis
(L-14210)

DE-11A72V Avian ulcerative enteritis
(L-14192)
Quail disease
(L-14192)

E-11B Glanders and Pseudoglanders

DE-11B00 Glanders 024.-
(L-23417)
Infection due to Pseudomonas mallei 024.-
(L-23417)
Malleus 024.-
(L-23417)
Infection due to Actinobacillus mallei 024.-
(L-23417)
Infection due to Malleomyces mallei 024.-
(L-23417)
Maliasmus 024.-
(L-23417)

DE-11B10 Cutaneous glanders 024.-
(L-23417)
Farcy 024.-
(L-23417)
Equine glanders
(L-23417)
Farcy buds
(L-23417)
Farcy pipes
(L-23417)
Farcy cords
(L-23417)

DE-11B50 Pseudoglanders 025.-
(L-23416)
Melioidosis 025.-
(L-23416)
Infection due to Pseudomonas pseudomallei 025.-
(L-23416)
Infection due to Malleomyces pseudomallei 025.-
(L-23416)
Infection due to Whitmore's bacillus 025.-
(L-23416)

E-11C Actinobacillus Infections

DE-11C00V Actinobacillus infection, NOS
(L-10600)
Actinobacillosis, NOS
(L-10600)

DE-11C10V Actinobacillosis due to Actinobacillus lignieresi
(L-10601)

E-11C Actinobacillus Infections — Continued

DE-11C11V Wooden tongue
(T-53000) (L-10601)

DE-11C12V Cutaneous actinobacillosis of sheep and cattle
(T-01000) (L-10601)

DE-11C13V Nasal actinobacillosis of sheep
(T-21000) (L-10601)

DE-11C14V Actinobacillosis of rumenoreticulum
(T-57A10) (L-10601)

DE-11C15V Pulmonary actinobacillosis
(T-28000) (L-10601)

DE-11C16V Actinobacillary mastitis
(T-04000) (L-10601)

DE-11C20V Actinobacillosis due to Actinobacillus equuli
(T-C2000) (L-10602)
Pyosepticemia neonatorum
(T-C2000) (L-10602)
Perinatal actinobacillosis of foals
(T-C2000) (L-10602)
Sleepy foal disease
(T-C2000) (L-10602)
Septicemia of foals
(T-C2000) (L-10602)

DE-11C30V Actinobacillosis due to Actinobacillus salpingitis
(L-10609)

DE-11C40V Actinobacillosis due to Actinobacillus seminis
(L-10606)

DE-11C50V Actinobacillosis due to Actinobacillus suis
(L-10605)

E-120 Gonorrhea

DE-12000 Gonorrhea, NOS 098.-
(L-22201) (DE-01600)
Gonococcal infection, NOS 098.-
(L-22201) (DE-01600)
Infection due to Neisseria gonorrhoeae 098.-
(L-22201) (DE-01600)

DE-12001 Acute gonorrhea of genitourinary tract, NOS 098.0
(T-70200) (M-41000) (L-22201) (DE-01600)

DE-12002 Acute gonorrhea of lower genitourinary tract, NOS 098.0
(T-70230) (M-41000) (L-22201) (DE-01600)

DE-12003 Acute gonorrhea of upper genitourinary tract, NOS 098.19
(T-70220) (M-41000) (L-22201) (DE-01600)

DE-12007 Gonococcemia 098.89
(T-C2000) (L-22201) (DE-01600)
Gonococcal septicemia 098.89
(T-C2000) (L-22201) (DE-01600)

DE-12010 Acute gonococcal bartholinitis 098.0
(T-81510) (M-41000) (L-22201) (DE-01600)

DE-12011 Acute gonococcal urethritis 098.0
(T-75000) (M-41000) (L-22201) (DE-01600)

DE-12012 Acute gonococcal vulvovaginitis 098.0
(T-81000) (T-82000) (M-41000) (L-22201) (DE-01600)

DE-12013 Acute gonococcal endometritis 098.16 —615.-*
(T-83400) (M-41000) (L-22201) (DE-01600)

DE-12014 Acute gonococcal salpingitis 098.17 —614.0*
(T-88000) (M-41000) (L-22201) (DE-01600)

DE-12015 Acute gonococcal cystitis 098.11 —595.4*
(T-74000) (M-41000) (L-22201) (DE-01600)

DE-12016 Acute gonococcal cervicitis 098.15 —616.0*
(T-83200) (M-41000) (L-22201) (DE-01600)

DE-12020 Acute gonococcal epididymo-orchitis 098.13 —604.9*
(T-95000) (T-94000) (M-41000) (L-22201) (DE-01600)

DE-12021 Acute gonococcal prostatitis 098.12 —601.4*
(T-92000) (M-41000) (L-22201) (DE-01600)

DE-12022 Acute gonococcal seminal vesiculitis 098.14 —608.0*
(T-93000) (M-41000) (L-22201) (DE-01600)

DE-12030 Chronic gonorrhea, NOS 098.2
(M-43000) (L-22201) (DE-01600)

DE-12031 Chronic gonorrhea of genitourinary tract, NOS 098.2
(T-70200) (M-43000) (L-22201) (DE-01600)

DE-12032 Chronic gonorrhea of lower genitourinary tract, NOS 098.2
(T-70230) (M-43000) (L-22201) (DE-01600)

DE-12033 Chronic gonorrhea of upper genitourinary tract, NOS 098.30
(T-70220) (M-43000) (L-22201) (DE-01600)

DE-12040 Chronic gonococcal bartholinitis 098.2
(T-81510) (M-43000) (L-22201) (DE-01600)

DE-12041 Chronic gonococcal urethritis 098.2
(T-75000) (M-43000) (L-22201) (DE-01600)

DE-12042 Chronic gonococcal vulvovaginitis 098.2
(T-81000) (T-82000) (M-43000) (L-22201) (DE-01600)

DE-12043 Chronic gonococcal salpingitis 098.37 —614.2*
(T-88000) (M-43000) (L-22201) (DE-01600)

DE-12044 Chronic gonococcal cystitis 098.31
(T-74000) (M-43000) (L-22201)
(DE-01600)

DE-12045 Chronic gonococcal cervicitis 098.35
(T-83200) (M-43000) (L-22201)
(DE-01600)

DE-12046 Chronic gonococcal endometritis 098.36
(T-83400) (M-43000) (L-22201)
(DE-01600)

DE-12051 Chronic gonococcal prostatitis 098.32
(T-92000) (M-43000) (L-22201)
(DE-01600)

DE-12052 Chronic gonococcal epididymo-orchitis 098.33
(T-95000) (T-94000) (M-43000)
(L-22201) (DE-01600)

DE-12053 Chronic gonococcal seminal vesiculitis 098.34
(T-93000) (M-43000) (L-22201)
(DE-01600)

DE-12060 Gonococcal infection of eye, NOS 098.49
(T-AA000) (M-40000) (L-22201)
(DE-01600)

DE-12061 Gonococcal conjunctivitis neonatorum 098.40 —372.0*
(T-AA860) (M-40000) (F-88000)
(L-22201) (DE-01600)

Gonococcal ophthalmia neonatorum 098.40 —372.0*
(T-AA000) (M-40000) (F-88000)
(L-22201) (DE-01600)

DE-12062 Gonococcal iridocyclitis 098.41 —364.0*
(T-AA500) (M-40000) (L-22201)
(DE-01600)

DE-12063 Gonococcal keratitis 098.43 —320.7*
(T-AA200) (M-40000) (L-22201)
(DE-01600)

Keratitis blennorrhagica
(T-AA200) (T-40000) (L-22201)
(DE-01600)

DE-12064 Gonococcal endophthalmia 098.42
(T-AA200) (T-D1480) (M-40000)
(L-22201) (DE-01600)

DE-12070 Gonococcal infection of joint, NOS 098.59
(T-15000) (M-40000) (L-22201)
(DE-01600)

Gonococcal arthritis 098.50 —711.4*
(T-15000) (M-40000) (L-22201)
(DE-01600)

Gonococcal rheumatism 098.59
(T-15000) (M-40000) (L-22201)
(DE-01600)

DE-12071 Gonococcal bursitis 098.52 —727.3*
(T-16000) (M-40000) (L-22201)
(DE-01600)

DE-12072 Gonococcal synovitis 098.51 —727.0*
(T-15003) (M-40000) (L-22201)
(DE-01600)

Gonococcal tenosynovitis 098.51 —727.0*
(T-17010) (T-15003) (M-40000)
(L-22201) (DE-01600)

DE-12073 Gonococcal spondylitis 098.53
(T-11510) (M-40000) (L-22201)
(DE-01600)

DE-12080 Gonorrhea of pharynx 098.6
(T-55000) (M-40000) (L-22201)
(DE-01600)

DE-12081 Gonorrhea of anus 098.7
(T-59900) (M-40000) (L-22201)
(DE-01600)

DE-12082 Gonorrhea of rectum 098.7
(T-59600) (M-40000) (L-22201)
(DE-01600)

Gonococcal proctitis 098.7
(T-59600) (M-40000) (L-22201)
(DE-01600)

DE-12091 Gonococcal meningitis 098.82 —320.7*
(T-A1110) (M-40000) (L-22201)
(DE-01600)

DE-12092 Gonococcal peritonitis 098.86 —567.0*
(T-D4400) (M-40000) (L-22201)
(DE-01600)

Fitz-Hugh-Curtis syndrome 098.86 —567.0*
(T-D4400) (M-40000) (L-22201)
(DE-01600)

DE-12093 Gonococcal keratosis 098.81
(T-01000) (M-72600) (L-22201)
(DE-01600)

DE-120A0 Gonococcal heart disease, NOS 098.85
(T-32000) (M-40000) (L-22201)
(DE-01600)

DE-120A1 Gonococcal endocarditis 098.84 —421.1*
(T-32060) (M-40000) (L-22201)
(DE-01600)

DE-120A2 Gonococcal pericarditis 098.83
(T-39000) (M-40000) (L-22201)
(DE-01600)

DE-120B0 Gonorrhea in mother complicating pregnancy, childbirth or puerperium, NOS 647.1

E-121 Granuloma Inguinale

DE-12100 Granuloma inguinale 099.2
(T-70260) (M-44000) (L-13401)
(DE-01600)

Granuloma venereum 099.2
(T-70260) (M-44000) (L-13401)
(DE-01600)

Donovanosis 099.2
(T-70260) (M-44000) (L-13401)
(DE-01600)

Ulcerating granuloma pudendi 099.2
(T-70260) (M-44000) (L-13401)
(DE-01600)

Infection due to Calymmatobacterium granulomatis 099.2
(T-70260) (M-44000) (L-13401)
(DE-01600)

E-121 Granuloma Inguinale — Continued

DE-12100 (cont.) Infection due to Donovania granulomatis 099.2
(T-70260) (M-44000) (L-13401) (DE-01600)
Pudendal ulcer 099.2
(T-70260) (M-44000) (L-13401) (DE-01600)

E-122 Impetigo

DE-12200 Impetigo, NOS 684.-
(T-01000) (M-41600) (M-41210) (L-24801) (L-25128)
Impetigo contagiosa 684.-
(T-01000) (M-41600) (M-41210) (L-24801) (L-25128)
DE-12210 Impetigo bullosa 684.-
(T-01000) (F-88000) (L-24801)
Pemphigus neonatorum 684.-
(T-01000) (F-88000) (L-24801)
Impetigo contagiosa bullosa 684.-
(T-01000) (F-88000) (L-24801)
Circinate impetigo 684.-
(T-01000) (F-88000) (L-24801)
Impetigo due to Staphylococcus aureus 684.-
(T-01000) (F-88000) (L-24801)
Impetigo neonatorum 684.-
(T-01000) (F-88000) (L-24801)
DE-12230 Bockhart impetigo 684.-
(T-01302) (T-D1160) (L-24801)
Superficial pustular perifolliculitis 684.-
(T-01302) (T-D1160) (L-24801)
DE-12240V Contagious porcine pyoderma
(T-01000) (M-41600) (M-41210) (L-24801) (L-25128)
Impetigo contagiosa suis
(T-01000) (M-41600) (M-41210) (L-24801) (L-25128)
Greasy pig disease
(T-01000) (M-41600) (M-41210) (L-24801) (L-25128)
Seborrhea oleosa suis
(T-01000) (M-41600) (M-41210) (L-24801) (L-25128)
Exudative epidermitis of swine
(T-01000) (M-41600) (M-41210) (L-24801) (L-25128)
DE-12242V Udder impetigo
(T-04700) (M-41600) (M-41210) (L-24801) (L-25128)

E-123 Leprosy

DE-12300 Leprosy, NOS 030.9
(T-01000) (T-A0500) (L-21827)
Hansen's disease 030.9
(T-01000) (T-A0500) (L-21827)
Infection due to Mycobacterium leprae 030.9
(T-01000) (T-A0500) (L-21827)
DE-12310 Lepromatous leprosy 030.0
(T-01000) (T-A0500) (L-21827)
Type L leprosy 030.0
(T-01000) (T-A0500) (L-21827)
DE-12320 Tuberculoid leprosy 030.1
(T-01000) (T-A0500) (L-21827)
Type T leprosy 030.1
(T-01000) (T-A0500) (L-21827)
DE-12330 Indeterminate leprosy 030.2
(T-01000) (T-A0500) (L-21827)
Group I leprosy 030.2
(T-01000) (T-A0500) (L-21287)
DE-12340 Borderline leprosy 030.3
(T-01000) (T-A0500) (L-21827)
Dimorphic leprosy 030.3
(T-01000) (T-A0500) (L-21827)
Group B leprosy 030.3
(T-01000) (T-A0500) (L-21827)
DE-12350 Lepromin reaction 030.8
(T-01000) (T-A0500) (L-21827)
DE-12360 Lucio phenomenon 030.8
(T-01000) (T-A0500) (L-21827)
DE-12370 Other specified leprosy 030.8
(T-01000) (T-A0500) (L-21827)
DE-12374 Leontiasis
(T-03120) (L-21827)
Leontiasis due to leprosy
(T-03120) (L-21827)
Leonine facies due to leprosy
(T-03120) (L-21827)
DE-12380V Infection due to Mycobacterium lepraemurium
(L-21828)
Murine leprosy
(L-21828)
Feline leprosy
(L-21828)

E-124 Leptospirosis

DE-12400 Leptospirosis, NOS 100.9
(L-20500) (DE-01750)
Infection due to Leptospira, NOS 100.9
(L-20500) (DE-01750)
DE-12401 Leptospirosis leptospiremic phase 100.9
(L-20500) (DE-01750)
DE-12402 Leptospirosis immune phase 100.9
(L-20500) (DE-01750)
DE-12410 Aseptic leptospiral meningitis 100.81 —321.8*
(T-A1110) (L-20500) (DE-01750)
DE-12420 Leptospirosis icterohaemorrhagica 100.0
(L-20503) (DE-01750)
Weil's disease 100.0
(L-20503) (DE-01750)

DE-12420 (cont.) Hemorrhagic spirochaetal jaundice 100.0
(L-20503) (DE-01750)
Hemorrhagic leptospiral jaundice 100.0
(L-20503) (DE-01750)
Infection due to Leptospira interrogans 100.0
(L-20503) (DE-01750)
Infection due to Leptospira icterohemorrhagiae 100.0
(L-20503) (DE-01750)

DE-12430 Fort Bragg Fever 100.89
(L-20505) (DE-01750)
Pretibial fever 100.89
(L-20505) (DE-01750)
Fever due to Leptospira autumnalis 100.89
(L-20505) (DE-01750)

DE-12440V Canine leptospirosis
(L-20508)
Canine typhus
(L-20508)
Stuttgart disease
(L-20508)
Infectious jaundice
(L-20508)

DE-12450V Bovine leptospirosis
(L-20518)
Redwater of calves
(L-20518)

DE-12460V Abortion due to Leptospira
(L-20518)

DE-12480 Leptospirosis due to other specific organisms 100.89
(L-205..) (DE-01750)
Leptospirosis due to other serogroups
(L-205..) (DE-01750)

DE-12481 Infection due to Leptospira australis 100.89
(L-20504) (DE-01750)

DE-12482 Infection due to Leptospira bataviae 100.89
(L-20507) (DE-01750)

DE-12483 Infection due to Leptospira pyrogenes 100.89
(L-20519) (DE-01750)

DE-12484 Infection due to Leptospira grippotyphosa 100.89
(L-20512) (DE-01750)

E-125 Listeriosis

DE-12500 Listeriosis, NOS 027.0
(L-20901)
Infection due to Listeria monocytogenes 027.0
(L-20901)
Circling disease
(L-20901)
Listerellosis
(L-20901)

DE-12510 Listeria meningitis 027.0 —320.7*
(T-A1110) (L-20901)

DE-12511 Listeria meningoencephalitis 027.0 —320.7*
(T-A1110) (T-A0100) (L-20901)

DE-12512V Listeria conjunctivitis
(L-20901)

DE-12520 Listeria septicemia 027.0
(T-C2000) (L-20901)

DE-12530 Disseminated infantile listeriosis 027.0
(L-20901)
Granulomatosis infantiseptica 027.0
(L-20901)

DE-12580 Congenital listeriosis 771.2
(L-20901) (DE-01900)

DE-12582V Listeria abortion
(L-20901)

E-126 Infections Due to Diphtheroid Bacteria

DE-12600 Infection due to Diphtheroid bacteria other than diphtheriae
(L-14400)
Infection due to Corynebacterium other than diphtheriae
(L-14400)

DE-12610V Canadian horsepox
(T-01000) (L-14405)
Acne contagiosa equi
(T-01000) (L-14405)
Contagious equine pustular dermatitis
(T-01000) (L-14405)
Contagious acne of horses
(T-01000) (L-14405)
Contagious pustular acne
(T-01000) (L-14405)

DE-12612V Caseous lymphadenitis
(L-14405)
Corynebacterial lymphadenitis
(L-14405)
Equine ulcerative lymphadenitis
(L-14405)

DE-12620V Infection due to Corynebacterium pyogenes
(L-10809)

DE-12621V Corynebacterial mastitis
(L-10809)
Summer mastitis
(L-10809)

DE-12625V Corynebacterial pneumonia of foals
(L-23703)

DE-12630V Contagious bovine pyelonephritis
(L-14407)

DE-12632V Balanoposthitis of bulls
(L-14407)

DE-12634V Ulcerative posthitis and vulvitis
(L-14407)
Pizzle rot
(L-14407)
Enzootic balanoposthitis in sheep
(L-14407)

E-126 Infections Due to Diphtheroid Bacteria — Continued

DE-12634V (cont.) Sheath-rot
(L-14407)

DE-12640V Bacterial kidney disease of fish
(L-26601)
Corynebacterium kidney disease
(L-26601)
Dee disease
(L-26601)

DE-12650V Porcine pyelonephritis
(L-1E832)

DE-12652V Infection due to Corynebacterium kutscheri
(L-14408)

E-127 Meningococcal Infections

DE-12700 Meningococcal infectious disease, NOS 036.9
(L-22202)
Meningococcal infection, NOS 036.9
(L-22202)
Infection due to Neisseria meningitidis 036.9
(L-22202)

DE-12710 Meningococcal meningitis 036.0 —320.5*
(T-A1110) (L-22202)
Cerebrospinal meningitis 036.0 —320.5*
(T-A1110) (L-22202)
Epidemic meningitis 036.0 —320.5*
(T-A1110) (L-22202)
Meningococcal cerebrospinal fever 036.0 —320.5*
(T-A1110) (L-22202)

DE-12711 Meningococcal encephalitis 036.1 —323.4*
(T-A0100) (L-22202)

DE-12720 Meningococcemia 036.2
(T-C2000) (L-22202)
Meningococcal septicemia 036.2
(T-C2000) (L-22202)

DE-12730 Meningococcal carditis, NOS 036.40
(T-32000) (L-22202)

DE-12731 Meningococcal endocarditis 036.42 —421.1*
(T-32060) (L-22202)

DE-12732 Meningococcal pericarditis 036.41 —420.0*
(T-39000) (L-22202)

DE-12733 Meningococcal myocarditis 036.43
(T-32020) (L-22202)

DE-12740 Waterhouse-Friderichsen syndrome, NOS 036.3
(T-B3000) (L-22202)
Waterhouse-Friderichsen disease 036.3
(T-B3000) (L-22202)
Meningococcal Waterhouse-Friderichsen syndrome 036.3 —255.5*
(T-B3000) (L-22202)
Meningococcal hemorrhagic adrenalitis 036.3
(T-B3000) (L-22202)
Meningococcal adrenal syndrome 036.3
(T-B3000) (L-22202)

DE-12750 Meningococcal optic neuritis 036.81 —377.3*
(T-A8040) (L-22202)

DE-12760 Meningococcal arthropathy 036.82
(T-15000) (L-22202)

DE-12780 Other specified meningococcal infection, NEC 036.89
(L-22202)

E-128 Mucopurulent Conjunctivitis

DE-12800 Mucopurulent conjunctivitis 372.03
(T-AA860) (L-1F712)
Koch-Weeks conjunctivitis 372.03
(T-AA860) (L-1F712)
Pink eye disease 372.03
(T-AA860) (L-1F712)
Conjunctivitis due to Haemophilus aegyptius 372.03
(T-AA860) (L-1F712)
Conjunctivitis due to Koch-Weeks bacillus 372.03
(T-AA860) (L-1F712)
Acute contagious conjunctivitis 372.03
(T-AA860) (L-1F712)
Acute epidemic conjunctivitis 372.03
(T-AA860) (L-1F712)

DE-12801 Catarrhal conjunctivitis, NOS 372.03
(T-AA860) (L-1F712)

E-129 Mycobacterioses

DE-12900 Mycobacteriosis, NOS 031.9
(L-21800)
Mycobacterial infectious disease, NOS (excluding tuberculosis and leprosy) 031.9
(L-21800)
Mycobacterial infection, NOS (excluding tuberculosis and leprosy) 031.9
(L-21800)
Atypical mycobacterial infection, NOS 031.9
(L-21840)

DE-12910 Pulmonary disease due to Mycobacteria, NOS 031.0
(T-28000) (L-21800)

DE-12911 Infection due to Mycobacterium kansasii 031.0
(L-21805)

DE-12912 Battey disease 031.0
(L-21814)
Infection due to Mycobacterium intracellulare 031.0
(L-21814)

DE-12930 Cutaneous infectious disease due to Mycobacteria 031.1
(T-00010) (L-21800)

DE-12931 Buruli ulcer 031.1
(L-21817)
Infection due to Mycobacterium ulcerans 031.1
(L-21817)

DE-12932 Swimming pool granuloma disease 031.1
(L-21806)
Infection due to Mycobacterium marinum 031.1
(L-21806)

DE-12936 Infection due to Mycobacterium scrofulaceum 031.8
(L-21813)

DE-12940V Infection due to Mycobacterium aquae
(L-21870)

DE-12941V Infection due to Mycobacterium fortuitum
(L-21822)

DE-12942V Infection due to Mycobacterium chelonei
(L-21823)

DE-12943V Infection due to Mycobacterium smegmatis
(L-21820)

DE-12944V Infection due to Mycobacterium vaccae
(L-21819)

DE-12945V Infection due to Mycobacterium xenopi
(L-21816)

DE-12980 Infection due to other mycobacteria, NOS 031.8
(L-21800)

E-12A Necrobacillosis

DE-12A00 Necrobacillosis, NOS 040.3
(M-54000) (L-1F306)

DE-12A01 Necrobacillosis due to Fusobacterium necrophorum 040.3
(M-54000) (L-1F306)
Infection due to Sphaerophorus necrophorus 040.3
(M-54000) (L-1F306)
Necrobacillosis due to Schmorl's bacillus 040.3
(M-54000) (L-1F306)

DE-12A02V Oral necrobacillosis
(L-1F306)
Calf diphtheria
(L-1F306)

DE-12A05 Infection due to Bacteroides 040.3
(M-54000) (L-12400)

DE-12A10V Hepatic necrobacillosis
(T-62000) (L-1F306)
Bovine liver abscess
(T-62000) (L-1F306)

DE-12A12V Phlegmonous stomatitis and cellulitis
(T-51000) (L-1F306)

DE-12A20V Interdigital necrobacillosis
(T-D9860) (L-1F306) (L-12417)
Infectious pododermatitis
(T-D9860) (L-1F306) (L-12417)
Bovine foot rot
(T-D9860) (L-1F306) (L-12417)
Foul-in-the-foot
(T-D9860) (L-1F306) (L-12417)

DE-12A22V Ovine interdigital dermatitis
(T-02925) (L-1F306) (L-10809)
OID
(T-02925) (L-1F306) (L-10809)
Foot scald
(T-02925) (L-1F306) (L-10809)

DE-12A24V Benign foot rot
(T-02925) (L-12413)
BFR
(T-02925) (L-12413)
Ovine foot rot
(T-02925) (L-12413)

DE-12A26V Virulent foot rot
(T-01730) (L-1F306) (L-12413)
Malignant foot rot
(T-01730) (L-1F306) (L-12413)
Contagious foot rot
(T-01730) (L-1F306) (L-12413)

DE-12A30V Infective bulbar necrosis
(T-15872) (L-1F306) (L-10809)
Foot abscess
(T-15872) (L-1F306) (L-10809)
Heel abscess
(T-15872) (L-1F306) (L-10809)

DE-12A32V Septic laminitis
(T-D9890) (L-1F306)
Lamellar suppuration
(T-D9890) (L-1F306) (L-10809)
Toe abscess
(T-D9890) (L-1F306) (L-10809)

DE-12A40V Calf diphteria
(T-24100) (L-1F306)
Necrotic laryngitis
(T-24100) (L-1F306)
Necrotic stomatitis
(T-53000) (L-1F306)

DE-12A42V Necrotic rhinitis
(T-21000) (L-1F306)
Bull nose
(T-21000) (L-1F306)

E-131 Pasteurelloses

DE-13100 Pasteurella infection, NOS 027.2
(L-22800)
Pasteurellosis, NOS 027.2
(L-22800)

DE-13110 Hemorrhagic septicemia due to Pasteurella multocida 027.2
(T-C2000) (L-22801)
Infection by Pasteurella multocida 027.2
(T-C2000) (L-22801)
Septicemic pasteurellosis
(T-C2000) (L-22801)

E-131 Pasteurelloses — Continued

DE-13112V Fowl cholera
(L-22801)

DE-13120 Mesenteric adenitis due to Pasteurella multocida 027.2
(T-C4510) (L-22801)

DE-13130 Localized septic infection by cat or dog bite due to Pasteurella multocida 027.2
(T-01000) (M-14360) (L-22801) (L-80A00) (L-80700)
Cat-bite fever
(T-01000) (M-41360) (L-22801) (L-80A00) (L-80700)

DE-13142V Anatipestifer infection
(L-22817)
New duck disease
(L-22817)
Goose influenza
(L-22817)
Avian infectious serositis
(L-22817)

DE-13150V Infection due to Pasteurella haemolytica
(L-22803)

DE-13151V Bovine pneumonic pasteurellosis
(T-28000) (L-22803)
Shipping fever of cattle
(T-28000) (L-22803)
Transit fever
(T-28000) (L-22803)

DE-13152V Enzootic pneumonia of sheep
(T-28000) (L-22803)
Pneumonic pasteurellosis
(T-28000) (L-22803)

DE-13160V Snuffles in rabbits
(L-22801)

DE-13162V Swine plague
(L-22801)

DE-13170V Infection due to Pasteurella pneumotropica
(L-22802)

DE-13180 Other pasteurellosis, NEC 027.8
(L-22800)

E-132 Bordetelloses

DE-13200 Bordetellosis, NOS
(L-12800)

DE-13210 Pertussis 033.9
(L-12801) (L-12802)
Whooping cough, NOS 033.9
(L-12801) (L-12802)
Infection due to Bordetella pertussis 033.0
(L-12801)

DE-13212 Pneumonia in pertussis 484.3
(T-28000) (M-40000)
Pneumonia in whooping cough 484.3
(T-28000) (M-40000)

DE-13214 Infection due to Bordetella parapertussis 033.1
(L-12802)

DE-13216 Infection due to Bordetella bronchiseptica
(L-12803)

DE-13230V Turkey coryza
(L-12804)
Turkey rhinotracheitis
(L-12804)
Infection due to Bordetella avium
(L-12804)

DE-13280 Whooping cough due to other specified organism 033.8
(L-128..)

E-133 Pinta

DE-13300 Pinta, NOS 103.9
(L-25902)
Azul 103.9
(L-25902)
Carate, NOS 103.9
(L-25902)
Infection by Treponema carateum 103.9
(L-25902)

DE-13310 Pinta, primary lesion 103.0
(L-25902)
Primary chancre of pinta 103.0
(M-40020) (L-25902)

DE-13311 Primary papule of pinta 103.0
(T-01000) (M-03130) (L-25902)

DE-13312 Pintid 103.0
(T-01000) (L-25902)

DE-13320 Pinta, intermediate lesion 103.1
(L-25902)

DE-13321 Erythematous plaques of pinta 103.1
(T-01000) (M-01790) (L-25902)

DE-13322 Hyperchromic lesions of pinta 103.1
(T-01000) (M-57170) (L-25902)

DE-13323 Hyperkeratosis of pinta 103.1
(T-01000) (M-72600) (L-25902)

DE-13340 Pinta, late lesion 103.2
(L-25902)

DE-13341 Cardiovascular lesions of pinta 103.2
(T-30000) (L-25902)

DE-13342 Cicatricial skin lesions of pinta 103.2
(T-01000) (M-78060) (L-25902)

DE-13343 Dyschromic skin lesions of pinta 103.2
(T-01000) (M-57120) (L-25902)

DE-13344 Vitiligo of pinta 103.2
(T-01000) (M-57160) (L-25902)

DE-13345 Achromic skin lesions of pinta 103.2
(T-01000) (M-57140) (L-25902)

DE-13350 Pinta, mixed lesions 103.3
(L-25902)

DE-13351 Achromic and hyperchromic skin lesions of pinta 103.3
(T-01000) (M-57140) (M-57170) (L-25902)

E-134 Yersinioses

DE-13400 Yersiniosis, NOS
(L-1E400)
DE-13410 Plague, NOS 020.9
(L-87000) (L-60025) (L-1E401)
(DE-01750)
Infection by Yersinia pestis 020.9
(L-87000) (L-60025) (L-1E401)
(DE-01750)
DE-13411 Abortive plague 020.8
(L-1E401) (DE-01750)
Ambulatory plague 020.8
(L-1E401) (DE-01750)
Pestis minor 020.8
(L-1E401) (DE-01750)
DE-13420 Bubonic plague 020.0
(L-1E401) (DE-01750)
DE-13430 Pneumonic plague, NOS 020.5
(T-28000) (L-1E401) (DE-01750)
DE-13431 Primary pneumonic plague 020.3
(T-28000) (L-1E401) (DE-01750)
DE-13432 Secondary pneumonic plague 020.4
(T-28000) (L-1E401) (DE-01750)
DE-13440 Septicemic plague 020.2
(T-C2000) (L-1E401) (DE-01750)
DE-13450 Cellulocutaneous plague 020.1
(T-01000) (T-03000) (L-1E401)
(DE-01750)
DE-13460 Pseudotuberculosis 027.2
(L-1E402) (L-87000)
Infection by Pasteurella pseudotuberculosis 027.2
(L-1E402) (L-87000)
Rodent pseudotuberculosis 027.2
(L-1E402) (L-87000)
Infection by Yersinia pseudotuberculosis 027.2
(L-1E402) (L-87000)
DE-13470V Infection by Yersinia enterocolitica
(L-1E403)
DE-13480V Enteric redmouth disease
(L-1E406)
Infection by Yersinia ruckeri
(L-1E406)

E-135 Pneumococcal Infections

DE-13500 Pneumococcal infectious disease, NOS 041.2
(L-25116)
Pneumococcal infection, NOS 041.2
(L-25116)
DE-13505 Pneumococcal tonsillitis 463.-
(T-C5100) (M-40000) (L-25116)
DE-13508 Pneumococcal pharyngitis 462.-
(T-55000) (M-40000) (L-25116)
DE-13509 Pneumococcal laryngitis 464.0
(T-24100) (M-40000) (L-25116)
DE-13510 Pneumococcal pneumonia 481.-
(T-28000) (M-40000) (L-25116)
DE-13511 Pneumococcal pleurisy 511.0
(T-29000) (M-40000) (L-25116)
DE-13512 Pneumococcal pleurisy with effusion 511.1
(T-29000) (M-40000) (L-25116)
(M-36700)
DE-13513 Pneumococcal bronchitis 466.0
(T-26000) (M-40000) (L-25116)
DE-13520 Pneumococcal meningitis 320.1
(T-A1110) (M-40000) (L-25116)
DE-13525 Pneumococcal peritonitis 567.1
(T-D4400) (M-40000) (L-25116)
DE-13530 Pneumococcal septicemia 038.2
(T-C2000) (L-25116)
Septicemia due to Streptococcus pneumonia 038.2
(T-C2000) (L-25116)
DE-13535 Pneumococcal arthritis 711.0
(T-15000) (M-40000) (L-25116)

E-136 Rat Bite Fevers

DE-13600 Rat bite fever, NOS 026.9
(M-14360) (L-81400)
DE-13610 Spirillary fever 026.0
(M-14360) (L-81400) (L-24501)
Sodoku 026.0
(M-14360) (L-81400) (L-24501)
Rat-bite fever due to Spirillum minus 026.0
(M-14360) (L-81400) (L-24501)
DE-13620 Streptobacillary fever 026.1
(M-14360) (L-81400) (L-25001)
Haverhill fever 026.1
(M-14360) (L-81400) (L-25001)
Rat-bite fever due to Streptobacillus moniliformis 026.1
(M-14360) (L-81400) (L-25001)
Epidemic arthritic erythema 026.1
(M-14360) (L-81400) (L-25001)

E-137 Relapsing Fevers

DE-13700 Relapsing fever, NOS 087.9
(L-12900)
Relapsing fever due to Borrelia 087.9
(L-12900)
Recurrent fever, NOS 087.9
(L-12900)
Recurrent fever due to Borrelia 087.9
(L-12900)
Borreliosis, NOS
(L-12900)
DE-13710 Louse-borne relapsing fever, NOS 087.0
(L-12902) (L-61521)
Relapsing fever due to Borrelia recurrentis 087.0
(L-12902) (L-61521)
DE-13720 Tick-borne relapsing fever, NOS 087.1
(L-12900) (L-60052)

E-137 Relapsing Fevers — Continued

DE-13721 Relapsing fever of Western North America 087.1
(L-12904) (L-66361)
Infection by Borrelia hermsii 087.1
(L-12904) (L-66361)

DE-13722 Relapsing fever of Asia and Africa 087.1
(L-12909) (L-66359)
Infection by Borrelia persica 087.1
(L-12909) (L-66359)

DE-13723 Relapsing fever of Iberian Peninsula and Northwest Africa 087.1
(L-12903) (L-66356)
Infection by Borrelia hispanica 087.1
(L-12903) (L-66356)

DE-13724 Relapsing fever of Central and South Africa 087.1
(L-12905) (L-66351)
Infection by Borrelia duttonii 087.1
(L-12905) (L-66351)

DE-13725 Relapsing fever of Southwest U.S. and Mexico 087.1
(L-12919) (L-66364)
Infection by Borrelia turicatae 087.1
(L-12919) (L-66364)

DE-13726 Relapsing fever of Central and South America 087.1
(L-12907) (L-66358)
Infection by Borrelia venezuelensis 087.1
(L-12907) (L-66358)

DE-13727 Relapsing fever of the Caucasus 087.1
(L-12910) (L-66363)
Infection by Borrelia caucasica 087.1
(L-12910) (L-66323)

DE-13728 Relapsing fever of North Africa 087.1
(L-12914) (L-12922) (L-66377)
Infection by Borrelia crocidurae 087.1
(L-12914) (L-66377)
Infection by Borrelia microti 087.1
(L-12922) (L-66377)

DE-13729 Relapsing fever of Western United States 087.1
(L-12906) (L-66372)
Infection by Borrelia parkeri 087.1
(L-12906) (L-66372)

DE-13731 Relapsing fever of Iran and Central Asia 087.1
(L-12915) (L-66371)
Infection by Borrelia latyschewii 087.1
(L-12915) (L-66371)

DE-13732 Relapsing fever of Southern U.S., Mexico, Central and South America 087.1
(L-12908) (L-66370)
Infection by Borrelia mazzottii 087.1
(L-12908) (L-66370)

DE-13741 Lyme disease 087.1
(L-12921) (L-66014)
Infection by Borrelia burgdorferi 087.1
(L-12921) (L-66014)

DE-13742 Lyme arthritis 087.1
(T-15000) (L-12921) (L-66014)

DE-13743 Lyme carditis 087.1
(T-32020) (L-12921) (L-66014)

DE-13748 Bannwarth syndrome
(T-A1110) (T-A0500) (M-40000) (L-12921) (L-66014)
Tick-borne meningopolyneuritis
(T-A1110) (T-A0500) (L-12921) (L-66014)

DE-13750V Avian borreliosis 087.1
(L-12901) (L-66300)
Infection by Borrelia anserina 087.1
(L-12901) (L-66300)
Avian spirochetosis
(L-12901) (L-66300)

DE-13760V Spirochetosis of cattle, horses and sheep 087.1
(L-12917) (L-66130) (L-66230)
Infection by Borrelia theileri 087.1
(L-12917) (L-66130) (L-66230)

E-138 Rhinoscleroma

DE-13800 Rhinoscleroma 040.1
(L-16008)
Infection by Klebsiella rhinoscleromatis 040.1
(L-16008)

E-139 Salmonelloses

DE-13900 Salmonellosis, NOS (except human typhoid & paratyphoid) 003.9
(L-17100)
Salmonella infection, NOS 003.9
(L-17100)

DE-13910 Salmonella gastroenteritis 003.0
(T-50100) (L-17100)
Salmonella food poisoning 003.0
(T-50100) (L-17100)

DE-13920 Salmonella septicemia 003.1
(T-C2000) (L-17100)

DE-13930 Localized Salmonella infection, NOS 003.20
(T-.....) (L-17100)

DE-13931 Salmonella arthritis 003.23 —711.3*
(T-15000) (L-17100)

DE-13932 Salmonella meningitis 003.21 —320.7*
(T-A1110) (L-17100)

DE-13933 Salmonella osteomyelitis 003.24 —730.2*
(T-11000) (L-17100)

DE-13934 Salmonella pneumonia 003.22 —484.8*
(T-28000) (L-17100)

DE-13940V Fowl typhoid
(L-18168)

DE-13942V Arizona infection
(L-17103)
Arizonosis
(L-17103)

DE-13942V (cont.) Paracolon infection
(L-17103)
Salmonella enteritis
(L-17103)

DE-13950V Avian paratyphoid infection
(L-17354)

DE-13970V Pullorum disease
(L-18168)

DE-13980 Other Salmonella infection, NEC 003.8
(T-.....) (L-17100)
Other specified localized Salmonella infection 003.29
(T-.....) (L-17100)

E-140 Shigelloses

DE-14000 Shigellosis, NOS 004.9
(L-1E100)
Bacillary dysentery 004.9
(L-1E100)

DE-14010 Infection due to Group A Shigella 004.0
(L-1E101)
Shigellosis due to Shigella dysenteriae 004.0
(L-1E101)

DE-14020 Infection due to Group B Shigella 004.1
(L-1E102)
Shigellosis due to Shigella flexneri 004.1
(L-1E102)

DE-14030 Infection due to Group C Shigella 004.2
(L-1E103)
Shigellosis due to Shigella boydii 004.2
(L-1E103)

DE-14040 Infection due to Group D Shigella 004.3
(L-1E104)
Shigellosis due to Shigella sonnei 004.3
(L-1E104)

DE-14080 Other specified Shigella infections 004.8
(L-1E100)

E-141 Staphylococcal Infections

DE-14100 Staphylococcal infectious disease, NOS 041.1
(L-24800)
Staphylococcosis 041.1
(L-24800)
Staphylococcal infection, NOS 041.1
(L-24800)

DE-14110 Staphylococcal enterocolitis 008.41
(T-50500) (L-24800)

DE-14111V Staphylococcal enteritis of chinchillas
(T-50500) (L-24801)

DE-14115 Staphylococcal tonsillitis 463.-
(T-C5100) (M-40000) (L-24801)

DE-14118 Staphylococcal pharyngitis 462.-
(T-55000) (M-40000) (L-24801)

DE-14120 Staphylococcal pneumonia 482.4
(T-28000) (L-24800)

DE-14121 Staphylococcal pleurisy 511.0
(T-29000) (M-40000) (L-24800)

DE-14122 Staphylococcal pleurisy with effusion 511.1
(T-29000) (M-40000) (L-24800)
(M-36700)

DE-14124 Sycosis vulgaris 704.8
(T-01400) (T-B0200) (M-41400)
Sycosis barbae, not parasitic 704.8
(T-01400) (T-B0200) (M-41400)
(L-24801)
Bacterial folliculitis 704.8
(T-01400) (T-B0200) (M-41400)
(L-24801)

DE-14125V Staphylococcal mastitis
(T-04000) (L-24801)

DE-14128 Staphylococcal arthritis 711.0
(T-15000) (M-40000) (L-24800)

DE-14130 Staphylococcal septicemia 038.1
(T-C2000) (L-24800)

DE-14135 Toxic epidermal necrolysis, subcorneal type 695.1
(T-01000) (L-24801)
Staphylococcal scalded skin syndrome
(T-01000) (L-24801)
Scalded skin syndrome 695.1
(T-01000) (L-24801)
Ritter's disease 695.81
(T-01000) (L-24801)
Dermatitis exfoliativa neonatorum 695.81
(T-01000) (L-24801)

DE-14140 Toxic shock syndrome 040.89
(T-82000) (L-24800) (L-10038)

DE-14170V Enzootic staphylococcosis
(T-C2000) (L-24801)
Staphylococcal pyaemia
(T-C2000) (L-24801)
Tick pyaemia
(T-C2000) (L-24801)

DE-14180V Bumblefoot
(T-D9700) (M-10000) (L-24800)

E-142 Streptococcal Infections

DE-14200 Streptococcal infectious disease, NOS 041.0
(L-25100)
Streptococcosis 041.0
(L-25100)
Streptococcal infection, NOS 041.0
(L-25100)

DE-14210 Streptococcal sore throat 034.0
(T-55000) (L-25100)
Streptococcal pharyngitis 034.0
(T-55000) (L-25100)
Septic sore throat 034.0
(T-55000) (L-25100)
Streptococcal angina 034.0
(T-55000) (L-25100)

DE-14211 Streptococcal laryngitis 034.0
(T-24100) (L-25100)

DE-14212 Streptococcal tonsillitis 034.0
(T-C5100) (L-25100)

E-142 Streptococcal Infections — Continued

DE-14213 Pneumonia due to Streptococcus 482.3
(T-28000) (M-40000) (L-25100)
Streptococcal pneumonia 482.3
(T-28000) (M-40000) (L-25100)

DE-14214 Streptococcal pleurisy 511.0
(T-29000) (M-40000) (L-25100)

DE-14215 Streptococcal pleurisy with effusion 511.1
(T-25100) (M-40000) (L-25100)
(M-36700)

DE-14216V Streptococcal meningitis
(T-A1110) (L-25168)

DE-14217V Streptococcal cervicitis
(T-83200) (L-25111)

DE-14218V Streptococcal arthritis 711.0
(T-15000) (L-25111)

DE-14220 Streptococcal septicemia 038.0
(T-C2000) (L-25100)
Streptococcaemia
(T-C2000) (L-25100)

DE-14221 Septicemia due to anaerobic streptococci 038.0
(T-C2000) (L-23000)
Septicemia due to Peptostreptococcus 038.0
(T-C2000) (L-23000)

DE-14240 Scarlet fever 034.1
(T-01000) (M-01710) (L-25128)
Scarlatina 034.1
(T-01000) (M-01710) (L-25128)

DE-14250 Erysipelas 035.-
(T-01000) (L-25124)

DE-14251 Postpartum or puerperal erysipelas 670.-
(T-01000) (F-84300) (L-25124)

DE-14255 Ecthyma 686.8
(T-01000) (M-41600) (L-25124)
(M-41750)

DE-14260V Streptococcal mastitis
(T-04000) (L-25107) (L-25108)

DE-14264V Strangles
(T-C4190) (L-25110)
Adenitis equorum
(T-C4190) (L-25110)

DE-14266V Streptococcal lymphadenitis of swine
(L-25132)
SLS
(L-25132)
Jowl abscess
(L-25132)
Cervical abscess
(L-25132)

DE-14268V Infection due to Streptococcus suis
(L-25168)

DE-14270V Avian streptococcosis
(L-25109)

E-143-145 Syphilis

DE-14300 Syphilis, NOS 097.9
(L-25901) (DE-01600)
Syphilis, stage unspecified 095.-
(L-25901) (DE-01600)
Lues 097.9
(L-25901) (DE-01600)
Infection by Treponema pallidum 097.9
(L-25901) (DE-01600)

DE-14301 Syphilis of bone 095.5 —730.8*
(T-11000) (L-25901) (DE-01600)

DE-14302 Syphilis of kidney 095.4 —583.8*
(T-71000) (L-25901) (DE-01600)

DE-14303 Syphilis of liver 095.3 —573.2*
(T-62000) (L-25901) (DE-01600)

DE-14304 Syphilis of lung 095.1 —517.8*
(T-28000) (L-25901) (DE-01600)

DE-14305 Syphilis of muscle 095.6 —728.0*
(T-13000) (L-25901) (DE-01600)

DE-14306 Syphilitic episcleritis 095.0 —379.0*
(T-AA110) (L-25901) (DE-01600)

DE-14307 Syphilitic peritonitis 095.2 —567.0*
(T-D4400) (L-25901) (DE-01600)

DE-14308 Syphilis of synovium 091.7
(T-15003) (L-25901) (DE-01600)

DE-14309 Syphilis of tendon 095.7
(T-17010) (L-25901) (DE-01600)

DE-14311 Syphilis of bursa 095.7
(T-16000) (L-25901) (DE-01600)

DE-14318 Syphilis in mother complicating pregnancy, childbirth or puerperium 647.0
(L-25901)

DE-14320 Symptomatic early syphilis, NOS 091.-
(L-25901) (DE-01600)

DE-14321 Primary symptomatic early syphilis 091.-
(L-25901) (DE-01600)

DE-14322 Primary genital syphilis 091.0
(T-70260) (L-25901) (DE-01600)
Genital chancre 091.0
(T-70260) (M-40020) (L-25901)
(DE-01600)

DE-14324 Primary anal syphilis 091.1
(T-59900) (L-25901) (DE-01600)

DE-14325 Primary syphilis of fingers 091.2
(T-D8800) (L-25901) (DE-01600)

DE-14326 Primary syphilis of lip 091.2
(T-52000) (L-25901) (DE-01600)

DE-14327 Primary syphilis of tonsils 091.2
(T-C5100) (L-25901) (DE-01600)

DE-14328 Primary syphilis of breast 091.2
(T-04000) (L-25901) (DE-01600)

DE-14340 Secondary symptomatic early syphilis 091.9
(L-25901) (DE-01600)

DE-14341 Secondary syphilis of skin 091.3
(T-01000) (L-25901) (DE-01600)

DE-14342 Secondary syphilis of mucous membrane 091.3
(T-00400) (L-25901) (DE-01600)

DE-14343 Condyloma latum 091.3
(T-70260) (M-76750) (L-25901)
(DE-01600)

DE-14344 Secondary syphilis of anus 091.3
(T-59900) (L-25901) (DE-01600)

DE-14345 Secondary syphilis of mouth 091.3
(T-51000) (L-25901) (DE-01600)

DE-14346 Secondary syphilis of pharynx 091.3
(T-55000) (L-25901) (DE-01600)

DE-14347 Secondary syphilis of tonsil 091.3
(T-C5100) (L-25901) (DE-01600)

DE-14348 Secondary syphilis of vulva 091.3
(T-81000) (L-25901) (DE-01600)

DE-14349 Secondary syphilitic adenopathy 091.4
(T-C4000) (L-25901) (DE-01600)
Secondary syphilitic lymphadenitis 091.4
(T-C4000) (L-25901) (DE-01600)

DE-14352 Secondary syphilitic chorioretinitis 091.51
—363.1*
(T-AA310) (T-AA610) (L-25901)
(DE-01600)

DE-14353 Secondary syphilitic iridocyclitis 091.52
—364.1*
(T-AA500) (T-AA400) (L-25901)
(DE-01600)

DE-14354 Secondary syphilitic uveitis 091.50
(T-AA570) (L-25901) (DE-01600)

DE-14355 Secondary syphilis of viscera 091.6
(T-D4030) (L-25901) (DE-01600)

DE-14356 Secondary syphilis of bone 091.6
(T-11000) (L-25901) (DE-01600)

DE-14357 Secondary syphilis of liver 091.62 —573.2*
(T-62000) (L-25901) (DE-01600)
Secondary syphilitic hepatitis 091.62
—573.2*
(T-62000) (L-25901) (DE-01600)

DE-14358 Secondary syphilitic periostitis 091.61
—730.3*
(T-11020) (L-25901) (DE-01600)

DE-14359 Acute syphilitic meningitis 091.81 —320.7*
(T-A1110) (L-25901) (DE-01600)

DE-14361 Syphilitic alopecia 091.82
(T-01400) (T-D1160) (M-58600)
(L-25901) (DE-01600)

DE-14362 Secondary syphilis of other viscera 091.69
(T-.....) (L-25901) (DE-01600)

DE-14370 Secondary syphilis, relapse 091.7
(L-25901) (DE-01600)

DE-14371 Secondary syphilis, relapse (treated) 091.7
(L-25901) (DE-01600)

DE-14372 Secondary syphilis, relapse (untreated) 091.7
(L-25901) (DE-01600)

DE-14390 Early syphilis, latent, NOS (+ sero., —
C.S.F., less than 2 years after) 092.9
(L-25901) (DE-01600)

DE-14392 Early syphilis, latent (+ sero., — C.S.F.,
relapse after treatment) 092.0
(L-25901) (DE-01600)

DE-14400 Late syphilis, NOS 097.0
(L-25901) (DE-01600)

DE-14401 Cardiovascular syphilis, NOS 093.9
(T-30000) (L-25901) (DE-01600)

DE-14402 Syphilitic aneurysm of aorta 093.0 —441.7*
(T-42000) (M-32400) (L-25901)
(DE-01600)
Syphilitic dilatation of aorta 093.0
—441.7*
(T-42000) (M-32400) (L-25901)
(DE-01600)

DE-14403 Syphilitic aortitis 093.1 —447.7*
(T-42000) (L-25901) (DE-01600)

DE-14404 Syphilitic endocarditis 093.2 —424.-*
(T-32060) (L-25901) (DE-01600)

DE-14405 Syphilitic aortic incompetence 093.22
—424.-*
(T-35400) (F-32400) (L-25901)
(DE-01600)

DE-14406 Syphilitic aortic stenosis 093.22 —424.-*
(T-35400) (M-34200) (L-25901)
(DE-01600)

DE-14407 Syphilitic ostial coronary disease 093.20
—424.-*
(T-43005) (L-25901) (DE-01600)

DE-14408 Syphilitic myocarditis 093.82 —422.0*
(T-32020) (L-25901) (DE-01600)

DE-14409 Syphilitic pericarditis 093.81 —420.0*
(T-39000) (L-25901) (DE-01600)

DE-14450 Neurosyphilis, NOS 094.9
(T-A0090) (L-25901) (DE-01600)
Syphilis of central nervous system, NOS
094.9
(T-A0090) (L-25901) (DE-01600)

DE-14451 Tabes dorsalis 094.0
(T-A0090) (F-A4580) (L-25901)
(DE-01600)
Progressive locomotor ataxia 094.0
(T-A0090) (F-A4580 (L-25901)
(DE-01600)
Syphilitic posterior spinal sclerosis 094.0
(T-A0090) (F-A4580) (L-25901)
(DE-01600)
Tabetic neurosyphilis 094.0
(T-A0090) (F-A4580) (L-25901)
(DE-01600)
Duchenne's disease 094.0
(T-A0090) (F-A4580) (L-25901)
(DE-01600)

DE-14452 General paresis 094.1
(T-A0090) (F-A0850) (L-25901)
(DE-01600)
Dementia paralytica 094.1
(T-A0090) (F-A0850) (L-25901)
(DE-01600)
Progressive general paresis 094.1
(T-A0090) (F-A0850) (L-25901)
(DE-01600)

E-143-145 Syphilis — Continued

DE-14452 (cont.) Paretic neurosyphilis 094.1
(T-A0090) (F-A0850) (L-25901) (DE-01600)

DE-14453 Taboparesis 094.1
(T-A0090) (F-A0850) (L-25901) (DE-01600)

DE-14455 Neurogenic arthropathy of Charcot 094.0 —713.5*
(T-15000) (L-25901) (DE-01600)
Tabetic arthropathy 094.0 —713.5*
(T-15000) (L-25901) (DE-01600)
Charcot's joint disease 094.0 —713.5*
(T-15000) (L-25901) (DE-01600)

DE-14456 Syphilitic meningitis 094.2 —320.7*
(T-A1110) (L-25901) (DE-01600)
Meningovascular syphilis 094.2 —320.7*
(T-A1110) (L-25901) (DE-01600)

DE-14457 Syphilitic acoustic neuritis 094.86 —388.5*
(T-A8500) (M-40000) (L-25901) (DE-01600)

DE-14458 Syphilitic disseminated retinochoroiditis 094.83 —363.1*
(T-AA310) (T-AA610) (L-25901) (DE-01600)

DE-14459 Syphilitic encephalitis 094.81 —323.4*
(T-A0100) (M-40000) (L-25901) (DE-01600)

DE-14461 Syphilitic optic atrophy 094.84 —377.1*
(T-AA000) (M-58000) (L-25901) (DE-01600)

DE-14462 Syphilitic parkinsonism 094.82 —332.1*
(T-A0090) (DA-21012) (L-25901) (DE-01600)

DE-14463 Syphilitic retrobulbar neuritis 094.85 —377.3*
(T-A8040) (T-D1480) (M-40000) (L-25901) (DE-01600)

DE-14464 Syphilitic ruptured cerebral aneurysm 094.87 —430.-*
(T-45510) (M-32201) (L-25901) (DE-01600)

DE-14471 Syphilitic gumma of central nervous system 094.9
(T-A0090) (M-44740) (L-25901) (DE-01600)

DE-14472 Syphilitic gumma of other sites 095.-
(T-.....) (M-44740) (L-25901) (DE-01600)

DE-14475 Syphilis of mitral valve 093.21
(T-35300) (L-25901) (DE-01600)

DE-14476 Syphilis of tricuspid valve 093.23
(T-35100) (L-25901) (DE-01600)

DE-14477 Syphilis of pulmonary valve 093.24
(T-35200) (L-25901) (DE-01600)

DE-14478 Other specified cardiovascular syphilis 093.89
(T-30000) (L-25901) (DE-01600)

DE-14480 Late syphilis, latent (+ sero., — C.S.F. 2 years after) 096.-
(L-25901) (DE-01600)

DE-14481 Asymptomatic neurosyphilis 094.3
(T-A0090) (L-25901) (DE-01600)

DE-14485 Latent syphilis, NOS (+ sero.) 097.1
(L-25901) (DE-01600)

DE-14500 Congenital syphilis, NOS 090.9
(L-25901) (DE-01900) (DE-01600)

DE-14510 Early congenital syphilis, NOS (less than 2 years) 090.2
(L-25901) (DE-01900) (DE-01600)
Early congenital syphilis, symptomatic (less than 2 years) 090.0
(L-25901) (DE-01900) (DE-01600)

DE-14511 Congenital syphilitic choroiditis 090.0
(T-AA310) (L-25901) (DE-01900) (DE-01600)

DE-14512 Congenital syphilitic coryza 090.0
(T-21010) (L-25901) (DE-01900) (DE-01600)

DE-14513 Congenital syphilitic hepatomegaly 090.0
(T-62000) (M-71000) (L-25901) (DE-01900) (DE-01600)

DE-14514 Congenital syphilitic mucous patches 090.0
(T-00400) (L-25901) (DE-01900) (DE-01600)

DE-14515 Congenital syphilitic periostitis 090.0
(T-11020) (L-25901) (DE-01900) (DE-01600)

DE-14516 Congenital syphilitic epiphysitis 090.0
(T-11035) (L-25901) (DE-01900) (DE-01600)

DE-14517 Congenital syphilitic osteochondritis 090.0
(T-11000) (T-1A700) (L-25901) (DE-01900) (DE-01600)

DE-14518 Congenital syphilitic splenomegaly 090.0
(T-C3000) (M-71000) (L-25901) (DE-01900) (DE-01600)

DE-14519 Congenital syphilitic pemphigus 090.0
(L-25901) (DE-01900) (DE-01600)

DE-14520 Early congenital syphilis, latent (+ sero. — C.S.F.) 090.1
(L-25901) (DE-01900) (DE-01600)

DE-14530 Late congenital syphilis, NOS (2 years or more) 090.7
(L-25901) (DE-01900) (DE-01600)
Late congenital syphilis, symptomatic (2 years or more) 090.5
(L-25901) (DE-01900) (DE-01600)

DE-14531 Congenital syphilis with gumma 090.5
(M-44740) (L-25901) (DE-01900) (DE-01600)

DE-14533 Syphilitic saddle nose 090.5
(T-21000) (M-02060) (L-25901) (DE-01900) (DE-01600)

DE-14534 Syphilitic interstitial keratitis 090.3 —370.5*
(T-AA200) (L-25901) (DE-01900) (DE-01600)

DE-14540 Late congenital syphilis, latent (+ sero., — C.S.F., 2 years or more) 090.6
(L-25901) (DE-01900) (DE-01600)

DE-14541 Juvenile neurosyphilis 090.4
(T-A0090) (L-25901) (DE-01900) (DE-01600)
Congenital neurosyphilis 090.4
(T-A0090) (L-25901) (DE-01900) (DE-01600)

DE-14542 Congenital syphilitic encephalitis 090.41 —323.4*
(T-A0100) (L-25901) (DE-01900) (DE-01600)

DE-14543 Congenital syphilitic meningitis 090.42 —320.7*
(T-A1110) (L-25901) (DE-01900) (DE-01600)

DE-14544 Dementia paralytica juvenilis 090.4
(T-A0090) (F-08040) (L-25901) (DE-01900) (DE-01600)
Juvenile general paresis 090.4
(T-A0090) (F-08040) (L-25901) (DE-01900) (DE-01600)

DE-14545 Juvenile tabes 090.4
(T-A0090) (F-08040) (L-25901) (DE-01900) (DE-01600)

DE-14546 Juvenile taboparesis 090.4
(T-A0090) (F-08040) (L-25901) (DE-01900) (DE-01600)

DE-14550V Treponematosis of rabbit
(L-25903)
Vent disease
(L-25903)
Rabbit syphilis
(L-25903)
Benign venereal spirochetosis
(L-25903)

DE-14560V Porcine ulcerative spirochaetosis
(L-25918)
Swine dysentery
(L-25918)
Bloody scours
(L-25918)

DE-14580 Non-venereal endemic syphilis 104.0
(L-25900)
Bejel 104.0
(L-25900)
Njovera 104.0
(L-25900)

E-146 Tetanus

DE-14600 Tetanus 037.-
(L-14158)
Lockjaw 037.-
(L-14158)
Infection due to Clostridium tetani 037.-
(L-14158)

DE-14610 Tetanus neonatorum 771.3
(F-88000) (L-14158)

DE-14620 Tetanus complicating abortion 639.0
(L-14158)

DE-14630 Tetanus complicating ectopic or molar pregnancy 639.0
(M-91000) (L-14158)

DE-14640 Puerperal tetanus 670.-
(F-84300) (L-14158)

DE-14642 Tetanus omphalitis 771.3
(T-F1800) (L-14158)

E-147 Tropical Phagedenic Ulcer

DE-14700 Tropical phagedenic ulcer 707.9
(L-12400)

DE-14710 Ulcer due to Bacteroides, NOS 707.9
(L-12400)

DE-14711 Ulcer due to Borrelia vincentii 707.9
(L-25915)
Ulcer due to Treponema vincentii 707.9
(L-25915)

DE-14750 Tropical pyomyositis 040.81 —728.0*
(T-13000) (L-24801)
Tropical myositis 040.81 —728.0*
(T-13000) (L-24801)

E-148-14B Tuberculosis

DE-14800 Tuberculosis, NOS 010.9
(L-21801)
Infection due to Mycobacterium tuberculosis 010.9
(L-21801)

DE-14801 Congenital tuberculosis 771.2
(L-21801) (DE-01900)

DE-14805 Tuberculosis in mother complicating pregnancy, childbirth or puerperium 647.3

DE-14810 Respiratory tuberculosis 011.9
(T-28000) (L-21801)
Pulmonary tuberculosis 011.9
(T-28000) (L-21801)

DE-14811 Infiltrative tuberculosis of lung 011.0
(T-28000) (M-44000) (L-21801)

DE-14812 Nodular tuberculosis of lung 011.1
(T-28000) (M-44000) (L-21801)

DE-14813 Tuberculosis of lung with cavitation 011.2
(T-28000) (M-39400) (L-21801)

DE-14814 Tuberculosis of lung with involvement of bronchus 011.3
(T-28000) (T-26000) (L-21801)

DE-14815 Tuberculous fibrosis of lung 011.4
(T-28000) (M-78000) (L-21801)

DE-14816 Tuberculous bronchiectasis 011.5
(T-26000) (M-32000) (L-21801)

DE-14817 Tuberculous pneumonia 011.6
(T-28000) (M-40000) (L-21801)

DE-14820 Tuberculosis of pleura 012.0
(T-29000) (L-21801)
Tuberculous pleurisy 012.0
(T-29000) (L-21801)

E-148-14B Tuberculosis — Continued

DE-14820 (cont.) Tuberculous pleuritis 012.0
(T-29000) (L-21801)
Pearly disease
(T-29000) (L-21801)

DE-14821 Tuberculous pneumothorax 011.7
(T-29050) (M-36670) (L-21801)

DE-14822 Tuberculous hydrothorax 012.0
(T-29050) (M-36700) (L-21801)

DE-14823 Tuberculous empyema 012.0
(T-29050) (M-41602) (L-21801)

DE-14828 Other specified pulmonary tuberculosis 011.8
(T-28000) (L-21801)

DE-14830 Tuberculosis of intrathoracic lymph nodes 012.1
(T-C4300) (L-21801)

DE-14831 Tuberculosis of hilar lymph nodes 012.1
(T-C4320) (L-21801)

DE-14832 Tuberculosis of mediastinal lymph nodes 012.1
(T-C4360) (L-21801)

DE-14833 Tuberculosis of tracheobronchial lymph nodes 012.1
(T-C4330) (L-21801)
Tuberculous tracheobronchial adenopathy 012.1
(T-C4330) (L-21801)

DE-14840 Isolated tracheal tuberculosis 012.2
(T-25000) (L-21801)

DE-14841 Isolated bronchial tuberculosis 012.2
(T-26000) (L-21801)

DE-14842 Tuberculous laryngitis 012.3
(T-24100) (M-44000) (L-21801)

DE-14843 Tuberculosis of glottis 012.3
(T-24440) (L-21801)

DE-14845 Tuberculosis of mediastinum 012.8
(T-D3300) (L-21801)

DE-14846 Tuberculosis of nasopharynx 012.8
(T-23000) (L-21801)

DE-14847 Tuberculosis of nose 012.8
(T-21000) (L-21801)

DE-14848 Tuberculosis of nasal septum 012.8
(T-21340) (L-21801)

DE-14849 Tuberculosis of nasal sinus 012.8
(T-22000) (L-21801)

DE-14860 Tuberculosis of central nervous system, NOS 013.9
(T-A0090) (L-21801)

DE-14861 Tuberculosis of meninges 013.0
(T-A1110) (L-21801)
Tuberculous meningitis 013.0 —320.4*
(T-A1110) (L-21801)

DE-14862 Tuberculosis of cerebral meninges 013.0
(T-A1112) (L-21801)

DE-14863 Tuberculosis of spinal meninges 013.0
(T-A1115) (L-21801)

DE-14864 Tuberculous leptomeningitis 013.0
(T-A1200) (L-21801)

DE-14865 Tuberculous meningoencephalitis 013.0
(T-A0100) (T-A1110) (L-21801)

DE-14866 Tuberculoma of meninges 013.1 —349.2*
(T-A1110) (M-44700) (L-21801)

DE-14867 Tuberculosis of brain 013.2 —348.8*
(T-A0100) (L-21801)

DE-14868 Tuberculoma of brain 013.2
(T-A0100) (M-44700) (L-21801)

DE-14869 Tuberculous abscess of brain 013.3 —324.0*
(T-A0100) (M-41610) (L-21801)

DE-14871 Tuberculous myelitis 013.6 —323.4*
(T-A7010) (L-21801)

DE-14880 Tuberculosis of intestines 014.-
(T-50500) (L-21801)

DE-14881 Tuberculosis of peritoneum 014.0
(T-D4400) (L-21801)

DE-14882 Tuberculosis of mesenteric glands 014.-
(T-C4510) (L-21801)

DE-14883 Tuberculosis of anus 014.8
(T-59900) (L-21801)

DE-14884 Tuberculosis of small intestine 014.8
(T-58000) (L-21801)

DE-14885 Tuberculosis of large intestine 014.8
(T-59000) (L-21801)

DE-14886 Tuberculosis of rectum 014.8
(T-59600) (L-21801)

DE-14887 Tuberculosis of retroperitoneal lymph nodes 014.8
(T-C4580) (L-21801)

DE-14888 Tuberculous ascites 014.0
(T-D4425) (M-36700) (L-21801)

DE-14891 Tuberculous enteritis 014.8
(T-50500) (L-21801)

DE-14892 Tuberculous peritonitis 014.0 —567.0*
(T-D4400) (L-21801)

DE-14900 Tuberculosis of bones and joints, NOS 015.9
(T-11000) (T-15000) (L-21801)

DE-14910 Tuberculosis of bone, NOS 015.7
(T-11000) (L-21801)

DE-14911 Tuberculous necrosis of bone 015.9 —730.-*
(T-11000) (M-54000) (L-21801)

DE-14912 Tuberculous osteitis 015.9 —730.-*
(T-11000) (L-21801)

DE-14913 Tuberculous osteomyelitis 015.9 —730.-*
(T-11000) (T-C1000) (L-21801)

DE-14914 Tuberculosis of vertebral column 015.0 —730.4*
(T-11500) (L-21801)
Pott's disease 015.0 —730.4*
(T-11500) (L-21801)

DE-14915 Pott's curvature 015.0 —734.4*
(T-11500) (M-31601) (L-21801)
Tuberculous kyphosis 015.0 —734.4*
(T-11500) (M-31601) (L-21801)

DE-14916 Tuberculous dactylitis 015.5
(T-D8800) (L-21801)

DE-14930 Tuberculosis of joint, NOS 015.9 —711.4*
(T-15000) (L-21801)
Tuberculous arthritis 015.9 —711.4*
(T-15000) (L-21801)
DE-14931 Tuberculous synovitis 015.9 —727.0*
(T-15003) (L-21801)
DE-14932 Tuberculous tenosynovitis 015.9 —727.0*
(T-17010) (L-21801)
DE-14934 Tuberculous spondylitis 015.0 —720.8*
(T-11500) (L-21801)
DE-14935 Tuberculosis of hip 015.1
(T-D2500) (L-21801)
DE-14936 Tuberculosis of knee 015.2
(T-D9200) (L-21801)
DE-14950 Tuberculosis of genitourinary system, NOS 016.9
(T-70200) (L-21801)
DE-14951 Tuberculosis of kidney 016.0
(T-71000) (L-21801)
DE-14952 Tuberculous pyelitis 016.0 —590.8*
(T-72000) (L-21801)
DE-14953 Tuberculous pyelonephritis 016.0 —590.8*
(T-71000) (T-72000) (L-21801)
DE-14954 Tuberculosis of bladder 016.1 —595.4*
(T-74000) (L-21801)
DE-14955 Tuberculosis of ureter 016.2 —593.8*
(T-73000) (L-21801)
DE-14961 Tuberculosis of epididymis 016.4 —604.9*
(T-95000) (L-21801)
DE-14962 Tuberculosis of prostate 016.5 —601.4*
(T-92000) (L-21801)
DE-14963 Tuberculosis of seminal vesicle 016.5 —608.8*
(T-93000) (L-21801)
DE-14964 Tuberculosis of testis 016.5 —608.8*
(T-94000) (L-21801)
DE-14970 Tuberculosis of female genital organs 016.6
(T-80000) (L-21801)
DE-14971 Tuberculous oophoritis 016.6 —614.2*
(T-87000) (L-21801)
DE-14972 Tuberculous salpingitis 016.6 —614.2*
(T-88000) (L-21801)
DE-14980 Tuberculosis of skin, NOS 017.0
(T-01000) (L-21801)
Tuberculosis cutis 017.0
(T-01000) (L-21801)
Tuberculoderma 017.0
(T-01000) (L-21801)
DE-14981 Scrofuloderma 017.0
(T-01000) (L-21801)
Tuberculosis colliquativa 017.0
(T-01000) (L-21801)
DE-14982 Tuberculosis cutis indurativa 017.1
(T-01000) (F-C3000) (L-21801)
Tuberculous erythema induratum 017.1
(T-01000) (F-C3000) (L-21801)
Tuberculous Bazin's disease 017.1
(T-01000) (F-C3000) (L-21801)
DE-14983 Tuberculosis cutis lichenoides 017.0
(T-01000) (M-44200) (L-21801)
Lichen scrofulosorum 017.0
(T-01000) (M-44200) (L-21801)
DE-14984 Tuberculosis orificialis of mouth 017.0
(T-D1204) (L-21801)
DE-14985 Tuberculosis orificialis of anus 017.0
(T-D2701) (L-21801)
DE-14986 Tuberculous chancre 017.0
(T-01000) (M-40020) (L-21801)
DE-14987 Tuberculosis papulonecrotica 017.0
(T-01000) (M-44200) (L-21801)
Papulonecrotic tuberculid 017.0
(T-01000) (M-44200) (L-21801)
DE-14988 Tuberculosis verrucosa cutis 017.0
(T-01000) (L-21801)
DE-14989 Tuberculous chancriform pyoderma 017.0
(T-01000) (M-40020) (M-41602)
(L-21801)
DE-14991 Lupus vulgaris 017.0
(T-01000) (L-21801)
Lupus exedens 017.0
(T-01000) (L-21801)
Tuberculosis cutis luposa 017.0
(T-01000) (L-21801)
DE-14992 Tuberculous erythema nodosum 017.1
(T-01000) (F-C3000) (L-21801)
Tuberculosis with erythema nodosum and hypersensitivity reaction 017.1
(T-01000) (F-C3000) (L-21801)
DE-149A0 Tuberculosis of subcutaneous cellular tissue, NOS 017.0
(T-03000) (L-21801)
DE-149A1 Scrofula 017.2
(T-C4200) (M-41610) (L-21801)
Scrofulous abscess 017.2
(T-C4200) (M-41610) (L-21801)
DE-149A2 Tuberculous adenitis, NOS 017.2
(T-C4000) (M-40000) (L-21801)
DE-149A3 Tuberculosis of peripheral lymph nodes 017.2
(T-C4000) (L-21801)
DE-149A5 Cervical tuberculous lymphadenitis 017.2
(T-C4200) (L-21801)
DE-14A00 Tuberculosis of eye, NOS 017.3
(T-AA000) (L-21801)
DE-14A01 Tuberculous disseminated chorioretinitis 017.3 —363.1*
(T-AA310) (T-AA610) (L-21801)
DE-14A02 Tuberculous episcleritis 017.3 —379.0*
(T-AA110) (L-21801)
DE-14A03 Tuberculous interstitial keratitis 017.3 —370.5*
(T-AA200) (L-21801)
DE-14A04 Chronic tuberculous iridocyclitis 017.3 —364.1*
(T-AA400) (T-AA500) (L-21801)
DE-14A05 Tuberculous phlyctenular keratoconjunctivitis 017.3 —370.3*
(T-AA860) (T-AA200) (L-21801)

E-148-14B Tuberculosis — Continued

DE-14A10 Tuberculosis of the ear, NOS 017.4 —382.3*
(T-AB000) (L-21801)

DE-14A11 Tuberculous otitis media 017.4 —382.3*
(T-AB300) (L-21801)

DE-14A21 Tuberculosis of thyroid gland 017.5
(T-B6000) (L-21801)

DE-14A23 Tuberculosis of adrenal glands 017.6 —255.4*
(T-B3000) (L-21801) (DB-70620)
Tuberculous Addison's disease 017.6 —255.4*
(T-B3000) (L-21801) (DB-70620)

DE-14A25 Tuberculosis of spleen 017.7
(T-C3000) (L-21801)

DE-14A26 Tuberculosis of esophagus 017.8 —530.1*
(T-56000) (L-21801)

DE-14A27 Tuberculosis of endocardium 017.9 —424.-*
(T-32060) (L-21801)

DE-14A28 Tuberculosis of myocardium 017.9 —422.0*
(T-32020) (L-21801)

DE-14A29 Tuberculosis of pericardium 017.9 —422.0*
(T-39000) (L-21801)

DE-14A31 Tuberculoma of spinal cord 013.4
(T-A7010) (M-44700) (L-21801)
Tuberculous abscess of spinal cord 013.5
(T-A7010) (M-41610) (L-21801)

DE-14A33 Tuberculous encephalitis 013.6
(T-A0100) (L-21801)

DE-14A35 Other specified tuberculosis of the central nervous system 013.8
(T-A0090) (L-21801)

DE-14A40 Tuberculosis of other specified bone 015.7
(T-11...) (L-21801)

DE-14A41 Tuberculosis of bones of arm 015.5
(T-11000) (T-D8200) (L-21801)

DE-14A42 Tuberculosis of bones of lower extremity 015.5
(T-11000) (T-D9000) (L-21801)

DE-14A43 Tuberculosis of mastoid process 015.6 —383.1*
(T-11133) (L-21801)
Tuberculous mastoiditis 015.6 —383.1*
(T-11133) (L-21801)

DE-14A44 Tuberculosis of other urinary organs 016.3
(T-.....) (L-21801)

DE-14A45 Tuberculous cervicitis 016.7
(T-83200) (L-21801)

DE-14A46 Tuberculous endometritis 016.7
(T-83400) (L-21801)

DE-14A47 Tuberculosis of other female genital organs 016.7
(T-80000) (L-21801)

DE-14A50 Tuberculosis of other specified joint 015.8
(T-15...) (L-21801)
Tuberculous arthropathy 015.9 —711.4*
(T-15...) (L-21801)

DE-14A60 Primary tuberculosis, NOS 010.9
(L-21801)
Primary tuberculous infection, NOS 010.9
(L-21801)

DE-14A61 Primary tuberculous complex 010.0
(M-44700) (L-21801)
Ghon tubercle 010.0
(M-44700) (L-21801)
Ghon complex 010.0
(M-44700) (L-21801)

DE-14A62 Primary progressive tuberculosis with tuberculous pleurisy 010.1
(T-29000) (L-21801)

DE-14A63 Other primary progressive tuberculosis 010.8
(L-21801)

DE-14A70 Acute tuberculosis 018.8
(M-41000) (L-21801)

DE-14A71 Acute miliary tuberculosis 018.0
(M-41000) (L-21801)
Disseminated tuberculosis 018.0
(L-21801)
Generalized tuberculosis 018.0
(L-21801)
Tuberculosis miliaris disseminata 018.0
(L-21801)

DE-14A72 Tuberculous polyserositis 018.0
(T-1A110) (L-21801)

DE-14A73 Acute diffuse tuberculosis 018.8
(M-41000) (L-21801)

DE-14A78 Miliary tuberculosis, NOS 018.9
(L-21801)

DE-14A80 Chronic tuberculosis 018.8
(M-43000) (L-21801)

DE-14A81 Chronic miliary tuberculosis 018.8
(M-43000) (L-21801)

DE-14A82 Chronic granulomatous tuberculosis 018.8
(M-44000) (L-21801)
Miliary granuloma of tuberculosis 018.8
(M-44000) (L-21801)

DE-14A90 Reinfection tuberculosis 018.8
(L-21801)

DE-14A92 Inactive tuberculosis 018.8
(L-21801)

DE-14B00V Avian tuberculosis
(T-28000) (L-21815)
Infection due to Mycobacterium avium 031.0
(L-21815)

DE-14B10V Bovine tuberculosis
(L-21803)
Infection due to Mycobacterium bovis
(L-21803)

DE-14B12V Bovine tuberculous mastitis
(T-04000) (M-40000) (L-21803)

DE-14B20V Fish tuberculosis due to Mycobacterium piscium
(L-21871)

DE-14B21V Fish tuberculosis due Mycobacterium marinum
(L-21806)

DE-14B22V Fish tuberculosis due to Mycobacterium fortuitum
(L-21822)

DE-14B30V Reptilian tuberculosis due to Mycobacterium ulcerans
(L-21817)

DE-14B31V Reptilian tuberculosis due to Mycobacterium chelonei
(L-21823)

DE-14B32V Reptilian tuberculosis due to Mycobacterium thamnophis
(L-21872)

DE-14B50V Johne's disease
(L-21826)
Infection due to Mycobacterium paratuberculosis
(L-21826)
Paratuberculosis
(L-21826)

E-150 Tularemia

DE-15000 Tularemia, NOS 021.9
(L-1F201)
Infection by Francisella tularensis 021.9
(L-1F201)
Deer fly fever 021.9
(L-1F201)
Rabbit fever 021.9
(L-1F201)
Ohara's disease
(L-1F201)
Yatobyo
(L-1F201)
Pahvant Valley fever
Pahvant Valley plague

DE-15010 Ulceroglandular tularemia 021.0
(T-C4000) (T-01000) (M-38000) (L-1F201)

DE-15011 Glandular tularemia 021.8
(T-C4130) (L-1F201)

DE-15015 Oculoglandular tularemia 021.3
(T-AA860) (T-AA200) (T-C4130) (M-38000) (L-1F201)

DE-15020 Enteric tularemia 021.1
(T-50500) (L-1F201)
Cryptogenic tularemia 021.1
(T-50500) (L-1F201)
Intestinal tularemia 021.1
(T-50500) (L-1F201)
Typhoidal tularemia 021.1
(T-55000) (T-50500) (T-C4200) (L-1F201)
Oropharyngeal tularemia 021.1
(T-55000) (T-50500) (T-C4200) (L-1F201)

DE-15030 Pulmonary tularemia 021.2
(T-28000) (L-1F201)
Bronchopneumonic tularemia 021.2
(T-26000) (T-28000) (L-1F201)

DE-15040 Generalized tularemia 021.8
(T-D0010) (L-1F201)
Disseminated tularemia 021.8
(T-D0010) (L-1F201)

DE-15080 Other specified tularemia
(L-1F201)

E-151 Human Typhoid and Paratyphoid Fevers

DE-15100 Typhoid fever 002.0
(L-18122)
Infection by Salmonella typhi 002.0
(L-18122)

DE-15104 Pneumonia in typhoid fever 484.8
(T-28000) (M-40000)

DE-15150 Paratyphoid fever, NOS 002.9
(L-17100)

DE-15160 Paratyphoid A fever 002.1
(L-17201)

DE-15170 Paratyphoid B fever 002.2
(L-17309)

DE-15180 Paratyphoid C fever 002.3
(L-17517)

E-152 Ulcerative Balanoposthitis

DE-15200 Ulcerative balanoposthitis 099.8
(T-91300) (T-91330) (L-25900)
Erosive balanitis 099.8
(T-91300) (T-91330) (L-25900)
Balanoposthitis due to Treponema, NOS 099.8
(T-91300) (T-91330) (L-25900)

E-153 Campylobacterioses

DE-15300 Campylobacteriosis, NOS
(L-13500)

DE-15310 Infection by Campylobacter fetus
(L-13502)
Infection by Vibrio fetus
(L-13502)

DE-15320V Bovine genital campylobacteriosis
(L-13504)
Bovine vibriosis
(L-13504)

DE-15322V Ovine genital campylobacteriosis
(L-13505)
Vibrionic abortion
(L-13505)

DE-15324V Enteric campylobacteriosis
(L-13505)

DE-15326V Bovine winter dysentery
(L-13505)
Winter scours
(L-13505)

E-153 Campylobacterioses — Continued

DE-15330V Canine vibriosis
(L-13505)

DE-15350V Avian vibrionic hepatitis
(L-13505)
Avian infectious hepatitis
(L-13505)

DE-15360V Porcine intestinal adenomatosis
(L-13515)
Porcine proliferative enteritis
(L-13515)
Porcine terminal ileitis
(L-13515)
Proliferative hemorrhagic enteropathy
(L-13515)

DE-15362V Proliferative enteritis of hamsters
(L-13505)
Wet tail of hamsters
(L-13505)

E-154 Vincent's Angina

DE-15400 Vincent's angina 101.-
(T-54910) (M-41750) (L-25915)
(L-1F301)
Acute necrotizing ulcerative gingivitis 101.-
(T-54910) (M-41750) (L-25915)
(L-1F301)
Acute necrotizing ulcerative stomatitis 101.-
(T-51000) (M-41750) (L-25915)
(L-1F301)
Fusospirochaetal pharyngitis 101.-
(T-55000) (M-41750) (L-25915)
(L-1F301)
Spirochaetal stomatitis 101.-
(T-51000) (M-41750) (L-25915)
(L-1F301)
Trench mouth 101.-
(T-51000) (M-41750) (L-25915)
(L-1F301)
Vincent's gingivitis 101.-
(T-54910) (M-41750) (L-25915)
(L-1F301)
Fusospirochetosis 101.-
(T-54910) (M-41750) (L-25910)
(L-1F301)
ANUG 101.-
(T-54910) (M-47150) (L-25925)
(L-1F301)

E-155 Yaws

DE-15500 Yaws, NOS 102.9
(L-25924)
Frambesia 102.9
(L-25924)
Pian 102.9
(L-25924)
Buba 102.9
(L-25924)
Infection by Treponema pertenue 102.9
(L-25924)

DE-15510 Initial lesion of yaws 102.0
(L-25924)
Primary stage of yaws 102.0
(L-25924)
Mother yaw 102.0
(L-25924)

DE-15511 Chancre of yaws 102.0
(T-01000) (M-40020) (L-25924)

DE-15512 Primary frambesia 102.0
(T-01000) (M-40020) (L-25924)

DE-15513 Initial frambesial ulcer 102.0
(T-01000) (M-40020) (M-38000)
(L-25924)

DE-15520 Secondary lesion of yaws 102.1
(L-25924)
Secondary stage of yaws 102.1
(L-25924)

DE-15521 Multiple papillomata of yaws 102.1
(M-80500) (L-25924)

DE-15522 Wet crab yaws 102.1
(L-25924)

DE-15523 Butter yaws 102.1
(L-25924)

DE-15524 Frambesioma 102.1
(L-25924)
Pianoma 102.1
(L-25924)

DE-15525 Plantar papilloma of yaws 102.1
(T-D9740) (M-80500) (L-25924)

DE-15526 Palmar papilloma of yaws 102.1
(T-D8740) (M-80500) (L-25924)

DE-15530 Early yaws 102.2
(T-01000) (L-25924)

DE-15531 Frambeside of early yaws 102.2
(T-01000) (M-40020) (L-25924)

DE-15532 Cutaneous yaws (less than 5 years) 102.2
(T-01000) (L-25924)

DE-15533 Hyperkeratosis of yaws 102.3
(T-01000) (M-72600) (L-25924)

DE-15534 Palmar hyperkeratosis of yaws 102.3
(T-D8740) (M-72600) (L-25924)
Ghoul hand 102.3
(T-D8700) (L-25924)

DE-15535 Plantar hyperkeratosis of yaws 102.3
(T-D9740) (M-72600) (L-25924)
Worm-eaten soles 102.3
(T-D9740) (M-72600) (L-25924)

DE-15540 Tertiary lesion of yaws 102.4
(L-25924)
Tertiary stage of yaws 102.4
(L-25924)

DE-15541 Gummata of yaws 102.4
(M-44740) (L-25924)

DE-15542 Ulcers of yaws 102.4
(M-38000) (L-25924)

DE-15543 Nodular late yaws 102.4
(M-03010) (L-25924)

DE-15544 Gummatous frambeside 102.4
(M-44740) (L-25924)

DE-15545 Gangosa of yaws 102.5
(T-23000) (M-44740) (L-25924)
Rhinopharyngitis mutilans of yaws 102.5
(T-23000) (M-44740) (L-25924)

DE-15546 Mucosal yaws 102.7
(T-00400) (L-25924)

DE-15550 Yaws of bone 102.6
(T-11000) (L-25924)

DE-15551 Goundou of yaws 102.6
(T-21000) (L-25924)

DE-15552 Yaws gumma of bone 102.6
(T-11000) (M-44740) (L-25924)

DE-15553 Gummatous osteitis of yaws 102.6
(T-11000) (M-44740) (L-25294)

DE-15554 Gummatous periostitis of yaws 102.6
(T-11020) (M-44740) (L-25924)

DE-15555 Osteitis of yaws 102.6
(T-11000) (M-40000) (L-25924)

DE-15556 Periostitis of yaws 102.6
(T-11020) (M-40000) (L-25924)

DE-15557 Hypertrophic periostitis of yaws 102.6
(T-11020) (M-40000) (M-71000)
(L-25294)

DE-15570 Yaws of joint 102.6
(T-15...) (L-25924)

DE-15571 Ganglion of yaws 102.6
(T-15003) (M-33600) (L-25924)

DE-15572 Hydrarthrosis of yaws 102.6
(T-15000) (M-36700) (L-25924)

DE-15573 Juxta-articular nodules of yaws 102.7
(T-15000) (M-03010) (L-25924)

DE-15580 Latent yaws (+ sero.) 102.8
(L-25924)

E-156 Haemophilus Infections

DE-15600 Haemophilus infection, NOS
(L-1F700)

DE-15610 Haemophilus influenzae infection, NOS 041.5
(L-1F701)

DE-15611 Haemophilus influenzae epiglottitis 464.3
(T-24000) (L-1F701)

DE-15612 Haemophilus influenzae laryngotracheobronchitis 464.2
(T-24100) (T-25000) (T-26000)
(L-1F701)

DE-15613 Haemophilus influenzae pneumonia 482.2
(T-28000) (L-1F701)

DE-15614 Haemophilus influenzae otitis media 382.0
(T-AB300) (L-1F701)

DE-15615 Haemophilus influenzae meningitis 320.0
(T-A1110) (L-1F701)

DE-15616 Haemophilus influenzae septicemia 038.41
(T-C2000) (L-1F701)

DE-15617 Haemophilus influenzae laryngitis 464.0
(T-24100) (L-1F701)

DE-15618 Haemophilus influenzae arthritis 711.0
(T-15000) (M-40000) (L-1F701)

DE-15620V Avian infectious coryza
(L-1F707)
Fowl coryza
(L-1F707)

DE-15630V Thromboembolic meningoencephalitis
(L-1F716)
TEME
(L-1F716)
Haemophilosis
(L-1F716)
Haemophilus septicemia of cattle
(T-C2000) (L-1F716)

DE-15632V Haemophilus septicemia in lambs
(T-C2000) (L-1F711)

DE-15635V Glasser's disease
(L-1F704)
Porcine polyserositis
(L-1F704)
Infectious polyarthritis
(L-1F704)

DE-15640V Porcine contagious pleuropneumonia
(L-1F715)

DE-15644V Contagious equine metritis
(L-1F719)
CEM
(L-1F719)

DE-15650V Finrot
(L-1F718) (L-11000)

E-157 Legionella Infections

DE-15700 Legionella infection, NOS
(L-20400)

DE-15710 Legionnaire's disease 482.8
(L-20401)
Infection by Legionella pneumophilia 482.8
(L-20401)

DE-15716 Pittsburg pneumonia
(L-20402)

E-158 Mycoplasma Infections

DE-15800 Disease caused by Mycoplasma, NOS 041.8
(L-22000)
Infection by Mycoplasma, NOS 041.8
(L-22000)
Infection by the Eaton agent, NOS 041.8
(L-22000)
Infection by PPLO, NOS 041.8
(L-22000)
Mycoplasmosis, NOS
(L-22000)

DE-15810 Mycoplasma pneumonia 483.-
(T-28000) (L-22018)
Primary atypical pneumonia due to Mycoplasma pneumoniae 483.-
(T-28000) (L-22018)

E-158 Mycoplasma Infections — Continued

DE-15810 (cont.) PAP due to Mycoplasma pneumoniae 483.- (T-28000) (L-22018)
Endemic pneumonia (T-28000) (L-22018)
EP (T-28000) (L-22018)

DE-15820 Mycoplasma arthritis 711.9 (T-15000) (L-22024)
Arthritis by Mycoplasma arthritidis 711.9 (T-15000) (L-22024)

DE-15830V Chronic respiratory disease due to Mycoplasma gallisepticum (T-20000) (L-22006)
Mycoplasma gallisepticum infection (T-20000) (L-22006)
Infectious sinusitis due to Mycoplasma gallisepticum (T-20000) (L-22006)

DE-15831V Mycoplasma meleagridis infection (L-22023)

DE-15832V Avian infectious synovitis due to Mycoplasma synoviae (T-15003) (M-40000) (L-22009)

DE-15838V Contagious bovine pleuropneumonia (L-22002)

DE-15840V Contagious caprine pleuropneumonia (L-22003)

DE-15841V Enzootic pneumonia of calves (L-22005)

DE-15842V Mycoplasma mastitis (T-04000) (M-40000) (L-22501)

DE-15844V Bovine granular vulvovaginitis (L-22019)

DE-15846V Contagious agalactia of goat and sheep (L-22020)

DE-15848V Murine respiratory mycoplasmosis (L-22011)
Chronic murine pneumonia (L-22011)
Murine chronic respiratory disease (L-22011)

DE-15852V Murine mycoplasmal arthritis (L-22024)

DE-15854V Mycoplasmal arthritis and polyserositis in swine (L-22016) (L-22028)

DE-15856V Enzootic mycoplasmal pneumonia of swine (L-22017)

E-159 Ureaplasma Nongonococcal Urethritis

DE-15900 Nongonococcal urethritis due to Ureaplasma urealyticum 099.4 (T-75000) (L-26001) (DE-01600)
NGU due to ureaplasma urealyticum 099.4 (T-75000) (L-26001) (DE-01600)

E-189 Miscellaneous Bacterial Intestinal Infections

DE-18900 Bacterial enteritis, NOS 008.5 (T-50500) (L-10000)

DE-18920 Intestinal infection due to Arizona group 008.1 (T-50500) (L-17103)

DE-18930 Intestinal infection due to Enterobacter aerogenes 008.2 (T-50500) (L-15802)

DE-18940 Intestinal infection due to Proteus mirabilis 008.3 (T-50500) (L-16802)

DE-18950 Intestinal infection due to Morganella morganii 008.3 (T-50500) (L-16501)

DE-18960 Intestinal infection due to Pseudomonas 008.42 (T-50500) (L-23400)

DE-18980 Intestinal infection due to other organisms 008.- (T-50500) (L-.....)
Intestinal infection due to other specified bacteria 008.49 (T-50500) (L-.....)

E-190 Miscellaneous Bacterial Septicemias

DE-19000 Bacterial septicemia, NOS 038.9 (T-C2000) (L-10000)
Bacterial sepsis, NOS 038.9 (T-C2000) (L-10000)
Bacteremia, NOS 790.7 (T-C2000) (L-10000)

DE-19010 Gram positive septicemia 038.8 (T-C2000) (L-10017)

DE-19020 Gram negative septicemia 038.40 (T-C2000) (L-10024)

DE-19030 Anaerobic septicemia 038.3 (L-C2000) (L-10034)

DE-19050 Other gram-negative septicemia 038.49 (T-C2000) (L-10024)

DE-19051 Septicemia due to Pseudomonas 038.43 (T-C2000) (L-23400)

DE-19052 Septicemia due to Serratia 038.44 (T-C2000) (L-1E000)

DE-19054 Septicemia due to Bacteroides 038.3 (T-C2000) (L-12400)

DE-19055V Septicemia due to Chromobacterium (T-C2000) (L-13800)

E-191 Miscellaneous Bacterial Infections

DE-19100 Bacterial infection, NEC 041.- (L-10000)

DE-19110 Bacterial infection due to Klebsiella pneumoniae 041.3 (L-16001)
Bacterial infection due to Friedlander's bacillus 041.3 (L-16001)

DE-19111 Pneumonia due to Klebsiella pneumoniae 482.0
(T-28000) (M-40000) (L-16001)

DE-19130 Bacterial infection due to Serratia 041.8
(L-1E000)

DE-19140 Bacterial infection due to Aerobacter aerogenes 041.8
(L-15802)

DE-19150 Bacterial infection due to Pseudomonas 041.7
(L-23400)

DE-19151 Pneumonia due to Pseudomonas 482.1
(T-28000) (M-40000) (L-23400)

DE-19152 Arthritis due to Pseudomonas 711.0
(T-15000) (M-40000) (L-23400)

DE-19155V Infection due to Pseudomonas aeruginosa
(L-23401)

DE-19156V Pseudomonas aeruginosa mastitis
(T-04000) (L-23401)

DE-19157 Malignant otitis media 380.14
(L-23401)
Otitis media due to Pseudomonas aeruginosa 380.14
(L-23401)

DE-19160 Bacterial infection due to Proteus mirabilis 041.6
(L-16802)

DE-19161 Bacterial infection due to Morganella morganii 041.6
(L-16501)
Bacterial infection due to Proteus morganii 041.6
(L-16501)

DE-19162 Pneumonia due to Proteus mirabilis 482.8
(T-28000) (M-40000) (L-16802)

DE-19170V Tyzzer's disease
(L-12252)
Infection due to Bacillus piliformis
(L-12252)

DE-19174V Cold water disease
(L-26A10)
Peduncle disease
(L-26A10)

DE-19176V Columnaris disease
(L-26A21)

DE-19180V Bacterial osteomyelitis
(L-10000)

E-192 Escherichia Coli Infections

DE-19200 Infection due to Escherichia coli, NOS 041.4
(L-15602)
Bacterial infection due to E. coli, NOS 041.4
(L-15602)
Colibacillosis
(L-15602)

DE-19202 Septicemia due to E. Coli 038.42
(T-C2000) (L-15602)
Septicemic colibacillosis
(T-C2000) (L-15601)

DE-19204 Pneumonia due to E. coli 482.8
(T-28000) (M-40000) (L-15602)

DE-19206 Arthritis due to E. coli 711.0
(T-15000) (M-40000) (L-15602)
Coliform arthritis 711.0
(T-15000) (M-40000) (L-15602)

DE-19210 Intestinal infection due to E. coli 008.0
(T-50500) (L-15602)
Enteric colibacillosis
(L-15602)

DE-19214V Neonatal colibacillosis
(L-15602)
Neonatal diarrhea in ruminants
(L-15602)

DE-19216V Edema disease
(L-15602)
E. coli enterotoxemia
(L-15602)
Enterotoxemic colibacillosis
(L-15602)

DE-19218V Cerebrospinal angiopathy
(L-15602)

DE-19220V Coliform mastitis
(L-15601)

DE-19222V Mastitis-metritis-agalactia syndrome
(L-15601)
MMA
(L-15601)

DE-19230V Coligranuloma
(L-15601)
Hjarre's disease
(L-15601)

DE-19240 Acute hemorrhagic colitis due to E. coli 008.0
(T-59300) (M-41790) (L-15602)

E-198 Infections Due to Unclassified Bacteria

DE-19800 Cat scratch disease 078.3
(L-29010)
Cat scratch fever 078.3
(L-29010)
Benign inoculation lymphoreticulosis 078.3
(L-29010)

DE-19820 Whipple's disease 040.2
(L-10000)
Intestinal lipodystrophy 040.2
(L-10000)

SECTION E-2 RICKETTSIAL INFECTIONS

E-200 Rickettsial Infections: General Terms

DE-20000 Disease caused by Rickettsia, NOS 083.9
(L-2A000)
Rickettsial infectious disease, NOS 083.9
(L-2A000)

E-200 Rickettsial Infections: General Terms — Continued

DE-20000 (cont.) Rickettsial infection, NOS 083.9
(L-2A000)

E-210 Bartonellosis

DE-21000 Bartonellosis 088.0
(L-2A401)
Verruga peruana 088.0
(L-2A401)
Carrion's disease 088.0
(L-2A401)
Oroya fever 088.0
(L-2A401)
Infection by Bartonella bacilliformis 088.0
(L-2A401)

E-212-216 CHLAMYDIAL INFECTIONS

E-212 Inclusion Conjunctivitis

DE-21200 Inclusion conjunctivitis of the adult 077.0 —372.0*
(T-AA860) (L-2A901)
Inclusion blennorrhea 077.0 —372.0*
(T-AA860) (L-2A901)
Paratrachoma 077.0 —372.0*
(T-AA860) (L-2A901)
Swimming pool conjunctivitis 077.0 —372.0*
(T-AA860) (L-2A901)
Inclusion conjunctivitis due to Chlamydia trachomatis 077.0 —372.0*
(T-AA860) (L-2A901)
Chronic conjunctivitis due to Chlamydia trachomatis 077.0 —372.0*
(T-AA860) (L-2A901)

DE-21220 Neonatal inclusion blennorrhea 771.6
(T-AA860) (F-88000) (L-2A901)

E-213 Trachoma

DE-21300 Trachoma, NOS 076.9
(L-2A901)

DE-21310 Trachoma, initial stage 076.0
(L-2A901)
Trachoma dubium 076.0
(L-2A901)

DE-21320 Trachoma, active stage 076.1
(L-2A901)

DE-21321 Trachomatous granular conjunctivitis 076.1
(T-AA860) (M-43020) (L-2A901)

DE-21322 Trachomatous follicular conjunctivitis 076.1
(T-AA860) (M-43020) (L-2A901)

DE-21323 Trachomatous pannus 076.1
(T-AA860) (M-40110) (L-2A901)

DE-21369 Late effects of trachoma 139.1
(L-2A901)

E-214 Lymphogranuloma Venereum

DE-21400 Lymphogranuloma venereum 099.1
(L-2A901) (DE-01600)
Lymphogranuloma inguinale 099.1
(L-2A901) (DE-01600)
Esthiomene 099.1
(L-2A901) (DE-01600)
Climatic or tropical bubo 099.1
(L-2A901) (DE-01600)
Nicolas-Favre disease 099.1
(L-2A901) (DE-01600)
Durand-Nicolas-Favre disease 099.1
(L-2A901) (DE-01600)

E-215 Chlamydial Urethritis

DE-21500 Nongonococcal urethritis due to Chlamydia trachomatis 099.4
(T-75000) (L-2A901) (DE-01600)
NGU due to Chlamydia trachomatis 099.4
(T-75000) (L-2A901) (DE-01600)
Urethritis due to Chlamydia trachomatis 099.4
(T-75000) (L-2A901) (DE-01600)

DE-21510 Pelvic inflammation with female sterility due to Chlamydia trachomatis
(T-D6221) (M-40000) (G-C008)
(F-80520) (G-C001) (L-2A901)
PID with female sterility due to Chlamydia trachomatis
(T-D6221) (M-40000) (G-C008)
(F-80520) (G-C001) (L-2A901)

E-216 Chlamydia Psitacci Infections

DE-21600 Chlamydia psitacci infection, NOS
(L-2A902)
Chlamydiosis
(L-2A902)

DE-21610 Ornithosis 073.9
(L-2A902)
Psittacosis 073.9
(L-2A902)
Parrot fever 073.9
(L-2A902)
Parrot fever due to Chlamydia psitacci 073.9
(L-2A902)

DE-21611 Ornithosis with pneumonia 073.0
(T-28000) (M-40000) (L-2A902)
Louisiana pneumonia
(T-28000) (M-40000) (L-2A902)

DE-21612 Ornithosis with specified complication 073.7
(L-2A902)

DE-21618 Ornithosis with unspecified complication 073.8
(L-2A902)

DE-21620V Endemic abortion of ewes
(L-2A902)
Chlamydial abortion of ewes
(L-2A902)

DE-21622V Epidemic bovine abortion
(L-2A902)
Foothill abortion of cattle
(L-2A902)

DE-21624V Sporadic bovine encephalomyelitis
(L-2A902)
Bovine SBE
(L-2A902)
Buss disease
(L-2A902)

DE-21626V Feline pneumonitis
(L-2A902)

DE-21630V Chlamydial polyarthritis
(L-2A902)
Transmissible serositis
(L-2A902)

DE-21632V Inclusion conjunctivitis of guinea pig
(L-2A902)

DE-21634V Follicular conjunctivitis of sheep
(L-2A902)

DE-21636V Chlamydial pneumonitis in all species except pig
(L-2A902)

DE-21640V Epizootic chlamydiosis
(L-2A902)

E-217 Q Fever

DE-21700 Q fever 083.0
(L-2A301)
Infection due to Coxiella burnetii 083.0
(L-2A301)

DE-21704 Pneumonia in Q fever 484.8
(T-28000) (M-40000)

E-218 Rickettsialpox

DE-21800 Rickettsialpox 083.2
(L-2A007)
Vesicular rickettsiosis 083.2
(L-2A007)
Rickettsialpox due to Rickettsia akari 083.2
(L-2A007)

E-219 Trench Fever

DE-21900 Trench fever 083.1
(L-2A201)
Quintan fever 083.1
(L-2A201)
Wolhynian fever 083.1
(L-2A201)
Fever due to Rochalimaea quintana 083.1
(L-2A201)

E-220 Typhus

DE-22000 Typhus, NOS 081.9
(L-2A001) (L-60007)

DE-22010 Louse-borne typhus 080.-
(L-2A001) (L-60007)
Epidemic typhus 080.-
(L-2A001) (L-60007)
Classical typhus 080.-
(L-2A001) (L-60007)
Typhus due to Rickettsia prowazekii 080.-
(L-2A001) (L-60007)
Exanthematic typhus, NOS 080.-
(L-2A001) (L-60007)

DE-22020 Murine typhus 081.0
(L-2A002) (L-60025)
Endemic typhus 081.0
(L-2A002) (L-60025)
Flea-borne typhus 081.0
(L-2A002) (L-60025)
Typhus due to Rickettsia typhi 081.0
(L-2A002) (L-60025)

DE-22030 Brill-Zinsser disease 081.1
(L-2A001) (L-60007)
Recrudescent typhus fever 081.1
(L-2A001) (L-60007)
Recrudescent typhus due to Rickettsia prowazekii 081.1
(L-2A001) (L-60007)
Brill's disease 081.1
(L-2A001) (L-60007)

DE-22040 Scrub typhus 081.2
(L-2A010) (L-60054)
Tsutsugamushi disease 081.2
(L-2A010) (L-60054)
Mite-borne typhus 081.2
(L-2A010) (L-60054)
Japanese river fever 081.2
(L-2A010) (L-60054)
Kedani fever 081.2
(L-2A010) (L-60054)
Mite-borne typhus due to Rickettsia tsutsugamushi 081.2
(L-2A010) (L-60054)

DE-22080 Tick-borne rickettsiosis, NOS 082.9
(L-2A000) (L-60052)
Tick-borne typhus, NOS 082.9
(L-2A000) (L-60052)

E-221 Rocky Mountain Spotted Fever

DE-22100 Rocky mountain spotted fever 082.0
(L-2A003) (L-66000)
Spotted fever due to Rickttsia rickettsii 082.0
(L-2A003) (L-66000)
Rocky mountain tick fever
(L-2A003)

E-221 Rocky Mountain Spotted Fever — Continued

DE-22110 Sao Paulo fever 082.0
(L-2A003) (L-66000)

E-222 Boutonneuse Fever

DE-22200 Boutonneuse fever 082.1
(L-2A005) (L-60052)
African tick-borne fever 082.1
(L-2A005) (L-60052)
African tick typhus 082.1
(L-2A005) (L-60052)
Marseilles fever 082.1
(L-2A005) (L-60052)
Kenya tick typhus 082.1
(L-2A005) (L-60052)
India tick fever 082.1
(L-2A005) (L-60052)
Mediterranean tick fever 082.1
(L-2A005) (L-60052)
Tick typhus due to Rickettsia conorii 082.1
(L-2A005) (L-60052)

E-223 North Asian Tick Fever

DE-22300 North Asian tick fever 082.2
(L-2A004) (L-60052)
Siberian tick typhus 082.2
(L-2A004) (L-60052)
Tick fever due to Rickettsia siberica 082.2
(L-2A004) (L-60052)

E-224 Queensland Tick Typhus

DE-22400 Queensland tick typhus 082.3
(L-2A006) (L-60052)
Tick typhus due to Rickettsia australis 082.3
(L-2A006) (L-60052)

E-225 Neorickettsioses

DE-22500V Neorickettsiosis, NOS
(L-2A800)

DE-22501V Salmon poisoning disease
(L-2A801) (L-59A21) (L-72811)
Canine neorickettsiosis
(L-2A801) (L-59A21) (L-72811)

DE-22508V Elokomin fluke fever
(L-2A802) (L-59A21) (L-72811)

E-226 Cowdrioses

DE-22610V Heartwater
(L-2A701) (L-66200)
Cowdriosis
(L-2A701) (L-66200)

E-227 Ehrlichioses

DE-22700V Ehrlichiosis, NOS
(L-2A600)

DE-22705V Tick-borne fever
(L-2A602) (L-66004)

DE-22710V Canine ehrlichiosis
(L-2A601) (L-66131)
Canine rickettsiosis
(L-2A601) (L-66131)
Tropical canine pancytopenia
(L-2A601) (L-66131)
Canine hemorrhagic fever
(L-2A601) (L-66131)
Tracker dog disease
(L-2A601) (L-66131)
Canine tick typhus
(L-2A601) (L-66131)
Nairobi bleeding disease
(L-2A601) (L-66131)
Lahore canine fever
(L-2A601) (L-66131)

DE-22712V Canine infectious cyclic thrombocytopenia
(L-2A606)

DE-22720V Equine ehrlichiosis
(L-2A603)

DE-22722V Potomac horse fever
(L-2A605)
Acute equine diarrhea syndrome
(L-2A605)
Equine monocytic ehrlichiosis
(L-2A605)

DE-22730V Bovine ehrlichiosis
(L-2A607) (L-66170)
Benign bovine rickettsiosis
(L-2A607) (L-66170)
Mild disease of cattle
(L-2A607) (L-66170)

DE-22734V Bovine petechial fever
(L-2A609)
Ondiri disease
(L-2A609)

DE-22740V Ovine ehrlichiosis
(L-2A608) (L-66136)
Benign ovine rickettsiosis
(L-2A608) (L-66136)
Mild disease of sheep
(L-2A608) (L-66136)

DE-22750V Jembrana disease
(L-2A600) (L-66234)

E-228 Grahamelloses

DE-22800V Grahamellosis, NOS
(L-2A500)

DE-22810V Infection by Grahamella peromysci
(L-2A501)

DE-22820V Infection by Grahamella talpae
(L-2A502)

E-229 Anaplasmoses

DE-22900V Anaplasmosis, NOS
(L-2B001)
Gallsickness
(L-2B001)

E-22A Haemobartonelloses

DE-22A00V Haemobartonellosis, NOS
(L-2B200)

DE-22A10V Feline infectious anemia
(L-2B201)
Feline haemobartonellosis
(L-2B201)

E-22B Eperythrozoonosis

DE-22B00V Eperythrozoonosis, NOS
(L-2B300)

SECTION E-3 VIRAL DISEASES

E-300 Viral Diseases: General Terms

DE-30000 Viral disease, NOS
(L-30000)
Disease caused by virus, NOS 079.9
(L-30000)
Viral infectious disease, NOS 079.9
(L-30000)
Viral illness, NOS 079.9
(L-30000)
Viral infection, NOS 079.9
(L-30000)

DE-30008 Viral disease in mother complicating pregnancy, childbirth or puerperium 647.6

DE-30010 Viremia, NOS 790.8
(T-C2000) (L-30000)
Viral sepsis 790.8
(T-C2000) (L-30000)

DE-30015 Viral pneumonia, NOS 480.9
(T-28000) (M-40000) (L-30000)

DE-30016 Viral myocarditis, NOS 079.9 —422.91
(T-32020) (L-30000)

DE-30017 Viral pericarditis, NOS 079.9 —420.91
(T-39000) (L-30000)

DE-30018 Acute viral pericarditis 079.9 —420.91
(T-39000) (M-41000) (L-30000)

DE-30020 Viral meningitis NOS 047.9 —321.7*
(T-A1110) (M-40000) (L-30000)
Aseptic meningitis 047.9 —321.7*
(T-A1110) (M-40000) (L-30000)
Abacterial meningitis 047.9 —321.7*
(T-A1110) (M-40000) (L-30000)
Viral meningitis, NEC 047.8
(T-A1110) (M-40000) (L-30000)

DE-30021 Viral encephalitis, NOS 049.9 —323.4*
(T-A0100) (M-40000) (L-30000)

DE-30023 Viral bronchitis, NOS 466.0
(T-26000) (M-40000) (L-30000)

DE-30024 Viral epiglottitis, NOS 464.3
(T-24000) (M-40000) (L-30000)

DE-30025 Viral pharyngitis, NOS 462.-
(T-55000) (M-40000) (L-30000)

DE-30026 Viral tonsillitis, NOS 463.-
(T-C5100) (M-40000) (L-30000)

DE-30027 Viral tracheitis, NOS 464.1
(T-25000) (M-40000) (L-30000)

DE-30028 Viral conjunctivitis, NOS 077.9 —372.0*
(T-AA860) (M-40000) (L-30000)

DE-30029 Viral labyrinthitis, NOS 386.35
(T-AB700) (L-30000)
Viral otitis interna, NOS 386.35
(T-AB700) (L-30000)

DE-30030 Viral enteritis, NOS 008.8
(T-50500) (M-40000) (L-30000)

DE-30032 Nonbacterial gastroenteritis 008.8
(T-50100) (M-40000) (L-30000)
Viral gastroenteritis 008.8
(T-50100) (M-40000) (L-30000)
Acute infectious nonbacterial gastroenteritis 008.8
(T-50100) (M-40000) (L-30000)

DE-30038 Viral gastroenteritis due to other viral agents 008.6
(T-50100) (M-40000) (L-30000)

DE-30040 Viral exanthem 057.9
(T-01000) (M-01710) (L-30000)
Viral exanthemata 057.9
(T-01000) (M-01710) (L-30000)

DE-30050 Non-arthropod-borne viral disease, NOS 079.9
(L-30000)

DE-30051 Non-arthropod-borne viral disease of the central nervous system, NOS 049.9
(T-A0090) (L-30000)

DE-30060 Arbovirus infection, NOS 066.9
(L-60000) (L-32200)
Arthropod-borne viral infection 066.9
(L-60000) (L-32200)

DE-30061 Arbovirus encephalitis, NOS 064.-
(T-A0100) (L-60000) (L-32200)
Arthropod-borne viral encephalitis, vector unknown 064.-
(T-A0100) (L-60000) (L-32200)

DE-30065 Arbovirus hemorrhagic fever, NOS 065.9
(L-60000) (L-32200)
Arthropod-borne hemorrhagic fever, NOS 065.9
(L-60000) (L-32200)

DE-30070 Other tick-borne hemorrhagic fever 065.3
(L-60052)

DE-30071 Mosquito-borne hemorrhagic fever 065.4
(L-32200) (L-60008)

DE-30072 Other specified arthropod-borne hemorrhagic fever 065.8
(L-60000) (L-.....)

DE-30073 Tick-borne viral encephalitis, NOS 063.9 —323.3*
(T-A0100) (L-60052) (L-30000)
Other tick-borne viral encephalitis 063.8 —323.3*
(T-A0100) (L-60052) (L-30000)

E-300 Viral Diseases: General Terms — Continued

DE-30074 Mosquito-borne viral encephalitis, NOS 062.9 —323.3*
(T-A0100) (L-60008) (L-30000)
Other mosquito-borne viral encephalitis 062.8 —323.3*
(T-A0100) (L-60008) (L-30000)

E-310 Diseases Due to Adenoviridae

DE-31000 Disease due to Adenovirus, NOS 079.0
(L-35800)
Adenovirus infection, NOS 079.0
(L-35800)

DE-31010 Adenoviral respiratory disease 480.0
(T-20000) (L-35800)
Respiratory disease due to Adenovirus 480.0
(T-20000) (L-35800)

DE-31011 Adenoviral pharyngitis 462.-
(T-55000) (L-35800)

DE-31012 Adenoviral bronchitis 466.0
(T-26000) (L-35800)

DE-31013 Adenoviral laryngotracheobronchitis 466.0
(T-24100) (T-25000) (T-26000) (L-35800)

DE-31014 Adenoviral bronchiolitis 466.1
(T-27000) (L-35800)

DE-31015 Adenoviral bronchopneumonia 480.0
(T-26000) (T-28000) (L-35800)

DE-31016 Adenoviral pneumonia 480.0
(T-28000) (L-35800)

DE-31030 Adenoviral pharyngoconjunctivitis 077.2 —372.0*
(T-55000) (T-AA860) (L-35823) (L-35827)
Pharyngoconjunctival fever 077.2 —372.0*
(T-55000) (T-AA860) (L-35823) (L-35827)

DE-31031 Acute adenoviral follicular conjunctivitis 077.3 —372.0*
(T-AA860) (M-43020) (L-35828)

DE-31032 Epidemic keratoconjunctivitis 077.1 —370.4*
(T-AA200) (T-AA860) (L-35828)
Shipyard eye 077.1 —370.4*
(T-AA200) (T-AA860) (L-35828)

DE-31060 Adenoviral encephalitis, NOS 049.8 —323.4*
(T-A0100) (L-35800)

DE-31061 Acute adenoviral encephalitis
(T-A0100) (M-41000) (L-35827)

DE-31062 Acute adenoviral meningoencephalitis 049.8 —323.4*
(T-A0100) (T-A1112) (M-41000) (L-35827)

DE-31063 Adenoviral meningitis 049.1 —321.7*
(T-A1110) (L-35800)

DE-31064 Subacute adenoviral encephalitis 049.8 —323.4*
(T-A0100) (M-42000) (L-35827) (L-35852)
Slow virus infection 049.8 —323.4*
(T-A0100) (M-42000) (L-35827) (L-35852)

DE-31065 Adenoviral enteritis 008.6
(T-50500) (L-35800)

DE-31068 Adenoviral myocarditis 079.0 —422.91*
(T-32020) (L-35800)

DE-31070V Avian inclusion body hepatitis
(L-36100)
Chicken hemorrhagic syndrome
(L-36100)

DE-31071V Turkey hemorrhagic enteritis
(L-36100)

DE-31072V Avian hemorrhagic enteritis
(L-36100)

DE-31074V Marble spleen disease
(L-36100)

DE-31076V Egg drop syndrome
(L-36100)

DE-31078V Quail bronchitis
(L-36100)

DE-31080V Infectious canine hepatitis
(L-36021)
ICH
(L-36021)
Hepatitis contagiosa canis
(L-36021)
Canine adenovirus infection
(L-36021)

DE-31082V Infectious canine tracheobronchitis
(L-36022)
Kennel cough
(L-36022)

DE-31084V Bovine adenovirus infection
(L-35900)

DE-31086V Murine adenovirus infection
(L-36019)

DE-31088V Equine adenovirus infection
(L-36016)

DE-31090V Porcine adenovirus infection
(L-36000)

DE-31092V Ovine adenovirus infection
(L-36010)

DE-31094V Caprine adenovirus infection
(L-36018)

DE-31096V Simian adenovirus infection
(L-35870)

E-314-31A DISEASES DUE TO POXVIRIDAE

E-314 Diseases Due to Orthopoxviridae

DE-31400 Disease due to orthopoxviridae, NOS
(L-37500)
DE-31410 Monkeypox 057.-
(L-37506)
Human monkeypox 057.-
(L-37506)
DE-31420 Vaccinia, NOS 999.0
(L-37501)
DE-31421 Progressive vaccina 051.-
(L-37501)
Vaccina gangrenosa 051.-
(L-37501)
DE-31422 Generalized vaccinia 999.0
(L-37501)
DE-31423 Eczema vaccinatum 999.0
(T-01000) (L-37501)
Kaposi's varicelliform eruption due to vaccinia virus 999.0
(T-01000) (L-37501)
DE-31428 Postvaccinal encephalomyelitis 325.5
(T-A0100) (T-A7010) (P.-.....) (L-37501)
DE-31430 Cowpox 051.0
(L-37504)
DE-31440 Smallpox, NOS 050.9
(T-01000) (M-01710) (L-37508)
Variola, NOS 050.9
(T-01000) (M-01710) (L-37508)
DE-31441 Variola major 050.0
(T-01000) (M-01710) (L-37508)
Classical smallpox 050.0
(T-01000) (M-01710) (L-37508)
DE-31442 Hemorrhagic smallpox 050.0
(T-01000) (M-01710) (L-37508)
Purpura variolosa 050.0
(T-01000) (M-01710) (L-37508)
Malignant smallpox 050.0
(T-01000) (L-01710) (L-37508)
DE-31447 Flat-type smallpox 050.0
(T-01000) (M-01710) (L-37508)
DE-31448 Smallpox without rash 050.-
(T-01000) (L-37508)
DE-31450 Alastrim 050.1
(L-37508)
Variola minor 050.1
(L-37508)
DE-31451 Modified smallpox 050.2
(L-37508)
DE-31456V Mousepox
(L-37505)
Infectious ectromelia
(L-37505)
DE-31458V Catpox
(L-37504)
DE-31463V Buffalopox
(L-37502)
DE-31464V Camelpox
(L-37503)
DE-31466V Horsepox
(L-37504)
DE-31467V Rabbitpox
(L-37507)

E-315 Diseases Due to Parapoxviridae

DE-31500 Disease due to Parapoxviridae, NOS 051.9
(L-37400)
DE-31510 Pseudocowpox 051.1
(L-37604)
Paravaccina 051.9
(L-37604)
Milker's node 051.1
(L-37604)
DE-31530 Orf virus disease 051.2
(L-37601)
Contagious pustular dermatitis 051.2
(L-37601)
Orf 051.2
(L-37601)
Contagious ovine ecthymaa
(L-37601)
DE-31532V Bovine papular stomatitis
(L-37602)
DE-31534V Chamois contagious ecthyma
(L-37603)
DE-31536V Sealionpox
(L-37605)
Sealpox
(L-37605)
DE-31542V Uasin gishu disease
(L-37400)
DE-31544V Viral papular dermatitis
(L-37400)

E-316 Diseases Due to Capripoxviridae

DE-31600V Disease due to Capripoxviridae, NOS
(L-37800)
DE-31610V Sheeppox
(L-37801)
DE-31620V Goatpox
(L-37802)
DE-31630V Lumpy skin disease
(L-37803)
DE-31640V Ulcerative dermatosis of sheep
(L-37804)
Ovine balanoposthitis
(L-37804)
Lip and leg ulceration
(L-37804)
Contagious venereal infection
(L-37804)

E-316 Diseases Due to Capripoxviridae — Continued

DE-31640V (cont.) Pisgoed (L-37804)

E-317 Diseases Due to Avipoxviridae

DE-31700V Disease due to Avipoxviridae, NOS (L-37700)

DE-31710V Fowlpox (L-37701)

DE-31712V Canarypox (L-37702)

DE-31714V Parrotpox (L-37711)

DE-31716V Sparrowpox (L-37706)

DE-31718V Starlingpox (L-37707)

DE-31722V Pigeonpox (L-37704)

DE-31724V Turkeypox (L-37708)

DE-31726V Juncopox (L-37703)

DE-31728V Quailpox (L-37703)

E-318 Diseases Due to Leporipoxviridae

DE-31800V Disease due to Leporipoxviridae, NOS (L-37900)

DE-31810V Infectious myxomatosis of rabbit (L-37901)

DE-31820V Shope fibroma (T-01000) (M-88100) (L-37903)
  Rabbit fibroma (T-01000) (M-88100) (L-37903)

DE-31822V Hare fibroma (T-01000) (M-88100) (L-37902)

DE-31824V Squirrel fibroma (T-01000) (M-88100) (L-37904)

E-319 Diseases Due to Suipoxviridae

DE-31900V Disease due to Suipoxviridae, NOS (L-38000)

DE-31910V Swinepox (L-38001)

E-31A Diseases Due to Unassigned Poxviridae

DE-31A00 Disease due to unassigned Poxviridae, NOS
  Poxvirus infection, NOS 079.8 (L-37400)

DE-31A10 Molluscum contagiosum infection 078.0 (T-01000) (M-76660) (L-38503)

DE-31A20 Tanapox 078.89 (L-38505)

DE-31A30 Yabapox 078.89 (L-38506)

DE-31A40V Elephantpox (L-38502)

DE-31A42V Raccoonpox (L-38504)

E-320-327 Diseases Due to Herpesviridae

DE-32000 Herpesvirus infection, NOS 054.9 (L-36200)
  Herpes infection, NOS 054.9 (L-36200)

DE-32010V Herpesvirus T infection (L-36200)
  Herpesvirus tamarinus infection (L-36200)
  Herpesvirus platyrrhinae infection (L-36200)

DE-32040V Marek's disease (L-36200)
  Neurolymphomatosis gallinarum (L-36200)

DE-32042V Pacheco's disease (L-36200)

E-321-324 Diseases Due to Alphaherpesvirinae

DE-32100 Disease due to Alphaherpesvirinae, NOS (L-36200)
  Alphaherpesviral disease, NOS (L-36200)

DE-32110 Herpes simplex, NOS 054.9 (L-36210)
  Herpes simplex without mention of complication 054.9 (L-36210)

DE-32111 Primary herpes simplex 054.9 (L-36210)

DE-32112 Recurrent herpes simplex 054.9 (L-36210)

DE-32113 Disseminated herpes simplex 054.5 (L-36210)

DE-32114 Herpes simplex septicemia 054.5 (T-C2000) (L-36210)
  Herpetic septicemia 054.5 (T-C2000) (L-36210)

DE-32115 Congenital herpes simplex 771.2 (F-88000) (L-36210) (DE-01900)
  Neonatal herpes simplex 771.2 (F-88000) (L-36210) (DE-01900)

DE-32120 Genital herpes simplex, NOS 054.10 (T-70260) (L-36210)

DE-32121 Herpetic vulvovaginitis 054.11 —616.1* (T-81000) (T-82000) (M-38000) (L-36210)

DE-32122 Herpetic ulceration of vulva 054.12 —616.1*
(T-81000) (M-38000) (L-36210)

DE-32127 Herpetic infection of penis 054.13
(T-91000) (L-36210)

DE-32131 Herpetic gingivostomatitis 054.2
(T-51000) (T-54910) (L-36210)

DE-32132 Herpes labialis 054.2
(T-52000) (L-36210)
Cold sores 054.2
(T-52000) (L-36210)
Fever blister 054.2
(T-52000) (L-36210)

DE-32141 Herpes encephalitis 054.3 —323.4*
(T-A0100) (L-36210)

DE-32142 Herpetic meningoencephalitis 054.3 —323.4*
(T-A1110) (T-A0100) (L-36210)

DE-32143 Herpes simplex meningitis 054.72 —321.4*
(T-A1110) (L-36210)

DE-32144 Herpetic acute necrotizing encephalitis 054.3 —323.4*
(T-A0100) (M-41700) (L-36210)

DE-32150 Herpes with ophthalmic complications 054.40
(T-AA000) (L-36210)

DE-32151 Herpes simplex dermatitis of eyelid 054.41 —373.5*
(T-AA810) (L-36210)
Herpesviral blepharitis 054.41 —373.5*
(T-AA810) (L-36210)

DE-32152 Herpes simplex keratitis 054.42 —370.4*
(T-AA200) (L-36210)

DE-32153 Herpes simplex keratoconjunctivitis 054.49 —370.4*
(T-AA200) (T-AA860) (L-36210)

DE-32154 Herpes simplex iritis 054.49 —364.0*
(T-AA500) (L-36210)

DE-32155 Herpes simplex dendritic keratitis 054.42 —370.2*
(T-AA200) (M-38190) (L-36210)

DE-32156 Herpes simplex disciform keratitis 054.43 —370.5*
(T-AA200) (M-38190) (L-36210)

DE-32157 Herpes simplex iridocyclitis 054.44
(T-AA400) (T-AA500) (L-36210)

DE-32160 Herpes simplex with other specified complications 054.79
(L-36210)

DE-32161 Herpes simplex otitis externa 054.73
(T-AB100) (L-36210)

DE-32162 Herpetic whitlow 054.6
(T-D8800) (L-36210)
Herpetic felon 054.6
(T-D8800) (L-36210)

DE-32165 Visceral herpes simplex 054.71
(T-D4030) (L-36210)

DE-32181 Eczema herpeticum 054.0
(T-01000) (L-36210)
Kaposi's varicelliform eruption due to herpes simplex virus 054.0
(T-01000) (L-36210)

DE-32190 Herpes simplex with unspecified complications 054.8
(L-36210)

DE-321A0V Duck viral enteritis
(L-36310)
Duck plague
(L-36310)

DE-321A2V Infectious avian laryngotracheitis
(L-36310)

DE-321B0V Lucke frog kidney carcinoma
(T-71000) (M-83123) (L-B1B06) (L-36210)
Renal adenocarcinoma in Rana pipiens
(T-71000) (M-83123) (L-B1B06) (L-36210)

DE-32200V Cercopithecus herpesvirus 1 disease
(L-36402)

DE-32210 Simian B disease 054.3
(L-36214)
Herpesvirus B infection 054.3
(L-36214)

DE-32211 Simian B encephalomyelitis 054.3
(T-A0100) (T-A7010) (L-36214)

DE-32214V Pigeon herpesvirus infection
(L-36200)

DE-32220V Herpesvirus disease of salmonids
(L-36200)

DE-32222V Herpesvirus disease of turbot
(L-36200)

DE-32224V Channel catfish virus disease
(L-36200)

DE-32226V Pseudorabies
(L-35301)
Aujesky's disease
(L-36301)
Infectious bulbar paralysis
(L-36301)
Mad itch
(L-36301)

DE-32228V Infectious bovine rhinotracheitis
(L-36220)
IBR
(L-36220)
Rednose
(L-36220)

DE-32230V Infectious pustular vulvovaginitis
(L-36220)
IPV
(L-36220)

DE-32232V Malignant catarrhal fever
(L-36230)
MCF
(L-36230)

E-321-324 Diseases Due to Alphaherpesvirinae — Continued

DE-32232V (cont.) Malignant head catarrh
(L-36230)
Snotsiekte
(L-36230)

DE-32234V Equine viral rhinopneumonitis
(L-36302)
EVR
(L-36302)
Equine virus abortion
(L-36302)
Equine herpesvirus 1 infection
(L-36302)

DE-32236V Feline viral rhinotracheitis
(L-36404)
FVR
(L-36404)

DE-32238V Equine coital exanthema
(L-36403)

DE-32240V Canine herpesvirus infection
(L-36406)

DE-32242V Bovine ulcerative mammillitis
(L-36221)
Bovine herpes mammillitis
(L-36221)
Pseudo-lumpy skin disease
(L-36221)

DE-32300 Varicella, NOS 052.9
(L-36401)
Chickenpox, NOS 052.9
(L-36401)

DE-32310 Postvaricella encephalitis 052.0
(T-A0100) (L-36401)
Postchickenpox encephalitis 052.0 —323.4*
(T-A0100) (L-36401)

DE-32320 Hemorrhagic varicella pneumonitis 052.1
(T-28000) (M-40000) (L-36401)

DE-32380 Chickenpox with other specified complications 052.7
(L-36401)

DE-32381 Acute cerebellar ataxia due to varicella 052.0 —334.3*
(T-A6000) (F-A4580) (L-36401)

DE-32390 Chickenpox with unspecified complication 052.8
(L-36401)

DE-32400 Herpes zoster, NOS 053.9
(L-36401)
Shingles 053.9
(L-36401)
Zona 053.9
(L-36401)
Herpes zoster without mention of complication 053.9
(L-36401)

DE-32405 Disseminated herpes zoster 053.7
(L-36401)

DE-32410 Herpes zoster ophthalmicus 053.29
(T-A8190) (L-36401)
Herpes zoster with ophthalmic complications 053.29
(T-A8190) (L-36401)
Zoster ocular disease 053.29
(T-A8190) (L-36401)

DE-32411 Herpes zoster dermatitis of eyelids 053.20 —375.5*
(T-AA810) (L-36401)

DE-32412 Herpes zoster iridocyclitis 053.22 —364.0*
(T-AA500) (T-AA400) (L-36401)

DE-32413 Herpes zoster keratoconjunctivitis 053.21 —370.4*
(T-AA200) (T-AA860) (L-36401)

DE-32430 Herpes zoster auricularis 053.11 —351.1*
(T-A8450) (L-36401)
Geniculate herpes zoster 053.11 —351.1*
(T-A8450) (L-36401)
Herpetic geniculate ganglionitis 053.11 —351.1*
(T-A8450) (L-36401)
Herpes zoster oticus 053.11 —351.1*
(T-A8450) (L-36401)

DE-32431 Post-herpetic polyneuropathy 053.13 —357.4*
(T-A0500) (L-36401)

DE-32432 Post-herpetic trigeminal neuralgia 053.12 —350.0*
(T-A8150) (L-36401)

DE-32438 Otitis externa due to Herpes zoster 053.71
(T-AB100) (L-36401)

DE-32450 Herpes zoster with other nervous system complications 053.10
(T-A0000) (L-36401)

DE-32451 Herpes zoster with meningitis 053.0 —321.3*
(T-A1110) (L-36401)

DE-32480 Herpes zoster with other complications 053.79
(L-36401)

DE-32490 Herpes zoster with unspecified complications 053.8
(L-36401)

E-326 Diseases Due to Betaherpesvirinae

DE-32600 Disease due to Betaherpesvirinae, NOS
(L-36500)

DE-32610 Cytomegalovirus infection, NOS 078.5
(L-36500)
Cytomegalic inclusion disease 078.5
(L-36500)
Salivary gland virus disease 078.5
(L-36500)

DE-32621 Congenital cytomegalovirus infection 771.1
(L-36500) (DE-01900)
Neonatal cytomegaloviral disease 771.1
(L-36500) (DE-01900)

DE-32631 Cytomegalic inclusion virus hepatitis 078.5 —573.1*
(T-62000) (L-36500)

DE-32641 Cytomegaloviral pneumonia 078.5 —484.1*
(T-28000) (L-36500)
Cytomegalic inclusion virus pneumonia 078.5 —484.1*
(T-28000) (L-36500)

DE-32651 Cytomegaloviral mononucleosis 075.-
(L-36500)

DE-32660V Inclusion body rhinitis of swine
(L-36500)

E-327 Diseases Due to Gammaherpesvirinae

DE-32700 Disease due to Gammaherpesvirinae, NOS
(L-36800)

DE-32710 Gammaherpesviral mononucleosis 075.-
(T-C4000) (M-71000) (L-36901)
Infectious mononucleosis 075.-
(T-C4000) (M-71000) (L-36901)
Glandular fever 075.-
(T-C4000) (M-71000) (L-36901)
Pfeiffer's disease 075.-
(T-C4000) (M-71000) (L-36901)
Monocytic angina 075.-
(T-C4000) (M-71000) (L-36901)

DE-32712 Infectious mononucleosis hepatitis 075.- —573.1*
(T-62000) (T-C4000) (M-71000) (L-36901)

DE-32720V Herpesvirus saimiri infection
(L-37101)

DE-32730V African swine fever
(L-37201)
ASF
(L-37201)
Wart hog disease
(L-37201)

DE-32740V Lymphocystis disease
(L-37301)

E-32A Diseases Due to Papovaviridae

DE-32A00 Disease due to Papilloma virus, NOS 078.1
(L-35600)

DE-32A10 Papovavirus infection subgroup A, NOS 078.1
(M-76600) (L-35620)
Human papilloma virus infection, NOS 078.1
(M-76600) (L-35620)
Viral warts due to papilloma virus 078.1
(M-76600) (L-35620)
Viral warts, NOS 078.1
(M-76600) (L-35620)
Infectious warts 078.1
(M-76600) (L-35620)

DE-32A11 Verruca vulgaris 078.1
(M-76630) (L-35620)

DE-32A12 Verruca plana 078.1
(M-76620) (L-35620)

DE-32A13 Verruca plantaris 078.1
(T-D9740) (M-76630) (L-35620)

DE-32A14 Verruca palmaris 078.1
(T-D8740) (M-76630) (L-35620)

DE-32A20 Condyloma acuminatum 078.1
(M-76720) (L-35620) (DE-01600)
Venereal wart 078.1
(M-76720) (L-35620) (DE-01600)
Anogenital wart 078.1
(M-76720) (L-35620) (DE-01600)

DE-32A30V Cutaneous papillomatosis, NOS
(T-01000) (M-80600) (L-35600)

DE-32A31V Bovine cutaneous papillomatosis
(T-01000) (M-80600) (L-36710)

DE-32A32V Equine cutaneous papillomatosis
(T-01000) (M-80600) (L-35600)

DE-32A33V Caprine cutaneous papillomatosis
(T-01000) (M-80600) (L-35600)

DE-32A34V Fibropapilloma of cattle
(T-91000) (L-35710) (DE-01600)

DE-32A35V Oral papillomatosis
(T-51030) (M-80600) (L-35600)

DE-32A36V Canine viral papillomatosis
(T-51030) (M-80600) (L-35600)
Canine oral papillomatosis
(T-51030) (M-80600) (L-35600)

DE-32A37V Oral lapine papillomatosis
(T-51030) (M-80600) (L-35600)
Oral papillomatosis of rabbit
(T-51030) (M-80600) (L-35600)

DE-32A38V Cutaneous papillomatosis of rabbit
(L-35601) (M-80600)
Shope papilloma
(L-35601) (M-80600)

DE-32A39V Teat papillomatosis
(T-04100) (M-80600) (L-35600)

DE-32A50 Disease due to Polyomavirus, NOS
(L-35740)

DE-32A51 Progressive multifocal leukoencephalopathy 046.3 —331.6*
(T-A0100) (L-35740)
Multifocal leukoencephalopathy, NOS 046.3 —331.6*
(T-A0100) (L-37540)

E-32B Diseases Due to Parvoviridae

DE-32B00 Disease due to Parvoviridae, NOS
(L-35400)

E-32B Diseases Due to Parvoviridae — Continued

DE-32B10 Aleutian disease
(L-35402)
Aleutian mink disease
(L-35402)

DE-32B12V Feline panleukemia
(L-35404)
Feline distemper
(L-35404)
Feline infectious enteritis
(L-35404)
Feline agranulocytosis
(L-35404)
Feline parvovirus infection
(L-35404)

DE-32B14V Canine parvovirus infection
(L-35407)

DE-32B16V Bovine parvovirus infection
(L-35403)

DE-32B18V Murine parvovirus infection
(L-35401)

DE-32B20V Mink parvovirus infection
(L-35406)
Mink enteritis
(L-35406)

E-330-334 Diseases Due to Togaviridae

DE-33000 Disease due to Togaviridae, NOS

E-331 Diseases Due to Alphavirus

DE-33100 Disease due to Alphavirus, NOS
(L-32200)

DE-33110 Chikungunya fever 066.3
(L-32206)

DE-33111 Chikungunya hemorrhagic fever 065.4
(L-32206)

DE-33120 Eastern equine encephalitis 062.2 —323.3*
(T-A0100) (L-32207)
EEE 062.1 —323.3
(T-A0100) (L-32207)
Eastern equine encephalomyelitis
(T-A0100) (L-32207)

DE-33130 Western equine encephalitis 062.1 —323.3*
(T-A0100) (L-32224)
WEE 062.1 —323.3*
(T-A0100) (L-32224)
Western equine encephalomyelitis 062.1
(T-A0100) (L-32223)

DE-33140 Venezuelan equine encephalitis 066.2
(T-A0100) (L-32223)
Venezuelan equine fever 066.2
(T-A0100) (L-32223)
VEE 066.2
(T-A0100) (L-32223)
Venezuelan equine encephalomyelitis 066.2
(T-A0100) (L-32223)

DE-33150 Ross river fever 066.3
(L-32218)
Epidemic Australian polyarthritis 066.3
(L-32218)

DE-33178 Bebaru fever
(L-32203)

DE-33180 Mayaro fever 066.3
(L-32212)
Uruma fever 066.3
(L-32212)

DE-33182 Mucambo fever 066.3
(L-32214)

DE-33184 O'nyong-nyong fever 066.3
(L-32216)

DE-33186 Sindbis fever 066.3
(L-32201)

DE-33188 Semliki forest fever 062.8
(L-32220)

DE-33192 Everglades virus disease 066.3
(L-32208)
Everglades fever 066.3
(L-32208)

E-332-333 Diseases Due to Flavivirus

DE-33200 Disease due to Flavivirus, NOS
(L-32300)

DE-33210 Yellow fever, NOS 060.9
(L-32301)

DE-33211 Jungle yellow fever 060.0
(L-32301)
Sylvan yellow fever 060.0
(L-32301)
Sylvatic yellow fever 060.0
(L-32301)

DE-33212 Urban yellow fever 060.1
(L-32301)

DE-33220 Zika virus disease 066.3
(L-32369)
Zika fever 066.3
(L-32369)

DE-33230 West Nile fever 066.3
(L-32368)

DE-33232 Uganda S fever 066.8
(L-32364)

DE-33235 Wesselsbron fever 066.3
(L-32367)

DE-33240 Spondweni fever 066.8
(L-32356)

DE-33250 Rio Bravo fever 049.8
(T-A0100) (L-32348)
Rio Bravo encephalitis 049.8 —323.4*
(T-A0100) (L-32348)

DE-33260 Central European encephalitis 063.2 —323.3*
(T-A0100) (L-32361) (L-66004)
Diphasic meningoencephalitis 063.8 —323.3*
(T-A0100) (L-32361) (L-66004)

DE-33260 (cont.) Biundulant meningoencephalitis 063.8 —323.3*
(T-A0100) (L-32361) (L-66004)
Central European tick-borne encephalitis 075.-
(T-A0100) (L-32361) (L-66004)
Diphasic milk fever 075.-
(T-A0100) (L-32361) (L-66004)

DE-33270 Louping ill 063.1 —323.3*
(L-32339)
Ovine encephalomyelitis 063.1 —323.3*
(T-A0100) (L-32339)

DE-33280 St. Louis encephalitis 062.3 —323.3*
(T-A0100) (L-32352)
St-Louis viral disease 062.3 —323.3*
(T-A0100) (L-32352)
SLE 062.3 —323.3*
(T-A0100) (L-32352)

DE-33290 Murray valley encephalitis 062.4 —323.3*
(T-A0100) (L-32342)
Australian encephalitis 062.4 —323.3*
(T-A0100) (L-32342)
Australian arboencephalitis 062.4 —323.3*
(T-A0100) (L-32342)
Australian X disease 062.4 —323.3*
(T-A0100) (L-32342)
MVE 062.4 —323.3*
(T-A0100) (L-32342)

DE-33300 Japanese encephalitis virus disease 062.0 —323.3*
(T-A0100) (L-32329)
Japanese encephalitis 062.0 —323.3*
(T-A0100) (L-32329)
Japanese B encephalitis 062.0 —323.3*
(T-A0100) (L-32329)

DE-33310 Ilheus virus encephalitis 062.8 —323.3*
(T-A0100) (L-32327)

DE-33320 Far Eastern tick-borne encephalitis 063.0 —323.3*
(T-A0100) (L-32362)
Russian spring-summer encephalitis 063.0 —323.3*
(T-A0100) (L-32362)
Forest-spring encephalitis 063.0 —323.3*
(T-A0100) (L-32362)

DE-33330 Dengue 061.-
(L-32320)
Dengue fever 061.-
(L-32320)
Breakbone fever 061.-
(L-32320)

DE-33338 Dengue hemorrhagic fever 065.4
(L-32320)

DE-33340 Powassan encephalitis 063.8 —323.3*
(T-A0100) (L-32347)

DE-33350 Kunjin fever
(L-32336)

DE-33360 Omsk hemorrhagic fever 065.1
(L-32345)

DE-33370 Kyasanur forest disease 065.2
(L-32337)

DE-33381 Banzi virus disease
(L-32305)
Banzi fever
(L-32305)

DE-33382 Bussuquara virus disease
(L-32309)
Bussuquara fever
(L-32309)

DE-33383 Koutango virus disease
(L-32335)

DE-33384 Rocio virus disease
(L-32349)

DE-33385 Encephalitis due to Langat virus 063.8 —323.3*
(L-32338)

E-334 Diseases Due to Rubivirus

DE-33400 Disease due to Rubivirus, NOS
(L-32500)

DE-33410 Rubella, NOS 056.9
(L-32501)
German measles 056.9
(L-32501)
Rubella without mention of complication 056.9
(L-32501)

DE-33411 Gestational rubella syndrome 771.0
(L-32501) (DE-01900)
Gregg's syndrome 771.0
(L-32501) (DE-01900)
Congenital rubella 771.0
(L-32501) (DE-01900)

DE-33412 Expanded rubella syndrome 771.0
(L-32501) (DE-01900)

DE-33413 Congenital rubella pneumonitis 771.0
(T-28000) (L-32501) (DE-01900)

DE-33418 Rubella in mother complicating pregnancy, childbirth or puerperium, NOS 647.5

DE-33420 Rubella with neurological complications, NOS 056.00
(T-A0000) (L-32501)
Rubella with other specified neurological complication 056.09
(T-A0000) (L-32501)

DE-33421 Progressive rubella panencephalitis 056.01 —323.4*
(T-A0100) (T-A7010) (L-32501)
Rubella encephalomyelitis 056.01 —323.4*
(T-A0100) (T-A7010) (L-32501)

DE-33422 Rubella meningoencephalitis 056.01
(T-A1110) (T-A0100) (L-32501)

DE-33430 Rubella with other specified complications 056.79
(L-32501)

E-334 Diseases Due to Rubivirus — Continued

DE-33431 Rubella arthritis 056.71 —711.5*
(T-15000) (L-32501)

DE-33436 Rubella myocarditis 056.79 —422.91*
(T-32020) (L-32501)

DE-33490 Rubella with unspecified complications 056.8
(L-32501)

E-335 Diseases Due to Pestivirus

DE-33500V Disease due to Pestivirus, NOS
(L-32600)

DE-33510V Hog cholera
(L-32603)
Classical swine fever
(L-32603)

DE-33514V Bovine viral diarrhea
(L-32601)
Bovine mucosal disease
(L-32601)

DE-33520V Border disease of sheep
(L-32602)
Fuzzy lamb
(L-32602)
Hairy shaker disease
(L-32602)
Hypomyelinosis congenita
(L-32602)

DE-33530V Equine viral arteritis
(L-32702)
Epidemic cellulitis
(L-32702)

DE-33540V Simian hemorrhagic fever
(L-32704)

E-337-33A DISEASES DUE TO PARAMYXOVIRIDAE

E-337-338 Diseases Due to Paramyxovirus

DE-33700 Disease due to Paramyxovirus, NOS 079.8
(L-32900)
Paramyxovirus infection, NOS 079.8
(L-32900)

DE-33710 Mumps, NOS 072.9
(T-61100) (L-32903)
Epidemic parotitis 072.9
(T-61100) (L-32903)
Infectious parotitis 072.9
(T-61100) (L-32903)
Mumps without mention of complication 072.9
(T-61100) (L-32903)

DE-33711 Mumps orchitis 072.0 —604.9*
(T-94000) (L-32903)

DE-33712 Mumps meningitis 072.1 —321.5*
(T-A1110) (L-32903)

DE-33713 Mumps encephalitis 072.2 —323.4*
(T-A0100) (L-32903)

DE-33714 Mumps meningoencephalitis 072.2 —323.4*
(T-A1110) (T-A0100) (L-32903)

DE-33715 Mumps pancreatitis 072.3 —577.0*
(T-65000) (L-32903)

DE-33716 Mumps hepatitis 072.71
(T-62000) (L-32903)

DE-33717 Mumps polyneuropathy 072.72
(T-A0500) (L-32903)

DE-33718 Mumps oophoritis 072.3 —577.0*
(T-87000) (L-32903)

DE-33721 Mumps thyroiditis 072.7 —245.0*
(T-B6000) (L-32903)

DE-33722 Mumps nephritis 072.7 —583.-*
(T-71000) (L-32903)

DE-33723 Mumps myocarditis 072.- —422.0*
(T-32020) (L-32903)

DE-33724 Mumps arthritis 072.- —711.5*
(T-15000) (L-32903)

DE-33730 Mumps with other specified complication 072.8
(L-32903)

DE-33740 Mumps with unspecified complication 072.8
(L-32903)

DE-33750 Newcastle disease 077.8 —372.0*
(T-AA860) (L-32901)
Newcastle conjunctivitis 077.8 —372.0*
(T-AA860) (L-32901)
Avian pneumoencephalitis
(L-32901)

DE-33800 Parainfluenza, NOS 078.8
(L-32910)

DE-33801 Infection due to Parainfluenza virus 1 079.8
(L-32911)
Sindai virus infection
(L-32911)

DE-33802 Infection due to Parainfluenza virus 2 079.8
(L-32912)

DE-33803 Infection due to Parainfluenza virus 3 079.8
(L-32913)

DE-33804 Infection due to Parainfluenza virus 4 079.8
(L-32914)

DE-33821 Parainfluenza virus pharyngitis 462.-
(T-55000) (L-32910)

DE-33822 Parainfluenza virus rhinopharyngitis 460.-
(T-23000) (L-32910)

DE-33823 Parainfluenza virus laryngitis 464.0
(T-24100) (L-32910)

DE-33824 Parainfluenza virus laryngotracheitis 464.2
(T-24100) (T-25000) (L-32910)

DE-33825 Parainfluenza virus bronchitis 466.0
(T-26000) (L-32910)

DE-33826 Parainfluenza virus laryngotracheobronchitis 490.-
(T-24100) (T-25000) (T-26000)
(L-32910)

DE-33827 Parainfluenza virus bronchopneumonia 480.2
(T-26000) (T-28000) (L-32910)

DE-33828 Parainfluenza virus pneumonia 480.2
(T-28000) (L-32910)

E-339 Diseases Due to Morbillivirus

DE-33900 Disease due to Morbillivirus, NOS
(L-33000)

DE-33910 Measles 055.9
(L-33001)
Rubeola 055.9
(L-33001)
Morbilli 055.9
(L-33001)
Measles without mention of complication 055.9
(L-33001)

DE-33911 Postmeasles encephalitis 055.0 —323.6*
(T-A0100) (L-33001)

DE-33912 Postmeasles pneumonia 055.1 —484.0*
(T-28000) (L-33001)

DE-33913 Postmeasles otitis media 055.2 —382.0*
(T-AB300) (L-33001)

DE-33920 Measles with other specified complications 055.79
(L-33001)

DE-33921 Measles keratoconjunctivitis 055.71
(T-AA200) (T-AA860) (L-33001)

DE-33922 Measles keratitis 055.71
(T-AA200) (L-33001)

DE-33926 Measles myocarditis 055.79 —422.91*
(T-32020) (L-33001)

DE-33950 Measles with unspecified complication 055.8
(L-33001)

DE-33960 Subacute sclerosing panencephalitis 046.2 —323.1*
(T-A0100) (L-33001)
Dawson's inclusion body encephalitis 046.2 —323.1*
(T-A0100) (L-33001)
Van Bogaert's sclerosing leukoencephalitis 046.2 —323.1*
(T-A0100) (L-33001)

DE-33970V Canine distemper
(L-33002)
Hardpad disease
(L-33002)
Carre's disease
(L-33002)
Old-dog encephalitis
(L-33002)

DE-33971V Mink distemper
(L-33002)

DE-33972V Rinderpest
(L-33004)
Cattle plague
(L-33004)
RP
(L-33004)

DE-33974V Peste des petits ruminants
(L-33003)
Pseudorinderpest
(L-33003)
PPR
(L-33003)

E-33A Diseases Due to Pneumovirus

DE-33A00 Disease due to Pneumovirus, NOS
(L-33100)

DE-33A10 Respiratory syncytial virus infection, NOS 480.1
(L-33101)

DE-33A11 Respiratory syncytial virus pneumonia 480.1
(T-28000) (L-33101)

DE-33A12 Respiratory syncitial virus bronchiolitis 466.1
(T-27000) (L-33101)

DE-33A13 Respiratory syncitial virus bronchitis 466.0
(T-26000) (L-33101)

DE-33A14 Respiratory syncitial virus pharyngitis 462.-
(T-55000) (L-33101)

DE-33A15 Respiratory syncitial virus laryngotracheobronchitis 466.0
(T-24100) (T-25000) (T-26000)
(L-33101)

E-340 Diseases Due to Orthomyxoviridae

DE-34000 Disease due to Orthomyxoviridae, NOS 079.8
(L-32800)
Orthomyxovirus infection, NOS 079.8
(L-32800)

DE-34010 Influenza, NOS 487.1
(L-32800)
Flu 487.1
(L-32800)
Grippe 487.1
(L-32800)

DE-34011 Influenza with pneumonia 487.0
(T-28000) (L-32800)
Influenzal pneumonia 487.0
(T-28000) (L-32800)

DE-34012 Influenzal bronchopneumonia 487.0
(T-26000) (T-28000) (L-32800)

DE-34020 Influenza with other respiratory manifestations 487.1
(T-20000) (L-32800)

DE-34021 Influenzal acute upper respiratory infection 487.1
(T-20100) (L-32800)

DE-34022 Influenzal pharyngitis 487.1
(T-55000) (L-32800)

DE-34023 Influenzal laryngitis 487.1
(T-24100) (L-32800)

DE-34030 Influenza with other manifestations 487.8
(L-32800)

E-340 Diseases Due to Orthomyxoviridae — Continued

DE-34031 Influenza with encephalopathy 487.8
(T-A0100) (L-32800)

DE-34032 Influenza with involvement of gastrointestinal tract 487.8
(T-50100) (L-32800)

DE-34034 Myocarditis due to influenza virus 079.9 —422.91*
(T-32020) (L-32800)

DE-34040 Influenza due to Influenza virus, type A, human 487.-
(L-32801)

DE-34041 Influenza due to Influenza virus, type A, porcine 487.-
(L-32801)

DE-34042 Influenza due to Influenza virus, type B 487.-
(L-32802)

DE-34043 Influenza due to Influenza virus, type C 487.-
(L-32803)

DE-34048 Influenza due to other Influenza virus 487.-
(L-32800)

DE-34050V Avian influenza
(L-32801)
Fowl plague
(L-32801)

DE-34052V Equine influenza
(L-32801)

DE-34054V Swine influenza
(L-32801)

E-342-344 DISEASES DUE TO RHABDOVIRIDAE

E-342 Diseases Due to Rhabdovirus

DE-34200 Disease due to Rhabdoviridae, NOS 079.8
(L-334A0)
Rhabdovirus infection, NOS 079.8
(L-334A0)

DE-34210V Bovine ephemeral fever
(L-33405)
Bovine epizootic fever
(L-33405)
Three-day sickness
(L-33405)
Stiff sickness
(L-33405)

DE-34222V Infectious hemopoietic necrosis
(L-33410)

DE-34224V Viral hemorrhagic septicemia of trout
(T-C2000) (L-33427)

DE-34228V Spring viremia of carp
(L-33433)

DE-34230V Pike fry rhabdovirus disease
(L-33426)

E-343 Diseases Due to Vesiculovirus

DE-34300 Disease due to Vesiculovirus, NOS 066.8
(L-33200)

DE-34310 Vesicular stomatitis, NOS 066.8
(L-33210)

DE-34311 Vesicular stomatitis Indiana virus disease 066.8
(L-33211)
Vesicular stomatitis fever 066.8
(L-33211)
Indiana fever 066.8
(L-33211)

DE-34312 Vesicular stomatitis New Jersey virus disease 066.8
(L-33215)

DE-34314 Vesicular stomatitis Alagoas virus disease 066.8
(L-33213)

DE-34320 Piry virus disease 066.8
(L-33218)
Piry fever 066.8
(L-33218)

DE-34330 Chandipura virus disease 066.8
(L-33216)
Chandipura fever 066.8
(L-33216)

E-344 Diseases Due to Lyssavirus

DE-34400 Disease due to Lyssavirus, NOS
(L-33300)

DE-34410 Rabies, NOS 071.-
(L-33301)
Hydrophobia 071.-
(L-33301)
Lyssa 071.-
(L-33301)

DE-34411 Urban rabies 071.-
(L-33301)

DE-34412 Sylvatic rabies 071.-
(L-33301)

DE-34420 Duvenhage virus disease 078.8
(L-33302)

DE-34430 Mokola virus disease 078.8
(L-33305)

DE-34440V Derriengue
(L-33304) (L-84C00)

E-345-348 DISEASES DUE TO BUNYAVIRIDAE

E-345 Diseases Due to Bunyavirus

DE-34500 Disease due to Bunyavirus, NOS 066.3
(L-33800)

DE-34510 Bunyamwera virus disease 066.3
(L-33801)
Bunyamwera fever 066.3
(L-33801)

DE-34515 Bwamba virus disease 066.3
(L-33828)
Bwamba fever 066.3
(L-33828)

DE-34517 Batai fever
(L-33809)

DE-34518 Catu virus disease 066.3
(L-33865)
Catu fever 066.3
(L-33865)

DE-34520 California encephalitis virus disease 062.5 —323.3*
(T-A0100) (L-33841)
California encephalitis 062.5 —323.3*
(T-A0100) (L-33841)
California meningoencephalitis virus disease 062.5 —323.3*
(T-A1110) (T-A0100) (L-33841)

DE-34527 La Crosse encephalitis 062.5 —323.3*
(T-A0100) (L-33846)

DE-34530V Akabane virus disease
(L-33884)
Enzootic bovine arthrogryposis
(L-33884)

DE-34531 Tahyna fever 062.5 —323.3*
(T-A0100) (L-33851)

DE-34532V Aino virus disease
(L-33833)

DE-34535 Guama virus disease 066.3
(L-33866)
Guama fever 066.3
(L-33866)

DE-34540 Germistan virus disease 066.3
(L-33813)
Germistan fever 066.3
(L-33813)

DE-34545 Guaroa virus disease 066.3
(L-33814)
Guaroa fever 066.3
(L-33814)

DE-34550 Oropouche virus disease 066.3
(L-33893)
Oropouche fever 066.3
(L-33893)

DE-34557 Wyeomyia virus disease 066.8
(L-33827)
Wyeomyia fever 066.8
(L-33827)

DE-34559 Shuni virus disease 066.8
(L-33899)

DE-34561 Jamestown Canyon virus disease 066.3
(L-33843)

DE-34563 Inkoo virus disease 066.3
(L-33842)

DE-34568 Restan virus disease 066.3
(L-33840)
Restan fever 066.3
(L-33840)

DE-34571 Ossa virus disease 066.3
(L-33839)
Ossa fever 066.3
(L-33839)

DE-34573 Oriboca virus disease 066.3
(L-33838)
Oriboca fever 066.3
(L-33838)

DE-34575 Nepuyo virus disease 066.3
(L-33837)

DE-34578 Murutucu virus disease 066.3
(L-33836)
Murutucu fever 066.3
(L-33836)

DE-34581 Marituba virus disease 066.3
(L-33835)
Marituba fever 066.3
(L-33835)

DE-34583 Madrid virus disease 066.3
(L-33834)
Madrid fever 066.3
(L-33834)

DE-34585 Itaqui virus disease 066.3
(L-33833)
Itaqui fever 066.3
(L-33833)

DE-34587 Caraparu virus disease 066.3
(L-33831)
Caraparu fever 066.3
(L-33831)

DE-34589 Apeu virus disease 066.3
(L-33830)

DE-34591 Tensaw virus disease 066.8
(L-33825)
Tensaw fever 066.8
(L-33825)

DE-34593 Ilesha virus disease 066.3
(L-33815)
Ilesha fever 066.3
(L-33815)

DE-34595 Calovo virus disease 066.3
(L-33812)
Calovo fever 066.3
(L-33812)

DE-34597 Tacaiuma virus disease 066.3
(L-33804)
Tacaiuma fever 066.3
(L-33804)

DE-34598 Lone star fever 082.8
(L-34517) (L-60052)
Bullis fever 082.8
(L-34517) (L-60052)

E-346 Diseases Due to Phlebovirus

DE-34600 Disease due to Phlebovirus, NOS
(L-34100)

DE-34610 Sandfly fever, NOS 066.0
(L-34101)
Pappataci 066.0
(L-34101)

E-346 Diseases Due to Phlebovirus — Continued

DE-34610 (cont.) Phlebotomus fever 066.0
(L-34101)

DE-34612 Sandfly fever due to SF-Naples virus 066.0
(L-34126)

DE-34614 Sandfly fever due to SF-Sicilian virus 066.0
(L-34127)

DE-34630 Rift valley fever 066.3
(T-62000) (L-34123)
Enzootic hepatitis 066.3
(T-62000) (L-34123)

DE-34640 Candidu virus disease 066.8
(L-34110)

DE-34650 Chagres virus disease 066.3
(L-34111)

DE-34660 Punta Toro virus disease 066.8
(L-34122)

E-347 Diseases Due to Nairovirus

DE-34700 Disease due to Nairovirus, NOS
(L-34200)

DE-34710 Congo-Crimean hemorrhagic fever 065.0
(L-34210)
Crimean hemorrhagic fever 065.0
(L-34210)
Central Asian hemorrhagic fever 065.0
(L-34210)

DE-34720 Nairobi sheep virus disease 066.1
(L-34201)
Nairobi sheep disease 066.1
(L-34201)

DE-34730 Ganjam virus disease 066.1
(L-34227)
Ganjam fever
(L-34227)

DE-34740 Dugbe virus disease 066.1
(L-34228)
Dugbe fever 066.1
(L-34228)

E-348 Diseases Due to Uukuvirus

DE-34800 Disease due to Uukuvirus, NOS
(L-34300)

DE-34810 Thogoto virus disease 066.1
(L-34511)
Thogoto fever 066.1
(L-34511)

DE-34820 Bhanja virus disease 066.1
(L-34513)

DE-34830 Tataguine virus disease 066.1
(L-34521)
Tataguine fever 066.1
(L-34521)

E-34A Diseases Due to Arenaviridae

DE-34A00 Disease due to Arenavirus, NOS
(L-35300)

DE-34A10 Lymphocytic choriomeningitis 049.0 —321.6*
(T-A1110) (L-35301)
Lymphocytic meningitis 049.0 —321.6*
(T-A1110) (L-35301)
Lymphocytic meningoencephalitis 049.0 —321.6*
(T-A0100) (T-A1110) (L-35301)

DE-34A20 Arenaviral hemorrhagic fever, NOS 078.7
(L-35300)

DE-34A21 South American hemorrhagic fever, NOS 078.7
(L-35300)

DE-34A22 Argentinian hemorrhagic fever 078.7
(L-35312)
Hemorrhagic fever due to Junin virus 078.7
(L-35312)

DE-34A23 Bolivian hemorrhagic fever 078.7
(L-35314)
Hemorrhagic fever due to Machupo virus 078.7
(L-35314)

DE-34A30 Lassa fever 078.89
(L-35302)

DE-34A70 Pichinde virus disease
(L-35316)

DE-34A80 Tacaribe virus disease
(L-35317)

E-350-353 DISEASES DUE TO PICORNAVIRIDAE

E-350-351 Diseases Due to Enterovirus

DE-35000 Disease due to Enterovirus, NOS
(L-30200)
Enterovirus infection, NOS
(L-30200)

DE-35010 Acute poliomyelitis, NOS 045.9 —323.2*
(L-30210)
Poliomyelitis, NOS 045.9 —323.2*
(L-30210)
Infantile paralysis, NOS 045.9 —323.2*
(L-30210)
Anterior acute poliomyelitis, NOS 045.9 —323.2*
(L-30210)
Epidemic acute poliomyelitis, NOS 045.9 —323.2*
(L-30210)

DE-35011 Acute paralytic poliomyelitis specified as bulbar 045.0 —323.2*
(T-A7010) (L-30210)
Acute infantile paralysis 045.0 —323.2*
(T-A7010) (L-30210)
Acute anterior poliomyelitis 045.0 —323.2*
(T-A7010) (L-30210)

DE-35011 (cont.) Acute bulbar polioencephalitis 045.0 —323.2*
(T-A7010) (L-30210)
Acute anterior bulbar polioencephalomyelitis 045.0 —323.2*
(T-A7010) (L-30210)

DE-35012 Acute poliomyelitis with other paralysis 045.1 —323.2*
(T-A7010) (L-30210)
Acute atrophic spinal paralysis 045.1 —323.2*
(T-A7010) (L-30210)
Infantile paralytic paralysis 045.1 —323.2*
(T-A7010) (L-30210)
Anterior acute poliomyelitis with paralysis except bulbar 045.1 —323.2*
(T-A7010) (L-30210)
Epidemic acute poliomyelitis with paralysis except bulbar 045.1 —323.2*
(T-A7010) (L-30210)

DE-35013 Acute nonparalytic poliomyelitis 045.2
(T-A7010) (L-30210)
Anterior acute poliomyelitis specified as nonparalytic 045.2 —323.2*
(T-A7010) (L-30210)
Epidemic acute poliomyelitis specified as non paralytic 045.2 —323.2*
(T-A7010) (L-30210)

DE-35030 Enteroviral vesicular pharyngitis
(T-55000) (L-30300) (L-30500)
Herpangina 074.0
(T-55000) (L-30300) (L-30500)
Vesicular pharyngitis 074.0
(T-55000) (L-30300) (L-30500)

DE-35040 Enteroviral vesicular stomatitis with exanthem 074.3
(T-51000) (M-01710) (L-30316)
Hand, foot and mouth disease 074.3
(T-51000) (M-01710) (L-30316)

DE-35045 Enteroviral lymphonodular pharyngitis 078.8
(T-55000) (L-30310)

DE-35049 Enterovirus enteritis 088.6
(T-50500) (L-30200)

DE-35050 Epidemic pleurodynia 074.1
(L-30401)
Bornholm disease 074.1
(L-30401)
Devil's grip 074.1
(L-30401)
Epidemic myalgia 074.1
(L-30401)
Epidemic myositis 074.1
(L-30401)

DE-35052V Poliomyelitis of mouse
(L-30606)
Mouse encephalomyelitis
(L-30606)
Theiler's disease
(L-30606)
Theiler's mouse encephalomyelitis
(L-30606)

DE-35060 Enteroviral hemorrhagic conjunctivitis
(T-AA860) (L-30603)
Epidemic hemorrhagic conjunctivitis 077.4 —372.0*
(T-AA860) (L-30603)
Apollo conjunctivitis 077.4 —321.2*
(T-AA860) (L-30603)
Apollo disease 077.4 —321.2*
(T-AA860) (L-30603)
Conjunctivitis due to enterovirus type 70 077.4 —321.2*
(T-AA860) (L-30603)

DE-35065 Enteroviral exanthematous fever
(L-30200)
Boston exanthem 048.-
(L-30200)
Meningoeruptive syndrome 079.1
(L-30200)

DE-35068V Viral hepatitis of turkeys
(L-30200)

DE-35070 Enteroviral encephalomyelitis 048.- —323.4
(T-A0100) (T-A7010) (L-30200)

DE-35071 Enterovirus meningitis 047.-
(T-A1110) (L-30200)

DE-35072 Coxsackie meningitis 047.0 —321.1*
(T-A1110) (L-30300)

DE-35080 Enterovirus heart infection, NOS
(T-32000) (L-30300)
Coxsackie carditis 074.20
(T-32000) (L-30300)

DE-35081 Coxsackie myocarditis 074.23 —422.0*
(T-32020) (L-30300)

DE-35082 Aseptic myocarditis of newborn 074.23 —433.0*
(T-32020) (F-88000) (L-30300)

DE-35083 Coxsackie endocarditis 074.22 —421.1*
(T-32060) (L-30300)

DE-35084 Coxsackie pericarditis 074.21 —420.0*
(T-39000) (L-30300)

DE-35088 Hepatitis in coxsackie viral disease —573.1*
(T-62000) (L-30300)

DE-35100 Viral hepatitis, type A 070.1 —573.1*
(T-62000) (L-30605)
Infectious hepatitis 070.1 —573.1*
(T-62000) (L-30605)
Viral hepatitis A without mention of hepatic coma 070.1 —573.1*
(T-62000) (L-30605)

DE-35101 Viral hepatitis A with hepatic coma 070.0 —573.1*
(T-62000) (D5-81120) (L-30605)

DE-35110 Acute type A viral hepatitis 070.1 —573.1*
(T-62000) (M-41000) (L-30605)

E-350-351 Diseases Due to Enterovirus — Continued

DE-35111 Chronic type A viral hepatitis 070.1 —573.1*
(T-62000) (M-43000) (L-30605)
DE-35112 Acute fulminating type A viral hepatitis 070.1 —573.1*
(T-62000) (M-41000) (L-30605)
DE-35113 Chronic active type A viral hepatitis 070.1 —573.1*
(T-62000) (M-42000) (L-30605)
DE-35114 Chronic persistent type A viral hepatitis 070.1 —573.1*
(T-62000) (M-43000) (L-30605)
DE-35115 Chronic aggressive type A viral hepatitis 070.1 —573.1*
(T-62000) (M-43000) (L-30605)
DE-35116 Anicteric type A viral hepatitis 070.1 —573.1*
(T-62000) (L-30605)
DE-35117 Relapsing type A viral hepatitis 070.1 —573.1*
(T-62000) (L-30605)
DE-35120V Duck viral hepatitis
(L-30290)
DE-35122V Infectious avian nephritis
(L-30200)
DE-35124V Avian encephalomyelitis
(L-30200)
DE-35125V Viral encephalomyelocarditis
(L-31001)
DE-35130V Porcine enteroviral encephalomyelitis
(L-30801)
Teschen disease
(L-30801)
Porcine polioencephalomyelitis
(L-30801)
Talfan disease
(L-30801)
Benign enzootic paresis of pig
(L-30801)
Canadian viral encephalomyelitis
(L-30801)
DE-35132V Swine vesicular disease
(L-30405)
SVD
(L-30405)
DE-35134V Murine encephalomyelitis
(L-31003)

E-352 Diseases Due to Rhinovirus

DE-35200 Disease due to Rhinovirus, NOS 079.3
(L-31100)
Rhinovirus infection, NOS 079.3
(L-31100)
DE-35210 Common cold 460.-
(T-23000) (M-41000) (L-31100)
Acute nasopharyngitis, NOS 460.-
(T-23000) (M-41000) (L-31100)
Acute coryza 460.-
(T-23000) (M-41000) (L-31100)
Acute nasal catarrh 460.-
(T-23000) (M-41000) (L-31100)
Infective nasopharyngitis, NOS 460.-
(T-23000) (M-41000) (L-31100)
Acute rhinitis 460.-
(T-23000) (M-41000) (L-31100)
Infective rhinitis 460.-
(T-23000) (M-41000) (L-31100)
DE-35220V Bovine rhinovirus infection
(L-31230)
DE-35222V Equine rhinovirus infection
(L-31510)

E-353 Diseases Due to Aphthovirus

DE-35300 Disease due to Aphthovirus, NOS
(L-31400)
DE-35310 Foot-and-mouth disease 078.4
(L-31401)
Epizootic aphtae 078.4
(L-31401)
Epizootic stomatitis 078.4
(L-31401)
Aphthous fever 078.4
(L-31401)

E-354 Diseases Due to Calicivirus

DE-35400V Disease due to Calicivirus, NOS
(L-31600)
DE-35410V Vesicular exanthema of swine
(L-31610)
VES
(L-31610)
DE-35420V Feline calcivirus infection
(L-31612)
DE-35422V Feline respiratory disease complex
(L-31612)
DE-35430V San Miguel sea lion virus disease
(L-31613)

E-355-357 DISEASES DUE TO REOVIRIDAE

E-355 Diseases Due to Reovirus

DE-35500 Disease due to Reovirus, NOS
(L-31700)
Reovirus infection, NOS 079.8
(L-31700)
DE-35510V Avian viral arthritis
(L-31704)
Avian tenosynovitis
(L-31704)
DE-35512V Avian malabsorption syndrome
(L-31704)
Pale bird syndrome
(L-31704)

E-356 Diseases Due to Orbivirus

DE-35600 Disease due to Orbivirus, NOS
(L-31800)
DE-35610 Changuinola virus disease 066.0
(L-31844)
Changuinola fever 066.0
(L-31844)
DE-35620 Colorado tick fever 066.1
(L-31851)
American mountain tick fever 066.1
(L-31851)
DE-35630 Kemerovo virus disease 066.1
(L-31868)
Kemerovo fever 066.1
(L-31868)
DE-35640 Tribec virus disease 066.1
(L-31879)
DE-35650 Lebombo virus disease 066.3
(L-31927)
DE-35660 Orunga virus disease 066.3
(L-31929)
DE-35670V Bluetongue of sheep
(L-32000)
Catarrhal fever of sheep
(L-32000)
Soremuzzle
(L-32000)
DE-35672V Epizootic hemorrhagic disease of deer
(L-31900)
DE-35674V African horse sickness
(L-31A00)

E-357 Diseases Due to Rotavirus

DE-35700 Disease due to Rotavirus, NOS
(L-32100)
DE-35710 Viral gastroenteritis due to Rotaviruses 008.6
(T-50100) (L-32100)
Rotaviral enteritis 008.6
(T-50500) (L-32100)
Nonbacterial gastroenteritis of infant 008.6
(T-50500) (L-32101)
Rotavirus infection of children 008.6
(T-50500) (L-32101)
Neonatal infantile diarrhea 008.6
(T-50500) (L-32101)
DE-35720V Neonatal calf diarrhea
(L-32104)
DE-35724V Epidemic diarrheal disease of infant mouse
(L-32103)
Murine epizootic diarrhea
(L-32103)
Epizootic diarrhea of infant mouse
(L-32103)
EDIM
(L-32103)
DE-35726V Lethal intestinal viral infection of mouse
(L-32103)
LIVIM
(L-32103)
DE-35730V Porcine rotaviral enteritis
(L-32105)

E-359 Diseases Due to Coronaviridae

DE-35900 Disease due to coronaviridae, NOS
(L-33500)
DE-35910V Bluecomb disease
(L-33601)
Coronaviral enteritis of turkey
(L-33601)
Transmissible enteritis of turkey
(L-33601)
DE-35920V Avian infectious bronchitis
(L-33501)
Gasping disease
(L-33501)
DE-35922V Transmissible gastroenteritis of swine
(L-33505)
TGE
(L-33505)
DE-35923V Epizootic catarrhal gastroenteritis of minks
(L-33500)
DE-35924V Porcine coronaviral encephalomyelitis
(L-33504)
Hemagglutinating encephalitis of pig
(L-33504)
Vomiting and wasting disease of piglet
(L-33504)
DE-35926V Feline infectious peritonitis and pleuritis
(L-33700)
Feline coronaviral infection
(L-33700)
FIP
(L-33700)
DE-35928V Rat coronaviral infection
(L-33605)
DE-35930V Sialodacryoadenitis of rat
(L-33604)
SDA
(L-33604)
DE-35932V Coronaviral calf diarrhea
(L-33602)
DE-35934V Murine hepatitis
(L-33503)
DE-35936V Canine coronaviral gastroenteritis
(L-33600)

E-36 DISEASES DUE TO RETROVIRIDAE

E-360 Diseases Due to Oncovirinae

DE-36000 Disease due to Oncovirus, NOS
(L-34610)
DE-36010V Avian leukosis
(L-34903) (L-34902)
Avian leukosis-sarcoma group
(L-34903) (L-34902)

E-360 Diseases Due to Oncovirinae — Continued

DE-36010V (cont.) Lymphoid leukosis
(L-34903) (L-34902)

DE-36012V Avian sarcoma
(L-34902)
Rous sarcoma
(L-34902)

DE-36014V Avian reticuloendotheliosis
(L-34901)

DE-36016V Lymphoproliferative disease of turkey
(L-34900)

DE-36020V Jaagziekte
(T-28000) (L-34600)
Jagziekte
(T-28000) (L-34600)
Pulmonary adenomatosis of sheep
(T-28000) (L-34600)
Lunger disease
(T-28000) (L-34600)

DE-36030V Feline leukemia virus infection
(L-34634)
Feline lymphosarcoma and leukemia
(L-34634)
Feline visceral lymphoma and leukemia
(L-34634)

DE-36032V Mouse mammary tumor virus infection
(L-34921)

DE-36034V Bovine viral leukosis
(L-34632)

E-361 Diseases Due to Spumavirinae

DE-36100 Disease due to Spumavirus, NOS
(L-35100)

E-362 Diseases Due to Lentivirinae

DE-36200 Disease due to Lentivirus, NOS
(L-35200)

DE-36210 Transmissible virus dementia 046.8
(L-35200)
Familial Alzheimer's disease 046.8
(L-35200)

DE-36220V Progressive pneumonia of sheep
(L-35201)
Maedi-Visna
(L-35201)
Zwoegersiekte
(L-35201)
Chronic viral encephalomyelitis of sheep
(L-35201)
Ovine progressive pneumonia
(L-35201)

DE-36222V Caprine arthritis-encephalitis
(L-35206)
Caprine leukoencephalomyelitis
(L-35206)
CAE
(L-35206)

DE-36230V Equine infectious anemia
(L-35205)
Swamp fever
(L-35205)
EIA
(L-35205)

E-363-365 Diseases Due to Immunodeficiency Virus

DE-36300 Human immunodeficiency virus infection, NOS 042.-
(L-34800) (DE-01600)

DE-36301 Human immunodeficiency virus I infection
(L-34801) (DE-01600)

DE-36302 Human immunodeficiency virus II infection
(L-34802) (DE-01600)

DE-36310 AIDS, NOS 042.-
(L-34800) (DE-01600)
Acquired immune deficiency syndrome, NOS 042.-
(L-34800) (DE-01600)
Acquired immunodeficiency syndrome, NOS 042.-
(L-34800) (DE-01600)

DE-36311 AIDS with candidiasis of lung 042.0
(L-34800) (L-43130) (DE-41051)

DE-36312 AIDS with coccidiosis 042.0
(L-34800) (L-52500) (DE-51000)
AIDS with isosporiasis 042.0
(L-34800) (L-52500) (DE-51000)

DE-36313 AIDS with cryptococcosis 042.0
(L-34800) (L-43165) (DE-41200)

DE-36314 AIDS with cryptosporidiosis 042.0
(L-34800) (L-52400) (DE-54800)

DE-36315 AIDS with pneumocystosis 042.0
(L-34800) (L-50F00) (DE-59100)

DE-36316 AIDS with progressive multifocal leukoencephalopathy 042.0
(L-34800) (L-35740) (DE-32A51)

DE-36317 AIDS with toxoplasmosis 042.0
(L-34800) (L-52801) (DE-51200)

DE-36318 AIDS with microsporidiosis 042.1
(L-34800) (DE-5A222) (L-54...)

DE-36319 AIDS with acute endocarditis 042.1
(T-32060) (L-34800) (M-41000)

DE-3631A AIDS with subacute endocarditis 042.1
(T-32060) (L-34800) (M-42000)

DE-3631B AIDS with acute myocarditis 042.1
(T-32020) (L-34800) (M-41000)

DE-3631C AIDS with subacute myocarditis 042.1
(T-32020) (L-34800) (M-42000)

DE-36321 AIDS with disseminated candidiasis of mouth 042.1
(L-34800) (L-43130) (DE-41012)

DE-36322 AIDS with disseminated candidiasis of skin and nails 042.1
(L-34800) (L-43130) (DE-41031) (DE-41032)

DE-36323 AIDS with disseminated candidiasis of other and unspecified sites 042.1
(L-34800) (L-43130) (DE-41002)

DE-36324 AIDS with coccidioidomycosis 042.1
(L-34800) (L-44181) (DE-40600)

DE-36325 AIDS with cytomegalic inclusion disease 042.1
(L-34800) (L-36500) (DE-32610)

DE-36326 AIDS with herpes simplex 042.1
(L-34800) (L-36210) (DE-32110)

DE-36327 AIDS with herpes zoster 042.1
(L-34800) (L-36401) (DE-32400)

DE-36328 AIDS with histoplasmosis 042.1
(L-34800) (L-44220) (DE-40700)

DE-36329 AIDS with other and unspecified mycobacteriosis 042.1
(L-34800) (L-21800) (DE-12900)

DE-3632A AIDS with bacterial pneumonia 042.1
(T-28000) (L-34800) (L-10000)

DE-3632B AIDS with pneumococcal pneumonia
(T-28000) (L-34800) (L-25100)

DE-36331 AIDS with Nocardia infection 042.1
(L-34800) (L-22300) (DE-11060)

DE-36332 AIDS with opportunistic mycosis 042.1
(L-34800) (DE-40010)

DE-36333 AIDS with pneumonia, NOS 042.1
(T-28000) (M-40000) (L-34800)

DE-36334 AIDS with viral pneumonia, NOS 042.1
(T-28000) (M-40000) (L-34800) (L-30000)

DE-36335 AIDS with Salmonella infection 042.1
(L-34800) (L-17100) (DE-13900)

DE-36336 AIDS with septicemia 042.1
(T-C2000) (L-34800) (DE-00020)

DE-36337 AIDS with strongyloidiasis 042.1
(L-34800) (L-55301) (DE-67B00)

DE-36338 AIDS with tuberculosis 042.1
(L-34800) (L-21801) (DE-14800)

DE-36340 AIDS with specified malignant neoplasm 042.2
(L-34800) (M-80003)

DE-36341 AIDS with Burkitt's tumor 042.2
(L-34800) (M-96873)

DE-36342 AIDS with Kaposi's sarcoma 042.2
(L-34800) (M-91403)

DE-36343 AIDS with immunoblastic sarcoma 042.2
(L-34800) (M-96843)

DE-36344 AIDS with primary lymphoma of the brain 042.2
(T-A0100) (L-34800) (M-95903)

DE-36345 AIDS with reticulosarcoma 042.2
(L-34800) (M-95933)

DE-36349 AIDS with or without other conditions 042.9
(L-34800)

DE-36351 AIDS with specified diseases of the central nervous system 043.1
(T-A0090) (L-34800) (DA-00000)

DE-36352 AIDS with central nervous system disorder, NOS 043.1
(T-A0090) (L-34800) (DA-00000)

DE-36353 AIDS with CNS demyelinating disease, NOS 043.1
(T-A0090) (L-34800) (DA-25000)

DE-36354 AIDS with non-arthropod-borne viral disease, NOS 043.1
(L-34800) (DE-30050)

DE-36355 AIDS with subacute adenoviral encephalitis
(T-A0100) (L-34800) (L-35827) (L-35852) (DE-31064)

AIDS with slow virus infection, NOS 043.1
(T-A0100) (L-34800) (L-35827) (L-35852) (DE-31064)

DE-36356 AIDS with dementia, NOS 043.1
(T-A0100) (L-34800)

DE-36357 AIDS with organic dementia 043.1
(T-A0100) (L-34800)

DE-36358 AIDS with presenile dementia 043.1
(T-A0100) (L-34800)

DE-36359 AIDS with encephalitis 043.1
(T-A0100) (L-34800)

DE-36361 AIDS with encephalomyelitis 043.1
(T-A0100) (T-A7010) (L-34800)

DE-36362 AIDS with encephalopathy 043.1
(T-A0100) (L-34800)

DE-36363 AIDS with myelitis 043.1
(T-A7010) (L-34800)

DE-36364 AIDS with myelopathy 043.1
(T-A7010) (L-34800)

DE-36365 AIDS with organic brain syndrome, NOS 043.1
(T-A0100) (L-34800)

DE-36367 AIDS with other disorders involving the immune mechanism 043.2
(L-34800)

DE-36368 AIDS with lymphadenopathy 043.0
(T-C4000) (L-34800) (M-71000)

DE-36370 AIDS with other specified conditions 043.3
(L-34800)

DE-36371 AIDS with abnormal weight loss 043.3
(L-34800) (F-01820)

DE-36372 AIDS with respiratory abnormality 043.3
(T-20000) (L-34800)

DE-36373 AIDS with agranulocytosis 043.3
(T-C1460) (L-34800)

DE-36374 AIDS with anemia, NOS 043.3
(L-34800)

DE-36375 AIDS with aplastic anemia 043.3
(L-34800)

DE-36376 AIDS with deficiency anemia 043.3
(L-34800)

DE-36377 AIDS with acquired hemolytic anemia 043.3
(L-34800)

DE-36378 AIDS with infective arthritis 043.3
(L-34800)

E-363-365 Diseases Due to Immunodeficiency Virus — Continued

DE-36379 AIDS with blindness 043.3
(L-34800)

DE-36381 AIDS with low vision 043.3
(L-34800)

DE-36382 AIDS with hematopoietic system disease, NOS 043.3
(L-34800)

DE-36383 AIDS with cachexia 043.3
(L-34800)

DE-36384 AIDS with dermatomycosis 043.3
(L-34800) (DE-45000)
AIDS with dermatophytosis 043.3
(L-34800) (DE-45000)

DE-36386 AIDS with salivary gland disease, NOS 043.3
(L-34800)

DE-36387 AIDS with skin disease, NOS 043.3
(L-34800)

DE-36388 AIDS with subcutaneous tissue disease, NOS 043.3
(L-34800)

DE-36389 AIDS with dyspnea 043.3
(L-34800)

DE-36391 AIDS with fatigue 043.3
(L-34800)

DE-36392 AIDS with fever 043.3
(L-34800)

DE-36393 AIDS with infectious gastroenteritis 043.3
(T-50100) (L-34800) (DE-B0130)

DE-36394 AIDS with noninfectious gastroenteritis 043.3
(T-50100) (L-34800)

DE-36395 AIDS with hepatomegaly 043.3
(T-62000) (M-71000) (L-34800)

DE-36396 AIDS with hyperhidrosis 043.3
(L-34800)

DE-36397 AIDS with hypersplenism 043.3
(L-34800)

DE-36398 AIDS with ill-defined intestinal infection 043.3
(T-50500) (L-34800) (DE-B0100)

DE-36399 AIDS with failure to thrive syndrome (in infant) 043.3
(L-34800)

DE-36401 AIDS with leukoplakia of oral mucosa (tongue) 043.3
(L-34800)

DE-36402 AIDS with intestinal malabsorption 043.3
(L-34800)

DE-36403 AIDS with malaise 043.3
(L-34800)

DE-36404 AIDS with neuralgia, NOS 043.3
(L-34800)

DE-36405 AIDS with neuritis, NOS 043.3
(L-34800)

DE-36406 AIDS with nutritional deficiency 043.3
(L-34800)

DE-36407 AIDS with polyneuropathy 043.3
(L-34800)

DE-36408 AIDS with pyrexia 043.3
(L-34800)

DE-36409 AIDS with radiculitis, NOS 043.3
(L-34800)

DE-36411 AIDS with rash, NOS 043.3
(T-01000) (M-01710) (L-34800)

DE-36412 AIDS with retinal vascular changes 043.3
(L-34800)

DE-36413 AIDS with background retinopathy 043.3
(L-34800)

DE-36414 AIDS with splenomegaly 043.3
(T-C3000) (M-71000) (L-34800)

DE-36415 AIDS with secondary thrombocytopenia 043.3
(L-34800)

DE-36416 AIDS with thrombocytopenia, NOS 043.3
(L-34800)

DE-36417 AIDS with volume depletion 043.3
(L-34800)

DE-36420 Other AIDS virus infection 044.-
(L-34800)
AIDS virus with specified acute infection 044.0
(L-34800)

DE-36421 AIDS virus with acute lymphadenitis 044.0
(T-C4000) (M-41000) (L-34800)

DE-36422 AIDS virus with aseptic meningitis 044.0
(T-01110) (L-34800) (DA-10011)

DE-36423 AIDS virus with viral infection 044.0
(L-34800) (L-30000)

DE-36424 AIDS virus with "infectious mononucleosis-like syndrome" 044.0
(L-34800) (L-36901) (DE-32710)

DE-36480 AIDS virus infection, NEC 044.9
(L-34800)

DE-36500 AIDS-like syndrome 043.9
(L-34800)
ARC 043.9
(L-34800)
AIDS-related complex 043.9
(L-34800)

DE-36510 AIDS-related complex with or without other conditions 043.9
(L-34800)

DE-36550 Positive serological or viral culture findings for human ummunodeficiency virus 795.8

DE-36570 AIDS with specified infection, NEC 042.0
(L-34800) (DE-.....)

DE-36580 HTLV-III/LAV infection, NOS 042.-
(L-34800) (DE-01600)

DE-36590V Simian acquired immune deficiency syndrome
(L-34807)
SAIDS
(L-34807)

E-38 DISEASES DUE TO UNCLASSIFIED VIRUSES

DE-38010 Type B viral hepatitis 070.3 —573.1*
(T-62000) (L-38601)
Serum hepatitis 070.3 —573.1*
(T-62000) (L-38601)
Viral hepatitis B without mention of hepatic coma 070.3 —573.1*
(T-62000) (L-38601)

DE-38011 Viral hepatitis B with hepatic coma 070.2 —573.1*
(T-62000) (L-38601) (D5-81120)

DE-38020 Acute type B viral hepatitis 070.3 —573.1*
(T-62000) (M-41000) (L-38601)

DE-38021 Chronic type B viral hepatitis 070.3 —573.1*
(T-62000) (M-43000) (L-38601)

DE-38022 Acute fulminating type B viral hepatitis 070.3 —573.1*
(T-62000) (M-41000) (L-38601)

DE-38023 Chronic active type B viral hepatitis 070.3 —573.1*
(T-62000) (M-42000) (L-38601)

DE-38024 Chronic persistent type B viral hepatitis 070.3 —573.1*
(T-62000) (M-43000) (L-38601)

DE-38025 Chronic aggressive type B viral hepatitis 070.3 —573.1*
(T-62000) (M-43000) (L-38601)

DE-38026 Anicteric type B viral hepatitis 070.3 —573.1*
(T-62000) (L-38601)

DE-38027 Relapsing type B viral hepatitis 070.3 —573.1*
(T-62000) (L-38601)

DE-38030 Marburg virus disease 078.89
(L-38711)
Vervet monkey disease 078.89
(L-38711)

DE-38050 Ebola virus disease
(L-38712)

DE-38060 Exanthema subitum 057.8
(L-38812)
Pseudorubella 057.8
(L-38812)
Sixth disease 057.8
(L-38812)
Roseola infantum 057.8
(L-38812)

DE-38070 Le Dantec virus disease
(L-38822)

DE-38080 Zinga virus disease
(L-38820)

DE-38090 Viral gastroenteritis due to Norwalk-like agents 008.6
(T-50100) (L-31615)

DE-38200 Viral hepatitis, NOS 070.9 —573.1*
(T-62000) (L-30000)
Unspecified viral hepatitis without mention of hepatic coma 070.9 —573.1*
(T-62000) (L-30000)

DE-38201 Neonatal hepatitis 070.5
(T-62000) (F-88000) (L-30000)

DE-38202 Viral hepatitis, carrier state 070.9 —573.1*
(T-62000) (L-30000) (F-06200)

DE-38203 Unspecified viral hepatitis with hepatic coma 070.6 —573.1*
(T-62000) (L-30000) (D5-81120)

DE-38210 Acute viral hepatitis 070.5 —573.1*
(T-62000) (M-41000) (L-30000)

DE-38220 Chronic viral hepatitis 070.5 —573.1*
(T-62000) (M-43000) (L-30000)

DE-38230 Acute fulminating viral hepatitis 070.5 —573.1*
(T-62000) (M-41000) (L-30000)

DE-38240 Chronic active viral hepatitis 070.5 —573.1*
(T-62000) (M-42000) (L-30000)

DE-38250 Chronic persistent viral hepatitis 070.5 —573.1*
(T-62000) (M-43000) (L-30000)

DE-38260 Chronic aggressive viral hepatitis 070.5 —573.1*
(T-62000) (M-43000) (L-30000)

DE-38270 Anicteric viral hepatitis 070.5 —573.1*
(T-62000) (L-30000)

DE-38280 Relapsing viral hepatitis 070.5 —573.1*
(T-62000) (L-30000)

DE-38290 Other specified viral hepatitis 070.5 —573.1*
(T-62000) (L-30000)

DE-38291 Other specified viral hepatitis without mention of hepatic coma 070.5 —573.1*
(T-62000) (L-30000)

DE-38292 Other specified viral hepatitis with hepatic coma 070.4 —573.1*
(T-62000) (L-30000) (D5-81120)

DE-38300V Infectious avian anemia
(L-30000)

DE-38302V Infectious bursal disease
(L-38805)
Gumboro disease
(L-38805)
Avian nephrosis
(L-38805)

DE-38310V Borna disease
(L-30000)
Near eastern equine encephalomyelitis
(L-30000)

DE-38900 Manzanilla fever
(L-33890)

DE-38901 Quaranfil fever 066.1
(L-38824)

E-39 DISEASES OF POSSIBLE VIRAL ORIGIN

DE-39030 Epidemic vertigo 078.81 —386.1*
(L-00004)
Vestibular neuronitis 078.81 —386.1*
(L-00004)

E-39 DISEASES OF POSSIBLE VIRAL ORIGIN — Continued

DE-39030 (cont.) Epidemic neurolabyrinthitis 078.81 —386.1*
(L-00004)

DE-39040 Hemorrhagic nephroso-nephritis 078.6 —581.8*
(L-00004)
Hemorrhagic fever with renal syndrome 078.6 —581.8*
(L-00004)
Epidemic hemorrhagic fever 078.6 —581.8*
(L-00004)
Korean hemorrhagic fever 078.6 —581.8*
(L-00004)
Russian hemorrhagic fever 078.6 —581.8*
(L-00004)

DE-39050 Encephalitis lethargica 049.8 —323.4*
(T-A0100) (L-30000)
Von Economo's disease 049.8 —323.4*
(T-A0100) (L-30000)
Epidemic encephalitis 049.8 —323.4*
(T-A0100) (L-30000)
Acute inclusion body encephalitis 049.8 —323.4*
(T-A0100) (L-30000)

DE-39058 Acute necrotizing encephalitis, NEC 049.8 —323.4*
(T-A0100) (L-30000)

DE-39060 Erythema infectiosum 057.0
(T-01000) (L-38811)
Fifth disease 057.0
(T-01000) (L-38811)
Erythema contagiosum 057.0
(T-01000) (L-38811)

DE-39070 Infectious lymphocytosis 078.89
(L-30000)

DE-39080 Viral hepatitis, non-A, non-B 070.5 —573.1*
(T-62000) (L-38801)

DE-39100 Rubeola scarlatinosa 057.8
(L-30000)
Rubella scarlatiniforma 057.8
(L-30000)
Fourth disease 057.8
(L-30000)

DE-39110 Dukes (Filatow) disease 057.8
(L-30000)
Parascarlatina 057.8
(L-30000)
Pseudoscarlatina 057.8
(L-30000)

E-3B0 Prion Diseases

DE-3B000 Prion disease, NOS
(L-30100)

DE-3B010 Kuru 046.0 —323.0*
(T-A0100) (L-30120)

DE-3B020 Jakob-Creutzfeld disease 046.1 —331.5*
(T-A0100) (L-30110)
Creutzfeld-Jakob disease 046.1 —331.5*
(T-A0100) (L-30110)
Subacute spongiform encephalopathy 046.1 —331.5*
(T-A0100) (L-30110)

DE-3B030 Gerstmann-Straussler-Scheinker syndrome
(L-30100)

DE-3B040 Fatal familial insomnia
(L-30100)

DE-3B100V Scrapie
(L-30102)

DE-3B110V Transmissible mink encephalopathy
(L-30100)
TEM

DE-3B120V Bovine spongiform encephalopathy
(L-30106)
BSE
(L-30106)

DE-3B130V Chronic wasting disease of captive mule, deer and elk
(L-30102)

SECTION E-4 MYCOSES

E-400 Mycoses: General Terms

DE-40000 Mycosis, NOS 117.9
(L-40000)
Disease caused by fungus, NOS 117.9
(L-40000)
Fungal infectious disease, NOS 117.9
(L-40000)
Fungus infection, NOS 117.9
(L-40000)

DE-40004 Allergy-sensitivity to fungi syndrome
(T-01000) (F-C3000) (L-40000)
Dermatophytid
(T-01000) (F-C3000) (L-40000)
Dermaphytid
(T-01000) (F-C3000) (L-40000)
Epidermophytid
(T-01000) (F-C3000) (L-40000)

DE-40010 Opportunistic mycosis, NOS 118.0
(L-40000)

DE-40020 Systemic mycosis, NOS
(T-D0010) (L-40000)

DE-40022 Pneumonia in systemic mycosis, NOS 484.7
(T-28000) (M-40000)

DE-40030 Otomycosis, NOS 111.9
(T-AB200) (L-40000)

DE-40031 Chronic mycotic otitis externa 380.15
(T-AB100) (L-40000)

DE-40036V Guttural pouch mycosis, NOS
(T-AB650) (L-40000)

DE-40040 Dermal mycosis, NOS
(T-01000) (L-40000)
Cutaneous mycosis, NOS
(T-01000) (L-40000)
DE-40050 Mycotic pericarditis, NOS 117.9
(T-39000) (L-40000)
DE-40060V Mycotic abortion
(L-40000)
DE-40070V Crop mycosis
(L-40000)

E-402 Aspergillosis

DE-40200 Aspergillosis, NOS 117.3
(L-44130)
DE-40210 Disseminated aspergillosis 117.3
(T-D0010) (L-44130)
DE-40220V Cutaneous aspergillosis
(T-01000) (L-44130)
DE-40230 Pulmonary aspergillosis 117.3
(T-28000) (L-44130)
DE-40231 Invasive pulmonary aspergillosis 117.3
(T-28000) (L-44130)
DE-40232 Pneumonia in aspergillosis 484.6
(T-28000) (M-40000)
DE-40234V Brooder pneumonia
(T-28850) (L-44136)
DE-40241 Infection by Aspergillus fumigatus 117.3
(L-44136)
DE-40242 Infection by Aspergillus nidulans 117.3
(L-44138)
DE-40243 Infection by Aspergillus niger 117.3
(L-44139)
DE-40244 Infection by Aspergillus flavus 117.3
(L-44135)
DE-40245 Infection by Aspergillus clavatus 117.3
(L-44133)
DE-40250V Equine gutturomycosis
(T-AB650) (L-44136)

E-404 Blastomycosis

DE-40400 Blastomycosis, NOS 116.-
(L-44170)
Infection by Blastomyces, NOS 116.-
(L-44170)
Blastomycotic infection, NOS 116.-
(L-44170)
DE-40410 North American blastomycosis 116.0
(L-44171)
Gilchrist's disease 116.0
(L-44171)
Infection by Blastomyces dermatitidis 116.0
(L-44171)
Chicago disease 116.0
(L-44171)
DE-40411 North American cutaneous blastomycosis 116.0
(T-01000) (L-44171)
North American blastomyycotic dermatitis 116.0
(T-01000) (L-44171)
DE-40412 North American pulmonary blastomycosis 116.0
(T-28000) (L-44171)
North American primary pulmonary blastomycosis 116.0
(T-28000) (L-44171)
DE-40414 North American ocular blastomycosis 116.0
(T-AA000) (L-44171)
DE-40416 North American urogenital blastomycosis 116.0
(T-70200) (L-44171)
DE-40419 North American disseminated blastomycosis 116.0
(T-D0010) (L-44171)

E-405 Paracoccidioidomycosis

DE-40500 Paracoccidioidomycosis 116.1
(L-44301)
South American blastomycosis 116.1
(L-44301)
Infection by Blastomyces brasiliensis 116.1
(L-44301)
Infection by Paracoccidioides brasiliensis 116.1
(L-44301)
Brazilian blastomycosis 116.1
(L-44301)
Lutz-Splendore-Almeida disease 116.1
(L-44301)
DE-40511 South American cutaneous blastomycosis 116.1
(T-01000) (L-44301)
DE-40512 South American oral blastomycosis 116.1
(T-51000) (L-44301)
DE-40513 South American visceral blastomycosis 116.1
(T-D4030) (L-44301)
Visceral paracoccidioidomycosis 116.1
(T-D4030) (L-44301)
DE-40514 South American lymphatic blastomycosis 116.1
(T-C6000) (L-44301)
DE-40515 Mucocutaneous-lymphangitic paracoccidioidomycosis 116.1
(T-00400) (T-01000) (T-C6000)
(L-44301)
DE-40516 Pulmonary paracoccidioidomycosis 116.1
(T-28000) (L-44301)
DE-40517 South American disseminated blastomycosis 116.1
(T-D0010) (L-44301)
DE-40550 Lobomycosis 116.2
(L-44511)
Keloidal blastomycosis 116.2
(L-44511)
Lobo's disease 116.2
(L-44511)
Infection by Paracoccidioides loboii 116.2
(L-44511)

E-405 Paracoccidioidomycosis — Continued

DE-40550 (cont.) Infection by Loboa loboii 116.2
(L-44511)

E-406 Coccidioidomycosis

DE-40600 Coccidioidomycosis, NOS 114.9
(L-44181)
Infection by Coccidioides immitis 114.9
(L-44181)
Posadas-Wernicke disease 114.9
(L-44181)

DE-40601 Disseminated coccidioidomycosis 114.3
(L-44181)

DE-40610 Primary pulmonary coccidioidomycosis 114.0
(T-28000) (L-44181)
San Joaquin Valley fever 114.0
(T-28000) (L-44181)
Coccidioidal pneumonitis 114.0
(T-28000) (L-44181)
Coccidioidomycotic pneumonitis 114.0
(T-28000) (L-44181)
Desert rheumatism 114.0
(T-28000) (L-44181)

DE-40611 Coccidioidal granuloma 114.3
(L-44181) (M-44000)

DE-40620 Primary extrapulmonary coccidioidomycosisis 114.1
(L-44181)

DE-40621 Primary cutaneous coccidioidomycosis 114.1
(T-01000) (L-44181)

DE-40622 Coccidioidomycosis with erythema nodosum 114.1
(T-01000) (L-44181)

DE-40623 Coccidioidomycosis with erythema multiforme 114.1
(T-01000) (L-44181)

DE-40624 Chancriform syndrome 114.1
(T-01000) (L-44181)

DE-40625 Coccidioidal meningitis 114.2
(T-A1110) (L-44181)

E-407 Histoplasmosis

DE-40700 Histoplasmosis, NOS 115.9
(L-44220)

DE-40710 African histoplasmosis 115.1
(L-44222)
Infection by Histoplasma duboisii 115.1
(L-44222)
Large form histoplasmosis 115.1
(L-44222)

DE-40720 American histoplasmosis 115.0
(L-44221)
Infection by Histoplasma capsulatum 115.0
(L-44221)
Darling's disease 115.0
(L-44221)
Small form histoplasmosis 115.0
(L-44221)

DE-40721 Reticuloendothelial cytomycosis 115.0
(L-44221)

DE-40722 American histoplasmosis with meningitis 115.01
(T-A1110) (M-40000) (L-44221)

DE-40723 American histoplasmosis with retinitis 115.02
(T-AA610) (M-40000) (L-44221)

DE-40724 American histoplasmosis with pericarditis 115.03
(T-39000) (M-40000) (L-44221)

DE-40725 American histoplasmosis with endocarditis 115.04
(T-32060) (M-40000) (L-44221)

DE-40726 American histoplasmosis with pneumonia 115.05
(T-28000) (M-40000) (L-44221)

DE-40730V Epizootic lymphadenitis
(L-44223)
Infection by Histoplasma farciminosus
(L-44223)

E-410 Candidiasis

DE-41000 Candidiasis, NOS 112.9
(L-43130)
Moniliasis, NOS 112.9
(L-43130)
Candidosis, NOS 112.9
(L-43130)
Infection by Candida species 112.9
(L-43130)

DE-41002 Disseminated candidiasis 112.5
(T-D0010) (L-43130)
Systemic candidiasis 112.5
(T-D0010) (L-43130)

DE-41010 Infection by Candida albicans 112.9
(L-43131)

DE-41011 Neonatal monilia infection 771.7
(L-43131)
Neonatal moniliasis 771.7
(L-43131)

DE-41012 Candidiasis of mouth 112.0
(T-51030) (L-43131)
Thrush 112.0
(T-51030) (L-43131)
Mycotic stomatitis
(T-51030) (L-43131)

DE-41013 Neonatal trush 771.7

DE-41021 Candidiasis of vulva 112.1 —616.1*
(T-81000) (L-43131)

DE-41022 Candidiasis of vagina 112.1 —616.1*
(T-82000) (L-43131)

DE-41023 Candidal vulvovaginitis 112.1 —616.1*
(T-81000) (T-82000) (L-43131)
Monilial vulvovaginitis 112.1 —616.1*
(T-81000) (T-82000) (L-43131)

DE-41025 Candidal balanitis 112.2
(T-91300) (L-43131)
DE-41029 Candidiasis of other urogenital sites 112.2
(T-.....) (L-43131)
DE-41031 Candidiasis of skin 112.3
(T-01000) (L-43131)
DE-41032 Candidiasis of nails 112.3
(T-01600) (L-43131)
DE-41033 Candidal intertrigo 112.3
(T-D8860) (L-43131)
Interdigital moniliasis 112.3
(T-D8860) (L-43131)
Erosio interdigitalis blastomycetica 112.3
(T-D8860) (L-43131)
DE-41034 Candidal paronychia 112.3
(T-01600) (L-43131)
Candidal onychia 112.3
(T-01600) (L-43131)
Candidal perionyxis 112.3
(T-01600) (L-43131)
DE-41038 Perleche with candidiasis 112.0
(T-52002) (L-43131)
DE-41039 Mucocutaneous candidiasis 112.3
(T-00400) (T-01000) (L-43131)
DE-41051 Candidiasis of lung 112.4 —484.7*
(T-28000) (L-43131)
Candidal pneumonia 112.4
(T-28000) (L-43131)
DE-41052 Candidal endocarditis 112.81 —421.1*
(T-32060) (L-43131)
DE-41053 Candidal otitis externa 112.82
(T-AB100) (L-43131)
Otomycosis in moniliasis 112.82
(T-AB100) (L-43131)
DE-41055 Candidal meningitis 112.83
(T-A1110) (L-43131)
DE-41069 Candidiasis of other specified sites 112.89
(T-.....) (L-43131)

E-412 Cryptococcosis

DE-41200 Cryptococcosis, NOS 117.5
(L-43165)
Torula 117.5
(L-43165)
European Blastomycosis 117.5
(L-43165)
Torulosis 117.5
(L-43165)
Infection by Cryptococcus neoformans 117.5
(L-43165)
DE-41202 Disseminated cryptococcosis 117.5
(T-D0010) (L-43165)
Systemic cryptococcosis 117.5
(T-D0010) (L-43165)
DE-41210 Pulmonary cryptococcosis 117.5
(T-28000) (L-43165)
DE-41231 Cryptococcal meningitis 117.5 —321.0*
(T-A1110) (L-43165)
DE-41241 Mucocutaneous cryptococcosis 117.5
(T-00400) (T-01000) (L-43165)
DE-41251 Osseous cryptococcosis
(T-11000) (L-43165)
Busse-Buschke's disease 117.5
(T-11000) (L-43165)

E-413 Geotrichosis

DE-41300 Geotrichosis 117.9
(L-43180)
Infection by Geotrichum, NOS 117.9
(L-43180)
DE-41310 Infection by Geotrichum candidum 117.9
(L-43181)

E-421 Chromomycosis

DE-42100 Chromomycosis 117.2
(L-45150) (L-45320)
Chromoblastomycosis 117.2
(L-45150) (L-45320)
Mossy foot disease 117.2
(L-45150) (L-45320)
DE-42105 Systemic chromomycosis 117.2
(T-D0010) (L-45150) (L-45320)
DE-42110 Cutaneous chromomycosis 117.2
(T-01000) (L-45150) (L-45320)
DE-42111 Infection by Phialophora verrucosa 117.2
(L-45325)
DE-42112 Infection by Fonsecaea pedrosoi 117.2
(L-45222)
DE-42113 Infection by Fonsecaea compacta 117.2
(L-45221)
DE-42114 Infection by Cladosporium carrionii 117.2
(L-45132)
DE-42115 Infection by Acrotheca aquaspersa 117.2
(L-45341)

E-430 Mycotic Mycetoma

DE-43000 Mycotic mycetoma 117.4
(T-D9700) (L-4....)
Mycotic madura foot 117.4
(T-D9700) (L-4....)
Mycotic maduromycosis 117.4
(T-D9700) (L-4....)
Eumycetoma 117.4
(T-D9700) (L-4....)
DE-43010 Infection by Ascomycetes 117.4
(L-41000)
DE-43020 Infection by Deuteromycetes 117.4
(L-43000)
DE-43031 Infection by Acremonium falciforme 117.4
(L-44101)
Infection by Cephalosporium falciforme 117.4
(L-44101)

E-430 Mycotic Mycetoma — Continued

DE-43032 Infection by Cephalosporium recifei 117.4
(L-44102)

DE-43033 Infection by Neotestudina rosatii 117.4
(L-41231)

DE-43034 Infection by Madurella grisea 117.4
(L-45291)

DE-43035 Infection by Madurella mycetomii 117.4
(L-45292)

DE-43036 Infection by Pyrenochaeta romeroi 117.4
(L-46012)

DE-43037 Infection by Leptosphaeria senegalensis 117.4
(L-41211)

E-431 Allescheriosis

DE-43100 Allescheriosis 117.6
(L-41241)
Allescheriasis 117.6
(L-41241)
Petriellidosis 117.6
(L-41241)
Infection by Allescheria boydii 117.6
(L-41241)
Infection by Petriellidium boydii 117.6
(L-41241)

DE-43101 Infection by Monosporium apiospermum 117.6
(L-45371)

E-432 Adiaspiromycosis

DE-43200 Adiaspiromycosis 136.8
(T-28000) (L-44122)
Adiaspirosis
(T-28000) (L-44122)
Haplosporangiosis
(T-28000) (L-44122)

DE-43210 Adiaspiromycosis due to Emmonsia crescens 136.8
(T-28000) (L-44122)

DE-43211 Pulmonary adiaspiromycosis
(T-28000) (L-44122)

DE-43220V Adiaspiromycosis due to Emmonsia parva 136.8
(T-28000) (L-44121)

E-433 Zygomycosis

DE-43300 Zygomycosis 117.7
(L-40100)
Phycomycosis 117.7
(L-40100)

DE-43310 Mucormycosis 117.7
(L-40150)

DE-43321 Infection by Absidia, NOS 117.7
(L-40120)

DE-43322 Infection by Basidiobolus, NOS 117.7
(L-40800)

DE-43323 Infection by Conidiobolus, NOS 117.7
(L-40820)
Infection by Entomophthora, NOS 117.7
(L-40820)

DE-43324 Infection by Cunninghamella, NOS 117.7
(L-40200)

DE-43326 Infection by Mucor, NOS 117.7
(L-40150)

DE-43327 Infection by Rhizopus, NOS 117.7
(L-40180)

DE-43328 Infection by Saksenaea, NOS 117.7
(L-40220)

DE-43331 Rhinophycomycosis due to Entomophthora coronata 117.7
(T-21000) (L-40821)

DE-43332 Subcutaneous phycomycosis due to Basidiobolus, NOS 117.7
(T-03000) (L-40800)

DE-43335V Mortierellosis
(L-40300)

DE-43336V Infection by Mortierella wolfii
(L-40301)

E-435 Phaeohyphomycosis

DE-43500 Phaeohyphomycosis, NOS 117.8
(L-45100)
Infection by dematiaceous fungi, NOS 117.8
(L-45100)

DE-43510 Cladosporiosis 117.8
(L-45161)
Infection by Cladosporium trichoides 117.8
(L-45161)

DE-43520 Infection by Drechlera hawaiiensis 117.8
(L-45182)

DE-43521 Infection by Phialophora gougerotii 117.8
(L-45241)
Infection by Phialophora jeanselmei 117.8
(L-45241)

E-436 Rhinosporidiosis

DE-43600 Rhinosporidiosis 117.0
(L-49091)
Rhinosporosis 117.0
(L-49091)
Infection by Rhinosporidium seeberi 117.0
(L-49091)

E-437 Sporotrichosis

DE-43700 Sporotrichosis 117.1
(L-45402)
Infection by Sporothrix schenkii 117.1
(L-45402)

DE-43701 Disseminated sporotrichosis 117.1
(T-D0010) (L-45402)

DE-43710 Cutaneous sporotrichosis 117.1
(T-01000) (L-45402)

DE-43712 Lymphocutaneous sporotrichosis 117.1
(T-C4000) (L-45402)

DE-43720 Pulmonary sporotrichosis 117.1
(T-28000) (L-45402)

DE-43730 Sporotrichosis of the bones 117.1
(T-11000) (L-45402)

DE-43750 Acladiosis 111.8
(L-45431)
Dermatomycosis by Acladium castellani 111.8
(L-45431)

E-45 DERMATOPHYTOSES

DE-45000 Dermatophytosis 110.9
(T-01000) (L-4....)
Tinea, NOS 110.9
(T-01000) (L-4....)
Ringworm, NOS 110.9
(T-01000) (L-4....)
Dermatomycosis 110.9
(T-01000) (L-4....)
Superficial mycosis 110.9
(T-01000) (L-4....)
Microsporic tinea, NOS 110.9
(T-01000) (L-4....)

DE-45001 Granulomatous dermatophytosis 110.6
(T-01000) (M-44000) (L-4....)

DE-45002 Disseminated dermatophytosis 110.6
(T-D0010) (L-4....)

DE-45010 Tinea barbae 110.0
(T-01000) (T-D1200) (L-44250) (L-44360)
Tinea sycosis 110.0
(T-01000) (T-D1200) (L-44250) (L-44360)
Barbers' itch
(T-01000) (T-D1200) (L-44250) (L-44360)

DE-45020 Tinea barbae due to Microsporum, NOS 110.0
(T-01000) (T-D1200) (L-44250)

DE-45021 Tinea barbae due to Microsporum canis 110.0
(T-01000) (T-D1200) (L-44252)

DE-45022 Tinea barbae due to Microsporum gypseum 110.0
(T-01000) (T-D1200) (L-44258)

DE-45030 Tinea barbae due to Trichophyton, NOS 110.0
(T-01000) (T-D1200) (L-44360)

DE-45031 Tinea barbae due to Trichophyton mentagrophytes 110.0
(T-01000) (T-D1200) (L-44366)

DE-45032 Tinea barbae due to Trichophyton verrucosum 110.0
(T-01000) (T-D1200) (L-44378)

DE-45033 Tinea barbae due to Trichophyton violaceum 110.0
(T-01000) (T-D1200) (L-44383)

DE-45100 Tinea capitis 110.0
(T-D1160) (L-44250) (L-44360)
Ringworm of the scalp 110.0
(T-D1160) (L-44250) (L-44360)

DE-45110 Tinea capitis due to Microsporum, NOS 110.0
(T-D1160) (L-44250)

DE-45120 Tinea capitis due to Trichophyton, NOS 110.0
(T-D1160) (L-44360)

DE-45121 Tinea capitis due to Trichophyton tonsurans 110.0
(T-D1160) (L-44375)

DE-45150 Tinea kerion 110.0
(L-44250) (L-44360)
Kerion 110.0
(L-44250) (L-44360)
Kerion celsi 110.0
(L-44250) (L-44360)

DE-45160 Kerion due to Microsporum, NOS 110.0
(L-44250)

DE-45162 Kerion due to Trichophyton, NOS 110.0
(L-44360)

DE-45200 Tinea corporis 110.5
(T-01000) (T-01400) (L-44250) (L-44360)
Tinea circinata 110.5
(T-01000) (T-01400) (L-44250) (L-44360)
Herpes circinatus 110.5
(T-01000) (T-01400) (L-44250) (L-44360)

DE-45210 Tinea corporis due to Microsporum, NOS 110.5
(L-44250)

DE-45220 Tinea corporis due to Trichophyton, NOS 110.5
(L-44360)

DE-45250 Tinea profunda 110.6
(L-44250) (L-44360)
Deep seated dermatophytosis 110.6
(L-44250) (L-44360)
Granuloma trichophyticum 110.6
(L-44250) (L-44360)
Majocchi's granuloma 110.6
(L-44250) (L-44360)

DE-45300 Tinea imbricata 110.5
(L-44361)
Tokelau 110.5
(L-44361)
Tinea due to Trichophyton concentricum 110.5
(L-44361)

DE-45400 Tinea cruris 110.3
(T-01000) (T-D7000) (L-44372) (L-44201)
Tinea inguinalis 110.3
(T-01000) (T-D7000) (L-44372) (L-44201)

E-45 DERMATOPHYTOSES — Continued

DE-45400 (cont.) Eczema marginatum 110.3
(T-01000) (T-D7000) (L-44372) (L-44201)
Tinea of groin 110.3
(T-01000) (T-D7000) (L-44372) (L-44201)
Tinea of perianal region 110.3
(T-01000) (T-D7000) (L-44372) (L-44201)
Dhobie itch 110.3
(T-01000) (T-D7000) (L-44372) (L-44201)
Jock itch
(T-01000) (T-D7000) (L-44372) (L-44201)

DE-45411 Tinea cruris due to Trichophyton rubrum 110.3
(T-01000) (T-D7000) (L-44372)

DE-45421 Tinea cruris due to Epidermophyton floccosum 110.3
(T-01000) (T-D7000) (L-44201)

DE-45500 Tinea favosa 110.0
(L-44373)
Favus 110.0
(L-44373)
Favus capitis 110.0
(L-44373)

DE-45510 Favus due to Trichophyton schoenleinii 110.0
(L-44373)

DE-45520V Favus due to Trichophyton gallinae
(L-44257)
Honeycomb ringworm
(L-44257)

DE-45600 Tinea nigra 111.1
(L-45244)
Infection by Cladosporium werneckii 111.1
(L-45244)
Keratomycosis nigricans palmaris 111.1
(L-45244)
Microsporosis nigra 111.1
(L-45244)
Pityriasis nigra 111.1
(L-45244)
Tinea palmaris nigra 111.1
(L-45244)

DE-45650 Black piedra 111.3
(L-41281)
Piedra due to Piedraia hortae 111.3
(L-41281)

DE-45680 White piedra 111.2
(L-43231)
Tinea blanca 111.2
(L-43231)
Piedra due to Trichosporon cutaneum 111.2
(L-43231)

DE-45700 Tinea pedis 110.4
(T-D9700) (L-44360) (L-44200)
Epidermophytosis pedis 110.4
(T-D9700) (L-44360) (L-44200)
Athlete's foot 110.4
(T-D9700) (L-44360) (L-44200)

DE-45710 Tinea pedis due to Trichophyton, NOS 110.4
(T-D9700) (L-44360)

DE-45720 Tinea pedis due to Epidermophyton, NOS 110.4
(T-D9700) (L-44200)

DE-45721 Tinea pedis due to Epidermophyton floccosum 110.4
(T-D9700) (L-44201)

DE-45740 Tinea manus 110.2
(T-D8700) (L-44360)
Tinea manuum 110.2
(T-D8700) (L-44360)

DE-45750 Tinea unguium 110.1
(T-01600) (L-44360) (L-44200)
Onychomycosis 110.1
(T-01600) (L-44360) (L-44200)
Dermatophytic onychia 110.1
(T-01600) (L-44360) (L-44200)

DE-45761 Onychomycosis due to Trichophyton rubrum 110.1
(T-01600) (L-44372)

DE-45762 Onychomycosis due to Trichophyton mentagrophytes 110.1
(T-01600) (L-44367)

DE-45771 Onychomycosis due to Epidermophyton floccosum 110.1
(T-01600) (L-44201)

DE-45800 Pityriasis versicolor 111.0
(L-43201)
Tinea versicolor 111.0
(L-43201)
Tinea flava 111.0
(L-43201)
Tinea versicolor due to Pityrosporum furfur 111.0
(L-43201)
Tinea versicolor due to Malassezia furfur 111.0
(L-43201)

DE-45850 Verrucous mycosis 111.8
(L-44501)
Infection by Cercospora apii 111.8
(L-44501)

E-480 Fusarium Infections

DE-48000 Fusarium infection, NOS
(L-45900)

DE-48010 Kashin-Bek disease 716.0
(T-15000) (L-45905)
Kaschin-Bek disease 716.0
(T-15000) (L-45905)

DE-48010 (cont.) Endemic generalized osteo-arthrosis 716.0
(T-15000) (L-45905)
Urov disease 716.0
(T-15000) (L-45905)
Infection by Fusarium sporotrichiella 716.0
(T-15000) (L-45905)
Endemic polyarthritis 716.0
(T-15000) (L-45905)

DE-48020 Otomycosis externa due to Fusarium, NOS
(T-AB100) (L-45900)

DE-48030 Mycotic keratitis due to Fusarium, NOS
(T-AA200) (L-45900)

DE-48031 Mycotic keratitis due to Fusarium oxysporum
(T-AA200) (L-45902)

DE-48032 Mycotic keratitis due to Fusarium solani
(T-AA200) (L-45903)

E-482 Miscellaneous Mycotic Infections

DE-48200V Dactylariosis
(L-45541)

DE-48210V Paecilomycosis
(L-44280)

DE-48211V Infection by Paecilomyces variotii
(L-44282)

SECTIONS E-5-7 PARASITIC DISEASES

SECTION E-5 PROTOZOAL INFECTIOUS DISEASES

E-500-501 Parasitic Diseases: General Terms

DE-50000 Disease caused by parasite, NOS 136.9
(L-50000)
Parasitic infectious disease, NOS 136.9
(L-50000)
Parasitic infection, NOS 136.9
(L-50000)
Parasite infestation, NOS 136.9
(L-50000)
Parasitic disease, NOS 136.9
(L-50000)
Parasitism, NOS 136.9
(L-50000)
Infestation, NOS 136.9
(L-50000)
Parasitosis, NOS
(L-50000)

DE-50008 Parasitic disease in mother complicating pregnancy, childbirth or puerperium, NOS 647.8

DE-50010 Intestinal parasitism, NOS 129.-
(T-50500) (L-50000)

DE-50020 Parasitic skin infestation, NOS 134.9
(T-01000) (L-50000)
Skin parasites, NOS 134.9
(T-01000) (L-50000)
Parasitic dermatitis 134.9
(T-01000) (L-50000)

DE-50030 Parasitic conjunctivitis, NOS 372.15
(T-AA860) (L-50000)

DE-50032 Parasitic infestation of orbit, NOS 376.13
(T-D1480) (L-50000)

DE-50040 Parasitic pericarditis, NOS
(T-39000) (L-50000)

DE-50100 Protozoal intestinal disease, NOS 007.9
(T-50500) (L-50001)
Protozoal diarrhea 007.9
(T-50500) (L-50001)
Protozoal dysentery, NOS 007.9
(T-50500) (L-50001)
Flagellate diarrhea, NOS 007.9
(T-50500) (L-50001)
Protozoal colitis, NOS 007.-
(T-59300) (L-50001)
Protozoosis, NOS
(L-50001)

DE-50108 Other protozoal intestinal disease, NEC 007.8
(T-50500) (L-50001)

DE-50110 Coccidiosis, NOS
(L-52500) (L-52600) (L-52870)
(L-52550) (L-52820)

DE-50120 Protozoan myocarditis, NOS 136.9
(T-32020) (L-50001)

DE-50130V Protozoal myelitis, NOS
(T-A7010) (L-50001)

E-502 Diseases Due to Endamoebidae

DE-50200 Amebiasis 006.9
(T-50500) (L-51511)
Amebic dysentery 006.9
(T-50500) (L-51511)
Infection due to Entamoeba histolytica, SAI 006.9
(T-50500) (L-51511)

DE-50210 Chronic amebiasis 006.1
(T-50500) (M-43000) (L-51511)
Chronic intestinal amebiasis without mention of abscess 006.1
(T-50500) (M-43000) (L-51511)
Chronic amebic dysentery 006.1
(T-50500) (M-43000) (L-51511)

DE-50211 Amebic nondysenteric colitis 006.2
(T-59300) (L-51511)

DE-50220 Acute amebiasis 006.0
(T-50500) (M-41000) (L-51511)
Acute amebic dysentery without mention of abscess 006.0
(T-50500) (L-51511)

DE-50230 Cutaneous amebiasis 006.6
(T-01000) (L-51511)
Amebic skin ulceration 006.6
(T-01000) (M-38000) (L-51511)

E-502 Diseases Due to Endamoebidae — Continued

DE-50251 Amebic liver abscess 006.3
(T-62000) (M-41610) (L-51511)

DE-50252 Amebic lung abscess 006.4
(T-28000) (M-41610) (L-51511)

DE-50253 Amebic brain abscess 006.5
(T-A0100) (M-41610) (L-51511)

DE-50254 Amebic appendicitis 006.8
(T-59200) (L-51511)

DE-50255 Amebic balanitis 006.8
(T-91300) (L-51511)

DE-50260 Amebic infection of other sites 006.8
(L-51511)

DE-50261 Ameboma 006.8
(M-44000) (L-51511)

DE-50270 Infection by Iodamoeba, NOS
(L-51570)
Iodamoebosis
(L-51570)

DE-50280 Infection by Entamoeba, NOS 136.2
(L-51510)
Entamoebosis 136.2
(L-51510)

DE-50281 Infection by Entamoeba coli 007.8
(L-51512)
Entamebiasis coli 007.8
(L-51512)
Entamoebosis coli 007.8
(L-51512)

DE-50290 Infection by Endolimax, NOS
(L-51590)
Endolimacosis
(L-51590)

E-505 Diseases Due to Balantidiidae

DE-50500 Balantidiasis 007.0
(L-53200)
Balantidiosis
(L-53200)

DE-50501 Infection by Balantidium coli 007.0
(L-53201)

E-507 Diseases Due to Chilomastigidae

DE-50700 Infection by Chilomastix, NOS 007.8
(L-50600)
Chilomastigiasis 007.8
(L-50600)

DE-50701 Infection by Chilomastix mesnili 007.8
(L-50601)

E-509 Diseases Due to Monocercomonadidae

DE-50900 Infection by Dientamoeba fragilis 007.8
(L-50811)
Dientamebal diarrhea 007.8
(L-50811)
Dientamoebosis 007.8
(L-50811)

DE-50920V Infection by Histomonas, NOS
(L-50800)
Histomoniasis
(L-50800)
Histomonosis
(L-50800)

DE-50922V Infectious enterohepatitis of turkeys
(L-50801)
Blackhead in turkeys
(L-50801)

E-510-511 Diseases Due to Eimeriidae

DE-51000 Isosporiasis 007.2
(L-52500)
Intestinal coccidiosis 007.2
(L-52500)
Isosporosis 007.2
(L-52500)
Human coccidiosis 077.2
(L-52500)

DE-51001 Infection by Isospora belli 007.2
(L-52501)

DE-51002 Infection by Isospora hominis 007.2
(L-52502)

DE-51100 Disease due to Eimeria, NOS
(L-52600)
Animal coccidiosis
(L-52600)
Eimeriosis
(L-52600)

DE-51110V Hepatic coccidiosis
(T-62000) (L-52724)

DE-51112V Renal coccidiosis
(T-71000) (L-52742)

E-512-517 Diseases Due to Sarcocystidae

DE-51200 Infection by Toxoplasma gondii 130.9
(L-52801)
Toxoplasmosis 130.9
(L-52801)

DE-51201 Multisystemic disseminated toxoplasmosis 130.8
(T-D0010) (L-52801)

DE-51202 Congenital toxoplasmosis 771.2
(L-52801) (DE-01900)

DE-51211 Focal chorioretinitis due to acquired toxoplasmosis 130.2 —363.0*
(T-AA610) (T-AA310) (M-40000)
(L-52801)

DE-51212 Hepatitis due to acquired toxoplasmosis 130.5 —573.2*
(T-62000) (M-40000) (L-52801)

DE-51213 Meningoencephalitis due to acquired toxoplasmosis 130.0 —323.4*
(T-A1110) (M-40000) (L-52801)

DE-51214 Myocarditis due to acquired toxoplasmosis 130.3 —422.0*
(T-32020) (M-40000) (L-52801)

DE-51215 Pneumonitis due to acquired toxoplasmosis 130.4 —484.8*
(T-28000) (M-40000) (L-52801)

DE-51216 Conjunctivitis due to acquired toxoplasmosis 130.1
(T-AA860) (M-40000) (L-52801)

DE-51228 Toxoplasmosis of other specified sites 130.7
(T-.....) (L-52801)

DE-51300V Infection by Cystoisospora, NOS
(L-52870)
Cystoisosporosis
(L-52870)

DE-51400 Sarcosporidiosis 136.5
(L-52840)
Sarcosporidiasis 136.5
(L-52840)
Sarcocystosis 136.5
(L-52840)
Sacocystiosis 136.5
(L-52840)

DE-51401 Infection by Sarcocystis lindemanni 136.5
(L-52854)

DE-51500 Infection by Besnoitia, NOS
(L-52820)
Besnoitiosis
(L-52820)

DE-51550 Infection by Hammondia, NOS
(L-52890)
Hammondiosis
(L-52890)

DE-51600 Infection by Frenkelia, NOS
(L-52880)
Frenkeliosis
(L-52880)

DE-51650 Infection by Tyzzeria, NOS
(L-52550)
Tyzzeriosis
(L-52550)

DE-51700 Infection by Caryospora, NOS
(L-52580)
Caryosporosis
(L-52580)

E-521 Diseases Due to Retortamonididae

DE-52100 Infection by Retortamonas intestinalis 007.8
(L-50621)
Embadomoniasis 007.8
(L-50621)
Retortamoniasis 007.8
(L-50621)

E-524 Diseases Due to Hexamitidae

DE-52400 Giardiasis 007.1
(L-50700)
Giardiosis 007.1
(L-50700)

DE-52401 Infection by Giardia lamblia 007.1
(L-50701)
Lambliasis 007.1
(L-50701)

DE-52420V Infection by Hexamita, NOS
(L-50720)
Hexamitosis
(L-50720)

DE-52430V Infection by Octomitus, NOS
(L-50730)
Octomitosis
(L-50730)

E-526 Diseases Due to Acanthamoebidae

DE-52600 Infection by Acanthoamoeba, NOS 136.2
(T-A1110) (T-A0100) (L-51700)
Primary amebic meningoencephalitis 136.2 —323.4*
(T-A1110) (T-A0100) (L-51700)
Acanthamoebiasis
(T-A1110) (T-A0100) (L-51700)
Acanthamoebosis
(L-51700)

DE-52610 Infection by Acanthamoeba castellani 136.2
(L-51702)

E-527 Diseases Due to Hartmannellidae

DE-52700 Infection by Hartmannella, NOS 136.2
(L-51800)
Hartmannellosis, NOS
(L-51800)

E-528 Diseases Due to Vahlkampfiidae

DE-52800 Infection by Naegleria, NOS 136.2 —323.4*
(L-51900)
Naegleriosis
(L-51900)

DE-52810 Infection by Naegleria gruberi 136.2 —323.4*
(L-51902)

DE-52820 Meningoencephalitis due to Naegleria 136.2 —323.4*
(T-A1110) (T-A0100) (L-51900)

DE-52830V Infection by Vahlkampfia, NOS
(L-51930)
Vahlkampfiosis
(L-51930)

E-531 Diseases Due to Trichomonadidae

DE-53100 Infection by Trichomonas, NOS 131.9
(T-50500) (L-50900)
Trichomoniasis 131.9
(T-50500) (L-50900)
Trichomonosis 131.9
(T-50500) (L-50900)

DE-53110 Intestinal infection by Trichomonas vaginalis 007.3
(T-50500) (L-50901)
Intestinal trichomoniasis 007.3
(T-50500) (L-50900)

DE-53120 Urogenital infection by Trichomonas vaginalis 131.00
(T-70200) (L-50901)
Urogenital trichomoniasis 131.00
(T-70200) (L-50901)

DE-53121 Trichomonal urethritis 131.02 —597.8*
(T-75000) (M-40000) (L-50901)

DE-53122 Trichomonal prostatitis 131.03 —601.4*
(T-92000) (M-40000) (L-50901)

DE-53130 Vaginal trichomoniasis 131.01
(T-82000) (L-50901)
Trichomonal fluor vaginalis 131.00
(T-82000) (L-50901)
Trichomonal leukorrhea vaginalis 131.00
(T-82000) (L-50901)
Trichomonal vaginitis 131.01 —616.1*
(T-82000) (M-40000) (L-50901)

DE-53131 Trichomonal vulvovaginitis 130.01 —616.1*
(T-81000) (T-82000) (M-40000)
(L-50901)

DE-53148 Trichomoniasis of other sites 131.8
(T-.....) (L-50901)

DE-53150V Avian trichomoniasis
(L-50904)
Infection by Trichomonas gallinae
(L-50904)
Avian canker
(L-50904)
Roup
(L-50904)
Frounce
(L-53152)

DE-53160V Infection by Tritrichomonas, NOS
(L-50920)
Tritrichomonosis
(L-50920)

DE-53161V Urogenital infection by Tritrichomonas foetus
(T-70200) (L-50921)
Bovine tritrichomonosis
(L-70200) (L-50921)

E-540 Diseases Due to Plasmodiidae

DE-54000 Malaria, NOS 084.6
(L-52900)
Paludism 084.6
(L-52900)
Plasmodiosis 084.6
(L-52900)

DE-54001 Congenital malaria 771.2
(L-52900) (DE-01900)

DE-54008 Malaria in mother complicating pregnancy, childbirth or puerperium, NOS 647.4

DE-54010 Falciparum malaria 084.0
(L-52901)
Malignant tertian malaria 084.0
(L-52901)
Malaria by Plasmodium falciparum 084.0
(L-52901)
Subtertian malaria 084.0
(L-52901)

DE-54013 Algid malaria 084.9
(T-50500) (L-52901)

DE-54014 Cerebral malaria 084.9
(T-A0100) (L-52901)

DE-54015 Malarial hepatitis 084.9 —573.2*
(T-62000) (L-52901)

DE-54017 Black water fever 084.8
(L-52901) (F-03003)
Malarial hemoglobinuria 084.8
(L-52901) (F-03003)
Hemoglobinuric fever 084.8
(L-52901) (F-03003)

DE-54030 Vivax malaria 084.1
(L-52904)
Benign tertian malaria 084.1
(L-52904)
Malaria by Plasmodium vivax 084.1
(L-52904)

DE-54050 Quartan malaria 084.2
(L-52902)
Malaria by Plasmodium malariae 084.2
(L-52902)
Malariae malaria 084.2
(L-52902)

DE-54051 Malarial nephrosis 084.9 —581.8*
(T-71000) (L-52901)

DE-54060 Ovale malaria 084.3
(L-52903)
Malaria by Plasmodium ovale 084.3
(L-52903)

DE-54070 Other malaria 084.4
(L-52900)

DE-54071 Simian malaria 084.4
(L-52917)
Malaria due to simian plasmodia
(L-52917)

DE-54072 Mixed malaria 084.5
(L-529..)
Malaria by more than one parasite 084.5
(L-529..)

DE-54080 Induced malaria 084.7
(L-52900)

DE-54081 Therapeutically induced malaria 084.7
(L-52900)

DE-54090V Infection by Cytauxzoon, NOS
(L-52960)
Cytauxzoonosis
(L-52960)

DE-54091V Infection by Cytauxzoon felis
(L-55961) (L-66000)
Feline cytauxzoonosis
(L-55961) (L-66000)

DE-54095V Avian malaria
(L-52900)

DE-54098V Infection by Leucocytozoon, NOS
(L-52A00)
Leucocytozoonosis
(L-52A00)

DE-54099V Infection by Haemoproteus, NOS
(L-52980)
Haemoproteosis
(L-52980)

E-541 Diseases Due to Adeleidae

DE-54100V Infection by Klossiella, NOS
(L-52060)
Klossiellosis
(L-52060)

E-542 Diseases Due to Haemogregarinidae

DE-54200V Infection by Hepatozoon, NOS
(L-52120)
Hepatozoonosis
(L-52120)

DE-54201V Infection by Hepatozoon canis
(L-52121) (L-66131)

E-543-544 Diseases Due to Babesiidae

DE-54300 Babesiosis 084.4
(L-52B00)
Piroplasmosis 084.4
(L-52B00)
Infection by Babesia, NOS 084.4
(L-52B00)

DE-54301 Infection by Babesia bovis 084.4
(L-52B01)

DE-54302 Infection by Babesia microti 084.4
(L-52B02)

DE-54303 Infection by Babesia divergens
(L-52B06)

DE-54310V Infection by Babesia bigemina
(L-52B03)
Bovine babesiosis
(L-52B03)
Bovine tick fever
(L-52B03)
Red water fever
(L-52B03)
Texas fever
(L-52B03)

DE-54312V Infection by Babesia equi
(L-52B07)
Equine babesiosis
(L-52B07)

DE-54314V Infection by Babesia canis
(L-52B05)
Canine babesiosis
(L-52B05)

DE-54400 Intraerythrocytic parasitosis by Nuttallia, NOS
(L-52B00)

DE-54450 Intraerythrocytic parasitosis by Entopolypoides, NOS
(L-52B50)

E-546 Diseases Due to Theileriidae

DE-54600V Infection by Theileria, NOS
(L-52C00)
Theileriosis
(L-52C00)

DE-54601V Infection by Theileria parva
(L-52C02) (L-66133)
East Coast fever
(L-52C02) (L-66133)
Turning disease
(L-52C02) (L-66133)
Turning sickness
(L-52C02) (L-66133)

DE-54602V Infection by Theileria lawrenci
(L-52C04) (L-66133)
Buffalo disease
(L-52C04) (L-66133)
Corridor disease
(L-52C04) (L-66133)

DE-54606V Infection by Theileria annulata
(L-52C08) (L-66170)
Tropical theileriosis
(L-52C08) (L-66170)

DE-54608V Infection by Theileria mutans
(L-52C05) (L-66133)
Tzaneen disease
(L-52C05) (L-66133)

DE-54620V Infection by Haematoxenus, NOS
(L-52C20)
Haematoxenosis
(L-52C20)

E-548 Diseases Due to Cryptosporidiidae

DE-54800 Infection by Cryptosporidium, NOS
(L-52400)
Cryptosporidiosis
(L-52400)

DE-54810V Infection by Cryptosporidium muris
(L-52401)

DE-54811V Infection by Cryptosporidium crotalis
(L-52406)

DE-54812V Infection by Cryptosporidium meleagridis
(L-52405)

E-548 Diseases Due to Cryptosporidiidae — Continued

DE-54813V Infection by Cryptosporidium parvum
(L-52408)

DE-54814V Infection by Cryptosporidium nasorum
(L-52407)

E-550-555 Diseases Due to Trypanosomatidae

DE-55000 Trypanosomiasis 086.9
(L-50400)
Trypanosomosis
(L-50400)

DE-55011 Trypanosomiasis with encephalitis 086.-
—323.2*
(T-A0100) (M-40000) (L-50400)

DE-55012 Trypanosomiasis with meningitis 086.-
—321.3*
(T-A1110) (M-40000) (L-50400)

DE-55020 Infection by Trypanosoma cruzi 086.2
(L-50405) (L-61300)
American trypanosomiasis 086.2
(L-50405) (L-61300)
Chagas' disease 086.2
(L-50405) (L-61300)
South American trypanosomiasis 086.2
(L-50405) (L-61300)

DE-55021 Chagas' disease without mention of organ involvement 086.2
(L-50405) (L-61300)

DE-55022 Chagas' disease with heart involvement 086.0 —425.6*
(T-32000) (L-50405) (L-61300)

DE-55028 Chagas' disease with other organ involvement 086.1
(T-.....) (L-50405) (L-61300)

DE-55030 African trypanosomiasis 086.5
(L-50402) (L-50403) (L-63800)
African sleeping sickness 086.5
(L-50402) (L-50403) (L-63800)
Sleeping sickness, NOS 086.5
(L-50402) (L-50403) (L-63800)

DE-55040 Infection by Trypanosoma gambiense 086.3
(L-50402) (L-63800)
Gambian trypanosomiasis 086.3
(L-50402) (L-63800)
Gambian sleeping sickness 086.3
(L-50402) (L-63800)
Chronic sleeping sickness
(L-50402) (L-63800)

DE-55050 Infection by Trypanosoma rhodesiense 086.4
(L-50403) (L-63800)
Rhodesian trypanosomiasis 086.4
(L-50403) (L-63800)
Rhodesian sleeping sickness 086.4
(L-50403) (L-63800)
Acute sleeping sickness
(L-50403) (L-63800)

DE-55100V Infection by Trypanosoma equiperdum
(F-9B900) (L-50408)
Dourine
(F-9B900) (L-50408)
Mal du coit
(F-9B900) (L-50408)

DE-55110V Infection by Trypanosoma brucei
(L-50401) (L-63800)
Nagana
(L-50401) (L-63800)
Tsetse fly disease
(L-50401) (L-63800)

DE-55120V Infection by Trypanosoma vivax
(L-50407) (L-63800)
Souma
(L-50407) (L-63800)

DE-55130V Infection by Trypanosoma evansi
(L-50409) (L-63000)
Surra
(L-50409) (L-63000)

DE-55140V Infection by Trypanosoma equinum
(L-50411)
Mal de caderas
(L-50411)

DE-55150V Infection by Trypanosoma hippicum
(L-50409)
Murrina de caderas
(L-50409)

DE-55160V Infection by Trypanosoma simiae
(L-50412)

DE-55170V Infection by Trypanosoma suis
(L-50413)

DE-55500 Leishmaniasis 085.9
(L-50460) (L-62100)
Leishmaniosis 085.9
(L-50460) (L-62100)

DE-55510 Infection by Leishmania donovani 085.0
(T-D4030) (L-50481) (L-62100)
Visceral leishmaniasis 085.0
(T-D4030) (L-50481) (L-62100)
Kala-azar 085.0
(T-D4030) (L-50481) (L-62100)
Dum-dum fever 085.0
(T-D4030) (L-50481) (L-62100)
Mediterranean leishmaniasis 085.0
(T-D4030) (L-50481) (L-62100)
Indian visceral leishmaniasis 085.0
(T-D4030) (L-50481) (L-62100)

DE-55511 Infection by Leishmania infantum 085.0
(L-50484) (L-62100)

DE-55519 Post-kala-azar dermal leishmaniasis 085.0
(T-01000) (L-50481) (L-62100)

DE-55520 Infection by Leishmania tropica minor 085.1
(T-01000) (L-50486) (L-62100)
Cutaneous urban leishmaniasis 085.1
(T-01000) (L-50486) (L-62100)
Oriental sore 085.1
(T-01000) (L-50486) (L-62100)

DE-55520 (cont.) Oriental leishmaniasis 085.1
(T-01000) (L-50486) (L-62100)
Aleppo boil 085.1
(T-01000) (L-50486) (L-62100)
Baghdad boil 085.1
(T-01000) (L-50486) (L-62100)
Delhi boil 085.1
(T-01000) (L-50486) (L-62100)

DE-55525 Dry form of cutaneous leishmaniasis 085.1
(T-01000) (L-50486) (L-62100)

DE-55526 Late cutaneous leishmaniasis 085.1
(T-01000) (L-50486) (L-62100)

DE-55527 Recurrent cutaneous leishmaniasis 085.1
(T-01000) (L-50486) (L-62100)

DE-55528 Ulcerating cutaneous leishmaniasis 085.1
(L-01000) (L-50486) (L-62100)

DE-55530 Infection by Leishmania tropica major 085.2
(T-01000) (L-50487) (L-62100)
Asian desert cutaneous leishmaniasis 085.2
(T-01000) (L-50487) (L-62100)

DE-55531 Disseminated anergic leishmaniasis 085.2
(T-01000) (L-50487) (L-62100)

DE-55532 Acute necrotizing cutaneous leishmaniasis 085.2
(T-01000) (L-50487) (L-62100)
Rural cutaneous leishmaniasis 085.2
(T-01000) (L-50487) (L-62100)

DE-55534 Wet form of cutaneous leishmaniasis 085.2
(T-01000) (L-50487) (L-62100)

DE-55535 Zoonotic form of cutaneous leishmaniasis 085.2
(T-01000) (L-50487) (L-62100)

DE-55540 Infection by Leishmania aethiopica 085.3
(T-01000) (L-50488) (L-62100)
Ethiopian cutaneous leishmaniasis 085.3
(T-01000) (L-50488) (L-62100)

DE-55541 Diffuse cutaneous leishmaniasis 085.3
(T-01000) (L-50488) (L-62100)

DE-55542 Lepromatous cutaneous leishmaniasis 085.3
(T-01000) (L-50488) (L-62100)

DE-55550 Infection by Leishmania mexicana 085.4
(T-01000) (L-50471) (L-62100)
American cutaneous leishmaniasis 085.4
(T-01000) (L-50471) (L-62100)
Chiclero ulcer 085.4
(T-01000) (L-50471) (L-62100)
Leishmaniasis tegumentaria diffusa 085.4
(T-01000) (L-50471) (L-62100)

DE-55560 Infection by Leishmania braziliensis 085.5
(T-00400) (T-01000) (L-50462) (L-62100)
American mucocutaneous leishmaniasis 085.5
(T-00400) (T-01000) (L-50462) (L-62100)
Espundia 085.5
(T-00400) (T-01000) (L-50462) (L-62100)
Mucocutaneous leishmaniasis 085.5
(T-00400) (T-01000) (L-50462) (L-62100)
Uta 085.5
(T-00400) (T-01000) (L-50462) (L-62100)

DE-55561 Disseminated mucocutaneous leishmaniasis 085.5
(T-00400) (T-01000) (L-50462) (L-62100)

E-558 Diseases Due to Enteromonadidae

DE-55800 Infection by Enteromonas, NOS
(T-50710)

DE-55801 Infection by Enteromonas hominis
(L-50711)

E-559 Diseases Due to Nosematidae

DE-55900 Infection by Nosema, NOS
(L-54000)
Nosemosis
(L-54000)

DE-55910 Infection by Nosema connori
(L-54006)

DE-55911V Infection by Nosema apis
(L-54001) (L-65201)

DE-55912V Infection by Nosema bombycis
(L-54002) (L-64B51)
Peprine
(L-54002) (L-64B51)
Fleckenkrankheit
(L-54002) (L-64B51)

DE-55950 Infection by Encephalitozoon, NOS
(L-54020)
Encephalitozoonosis
(L-54020)

DE-55960 Infection by Encephalitozoon cuniculi
(L-54031)

DE-55970V Infection by Glugea, NOS
(L-54080)
Glugeosis
(L-54080)

E-55A Diseases Due to Other Ciliate Protozoa, NEC

DE-55A10 Infection by Diplodinium, NOS
(L-53410)

DE-55A20 Infection by Ophryoscolex, NOS
(L-53420)

DE-55A30 Infection by Buxtonella, NOS
(L-53B50)
Buxtonellosis
(L-53B50)

DE-55A40 Infection by Entodinium, NOS
(L-53400)

E-55A Diseases Due to Other Ciliate Protozoa, NEC — Continued

DE-55A50 Infection by Ichthyophthirius, NOS
(L-53B00)
Ichthyophthiriosis
(L-53B00)

E-55C Diseases Due to Myxozoa

DE-55C00 Infection by Myxobolus, NOS
(L-54200)
Myxobolosis
(L-54200)
DE-55C20 Infection by Henneguya, NOS
(L-54220)
Henneguyosis
(L-54220)
DE-55C30 Infection by Lentospora, NOS
(L-54250)
Lentosporosis
(L-54250)

E-59 INCERTA SEDIS

DE-59100 Pneumocytosis 136.3
(L-50F00)
DE-59101 Infection by Pneumocystis carinii 136.3
(L-50F00)
DE-59102 Infection by Pneumocystis jiroveci
(L-50F01)
DE-59110 Pulmonary pneumocystosis 136.3 —484.8*
(T-28000) (M-40000) (L-50F00)
Pneumonia due to Pneumocystis carinii 136.3 —484.8*
(T-28000) (M-40000) (L-50F00)

E-5A0 Diseases Due to Oomycetes

DE-5A000 Infection by Oomycetes, NOS
DE-5A010V Infection by Pythium, NOS
(L-54600)
Infection by Hyphomyces, NOS
(L-54600)
DE-5A020V Infection by Pythium insidiosum
(L-54601)
Infection by Hyphomyces destruens
(L-54601)
Pythiosis
(L-54601)
Swamp cancer
(L-54601)
Hyphomycosis destruens equi
(L-54601)
Equine dermal granuloma
(L-54601)
DE-5A030V Infection by Saprolegnia, NOS
(L-54620)
Saprolegniosis
(L-54620)

E-5A2 Diseases Due to Microspora

DE-5A200 Infection by Microspora, NOS
(L-54...)
Infection by Cnidospora, NOS
(L-54...)
DE-5A210 Infection by Rudimicrosporea, NOS
(L-54...)
DE-5A220 Infection by Microsporea, NOS
(L-54...)
DE-5A222 Infection by Microsporida
(L-54...)
Infection by Microsporidia
(L-54...)
Infection by Cnidosporidia
(L-54...)
Microsporidiosis
(L-54...)

SECTION E-6 HELMINTHIC INFECTIOUS DISEASES

E-600 Helminthic Infections: General Terms

DE-60000 Helminth infection, NOS 128.9
(L-55000)
Helminthiasis 128.9
(L-55000)
Worms, NOS 128.9
(L-55000)
Helminthosis 128.9
(L-55000)
DE-60010 Cestode infection, NOS 123.9
(L-5B000)
Tapeworm infection, NOS 123.9
(L-5B000)
Cestodosis 123.9
(L-5B000)
Cestodiasis 123.9
(L-5B000)
DE-60020 Intestinal helminthiasis, NOS 127.9
(T-50500) (L-55000)
DE-60030 Mixed intestinal helminthiasis 127.8
(T-50500) (L-55000)
DE-60040 Nematode infection, NOS 127.9
(L-55100)
Nematodiasis 127.9
(L-55100)
DE-60041 Intestinal nematode infection, NOS 127.9
(T-50500) (L-55100)
DE-60042V Cutaneous nematodiasis
(L-55100)
DE-60043V Cerebrospinal nematodiasis
(L-55100)
DE-60045 Pulmonary nematodiasis
(T-28000) (L-55100)
DE-60050 Trematode infection, NOS 121.9
(L-58000)
Infection by Trematode, NOS 121.9
(L-58000)

DE-60050V (cont.) Trematodosis 121.9
(L-58000)

DE-60080 Fluke disease, NOS 121.9
(L-58000)
Distomiasis 121.9
(L-58000)

E-60-62 DISEASES DUE TO TREMATODA

E-601-603 Diseases Due to Schistosomatidae

DE-60100 Infection by Schistosoma, NOS 120.9
(L-58120)
Schistosomiasis 120.9
(L-58120)
Bilharziasis 120.9
(L-58120)
Blood flukes, NOS 120.9
(L-58120)
Hemic distomiasis 120.9
(L-58120)
Schistosomosis 120.9
(L-58120)

DE-60110 Schistosoma hematobium infection 120.0
(T-74000) (L-58123)
Vesical schistosomiasis 120.0
(T-74000) (L-58123)

DE-60120 Schistosoma mansonii infection 120.1
(T-50500) (L-58121)
Intestinal schistosomiasis 120.1
(T-50500) (L-58121)

DE-60130 Schistosoma japonicum infection 120.2
(L-58122)
Katayama disease 120.2
(L-58122)
Katamaya syndrome 120.2
(L-58122)
Katamaya fever 120.2
(L-58122)
Asiatic schistosomiasis 120.2
(L-58122)

DE-60132 Cardiopulmonary schistosomiasis 120.2
(T-32000) (L-58122)

DE-60133 Pulmonary schistosomiasis 120.2
(T-28000) (L-58122)

DE-60200 Infection by cercariae of schistosoma 120.3
(T-01000) (L-58120)
Marine dermatitis 120.3
(T-01000) (L-58120)
Sea bather's eruption 120.3
(T-01000) (L-58120)
Cercarial dermatitis 120.3
(T-01000) (L-58120)
Swimmer's itch 120.3
(T-01000) (L-58120)
Schistosome dermatitis 120.3
(T-01000) (L-58120)
Clam digger's itch 120.3
(T-01000) (L-58120)
Cutaneous schistosomiasis 120.3
(T-01000) (L-58120)
Swamp itch

DE-60210 Cercarial dermatitis of freshwater avian type 120.3
(T-01000) (L-58120)

DE-60220 Cercarial dermatitis of sea water avian type 120.3
(T-01000) (L-58120)

DE-60230 Cercarial dermatitis of freshwater mammalian type 120.3
(T-01000) (L-58120)

DE-60250 Infection by other schistosoma 120.8
(L-581..)

DE-60251 Infection by Schistosoma bovis 120.8
(L-58129)

DE-60252 Infection by Schistosoma intercalatum 120.8
(L-58124)

DE-60253 Infection by Schistosoma mattheii 120.8
(L-58126)

DE-60254 Infection by Schistosoma spindale 120.8
(L-58128)

DE-60255 Infection by Schistosoma chestermani 120.8
(L-58139)

DE-60256V Infection by Schistosoma hippopotami
(L-58137)

DE-60257V Infection by Schistosoma incognitum
(L-58127)

DE-60258V Infection by Schistosoma nasalis
(L-58134)
Nasal schistosomiasis
(L-58134)

DE-60259V Infection by Schistosoma indicum
(L-58133)

DE-60300V Infection by Ornithobilharzia, NOS
(L-58170)
Ornithobilharziosis
(L-58170)

DE-60310V Infection by Trichobilharzia, NOS
(L-58210)
Trichobilharziosis
(L-58210)

DE-60311V Infection by Trichobilharzia ocellata
(L-58211)

DE-60312V Infection by Trichobilharzia stagnicolae
(L-58213)

DE-60313V Infection by Trichobilharzia physellae
(L-58212)

DE-60318V Trichobilharzia cercarial dermatitis
(T-01000) (L-58210)

DE-60320V Infection by Austrobilharzia, NOS
(L-58190)
Austrobilharziosis
(L-58190)

DE-60330V Infection by Gigantobilharzia, NOS
(L-58200)
Gigantobilharziosis
(L-58200)

E-601-603 Diseases Due to Schistosomatidae — Continued

DE-60340V Infection by Bilharziella, NOS
(L-58220)
Bilharziellosis
(L-58220)

DE-60350V Infection by Schistosomatium, NOS
(L-58160)

DE-60351V Infection by Schistosomatium douthitti
(L-58161)

DE-60360V Infection by Heterobilharzia, NOS
(L-58140)
Heterobilharziosis
(L-58140)

DE-60361V Infection by Heterobilharzia americanum
(L-58141)

DE-60370V Infection by Orientobilharzia, NOS
(L-58170)
Orientobilharziosis
(L-58170)

DE-60371V Infection by Orientobilharzia harinasutai
(L-58173)

E-604 Diseases Due to Fasciolidae

DE-60400 Infection by Fasciola, NOS 121.3
(L-59300)
Fascioliasis 121.3
(L-59300)
Liver flukes, NOS 121.3
(L-59300)
Fasciolosis 121.3
(L-59300)

DE-60410 Fasciola gigantica infection 121.3
(L-59302)

DE-60420 Fasciola hepatica infection 121.3
(L-59301)
Sheep liver fluke infection 121.3
(L-59301)

DE-60450 Infection by Fasciolopsis buski 121.4
(T-50500) (L-59311)
Fasciolopsiasis 121.4
(T-50500) (L-59311)
Giant intestinal fluke infection 121.4
(T-50500) (L-59311)
Intestinal distomiasis 121.4
(T-50500) (L-59311)
Fasciolopsiosis 121.4
(T-50500) (L-59311)

DE-60460V Infection by Fascioloides, NOS
(L-59320)
Fascioloidosis
(L-59320)

DE-60461V Infection by Fascioloides magna
(L-59321)

E-605 Diseases Due to Diplostomatidae

DE-60500V Infection by Alaria, NOS
(L-58410)
Alariosis
(L-58410)

DE-60510V Infection by Diplostomum, NOS
(L-58400)

E-606 Diseases Due to Echinostomatidae

DE-60600 Echinostomiasis 121.8
(L-59100)
Echinostomosis 121.8
(L-59100)

DE-60601 Infection by Echinostoma ilocanum 121.8
(L-59101)

DE-60602 Infection by Echinostoma lindoense 121.8
(L-59102)

DE-60610 Infection by Echinochasmus, NOS
(L-59140)
Echinochasmosis
(L-59140)

DE-60611 Infection by Echinochasmus perfoliatus 121.8
(L-59141)

DE-60620V Infection by Echinoparyphium, NOS
(L-59120)
Echinoparyphiosis
(L-59120)

DE-60630V Infection by Hypoderaerum, NOS
(L-59210)
Hypoderaerosis
(L-59210)

DE-60640V Infection by Euparyphium, NOS
(L-59130)
Euparyphiosis
(L-59130)

E-607 Diseases Due to Strigeidae

DE-60700V Infection by Strigea, NOS
(L-58300)

DE-60710V Infection by Apatemon, NOS
(L-58330)
Apatemosis
(L-58330)

DE-60720V Infection by Cotylurus, NOS
(L-58320)
Cotylurosis
(L-58320)

E-608 Diseases Due to Paramphistomatidae

DE-60800V Infection by Paramphistomum, NOS
(L-59400)
Paramphistomosis
(L-59400)

DE-60810V Infection by Gigantocotyle, NOS
(L-59430)
Gigantocotylosis
(L-59430)

DE-60820V Infection by Calicophoron, NOS
(L-59440)
DE-60830V Infection by Cylonocotyle, NOS
(L-59470)
DE-60840V Infection by Cotylophoron, NOS
(L-59480)

E-609 Diseases Due to Gastrodiscidae

DE-60900 Gastrodiscoidiasis 121.8
(L-59410)
DE-60901 Infection by Gastrodiscoides hominis 121.8
(L-59411)

E-611 Diseases Due to Dicrocoeliidae

DE-61100 Dicrocoeliasis 121.8
(L-59600)
Dicrocoeliosis 121.8
(L-59600)
DE-61101 Infection by Dicrocoelium dendriticum 121.8
(L-59601)
DE-61110V Infection by Eutrema, NOS
(L-59610)
DE-61111V Infection by pancreaticum
(L-59611)
DE-61120V Infection by Athesmia, NOS
(L-59630)
DE-61121V Infection by Athesmia foxi
(L-59631)
DE-61130V Infection by Platynosomum, NOS
(L-59640)
DE-61131V Infection by Platynosomum concinnum
(L-59642)
DE-61132V Infection by Platynosomum fastosum
(L-59641)
Lizard poisoning
(L-59641)

E-612 Diseases Due to Plagiorchiidae

DE-61200V Infection by Plagiorchis, NOS
(L-59800)
Plagiorchiosis
(L-59800)
DE-61220V Infection by Prosthogonimus, NOS
(L-59810)
Prosthogonimosis
(L-59810)
DE-61221V Infection by Prosthogonimus macrorchis
(L-59812)

E-613 Diseases Due to Paragonimidae

DE-61300 Infection by Paragonimus, NOS 121.2
(T-28000) (L-59A00)
Paragonimiasis 121.2
(T-28000) (L-59A00)
Oriental lung fluke disease 121.2
(T-28000) (L-59A00)
Pulmonary distomiasis 121.2
(T-28000) (L-59A00)
Paragonimosis 121.2
(T-28000) (L-59A00)
DE-61301 Infection by Paragonimus westermanii 121.2
(T-28000) (L-59A01)
DE-61302V Infection by Paragonimus kellicotti
(L-59A02)
DE-61320V Infection by Collyricum, NOS
(L-59A30)
Collyriclosis
(L-59A30)
DE-61321V Infection by Collyricum faba
(L-59A31)

E-614 Diseases Due to Cyclocoelidae

DE-61410V Infection by Typhlocoelum, NOS
(L-5A600)
Typhlocoelosis
(L-5A600)
Infection by Tracheophilus
(L-5A600)

E-615-616 Diseases Due to Opisthorchiidae

DE-61500 Opisthorchiasis 121.0
(L-5A000)
Cat liver fluke infection 121.0
(L-5A000)
Opisthorchiosis 121.0
(L-5A000)
DE-61501 Infection by Opisthorchis felineus 121.0
(L-5A001)
Infection by Opisthorchis tenuicollis 121.0
(L-5A001)
DE-61503 Infection by Opisthorchis viverrini 121.0
(L-5A002)
DE-61504V Infection by Opisthorchis caninus
(L-5A004)
DE-61505V Infection by Opisthorchis noverca
(L-5A005)
DE-61600 Clonorchiasis 121.1
(T-62000) (L-5A040)
Chinese liver fluke disease 121.1
(T-62000) (L-5A041)
Oriental liver fluke disease 121.1
(T-62000) (L-5A041)
Hepatic distomiasis due to Clonorchis sinensis 121.1
(T-62000) (L-5A041)
Clonorchiosis 121.1
(L-5A041)
DE-61610 Clonorchiasis with biliary cirrhosis 121.1
(T-62000) (T-60610) (M-78000)
(L-5A040)

E-615-616 Diseases Due to Opisthorchiidae — Continued

DE-61620V Infection by Amphimerus, NOS
(L-5A030)

DE-61621V Infection by Amphimerus pseudofelineus
(L-5A031)

DE-61622V Infection by Amphimerus elongatus
(L-5A032)

DE-61650V Infection by Metorchis, NOS
(L-5A010)
Metorchiosis
(L-5A010)

E-617 Diseases Due to Notocotylidae

DE-61700V Infection by Notocotylus, NOS
(L-5A500)
Notocotylosis
(L-5A500)

DE-61710V Infection by Catatropis, NOS
(L-5A510)
Catatropiosis
(L-5A510)

E-620-621 Diseases Due to Heterophyidae

DE-62000 Infection by Heterophyes heterophyes 121.6
(L-5A201)
Heterophyiasis 121.6
(L-5A201)
Heterophyosis 121.6
(L-5A201)

DE-62050 Infection by Stellantchasmus falcatus 121.6
(L-5AD02)

DE-62100 Infection by Metagonimus yokogawai 121.5
(L-5A231)
Metagonimiasis 121.5
(L-5A231)
Metagonimosis
(L-5A231)

DE-62120V Infection by Apophallus, NOS
(L-5A220)
Apophallosis
(L-5A220)

DE-62130V Infection by Cryptocotyle, NOS
(L-5A210)
Cryptocotylosis
(L-5A210)

E-623 Diseases Due to Dactylogyridae

DE-62300V Infection by Dactylogyrus, NOS
(L-5A800)
Dactylogyrosis
(L-5A800)
Infection by Gyrodactylus, NOS
(L-5A800)
Gyrodactylosis
(L-5A800)

E-624 Diseases Due to Sanguinicolidae

DE-62400V Infection by Sanguinicola, NOS
(L-58600)
Sanguinicolosis
(L-58600)

E-64-66 DISEASES DUE TO CESTODA

E-640-643 DISEASES DUE TO CESTODES OF THE ORDER PSEUDOPHYLLIDEA

E-640-643 Diseases Due to Diphyllobothriidae

DE-64000 Infection by Diphyllobothrium, NOS 123.4
(T-50500) (L-5C000)
Diphyllobothriasis 123.4
(T-50500) (L-5C000)
Intestinal diphyllobothriasis 123.4
(T-50500) (L-5C000)
Fish tapeworm infection 123.4
(T-50500) (L-5C000)
Diphyllobothriosis 123.4
(T-50500) (L-5C000)

DE-64010 Infection by Diphyllobothrium latum 123.4
(T-50500) (L-5C001)

DE-64012 Infection by Diphyllobothrium pacificum 123.4
(T-50500) (L-5C004)

DE-64230 Infection by Digramma, NOS
(L-5C030)
Digrammosis
(L-5C030)

DE-64250 Infection by Ligula, NOS
(L-5C050)
Ligulosis
(L-5C050)

DE-64270 Infection by Braunia, NOS
(L-5C090)

DE-64280V Infection by Bothriocephalus, NOS
(L-5C060)
Bothriocephalosis
(L-5C060)

DE-64290V Infection by Triaenophorus, NOS
(L-5C070)
Triaenophorosis
(L-5C070)

DE-64300V Infection by Diplogonoporus, NOS
(L-5C080)

DE-64301 Infection by Diplogonoporus grandis 123.8
(L-5C081)

DE-64310V Infection by Schistocephalus, NOS
(L-5C100)

DE-64320V Infection by Cyathocephalus, NOS
(L-5C110)

E-645-65C DISEASES DUE TO CESTODES OF THE ORDER CYCLOPHYLLIDEA

E-645 Diseases Due to Dilepididae

DE-64500 Infection by Dipylidium caninum 123.8
(L-5B501)
Dipylidiasis 123.8
(L-5B501)
Dog tapeworm infection 123.8
(L-5B501)
Dipylidiosis 123.8
(L-5B501)

DE-64510V Infection by Amoebotaenia, NOS
(L-5B510)
Amoebotaeniosis
(L-5B510)

DE-64520V Infection by Choanotaenia, NOS
(L-5B520)
Choanotaeniosis
(L-5B520)

DE-64530V Infection by Metroliasthes, NOS
(L-5B530)

E-647 Diseases Due to Hymenolepididae

DE-64700 Hymenolepiasis 123.6
(L-5B300)
Hymenolepiosis 123.6
(L-5B300)

DE-64710 Hymenolepis diminuta infection 123.6
(L-5B302)
Rat tapeworm infection 123.6
(L-5B302)

DE-64720 Hymenolepis nana infection 123.6
(L-5B301)
Dwarf tapeworm infection 123.6
(L-5B301)

DE-64730V Infection by Diorchis, NOS
(L-5B310)
Diorchiosis
(L-5B310)

DE-64740V Infection by Microsomacanthus, NOS
(L-5B330)
Microsomacanthosis
(L-5B330)

DE-64750V Depranidotaeniosis
(L-5B320)

DE-64751V Infection due to Drepanidotaenia lanceolata
(L-5B321)

DE-64760V Infection by Echinolepis, NOS
(L-5B340)
Echinolepiosis
(L-5B340)

DE-64770V Infection by Stachylepis, NOS
(L-5B350)
Stachylepiosis
(L-5B350)

DE-64780V Infection by Vampirolepis, NOS
(L-5B360)
Vampirolepiosis
(L-5B360)

E-650-651 Diseases Due to Taeniidae

DE-65000 Echinococciasis 122.9
(L-5B140)
Echinococcosis 122.9
(L-5B140)
Hydatid disease 122.9
(I-5B140)
Hydatidosis 122.9
(L-5B140)

DE-65005 Echinococcosis of liver, NOS 122.8
(T-62000) (L-5B140)

DE-65010 Echinococcus granulosus infection 122.4
(L-5B141)
Unilocular hydatid disease 122.4
(L-5B141)

DE-65011 Echinococcus granulosus infection of liver 122.0
(T-62000) (L-5B141)

DE-65012 Echinococcus granulosus infection of lung 122.1
(T-28000) (L-5B141)

DE-65013 Echinococcus granulosus infection of thyroid 122.2
(T-B6000) (L-5B141)

DE-65018 Echinococcus granulosus infection of other site 122.3
(T-.....) (L-5B141)

DE-65020 Echinococcus multilocularis infection 122.7
(L-5B142)
Alveolar hydatid disease 122.7
(L-5B142)

DE-65021 Echinococcus multilocularis infection of liver 122.5
(T-62000) (L-5B142)

DE-65029 Echinococcus multilocularis infection of other site 122.6
(T-.....) (L-5B142)

DE-65030 Echinococcus oligarthrus infection
(L-5B144)

DE-65040 Echinococcus vogeli infection
(L-5B143)

DE-65100 Infection by Taenia, NOS 123.3
(L-5B100)
Taeniasis 123.3
(L-5B100)
Taeniosis 123.3
(L-5B100)

DE-65110 Taenia saginata infection 123.2
(L-5B102)
Beef tapeworm infection 123.2
(L-5B102)

E-650-651 Diseases Due to Taeniidae — Continued

DE-65110 (cont.) Infection by Taenia saginata 123.2
(L-5B102)

DE-65120 Taenia solium infection, intestinal form 123.0
(T-50500) (L-5B101)
Pork tapeworm infection 123.0
(T-50500) (L-5B101)
Infection by Taenia solium 123.0
(T-50500) (L-5B101)

DE-65122V Infection by Taenia hydatigena
(L-5B106)

DE-65124V Infection by Taenia ovis
(L-5B109)

DE-65126V Infection by Taenia pisiformis
(L-5B111)

DE-65128V Infection by Taenia taeniaeformis
(L-5B105)

DE-65130V Multicepsosis
(L-5B180)

DE-65131 Infection by Multiceps multiceps 123.8
(L-5B181)

E-652 Infections by Tapeworm Larvae

DE-65200 Cysticercosis 123.1
(L-5B210)
Cysticerciasis 123.1
(L-5B210)

DE-65201 Infection by Cysticercus cellulosae 123.1
(L-5B213) (L-5B101)
Infection by larvae of taenia solium 123.1
(L-5B213) (L-5B101)
Pork measles
(L-5B213) (L-5B101)

DE-65202V Infection by Cysticercus bovis
(L-5B211) (L-5B102)
Beef measles
(L-5B211) (M-5B102)

DE-65203V Infection by Cysticercus fasciolaris
(L-5B215) (L-5B105)

DE-65206V Infection by Cysticercus ovis
(L-5B212) (L-5B109)

DE-65208V Infection by Cysticercus pisiformis
(L-5B216) (L-5B211)

DE-65210V Infection by Cysticercus tarandi
(L-5B217) (L-5B117)

DE-65212V Infection by Cysticercus tenuicollis
(L-5B214) (L-5B106)

DE-65230V Coenurosis 123.8
(L-5B230) (L-5B180)
Infection by larvae of dog tapeworm 123.8
(L-5B230) (L-5B180)
Infection by larvae of Multiceps 123.8
(L-5B230) (L-5B180)

DE-65231V Infection by Coenurosis cerebralis
(L-5B231) (L-5B181)

DE-65232V Infection by Coenurosis serialis
(L-5B232) (L-5B183)

DE-65250 Infection by Spirometra larvae 123.5
(L-5C020)
Sparganosis 123.5
(L-5C020)
Larval diphyllobothriasis 123.5
(L-5C020)
Spirometriosis 123.5
(L-5C020)
Spirometrosis 123.5
(L-5C020)

DE-65251 Infection by Sparganum proliferum 123.5
(L-5C041)

DE-65252 Infection by Sparganum mansoni 123.5
(L-5C021)

E-653 Diseases Due to Fimbriariidae

DE-65300V Infection by Fimbriaria, NOS
(L-5B400)
Fimbriariosis
(L-5B400)

E-654 Diseases Due to Anoplocephalidae

DE-65400V Infection by Anoplocephala, NOS
(L-5B600)
Anoplocephalosis
(L-5B600)

DE-65401V Infection by Anoplocephala magna
(L-5B601)

DE-65402V Infection by Anoplocephala perfoliata
(L-5B602)

DE-65410V Infection by Moniezia, NOS
(L-5B610)
Monieziosis
(L-5B610)

DE-65411V Infection by Moniezia expansa
(L-5B611)

DE-65412V Infection by Moniezia benedeni
(L-5B612)

DE-65420V Infection by Paranoplocephala, NOS
(L-5B650)
Paranoplocephalosis
(L-5B650)

DE-65421V Infection by Paranoplocephala mammillana
(L-5B651)

DE-65430V Infection by Cittotaenia, NOS
(L-5B660)
Cittotaeniosis
(L-5B660)

DE-65440V Infection by Andrya, NOS
(L-5B690)
Andryosis
(L-5B690)

DE-65450V Infection by Bertiella, NOS
(L-5B620)

DE-65460V Infection by Mosgovoyia, NOS
(L-5B6A0)
Mosgovoyiosis
(L-5B6A0)

DE-65470V Infection by Neoctenotaenia, NOS
(L-5B6B0)
Neoctenotaeniosis
(L-5B6B0)

E-656 Diseases Due to Thysanosomidae

DE-65600V Infection by Thysanosoma, NOS
(L-5B700)
Thysanosomosis
(L-5B700)

DE-65601V Infection by Thysanosoma actinioides
(L-5B701)

DE-65610V Infection by Thysaniezia, NOS
(L-5B710)
Thysanieziosis
(L-5B710)

DE-65620V Infection by Stilesia, NOS
(L-5B720)
Stilesiosis
(L-5B720)

DE-65621V Infection by Stilesia hepatica
(L-5B721)

DE-65622V Infection by Stilesia globipunctata
(L-5B722)

DE-65630V Infection by Avitellina, NOS
(L-5B740)
Avitellinosis
(L-5B740)

E-658 Diseases Due to Davaineidae

DE-65800V Infection by Davainea, NOS
(L-5B800)
Davaineosis
(L-5B800)

DE-65810V Infection by Raillietina, NOS
(L-5B810)
Raillietinosis
(L-5B810)

DE-65820V Infection by Cotugnia, NOS
(L-5B840)
Cotugniosis
(L-5B840)

DE-65830V Infection by Houttuynia, NOS
(L-5B830)

E-65A Diseases Due to Mesocestoididae

DE-65A00V Infection by Mesocestoides, NOS
(L-5BA00)
Mesocestoidosis
(L-5BA00)

DE-65A01V Infection by Mesocestoides corti
(L-5BA03)

DE-65A02V Infection by Mesocestoides lineatus
(L-5BA02)

E-65C Diseases Due to Linstowiidae

DE-65C00V Infection by Oochoristica, NOS
(L-5B900)

DE-65C10V Infection by Inermicapsifer, NOS
(L-5B910)

E-66 DISEASES DUE TO CESTODES OF THE ORDER CARYOPHYLLIDEA

E-660 Diseases Due to Caryophyllaeidae

DE-66000V Infection by Caryophyllaeus, NOS
(L-5C400)
Caryophyllaeosis
(L-5C400)

DE-66010V Infection by Khawia, NOS
(L-5C410)
Khawiosis
(L-5C410)

E-67-6A DISEASES DUE TO NEMATODA

E-670 Diseases Due to Superfamily Ancylostomatoidea

DE-67000 Ancylostomiasis 126.9
(L-55810)
Hookworm disease, NOS 126.9
(L-55810)
Ancylostomosis 126.9
(L-55810)

DE-67010 Ancylostomiasis due to Ancylostoma duodenale 126.0
(L-55811)

DE-67011 Ancylostomiasis due to Ancylostoma braziliense 126.2
(L-55812)

DE-67012 Ancylostomiasis due to Ancylostoma ceylonicum 126.3
(L-55815)

DE-67013V Infection by Ancyclostoma caninum
(L-55814)

DE-67020 Necatoriasis 126.9
(L-55840)
Necatorosis 126.9
(L-55840)

DE-67021 Necatoriasis due to Necator americanus 126.1
(L-55841)

DE-67030V Infection by Uncinaria, NOS 126.9
(L-55850)
Uncinariasis 126.9
(L-55850)
Uncinariosis 126.9
(L-55850)

DE-67031V Infection by Uncinaria stenocephala
(L-55851)

E-670 Diseases Due to Superfamily Ancylostomatoidea — Continued

DE-67040 Cutaneous larva migrans 126.9
(T-01000) (L-55841)
Creeping eruption 126.9
(T-01000) (L-55841)
Uncinarial dermatitis 126.9
(T-01000) (L-55841)
Ground itch 126.9
(T-01000) (L-55841)

DE-67041 Cutaneous larva migrans by Ancylostoma braziliense 126.2
(T-01000) (L-55812)

DE-67042 Cutaneous larva migrans by Ancylostoma caninum 126.8
(T-01000) (L-55814)

DE-67050V Infection by Bunostomum, NOS
(L-55830)
Bunostomosis
(L-55830)

DE-67051V Infection by Bunostomum phlebotomum
(L-55831)

DE-67052V Infection by Bunostomum trigonocephalum
(L-55832)

DE-67060V Infection by Globocephalus, NOS
(L-55870)
Globocephalosis
(L-55870)

DE-67061V Infection by Globocephalus urosubulatus
(L-55871)

E-672-673 Diseases Due to Superfamily Protostrongyloidea

DE-67200 Infection by Angiostrongylus 128.8
(L-56000)
Angiostrongyliasis 128.8
(L-56000)
Angiostrongylosis 128.8
(L-56000)

DE-67210 Infection by Angiostrongylus cantonensis 128.8
(L-56001)

DE-67212 Eosinophilic meningoencephalitis 128.8
(T-A1110) (L-56001)

DE-67220V Infection by Aelurostrongylus, NOS
(L-56040)
Aelurostrongylosis
(L-56040)

DE-67230V Infection by Spiculocaulus, NOS
(L-56080)
Spiculocaulosis
(L-56080)

DE-67240V Infection by Elaphostrongylus
(L-56030)
Elaphostrongylosis
(L-56030)

DE-67250V Infection by Pneumostrongylus, NOS
(L-56020)
Pneumostrongylosis
(L-56020)

DE-67260V Infection by Bicaulus, NOS
(L-56050)
Bicaulosis
(L-56050)

DE-67270V Infection by Capreocaulus, NOS
(L-56060)
Capreocaulosis
(L-56060)

DE-67280V Infection by Pneumocaulus, NOS
(L-56140)
Pneumocaulosis
(L-56140)

DE-67290V Infection by Neostrongylus, NOS
(L-56070)
Neostrongylosis
(L-56070)

DE-67300V Infection by Cystocaulus, NOS
(L-56130)
Cystocaulosis
(L-56130)

DE-67310V Infection by Muellerius, NOS
(L-56010)
Muelleriosis
(L-56010)

E-674-676 Diseases Due to Superfamily Ascaridoidea

DE-67400 Ascariasis 127.0
(L-56200)
Round worm infection 127.0
(L-56200)
Ascariosis 127.0
(L-56200)

DE-67401 Infection by Ascaris lumbricoides 127.0
(L-56201)

DE-67402V Infection by Ascaris suum
(L-56202)

DE-67420V Infection by Parascaris, NOS
(L-56250)
Parascariosis
(L-56250)

DE-67421V Infection by Parascaris equorum
(L-56251)

DE-67430V Infection by Ascaridia, NOS
(L-56210)
Ascaridiosis
(L-56210)

DE-67431V Infection by Ascaridia galli
(L-56212)

DE-67432V Infection by Ascaridia dissimilis
(L-56215)

DE-67440V Infection by Baylisascaris, NOS
(L-56260)

DE-67441V Infection by Baylisascaris columnaris
(L-56261)

DE-67450V Infection by Neoascaris, NOS
(L-56230)
Neoascarosis
(L-56230)

DE-67451V Infection by Neoascaris vitulorum
(L-56231)
DE-67500 Toxocariasis 128.0
(L-56220)
Toxocarosis 128.0
(L-56220)
DE-67510 Infection by Toxocara canis 128.0
(L-56221)
DE-67520 Infection by Toxocara cati 128.0
(L-56222)
DE-67540 Visceral larva migrans syndrome 128.0
(T-D4030) (L-56222) (L-56221)
DE-67600 Infection by Lagochilascaris, NOS
(L-56290)
DE-67620 Infection by Toxascaris, NOS
(L-56240)
Toxascariosis
(L-56240)
DE-67621V Infection by Toxascaris leonina
(L-56241)

E-679 Diseases Due to Superfamily Heterocheiloidea

DE-67900 Infection by Anisakis larva 127.1
(T-50100) (L-56410)
Anisakiasis 127.1
(T-50100) (L-56410)
Herringworm disease 127.1
(T-50100) (L-56410)
Eosinophilic gastroenteritis 127.1
(T-50100) (L-56410)
Anisakiosis 127.1
(T-50100) (L-56410)
DE-67910 Anisakiasis due to Anisakis marina 127.1
(L-56411)
DE-67911 Anisakiasis due to Anisakis simplex 127.1
(L-56412)
DE-67920V Infection by Porrocaecum, NOS
(L-56440)
Porrocaecosis
(L-56440)
DE-67930 Infection by Contracaecum, NOS
(L-56420)
Contracaecosis
(L-56420)
DE-67940V Infection by Cucullanus, NOS
(L-56480)
Cucullanosis
(L-56480)
DE-67950 Infection by Pseudoterranova, NOS
(L-56490)

E-67A-67B Diseases Due to Superfamily Spiruroidea

DE-67A00 Infection by Physaloptera, NOS 127.7
(L-56840)
Physalopteriasis 127.7
(L-56840)
Physalopterosis 127.7
(L-56840)
DE-67A10 Infection by Physaloptera mordens 127.7
(L-56841)
Infection by Physaloptera caucasica 127.7
(L-56841)
DE-67A20V Infection by Gongylonema, NOS
(L-56800)
Gongylonemosis
(L-56800)
DE-67A21V Infection by Gongylonema ingluvicola
(L-56803)
DE-67A22V Infection by Gongylonema pulchrum
(L-56801)
DE-67A23V Infection by Gongylonema verrucosum
(L-56804)
DE-67A24V Infection by Gongylonema neoplasticum
(L-56802)
DE-67A30V Infection by Habronema, NOS
(L-56810)
Habronemosis
(L-56810)
DE-67A32V Cutaneous habronemiasis
(T-01000) (L-56810)
Summer sores
(T-01000) (L-56810)
Jack sores
(T-01000) (L-56810)
Bursatti
(T-01000) (L-56810)
DE-67A40V Infection by Tetrameres, NOS
(L-56820)
Tetramerosis
(L-56820)
DE-67A50V Infection by Camallanus, NOS
(L-56830)
Camallanosis
(L-56830)
DE-67A60V Infection by Spirura, NOS
(L-56860)
Spirurosis
(L-56860)
DE-67A70V Infection by Protospirura, NOS
(L-56870)
Protospirurosis
(L-56870)
DE-67A80V Infection by Pneumospirura, NOS
(L-56880)
Pneumospirurosis
(L-56880)
DE-67A90V Infection by Acuaria, NOS
(L-56900)
Acuariosis
(L-56900)
DE-67B00V Infection by Physocephalus, NOS
(L-56910)
Physocephalosis
(L-56910)

E-67A-67B Diseases Due to Superfamily Spiruroidea — Continued

DE-67B10V Infection by Ascarops, NOS
(L-56920)
Ascaropsosis
(L-56920)

DE-67B20V Infection by Draschia, NOS
(L-56930)
Draschiosis
(L-56930)

DE-67B22V Cutaneous draschiasis
(T-01000) (L-56930)

DE-67B30V Infection by Dispharynx, NOS
(L-56940)
Dispharyngosis
(L-56940)

DE-67B40V Infection by Streptocara, NOS
(L-56950)
Streptocarosis
(L-56950)

E-67C Diseases Due to Superfamily Thelazioidea

DE-67C00V Infection by Thelazia, NOS
(L-56A00)
Thelaziosis
(L-56A00)
Verminous ophthalmia
(T-AA000) (L-56A00) (L-63700)

DE-67C01V Infection by Thelazia californiensis
(L-56A02) (L-63700)

DE-67C02V Infection by Thelazia callipaeda
(L-56A01) (L-63700)

DE-67C10V Infection by Spirocerca, NOS
(L-56A20)
Spirocercosis
(L-56A20)

DE-67C11V Infection by Spirocerca arctica
(L-56A23)

DE-67C12V Infection by Spirocerca lupi
(L-56A22)

DE-67C13V Infection by Spirocerca sanguinolenta
(L-56A21)

DE-67C20V Infection by Oxyspirura, NOS
(L-56A30)
Oxyspirurosis
(L-56A30)

DE-67C30V Infection by Simondsia, NOS
(L-56A40)
Simondsiosis
(L-56A40)

DE-67C40 Infection by Gnathostoma, NOS 128.1
(L-56A50)
Gnathostomiasis 128.1
(L-56A50)
Gnathomiasis 128.1
(L-56A50)
Gnathostomosis 128.1
(L-56A50)

DE-67C41 Infection by Gnathostoma dolorosi 128.1
(L-56A53)

DE-67C42 Infection by Gnathostoma nipponicum 128.1
(L-56A54)

DE-67C43 Infection by Gnathostoma spinigerum 121.1
(L-56A51)

E-680-682 Diseases Due to Superfamily Trichinelloidea

DE-68000 Capillaria infection, NOS 127.5
(L-57100)
Capillariasis 127.5
(L-57100)
Capillariosis 127.5
(L-57100)

DE-68001 Capillaria hepatica infection 128.8
(L-57111)

DE-68002 Capillaria philippinensis infection 127.5
(L-57115)

DE-68100 Trichuriasis 127.3
(L-57150)
Trichocephaliasis 127.3
(L-57150)
Whipworm infection 127.3
(L-57150)
Trichuriosis 127.3
(L-57151)

DE-68101 Infection by Trichuris trichura 127.3
(L-57151)
Infection by Trichocephalus trichiura 127.3
(L-57151)

DE-68102V Infection by Trichuris ovis
(L-57152)

DE-68103V Infection by Trichuris globulosa
(L-57153)

DE-68104V Infection by Trichuris suis
(L-57155)

DE-68105V Infection by Trichuris vulpis
(L-57156)

DE-68150 Infection by Anatrichosoma, NOS
(L-57190)

DE-68160V Infection by Trichosomoides, NOS
(L-57170)
Trichosomoidosis
(L-57170)

DE-68200 Infection by larvae of Trichinella spiralis 124.-
(L-57181)
Trichiniasis 124.-
(L-57181)
Trichinosis 124.-
(L-57181)
Trichinellosis 124.-
(L-57181)

E-684 Diseases Due to Superfamily Dioctophymatoidea

DE-68400 Dioctophyma renale infection 128.8
(L-57301)
Dioctophymosis 128.8
(L-57301)

DE-68410V Infection by Histrichis, NOS
(L-57320)
Histrichiosis
(L-57320)

DE-68420V Infection by Eustrongylides, NOS
(L-57310)
Eustrongylidosis
(L-57310)

E-685 Diseases Due to Superfamily Oxyuroidea

DE-68500 Infection by Enterobius vermicularis 127.4
(L-56601)
Enterobiasis 127.4
(L-56601)
Pinworm infection 127.4
(L-56601)
Oxyuriasis 127.4
(L-56601)
Pinworm disease 127.4
(L-56601)
Threadworm infection 127.4
(L-56601)
Oxyuris vermicularis infection 127.4
(L-56601)
Enterobiosis 127.4
(L-56601)

DE-68510V Infection by Skrjabinema, NOS
(L-56640)
Skrjabinemosis
(L-56640)

DE-68520V Infection by Probstmayria, NOS
(L-56650)
Probstmayriosis
(L-56650)

E-686 Diseases Due to Superfamily Syphacioidea

DE-68600 Infection by Syphacia, NOS
(L-56720)
Syphaciosis
(L-56720)

DE-68610V Infection by Aspiculuris, NOS
(L-56700)
Aspiculuriosis
(L-56700)

DE-68620V Infection by Passalurus, NOS
(L-56710)
Passalurosis
(L-56710)

E-687-689 Diseases Due to Superfamily Strongyloidea

DE-68700 Esophagostomiasis 127.7
(L-55540)
Esophagostomosis 127.7
(L-55540)
Oesophagostomiasis 127.7
(L-55540)
Oesophagostomosis 127.7
(L-55540)
Nodular worm disease 127.7
(L-55540)

DE-68701 Infection by Oesophagostomum apiostomum 127.7
(L-55541)

DE-68702 Infection by Oesophagostomum stephanostomum 127.7
(L-55542)

DE-68703V Infection by Oesophagostomum radiatium
(L-55544)

DE-68704V Infection by Oesophagostomum columbianum
(L-55543)

DE-68705V Infection by Oesophagostomum dentatum
(L-55545)

DE-68720V Infection by Amidostomum, NOS
(L-55620)
Amidostomosis
(L-55620)

DE-68730V Infection by Strongylus, NOS
(L-55500)
Strongylosis
(L-55500)
Redworm infestation
(L-55500)
Mal seco
(L-55500)
Large-strongyle infection
(L-55500)

DE-68732V Infection by Strongylus vulgaris
(T-46510) (M-40000) (L-55504)
Verminous arteritis
(T-46510) (M-40000) (L-55504)
Verminous aneurysm
(T-46510) (M-32200) (L-55504)

DE-68734V Infection by Strongylus edentatus
(L-55502)

DE-68736V Infection by Strongylus equinus
(L-55503)

DE-68740V Infection by Triodontophorus, NOS
(L-55510)
Triodontophorosis
(L-55510)

DE-68750V Infection by Oesophagodontus, NOS
(L-555B0)
Oesophagodontosis
(L-555B0)

DE-68760V Infection by Cyathostomum, NOS
(L-55520)
Cyathostomosis
(L-55520)

E-687-689 Diseases Due to Superfamily Strongyloidea — Continued

DE-68770V Infection by Chabertia, NOS
(L-55560)
Chabertiosis
(L-55560)

DE-68780 Ternidens deminutus infection 127.7
(L-56611)

DE-68790V Infection by Posteriostomum, NOS
(L-555C0)
Posteriostomosis
(L-555C0)

DE-687A0V Infection by Craterostomum, NOS
(L-555D0)
Craterostomosis
(L-555D0)

DE-687B0V Infection by Gyalocephalus, NOS
(L-55600)
Gyalocephalosis
(L-55600)

DE-687C0V Infection by Caballonema, NOS
(L-55570)
Caballonemosis
(L-55570)

DE-68940V Infection by Cylicodontophorus, NOS
(L-55580)
Cylicodontophorosis
(L-55580)

DE-68950V Infection by Cylicostephanus, NOS
(L-55590)
Cylicostephanosis
(L-55590)

DE-68960V Infection by Cylicocyclus, NOS
(L-555A0)
Cylicocyclosis
(L-555A0)

E-68A Diseases Due to Superfamily Heterakoidea

DE-68A00V Infection by Heterakis, NOS
(L-56500)
Heterakiosis
(L-56500)

DE-68A10V Infection by Subulura, NOS
(L-56520)
Subulurosis
(L-56520)

E-690-695 Diseases Due to Superfamily Filarioidea

DE-69000 Filariasis 125.9
(L-56D00)
Filariosis 125.9
(L-56D00)

DE-69100 Infection by Dipetalonema, NOS 125.4
(L-56D80)
Dipetalonemiasis 125.4
(L-56D80)
Dipetalonemosis 125.4
(L-56D80)

DE-69110 Infection by Dipetalonema perstans 125.4
(L-56D88)
Acanthocheilonemiasis 125.4
(L-56D88)
Acanthocheilonema perstans infection 125.4
(L-56D88)

DE-69111V Infection by Dipetalonema reconditum
(L-56D81)

DE-69120 Infection by Dipetalonema streptocerca 125.6
(L-56D91)
Streptocerciasis 125.6
(L-56D91)
Acanthocheilonema streptocerca infection 125.6
(L-56D91)

DE-69200 Infection by Wuchereria bancrofti 125.0
(M-40000) (L-56E41)
Bancroftian filariasis 125.0
(M-40000) (L-56E41)
Wuchereriasis 125.0
(M-40000) (L-56E41)
Wuchereriosis 125.0
(M-40000) (L-56E41)

DE-69201 Bancroftian elephantiasis 125.0
(T-C4000) (M-40000) (L-56E41)
Chyluria due to Wuchereria bancrofti 125.0
(T-C4000) (M-40000) (L-56E41)
Lymphadenitis due to Wuchereria bancrofti 125.0
(T-C4000) (M-40000) (L-56E41)
Lymphangitis due to Wuchereria bancrofti 125.0
(T-C6010) (M-40000) (L-56E41)

DE-69210 Tropical eosinophilia 518.3
(T-28000) (M-43040) (L-56D11)
(L-56141)
Eosinophilic lung
(T-28000) (M-43040) (L-56D11)
(L-56141)
Filarial hypereosinophilia
(T-28000) (M-43040) (L-56D11)
(L-56141)
Weingarten's syndrome
(T-28000) (M-43040) (L-56D11)
(L-56141)

DE-69220 Infection by Brugia malayi 125.1
(L-56D11)
Malayan filariasis 125.1
(L-56D11)
Brugia filariasis 125.1
(L-56D11)
Brugiosis 125.1
(L-56D11)

DE-69221 Malayan elephantiasis 125.1
(T-C4000) (M-40000) (L-56D11)
Chyluria due to Brugia malayi 125.1
(T-C4000) (M-40000) (L-56D11)
Lymphadenitis due to Brugia malayi 125.1
(T-C4000) (M-40000) (L-56D11)
Lymphangitis due to Brugia malayi 125.1
(T-C6010) (M-40000) (L-56D11)

DE-69240 Ozzardian filariasis 125.5
(L-56D61)
Mansonella ozzardi infection 125.5
(L-56D61)
Filariasis ozzardi 125.5
(L-56D61)

DE-69300 Infection by Onchocerca volvulus 125.3
(L-56D31)
Onchocerciasis 125.3
(L-56D31)
Onchocercosis 125.3
(L-56D31)

DE-69301V Infection by Onchocerca gutturosa
(L-56D37)

DE-69302V Infection by Onchocerca cervicalis
(L-56D32)

DE-69303V Infection by Onchocerca reticulata
(L-56D34)

DE-69304V Infection by Onchocerca gibsoni
(L-56D33)

DE-69305V Infection by Onchocerca armillata
(L-56D36)

DE-69310V Infection by Setaria, NOS
(L-56DA0)
Setariosis
(L-56DA0)

DE-69320V Infection by Parafilaria, NOS
(L-56DB0)
Parafilariosis
(L-56DB0)

DE-69330V Infection by Stephanofilaria, NOS
(L-56E00)
Stephanofilariosis
(L-56E00)

DE-69331V Infection by Stephanofilaria stilesi
(T-01000) (M-40000) (L-56E01)
Filarial dermatitis of cattle
(T-01000) (M-40000) (L-56E01)

DE-69332V Infection by Stephanofilaria deodesi
(L-56E02)
Cascado
(L-56E02)

DE-69333V Infection by Stephanofilaria assamensis
(L-56E03)
Hump sore
(L-56E03)

DE-69334V Infection by Stephanofilaria kaeli
(L-56E04)

DE-69340V Infection by Wehrdikmansia, NOS
(L-56E30)
Wehrdikmansiosis
(L-56E30)

DE-69350V Infection by Elaeophora, NOS
(L-56D70)
Elaeophorosis
(L-56D70)

DE-69351V Infection by Elaeophora schneideri
(L-56D71) (L-63000) (L-63070)
Filarial dermatosis
(T-01000) (L-56D71) (L-63000)
(L-63070)
Sore head
(L-56D71) (L-63000) (L-63070)
Clear-eyed blindness
(T-AA000) (L-56D71) (L-63000)
(L-63070)

DE-69400 Infection by Dirofilaria, NOS 125.6
(L-56D20)
Dirofilariasis 125.6
(L-56D20)
Dirofilariosis 125.6
(L-56D20)

DE-69402 Pulmonary dirofilariasis 125.6
(T-28000) (L-56D20)

DE-69404 Subcutaneous dirofilariasis 125.6
(T-03000) (L-56D22)
Infection by Dirofilaria conjunctivae 125.6
(T-03000) (L-56D22)

DE-69410 Infection by Dirofilaria immitis 125.6
(L-56D21)
Canine filariasis 125.6
(L-56D21)
Heartworm disease 125.6
(L-56D21)

DE-69500 Infection by Loa loa 125.2
(T-AA000) (L-56D51)
Loiasis 125.2
(T-AA000) (L-56D51)
Eyeworm disease of Africa 125.2
(T-AA000) (L-56D51)
Loasis 125.2
(T-AA000) (L-56D51)

DE-69550 Infection by Meningonema, NOS
(L-56E50)
Meningonemiasis
(L-56E50)

DE-69551 Infection by Meningonema peruzzi
(L-56E51)

E-697 Diseases Due to Superfamily Dracunculoidea

DE-69700 Infection by Dracunculus medinensis 125.7
(L-56C01)
Dracontiasis 125.7
(L-56C01)
Dracunculiasis 125.7
(L-56C01)
Guinea worm disease 125.7
(L-56C01)

E-697 Diseases Due to Superfamily Dracunculoidea — Continued

DE-69700V (cont.) Dracunculosis 125.7
(L-56C01)

DE-69702V Infection by Dracunculus insignis
(L-56C02)

DE-69720V Infection by Philometroides, NOS
(L-56C20)
Philometroidosis
(L-56C20)

E-698-699 Diseases Due to Superfamily Trichostrongyloidea

DE-69800 Trichostrongyliasis 127.6
(L-55A00)
Trichostrongylosis 127.6
(L-55A00)

DE-69801 Infection by Trichostrongylus orientalis 127.6
(L-55A02)

DE-69802 Infection by Trichonstrongylus colubriformis 127.6
(L-55A01)

DE-69803V Infection by Trichostrongylus axei
(L-55A06)

DE-69830V Infection by Haemonchus, NOS
(L-55A20)
Haemonchosis
(L-55A20)

DE-69831V Infection by Haemonchus contortus
(L-55A21)

DE-69832V Infection by placei
(L-55A22)

DE-69840V Infection by Ostertagia, NOS
(L-55A50)
Ostertagiosis
(L-55A50)

DE-69841V Infection by Ostertagia ostertagi
(L-55A51)

DE-69842V Infection by Ostertagia circumcincta
(L-55A52)

DE-69850V Infection by Cooperia, NOS
(L-55B00)
Cooperiosis
(L-55B00)

DE-69851V Infection by Cooperia punctata
(L-55B01)

DE-69852V Infection by Cooperia curticei
(L-55B02)

DE-69860V Infection by Nematodirus, NOS
(L-55A30)
Nematodirosis
(L-55A30)

DE-69861V Infection by Nematodiirus filicollis
(L-55A33)

DE-69862V Infection by Nematodirus spathiger
(L-55A32)

DE-69870V Infection by Marshallagia, NOS
(L-55C00)
Marshallagiosis
(L-55C00)

DE-69880V Infection by Skrjabinagia, NOS
(L-55AA0)
Skrjabinagiosis
(L-55AA0)

DE-69890V Infection by Grosspiculagia, NOS
(L-55AB0)
Grosspiculagiosis
(L-55AB0)

DE-698A0V Infection by Ollulamus, NOS
(L-55C70)
Ollulanosis
(L-55C70)

DE-698B0V Infection by Molineus, NOS
(L-55B70)
Molineosis
(L-55B70)

DE-698C0V Infection by Nippostrongylus, NOS
(L-55D00)
Nippostrongylosis
(L-55D00)

DE-69900V Infection by Spiculopteragia, NOS
(L-55AC0)
Spiculopteragiosis
(L-55AC0)

DE-69910V Infection by Camelostrongylus, NOS
(L-55C30)
Camelostrongylosis
(L-55C30)

DE-69920V Infection by Mecistocirrus, NOS
(L-55C80)
Mecistocirrosis
(L-55C80)

DE-69930V Infection by Hyostrongylus, NOS
(L-55A90)
Hyostrongylosis
(L-55A90)

DE-69940V Infection by Dictyocaulus, NOS
(L-55A70)
Dictyocaulosis
(L-55A70)

DE-69950V Infection by Obeliscoides, NOS
(L-55A80)
Obeliscoidosis
(L-55A80)

DE-69960V Infection by Ornithostrongylus, NOS
(L-55C10)
Ornithostrongylosis
(L-55C10)

DE-69970V Infection by Graphidium, NOS
(L-55C40)
Graphidiosis
(L-55C40)

DE-69980V Infection by Epomidiostomum, NOS
(L-55C60)
Epomidiostomosis
(L-55C60)

E-69A Diseases Due to Superfamily Rhabdiasoidea

DE-69A00 Infection by Strongyloides, NOS 127.2
(L-55300)
Strongyloidiasis 127.2
(L-55300)
Strongyloidosis 127.2
(L-55300)

DE-69A01 Infection by Strongyloides stercoralis 127.2
(L-55301)

DE-69A03V Infection by Strongyloides westeri
(L-55304)

DE-69A04V Infection by Strongyloides ransomi
(L-55305)

DE-69A05V Infection by Strongyloides papillosus
(L-55302)

DE-69A06V Infection by Strongyloides ratti
(L-55307)

DE-69A07V Infection by Strongyloides simiae
(L-55309)

DE-69A08V Infection by Strongyloides fulleborni
(L-55306)

DE-69A09V Infection by Strongyloides cebus
(L-55312)

DE-69A11V Infection by Strongyloides tumefaciens
(L-55313)

DE-69A12V Infection by Strongyloides canis
(L-55311)

E-69B Diseases Due to Superfamily Rhabditoidea

DE-69B00V Infection by Rhabditis, NOS
(L-55400)

DE-69B01V Infection by Rhabditis strongyloides
(T-01000) (M-40000) (L-55405)
Rhabditic dermatitis
(T-01000) (M-40000) (L-55405)
Pelodera dermatitis
(T-01000) (M-40000) (L-55405)

DE-69B10V Infection by Micronema, NOS
(L-55450)

E-6A0 Diseases Due to Superfamily Metastrongyloidea

DE-6A000V Infection by Metastrongylus, NOS
(L-55E00)
Metastrongylosis
(L-55E00)

DE-6A010V Infection by Protostrongylus, NOS
(L-55E10)
Protostrongylosis
(L-55E10)

DE-6A020V Infection by Filaroides, NOS
(L-55E30)
Filaroidosis
(L-55E30)

DE-6A030V Infection by Parafilaroides, NOS
(L-55E40)
Parafilaroidosis
(L-55E40)

DE-6A040V Infection by Troglostrongylus, NOS
(L-55E50)
Troglostrongylosis
(L-55E50)

DE-6A050V Infection by Crenosoma, NOS
(L-55E60)
Crenosomosis
(L-55E60)

E-6A2 Diseases Due to Superfamily Syngamoidea

DE-6A200V Infection by Syngamus, NOS
(L-55700)
Syngamosis
(L-55700)

DE-6A210V Infection by Stephanurus, NOS
(L-55710)
Stephanurosis
(L-55710)

DE-6A211V Infection by Strephanurus dentatus
(T-71000) (L-55711)
Kidney worm infection
(T-71000) (L-55711)

DE-6A220V Infection by Cyathostoma, NOS
(L-55720)

DE-6A230V Infection by Mammomonogamus, NOS
(L-55750)

E-6C DISEASES DUE TO ACANTHOCEPHALA

DE-6C000V Infection by Acanthocephala, NOS
(L-5E000)

DE-6C100V Infection by Macracanthorhynchus, NOS
(L-5E810)
Macracanthorhynchosis
(L-5E810)

DE-6C101V Infection by Macracanthorhynchus hirudinaceus
(L-5E811)

DE-6C120V Infection by Moniliformis, NOS
(L-5E830)
Moniliformiosis
(L-5E830)

DE-6C130V Infection by Acanthocephalus, NOS
(L-5E400)
Acanthocephalosis
(L-5E400)

DE-6C140V Infection by Echinorhynchus, NOS
(L-5E420)
Echinorhynchosis
(L-5E420)

DE-6C150V Infection by Polymorphus, NOS
(L-5E540)
Plymorphosis
(L-5E540)

DE-6C160V Infection by Filicollis, NOS
(L-5E550)
Filicolliosis
(L-5E550)

E-6C DISEASES DUE TO ACANTHOCEPHALA — Continued

DE-6C200V Infection by Pomphorhynchus, NOS
(L-5E300)
Pomphorhynchosis
(L-5E300)

DE-6C250V Infection by Neoechinorhynchus, NOS
(L-5E700)
Neoechinorhynchosis
(L-5E700)

DE-6C260V Infection by Prosthenorchis, NOS
(L-5E850)
Prosthenorchosis
(L-5E850)

DE-6C261V Infection by Prosthenorchis elegans
(L-5E851)

SECTION E-7 DISEASES DUE TO ARTHROPODS

E-70-74 DISEASES DUE TO ARTHROPODS

DE-70000 Disease due to Arthropod, NOS
(L-60000)
Arthropod infestation, NOS
(L-60000)
Arthropodosis
(L-60000)

DE-70010 Infestation by insect, NOS
(L-60001)

DE-70020 Infestation by cockroach, NOS
(L-60002)

DE-70030 Infestation by beetle, NOS 134.1
(L-60003)
Scarabiasis 134.1
(L-60003)

DE-70040 Infestation by bed bug, NOS
(L-61100)
Infestation by Cimex, NOS
(L-61100)

DE-70041 Infestation by Cimex lectularius
(L-61101)

DE-70100 Infestation by Anoplura, NOS
(L-61500)
Infestation by sucking lice, NOS
(L-61500)
Anoplurosis
(L-61500)

DE-70110 Infestation by Haematopinus, NOS
(L-61510)
Haematopinosis
(L-61510)

DE-70120 Infestation by Linognathus, NOS
(L-61540)
Linognathosis
(L-61540)

DE-70130 Infestation by Pediculus, NOS 132.9
(L-61520)
Pediculosis 132.9
(L-61520)

DE-70131 Pediculosis capitis 132.0
(T-01400) (T-D1160) (L-61523)

DE-70132 Pediculosis corporis 132.1
(T-01400) (T-D2000) (L-61521)

DE-70138 Mixed pediculosis 132.3
(L-.....)

DE-70140 Infestation by Phthirus, NOS
(L-61530)
Phthiriasis
(L-61530)
Phthiriosis
(L-61530)

DE-70141 Infestation by Phthirus pubis 132.2
(T-01400) (T-12360) (L-61531)
Pediculosis pubis 132.2
(T-01400) (T-12360) (L-61531)

DE-70150 Infestation by Solenopotes, NOS
(L-61550)

DE-70200 Infestation by Mallophaga, NOS
(L-61800)
Infestation by biting lice, NOS
(L-61800)
Mallophagosis
(L-61800)

DE-70300 Infestation by Siphonaptera, NOS
(L-60025)
Infestation by fleas, NOS
(L-60025)
Siphonapterosis
(L-60025)

DE-70310 Tunga penetrans infestation 134.1
(L-64001)
Tungiasis 134.1
(L-64001)
Jigger disease 134.1
(L-64001)
Chigoe disease 134.1
(L-64001)
Infestation by sand flea 134.1
(L-64001)
Sarcopsyllosis 134.1
(L-64001)

DE-70320 Infestation by Pulex, NOS
(L-64100)
Pulicosis
(L-64100)

DE-70321 Infestation by Pulex irritans
(L-64101)
Infestation by human flea
(L-64101)

DE-70330 Infestation by Xenopsylla, NOS
(L-64110)
Xenopsyllosis
(L-64110)

DE-70340 Infestation by Ceratophyllus, NOS
(L-64220)
Ceratophyllosis
(L-64220)

DE-70350 Infestation by Ctenocephalides, NOS
(L-64130)
Ctenocephalidosis
(L-64130)

DE-70352V Allergic dermatitis due to bite of Ctenocephalides felis
(T-01000) (M-40000) (F-C3000)
(G-C001) (M-14360) (L-64132)

DE-70354V Allergic dermatitis due to bite of Ctenocephalides canis
(T-01000) (M-40000) (F-C3000)
(G-C001) (M-14360) (L-64131)

DE-71000 Infestation by Diptera, NOS
(L-60008)
Infestation by biting gnats, NOS
(L-60008)
Dipterosis
(L-60008)

DE-71100V Infestation by Simuliidae, NOS
(L-62000)
Simuliidosis
(L-62000)

DE-71150V Infestation by Psychodidae, NOS
(T-01000) (L-62100)

DE-71152V Harara
(T-01000) (M-14360) (L-62100)
(M-36320) (M-01730) (F-C3000)
Allergic skin reaction due to sand fly bite
(T-01000) (M-14360) (L-62100)
(M-36320) (M-01730) (F-C3000)
Urticaria multiformis endemica
(T-01000) (M-14360) (L-62100)
(M-36320) (M-01730) (F-C3000)

DE-71200V Infestation by Ceratopogonidae, NOS
(L-62200)
Ceratopogonidosis
(L-62200)

DE-71300V Infestation by Culicidae, NOS
(L-62600)
Culicidosis
(L-62600)

DE-71302V Culicoides brevitarsus hypersensitivity reaction of skin
(T-01000) (F-C3000) (L-62218)
Sweet itch in horses
(T-01000) (F-C3000) (L-62218)
Queensland itch
(T-01000) (F-C3000) (L-62218)
Kasen
(T-01000) (F-C3000) (L-62218)
Equine allergic dermatitis
(T-01000) (F-C3000) (L-62218)

DE-71400 Infestation by fly larvae, NOS 134.0
(L-60020)
Myiasis, NOS 134.0
(L-60020)
Infestation by maggots 134.0
(L-60020)

DE-71401 Dermal myiasis 134.0
(T-01000) (L-60020)
Creeping myiasis 134.0
(T-01000) (L-60020)
Congo floor maggot disease 134.0
(T-01000) (L-60020)
Cutaneous myiasis 134.0
(T-01000) (L-60020)

DE-71402 Ophthalmic myiasis 134.0
(T-AA000) (L-60020)
Ophthalmomyiasis 134.0
(T-AA000) (L-60020)

DE-71403 Genitourinary myiasis 134.0
(T-70200) (L-60020)

DE-71404 Intestinal myiasis 134.0
(T-50500) (L-60020)

DE-71405 Rectal myiasis 134.0
(T-59600) (L-60020)

DE-71500V Infestation by Tabanidae, NOS
(L-63000)
Tabanidosis
(L-63000)

DE-71600V Infestation by Muscidae, NOS
(L-63700)
Muscidosis
(L-63700)

DE-71700V Infestation by Calliphoridae, NOS
(L-63900)
Infestation by blow flies, NOS
(L-63900)
Calliphoridosis
(L-63900)

DE-71702V Cutaneous blowfly myiasis
(T-01000) (L-63960) (L-63920)
(L-63900)
Calliphorine myiasis
(T-01000) (L-63960) (L-63920)
(L-63900)
Blowfly strike
(T-01000) (L-63960) (L-63920)
(L-63900)

DE-71710V Infestation by Calliphora, NOS
(L-63900)
Calliphorosis
(L-63900)

DE-71720V Infestation by Lucilia, NOS
(L-63960)
Luciliosis
(L-63960)

DE-71730V Infestation by Phormia, NOS
(L-63920)
Phormiosis
(L-63920)

DE-71740V Infestation by Chrysomya, NOS
(L-63A00)
Chrysomyosis
(L-63A00)

E-70-74 DISEASES DUE TO ARTHROPODS — Continued

DE-71742V Cutaneous screw-worm myiasis
(T-01000) (L-63980) (L-63A00)
DE-71750V Infestation by Cochliomyia, NOS
(L-63980)
Cochliomyiosis
(L-63980)
Infestation by Callitroga, NOS
(L-63980)
Callitrogosis
(L-63980)
DE-71800V Infestation by Sarcophagidae, NOS
(L-63D00)
Infestation by flesh flies, NOS
(L-63D00)
Sarcophagidosis
(L-63D00)
DE-71810V Infestation by Sarcophaga, NOS
(L-63D00)
Sarcophagosis
(L-63D00)
DE-71820V Infestation by Wohlfahrtia, NOS
(L-63D20)
Wohlfahrtiosis
(L-63D20)
DE-71900V Infestation by Hypodermatidae, NOS
(L-63B00)
Hypodermatidosis
(L-63B00)
DE-71910V Infestation by Hypoderma, NOS
(L-63B00)
Hypodermosis
(L-63B00)
Hypodermal rash
(L-63B00)
DE-71911V Infestation by Hypoderma bovis
(L-63B02)
Ox warble
(L-63B02)
DE-71912V Infestation by Hypoderma lineatum
(L-63B01)
DE-71920V Infestation by Oedemagena, NOS
(L-63B10)
Oedemagenosis
(L-63B10)
DE-72000V Infestation by Gasterophilus, NOS
(L-63C00)
Gasterophilosis
(L-63C00)
DE-72001 Infestation by Gasterophilus intestinalis 134.0
(L-63C01)
Horse bots
(L-63C01)
DE-72002V Infestation by Gasterophilus haemorrhoidalis
(L-63C02)
DE-72003V Infestation by Gasterophilus nasalis
(L-63C03)
DE-72004V Infestation by Gasterophilus pecorum
(L-63C05)
DE-72005V Infestation by Gasterophilus inermis
(L-63C04)
DE-72010V Infestation by Oestrus, NOS
(L-63B20)
Oestrosis
(L-63B20)
DE-72011 Infestation by Oestrus ovis 134.0
(L-63B21)
DE-72020V Infestation by Rhinoestrus, NOS
(L-63B30)
Rhinoestrosis
(L-63B30)
DE-72030V Infestation by Cephenemyia, NOS
(L-63B50)
Cephenemyiosis
(L-63B50)
DE-72040 Infestation by Dermatobia, NOS
(L-63B70)
DE-72041 Infestation by Dermatobia hominis 134.0
(L-63B71)
DE-72100V Infestation by Hippoboscidae, NOS
(L-63300)
Infestation by louse flies, NOS
(L-63300)
DE-72110V Infestation by Hippobosca, NOS
(L-63300)
Hippoboscosis
(L-63300)
DE-72120V Infestation by Melophagus, NOS
(L-63370)
Melophagosis
(L-63370)
DE-72130V Infestation by Cuterebra, NOS
(L-63E50)
Cuterebrosis
(L-63E50)
DE-74000 Infestation by Acarina, NOS 133.9
(L-60054)
Acariasis 133.9
(L-60054)
Mite infestation, NOS 133.9
(L-60054)
Acarinosis 133.9
(L-60054)
DE-74010V Infection by Tyrophagus, NOS
(L-67030)
DE-74080 Tick fever, NOS
DE-74090 Tick paralysis 989.5
DE-74100 Infestation by Ixodidae, NOS
(L-66000)
Ixodidosis
(L-66000)
Infestation by hard tick
(L-66000)
DE-74110 Infestation by Ixodes, NOS
(L-66000)
Ixodosis
(L-66000)

DE-74120V Infestation by Dermacentor, NOS
(L-66050)
Dermacentorosis
(L-66050)
DE-74130V Infestation by Haemaphysalis, NOS
(L-66080)
Haemaphysalosis
(L-66080)
DE-74140V Infestation by Rhipicephalus, NOS
(L-66130)
Rhipicephalosis
(L-66130)
DE-74150V Infestation by Hyalomma, NOS
(L-66170)
Hyalommosis
(L-66170)
DE-74160V Infestation by Amblyomma, NOS
(L-66200)
Amblyommosis
(L-66200)
DE-74170V Infestation by Boophilus, NOS
(L-66230)
Boophilosis
(L-66230)
DE-74300V Infestation by Argasidae, NOS
(L-66300)
Argasidosis
(L-66300)
Infestation by soft tick
(L-66300)
DE-74310V Infestation by Argas, NOS
(L-66300)
Argasosis
(L-66300)
DE-74320V Infestation by Ornithodorus, NOS
(L-66350)
Ornithodorosis
(L-66350)
DE-74330V Infestation by Otobius, NOS
(L-66330)
Otobiosis
(L-66330)
DE-74400V Infestation by Dermanyssidae, NOS
(L-66600)
DE-74410V Infestation by Dermanyssus, NOS
(L-66600)
Dermanyssosis
(L-66600)
DE-74411V Infestation by Dermanyssus gallinae
(L-66601)
DE-74420V Infestation by Pneumonyssus, NOS
(L-66640)
Pneumonyssosis, NOS
(L-66640)
DE-74421V Infestation by Pneumonyssus simicola
(T-28000) (L-66641)
Pulmonary acariasis
(T-28000) (L-66641)
DE-74422V Infestation by Pneumonyssus caninum
(L-66651)
Nasal acariasis
(L-66651)
DE-74430V Infestation by Rhinophaga, NOS
(L-66680)
DE-74500V Infestation by Macronyssidae, NOS
(L-66700)
DE-74510V Infestation by Ornithonyssus, NOS
(L-66720)
Ornithonyssosis
(L-66720)
DE-74600V Infestation by Varroidae, NOS
(L-66A00)
DE-74610V Infestation by Varroa, NOS
(L-66A00)
Varroosis
(L-66A00)
DE-74700V Infestation by Tarsonemidae, NOS
(L-66B00)
DE-74710V Infestation by Acarapis, NOS
(L-66B10)
Acarapisosis
(L-66B10)
DE-74800V Infestation by Demodex, NOS
(L-67500)
Demodicosis
(L-67500)
Demodectic mange
(L-67500)
Follicular mange
(L-67500)
Demodectic red mange
(L-67500)
DE-74801 Infestation by Demodex folliculorum 133.8
(L-67501)
DE-74802V Infestation by Demodex canis
(L-67502)
DE-74803V Infestation by Demodex cati
(L-67507)
DE-74804V Infestation by Demodex criceti
(L-67511)
DE-74805V Infestation by Demodex phylloides
(L-67504)
DE-74850V Infestation by Trombicula, NOS 133.8
(L-67600)
Chiggers 133.8
(L-67600)
Trombiculosis 133.8
(L-67600)
DE-74860V Infestation by Neotrombicula
(L-67604)
Neotrombiculosis
(L-67604)
DE-74870V Infestation by Cheyletiella, NOS
(L-67900)
Cheyletiellosis
(L-67900)

E-70-74 DISEASES DUE TO ARTHROPODS — Continued

DE-74870V (cont.) Cheyletiella dermatitis
(L-67900)

DE-74871V Infestation by Cheyletiella parasitivorax
(L-67901)

DE-74872V Infestation by Cheyletiella yasguri
(L-67902)

DE-74880V Infestion by Cytodites, NOS
(L-67490)
Cytoditosis
(L-67490)

DE-74881V Infestation by Cytodites nudus
(L-67491)

DE-74890V Infestation by Psorergates, NOS
(L-67930)
Psorergatosis
(L-67930)

DE-74891V Infestation by Psorergates ovis
(L-67931)
Itch mite infestation
(L-67931)

DE-74892V Infestation by Psorergates simplex
(L-67932)

DE-74900V Infestation by Myobia, NOS
(L-67A00)
Myobiosis
(L-67A00)

DE-74901V Infection by Myobia musculi
(L-67A01)

DE-74910V Infestation by Acarus, NOS
(L-67000)

DE-74920 Infestation by Pyemotes, NOS
(L-67700)

DE-74921 Infestation by Pyemotes ventricosus 133.8
(L-67702)
Infestation by Grain mite, NOS 133.8
(L-67702)
Grain itch 133.8
(L-67702)

DE-74930 Infestation by Sarcoptes, NOS 133.0
(L-67200)
Sarcoptosis 133.0
(L-67200)

DE-74931 Infestation by Sarcoptes scabiei 133.0
(L-67201)
Scabies 133.0
(L-67201)
Sarcoptic itch 133.0
(L-67201)
Mange 133.0
(L-67201)
Sarcoptic mange 133.0
(L-67201)
Cutaneous acariasis 133.0
(T-01000) (L-67201)
Sarcoptic red mange 133.0
(L-67201)
Norwegian scabies 133.0
(L-67201)

DE-74932V Infestation by Sarcoptes scabiei var bovis
(L-67205)
Barn itch
(L-67205)

DE-74933V Infestation by Sarcoptes scabiei var equi
(L-67204)

DE-74934V Infestation by Sarcoptes scabiei var suis
(L-67203)

DE-74935V Infestation by Sarcoptes scabiei var canis
(L-67206)

DE-74936V Infestation by Sarcoptes scabiei var ovis
(L-67207)

DE-74940V Infestation by Notoedres, NOS
(L-67230)
Notoedrosis
(L-67230)
Notoedric mange
(L-67230)
Head mange
(L-67230)

DE-74941V Infestation by Notoedres cati
(L-67231)

DE-74950V Infestation by Knemidokoptes, NOS
(L-67250)
Knemidokoptosis
(L-67250)

DE-74951V Infestation by Knemidokoptes mutans
(L-67251)
Scaly leg
(L-67251)

DE-74952V Infestation by Knemidokoptes gallinae
(L-67252)
Depluming itch
(L-67252)

DE-74953V Infestation by Knemidokoptes pilae
(L-67253)
Scaly face
(L-67253)

DE-74960V Infestation by Psoroptes, NOS
(L-67400)
Psoroptosis
(L-67400)
Psoroptic mange
(L-67400)
Psotoptic scabies
(L-67400)
Scab
(L-67400)

DE-74961V Infestation by Psoroptes ovis
(L-67402)
Sheep scab
(L-67402)

DE-74962V Infestation by psotoptes cuniculi
(L-67401)
Psoroptic ear mange in goat
(L-67401)

DE-74962V (cont.) Otoacariasis
(L-67401)

DE-74970V Infestation by Chorioptes, NOS
(L-67420)
Chorioptosis
(L-67420)
Chorioptic mange
(L-67420)

DE-74971V Infestation by Chorioptes bovis
(L-67421)
Leg mange
(L-67421)

DE-74972V Infestation by Chorioptes texanus
(L-67422)

DE-74980V Infestation by Otodectes, NOS
(L-67450)
Otodectosis
(L-67450)
Otodectic mange
(L-67450)
Ear mange
(L-67450)

DE-74981V Infestation by Otodectes cynotis
(L-67451)

DE-74990V Infestation by Myocoptes, NOS
(L-67350)
Myocoptosis
(L-67350)

DE-74991V Infestation by Mycoptes musculinus
(L-67351)

E-780 Diseases Due to Pentastomida

DE-78000 Disease due to Pentastomida, NOS 134.8
(L-69320)

DE-78010 Linguatulosis 134.8
(L-69400)
Disease due to Linguatula, NOS 134.8
(L-69400)

DE-78011 Disease due to Linguatula serrata 134.8
(L-69401)

DE-78012 Nasopharyngeal linguatulosis 134.8
(T-23000) (L-69400)

DE-78020 Disease due to Pentastoma, NOS 134.8
(L-69320)

DE-78021 Infection by Pentastoma denticulatum 134.8
(L-69321)

DE-78022 Infection by Pentastoma najae 134.8
(L-69325)

DE-78030 Disease due to Armillifer, NOS 134.8
(L-69300)

DE-78031 Infection by Armillifer armillatus 134.8
(L-69301)
Infection by Porocephalus armillatus 134.8
(L-69301)

DE-78032 Infection by Armillifer grandi 134.8
(L-69302)

DE-78040 Porocephaliasis 134.8
(L-69340)
Porocephalosis 134.8
(L-69340)
Porcephalosis 134.8
(L-69340)

DE-78041 Infection by Porocephalus moniliformis 134.8
(L-69303)

DE-78042 Infection by Porocephalus crotali 134.8
(L-69344)

E-790 Diseases Due to Annelida

DE-79000 Disease due to Annelid worms, NOS

DE-79010 Leech infestation, NOS 134.2
(L-5F100)
Hirudiniasis, NOS 134.2
(L-5F100)
Leeches, NOS 134.2
(L-5F100)

DE-79011 Infestation by Hirudo medicinalis 134.2
(L-5F102)

SECTION E-8 INFECTIOUS DISEASES DUE TO PLANTS

DE-80100 Infection by Algae, NOS 136.8
(L-DD110)
Protothecosis, NOS 136.8
(L-DD110)

DE-80110 Infection by Prototheca segbwema 136.8
(L-DD116)

DE-80120 Infection by Prototheca wickerhamii 136.8
(L-DD113)

DE-80130 Infection by Prototheca zopfi 136.8
(L-DD111)

SECTION E-9 INFECTIONS DUE TO CHORDATES

DE-90100 Icthyoparasitism, NOS 136.8
(L-C0000)

DE-90110 Candiru infestation 136.8
(L-C0000)

DE-90120 Icthyoparasitism due to Vandellia cirrhosa 136.8
(L-C0000)

SECTION E-A INFECTIOUS DISEASES OF UNDETERMINED ETIOLOGY

DE-A0000 Infectious or communicable disease of undetermined etiology, NOS 136.9
(L-00004)

DE-A0100 Acute infective gastroenteritis, NOS 009.0
(T-50100) (L-00004)

DE-A0200 Acute mesenteric adenitis 289.2
(T-C4510) (L-00004)
Acute mesenteric lymphadenitis 289.2
(T-C4510) (L-00004)

SECTION E-A INFECTIOUS DISEASES OF UNDETERMINED ETIOLOGY — Continued

DE-A0300 Ainhum 136.0
(M-17050) (L-00004)
Dactylolysis spontanea 136.0
(M-17050) (L-00004)

DE-A0350 Nongonococcal urethritis, NOS 099.4
(T-75000) (L-00004) (DE-01600)
Nonspecific urethritis, NOS 099.4
(T-75000) (L-00004) (DE-01600)
NGU, NOS 099.4
(T-75000) (L-00004) (DE-01600)

DE-A0400 Behcet's syndrome, NOS 136.1
(L-00004)
Behcet's disease, NOS 136.1
(L-00004)
Generalized aphthosis 136.1
(L-00004)

DE-A0401 Behcet's syndrome, complete type 136.1
(L-00004)

DE-A0402 Behcet's syndrome, incomplete type 136.1
(L-00004)

DE-A0403 Behcet's syndrome, vascular type 136.1
(L-00004)

DE-A0404 Behcet's syndrome, intestinal type 136.1
(L-00004)

DE-A0405 Behcet's syndrome, neurologic type 136.1
(L-00004)

DE-A0600 Bilateral hilar adenopathy syndrome 785.6
(L-00004)
Lofgren's syndrome 785.6
(L-00004)

DE-A0650 Benign multirecurrent endothelioleukocytal meningitis 322.9
(L-00004)
Mollaret's meningitis 322.9
(L-00004)

DE-A0700 Chronic benign lymphocytic meningitis 047.8 —321.7*
(L-00004)

DE-A0800 Epidemic cervical myalgia 078.89
(L-00004)

DE-A1000 Fisher's syndrome
(L-00004)
Ophthalmoplegia, ataxia, areflexia syndrome
(L-00004)

DE-A1100 Hakuri
(L-00004)
Sakamoto's disease
(L-00004)
Pseudocholera infantum
(L-00004)

DE-A1200 Iceland disease 049.8 —323.4*
(L-00004)
Epidemic neuromyasthenia 049.8 —323.4*
(L-00004)
Akureyri disease 049.8 —323.4*
(L-00004)
Benign myalgic encephalomyelitis 049.8 —323.4*
(L-00004)

DE-A1300 Infectious neuronitis 357.0
(L-00004)
Landry-Guillain-Barré syndrome 357.0
(L-00004)
Ascending paralysis 357.0
(L-00004)
PNS neuronitis 357.0
(L-00004)
Guillain-Barré syndrome 357.0
(L-00004)
Acute infective polyneuritis 357.0
(L-00004)

DE-A1306V Canine polyradiculoneuritis
Coonhound paralysis

DE-A1320 Izumi fever
(L-00004)

DE-A1350 Ozena 472.0
(L-00004)
Severe chronic rhinitis 472.0
(L-00004)

DE-A1400 Reiter's disease 099.3
(L-00004)
Urethrooculoarticular syndrome 099.3
(L-00004)
Reiter's syndrome 099.3
(L-00004)

DE-A1420 Sarcoidosis, NOS 135.-
(L-00004)
Boeck's sarcoid 135.-
(L-00004)
Besnier-Boeck-Schaumann syndrome 135.-
(L-00004)
Miliary lupoid of Boeck 135.-
(L-00004)
Lupus pernio of Besnier 135.-
(L-00004)
Benign lymphogranulomatosis of Schaumann 135.-
(L-00004)
Darier-Roussy sarcoid 135.-
(L-00004)
Uveoparotid fever 135.-
(L-00004)

DE-A1421 Pulmonary sarcoidosis 135.-
(T-28000) (L-00004)

DE-A1422 Splenic sarcoidosis 135.-
(T-C3000) (L-00004)

DE-A1423 Lymph node sarcoidosis 135.-
(T-C4000) (L-00004)

DE-A1424 Cutaneous sarcoidosis 135.-
(T-01000) (L-00004)

DE-A1425 Subcutaneous sarcoidosis 135.-
(T-03000) (L-00004)

DE-A1430 Sarcoidosis, anular type 135.-
(L-00004)

DE-A1431 Sarcoidosis, nodular type 135.-
(L-00004)

DE-A1432 Sarcoidosis, plaque type 135.-
(L-00004)

DE-A1433 Sarcoidosis, erythrodermic type 135.-
(L-00004)

DE-A1434 Sarcoidosis, lupus pernio type 135.-
(L-00004)

DE-A1435 Sarcoidosis, angiolupoid type 135.-
(L-00004)

DE-A1436 Sarcoidosis, Darier-Roussy type 135.-
(L-00004)

DE-A1500 Summer diarrhea of infants 009.3
(L-00004)
Infantile diarrhea 009.3
(L-00004)

DE-A1520 Epidemic vomiting syndrome 078.82
—386.1*
(L-00004)
Winter vomiting disease 078.82
(L-00004)

DE-A1550 Myospherulosis 136.8
(L-00004)

DE-A2000V Transmissible canine venereal tumor
Transmissible venereal tumor of dog
Infectious granuloma
Venereal granuloma
Sticker tumor
Transmissible sarcoma

SECTION E-B ILL-DEFINED AND PRESUMED INFECTIOUS DISEASES

DE-B0000 Ill-defined infectious disease, NOS
(L-00004)

DE-B0100 Ill-defined intestinal infection, NOS 009.-
(T-50500) (L-00004)

DE-B0110 Infectious colitis, NOS 009.0
(T-59300) (L-00004)
Septic colitis, NOS 009.0
(T-59300) (L-00004)

DE-B0120 Infectious enteritis, NOS 009.0
(T-50500) (L-00004)
Septic enteritis, NOS 009.0
(T-50500) (L-00004)

DE-B0130 Infectious gastroenteritis, NOS 009.0
(T-50100) (L-00004)
Septic gastroenteritis, NOS 009.0
(T-50100) (L-00004)

DE-B0200 Infectious diarrheal disease, NOS 009.2
(T-50500) (L-00004)
Infectious diarrhea 009.2
(T-50500) (L-00004)

DE-B0210 Dysenteric diarrhea 009.2
(T-50500) (L-00004)

DE-B0220 Epidemic diarrhea 009.2
(T-50500) (L-00004)

DE-B0230 Traveler's diarrhea
(T-50500) (L-00004)
Turista
(T-50500) (L-00004)

DE-B0300 Dysentery, NOS 009.0
(T-50500) (L-00004)

DE-B0310 Catarrhal dysentery 009.0
(T-50500) (L-00004)

DE-B0320 Hemorrhagic dysentery 009.0
(T-50500) (L-00004)

DE-B2000 Disease of presumed infectious origin, NOS
(L-00004)

DE-B2100 Diarrhea of presumed infectious origin 009.3
(T-50500) (L-00004)
Diarrheal disease, NOS 009.3
(T-50500) (L-00004)

DE-B2110 Colitis presumed infectious 009.1
(T-59300) (L-00004)

DE-B2120 Enteritis presumed infectious 009.1
(T-50500) (L-00004)

DE-B2130 Gastroenteritis presumed infectious 009.1
(T-50100) (L-00004)

CHAPTER F — GENERAL DISEASE CLASSES, VICTIM STATUS AND DEATH

SECTION F-0 GENERAL CONVENIENCE DISEASE TERMS

DF-00000 Disease, NOS
  Disease or syndrome present, NOS
  Clinical disease or syndrome present, NOS
  Clinical disease or syndrome, NOS
DF-00001 Acute disease, NOS
DF-00002 Subacute disease, NOS
DF-00003 Chronic disease, NOS
DF-00009 Ill-defined disease 799.8
  Ill-defined condition 799.8
DF-00010 Disease, alleged but not proven
DF-00020 Disease suspected
DF-00030 Disease ruled out after examination
DF-00050 Organic disease present
DF-00060 Functional disease present
  Clinical disease or syndrome present, related to functional disturbance
DF-00090 Subclinical disease or syndrome
DF-000A0 Disease type or category unknown 799.9
  Undiagnosed disease or syndrome present 799.9
DF-000B0 Disease type or category not applicable
DF-000C0 Disease type or category not assigned
DF-00100 Systemic disease, NOS
DF-00110 Epidemic disease, NOS
DF-00114 Epizootic disease
DF-00120 Endemic disease, NOS
DF-00124 Enzootic disease
DF-00130 Idiopathic disease, NOS
DF-00140 Primary disease, NOS
DF-00150 Secondary disease, NOS
DF-00160 Recurrent disease, NOS
DF-00170 Intercurrent disease, NOS
DF-00180 Hereditary disease, NOS
  Inherited disease, NOS
  Genetic disease, NOS
DF-00190 Familial disease, NOS
DF-00200 Neonatal disease, NOS
  Perinatal disease, NOS
DF-00210 Infantile disease, NOS
DF-00220 Juvenile disease, NOS
DF-00230 Adult disease, NOS
DF-00280 Local disease, NOS
  Localized disease, NOS
DF-00300 Environment related disease, NOS
DF-00320 Social environment related disease
DF-00330 Nature environment related disease
DF-00340 Industrial environment related disease
DF-00350 Institutional environment related disease
DF-00360 Home environment related disease
DF-00380 Radiation disease, NOS
DF-00400 Neoplastic disease, NOS
  Neoplastic syndrome, NOS
DF-00410 Benign neoplastic disease
DF-00430 Malignant neoplastic disease
DF-00440 Familial neoplastic disease
DF-00450 Paraneoplastic syndrome
DF-00500V Psychic disease, NOS

SECTION F-1 DRUG-RELATED DISORDERS

DF-10000 Drug-related disorder, NOS
DF-10010 Drug reaction, NOS
  Adverse drug effect, NOS
DF-10012 Idiosyncratic drug effect
  Drug idiosyncratic effect
DF-10020 Drug interaction
DF-10030 Allergic drug reaction
DF-10100 Drug overdose, NOS
  (C-50000)
DF-10200 Drug abuse, NOS
  (C-50000)
DF-10202 Dependent drug abuse
  Drug addiction
DF-10204 Non dependent drug abuse
DF-10300 Drug tolerance, NOS
  (C-50000)
DF-10350 Drug intolerance, NOS
  (C-50000)
DF-10352 Oral contraceptive intolerance
  (C-A0700)
DF-10400 Drug resistance, NOS
  (C-50000)
DF-10402 Drug resistance to insulin
  (C-A2200)

SECTION F-D DEATHS, VICTIM STATUS AND BODY IDENTIFICATION

F-D0 DEATHS

F-D00 Types of Deaths

DF-D0000 Death, NOS
DF-D0005 Death of unknown cause 799.9
DF-D0006 Death in less then 24 hours from onset of symptoms 798.2
  Died without sign of disease 798.2
DF-D0010 Sudden death, NOS 798.-
DF-D0012 Instantaneous death 798.1
DF-D0020 Unexpected death, NOS
DF-D0021V Sudden death syndrome of feeder cattle
DF-D0022 Unexpected sudden death of adult
DF-D0024 Sudden infant death syndrome 798.0
  Unexpected sudden death of infant 798.0
  SIDS 798.0
  Crib death 798.0
  Cot death 798.0
DF-D0030 Unattended death, NOS 798.9
  Found dead 798.9
DF-D0032 Death unattended by physician
DF-D0040 Iatrogenic death, NOS
DF-D0042 Death during anesthetic induction

DF-D0044 Anesthetic death
DF-D0046 Intraoperative death
DF-D0048 Postoperative death
DF-D0050 Death by fire, NOS
DF-D0052 Death by cremation
DF-D0054 Death by immolation
  Immolation
DF-D0060 Maternal death, NOS
DF-D0062 Antepartum maternal death
DF-D0064 Intrapartum maternal death
DF-D0066 Postpartum maternal death
DF-D0080 Death in hospital, NOS
DF-D0090 Dead on arrival
  D.O.A.

F-D01 Natural Deaths

DF-D0100 Natural death, NOS
  Death due to natural causes, NOS
DF-D0110 Natural death with proved cause, NOS
DF-D0120 Natural death with proved cause by autopsy
DF-D0122 Natural death with proved cause without autopsy
DF-D0130 Natural death with probable cause suspected
  Natural death with suspected cause
DF-D0140 Natural death with unknown cause
DF-D0160 Natural death reportable to medicolegal authority

F-D02 Deaths by Asphyxiation and Drowning

DF-D0200 Asphyxiation, NOS 994.7
  Suffocation, NOS 994.7
  Death by asphyxiation, NOS 994.7
  Death by suffocation, NOS 994.7
DF-D0210 Traumatic asphyxiation 994.7
  Traumatic asphyxial state 994.7
  Smothering 994.7
DF-D0220 Asphyxiation by injury to air passages
DF-D0222 Asphyxiation by sustained compression of chest
DF-D0230 Asphyxiation by environmental gas exposure, NOS
DF-D0232 Asphyxiation by environmental toxic gas
DF-D0234 Asphyxiation by environmental toxic vapors
DF-D0238 Asphyxiation by environmental oxygen lack
DF-D0241 Suffocation by bedclothes 994.7
DF-D0242 Suffocation by cave-in 994.7
DF-D0243 Suffocation by constriction 994.7
DF-D0244 Suffocation by plastic bag 994.7
DF-D0245 Suffocation by pressure 994.7
DF-D0260 Death by strangulation 994.7
  Strangulation 994.7
DF-D0264 Garrotment 994.7
DF-D0270 Death by hanging
DF-D0290 Drowning, NOS 994.1
  Fatal submersion-immersion
DF-D0292 Drowning in fresh water
DF-D0294 Drowning in salt water
DF-D0296 Drowning in brackish water
DF-D0298 Drowning in other liquid

F-D03 Accidental Deaths

DF-D0300 Accidental death, NOS
DF-D0310 Accidental death in home
DF-D0320 Accidental death in industrial place
  Accidental death in work place
DF-D0330 Accidental death in public place
DF-D0340 Traffic vehicular accidental death
DF-D0342 Non-traffic vehicular accidental death
DF-D0350 Death by electrocution 994.8
  Electrocution 994.8

F-D05 Homicides

DF-D0500 Homicide, NOS
DF-D0510 Murder, NOS
DF-D0511 First degree murder
DF-D0512 Second degree murder
DF-D0514 Manslaughter
DF-D0516 Justifiable homicide
DF-D0520 Matricide
DF-D0522 Patricide
DF-D0524 Fratricide
DF-D0526 Sororicide
DF-D0528 Infanticide
DF-D0530 Murder of spouse
DF-D0540 Murder of relative
DF-D0550 Murder of friend
DF-D0552 Murder of acquaintance
DF-D0554 Murder of stranger
DF-D0560 Murder by hired killer
DF-D0562 Gangland style homicide
  Gangland execution
DF-D0570 Homicide attempt
DF-D0590 Euthanasia
  Mercy killing

F-D06 Suicides

DF-D0600 Suicide, NOS
DF-D0610 Suicide by self-administered drug
DF-D0630 Suspected suicide
  Probable suicide
DF-D0640 Suicide attempt, NOS
DF-D0641 First known suicide attempt
DF-D0642 Previous known suicide attempt
DF-D0643 Suicide attempt by adequate means
DF-D0644 Suicide by multiple means
DF-D0646 Suicide attempt by inadequate means
  Unsuccessful suicide attempt
  Suicide gesture
DF-D0680 Suicide while incarcerated
  Suicide under legal jurisdiction

F-D07 Legal Executions

DF-D0700 Execution, NOS
DF-D0710 Judicial execution, NOS
  Legal execution, NOS

F-D07 Legal Executions — Continued

DF-D0720 Judicial execution by hanging
DF-D0730 Judicial execution by electric chair
DF-D0740 Judicial execution by gas chamber
DF-D0750 Judicial execution by guillotine
DF-D0760 Judicial execution by firing squad

F-D09 Undetermined Manner of Death

DF-D0900 Undetermined manner of death, NOS
  Open verdict
DF-D0910 Undetermined manner of death, natural causes suspected
DF-D0920 Undetermined manner of death, accidental cause suspected
DF-D0922 Undetermined manner of death, accidental means suspected
DF-D0930 Undetermined manner of death, homicide suspected
DF-D0940 Undetermined manner of death, suicide suspected

F-D1 VICTIM STATUS AND IDENTIFICATION

F-D10 Victim Status: General Terms

DF-D1000 Victim status, NOS
DF-D1010 Victim of physical trauma, NOS
DF-D1020 Victim of trauma with multiple injuries, NOS

F-D11 Vehicular Traffic Accident Victims

DF-D1100 Victim of vehicular or traffic accident, NOS
DF-D1102 Driver in vehicular or traffic accident
DF-D1104 Passenger in vehicular or traffic accident, NOS
DF-D1106 Front seat passenger in vehicular or traffic accident
DF-D1108 Rear seat passenger in vehicular or traffic accident
DF-D1120 Victim, pedestrian in vehicular or traffic accident
DF-D1130 Victim, cyclist in vehicular or traffic accident
DF-D1140 Victim, motorcycle rider in vehicular or traffic accident
DF-D1152 Victim in two vehicle accident
DF-D1158 Victim in more than two vehicle accident
  Multiple vehicle crash victim

F-D12 Aircraft Accident Victims

DF-D1200 Victim of aircraft accident, NOS
DF-D1210 Pilot in aircraft accident
DF-D1212 Crewmember in aircraft accident
DF-D1216 Steward in aircraft accident
DF-D1220 Passenger in aircraft accident
DF-D1250 On ground bystander victim in aircraft accident
DF-D1280 Victim of spacecraft accident

F-D13 Watercraft Accident Victims

DF-D1300 Victim of watercraft accident, NOS
DF-D1310 Driver in watercraft accident
DF-D1320 Passenger in watercraft accident
DF-D1330 Water-skier in watercraft accident
DF-D1340 Bystander in watercraft accident

F-D14 Sports Activities Victims

DF-D1400 Victim of sports activities, NOS
DF-D1410 Player in sports activity accident
  Participant in sports activity accident
DF-D1420 Coach in sports activity accident
DF-D1430 Bystander in sports activity accident

F-D15 Work-Related Accident Victims

DF-D1500 Work-related activity accident, NOS
DF-D1510 Worker in work-related accident
DF-D1520 Co-worker in work-related accident
DF-D1530 Employer in work-related accident
DF-D1540 Visitor in work related accident

F-D16 Victims of Physical Assault

DF-D1600 Victim of physical assault, NOS
DF-D1610 Child maltreatment syndrome 995.5
  Victim of infant/child abuse
  Battered baby or child syndrome, NOS 995.5
DF-D1616 Emotional and/or nutritional maltreatment of child 995.5
  Victim of infant/child neglect
DF-D1620 Adult maltreatment syndrome 995.81
  Abused person, NOS 995.81
  Battered person syndrome, NOS 995.81
DF-D1622 Battered spouse syndrome 995.81
DF-D1626 Battered woman syndrome 995.81
DF-D1630 Victim of sexual aggression
DF-D1634 Victim of rape
  Rape victim
DF-D1636 Victim of statutory rape
  Statutory rape victim
DF-D1640 Victim of homosexual agression

F-D17 Victims of Armed Conflict

DF-D1700 Victim of armed conflict, NOS
DF-D1710 Victim of civil disturbance
DF-D1712 Victim of civil insurrection
DF-D1714 Victim of civil warfare
DF-D1720 Victim of ambush
DF-D1722 Victim of guerrilla warfare
DF-D1730 Victim of land warfare
DF-D1740 Victim of naval warfare
DF-D1750 Victim of aerial warfare
DF-D1760 Victim of international warfare
DF-D1770 Victim of international action
  Victim of military action
  Victim of peacekeeping action

F-D18 Conditions and Status of Human Remains

DF-D1800 Body condition unknown
DF-D1810 Body recently dead and well preserved
DF-D1820 Embalmed body
DF-D1830 Body examined by medicolegal authority
DF-D1840 Autopsied body, NOS
DF-D1842 Body autopsied twice
DF-D1844 Body autopsied three or more times
DF-D1850 Body claimed by anatomic board
DF-D1856 Unclaimed body
DF-D1860 Decomposed body, NOS
DF-D1862 Decomposed body with immersion
Wet floater
DF-D1864 Decomposed body without immersion
Dry floater
DF-D1870 Mummified body
DF-D1872 Partially skeletonized body
DF-D1874 Skeletonized body
DF-D1880 Remains of cremated body
DF-D1890 Body with missing parts, NOS
DF-D1894 Body parts for identification
(T-.....)
DF-D1896 Human bone for identification
(T-.....)
DF-D1898 Human tissue for identification
(T-.....)
DF-D18A0V Animal body parts for identification

F-D19 Body Identification

DF-D1900 Body identification, NOS
DF-D1910 Unidentified body, NOS
DF-D1912 Unidentified body but identity suspected
DF-D1920 Body identified by finger prints
DF-D1922 Body identified by scars
DF-D1923 Body identified by specific x-ray details
DF-D1924 Body identified by dental examination
DF-D1930 Body with presumptive identification by family
DF-D1932 Body with presumptive identification by personal objects

F-D1A Burial and Disinterment

DF-D1A00 Burial, NOS
DF-D1A10 Burial alive
Live burial
Buried alive
DF-D1A50 Disinterment, NOS
Exhumation, NOS
DF-D1A52 Disinterment for identification
DF-D1A54 Disinterment for establishment of cause of death
DF-D1A55 Disinterment for recovery of objects
DF-D1A56 Disinterment for recovery of evidence
DF-D1A57 Disinterment for recovery of tissues

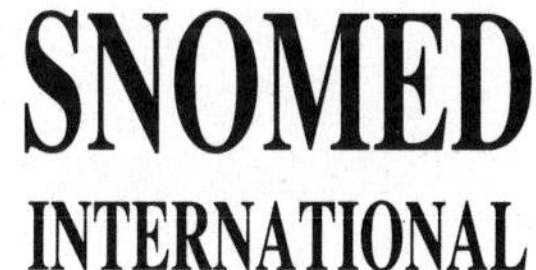

Procedures

A classification of health care procedures

The Procedures Module contains both generic and specific administrative, medical, surgical, and nursing procedures as well as those performed by paraprofessionals and other providers from the entire health care field. Procedures organized in this manner will facilitate the full integration of the actions taken by all health professionals that are deemed necessary to provide care to patients.

P

Introduction to Procedures

The Procedures Module of SNOMED International consists of an ordered set of terms that describe and name in a precise and specific manner the procedural activities utilized by the entire array of providers who contribute to the care of patients.

An enumeration of the chapter headings of this module provides an overview of the extent of provider services that are included. In alphabetical order, these include: Administrative Procedures and Services; Anesthesia; Dental; Laboratory; Medical Invasive and Medical Non invasive; Nursing; Operative; Physical Medicine Procedures and Activities; Psychiatric and Psychologic; and Radiologic including Ultrasound and Nuclear Medicine. In each of these professional areas, the full range of procedures and services provided are assigned a standardized termcode that is unique for each service or activity. This provides a single unified representation in the record for all medical specialties and for all other providers, including institutions.

There are approximately 27,000 terms each with its specifically assigned termcode. Multiple national and international documents were used as sources for this module.

The first chapter, P0, includes administrative procedures such as hospital admissions, discharges, transfers, and referrals, as well as patient status determinations, disability evaluations, chart reviews and audits, and medico-legal procedures.

Operative procedures are found in Chapter P1, which is the largest section of the module containing more than 18,000 entries. The first section (0) of the Operative Procedures chapter (P1) is devoted solely to generic procedures. These are the basic procedures that are performed on virtually all organ systems. Each generic procedure is assigned to one of nine categories: General and Miscellaneous Operative Procedures; Incisions; Excisions; Injections-Implantations; Endoscopy; Surgical Repairs, Closures, and Reconstructions; Destructive Procedures; Transplantations-Transpositions; and Manipulations. The same nine major categories are used to divide the operative procedures performed on each organ system. The subsequent sections devoted to Operative Procedures contain the site specific operations presented in a standardized organ-system format which to a large extent encompasses the operations performed by each surgical specialty. Chapter P1–1 is devoted to the Musculoskeletal System procedures; P1–2 to the Respiratory System Procedures; P1–3 to the Cardiovascular System Procedures, etc. It should be noted that the Topography and Diseases/Diagnoses Modules are similarly constructed in their organ system assignment.

Operative Procedures can also be cross-referenced back to the site of the operation as well as to the generic procedure creating a polyhierarchial data structure that is rich in detail. For example, the generic operation, **Incision, NOS** is found in the **P1-0** section as **-01000.** If the incision is of a specific anatomical site the first **0** is replaced by a two-digit topography code and the **1** for incision is moved back to the third position.; thus, **P1-52100 = Incision of tongue,** NOS. In the same manner, the code for the generic term **Excision, NOS** is **P1-03000** and **Excision of tongue, NOS** is **P1-52300.**

Qualifying terms describing the approach used in performing a specific procedure such as transabdominal vs transthoracic are found in the General Linkage–Modifiers module of SNOMED International. In this way any procedure that is performed can be linked by cross reference to designate a specific approach. This is unlike previous editions of SNOMED where a fifth digit modifier was used to describe approaches for a select number of procedures. The advantage of using the General Linkage–Modifiers module is that these terms become available for the entire set of procedural terms on an as-needed basis.

This edition of the Procedures Module does not provide references to other procedural coding schemes. In the Diseases/Diagnoses Module, for example, corresponding ICD–9–CM codes are provided when applicable for each SNOMED entry; in the Function Module, the International Union of Biochemistry (IUB) codes are referenced for each enzyme; and in the Topography Module, the ICD–O site codes for neoplasms are referenced.

Veterinary terms and procedures are integrated and intermingled into each of the chapters. Some categories such as feed analysis and animal grooming require separate sections.

Laboratory services are the second largest section of the Procedures Module. This is a comprehensive compilation of services performed by clinical laboratories, research laboratories, and specialty laboratories throughout the world. Whether it is a rare hemoglobin type or an unusual enzyme, a precise procedure termcode is provided and available by cross referencing between the Function and Procedures Modules of SNOMED International. The other chapters contain Medical Procedures and Services; Physical Medicine Procedures, including Osteopathic and Chiropractic Manipulations; Psychiatric and Psychologic Tests and Services; Dental Services and Procedures; Radiology Procedures with Radiotherapy, Nuclear Medicine, and Ultrasound; and a final Chapter that attempts to list and categorize all patient-related procedures and activities of the nursing staff that are essential to the overall care of the patient.

This Procedures Module represents a significant expansion from its predecessor in the second edition of SNOMED. It is intended to fully and precisely describe procedures performed by all health care personnel. As currently elaborated, it is not intended to function as a billing system.

As the need to computerize the entire medical record increases, not only physician services but all services will need to be defined, captured, and analyzed. A single unified representation of all of these activities is essential. This Procedures Module is a first step in that process.

CHAPTER 0 — ADMINISTRATIVE PROCEDURES AND PHYSICIAN SERVICES

SECTION 0-0 PROCEDURES: GENERAL TERMS

P0-00000 Procedure, NOS
P0-00010 Unknown procedure
P0-00020 Procedure code not applicable
P0-00030 Procedure code not assigned
P0-00100 Administrative procedure, NOS

SECTION 0-1 HOSPITAL ADMISSIONS

P0-10000 Hospital admission, NOS
P0-10010 Hospital admission, elective, NOS
  Hospital admission, planned, NOS
P0-10020 Hospital admission, elective, with complete pre-admission work-up
P0-10030 Hospital admission, elective, with partial pre-admission work-up
P0-10040 Hospital admission, elective, without pre-admission work-up
P0-10050 Hospital admission, precertified by medical audit action
P0-10060 Hospital admission, urgent, 48 hours
P0-10100 Hospital admission, emergency, NOS
P0-10110 Hospital admission, emergency, direct
P0-10120 Hospital admission, emergency, indirect
P0-10130 Hospital admission, emergency, from emergency room, NOS
P0-10140 Hospital admission, emergency, from emergency room, medical nature
P0-10150 Hospital admission, emergency, from emergency room, accidental injury
P0-10160 Hospital admission for isolation
P0-10200 Hospital admission, special, NOS
P0-10210 Hospital admission, transfer from other hospital or health care facility
P0-10230 Hospital admission, boarder, for social reasons
P0-10240 Hospital admission, parent, for in-hospital child care
P0-10250 Hospital admission, for observation
P0-10260 Hospital admission, involuntary
P0-10270 Hospital admission, under police custody
P0-10280 Hospital admission, by legal authority (commitment)
P0-10290 Hospital admission, from remote area, by means of special transportation
P0-10300 Hospital admission, limited to designated procedures
P0-10310 Hospital admission, for research investigation
P0-10320 Hospital admission, donor for transplant organ
P0-10330 Hospital admission, mother, for observation, delivered outside of hospital
P0-10340 Hospital admission, infant, for observation, delivered outside of hospital
P0-10410 Hospital admission, blood donor
P0-10420 Hospital admission, for laboratory work-up, radiography, etc.
P0-10430 Hospital admission, pre-nursing home placement
P0-10450 Hospital admission, short-term, NOS
P0-10460 Hospital admission, short-term, day care
P0-10470 Hospital admission, short-term, 24 hours
P0-10500 Admission certification, NOS
  Certification of admission, NOS
  Admission review, NOS
P0-10510 Admission certification approved
P0-10520 Admission certification denied
P0-10600 Procurement of patient informed consent, NOS
  Assurance of patient protection
P0-10610 Procurement of patient informed consent, investigational study
P0-10800 Emergency room admission, NOS
P0-10810 Emergency room admission, followed by release
P0-10820 Emergency room admission, dead on arrival (DOA)
P0-10830 Emergency room admission, died in emergency room
P0-10850 Hospital re-admission
P0-10890 Hospital admission, type unclassified, explain by report
P0-10900 General outpatient clinic admission, NOS
P0-10950 Specialty clinic admission, NOS

SECTION 0-2 PATIENT DISCHARGES, TRANSFERS AND REFERRALS

0-200-202 Patient Discharges

P0-20000 Patient discharge, NOS
P0-20030 Patient discharge, to home, routine
P0-20050 Patient discharge, to home, ambulatory
P0-20070 Patient discharge, to home, with assistance
P0-20090 Patient discharge, to legal custody
P0-20100 Patient discharge, signed out against medical advice
  Self-discharged patient
P0-20120 Patient discharge, elopement
P0-20130 Patient discharge, escaped from custody
P0-20180 Patient discharge, deceased, autopsy
P0-20190 Patient discharge, deceased, no autopsy
P0-20210 Patient discharge, deceased, medicolegal case
P0-20260 Patient discharge, deceased, donation of body
P0-20270 Patient discharge, deceased, to anatomic board
P0-20280 Patient on pass
P0-20290 Patient discharge, type unclassified, explain by report

0-203-204 Patient Transfers

P0-20300 Patient transfer, to another health care facility, NOS
P0-20310 Patient transfer, to another health care facility, definitive
P0-20320 Patient transfer, to another health care facility, temporary
P0-20330 Patient transfer to skilled nursing facility (SNF)
P0-20331 Patient transfer to skilled nursing facility for level 1 care
P0-20332 Patient transfer to skilled nursing facility for level 2 care
P0-20333 Patient transfer to skilled nursing facility for level 3 care
P0-20334 Patient transfer to skilled nursing facility for level 4 care
P0-20390 Patient transfer, to another health care facility, type unclassified, explain by report
P0-20400 Patient transfer, in-hospital, NOS
P0-20410 Patient transfer, in-hospital, bed-to-bed
P0-20420 Patient transfer, in-hospital, unit-to-unit
P0-20430 Patient transfer, in-hospital, service-to-service

0-205-206 Patient Referrals

P0-20500 Patient referral, NOS
P0-20510 Patient referral for consultation, NOS
  Request for consultation, NOS
P0-20520 Patient referral for medical consultation, NOS
P0-20530 Patient referral for specialized institutional services, NOS
P0-20540 Patient referral for rehabilitation, physical
P0-20550 Patient referral for rehabilitation, psychological
P0-20551 Patient referral for psychotherapy
P0-20552 Patient referral for psychiatric aftercare
P0-20553 Patient referral for alcoholism rehabilitation
P0-20554 Patient referral for drug addiction rehabilitation
P0-20555 Patient referral for vocational rehabilitation
P0-20580 Patient referral for special education
P0-20590 Patient referral for specialized training
P0-20600 Patient referral for socioeconomic factors
P0-20610 Patient referral for family planning
P0-20670 Patient referral for evaluation, aging problem
P0-20680 Patient referral for special care, aging problem

SECTION 0-3 DISPOSITIONS, DETERMINATIONS AND OUTCOMES

0-300 Patient Dispositions

P0-30000 Routine patient disposition, no follow-up planned
P0-30010 Patient follow-up planned and scheduled
  Patient follow-up appointment scheduled
P0-30020 Patient follow-up to return when and if necessary

0-302-303 Patient Status Determinations

P0-30200 Patient status determination, NOS
  Patient condition determination, NOS
P0-30210 Patient status determination, unchanged
  Patient status stable
P0-30220 Patient status determination, slightly improved
P0-30230 Patient status determination, moderately improved
P0-30240 Patient status determination, greatly improved
P0-30270 Patient status determination, slightly worse
P0-30280 Patient status determination, moderately worse
P0-30290 Patient status determination, much worse
P0-30300 Patient status determination, critical
P0-30320 Patient status determination, pre-terminal
P0-30350 Patient status determination, deceased
  Patient pronounced dead

0-304 Disease Condition Determinations

P0-30400 Disease condition determination, NOS
P0-30410 Disease condition determination, uncontrolled
P0-30420 Disease condition determination, slightly controlled
P0-30430 Disease condition determination, moderately controlled
P0-30440 Disease condition determination, fairly well controlled
P0-30450 Disease condition determination, well controlled
P0-30460 Disease condition determination, arrested
P0-30470 Disease condition determination, cured

0-305 Treatment Response Determinations

P0-30500 Treatment response determination, NOS
P0-30510 Treatment response determination, no response
P0-30520 Treatment response determination, minimal
  Treatment response determination, slight
P0-30530 Treatment response determination, fair
P0-30540 Treatment response determination, good
P0-30550 Treatment response determination, excellent

0-306-308 Outcome Determinations

P0-30600 Determination of outcome, NOS
P0-30610 Determination of outcome, satisfactory to patient
P0-30620 Determination of outcome, unsatisfactory to patient
P0-30630 Determination of outcome, satisfactory to physician
P0-30640 Determination of outcome, unsatisfactory to physician

P0-30700 Determination of outcome, complication unavoidable
P0-30710 Determination of outcome, complication avoidable, NOS
  Therapeutic misadventure
P0-30720 Determination of outcome, complication avoidable, error in diagnosis
P0-30730 Determination of outcome, complication avoidable, error in judgement
P0-30740 Determination of outcome, complication avoidable, error in technique
P0-30800 Determination of outcome, death unavoidable
P0-30810 Determination of outcome, death avoidable, NOS
P0-30820 Determination of outcome, death avoidable, error in diagnosis
P0-30830 Determination of outcome, death avoidable, error in judgement
P0-30840 Determination of outcome, death avoidable, error in technique
P0-30850 Determination of outcome, death avoidable, chart audit required

SECTION 0-8 CHART RELATED PROCEDURES

0-800-801 Chart Reviews and Audits

P0-80000 Chart review by physician, NOS
P0-80010 Chart review by physician, complete
P0-80012 Chart review by physician and preparation of abstract or summary
  Preparation of discharge summary
P0-80020 Chart review by physician, update
  Progress note by physician
P0-80040 Chart review by physician and preparation of detailed report for other physician or institution
  Chart review by physician and preparation of referral report
P0-80050 Chart review by physician with change in entry

0-805-806 Medical Audit and Quality of Care Procedures

P0-80500 Quality of care or medical audit procedure, NOS
  Medical evaluation, quality of care
P0-80510 Medical evaluation, quality of care, review of exception case
P0-80520 Medical evaluation, utilization review
  Medical evaluation, extended stay review
P0-80600 Medical audit procedure, NOS
P0-80610 Concurrent audit
P0-80620 Primary audit
P0-80630 Process audit
P0-80640 Prospective audit
P0-80650 Retrospective audit
  Outcome audit
P0-80660 Medical service audit
P0-80670 Nursing service audit
P0-80680 Planning audit
P0-80690 Ancillary service audit
P0-806A0 Financial audit
  Disease costing audit

0-808 Chart Evaluation by Medical Records

P0-80800 Chart evaluation, NOS
  Chart evaluation by medical records department
P0-80820 Chart review, verification of charges
P0-80830 Chart review, verification of procedures
P0-80850 Chart opening
P0-80860 Chart abstracting
P0-80870 Chart abstracting by exception
P0-80890 Chart completion by medical records

SECTION 0-9 MEDICO-LEGAL PROCEDURES AND DISABILITY EVALUATIONS

0-900 Medical Testimony and Reports

P0-90000 Medical testimony, NOS
P0-90010 Preparation of written report for lawyer
P0-90020 Legal deposition regarding patient's problem or condition
P0-90030 Legal court testimony concerning aspects of patient's problem or condition
P0-90040 Chain of custody procedure
P0-90050 Preparation of routine medical insurance claim
P0-90080 Consultation for paternity case

0-902-904 Disability Evaluation Procedures

P0-90200 Disability evaluation procedure, NOS
P0-90201 Disability evaluation, disability 1%
P0-90202 Disability evaluation, disability 2%
P0-90203 Disability evaluation, disability 3%
P0-90204 Disability evaluation, disability 4%
P0-90205 Disability evaluation, disability 5%
P0-90206 Disability evaluation, disability 6%
P0-90207 Disability evaluation, disability 7%
P0-90208 Disability evaluation, disability 8%
P0-90209 Disability evaluation, disability 9%
P0-90210 Disability evaluation, disability 10%
P0-90212 Disability evaluation, disability 12%
P0-90215 Disability evaluation, disability 15%
P0-90218 Disability evaluation, disability 18%
P0-90220 Disability evaluation, disability 20%
P0-90225 Disability evaluation, disability 25%
P0-90230 Disability evaluation, disability 30%
P0-90235 Disability evaluation, disability 35%
P0-90240 Disability evaluation, disability 40%
P0-90245 Disability evaluation, disability 45%

0-902-904 Disability Evaluation Procedures — Continued

P0-90250 Disability evaluation, disability 50%
P0-90255 Disability evaluation, disability 55%
P0-90260 Disability evaluation, disability 60%
P0-90265 Disability evaluation, disability 65%
P0-90270 Disability evaluation, disability 70%
P0-90275 Disability evaluation, disability 75%
P0-90280 Disability evaluation, disability 80%
P0-90285 Disability evaluation, disability 85%
P0-90290 Disability evaluation, disability 90%
P0-90295 Disability evaluation, disability 95%
P0-90298 Disability evaluation, disability 98%
P0-90299 Disability evaluation, disability 99%
P0-90300 Disability evaluation, disability 100%
P0-90350 Preparation of disability evaluation report
P0-90370 Preparation of detailed report for patient's disability including corrective recommendations
P0-90380 Preparation of workmen's compensation claim for occupational/industrial disease or condition
P0-90400 Disability evaluation, normal, no disability, no impairment
P0-90410 Disability evaluation, impairment, class 1
P0-90420 Disability evaluation, impairment, class 2
P0-90430 Disability evaluation, impairment, class 3
P0-90440 Disability evaluation, impairment, class 4
P0-90450 Disability evaluation, impairment, class 5
P0-90460 Disability evaluation, impairment, class 6
P0-90470 Disability evaluation, impairment, class 7
P0-90480 Disability evaluation, impairment, class 8
P0-90490 Disability evaluation, impairment, class 9

CHAPTER 1 — OPERATIONS AND ANESTHESIA PROCEDURES

SECTION 1-0 GENERIC OPERATIVE PROCEDURES

1-00 GENERAL OPERATIVE PROCEDURES

P1-00000 Operative procedure, NOS
Operation, NOS
P1-00010 Routinely scheduled operation, NOS
P1-00020 Emergency operation, NOS
P1-00030 Revisional operation, NOS
Surgical revision, NOS
Revision, NOS
P1-00050 Incision, exploration and biopsy for determination of stage of disease, NOS
Staging operation, NOS
P1-00052 Incision and reexploration for second look
Second look operation
Incision and reexploration of recent operation
P1-00100 First stage of staged operation
P1-00102 Subsequent stage of staged operation
P1-00200 Laser surgery, NOS
Laser surgical technique, NOS

1-01 INCISIONS

P1-01000 Incision, NOS
Dissection, NOS
P1-01001 Exploratory incision
Incision and exploration
Surgical exploration
P1-01005 Preliminary incision
Preparatory incision
P1-01006 Preventive incision
P1-01007 Incision and packing of wound
P1-01008 Decompressive incision
Decompression
P1-01010 Incision and drainage
I and D
Incision and evacuation
P1-01011 Drilling
P1-01020 Transection, NOS
Release, NOS
Division, NOS
Cutting, NOS
Section, NOS
Severing, NOS
P1-01021 Discission
P1-01023 Slitting
P1-01025 Bisection
P1-01026 Bifurcation
P1-01100 Puncture, NOS
Piercing, NOS
Perforation, NOS
P1-01105 Scarification
P1-01130 Centesis, NOS
Paracentesis
Puncture and aspiration
Puncture and drainage
Needling and drainage
Tap

1-03 EXCISIONS

P1-03000 Excision, NOS
Resection, NOS
Incision and removal, NOS
Extirpation, NOS
Ablation, NOS
Abscission, NOS
P1-03001 Partial excision
Subtotal excision
Incision and partial removal
P1-03002 Complete excision
Complete incision and removal
P1-03004 Wedge excision, NOS
Wedge resection, NOS
V excision, NOS
P1-03005 Tylectomy, NOS
Lumpectomy, NOS
P1-03007 Hemi-excision
Partial excision of one half of organ
Partial excision of one half of structure
Hemi-resection
P1-03008 Segmental excision and ligation, NOS
P1-03009 Excision incidental to other operation
Incidental operation
P1-03020 Reexcision, NOS
P1-03030 Amputation, NOS
P1-03032 Plastic amputation
Kineplasty
P1-03033 Radical amputation
P1-03034 Transfixion
P1-03035 Reamputation, NOS
P1-03038 Disarticulation, NOS
P1-03050 Radical excision
Extended excision
P1-03051 Radical excision with lymph node dissection
Extended excision with lymph node dissection
P1-03052 Radical excision with en bloc resection of regional organs and tissues
P1-03053 Evisceration
Exenteration
Evidement
P1-03056 Enucleation
P1-03080 Trephination, NOS
P1-03100 Biopsy, NOS
P1-03101 Excisional biopsy
P1-03102 Incisional biopsy
Incision and biopsy
Open biopsy
P1-03110 Shave biopsy
P1-03112 Punch biopsy
P1-03114 Trephine biopsy

1-03 EXCISIONS — Continued

P1-03116 Trocar biopsy
P1-03120 Needle biopsy, NOS
  Core needle biopsy, NOS
P1-03122 Fine needle biopsy, NOS
  Aspiration biopsy, NOS
  Fine needle aspiration biopsy, NOS
P1-03123 Superficial fine needle aspiration biopsy
P1-03124 Deep fine needle aspiration biopsy under radiologic guidance
P1-03125 Combined needle and aspiration biopsy
P1-03126 Loop electrosurgical excision procedure, NOS
  LEEP
P1-03130 Removal by suction
  Aspiration procedure
P1-03140 Debridement, NOS
P1-03142 Saucerization, NOS
P1-03150 Curettage, NOS
  Curettement, NOS
P1-03151 Dilation and curettage
P1-03154 Grattage
  Removal by scraping
  Scraping
P1-03156 Filleting
P1-03160 Excision and replacement, NOS
P1-03170 Removal of suture, NOS
P1-03176 Removal of foreign body, NOS
P1-03177 Incision and removal by magnet
  Incision and removal of foreign body by magnet
P1-03180 Excision and storage of tissue, organ or cells

1-05 INJECTIONS AND IMPLANTATIONS

1-050 Injections

P1-05000 Injection, NOS
P1-05001 Intralesional injection
P1-05002 Intravenous injection
P1-05003 Intra-arterial injection
P1-05004 Intramuscular injection
P1-05005 Subcutaneous injection
P1-05006 Intradermal injection
P1-05007 Intraperitoneal injection
P1-05008 Intramedullary injection
P1-05009 Intrathecal injection
P1-05011 Intra-articular injection
P1-05012 Intracavitary injection
P1-05015 Tattooing
P1-05020 Injection of prophylactic substance, NOS
P1-05022 Injection of therapeutic agent, NOS
P1-05024 Injection of sclerosing agent, NOS
P1-05026 Injection of air
P1-05027 Injection of gas
P1-05028 Politzerization, NOS
P1-05030 Infusion, NOS
P1-05031 Intravenous infusion, NOS
P1-05032 Intra-arterial infusion, NOS
P1-05033 Intra-arterial infusion of prophylactic substance, NOS
P1-05034 Intra-arterial infusion of therapeutic substance, NOS
P1-05035 Intra-arterial infusion of thrombolytic agent
P1-05036 Intra-arterial infusion of antineoplastic agent
  Intra-arterial infusion of cancer chemotherapy agent
P1-05040 Perfusion, NOS
P1-05041 In situ perfusion
P1-05042 Extracorporeal perfusion
P1-05050 Irrigation, NOS
  Lavage, NOS
P1-05052 Irrigation following insertion of catheter
  Lavage following intubation
  Irrigation following insertion of tube
  Irrigation following intubation
P1-05054 Irrigation following insertion of cannula
P1-05055 Irrigation with syringe
  Syringing
P1-05056 Toilet, NOS
P1-05060 Insufflation, NOS
P1-05070 Instillation, NOS

1-055 Implantations

P1-05500 Implantation, NOS
  Insertion, NOS
  Implant, NOS
P1-05501 Reimplantation, NOS
  Reinsertion, NOS
P1-05506 Implantation of therapeutic agent, NOS
P1-05510 Insertion of therapeutic device, NOS
  Implantation of therapeutic device, NOS
P1-05511 Closed insertion of therapeutic device
  Closed implantation of therapeutic device
P1-05512 Open insertion of therapeutic device
  Open implantation of therapeutic device
P1-05513 Removal of therapeutic device, NOS
P1-05514 Replacement of device, NOS
  Removal and replacement of prosthetic device, NOS
  Replacement of appliance, NOS
  Removal and reapplication of therapeutic device, NOS
P1-05516 Removal of external immobilization device
P1-05520 Insertion of pack
P1-05522 Insertion of tissue expander
P1-05524 Insertion of infusion pump
P1-05530 Intubation, NOS
P1-05532 Intubation and aspiration
P1-05535 Catheterization
  Insertion of catheter
P1-05540 Cannulation, NOS
  Insertion of cannula

1-07 ENDOSCOPY

P1-07000 Endoscopy, NOS
P1-07001 Endoscopy with surgical procedure, NOS
  Endoscopic surgical procedure, NOS
P1-07002 Endoscopy and calibration

P1-07004 Endoscopy and photography
P1-07006 Endoscopy and removal of foreign material
P1-07008 Endoscopy and control of hemorrhage
P1-07010 Endoscopy and fulguration
P1-07012 Endoscopy and chemocautery
P1-07014 Endoscopy and cryocautery
P1-07020 Endoscopy and catheterization
Endoscopic catheterization
P1-07030 Endoscopy and biopsy
Endoscopic biopsy
P1-07032 Endoscopy and brush biopsy
Endoscopic brush biopsy
P1-07034 Endoscopy and washing
Endoscopic washing
P1-07036 Endoscopy with brush biopsy and washing
Endoscopic brush biopsy and washing

1-08 SURGICAL REPAIRS, CLOSURES AND RECONSTRUCTIONS

1-080 Surgical Repairs

P1-08000 Surgical repair, NOS
Plastic repair, NOS
P1-08002 Plastic repair with lengthening
P1-08004 Plastic repair with shortening
Cinching
P1-08006 Plastic repair with augmentation
P1-08008 Plastic repair with reduction
Plastic repair with diminution
P1-08012 Plastic repair with reconstruction
P1-08014 Plastic repair with prosthetic implant
P1-08018 Plastic repair with excision of tissue
P1-08022 Plastic repair with radial incision
P1-08024 Plastic repair and transfer of tissue
P1-08026 Plastic repair and revision of injury
Plastic repair and revision of deformity
P1-08028 Plastic repair and revision with revascularization
P1-08032 Plastic revision of recent operation
P1-08034 Plastic repair by z plasty
Z plasty
P1-08050 Suspension and fixation, NOS
P1-08060 Exteriorization
Marsupialization
P1-08080 Repair by nailing
Nailing
Pinning
P1-08090 Reinforcement, NOS

1-084 Closures

P1-08400 Closure, NOS
Surgical closure, NOS
P1-08401 Suture, NOS
Closure by suture, NOS
P1-08402 Debridement and suture
Suture of wound following debridement
P1-08403 Resuture of wound dehiscence
P1-08405 Delayed suture of wound
Secondary closure of wound by suture
Closure of granulating wound
P1-08407 Repair with closure of non-surgical wound
P1-08408 Incision and resuture of wound
P1-08410 Closure by tape
P1-08411 Closure by clip
P1-08412 Closure by clamp
P1-08413 Closure by staple
Stapling
P1-08416 Closure by buckling
Buckling procedure
P1-08417 Banding, NOS
P1-08418 Cerclage, NOS
P1-08420 Ligation, NOS
Closure by ligation, NOS
P1-08421 Suture ligature, NOS
P1-08431 Surgical closure of anastomosis
P1-08432 Surgical closure of shunt
P1-08433 Surgical closure of stoma
P1-08434 Surgical closure of window
P1-08435 Surgical closure of pouch
P1-08440 Closure with prosthetic implant
P1-08450 Hernia repair, NOS
Herniorrhaphy, NOS
P1-08460 Fixation, NOS
Attachment, NOS
P1-08462 Cryopexy, NOS
P1-08464 Laserpexy, NOS
P1-08470 Plication
Folding
Pleating
Tucking
P1-08480 Imbrication
Overlapping

1-086-087 Surgical Constructions

P1-08600 Surgical construction, NOS
Surgical reconstruction, NOS
P1-08610 Surgical construction of anastomosis
P1-08611 Surgical construction of shunt
P1-08612 Surgical construction of stoma
P1-08613 Surgical construction of window
Fenestration
P1-08614 Surgical construction of pouch
P1-08615 Surgical construction of fistula
Fistulization
P1-08620 Microvascular anastomosis
P1-08640 Surgical repair and revision of anastomosis
Surgical reanastomosis
P1-08641 Surgical repair and revision of shunt
P1-08642 Surgical repair and revision of stoma
P1-08643 Surgical repair and revision of window
P1-08644 Surgical repair and revision of pouch
P1-08650 Surgical sequestration
P1-08700 Fusion-stabilization and immobilization
P1-08710 Refixation
Reattachment

1-0C DESTRUCTIVE PROCEDURES

P1-0C000 Destruction, NOS
  Destructive procedure, NOS
  Obliteration, NOS
P1-0C002 Avulsion, NOS
  Evulsion, NOS
P1-0C003 Partial avulsion
P1-0C004 Complete avulsion
P1-0C010 Lysis of adhesions, NOS
  Freeing and lysis, NOS
  Division and lysis, NOS
  Adhesiolysis, NOS
P1-0C012 Decortication, NOS
P1-0C015 Stripping, NOS
P1-0C016 Stripping and ligation
P1-0C020 Surgical abrasion, NOS
P1-0C021 Salabrasion
P1-0C024 Removal by grinding
  Grinding
P1-0C080 Cauterization, NOS
P1-0C100 Cryosurgery, NOS
  Cryocautery, NOS
  Destruction of lesion or structure by cold application
P1-0C104 Cryoextraction
P1-0C110 Cryosurgery with thermocouple control
  Cryosurgery with thermocouple control with liquid nitrogen
P1-0C200 Thermocautery, NOS
  Destruction of lesion or structure by heat application, NOS
  Thermocauterization, NOS
P1-0C220 Destruction of lesion or structure by electrocautery, NOS
  Fulguration, NOS
P1-0C221 Electrodesiccation
  Destruction of lesion or structure by monoterminal monopolar fulguration
P1-0C222 Electrocoagulation
  Destruction of lesion or structure by biterminal bipolar fulguration
  Electrosection cutting
P1-0C240 Destruction of lesion or structure by radiofrequency
P1-0C300 Electrodesiccation with curettage
P1-0C310 Electrocoagulation with curettage
P1-0C400 Crushing, NOS
P1-0C410 Litholapaxy
  Lithotrity
  Lithotripsy
P1-0C420 Fragmentation, NOS
  Destruction of lesion or structure by fragmentation, NOS
P1-0C430 Emulsification, NOS
  Destruction of lesion or structure by emulsification, NOS
P1-0C440 Destruction of lesion by ultrasound, NOS
P1-0C442 Extracorporeal shockwave lithotripsy, NOS
P1-0C500 Chemosurgery, NOS
  Chemocautery, NOS
  Destruction of lesion or structure by chemical application, NOS
  Chemocauterization, NOS
P1-0C504 Chemodenervation, NOS
P1-0C510 Cosmetic chemosurgery, NOS
P1-0C512 Partial cosmetic chemosurgery
P1-0C514 Complete cosmetic chemosurgery
P1-0C600 Photocoagulation, NOS
  Destruction or coagulation of lesion or structure by photocoagulation, NOS
P1-0C620 Laser beam photocoagulation, NOS
P1-0C621 Ion laser photocoagulation, NOS
P1-0C622 Argon laser photocoagulation
P1-0C623 Carbon dioxide laser photocoagulation
P1-0C624 Krypton laser photocoagulation
P1-0C625 Neodynium, yttrium, aluminum garnet laser photocoagulation
  Nd:YAG laser photocoagulation

1-0D TRANSPLANTATIONS AND TRANSPOSITIONS

P1-0D000 Transplantation, NOS
  Graft, NOS
  Grafting, NOS
P1-0D001 Pinch transplantation
P1-0D002 Split thickness transplantation
P1-0D004 Full thickness transplantation
P1-0D006 Full thickness transplantation with tube
P1-0D007 Full thickness transplantation with tube and pedicle
  Incision and tubing pedicle graft
P1-0D008 Myocutaneous transplantation
P1-0D009 Myocutaneoosseous transplantation
P1-0D010 Autogenous transplantation
  Autotransplantation
P1-0D012 Syngeneic transplantation
  Isogeneic transplantation
P1-0D016 Allogeneic transplantation
  Homotransplantation
P1-0D018 Xenogeneic transplantation
  Animal-human transplantation
  Xenotransplantation
  Heterologous transplantation
P1-0D020 Heteroautogenous transplantation, NOS
P1-0D022 Immediate allogeneic transplantation, living donor
P1-0D023 Immediate allogeneic transplantation, cadaver donor
P1-0D024 Delayed allogeneic transplantation, living donor
P1-0D025 Delayed allogeneic transplantation, cadaver donor
P1-0D026 Immediate isogeneic transplantation, living donor
P1-0D027 Immediate isogeneic transplantation, cadaver donor

P1-0D028 Delayed isogeneic transplantation, living donor
P1-0D029 Delayed isogeneic transplantation, cadaver donor
P1-0D050 Excision of tissue or organ for grafting from donor site
P1-0D052 Excision of tissue or organ for grafting from recipient site
P1-0D054 Excision of transplanted tissue or organ
P1-0D056 Excision and reimplantation of organ for extracorporeal surgery
  Bench surgery procedure
P1-0D059 Tissue graft, NOS
P1-0D100 Bypass graft, NOS
P1-0D101 Heteroautogenous bypass transplantation
P1-0D104 Bypass transplantation with xenogeneic transplant
P1-0D106 Bypass transplantation with allogeneic transplant
P1-0D108 Bypass transplantation with isogeneic transplant
P1-0D109 Repeat heteroautogenous transplantation bypass
P1-0D150 Artificial graft, NOS
  Synthetic graft, NOS
P1-0D152 Bypass graft with artificial transplant, NOS
P1-0D200 Transposition, NOS
  Surgical transfer, NOS
  Transection and repositioning
P1-0D230 Repair with advancement, NOS
  Surgical transfer with flap advancement
P1-0D235 Surgical transfer with flap construction
P1-0D237 Repair with recession, NOS
P1-0D239 Repair with resection-recession, NOS
P1-0D300 Harvesting of tissue, NOS

1-0E MANIPULATIONS

P1-0E000 Manipulation, NOS
P1-0E100 Mobilization, NOS
P1-0E110 Remobilization, NOS
P1-0E200 Manual reduction, NOS
  Taxis, NOS
P1-0E300 Extraction, NOS
  Manual extraction
P1-0E320 Epilation, NOS
P1-0E322 Epilation by forceps
P1-0E350 Expression, NOS
P1-0E400 Dilation, NOS
P1-0E410 Dilation and stretching, NOS
P1-0E420 Manual dilation and stretching
P1-0E430 Instrumental dilation and stretching
P1-0E440 Probing, NOS
  Insertion of probe, NOS
P1-0E450 Bougienage, NOS
P1-0E500 Fitting of prosthesis, NOS
  Fitting of prosthetic device, NOS
  Application of prosthesis, NOS
P1-0E600 Application, NOS
P1-0E650 Adjustment, NOS

SECTION 1-1 OPERATIVE PROCEDURES ON THE MUSCULOSKELETAL SYSTEM

1-10 GENERAL OPERATIVE PROCEDURES ON THE MUSCULOSKELETAL SYSTEM

1-100 Musculoskeletal System: General and Miscellaneous Operative Procedures

P1-10000 Operation on musculoskeletal system, NOS
P1-10001 Operation on bone, NOS
P1-10002 Operation on joint, NOS
  Operation on joint structures, NOS
P1-10003 Operation on muscle, NOS
P1-10004 Operation on tendon, NOS
P1-10005 Operation on tendon sheath, NOS
P1-10006 Operation on ligament, NOS
P1-10007 Operation on fascia, NOS
P1-10008 Operation on bursa, NOS
P1-10009 Operation on soft tissue, NOS
P1-10010 Diagnostic procedure on musculoskeletal system, NOS
P1-10011 Diagnostic procedure on bone, NOS
P1-10012 Diagnostic procedure on joint structures, NOS
P1-10013 Diagnostic procedure on muscle, NOS
P1-10014 Diagnostic procedure on tendon, NOS
P1-10015 Diagnostic procedure on tendon sheath, NOS
P1-10016 Diagnostic procedure on ligament, NOS
P1-10017 Diagnostic procedure on fascia, NOS
P1-10018 Diagnostic procedure on bursa, NOS
P1-10019 Diagnostic procedure on soft tissue, NOS
P1-10020 Operation on bone injury, NOS

1-101 Musculoskeletal System: Incisions

P1-10100 Incision of bone, NOS
  Incision of bone without division, NOS
P1-10102 Division of bone, NOS
  Transection of bone, NOS
  Osteotomy, NOS
P1-10104 Wedge osteotomy, NOS
P1-10105 Drilling of bone, NOS
P1-10106 Exploration of bone, NOS
P1-10107 Bifurcation of bone, NOS
P1-10108 Periosteotomy, NOS
  Periostal release
P1-10109 Reopening of osteotomy site
P1-10110 Osteoarthrotomy, NOS
P1-10112 Arthrotomy, NOS
  Arthrostomy, NOS
  Exploration of joint structures by incision
  Incision of joint structures
P1-10115 Division of joint cartilage, NOS
  Joint chondrotomy, NOS
P1-10116 Condylotomy, NOS
P1-10117 Division of joint capsule, NOS
  Capsulotomy of joint, NOS

1-101 Musculoskeletal System: Incisions — Continued

P1-10118 Division of joint ligament, NOS
P1-10120 Arthrocentesis, NOS
  Aspiration of joint, NOS
  Puncture of joint, NOS
  Tap of joint, NOS
P1-10122 Arthrocentesis with aspiration of small joint, bursa or ganglion cyst
P1-10124 Arthrocentesis with aspiration of intermediate joint, bursa or ganglion cyst
P1-10126 Arthrocentesis with aspiration of major joint or bursa
P1-10130 Incision of tendon, NOS
P1-10131 Incision of tendon sheath, NOS
P1-10132 Exploration of tendon, NOS
P1-10133 Exploration of tendon sheath, NOS
P1-10134 Decompression of tendon or tendon sheath, NOS
P1-10136 Drainage of tendon or tendon sheath, NOS
P1-10138 Aspiration of tendon, NOS
P1-10139 Aspiration of tendon sheath, NOS
P1-10140 Tenotomy, NOS
  Division of tendon, NOS
  Incision of tendon with division, NOS
  Myotenotomy, NOS
  Release of tendon, NOS
  Transection of tendon, NOS
P1-10141 Division of tendon sheath, NOS
  Release of tendon sheath, NOS
  Transection of tendon sheath, NOS
P1-10145 Release of tenosynovitis, NOS
P1-10148 Incision of ligament, NOS
  Release of ligament, NOS
  Syndesmotomy, NOS
  Division of ligament, NOS
  Desmotomy, NOS
P1-1014B Retinaculotomy, NOS
P1-10160 Incision of muscle, NOS
  Myotomy, NOS
P1-10161 Exploration of muscle, NOS
P1-10162 Decompression of muscle, NOS
P1-10165 Division of muscle, NOS
  Incision of muscle with division, NOS
  Myotomy with division, NOS
  Release of muscle by division, NOS
  Transection of muscle, NOS
P1-10168 Aspiration of muscle, NOS
P1-10170 Incision of fascia, NOS
P1-10171 Exploration of fascia, NOS
P1-10172 Division of fascia, NOS
  Fasciotomy, NOS
  Incision of fascia with division
P1-10173 Lateral fasciotomy
P1-10174 Medial fasciotomy
P1-10175 Fasciotomy for release of Volkmann contracture
P1-10176 Aspiration of fascia, NOS
P1-10178 Incision of aponeurosis, NOS
  Aponeurotomy, NOS
P1-1017A Division of aponeurosis, NOS
P1-10180 Incision of bursa, NOS
  Bursotomy, NOS
P1-10181 Exploration of bursa, NOS
P1-10182 Drainage of bursa, NOS
P1-10183 Drainage of bursa by aspiration, NOS
  Aspiration of bursa, NOS
  Bursocentesis, NOS
  Puncture of bursa, NOS
P1-101A0 Incision of soft tissue, NOS
P1-101A1 Exploration of soft tissue, NOS
P1-101A4 Division of soft tissue, NOS
  Incision of soft tissue with division, NOS

1-103-104 Musculoskeletal System: Excisions

P1-10300 Biopsy of bone, NOS
  Excisional biopsy of bone, NOS
P1-10301 Excisional biopsy of bone, superficial
P1-10302 Excisional biopsy of bone, deep
P1-10310 Needle bone biopsy, NOS
P1-10312 Needle bone biopsy, superficial
P1-10313 Needle bone biopsy, deep
P1-10314 Trocar biopsy of bone, NOS
P1-10315 Trocar biopsy of bone, superficial
P1-10316 Trocar biopsy of bone, deep
P1-10320 Partial ostectomy, NOS
  Partial ostectomy, except facial
P1-10321 Partial excision of bone, superficial
P1-10322 Partial excision of bone, deep
P1-10323 Symphysiectomy of bone, NOS
P1-10324 Excision of condyle of bone, NOS
  Condylectomy of bone, NOS
P1-10325 Diaphysectomy of bone, NOS
P1-10326 Sequestrectomy
  Excision of necrotic bone fragments
  Removal of necrotic bone fragment
P1-10327 Excision of bone fragments
  Removal of bone chips
P1-10328 Removal of foreign body from bone, except fixation device
P1-10329 Debridement of skin, subcutaneous tissue and muscle
P1-1032A Debridement of skin, subcutaneous tissue, muscle and bone
P1-1032B Debridement of bone
P1-10330 Local excision of tissue of bone, NOS
  Local excision of bone, NOS
P1-10332 Excision of bone for graft, NOS
  Excision of bone for graft, autograft or homograft
  Ostectomy for graft, NOS
P1-10334 Excision of benign tumor of bone, superficial with autograft
P1-10335 Excision of benign tumor of bone, superficial without autograft

P1-10336 Excision of bone cyst, superficial with autograft
P1-10337 Excision of bone cyst, superficial without autograft
P1-10338 Excision of benign tumor of bone, deep with autograft
P1-10339 Excision of benign tumor of bone, deep without autograft
P1-1033A Excision of bone cyst, deep, with autograft
P1-1033B Excision of bone cyst, deep, without autograft
P1-1033C Excision of benign tumor of bone with autograft requiring separate incision
P1-1033D Excision of bone cyst with autograft requiring separate incision
P1-10340 Total ostectomy, NOS
  Ostectomy, NOS
  Total excision of bone, except facial
  Total ostectomy, except facial
P1-10345 Debridement of open fracture, NOS
P1-10346 Debridement of open fracture of bone, except facial bones
P1-10348 Harvesting of bone autograft for arthrodesis
P1-10350 Curettage of bone
  Shaving of bone
P1-10352 Craterization of bone
  Guttering of bone
  Saucerization of bone
P1-10355 Fistulectomy of bone
P1-10356 Excision of lesion of bone
P1-10357 Excision of exostosis of bone
  Exostectomy
P1-10358 Obliteration of bone cavity
P1-10359 Excision of ectopic bone tissue from muscle
P1-10370 Excision of joint, NOS
  Arthrectomy, NOS
  Chondrectomy of joint
  Excision of cartilage of joint, NOS
P1-10371 Excision of bone fragments of joint
  Removal of bone fragment from joint
P1-10372 Removal of necrotic bone fragment from joint
P1-10373 Removal of foreign body from joint structures
P1-10374 Removal of osteocartilagenous loose body from joint structures
  Excision of osteochondritis dissecans of joint
P1-10375 Biopsy of joint structure, NOS
  Excisional biopsy of joint structure, NOS
P1-10376 Excision of lesion of joint, NOS
  Local excision of lesion of joint, NOS
P1-10379 Capsulectomy of joint
P1-1037B Fistulectomy of joint
P1-1037C Excision of lesion of ligament of joint
P1-1037D Curettage of joint
  Curettage of cartilage of joint
P1-1037E Excision of ligament of joint
  Resection of ligament of joint
P1-10380 Excision of tendon, NOS
P1-10381 Excision of tendon sheath, NOS
P1-10382 Tenonectomy, NOS
P1-10384 Excision of tendon for graft
  Tenonectomy for graft
P1-10390 Excisional biopsy of tendon
P1-10391 Curettage of tendon
P1-10392 Curettage of tendon sheath
P1-10394 Excision of lesion of tendon, NOS
  Tenectomy of tendon, NOS
P1-10397 Excision of lesion of tendon sheath, NOS
  Tenectomy of tendon sheath, NOS
P1-103A0 Removal of foreign body of tendon or sheath, NOS
P1-103A1 Removal of foreign body of tendon sheath, simple
P1-103A2 Removal of rice bodies from tendon sheath
P1-103A3 Removal of foreign body of tendon sheath, complicated
P1-103A4 Removal of foreign body of tendon sheath, deep
P1-103A5 Removal of intratendinous calcareous deposits, open method
P1-103B0 Excision of ganglion site, NOS
P1-103B2 Ganglionectomy of tendon sheath site
P1-10400 Excision of soft tissue, NOS
  Resection of soft tissue, NOS
P1-10401 Aspiration of soft tissue, NOS
P1-10404 Biopsy of soft tissue, NOS
  Excisional biopsy of soft tissue, NOS
P1-10406 Excision of lesion of soft tissue, NOS
P1-10407 Excision of xanthoma site, NOS
P1-10408 Removal of foreign body from soft tissue, NOS
P1-10420 Myectomy, NOS
  Excision of muscle, NOS
  Resection of muscle, NOS
P1-10422 Myectomy for graft
  Excision of muscle for graft
  Resection of muscle for graft
P1-10423 Debridement of muscle
P1-10424 Curettage of muscle
P1-10425 Biopsy of muscle, NOS
  Excisional biopsy of muscle, NOS
P1-10426 Superficial biopsy of muscle
P1-10427 Deep biopsy of muscle
P1-10428 Percutaneous needle biopsy of muscle
P1-10430 Excision of lesion of muscle, NOS
P1-10431 Excision of myositis ossificans
  Excision of heterotopic bone from muscle
P1-10434 Removal of foreign body from muscle, NOS
P1-10435 Removal of foreign body from muscle, complicated
P1-10436 Removal of foreign body from muscle, deep
P1-10440 Fasciectomy, NOS
  Excision of fascia, NOS
  Resection of fascia, NOS
P1-10441 Excision of fascia for graft
  Fasciectomy for graft
  Resection of fascia for graft

1-103-104 Musculoskeletal System: Excisions — Continued

P1-10443 Excisional biopsy of fascia
P1-10444 Excision of lesion of fascia
P1-10445 Removal of foreign body from fascia
P1-10448 Aponeurectomy, NOS
  Excision of aponeurosis
P1-10450 Bursectomy, NOS
  Excision of bursa, NOS
  Resection of bursa, NOS
P1-10452 Excisional biopsy of bursa
P1-10453 Curettage of bursa
P1-10454 Aspiration of bursa
P1-10455 Removal of foreign body from bursa
P1-10456 Removal of calcareous deposit from bursa
P1-10460 Synovectomy, NOS
  Synoviectomy, NOS
  Villusectomy, NOS
P1-10462 Excision of synovial cyst
  Resection of synovial membrane
P1-10464 Synovectomy of tendon sheath
  Tenosynovectomy
P1-10480 Removal of internal fixation device from bone, NOS
P1-10490 Musculoskeletal system amputation, NOS
P1-10494 Musculoskeletal system disarticulation, NOS

1-105 Musculoskeletal System: Injections and Implantations

P1-10500 Implantation of prosthetic limb device, NOS
  Insertion of prosthesis or prosthetic device of extremity, bioelectric or cineplastic
P1-10501 Replacement of prosthesis of extremity, bioelectric or cineplastic
P1-10502 Insertion of metal staples into epiphyseal plate
P1-10504 Removal of internal fixation device
P1-10505 Reinsertion of internal fixation device
P1-10506 Revision of fixation device, broken or displaced
P1-10508 Implantation of joint prosthesis, NOS
P1-10509 Implantation of prosthesis or prosthetic device of acetabulum of joint, NOS
P1-1050A Insertion of rod through fracture
P1-10510 Insertion of bone growth stimulator, NOS
P1-10511 Transcutaneous stimulation of bone growth
P1-10513 Electrical stimulation to aid bone healing, noninvasive
P1-10514 Electrical stimulation to aid bone healing, invasive
P1-10515 Electrical stimulation to aid bone healing by percutaneous insertion of electrodes
P1-10516 Insertion of osteogenic pins for bone growth stimulation
P1-10517 Removal of bone growth stimulator
  Removal of electronic bone stimulator
P1-10518 Removal of electrodes of bone growth stimulator
P1-10520 Insertion of skeletal muscle stimulator
  Implantation of electronic stimulator of skeletal muscle
P1-10522 Replacement of skeletal muscle stimulator
  Removal of electronic stimulator of skeletal muscle with synchronous replacement
P1-10524 Removal of skeletal muscle stimulator
  Removal of electronic stimulator from skeletal muscle
P1-10530 Injection of therapeutic substance into joint, NOS
  Arthrotomy with injection of drug, NOS
  Introduction of therapeutic substance into joint, NOS
P1-10531 Introduction of therapeutic substance into ligament of joint, NOS
P1-10532 Injection of therapeutic substance into bursa
P1-10534 Therapeutic injection of sinus tract
P1-10535 Diagnostic injection of sinus tract
P1-10536 Injection of therapeutic substance into tendon
  Introduction of therapeutic substance into tendon
P1-10540 Injection of ganglion cyst
P1-10542 Injection of ligament, NOS
P1-10543 Injection of tendon sheath, NOS
P1-10544 Injection of trigger points
P1-10545 Injection of tendon, NOS
P1-10546 Injection of fascia, NOS
P1-10550 Arthrocentesis with aspiration and injection of small joint, bursa or ganglion cyst
P1-10551 Arthrocentesis with injection of small joint, bursa or ganglion cyst
P1-10552 Arthrocentesis with aspiration and injection of intermediate joint, bursa or ganglion cyst
P1-10553 Arthrocentesis with injection of intermediate joint, bursa or ganglion cyst
P1-10554 Arthrocentesis with aspiration and injection of major joint or bursa
P1-10555 Arthrocentesis with injection of major joint or bursa
P1-10556 Arthrotomy with removal of prosthesis, NOS
  Removal of prosthesis from joint structures, NOS
P1-10558 Aspiration and injection for treatment of bone cyst
P1-10560 Irrigation of tendon, NOS
P1-10561 Irrigation of tendon sheath, NOS
P1-10563 Irrigation of muscle, NOS
P1-10568 Introduction of therapeutic substance into fascia
P1-10570 Intramuscular chemotherapy administration with local anesthesia
P1-10572 Intramuscular chemotherapy administration without local anesthesia
P1-10580 Injection of soft tissue, NOS
P1-10582 Introduction of therapeutic substance into soft tissue, NOS

P1-10584 Removal of implant from superficial soft tissues
P1-10585 Removal of implant from deep soft tissues

1-107 Musculoskeletal System: Endoscopy

P1-10700 Arthroscopy, NOS

1-108-10A Musculoskeletal System: Surgical Repairs, Closures and Reconstructions

P1-10800 Reconstructive orthopedic procedure, NOS
P1-10804 Osteoplasty, NOS
 Repair of bone, NOS
 Fusion of bone, NOS
 Repair or plastic operation on bone, NOS
P1-10805 Repair or plastic operation on bone, except facial bones
 Reconstruction of bone, except facial
P1-10808 Banding of bone, NOS
P1-10810 Change in bone length, NOS
P1-10811 Epiphysiodesis
 Epiphyseal arrest of bone growth
 Epiphyseal-diaphyseal fusion
 Fusion epiphysiodesis
P1-10812 Epiphyseal stapling, NOS
 Stapling of diaphysis
 Stapling of epiphyseal plate
P1-10814 Lengthening of bone with bone graft
P1-10816 Shortening of bone by fusion
P1-10820 Internal fixation of bone without fracture reduction, NOS
P1-10821 Open reduction of fracture, NOS
 Open reduction of fracture without internal fixation, NOS
P1-10822 Open reduction of fracture with internal fixation, NOS
P1-10823 Repair of fracture with sequestrectomy
P1-10824 Repair of fracture with osteotomy and correction of alignment
P1-10825 Repair of fracture with osteotomy and correction of alignment with internal fixation device
P1-10826 Repair of fracture with osteotomy and correction of alignment with intramedullary rod
P1-10827 Repair of fracture with Sofield type procedure
P1-10829 Repair of macrodactyly, NOS
P1-10832 Intramedullary nailing
P1-10835 Open reduction of separation of epiphysis, NOS
P1-10840 Arthroplasty, NOS
P1-10841 Arthroplasty with fixation device, prosthesis or traction
P1-10842 Arthrodesis of joint, NOS
P1-10843 Fusion of joint with bone graft
P1-10844 Replacement of joint, NOS
P1-10846 Revision of joint replacement, NOS
P1-10847V Imbrication of joint, NOS
P1-10848 Stabilization of joint, NOS
P1-10850 Reattachment of joint capsule
P1-10851 Reefing of joint capsule
P1-10854 Joint capsuloplasty, NOS
P1-10856 Joint capsulodesis, NOS
P1-10860 Open reduction of dislocation, NOS
P1-10861 Open reduction of dislocation, except temporomandibular
P1-10862 Open reduction of dislocation with external fixation
P1-10863 Open reduction of dislocation with internal fixation
P1-10864 Tendon pulley reconstruction
P1-10865 Reconstruction of tendon pulley with graft or local tissue
P1-10868 Reattachment of tendon
P1-10870 Plastic operation on tendon, NOS
 Tenoplasty
 Duvries operation
 Lindholm operation
 Repair of ruptured tendon, NOS
 Tenomyoplasty
 Watson-Jones operation
P1-10872 Change in muscle or tendon length, NOS
P1-10874 Repair of tendon by direct suture
P1-10875 Repair of tendon sheath by direct suture
P1-10876 Repair of tendon by transfer or transplantation
P1-10877 Repair of tendon by graft or implant of tendon
P1-10878 Repair of tendon by graft or implant of fascia
P1-10879 Repair of tendon by graft or implant of muscle
P1-10880 Change of length of tendon
P1-10881 Lengthening of tendon
P1-10882 Shortening of tendon
P1-10883 Fixation of tendon
P1-10884 Myotenoplasty
P1-10885 Myotenontoplasty
P1-10886 Reattachment of tendon to skeletal attachment
P1-10900 Plastic operation on muscle, NOS
 Myoplasty
 Musculoplasty
 Repair of muscle, NOS
P1-10904 Reattachment of muscle
P1-10912 Plication of ligament
P1-10914 Repair of ligament
P1-10916 Repair of muscle by direct suture
P1-10918 Repair of muscle by graft or implant of tendon
P1-10919 Repair of muscle by graft or implant of fascia
P1-10920 Change of length of muscle
P1-10922 Lengthening of muscle
P1-10924 Shortening of muscle
P1-10930 Plastic operation on fascia, NOS
 Repair of fascia

1-108-10A Musculoskeletal System: Surgical Repairs, Closures and Reconstructions — Continued

P1-10930 (cont.) Fascioplasty
P1-10932 Repair of fascia by suture
P1-10933 Repair of fascia by graft of tendon
P1-10934 Repair of fascia with graft of fascia
P1-10935 Repair of fascia with graft of muscle
P1-10936 Repair of hernia of fascia
P1-10939 Lengthening of fascia
P1-10940 Reattachment of extremity
P1-10942 Reamputation of stump
  Revision of amputation stump
P1-10943 Trimming of amputation stump
P1-10944 Cineplasty or cineplastic prosthesis of extremity
P1-10946 Secondary closure of amputation stump
P1-10950 Separation of unequal conjoined twins
P1-10954 Separation of siamese twins
P1-10A00 Osteorrhaphy
P1-10A04 Capsulorrhaphy of joint, NOS
  Joint capsulorrhaphy, NOS
P1-10A10 Periosteal suture, NOS
  Suture of periosteum, NOS
P1-10A20 Tenorrhaphy
  Suture of tendon
  Tendinosuture
  Tenosuture
P1-10A21 Delayed suture of tendon
P1-10A22 Suture of tendon sheath
P1-10A23 Suture of tendon to skeletal attachment
  Tenodesis
  Tenosuspension
  Tenosuture to skeletal attachment
  Tenorrhaphy to skeletal attachment
P1-10A24 Suture of joint capsule
P1-10A26 Reattachment of tendon to tendon
P1-10A27 Plication of tendon
P1-10A30 Suture of muscle, NOS
  Myorrhaphy, NOS
  Myosuture, NOS
P1-10A38 Suture of ligament, NOS
P1-10A40 Suture of fascia, NOS
  Fasciorrhaphy, NOS
  Suture of lacerated fascia, NOS
P1-10A42 Suture of aponeurosis
  Aponeurorrhaphy
P1-10A45 Plication of fascia
P1-10A46 Suture of fascia to skeletal attachment
  Fasciodesis
P1-10A50 Suture of bursa, NOS

1-10C Musculoskeletal System: Destructive Procedures

P1-10C00 Destructive procedure of musculoskeletal system, NOS
P1-10C04 Osteoclasis, NOS
  Surgical fracture
P1-10C05 Stripping of bone
P1-10C06 Epiphysiolysis
P1-10C08 Fracturing-refracturing, NOS
P1-10C09 Refracture of bone for faulty union
P1-10C10 Local destruction of lesion of joint, NOS
P1-10C12 Lysis of adhesions of joint
P1-10C13 Lysis of adhesions of muscle
  Myoclasis
P1-10C14 Lysis of adhesions of tendon
  Tendolysis
  Tenolysis
P1-10C15 Lysis of adhesions of fascia
P1-10C16 Stripping of fascia
P1-10C18 Lysis of adhesions of bursa

1-10D Musculoskeletal System: Transplantations and Transpositions

P1-10D00 Bone graft, NOS
  Transplantation of bone, NOS
P1-10D02 Grafting of bone, autogenous or bone bank
P1-10D04 Tendon transplantation
  Tendon transfer
P1-10D05 Tendon graft
  Grafting of tendon
P1-10D06 Advancement of tendon
P1-10D07 Recession of tendon
P1-10D08 Transposition of joint capsule
P1-10D10 Muscle transplantation, NOS
P1-10D11 Release of Volkmann's contracture by muscle transplantation
P1-10D12 Muscle transfer
  Transfer of muscle origin
P1-10D14 Graft of muscle, NOS
P1-10D16 Muscle transposition, NOS
P1-10D20 Graft of fascia, NOS
  Transplantation of fascia, NOS
P1-10D22 Fascia lata graft by stripper
P1-10D23 Fascia lata graft by incision and area exposure, complex
P1-10D24 Fascia lata graft by incision and area exposure, sheet
P1-10D50 Harvesting of bone
P1-10D52 Harvesting of muscle
P1-10D53 Harvesting of ligament
P1-10D54 Harvesting of tendon
P1-10D56 Harvesting of fascia

1-10E Musculoskeletal System: Manipulations

P1-10E08 Application of sling
P1-10E10 Application of halo type body cast
P1-10E11 Removal or bivalving of body cast
P1-10E12 Removal or bivalving of gauntlet cast
P1-10E13 Windowing of cast
P1-10E14 Wedging of cast, except clubfoot cast
P1-10E15 Bivalving of cast, NOS
P1-10E20 Application of Risser jacket, localizer, body only

P1-10E21 Application of Risser jacket, localizer, body, including head
P1-10E22 Application of turnbuckle jacket, body only
P1-10E23 Application of turnbuckle jacket, body including head
P1-10E24 Removal or bivalving of Minerva jacket
P1-10E25 Removal or bivalving of Risser jacket
P1-10E26 Removal or bivalving of turnbuckle jacket
P1-10E27 Denis-Browne splint strapping
P1-10E30 Closed reduction of fracture, NOS
P1-10E32 Closed reduction of fracture without internal fixation, NOS
P1-10E33 Closed reduction of fracture with internal fixation, NOS
P1-10E35 Closed reduction of separated epiphysis, NOS
P1-10E36 Closed reduction of dislocation, NOS
P1-10E40 Casting or strapping procedure, NOS
P1-10E41 Application of plaster figure of eight
P1-10E42 Application of plaster, Velpeau type
P1-10E48 Repair of spica, body cast or jacket
P1-10E50 Fitting of artificial limb, NOS
Fitting of prosthesis or prosthetic device of limb, NOS
P1-10E54V Fitting of shoe, NOS
Shoeing, NOS
P1-10E60 Insertion of wire or pin with application of skeletal traction
P1-10E62V Application of Kirschner-Ehmer splint
P1-10E63V Application of Kirschner wire

1-11 OPERATIVE PROCEDURES ON THE FACIAL BONES

1-110 Facial Bones: General and Miscellaneous Operative Procedures

P1-11000 Orthopedic procedure on head, NOS
P1-11010 Operation on facial bone, NOS
P1-11012 Operation on mandible, NOS
P1-11014 Operation on facial joint, NOS
P1-11018 Operation on temporal bone, middle fossa approach, NOS
P1-11020 Diagnostic procedure on facial bone, NOS
P1-11022 Diagnostic procedure on facial joint, NOS

1-111 Facial Bones: Incisions

P1-11100 Incision of facial bone, NOS
P1-11102 Osteotomy of facial bone, NOS
P1-11104 Periosteotomy of facial bone
P1-11106 Reopening of osteotomy site of facial bone
P1-11110 Osteotomy of mandible, NOS
P1-11111 Total osteotomy of mandible
P1-11112 Horizontal osteotomy of mandible
P1-11113 Segmental osteotomy of mandible
P1-11114 Subapical osteotomy of mandible
P1-11115 Osteotomy of body of mandible
Osteotomy of mandibular body
P1-11116 Smith operation, open osteotomy of mandible
P1-11117 Osteotomy of mandible by Gigli saw
P1-11120 Osteotomy of mandibular ramus
P1-11122 Open osteotomy of mandibular ramus
P1-11124 Closed osteotomy of mandibular ramus
P1-11126 Condylotomy of mandible, NOS
P1-11127 Open condylotomy of mandible
P1-11128 Closed condylotomy of mandible
P1-11131 Closed osteotomy of mandibular angle
Closed division of angle of mandible
P1-11132 Open osteotomy of mandibular angle
Open division of angle of mandible
P1-11140 Arthrotomy of temporomandibular joint
P1-11151 Total osteotomy of maxilla
P1-11152 Segmental osteotomy of maxilla
P1-11190 Drainage of facial region, NOS
P1-11192 Incision of fascial compartments of head
P1-11193 Drainage of fascial compartments of head
P1-11194 Incision of postzygomatic space
P1-11195 Drainage of postzygomatic space
P1-11196 Incision of pterygopalatine fossa
P1-11197 Drainage of pterygopalatine fossa
P1-11198 Incision of infratemporal fossa
P1-11199 Drainage of infratemporal fossa
P1-111A0 Incision of temporal pouches
P1-111A1 Drainage of temporal pouches
P1-111A2 Incision of submental space
Incision of submandibular space

1-113 Facial Bones: Excisions

P1-11300 Excision of bone from facial bones, NOS
Excision of facial bone, NOS
Facial ostectomy, NOS
P1-11302 Total ostectomy of facial bone, NOS
Total excision of facial bone, NOS
Total ostectomy of facial bone, except mandible
P1-11304 Partial ostectomy of facial bone
P1-11305 Excisional biopsy of facial bone
P1-11310 Excision of lesion from facial bone
P1-11311 Excision of benign tumor of facial bone, except mandible
P1-11312 Excision of malignant tumor of facial bone, except mandible
P1-11314 Excision of cyst of facial bone, except mandible
P1-11316 Excision of exostosis of facial bone
P1-11318 Sequestrectomy of facial bone
P1-11320 Excision of mandible, NOS
Total mandibulectomy
Total ostectomy of mandible
P1-11322 Hemimandibulectomy
P1-11324 Partial mandibulectomy
P1-11330 Mandibular condylectomy
Excision of condyle of mandible
Condylectomy of temporomandibular joint
P1-11334 Mandibular coronoidectomy
P1-11340 Excision of lesion of jaw bone, NOS
P1-11341 Excision of lingual torus
Excision of torus mandibularis

1-113 Facial Bones: Excisions — Continued

P1-11343 Simple excision of benign cyst or tumor of mandible
P1-11344 Complex excision of benign cyst or tumor of mandible
P1-11350 Excision of malignant tumor of mandible
P1-11352 Excision of malignant tumor of mandible by radical resection
P1-11360 Excision of meniscus of jaw bone
  Meniscectomy of temporomandibular joint
  Excision of meniscus of temporomandibular joint
P1-11362 Complete meniscectomy of temporomandibular joint
P1-11364 Partial meniscectomy of temporomandibular joint
P1-11370 Excision of maxillary torus palatinus
P1-11390 Removal of foreign body from alveolus
  Removal of foreign body from alveolar bone
P1-11395 Excision of lesion from soft tissue of face, NOS

1-115 Facial Bones: Injections and Implantations

P1-11500 Implantation of facial bone, synthetic or alloplastic, NOS
  Insertion of facial bone implant, alloplastic or synthetic, NOS
  Insertion of synthetic implant in facial bone
P1-11502 Removal of internal fixation device from facial bone
P1-11506 Implantation of premaxilla
P1-11510 Insertion of prosthesis or prosthetic device of chin, polyethylene or silastic
  Implantation of chin, polyethylene or silastic
P1-11540 Injection of temporomandibular joint, NOS
P1-11542 Injection of therapeutic substance into temporomandibular joint
P1-11550 Injection procedure for temporomandibular joint arthrography
P1-11560V Insertion of metal device into nasal cartilage

1-118-11A Facial Bones: Surgical Repairs, Closures and Reconstructions

P1-11800 Osteoplasty of facial bones, NOS
  Repair of facial bone, NOS
P1-11802 Reduction of fracture of facial bone, NOS
P1-11803 Open reduction of fracture of facial bone, NOS
  Open reduction of facial fracture, NOS
P1-11805 Reconstruction of facial bones, NOS
  Reconstruction of facial bone, except mandible, NOS
P1-11806 Augmentation osteoplasty of facial bones
P1-11807 Reduction osteoplasty of facial bones
P1-11810 Total facial ostectomy with reconstruction
  Total ostectomy of facial bone, except mandible, with synchronous reconstruction
  Total facial bone excision with reconstruction
  Grafting of facial bone with total ostectomy
  Reconstruction of facial bone with total ostectomy
P1-11812 Osteoplasty of facial bones, except maxilla, for midface hypoplasia or retrusion
P1-11814 Osteoplasty of facial bones, except maxilla, for midface hypoplasia or retrusion with bone graft
P1-11821 Open treatment of craniofacial separation, Lefort III type with wiring and/or local fixation
  Open reduction of craniofacial separation with local fixation, Lefort III type
  Open reduction of craniofacial separation with wiring, Lefort III type
P1-11822 Open treatment of craniofacial separation, complicated, by multiple approaches
  Open treatment of craniofacial separation, Lefort III type, with wiring and/or local fixation, complicated
P1-11823 Open treatment of craniofacial separation, Lefort III type with wiring and/or local fixation, complicated, fixation by head cap, halo device, multiple surgical approaches, internal fixation, and/or wiring of teeth
P1-11842 Repair for facial weakness
P1-11850 Open reduction of orbital floor blowout fracture by transantral approach
P1-11851 Open treatment of orbital floor blowout fracture, Caldwell-Luc type operation
P1-11852 Open reduction of orbital floor blowout fracture by periorbital approach
P1-11853 Open reduction of orbital floor blowout fracture by combined approach
P1-11854 Open reduction of orbital floor blowout fracture by periorbital approach with alloplastic or other implant
P1-11855 Open reduction of orbital floor blowout fracture by periorbital approach with bone graft
P1-11856 Periorbital osteotomies for orbital hypertelorism with bone grafts by extracranial approach
P1-11857 Periorbital osteotomies for orbital hypertelorism with bone grafts by combined intra- and extracranial approach
P1-11858 Periorbital osteotomies for orbital hypertelorism with bone grafts and with forehead advancement
P1-11859 Orbital repositioning, periorbital osteotomies, unilateral with bone grafts by extracranial approach
P1-1185A Orbital repositioning, periorbital osteotomies, unilateral, with bone grafts by combined intra- and extracranial approach

P1-11860 Open reduction of fracture of orbit
P1-11861 Elevation of bone fragments for fracture of orbit
P1-11862 Reduction of fracture of orbit, except blowout without manipulation
P1-11863 Reduction of fracture of orbit, except blowout with manipulation
P1-11864 Open reduction of fracture of orbit, except blowout without implant
P1-11865 Open reduction of fracture of orbit, except blowout with implant
P1-11868 Secondary revision of orbitocraniofacial reconstruction
P1-11870 Orthognathic operation of mandible, NOS
P1-11871 Recession of prognathic jaw
  Correction of mandibular prognathism
  Prognathic recession
P1-11872 Osteoplasty of mandible, NOS
P1-11873 Repair of mandibular ridge
P1-11890 Reduction of open nasal fracture without manipulation
P1-11891 Uncomplicated open reduction of nasal fracture
P1-11892 Complicated open reduction of nasal fracture with external skeletal fixation
P1-11893 Complicated open reduction of nasal fracture with internal and external skeletal fixation
P1-11894 Complicated open reduction of nasal fracture with internal skeletal fixation
P1-11895 Open reduction of nasal fracture with concomitant open treatment of fractured septum
P1-118A0 Open reduction of nasoethmoid fracture without external fixation
P1-118A1 Open reduction of nasoethmoid fracture with external fixation
P1-118A2 Reduction of closed nasoethmoid complex fracture with headcap fixation including repair of canthal ligaments and nasolacrimal apparatus
P1-118A3 Reduction of closed nasoethmoid complex fracture with splint fixation including repair of canthal ligaments and nasolacrimal apparatus
P1-118A4 Reduction of closed nasoethmoid complex fracture with wire fixation including repair of canthal ligaments and nasolacrimal apparatus
P1-118A5 Reduction of open nasoethmoid complex fracture with headcap fixation including repair of canthal ligaments and nasolacrimal apparatus
P1-118A6 Reduction of open nasoethmoid complex fracture with splint fixation including repair of canthal ligaments and nasolacrimal apparatus
P1-118A7 Reduction of open nasoethmoid complex fracture with wire fixation including repair of canthal ligaments and nasolacrimal apparatus
P1-118B0 Treatment of nasomaxillary complex fracture, Lefort II type
P1-118B1 Reduction of nasomaxillary complex fracture with fixation of denture or splint
P1-118B2 Open treatment of nasomaxillary complex fracture, Lefort II type
P1-118B3 Open reduction of nasomaxillary complex fracture with wiring and local fixation
P1-118B4 Open reduction of nasomaxillary complex fracture with local fixation
P1-118B5 Open reduction of nasomaxillary complex fracture with wiring
P1-118B6 Open reduction of nasomaxillary complex fracture by multiple approaches
  Open treatment of nasomaxillary complex fracture, Lefort II type by multiple approaches
P1-11900 Total osteoplasty of maxilla
P1-11902 Segmental osteoplasty of maxilla
P1-11903 Partial reconstruction of maxilla with subperiosteal implant
P1-11904 Complete reconstruction of maxilla with subperiosteal implant
P1-11905 Partial reconstruction of maxilla with endosteal implant
P1-11906 Complete reconstruction of maxilla with endosteal implant
P1-11910 Osteoplasty of maxilla and facial bones for midface hypoplasia or retrusion
P1-11912 Osteoplasty of maxilla for midface hypoplasia or retrusion
  Osteoplasty of maxilla, Lefort type operation
P1-11913 Osteoplasty of maxilla and facial bones for midface hypoplasia or retrusion with bone graft
  Osteoplasty of maxilla for midface hypoplasia or retrusion with bone graft
P1-11914 Open reduction of closed malar fracture, including zygomatic arch and malar tripod
  Open reduction of depressed malar fracture, including zygomatic arch and malar tripod
P1-11915 Open reduction of closed fracture of malar area, including zygomatic arch and malar tripod with internal skeletal fixation, multiple surgical approaches
P1-11916 Open reduction of complicated open fracture of malar area, including zygomatic arch and malar tripod with internal skeletal fixation, multiple surgical approaches
P1-11920 Malar augmentation with alloplastic material
P1-11921 Malar augmentation with bone
P1-11923 Hemimaxillectomy with bone graft or with prosthesis
P1-11930 Open reduction of maxillary fracture
P1-11931 Open reduction of malar fracture
P1-11932 Open reduction of malar and zygomatic fracture
P1-11933 Open reduction of fracture of alveolar process of maxilla

1-118-11A Facial Bones: Surgical Repairs, Closures and Reconstructions — Continued

P1-11940 Reconstruction of mandible, extraoral, with transosteal bone plate
P1-11941 Partial reconstruction of mandible with subperiosteal implant
P1-11942 Complete reconstruction of mandible with subperiosteal implant
P1-11944 Partial reconstruction of mandible with endosteal implant
P1-11945 Complete reconstruction of mandible with endosteal implant
P1-11950 Ostectomy for graft of mandible
P1-11951 Total ostectomy for graft of mandible
P1-11952 Total mandibulectomy with reconstruction
  Total ostectomy for graft of mandible with reconstruction
  Grafting of bone of mandible with total mandibulectomy
  Total ostectomy of mandible with reconstruction
  Total excision of bone of mandible with reconstruction
  Total mandibulectomy with synchronous reconstruction
  Reconstruction of bone of mandible with total mandibulectomy
P1-11954 Excision of bone of mandible with arthrodesis
P1-11955 Excision of bone of mandible with arthrodesis and reconstruction
P1-11956 Reconstruction of mandible, NOS
  Reconstruction of bone of mandible
P1-11958 Extension of mandibular ridge
P1-11960 Reduction of open mandibular fracture without manipulation
  Open reduction of mandibular fracture
P1-11961 Reduction of open mandibular fracture with manipulation
P1-11962 Reduction of open mandibular fracture with manipulation and with external fixation
P1-11963 Open reduction of closed mandibular fracture with external fixation
P1-11964 Open reduction of open mandibular fracture with external fixation
P1-11965 Open reduction of closed mandibular fracture without interdental fixation
P1-11966 Open reduction of open mandibular fracture without interdental fixation
P1-11967 Open reduction of closed mandibular fracture with interdental fixation
P1-11968 Closed osteoplasty of mandibular ramus
P1-11969 Osteoplasty of mandibular body
  Osteoplasty of body of mandible
P1-1196A Open osteoplasty of mandibular ramus
P1-11970 Open reduction of open mandibular fracture with interdental fixation
P1-11971 Open reduction of mandibular condylar fracture
P1-11972 Open reduction of complicated closed mandibular fracture by multiple surgical approaches including internal fixation, interdental fixation, and/or wiring of dentures or splints
P1-11973 Open reduction of complicated open mandibular fracture by multiple surgical approaches including internal fixation, interdental fixation, and/or wiring of dentures or splints
P1-11975 Reduction genioplasty
  Reduction mentoplasty
  Reduction of chin
P1-11976 Augmentation genioplasty
  Augmentation of chin
  Augmentation mentoplasty
P1-11978 Augmentation genioplasty with graft and implant
  Augmentation mentoplasty with graft and implant
P1-11980 Open reduction of alveolar fracture of mandible
  Open reduction of fracture of alveolar process of mandible
P1-11983 Open reduction of closed depressed frontal sinus fracture
P1-11984 Open reduction of open depressed frontal sinus fracture
P1-11989 Invasive repair of fracture of facial bone with insertion of bone growth stimulator
P1-11A00 Open reduction of alveolar ridge fracture, NOS
P1-11A01 Open treatment of palatal and alveolar ridge fractures, Lefort I type
P1-11A02 Reduction of alveolar ridge fractures, open treatment, Lefort I type
P1-11A03 Reduction of palatal fractures, open treatment, Lefort I type
P1-11A05 Open reduction of fracture of zygoma or zygomatic arch
P1-11A20 Arthroplasty of temporomandibular joint, NOS
  Temporomandibular arthroplasty, NOS
P1-11A21 Arthroplasty of temporomandibular joint with autograft
P1-11A22 Arthroplasty of temporomandibular joint with allograft
P1-11A23 Arthroplasty of temporomandibular joint with prosthetic joint replacement
P1-11A26 Open reduction of temporomandibular dislocation

1-11C Facial Bones: Destructive Procedures

P1-11C00 Destructive procedure of facial bone, NOS
P1-11C02 Local destruction of lesion of facial bone

1-11D Facial Bones: Transplantations and Transpositions

P1-11D00 Bone graft to facial bone, NOS
  Grafting of facial bone, NOS
P1-11D10 Transplantation of temporalis muscle
P1-11D20 Autogenous graft of rib cartilage to face
P1-11D21 Autogenous graft of rib cartilage to nose
P1-11D22 Cartilage graft to nasal septum
P1-11D23 Bone graft to nose
P1-11D24 Autogenous graft of ear cartilage to nose
P1-11D30 Bone graft to malar areas
P1-11D32 Bone graft to maxilla
P1-11D36 Bone graft to mandible
  Grafting of bone to mandible
P1-11D38 Autogenous graft of rib cartilage to chin
P1-11D40 Graft for facial nerve paralysis, free muscle graft
P1-11D41 Graft for facial nerve paralysis, free muscle graft by microsurgical technique
P1-11D42 Graft for facial nerve paralysis by regional muscle transfer

1-11E Facial Bones: Manipulations

P1-11E00 Closed reduction of fracture of facial bones, NOS
P1-11E01 Closed reduction of facial fracture, except mandible
P1-11E04 Interdental wiring for condition other than fracture
P1-11E10 Reduction of craniofacial separation using interdental wire fixation of denture, Lefort III type
  Treatment of craniofacial separation, Lefort III type using interdental wire fixation of denture or splint
P1-11E13 Reduction of alveolar ridge fractures, closed manipulation with interdental wire fixation
  Reduction of alveolar ridge fractures, closed manipulation with fixation of denture or splint
P1-11E20 Mobilization of mandible
P1-11E21 Initial uncomplicated reduction of temporomandibular dislocation
  Closed reduction of temporomandibular dislocation
P1-11E22 Subsequent uncomplicated reduction of temporomandibular dislocation
P1-11E23 Initial complicated manipulative reduction of temporomandibular dislocation
P1-11E24 Subsequent complicated manipulative reduction of temporomandibular dislocation
P1-11E30 Closed reduction of mandibular fracture, NOS
P1-11E31 Reduction of closed mandibular fracture without manipulation
P1-11E32 Reduction of closed mandibular fracture with manipulation and with external fixation
P1-11E33 Closed manipulative reduction by interdental fixation of closed mandibular fracture
  Closed reduction of fracture of mandible with dental wiring
P1-11E34 Closed manipulation reduction by interdental fixation of open mandibular fracture
P1-11E36 Closed reduction of fracture of orbit, rim or wall
P1-11E40 Reduction of masseter muscle by extraoral approach
P1-11E41 Reduction of masseter muscle by intraoral approach
P1-11E42 Reduction of closed nasal fracture without manipulation
P1-11E43 Manipulative reduction of nasal bone fracture without stabilization
P1-11E44 Manipulative reduction of nasal bone fracture with stabilization
P1-11E45 Reduction of closed nasal septal fracture
P1-11E46 Application of interdental fixation device for conditions other than fracture or dislocation
P1-11E47 Manipulative treatment of closed or open fracture of malar area, towel clip technique
P1-11E48 Manipulative reduction of closed fracture of malar area, including zygomatic arch and malar tripod, towel clip technique
P1-11E49 Manipulative reduction of open fracture of malar area, including zygomatic arch and malar tripod, towel clip technique
P1-11E4A Closed reduction of palatal fractures by manipulation with fixation of denture or splint
  Closed reduction of palatal fractures by manipulation with interdental wire fixation
P1-11E4B Treatment of palatal or alveolar ridge fractures, Lefort I type, closed manipulation with interdental wire fixation or splint
P1-11E50 Closed reduction of malar fracture
P1-11E51 Closed reduction of malar and zygomatic fracture
P1-11E52 Closed reduction of fracture of zygoma or zygomatic arch
P1-11E53 Closed reduction of maxillary fracture
P1-11E54 Closed reduction of fracture of maxilla with dental wiring
P1-11E55 Reduction of nasomaxillary complex fracture with interdental wire fixation
P1-11E70 Manipulative reduction of alveolar ridge fracture, NOS
P1-11E71 Closed reduction of fracture of alveolar process of maxilla
P1-11E72 Closed reduction of fracture of alveolar process of mandible
P1-11E90 Manipulation of temporomandibular joint, NOS
P1-11E91 Manipulation of joint adhesions of temporomandibular joint

1-12 OPERATIVE PROCEDURES ON THE NECK AND TRUNK

1-120 Neck and Trunk: General and Miscellaneous Operative Procedures

P1-12000 Operation on neck and trunk, NOS
P1-12010 Operation on neck, NOS
  Unlisted procedure on neck, NOS
P1-12030 Operation on trunk, NOS
P1-12050 Diagnostic procedure on thorax, ribs and sternum, NOS
P1-12070 Musculoskeletal system procedure on abdomen, NOS

1-121 Neck and Trunk: Incisions

P1-12100 Incision and exploration of neck, NOS
P1-12110 Incision and drainage of deep abscess of soft tissues of neck
P1-12112 Incision and drainage of deep hematoma of soft tissues of neck
P1-12114 Incision and drainage of deep abscess of soft tissues of thorax
P1-12115 Incision and drainage of deep hematoma of soft tissues of thorax
P1-12116 Incision and drainage of deep abscess of soft tissues of thorax with partial rib ostectomy
P1-12117 Incision and drainage of deep hematoma of soft tissues of thorax with partial rib ostectomy
P1-12118 Incision of bone of thorax, ribs or sternum, NOS
P1-12119 Division of bone of thorax, ribs or sternum, NOS
  Osteotomy of thorax, ribs or sternum, NOS
P1-12122 Wedge osteotomy of thorax, ribs or sternum
P1-12126 Deep incision with opening of bone cortex of thorax
P1-12130 Decompression of thoracic outlet by tenotomy
  Tenotomy of pectoralis minor tendon for decompression of thoracic outlet
P1-12132 Decompression of thoracic outlet by myotomy of scalenus anticus muscle
  Division of scalenus anticus muscle
  Scalenotomy
  Division of scalenus anticus without resection of cervical rib
P1-12136 Costotomy
P1-12137 Sternotomy
P1-12138 Cleidotomy
P1-12150 Incision of fascial compartments of neck
P1-12152 Drainage of fascial compartments of neck
P1-12160 Division of sternocleidomastoid for torticollis, open operation without cast application
P1-12162 Division of sternocleidomastoid for torticollis, open operation with cast application
P1-12170V Incision and drainage of atlantal bursa
P1-12174V Ventral slot cervical decompression
P1-12178V Transection of muscle of trunk

1-123-124 Neck and Trunk: Excisions

P1-12310 Biopsy of soft tissue of neck
P1-12312 Excision of tumor of soft tissue of neck, subcutaneous
P1-12314 Excision of tumor of soft tissue of neck, deep, subfascial, intramuscular
P1-12315 Radical neck dissection, NOS
P1-12316 Radical resection of tumor of soft tissue of neck
P1-12320 Removal of foreign body from neck, NOS
P1-12321 Removal of foreign body without incision from neck
P1-12324 Removal of therapeutic device from neck
P1-12330 Local excision of lesion or tissue of clavicle
P1-12332 Excision of clavicle for graft
P1-12340 Biopsy of soft tissue of thorax
P1-12342 Excision of tumor of soft tissue of thorax, subcutaneous
P1-12344 Excision of tumor of soft tissue of thorax, deep, subfascial, intramuscular
P1-12345 Radical resection of tumor of soft tissue of thorax
P1-12348 Removal of internal fixation device of thorax, ribs or sternum
P1-12350 Excisional biopsy of bone of thorax, ribs or sternum
  Biopsy of thorax, ribs or sternum
P1-12351 Sequestrectomy of bone of thorax, ribs or sternum
P1-12352 Excision of lesion of bone of thorax, ribs or sternum
P1-12354 Local excision of lesion or tissue of thorax, ribs or sternum
P1-12356 Excision of bone of thorax, ribs or sternum for graft
P1-12357 Partial ostectomy of thorax, ribs or sternum
P1-12358 Total ostectomy of thorax, ribs or sternum
P1-12359 Removal of foreign body of trunk, NOS
P1-12360 Forequarter amputation, NOS
  Interscapulothoracic amputation
  Interthoracoscapular amputation
  Littlewood amputation
P1-12361 Forequarter amputation, right
P1-12362 Forequarter amputation, left
P1-12370 Costectomy
  Resection of rib
P1-12371 Costochondrectomy
  Excision of costal cartilage
P1-12373 Costotransversectomy
P1-12374 Partial excision of rib
P1-12380 Excision of first rib for outlet compression syndrome
P1-12382 Excision of first rib for outlet compression syndrome with sympathectomy
P1-12384 Excision of first rib for unlisted cause
P1-12385 Excision of first rib for other cause with sympathectomy

P1-12390 Excision of cervical rib for outlet compression syndrome
P1-12392 Excision of cervical rib for outlet compression syndrome with sympathectomy
P1-12394 Excision of cervical rib for unlisted cause
P1-12395 Excision of cervical rib for other cause with sympathectomy
P1-12396 Excision of first and cervical rib for outlet compression syndrome
P1-12397 Excision of first and cervical rib for outlet compression syndrome with sympathectomy
P1-12398 Excision of first and cervical rib for unlisted cause
P1-12399 Excision of first and cervical rib for other cause with sympathectomy
P1-123A0 Excision of rib by cervical approach
P1-123A2 Resection of rib by transaxillary approach
P1-123A4 Division of scalenus anticus with resection of cervical rib
P1-12400 Resection of sternum, NOS
P1-12401 Xiphoidectomy
P1-12402 Sternal debridement
P1-12404 Partial ostectomy of sternum
P1-12410 Radical resection of sternum for tumor
P1-12412 Radical resection of sternum with mediastinal lymphadenectomy
P1-12414 Radical resection of sternum for osteomyelitis
P1-12418 Scalenectomy
Excision of scalenus muscle
P1-12420 Superficial biopsy of soft tissue of back
P1-12421 Deep biopsy of soft tissue of back
P1-12422 Excision of tumor of soft tissue of back
P1-12423 Radical resection of tumor of soft tissue of back
P1-12430 Superficial biopsy of soft tissue of flank
P1-12431 Deep biopsy of soft tissue of flank
P1-12432 Excision of tumor of soft tissue of flank
P1-12433 Radical resection of tumor of soft tissue of flank

1-125 Neck and Trunk: Injections and Implantations

P1-12500 Injection procedure on neck or trunk, NOS
P1-12502 Injection of costochondral junction
P1-12504 Insertion of bone growth stimulator into thorax, ribs or sternum

1-128 Neck and Trunk: Surgical Repairs, Closures and Reconstructions

P1-12800 Osteoplasty of thorax, ribs or sternum, NOS
Repair or plastic operation on thorax, ribs or sternum
P1-12801 Internal fixation of bone of thorax, ribs or sternum
P1-12802 Internal fixation of thorax, ribs or sternum without fracture reduction
P1-12803 Internal fixation of clavicle without fracture reduction
P1-12805 Internal fixation of scapula without fracture reduction
P1-12820 Reconstructive repair of pectus carinatum
P1-12822 Reconstructive repair of pectus excavatum
P1-12830 Open reduction of rib fracture, each
P1-12832 Open reduction of rib fracture requiring external fixation
P1-12834 Open reduction of sternum fracture
P1-12840 Repair of sternal defect
P1-12842 Repair of diastasis recti
P1-12846 Repair of serratus anterior muscle
Whitman operation on serratus anterior muscle
P1-12850 Reduction of open hyoid fracture without manipulation
P1-12852 Reduction of open hyoid fracture with manipulation
P1-12854 Open reduction of closed hyoid fracture
P1-12856 Open reduction of open hyoid fracture
P1-12860 Periosteal suture of thorax, ribs or sternum
Suture of periosteum of thorax, ribs or sternum
P1-12890 Change in bone length of thorax, ribs or sternum, NOS

1-12C Neck and Trunk: Destructive Procedures

P1-12C04 Osteoclasis of thorax, ribs or sternum

1-12D Neck and Trunk: Transplantations and Transpositions

P1-12D02 Bone graft of thorax, ribs or sternum
Grafting of bone of thorax, ribs or sternum
P1-12D04 Costochondral cartilage graft
P1-12D10 Bone graft of rib with microvascular anastomosis
P1-12D12 Free osteocutaneous flap with microvascular anastomosis of rib
P1-12D20 Transfer of pectoralis major tendon
Seddon-Brooks operation
P1-12D22 Transfer of iliopsoas muscle
Sharrard operation

1-12E Neck and Trunk: Manipulations

P1-12E00 Manipulation of neck or trunk, NOS
P1-12E10 Uncomplicated closed reduction of rib fracture, each
P1-12E11 Complicated closed reduction of rib fracture, each
P1-12E12 Closed reduction of rib fracture requiring external fixation
P1-12E14 Closed treatment of fracture of sternum
P1-12E20 Application of body cast, shoulder to hips
P1-12E22 Application of body cast, shoulder to hips including head, Minerva type
P1-12E24 Application of body cast, shoulder to hips including one thigh

1-12E Neck and Trunk: Manipulations — Continued

P1-12E26 Application of body cast, shoulder to hips including both thighs
P1-12E28 Strapping of thorax
P1-12E40 Reduction of closed hyoid fracture without manipulation
P1-12E42 Reduction of closed hyoid fracture with manipulation

1-13 OPERATIVE PROCEDURES ON THE VERTEBRAL COLUMN

1-130 Vertebral Column: General and Miscellaneous Operative Procedures

P1-13001 Procedure on spine, NOS
P1-13020 Operation on vertebra, NOS
P1-13022 Repair of vertebral fracture, NOS
P1-13028 Diagnostic procedure on bone of vertebrae, NOS

1-131 Vertebral Column: Incisions

P1-13100 Incision of bone of vertebra
  Osteotomy of vertebra
P1-13102 Arthrotomy of spine
P1-13104 Division of cartilage of spine
P1-13106 Division of ligament of spine
  Section of spinal ligament
P1-13110 Exploration of spinal fusion
P1-13120V Fenestration of intervertebral disc
P1-13130V Incision and drainage of sacrococcygeal region
P1-13132V Transection of muscle of tail

1-133 Vertebral Column: Excisions

P1-13300 Excisional biopsy of bone of vertebra
P1-13302 Wedge osteotomy of vertebra
P1-13304 Excision of lesion of bone of vertebra
P1-13306 Sequestrectomy of vertebra
P1-13308 Removal of foreign body from vertebra, NOS
P1-13310 Excision of spinous process of vertebra
P1-13312 Facetectomy of vertebra
P1-13320 Arthrectomy of spine, NOS
P1-13322 Chondrectomy of spine
  Chondrectomy of intervertebral cartilage
  Excision of intervertebral cartilage
  Excision of intervertebral disc
  Arthrectomy of intervertebral disc
  Intervertebral discectomy
P1-13328 Excisional biopsy of joint structure of spine
P1-13330 Discectomy for intervertebral herniated disc, nucleus pulposus
  Excision of disc for intervertebral herniated disc, nucleus pulposus
P1-13336 Harvesting of bone autograft for vertebral reconstruction following vertebral corpectomy
P1-13337 Laminectomy with excision of herniated intervertebral disc, nucleus pulposus
P1-13338 Synovectomy of spine
P1-13339V Deroofing procedure on vertebra
P1-13340 Excision of lesion from joint of spine
P1-13350 Open biopsy of vertebral body of cervical region
P1-13351 Partial excision of vertebra of cervical region
P1-13352 Partial resection of vertebral component, spinous process of cervical region
P1-13353 Partial resection of vertebral component for tumor of cervical region
P1-13360 Open biopsy of vertebral body of thoracic region
P1-13362 Partial resection of vertebral component, spinous process of thoracic region
P1-13364 Partial resection of vertebral component for tumor of thoracic region
P1-13366 Partial excision of vertebra of thoracic region
P1-13370 Open biopsy of vertebral body of lumbar region
P1-13371 Partial excision of vertebra of lumbar region
P1-13372 Partial resection of vertebral component, spinous process of lumbar region
P1-13374 Partial resection of vertebral component for tumor of lumbar region
P1-13380 Total sacrectomy
P1-13382 Partial sacrectomy
P1-13384 Total coccygectomy
  Amputation of coccygeal vertebra
P1-13386 Partial coccygectomy
P1-13390V Amputation of tail
  Tail docking
P1-13392V Open biopsy of sacrococcygeal region
P1-13393V Excision of lesion of sacrococcygeal region

1-135 Vertebral Column: Injections and Implantations

P1-13500 Injection of intervertebral space, NOS
P1-13510 Reinsertion of spinal fixation device
P1-13520 Removal of prosthesis of joint structure of spine
P1-13524 Removal of internal fixation device of vertebra
P1-13530 Removal of anterior instrumentation of spine
P1-13532 Removal of posterior nonsegmental instrumentation of spine
P1-13534 Removal of posterior segmental instrumentation of spine

1-138-139 Vertebral Column: Surgical Repairs, Closures and Reconstructions

P1-13800 Surgical repair of vertebral column, NOS
  Osteoplasty of vertebrae, NOS
P1-13810 Internal fixation of bone of vertebra
P1-13811 Posterior spinal instrumentation without segmental fixation
P1-13812 Posterior spinal instrumentation with segmental fixation
P1-13813 Anterior spinal instrumentation

P1-13814 Osteotomy of spine for correction of deformity, each additional segment
P1-13820 Spinal arthrodesis, NOS
  Fixation of spine with fusion
  Fusion of spinal joint, NOS
  Spinal fusion, NOS
  Spondylosyndesis, NOS
P1-13822 Spinal fusion with graft, NOS
P1-13824 Laminectomy with spinal fusion
  Girdlestone operation for spinal fusion
P1-13825 Correction of spinal pseudoarthrosis
  Bosworth operation for pseudoarthrosis of spine
P1-13830 Spinal arthrodesis, anterior technique, each additional interspace
P1-13831 Spinal arthrodesis, anterolateral technique, each additional interspace
P1-13832 Spinal arthrodesis, lateral transverse process technique, each additional interspace
P1-13833 Spinal arthrodesis, posterior technique, each additional interspace
P1-13834 Spinal arthrodesis, posterolateral technique, each additional interspace
P1-13835 Arthrodesis, posterior, for spinal deformity, with cast, with bone graft, 6 or fewer vertebrae
P1-13836 Arthrodesis, posterior, for spinal deformity, without cast, with bone graft, 6 or fewer vertebrae
P1-13837 Arthrodesis, posterior, for spinal deformity, with cast, with bone graft, 7 or more vertebrae
P1-13838 Arthrodesis, posterior, for spinal deformity, without cast, with bone graft, 7 or more vertebrae
P1-13839 Arthrodesis, anterior, for spinal deformity, with cast, with bone graft, 4 to 7 vertebrae
P1-1383A Arthrodesis, anterior, for spinal deformity, without cast, with bone graft, 4 to 7 vertebrae
P1-1383B Arthrodesis, anterior, for spinal deformity, with cast, with bone graft, 8 or more vertebrae
P1-1383C Arthrodesis, anterior, for spinal deformity, without cast, with bone graft, 8 or more vertebrae
P1-13840 Refusion of spine, NOS
  Refusion of spine, unlisted level or technique
P1-13842 Reconstruction of spine with bone graft following resection of single vertebral body of cervical region
P1-13843 Reconstruction of spine with prefabricated prosthetic replacement following resection of one or more vertebral bodies of cervical region
P1-13844 Osteotomy of spine by posterior approach for correction of deformity, single segment of cervical region
P1-13845 Open reduction of vertebral dislocation of cervical region, each
P1-13846 Open reduction of vertebral fracture of cervical region, each
P1-13847 Open reduction of vertebral fracture and dislocation of cervical region, each
P1-13848 Osteotomy of spine by anterior approach for correction of deformity, single segment of cervical region
P1-13849 Reconstruction of spine following vertebral body resection, each additional vertebral body
P1-13851 Arthrodesis by anterior extraoral technique, clivus-C1-C2, with bone graft and excision of odontoid process
P1-13852 Arthrodesis by anterior extraoral technique, clivus-C1-C2, with bone graft, without excision of odontoid process
P1-13853 Arthrodesis by anterior transoral technique, clivus-C1-C2, with bone graft and excision of odontoid process
P1-13854 Arthrodesis by anterior transoral technique, clivus-C1-C2, with bone graft, without excision of odontoid process
P1-13855 Arthrodesis by anterior interbody technique of cervical region below C2 with bone graft
P1-13857 Arthrodesis by posterior technique, craniocervical, with bone graft and internal fixation
P1-13858 Spinal fusion of atlas-axis
P1-13859 Arthrodesis by posterior technique of atlas-axis with bone graft
P1-1385A Arthrodesis by posterior technique of atlas-axis with bone graft and internal fixation
P1-1385B Arthrodesis by posterior technique of atlas-axis with internal fixation
P1-1385C Arthrodesis by posterior technique of cervical region below C2, local bone or bone allograft and internal fixation
P1-13860 Cervical spinal fusion, NOS
P1-13861 Cervical spinal fusion by anterior technique, NOS
P1-13862 Cervical spinal fusion by posterior technique, NOS
P1-13863 Spinal fusion of atlas-axis for pseudoarthrosis
P1-13864 Cervical spinal fusion for pseudoarthrosis
P1-13865 Craniocervical spinal fusion, NOS
P1-13866 Craniocervical spinal fusion for pseudoarthrosis
P1-13870 Reconstruction of spine with bone graft following resection of single vertebral body of thoracic region
P1-13871 Reconstruction of spine with prefabricated prosthetic replacement following resection of one or more vertebral bodies of thoracic region
P1-13872 Osteotomy of spine by posterior approach for correction of deformity, single segment of thoracic region

1-138-139 Vertebral Column: Surgical Repairs, Closures and Reconstructions — Continued

P1-13873 Open reduction of vertebral dislocation of thoracic region, each
P1-13874 Osteotomy of spine by anterior approach for correction of deformity, single segment of thoracic region
P1-13875 Open reduction of vertebral fracture and dislocation of thoracic region, each
P1-13876 Open reduction of vertebral fracture of thoracic region, each
P1-13877 Arthrodesis by anterior interbody technique of thoracic region with local bone and bone allograft
P1-13880 Dorsal spinal fusion, NOS
P1-13881 Dorsal spinal fusion for pseudoarthrosis
P1-13882 Arthrodesis by posterior technique with local bone or bone allograft and internal fixation of thoracic region
P1-13883 Arthrodesis by posterolateral technique with local bone or bone allograft and internal fixation of thoracic region
P1-13890 Reconstruction of spine with bone graft following resection of single vertebral body of lumbar region
P1-13891 Open reduction of vertebral dislocation of lumbar region, each
P1-13892 Open reduction of vertebral fracture and dislocation of lumbar region, each
P1-13893 Reconstruction of spine with prefabricated prosthetic replacement following resection of one or more vertebral bodies of lumbar region
P1-13894 Open reduction of vertebral fracture of lumbar region, each
P1-13895 Osteotomy of spine by posterior approach for correction of deformity, single segment of lumbar region
P1-13896 Osteotomy of spine by anterior approach for correction of deformity, single segment of lumbar region
P1-13897 Arthrodesis by anterior interbody technique of lumbar region with bone graft
P1-138A0 Arthrodesis by posterior technique with local bone or bone allograft and internal fixation of lumbar region
P1-138A1 Arthrodesis by posterolateral technique with local bone or bone allograft and internal fixation of lumbar region
P1-138A2 Arthrodesis by lateral transverse process technique with local bone or bone allograft and internal wire fixation of lumbar region
P1-138A3 Arthrodesis by posterior interbody technique with local bone or bone allograft and internal wire fixation of lumbar region
P1-13900 Dorsolumbar fusion, NOS
  Dorsolumbar spinal fusion, NOS
P1-13902 Dorsal and dorsolumbar fusion by anterior technique
P1-13903 Dorsolumbar spinal fusion with Harrington rod
  Insertion of Harrington rod for dorsolumbar fusion
P1-13908 Dorsal and dorsolumbar fusion by posterior technique
P1-13912 Lumbar spinal fusion
  Hibbs operation
P1-13913 Fusion of posterior lumbar spine
  Bosworth operation on lumbar spine
P1-13914 Dorsolumbar fusion for pseudoarthrosis
  Dorsolumbar spinal fusion for pseudoarthrosis
P1-13918 Lumbar and lumbosacral fusion by anterior technique
P1-13920 Lumbosacral arthrodesis
  Lumbosacral fusion
  Lumbosacral spinal fusion
P1-13922 Lumbar and lumbosacral fusion by lateral transverse process technique
P1-13924 Lumbosacral fusion for pseudoarthrosis
  Lumbar spinal fusion for pseudoarthrosis
  Lumbosacral spinal fusion for pseudoarthrosis
P1-13928 Lumbar and lumbosacral fusion by posterior technique
P1-13930 Sacroiliac arthrodesis
  Arthrodesis of sacroiliac joint
P1-13940 Open reduction of closed sacral fracture
P1-13942 Open reduction of open sacral fracture
P1-13990 Suture of periosteum of vertebra, NOS

1-13C Vertebral Column: Destructive Procedures

P1-13C00 Osteoclasis of vertebrae, NOS
P1-13C01 Destruction of intervertebral disc, NOS
P1-13C10 Destruction of intervertebral disc by injection
  Discolysis by injection
  Injection of intervertebral space for herniated disc
P1-13C11 Chemonucleolysis
  Intervertebral chemonucleolysis
P1-13C16 Injection of spinal intervertebral space with chemopapain
P1-13C17 Injection of spinal intervertebral space with chymotrypsin
P1-13C18 Injection of spinal intervertebral space with chymodiactin
P1-13C28 Destruction of intervertebral disc by other specified method

1-13D Vertebral Column: Transplantations and Transpositions

P1-13D10 Grafting of bone of spine
  Grafting of bone of vertebra

1-13E Vertebral Column: Manipulations

P1-13E10 Manipulation of back, NOS
P1-13E11 Manipulation of spine requiring anesthesia, any region
P1-13E14 Strapping of lower back
P1-13E20 Reduction of fracture of spine, NOS
  Reduction of fracture of vertebra, NOS
  Closed repair of fracture of vertebra, NOS
P1-13E21 Closed reduction of vertebral process fracture
P1-13E22 Closed reduction of vertebral body fracture without manipulation
P1-13E23 Closed reduction of vertebral fracture and/or dislocation, with anesthesia, by manipulation or traction, each
P1-13E25 Closed reduction of vertebral fracture and/or dislocation, without anesthesia, by manipulation or traction, each
P1-13E30V Manipulation of tail with application of splint

1-14 OPERATIVE PROCEDURES ON THE PELVIS AND HIP

1-140 Pelvis and Hip: General and Miscellaneous Operative Procedures

P1-14010 Operative procedure on the pelvis and hip, NOS
P1-14020 Operative procedure on pelvis, NOS
P1-14030 Operative procedure on hip joint, NOS
P1-14050 Diagnostic procedure on pelvic bone, NOS

1-141 Pelvis and Hip: Incisions

P1-14100 Pelvic osteotomy
  Incision of pelvic bone
  Pelviotomy
P1-14108V Transection of muscle of pelvis, NOS
P1-14110 Incision and drainage of pelvis for deep abscess
P1-14111 Incision and drainage of hematoma of pelvis
P1-14112 Incision and drainage of infected bursa of pelvis
P1-14114 Deep incision with opening of bone cortex of pelvis and hip joint
P1-14115 Deep incision with opening of bone cortex of hip joint
P1-14116 Deep incision with opening of bone cortex of pelvis
P1-14117 Bilateral osteotomy of pelvis for congenital malformation
P1-14118V Pectinotomy
P1-14120 Arthrotomy of hip, NOS
  Arthrotomy of hip for exploration
P1-14121 Division of cartilage of hip
  Division of joint cartilage of hip
P1-14122 Arthrotomy of hip for infection with drainage
P1-14123 Division of ligament of hip
  Division of joint ligament of hip
P1-14124 Hanging hip operation
  Voss operation
P1-14125 Incision and drainage of hip joint area for deep abscess
P1-14126 Incision and drainage of hematoma of hip joint area
P1-14127 Incision and drainage of infected bursa of hip joint area
P1-14128 Division of joint capsule of hip
P1-14129 Adductor tenotomy of hip
  Division of adductor tendon of hip
P1-1412A First stage adductor tenotomy of hip
  Colonna adductor tenotomy of hip
P1-1412B Tenotomy of adductor of hip, subcutaneous, closed
P1-1412C Tenotomy of adductor of hip, subcutaneous, open
P1-1412D Tenotomy of adductor of hip, subcutaneous, open, with obturator neurectomy
P1-1412E Tenotomy of abductor of hip, open
P1-1412F Open tenotomy of iliopsoas
P1-14130 Osteotomy of innominate bone
  Salter operation
  Innominate osteotomy
P1-14131 Osteotomy of innominate bone with open reduction of hip
P1-14132 Osteotomy of innominate bone with femoral osteotomy
P1-14133 Osteotomy of iliac bone
P1-14134 Osteotomy of iliac bone with open reduction of hip
P1-14135 Osteotomy of iliac bone with femoral osteotomy
P1-14136 Osteotomy of acetabular bone
P1-14137 Osteotomy of acetabular bone with open reduction of hip
P1-14138 Osteotomy of acetabular bone with femoral osteotomy
P1-14139 Osteotomy of innominate bone with femoral osteotomy and open reduction of hip
P1-1413A Osteotomy of iliac bone with femoral osteotomy and open reduction of hip
P1-1413B Osteotomy of acetabular bone with femoral osteotomy and open reduction of hip
P1-14140 Iliac crest fasciotomy, Soutter or Campbell type procedure with stripping of ilium
  Campbell operation fasciotomy of iliac crest
  Soutter operation fasciotomy of iliac crest
P1-14142 Coccygotomy
P1-14144 Ischiopubiotomy
  Farabeuf operation
P1-14146 Pubiotomy
P1-14148 Synchondrotomy
P1-14149 Symphysiotomy
P1-14150 Gluteal-iliotibial fasciotomy, Ober type procedure
  Ober-Yount fasciotomy operation
P1-14154 Ober-Yount fasciotomy, combined with spica cast, pins in tibia and wedging the cast

1-141 Pelvis and Hip: Incisions — Continued

P1-14158 Pemberton osteotomy operation of ilium

1-143 Pelvis and Hip: Excisions

P1-14300 Excisional biopsy of pelvic bone
P1-14301 Excision of lesion of pelvic bone
P1-14302 Wedge osteotomy of pelvic bone
P1-14304 Sequestrectomy of pelvic bone
P1-14306 Local excision of lesion of hip joint, NOS
P1-14308 Excisional biopsy of joint structure of hip
P1-14310 Biopsy of soft tissue of pelvis and hip area, superficial
P1-14312 Biopsy of soft tissue of pelvis and hip area, deep
P1-14314 Excision of tumor of pelvis and hip area, subcutaneous
P1-14316 Excision of tumor of pelvis and hip area, deep, subfascial, intramuscular
P1-14318 Radical resection of tumor of soft tissue of pelvis and hip area
P1-14320 Radical resection for infection of pelvis
P1-14322 Radical resection for tumor of pelvis
P1-14324 Removal of foreign body of pelvis from subcutaneous tissue
P1-14326 Removal of foreign body of pelvis, deep
P1-14330 Abdominopelvic amputation
Interpelviabdominal amputation
Hindquarter amputation
Hemipelvectomy
Jaboulay's amputation
P1-14332 Gordon-Taylor hindquarter operation
P1-14333 King-Steelquist hindquarter operation
P1-14334 Sorondo-Ferré hindquarter operation
P1-14350 Arthrotomy of hip for removal of foreign body
Arthrotomy of hip for removal of loose body
P1-14351 Removal of foreign body of hip from subcutaneous tissue
P1-14352 Removal of foreign body of hip, deep
P1-14356 Arthrectomy of hip, NOS
P1-14357 Synovectomy of hip
P1-14358 Chondrectomy of hip
P1-14360 Disarticulation of hip
Amputation by hip disarticulation
Amputation of leg through hip by disarticulation
P1-14361 Boyd operation for hip disarticulation
P1-14362 Dieffenbach operation for hip disarticulation
P1-14370 Excision of trochanteric bursa or calcification
Excision of trochanteric calcification
P1-14371 Excision of ischial bursa
P1-14372 Radical resection for infection of ischium and acetabulum
P1-14373 Radical resection for tumor of ischium and acetabulum
P1-14374 Radical resection for infection of ischial tuberosity and greater trochanter of femur
P1-14375 Radical resection for tumor of ischial tuberosity and greater trochanter of femur
P1-14376 Radical resection for infection of ischial tuberosity and greater trochanter of femur, with skin flaps
P1-14377 Radical resection for tumor of ischial tuberosity and greater trochanter of femur, with skin flaps
P1-14380 Total ischiectomy
P1-14381 Partial ischiectomy
P1-14382 Acetabulectomy
P1-14385 Radical resection for infection of innominate bone, total
P1-14386 Radical resection for tumor of innominate bone, total
P1-14388 Primary coccygectomy
P1-14390 Arthrotomy with biopsy of sacroiliac joint
P1-14392 Arthrotomy with biopsy of hip joint
P1-14393 Arthrotomy for synovectomy of hip joint
P1-14396 Debridement of sacral decubitus ulcer

1-145 Pelvis and Hip: Injections and Implantations

P1-14500 Insertion of hip prosthesis, NOS
Insertion of prosthesis or prosthetic device of hip, NOS
P1-14502 Insertion of hip prosthesis, total
Insertion of prosthesis or prosthetic device of hip, total
Implantation of hip joint, total
P1-14510 Insertion of prosthesis or prosthetic device of hip, total, with use of methyl methacrylate
Implantation of hip joint, total, with use of methyl methacrylate
Implantation of prosthesis or prosthetic device of acetabulum and femoral head with use of methyl methacrylate
Implantation of prosthesis or prosthetic device of acetabulum and femoral head, Austin-Moore, Eicher, or Thompson
P1-14511 Implantation of prosthesis or prosthetic device of acetabulum of hip joint
P1-14512 Implantation of prosthesis or prosthetic device of acetabulum of hip joint with use of methyl methacrylate
Insertion of prosthesis or prosthetic device of acetabulum of hip joint with use of methyl methacrylate
P1-14513 Implantation of prosthesis or prosthetic device of acetabulum of hip joint, Aufranc-Turner
Insertion of prosthesis or prosthetic device of acetabulum of hip joint, Aufranc-Turner
P1-14520 Implantation of hip joint, partial, NOS
P1-14530 Removal of prosthesis of joint structures of hip
Removal of hip prosthesis
Arthrotomy for removal of prosthesis of hip
P1-14534 Removal of hip prosthesis, complicated, with methyl methacrylate

P1-14538 Removal of internal fixation device from pelvis
P1-14550 Injection of hip joint, NOS
  Injection of coxofemoral joint, NOS
P1-14551 Injection procedure for hip arthrography without anesthesia
P1-14552 Injection procedure for hip arthrography with anesthesia

1-147 Pelvis and Hip: Endoscopy

P1-14700 Arthroscopy of hip, NOS

1-148-149 Pelvis and Hip: Surgical Repairs, Closures and Reconstructions

P1-14800 Pelvic osteoplasty, NOS
P1-14802 Repair of hip, NOS
  Arthroplasty of coxofemoral joint, NOS
P1-14804 Internal pelvic fixation of bone
P1-14811 Partial hip replacement by prosthesis
  Partial hip replacement
P1-14812 Partial hip replacement by cup
  Cup arthroplasty of hip
P1-14813 Partial hip replacement by cup with acetabuloplasty
P1-14814 Cup arthroplasty of hip with use of methyl methacrylate
P1-14815 Total replacement of hip
  Total reconstruction of hip with prosthesis
P1-14817 Revision of hip replacement, NOS
P1-14818 Revision of total hip replacement
  Revision of total hip prosthesis
P1-14820 Revision of total hip arthroplasty, both components, with autograft
P1-14821 Revision of total hip arthroplasty, both components, without autograft or allograft
P1-14822 Revision of total hip arthroplasty, both components, with allograft
P1-14823 Reconstruction of hip with use of methyl methacrylate
  Total replacement of hip with use of methyl methacrylate
  Arthroplasty of hip, total, with use of methyl methacrylate
P1-14824 Total revision of hip replacement with use of methyl methacrylate
  Revision of prosthesis of hip with use of methyl methacrylate
P1-14826 Conversion of previous hip surgery to total hip replacement without autograft or allograft
P1-14827 Conversion of previous hip surgery to total hip replacement with allograft
P1-14828 Conversion of previous hip surgery to total hip replacement with autograft
P1-14830 Revision of total hip arthroplasty, acetabular component only, without autograft or allograft
P1-14831 Revision of total hip arthroplasty, acetabular component only, with autograft
P1-14832 Revision of total hip arthroplasty, acetabular component only, with allograft
P1-14833 Revision of total hip arthroplasty, femoral component only, without allograft
P1-14834 Revision of total hip arthroplasty, femoral component only, with allograft
P1-1483A Open reduction of coxofemoral joint dislocation, NOS
P1-14840 Open reduction of closed or open traumatic hip dislocation with acetabular lip fixation, with external skeletal fixation
P1-14841 Open reduction of closed or open traumatic hip dislocation with acetabular lip fixation, with internal skeletal fixation
P1-14842 Open reduction of closed or open traumatic hip dislocation with acetabular lip fixation, with external skeletal fixation, complicated
P1-14843 Open reduction of closed or open traumatic hip dislocation with acetabular lip fixation, with external skeletal fixation, late
P1-14844 Open reduction of closed or open traumatic hip dislocation with acetabular lip fixation, with internal skeletal fixation, complicated
P1-14845 Open reduction of closed or open traumatic hip dislocation with acetabular lip fixation, with internal skeletal fixation, late
P1-14846 Open reduction of closed or open traumatic hip dislocation with acetabular lip fixation, complicated
P1-14847 Open reduction of closed or open traumatic hip dislocation with acetabular lip fixation, late
P1-14848 Arthrodesis of hip, NOS
  Arthrodesis of hip joint, NOS
  Ischiofemoral arthrodesis, NOS
  Fusion of hip joint, NOS
  Fusion of ischiofemoral joint, NOS
P1-14849 Chandler operation for hip fusion
P1-1484A Charnley operation for hip fusion
P1-1484B Ghormley operation for hip fusion
P1-1484C Watson-Jones operation for hip fusion
P1-1484D Albee operation for hip fusion
P1-14850 Open reduction of dislocation of hip
P1-14852 Open reduction of congenital hip dislocation, replacement of femoral head in acetabulum
P1-14854 Open reduction of congenital hip dislocation with femoral shaft shortening
P1-14856 Total arthroplasty of hip, low friction
P1-14857 Partial replacement of hip with fixation device or with prosthesis, with traction
P1-14858 Arthroplasty of hip with bone graft
P1-14859 Shelf operation, arthroplasty of hip
  Bosworth shelf operation of hip
P1-14860 Fixation of hip, NOS
P1-14864 Open reduction of closed or open ischial fracture
P1-14865 Open reduction of closed or open ischial fracture with internal skeletal fixation

1-148-149 Pelvis and Hip: Surgical Repairs, Closures and Reconstructions — Continued

P1-14867 Arthrodesis of symphysis pubis
P1-14871 Arthrodesis of hip joint with subtrochanteric osteotomy
P1-14880 Reduction of open coccygeal fracture
P1-14881 Open reduction of closed coccygeal fracture
P1-14882 Open reduction of open coccygeal fracture
P1-14883 Reduction of open iliac fracture with uncomplicated soft tissue closure
P1-14884 Reduction of open ischial fracture with uncomplicated soft tissue closure
P1-14885 Reduction of open pubic fracture with uncomplicated soft tissue closure
P1-14886 Open reduction of closed or open iliac fracture
P1-14887 Open reduction of closed or open iliac fracture with internal skeletal fixation
P1-14888 Open reduction of closed or open pubic fracture
P1-14889 Open reduction of closed or open pubic fracture with internal skeletal fixation
P1-1488A Open reduction of closed traumatic hip dislocation
P1-1488B Open reduction of open traumatic hip dislocation
P1-1488C Open reduction of closed or open traumatic hip dislocation with acetabular lip fixation
P1-14890 Acetabuloplasty
P1-14891 Acetabuloplasty with resection of femoral head
P1-14892 Arthroplasty, acetabular and proximal femoral, prosthetic replacement
P1-14893 Acetabuloplasty, Colonna type procedure
Colonna operation hip arthroplasty, second stage
Colonna operation for reconstruction of hip, second stage
P1-14894 Arthroplasty, acetabular and proximal femoral prosthetic replacement, with allograft
P1-14895 Acetabuloplasty, Whitman type procedure
Whitman operation for hip reconstruction
P1-14896 Arthroplasty, acetabular and proximal femoral prosthetic replacement, with autograft
P1-14897 Open reduction of closed or open acetabulum fractures with external skeletal fixation, simple
P1-14899 Open reduction of closed or open acetabulum fractures, simple
P1-1489A Open reduction of closed or open acetabulum fractures with external skeletal fixation, complicated, by intrapelvic approach
P1-1489B Open reduction of closed or open acetabulum fractures with internal skeletal fixation, complicated, by intrapelvic approach
P1-1489C Open reduction of closed or open acetabulum fractures, complicated, by intrapelvic approach
P1-148A0 Replacement of acetabulum of hip
Replacement of acetabulum with prosthesis
P1-148A1 Replacement of acetabulum with use of methyl methacrylate
P1-148A3 Replacement of prosthesis of acetabulum
P1-148A4 Replacement of prosthesis of acetabulum with use of methyl methacrylate
P1-148A5 Acetabular augmentation
P1-14910 Suture of pelvic periosteum
P1-14920V Suture of wound of coxofemoral joint capsule

1-14C Pelvis and Hip: Destructive Procedures

P1-14C00 Destructive procedure of pelvis and hip, NOS
P1-14C10 Pelvic osteoclasis
P1-14C20 Local destruction of lesion of hip joint

1-14D Pelvis and Hip: Transplantations and Transpositions

P1-14D00 Grafting of pelvic bone, NOS
P1-14D10 Free osteocutaneous flap with microvascular anastomosis, iliac crest
P1-14D20 Adductor transfer to ischium
P1-14D24 Transfer of external oblique muscle to greater trochanter including fascial or tendon extension
P1-14D26 Transfer of paraspinal muscle to hip
P1-14D28 Transfer of iliopsoas to greater trochanter
P1-14D29 Transfer of iliopsoas to femoral neck
P1-14D32 Proximal hamstring recession
P1-14D40V Trochanteric transplant

1-14E Pelvis and Hip: Manipulations

P1-14E04 Closed manipulation of dislocation of hip
P1-14E06 Manipulation of hip joint with general anesthesia
P1-14E10 Reduction of sacroiliac and symphysis pubis dislocation without manipulation
P1-14E11 Reduction of sacroiliac dislocation without manipulation
P1-14E12 Reduction of sacroiliac and symphysis pubis dislocation with anesthesia and with manipulation
P1-14E13 Reduction of sacroiliac dislocation with anesthesia and with manipulation
P1-14E15 Reduction of symphysis pubis dislocation without manipulation
P1-14E16 Reduction of symphysis pubis dislocation with anesthesia and with manipulation
P1-14E20 Reduction of closed sacral fracture
P1-14E21 Reduction of closed pubic fracture
P1-14E22 Reduction of closed coccygeal fracture
P1-14E24 Reduction of closed iliac fracture
P1-14E25 Reduction of closed ischial fracture
P1-14E30 Reduction of closed acetabulum fractures without manipulation

P1-14E31 Reduction of closed acetabulum fractures with manipulation
P1-14E34 Reduction of closed acetabulum fractures with manipulation and skeletal traction
P1-14E40 Reduction of closed traumatic hip dislocation
P1-14E41 Reduction of closed traumatic hip dislocation with anesthesia
P1-14E42 Reduction of congenital hip dislocation by abduction, unlisted method
P1-14E43 Reduction of congenital hip dislocation by splint, unlisted method
P1-14E44 Reduction of congenital hip dislocation by traction, unlisted method
P1-14E45 Reduction of congenital hip dislocation by abduction with manipulation and anesthesia
P1-14E46 Reduction of congenital hip dislocation by splint with manipulation and anesthesia
P1-14E47 Reduction of congenital hip dislocation by traction with manipulation and anesthesia
P1-14E48 Reduction of atraumatic hip dislocation
P1-14E49 Reduction of atraumatic hip dislocation with general anesthesia
P1-14E50V Closed reduction of coxofemoral joint with splint
P1-14E52V Manipulation of coxofemoral joint

1-16-17 OPERATIVE PROCEDURES ON THE UPPER EXTREMITY

1-16 OPERATIVE PROCEDURES ON THE UPPER EXTREMITY: SHOULDER AND ARM

1-160 Shoulder and Arm: General and Miscellaneous Operative Procedures

P1-16010 Operative procedure on shoulder, NOS
P1-16012 Diagnostic procedure on clavicle, NOS
P1-16014 Diagnostic procedure on scapula, NOS
P1-16016 Operative procedure on humerus, NOS
P1-16018 Diagnostic procedure on humerus, NOS
P1-16019 Operation on bone injury of humerus, NOS
P1-16020 Operative procedure on elbow, NOS
P1-16022 Operative procedure on forearm, NOS
P1-16024 Diagnostic procedure on radius and ulna, NOS
P1-16026 Diagnostic procedure on radius, NOS
P1-16028 Diagnostic procedure on ulna, NOS
P1-16029 Operation for injury of radius and ulna, NOS

1-161 Shoulder and Arm: Incisions

P1-16102 Arthrotomy of shoulder, NOS
P1-16103 Division of cartilage of shoulder
  Division of joint cartilage of shoulder
P1-16104 Division of joint capsule of shoulder
P1-16105 Division of ligament of shoulder
  Division of joint ligament of shoulder
P1-16108V Incision and drainage of forelimb
P1-16110 Incision and drainage of shoulder area for deep abscess
P1-16111 Incision and drainage of hematoma of shoulder area
P1-16112 Incision and drainage of infected bursa of shoulder area
P1-16113 Deep incision with opening of bone cortex of shoulder area
P1-16114 Arthrotomy of glenohumeral joint for infection with exploration
P1-16115 Arthrotomy of glenohumeral joint for infection with drainage
P1-16117 Arthrotomy of glenohumeral joint for infection with removal of foreign body
P1-16118 Arthrotomy of acromioclavicular joint for infection with drainage
P1-16119 Arthrotomy of sternoclavicular joint for infection with drainage
P1-1611A Arthrotomy of acromioclavicular joint for infection with exploration
P1-1611B Arthrotomy of sternoclavicular joint for infection with exploration
P1-1611C Arthrotomy of glenohumeral joint with joint exploration without removal of loose or foreign body
P1-16121 Capsular contracture release for Erb's palsy
  Sever operation for capsular contracture release for Erb's palsy
P1-16122 Open tenotomy, elbow to shoulder, single, each
P1-16123 Tenomyotomy of shoulder area, multiple, through same incision
P1-16124 Coracoacromial ligament release without acromioplasty for chronic ruptured supraspinatus tendon
P1-16125 Tenomyotomy of shoulder area, single
P1-16130 Clavicotomy
  Incision of bone of clavicle
  Incision of clavicle without division
P1-16131 Osteotomy of clavicle
  Division of clavicle
P1-16132 Wedge osteotomy of clavicle
P1-16133 Incision of bone of scapula
  Incision of scapula without division
P1-16134 Osteotomy of scapula
  Division of scapula
P1-16140 Incision and drainage of infected bursa of upper arm
P1-16141 Deep incision with opening of bone cortex of humerus
P1-16142 Incision of bone of humerus
  Incision of humerus without division
P1-16143 Osteotomy of humerus
  Division of humerus
P1-16144 Osteotomy of humerus without internal fixation
P1-16150 Arthrotomy of elbow, NOS
P1-16152 Incision and drainage of infected bursa of elbow area
P1-16153 Arthrotomy of elbow for infection with exploration

1-161 Shoulder and Arm: Incisions — Continued

P1-16154 Arthrotomy of elbow with joint exploration and without biopsy
P1-16155 Arthrotomy of elbow with joint exploration and without removal of loose or foreign body
P1-16156 Arthrotomy of elbow for infection with drainage
P1-16157 Deep incision with opening of bone cortex of elbow
P1-16160 Division of cartilage of elbow
  Division of joint cartilage of elbow
P1-16161 Division of joint capsule of elbow
P1-16163 Division of ligament of elbow
  Division of joint ligament of elbow
P1-16165 Lateral fasciotomy with extensor origin detachment
P1-16166 Medial fasciotomy with extensor origin detachment
P1-16167 Decompression fasciotomy of forearm with brachial artery exploration
P1-16168 Tendon sheath incision at radial styloid for de Quervain's disease
P1-16169 Decompression fasciotomy of extensor compartment
P1-1616A Decompression fasciotomy of flexor compartment
P1-16170 Incision and drainage of forearm for deep abscess
P1-16171 Incision and drainage of hematoma of forearm
P1-16172 Incision and drainage of infected bursa of forearm
P1-16173 Deep incision with opening of bone cortex of forearm
P1-16174 Drainage of palmar bursa, single, radial
  Drainage of radial bursa
P1-16175 Drainage of palmar bursa, single, ulnar
  Drainage of ulnar bursa
P1-16180 Incision of bone of radius
P1-16181 Osteotomy of radius
P1-16182 Osteotomy of radius, distal third
P1-16183 Osteotomy of radius, middle or proximal third
P1-16184 Incision of bone of ulna
P1-16185 Osteotomy of ulna
P1-16186 Incision of radius and ulna without division, NOS
P1-16187 Osteotomy of radius and ulna, NOS
  Division of radius and ulna, NOS
P1-16188 Open tenotomy of flexor tendon of forearm
P1-16189 Open tenotomy of extensor tendon of forearm

1-163-164 Shoulder and Arm: Excisions

P1-16300 Upper limb amputation, NOS
  Amputation of arm, NOS
  Amputation of upper limb, NOS
  Amputation of forelimb, NOS
P1-16302V Biopsy of forelimb, NOS
P1-16304 Lateral fasciotomy with partial ostectomy
P1-16306 Medial fasciotomy with partial ostectomy
P1-16307 Debridement of open fracture of arm, NOS
P1-16308V Debridement of forelimb, NOS
P1-16310 Removal of foreign body from upper limb, except hand
  Removal of foreign body without incision from upper limb, except hand
  Removal of foreign body of forelimb
P1-16311 Removal of subdeltoid calcareous deposits, open method
P1-16312V Excision of lesion of forelimb, NOS
P1-16314 Biopsy of soft tissue of shoulder area, superficial
P1-16315 Biopsy of soft tissue of shoulder area, deep
P1-16316 Excision of tumor from shoulder area, deep, intramuscular
P1-16317 Excision of tumor from shoulder area, deep, subfascial
P1-16318 Radical resection of tumor of soft tissue of shoulder area
P1-16319 Arthrotomy for synovial biopsy of glenohumeral joint
P1-16320 Arthrotomy of glenohumeral joint for infection with exploration, drainage and removal of foreign body
P1-16321 Arthrotomy of acromioclavicular or sternoclavicular joint for infection with removal of foreign body
P1-16322 Arthrotomy for excision of torn cartilage of sternoclavicular joint
P1-16323 Arthrotomy for excision of torn cartilage of acromioclavicular joint
P1-16324 Arthrotomy for synovectomy of glenohumeral joint
  Synovectomy of shoulder
P1-16325 Arthrotomy for synovectomy of sternoclavicular joint
P1-16326 Arthrotomy of glenohumeral joint with joint exploration and with removal of loose or foreign body
P1-16328 Removal of foreign body of shoulder, deep
P1-16329 Removal of foreign body of shoulder, complicated
P1-16335 Excisional biopsy of joint structure of shoulder
  Biopsy of joint structure of shoulder
P1-16336 Excision of lesion of joint of shoulder, NOS
  Local excision of lesion of shoulder joint, NOS
P1-16340 Arthrectomy of shoulder, NOS
  Excision of shoulder joint, NOS
P1-16341 Chondrectomy of shoulder
P1-16342 Excision of meniscus of acromioclavicular joint
  Meniscectomy of acromioclavicular joint
P1-16350 Amputation of arm through shoulder
  Amputation at shoulder

P1-16350 (cont.) Disarticulation at shoulder

P1-16351 Larry shoulder disarticulation
Larry operation

P1-16352 Lisfranc shoulder disarticulation
Lisfranc amputation
Lisfranc operation

P1-16353 Dupuytren shoulder disarticulation
Dupuytren operation

P1-16354 Disarticulation of shoulder, secondary closure or scar revision

P1-16360 Removal of foreign body from axilla

P1-16370 Resection of clavicle

P1-16371 Partial claviculectomy
Partial excision of bone of clavicle
Mumford operation
Partial ostectomy of clavicle

P1-16372 Total claviculectomy
Total excision of clavicle
Total ostectomy of clavicle

P1-16380 Excisional biopsy of bone of clavicle
Biopsy of clavicle
Excision of lesion of bone of clavicle

P1-16381 Curettage of benign tumor of clavicle
Excision of benign tumor of clavicle

P1-16382 Curettage of cyst of clavicle
Excision of cyst of clavicle

P1-16385 Sequestrectomy of clavicle

P1-16388 Radical resection for tumor of clavicle

P1-16390 Excision of meniscus of sternoclavicular joint
Meniscectomy of sternoclavicular joint

P1-16392 Removal of foreign body from supraclavicular fossa

P1-16394 Partial acromionectomy

P1-16395 Curettage of benign tumor of scapula
Excision of benign tumor of scapula

P1-16396 Curettage of cyst of scapula
Excision of cyst of scapula

P1-16397 Sequestrectomy of scapula

P1-16398 Partial excision of bone of scapula
Partial ostectomy of scapula
Partial scapulectomy

P1-16399 Radical resection for tumor of scapula

P1-1639A Excision of scapula for graft

P1-163A0 Excisional biopsy of bone of scapula
Biopsy of scapula

P1-163A1 Wedge osteotomy of scapula

P1-163A2 Excision of lesion of bone of scapula
Local excision of lesion or tissue of scapula

P1-163A3 Total scapulectomy

P1-163A4 Acromionectomy

P1-163A7 Radical resection for tumor of proximal humerus with prosthetic replacement

P1-163A8 Excision or curettage of bone cyst of proximal humerus

P1-163A9 Excision or curettage of benign tumor of proximal humerus

P1-163B2 Sequestrectomy of humeral head to surgical neck

P1-163B3 Partial excision of bone of proximal humerus

P1-163B4 Resection of humeral head

P1-163B5 Radical resection for tumor of proximal humerus

P1-163B6 Resection of long tendon of biceps for chronic tenosynovitis

P1-163B7 Biopsy of soft tissue of upper arm, superficial

P1-163B8 Biopsy of soft tissue of upper arm, deep

P1-163C0 Excision of tumor of upper arm, deep, intramuscular

P1-163C1 Excision of tumor of upper arm, deep, subfascial

P1-163C2 Radical resection of tumor of soft tissue of upper arm

P1-163C3 Excision or curettage of benign tumor of humerus

P1-163C4 Excision or curettage of bone cyst of humerus

P1-163C5 Sequestrectomy of shaft or distal humerus

P1-163C6 Sequestrectomy of bone of humerus

P1-163C7 Partial excision of bone of humerus

P1-163C8 Radical resection for tumor of shaft or distal humerus

P1-163C9 Removal of foreign body of upper arm, deep

P1-163D0 Amputation of upper arm
Amputation above-elbow
Amputation of arm through humerus
Amputation through humerus

P1-163D1 Amputation of arm through humerus, open, circular

P1-163D2 Amputation of arm through humerus with primary closure

P1-163D4 Amputation of arm through humerus, secondary closure or scar revision

P1-163D5 Amputation of arm through humerus, reamputation

P1-163D6 Amputation of arm through humerus with implant

P1-16400 Wedge osteotomy of humerus

P1-16402 Excisional biopsy of bone of humerus, NOS
Biopsy of humerus, NOS

P1-16403 Excision of lesion of bone of humerus

P1-16404 Local excision of lesion or tissue of humerus

P1-16405 Partial ostectomy of humerus, NOS

P1-16406 Total ostectomy of humerus

P1-16407 Excision of humerus for graft

P1-16409 Debridement of open fracture of humerus

P1-16412 Arthrotomy of elbow for infection with exploration and drainage and removal of foreign body

P1-16413 Arthrotomy of elbow for infection with removal of foreign body

P1-16414 Arthrotomy of elbow for synovial biopsy only

P1-16416 Arthrotomy of elbow with joint exploration and with biopsy
Excisional biopsy of joint structure of elbow
Biopsy of joint structure of elbow

P1-16417 Arthrotomy of elbow with joint exploration and with removal of loose or foreign body

1-163-164 Shoulder and Arm: Excisions — Continued

P1-16418 Arthrotomy of elbow for synovectomy
Synovectomy of elbow
P1-16419 Excision of lesion of elbow joint, NOS
Local excision of lesion of elbow joint, NOS
P1-1641A Removal of foreign body from antecubital fossa
P1-16420 Biopsy of soft tissue of elbow area, superficial
P1-16421 Biopsy of soft tissue of elbow area, deep
P1-16422 Excision of tumor from elbow area, deep, intramuscular
P1-16423 Excision of tumor from elbow area, deep, subfascial
P1-16424 Radical resection of tumor of soft tissue of elbow area
P1-16426 Resection of elbow joint, NOS
Arthrectomy of elbow, NOS
Chondrectomy of elbow, NOS
Excision of elbow joint, NOS
P1-16428 Removal of foreign body from elbow area, deep
P1-16430 Amputation of arm through elbow
Amputation of elbow
Disarticulation of elbow
P1-16435 Excision of olecranon bursa
P1-16436 Excision or curettage of benign tumor of head or neck of radius or olecranon process
P1-16437 Excision or curettage of bone cyst of head or neck of radius or olecranon process
P1-16438 Excision of radial head
Resection of radial head
P1-16439 Exploration for removal of deep foreign body of forearm
P1-16440 Sequestrectomy of radial head or neck
P1-16441 Sequestrectomy of olecranon process
P1-16442 Partial excision of radial head or neck
P1-16443 Partial excision of bone of olecranon process
P1-16444 Radical resection for tumor of radial head or neck
P1-16445 Biopsy of soft tissue of forearm, superficial
P1-16446 Biopsy of soft tissue of forearm, deep
P1-16447 Excision of tumor from forearm area, deep, intramuscular
P1-16448 Excision of tumor from forearm area, deep, subfascial
P1-16449 Radical resection of tumor of soft tissue of forearm area
P1-16450 Excision of lesion of tendon sheath of forearm
P1-16451 Radical excision of forearm flexor tendon sheaths
P1-16452 Radical excision of forearm extensor tendon sheaths
P1-16453 Excision or curettage of benign tumor of radius
P1-16454 Excision or curettage of benign tumor of ulna
P1-16455 Wedge osteotomy of radius and ulna
P1-16456 Excision or curettage of bone cyst of radius
P1-16457 Excision or curettage of bone cyst of ulna
P1-16460 Sequestrectomy of forearm, NOS
P1-16461 Sequestrectomy of bone of radius
P1-16462 Sequestrectomy of bone of ulna
P1-16463 Partial excision of ulna
P1-16464 Partial excision of radius
P1-16465 Radical resection for tumor of radius
P1-16466 Radical resection for tumor of ulna
P1-16467 Radial styloidectomy
P1-16468 Excision of distal ulna
P1-16469 Excision of radius and ulna for graft
P1-16470 Amputation of forearm through radius and ulna
Amputation of arm through forearm
Amputation of forearm
Amputation through forearm
P1-16472 Amputation of forearm through radius and ulna, open, circular
P1-16473 Amputation of forearm through radius and ulna, secondary closure or scar revision
P1-16474 Amputation of forearm through radius and ulna, reamputation
P1-16476 Excisional biopsy of bone of radius
P1-16477 Excisional biopsy of bone of ulna
P1-16478 Wedge osteotomy of radius
P1-16479 Wedge osteotomy of ulna
P1-1647A Biopsy of radius and ulna
P1-16480 Excision of lesion of bone of radius
P1-16481 Excision of lesion of bone of ulna
P1-16482 Local excision of lesion or tissue of radius and ulna
P1-16484 Resection of ulna
Darrach operation
P1-16485 Partial ostectomy of radius and ulna, NOS
P1-16486 Total excision of radius
P1-16487 Total ostectomy of radius and ulna
P1-16488 Debridement of open fracture of radius and ulna
P1-16490 Debridement of open fracture of radius
P1-16491 Debridement of open fracture of ulna
P1-16492 Resection of radial head ligaments for tennis elbow
Bosworth operation for tennis elbow

1-165 Shoulder and Arm: Injections and Implantations

P1-16500 Injection procedure for shoulder arthrography
P1-16501 Injection procedure for elbow arthrography
P1-16510 Insertion of prosthesis or prosthetic device of arm, bioelectric or cineplastic
Implantation of prosthetic device of arm
Insertion of prosthesis or prosthetic device of upper extremity
P1-16512 Replacement of prosthesis of upper extremity
Replacement of prosthesis of arm, bioelectric or cineplastic
P1-16514 Implantation of shoulder joint, NOS

P1-16515 Implantation of prosthesis or prosthetic device of acetabulum of shoulder joint
Implantation of prosthesis or prosthetic device of acetabulum of arm, bioelectric or cineplastic
Implantation of prosthesis or prosthetic device of acetabulum of upper extremity
P1-16518 Removal of prosthesis of joint structures of shoulder
Arthrotomy for removal of prosthesis of shoulder
P1-16519 Removal of internal fixation device from scapula
P1-16520 Prophylactic treatment of clavicle with methyl methacrylate
P1-16521 Insertion of bone growth stimulator into clavicle
P1-16522 Insertion of bone growth stimulator into scapula
P1-16523 Prophylactic treatment of humerus with methyl methacrylate
P1-16524 Prophylactic treatment of proximal humerus and humeral head with methyl methacrylate
P1-16525 Insertion of bone growth stimulator into humerus
P1-16527 Removal of internal fixation device from clavicle
P1-16528 Removal of internal fixation device from humerus
P1-16540 Implantation of elbow joint, NOS
P1-16541 Implantation of prosthesis or prosthetic device of acetabulum of elbow joint
P1-16542 Prophylactic treatment of radius with methyl methacrylate
P1-16543 Prophylactic treatment of ulna with methyl methacrylate
P1-16544 Prophylactic treatment of radius and ulna with methyl methacrylate
P1-16545 Insertion of bone growth stimulator into radius and ulna
P1-16546 Removal of prosthesis of joint structures of elbow
Arthrotomy of elbow for removal of prosthesis
P1-16547 Implant removal of elbow joint
P1-16548 Implant removal of radial head
P1-16549 Removal of internal fixation device of radius
P1-1654A Removal of internal fixation device of ulna
P1-1654B Removal of internal fixation device from radius and ulna

1-167 Shoulder and Arm: Endoscopy

P1-16700 Arthroscopy of shoulder, NOS
Diagnostic arthroscopy of shoulder, NOS
P1-16702 Arthroscopy of shoulder with partial synovectomy
Diagnostic arthroscopy of shoulder with synovial biopsy
P1-16703 Arthroscopy of shoulder with complete synovectomy
P1-16705 Arthroscopy of shoulder with limited debridement
P1-16706 Arthroscopy of shoulder with extensive debridement
P1-16707 Arthroscopy of shoulder with removal of foreign body
Arthroscopy of shoulder with removal of loose body
P1-16710 Arthroscopy of shoulder with lysis and resection of adhesions with manipulation
P1-16712 Arthroscopy of shoulder with lysis and resection of adhesions without manipulation
P1-16715 Arthroscopy of shoulder for decompression of subacromial space with partial acromioplasty and coracoacromial release
P1-16716 Arthroscopy of shoulder for decompression of subacromial space with partial acromioplasty without coracoacromial release
P1-16720 Arthroscopy of elbow, NOS
Diagnostic arthroscopy of elbow, NOS
P1-16721 Diagnostic arthroscopy of elbow with synovial biopsy
P1-16722 Arthroscopy of elbow with partial synovectomy
P1-16723 Arthroscopy of elbow with complete synovectomy
P1-16724 Arthroscopy of elbow with limited debridement
P1-16725 Arthroscopy of elbow with extensive debridement
P1-16726 Arthroscopy of elbow with removal of foreign body
Arthroscopy of elbow with removal of loose body

1-168-16B Shoulder and Arm: Surgical Repairs, Closures and Reconstructions

P1-16800 Plastic amputation of upper extremity, NOS
P1-16801 Cineplasty or cineplastic prosthesis of upper extremity
Cineplasty of upper extremity, complete procedure
P1-16802 Cineplasty or cineplastic prosthesis of arm
P1-16803 Cineplasty or cineplastic prosthesis of biceps
P1-16804 Reattachment of upper extremity
Replantation of arm after complete amputation
Reattachment of arm
P1-16805 Replantation of arm after incomplete amputation
P1-16806 Stump elongation of upper extremity, NOS
P1-16807 Suture of joint capsule with arthroplasty of upper extremity, NOS
P1-16808 Open reduction of fracture of arm
P1-16809 Open reduction of fracture of arm with internal fixation

1-168-16B Shoulder and Arm: Surgical Repairs, Closures and Reconstructions — Continued

P1-16811 Open reduction of closed sternoclavicular dislocation, chronic with fascial graft
P1-16812 Repair of ruptured musculotendinous cuff, acute
P1-16813 Repair of ruptured supraspinatus tendon, acute
P1-16814 Repair of ruptured musculotendinous cuff, chronic
P1-16815 Repair of ruptured supraspinatus tendon, chronic
P1-16816 Coracoacromial ligament release with acromioplasty for chronic ruptured supraspinatus tendon
P1-16817 Arthroplasty of shoulder with synthetic joint prosthesis, NOS
P1-16818 Acromioplasty with synthetic joint prosthesis
P1-16819 Glenoplasty of shoulder with synthetic joint prosthesis
P1-16821 Repair of complete shoulder cuff avulsion, chronic
P1-16822 Arthroplasty with glenoid and proximal humeral replacement
P1-16823 Open reduction of closed sternoclavicular dislocation, acute
P1-16824 Open reduction of closed sternoclavicular dislocation, chronic
P1-16825 Open reduction of open sternoclavicular dislocation, acute
P1-16826 Open reduction of open sternoclavicular dislocation, chronic
P1-16827 Open reduction of closed sternoclavicular dislocation, acute, with fascial graft
P1-16828 Open reduction of open sternoclavicular dislocation, acute, with fascial graft
P1-16829 Open reduction of open sternoclavicular dislocation, chronic, with fascial graft
P1-16830 Open reduction of closed acromioclavicular dislocation, acute
P1-16831 Open reduction of closed acromioclavicular dislocation, chronic
P1-16832 Open reduction of open acromioclavicular dislocation, acute
P1-16833 Open reduction of open acromioclavicular dislocation, chronic
P1-16834 Open reduction of closed acromioclavicular dislocation, chronic, with fascial graft
P1-16835 Open reduction of open acromioclavicular dislocation, acute, with fascial graft
P1-16836 Open reduction of open acromioclavicular dislocation, chronic, with fascial graft
P1-16837 Open reduction of closed acromioclavicular dislocation, acute, with fascial graft
P1-16840 Open reduction of dislocation of shoulder
  Reduction of open shoulder dislocation with uncomplicated soft tissue closure
P1-16841 Open reduction of closed shoulder dislocation
P1-16842 Open reduction of open shoulder dislocation
P1-16843 Open reduction of closed shoulder dislocation with fracture of greater tuberosity
P1-16844 Open reduction of open shoulder dislocation with fracture of greater tuberosity
P1-16845 Open reduction of closed shoulder dislocation with surgical or anatomical neck fracture
P1-16846 Open reduction of open shoulder dislocation with surgical or anatomical neck fracture
P1-16847 Arthrodesis of shoulder, NOS
P1-16848 Arthrodesis of shoulder joint without local bone graft
P1-16849 Arthrodesis of shoulder joint with local bone graft
P1-1684A Arthrodesis of shoulder joint with primary autogenous graft
P1-1684B Gill operation for arthrodesis of shoulder
P1-1684C Watson-Jones operation for shoulder arthrodesis, extra-articular
P1-16850 Zancolli operation capsuloplasty
P1-16851 Total shoulder replacement
P1-16852 Partial shoulder replacement
P1-16853 Arthroplasty of shoulder for recurrent dislocation
  Repair of recurrent dislocation of shoulder
P1-16854 Acromioplasty for recurrent dislocation of shoulder
P1-16856 Glenoplasty for recurrent dislocation of shoulder
P1-16860 Arthroplasty of shoulder, NOS
  Repair of shoulder, NOS
P1-16861 Acromioplasty of shoulder, NOS
P1-16862 Bosworth operation arthroplasty for acromioclavicular separation
P1-16863 Glenoplasty of shoulder, NOS
P1-16870 Repair of musculotendinous cuff of shoulder
P1-16871 Repair of rotator cuff by suture
  Repair of tendon rotator of cuff by direct suture
  Rotator cuff repair
  Suture of tendon of rotator cuff
  Suture of supraspinatus tendon for rotator cuff repair
P1-16873 Osteoplasty of clavicle, NOS
  Repair or plastic operation on clavicle, NOS
P1-16874 Internal fixation of bone of clavicle
P1-16875 Prophylactic treatment of clavicle without methyl methacrylate
P1-16878 Change in bone length of clavicle
P1-16880 Excision or curettage of benign tumor of clavicle with autograft
P1-16881 Excision or curettage of bone cyst of clavicle with autograft
P1-16882 Excision or curettage of benign tumor of clavicle with allograft
P1-16883 Excision or curettage of bone cyst of clavicle with allograft
P1-16885 Osteotomy of clavicle with internal fixation

P1-16886 Osteotomy of clavicle with internal fixation and bone graft for nonunion or malunion
P1-16887 Osteotomy of clavicle with bone graft for nonunion or malunion
P1-16890 Reduction of open clavicular fracture with uncomplicated soft tissue closure
P1-16891 Open reduction of closed clavicular fracture
P1-16892 Open reduction of closed clavicular fracture with internal or external skeletal fixation
P1-16893 Open reduction of open clavicular fracture
P1-16894 Open reduction of open clavicular fracture with internal or external skeletal fixation
P1-16895 Radical resection for tumor of radial head or neck with autograft
P1-16896 Osteoplasty of scapula, NOS
  Repair or plastic operation on scapula, NOS
P1-16897 Internal fixation of scapula
P1-16898 Change in bone length of scapula
P1-1689A Partial acromioplasty
P1-168A0 Scapulopexy
  Green operation
P1-16900 Excision or curettage of benign tumor of scapula with autograft
P1-16901 Excision or curettage of benign tumor of scapula with allograft
P1-16902 Excision or curettage of bone cyst of scapula with autograft
P1-16903 Excision or curettage of bone cyst of scapula with allograft
P1-16905 Reduction of open scapular fracture with uncomplicated soft tissue closure
P1-16906 Open reduction of closed scapular fracture, juxta-articular
P1-16907 Open reduction of open scapular fracture, juxta-articular
P1-16909 Glenoid bone block
  Eden-Hybinette operation
P1-1690A Release of high riding scapula
  Woodward operation
P1-16912 Internal fixation of bone of humerus
P1-16913 Tenodesis for rupture of long tendon of biceps
P1-16914 Arthroplasty with proximal humeral implant
P1-16916 Intramedullary nailing of humerus
P1-16920 Excision or curettage of benign tumor of proximal humerus with autograft
P1-16921 Excision or curettage of benign tumor of proximal humerus with allograft
P1-16922 Excision or curettage of bone cyst of proximal humerus with autograft
P1-16924 Excision or curettage of bone cyst of proximal humerus with allograft
P1-16925 Prophylactic treatment of proximal humerus and humeral head without methyl methacrylate
P1-16928 Radical resection for tumor of proximal humerus with autograft
P1-16930 Reduction of open humeral fracture with uncomplicated soft tissue closure
P1-16931 Open reduction of closed humeral fracture with external skeletal fixation
P1-16932 Open reduction of closed humeral fracture with internal skeletal fixation
P1-16933 Open reduction of open humeral fracture with external skeletal fixation
P1-16934 Open reduction of open humeral fracture with internal skeletal fixation
P1-16935 Open reduction of closed greater tuberosity fracture
P1-16936 Open reduction of closed greater tuberosity fracture with external skeletal fixation
P1-16937 Open reduction of closed greater tuberosity fracture with internal skeletal fixation
P1-16938 Open reduction of open greater tuberosity fracture with external skeletal fixation
P1-16939 Open reduction of open greater tuberosity fracture with internal skeletal fixation
P1-16940 Excision or curettage of benign tumor of humerus with autograft
P1-16941 Excision or curettage of bone cyst of humerus with autograft
P1-16942 Excision or curettage of benign tumor of humerus with allograft
P1-16943 Excision or curettage of bone cyst of humerus with allograft
P1-16945 Tendon lengthening of upper arm, single, each
P1-16946 Tenoplasty with muscle transfer with free graft, elbow to shoulder, single
P1-16947 Tenoplasty with muscle transfer without free graft, elbow to shoulder, single
P1-16948 Radical resection for tumor of shaft or distal humerus with autograft
P1-16949 Reinsertion of ruptured biceps tendon, distal, without tendon graft
P1-1694A Reinsertion of ruptured biceps tendon, distal, with tendon graft
P1-16950 Osteotomy of humerus with internal fixation
P1-16952 Multiple osteotomies with realignment on intramedullary rod of humeral shaft
P1-16953 Osteoplasty of humerus, NOS
P1-16954 Repair of malunion of humerus without graft
P1-16955 Repair of nonunion of humerus without graft
P1-16956 Repair of malunion of humerus with iliac autograft
P1-16957 Repair of malunion of humerus with other autograft
P1-16958 Repair of nonunion of humerus with iliac autograft
P1-16959 Repair of nonunion of humerus with other autograft
P1-16960 Reduction of open humeral shaft fracture with uncomplicated soft tissue closure
P1-16961 Open reduction of closed humeral shaft fracture with external skeletal fixation

1-168-16B Shoulder and Arm: Surgical Repairs, Closures and Reconstructions — Continued

P1-16962 Open reduction of closed humeral shaft fracture with internal skeletal fixation
P1-16963 Open reduction of closed humeral shaft fracture without skeletal fixation
P1-16964 Open reduction of open humeral shaft fracture with external skeletal fixation
P1-16965 Open reduction of open humeral shaft fracture with internal skeletal fixation
P1-16966 Open reduction of open humeral shaft fracture without skeletal fixation
P1-16967 Reduction of open humeral supracondylar fracture with uncomplicated soft tissue closure
P1-16968 Reduction of open humeral transcondylar fracture with uncomplicated soft tissue closure
P1-16969 Reduction of open humeral supracondylar fracture with uncomplicated soft tissue closure with traction
P1-16970 Reduction of open humeral transcondylar fracture with uncomplicated soft tissue closure with traction
P1-16971 Open reduction of closed or open humeral supracondylar fracture with internal skeletal fixation
P1-16972 Open reduction of closed or open humeral supracondylar fracture without internal or external skeletal fixation
P1-16973 Open reduction of closed or open humeral transcondylar fracture with external skeletal fixation
P1-16974 Open reduction of closed or open humeral transcondylar fracture with internal skeletal fixation
P1-16975 Open reduction of closed or open humeral transcondylar fracture without internal or external skeletal fixation
P1-16976 Reduction of open humeral epicondylar fracture, lateral, with uncomplicated soft tissue closure
P1-16977 Reduction of open humeral epicondylar fracture, medial, with uncomplicated soft tissue closure
P1-16978 Open reduction of closed or open humeral epicondylar fracture, lateral, with external skeletal fixation
P1-16979 Open reduction of closed or open humeral epicondylar fracture, lateral, with internal skeletal fixation
P1-16980 Open reduction of closed or open humeral epicondylar fracture, lateral, without internal or external skeletal fixation
P1-16981 Open reduction of closed or open humeral epicondylar fracture, medial, with external skeletal fixation
P1-16982 Open reduction of closed or open humeral epicondylar fracture, medial, with internal skeletal fixation
P1-16983 Open reduction of closed or open humeral epicondylar fracture, medial, without internal or external skeletal fixation
P1-16984 Reduction of open humeral condylar fracture, lateral, with uncomplicated soft tissue closure
P1-16985 Reduction of open humeral condylar fracture, medial, with uncomplicated soft tissue closure
P1-16986 Open reduction of closed or open humeral condylar fracture, lateral, without external skeletal fixation
P1-16987 Open reduction of closed or open humeral condylar fracture, lateral, without internal or external skeletal fixation
P1-16988 Open reduction of closed or open humeral condylar fracture, lateral, without internal skeletal fixation
P1-16989 Open reduction of closed or open humeral condylar fracture, medial, without internal or external skeletal fixation
P1-1698A Open reduction of closed or open humeral condylar fracture, medial, with external skeletal fixation
P1-1698B Open reduction of closed or open humeral condylar fracture, medial, with internal skeletal fixation
P1-16993 Repair or plastic operation on humerus, NOS
P1-16994 Internal fixation of humerus without fracture reduction
P1-16995 Open reduction of fracture of humerus
  Open reduction of fracture of humerus without internal fixation
P1-16996 Open reduction of fracture of humerus with internal fixation
P1-16997 Open reduction of separated epiphysis of humerus
P1-16998 Anchoring of tendon of biceps
  Hitchcock operation
P1-169A0 Change in bone length of humerus, NOS
P1-169A1 Arrest of bone growth of humerus, NOS
P1-169A2 Epiphyseal arrest by stapling of epiphyseal plate of humerus
  Epiphyseal stapling of humerus
P1-169A3 Hemiepiphyseal arrest of distal humerus
P1-16A00 Arthroplasty of elbow, NOS
  Repair of elbow, NOS
P1-16A01 Total elbow replacement
  Arthroplasty of elbow with synthetic joint prosthesis
P1-16A02 Arthroplasty of elbow with membrane
P1-16A03 Arthroplasty of elbow with distal humeral prosthetic replacement
P1-16A04 Arthroplasty of elbow with implant and fascia lata ligament reconstruction
P1-16A05 Arthroplasty of elbow with distal humeral and proximal ulnar prosthetic replacement
P1-16A06 Tendon lengthening of elbow, single, each
P1-16A07 Flexorplasty of elbow
  Steindler operation flexorplasty of elbow

P1-16A07 (cont.) Steindler operation muscle transfer
Steindler type advancement
P1-16A08 Flexorplasty of elbow with extensor advancement
P1-16A09 Tenodesis for rupture of biceps tendon at elbow
P1-16A10 Arthrodesis of elbow, NOS
P1-16A11 Arthrodesis of elbow joint with autograft
P1-16A12 Reduction of open comminuted elbow fracture with uncomplicated soft tissue closure
P1-16A13 Open reduction of dislocation of elbow
P1-16A14 Open reduction of closed elbow dislocation
P1-16A15 Open reduction of open elbow dislocation
P1-16A16 Reduction of open elbow dislocation with uncomplicated soft tissue closure
P1-16A1A Replantation of forearm, complete amputation
P1-16A1B Replantation of forearm, incomplete amputation
P1-16A22 Internal fixation of bone of radius
P1-16A23 Internal fixation of bone of ulna
P1-16A24 Intramedullary nailing of radius
P1-16A25 Intramedullary nailing of ulna
P1-16A30 Excision or curettage of benign tumor of head or neck of radius or olecranon process with autograft
P1-16A31 Excision or curettage of bone cyst of head or neck of radius or olecranon process with autograft
P1-16A32 Excision or curettage of benign tumor of head or neck of radius or olecranon process with allograft
P1-16A33 Excision or curettage of bone cyst of head or neck of radius or olecranon process with allograft
P1-16A34 Arthroplasty of radial head
P1-16A35 Arthroplasty of radial head with implant
P1-16A36 Radical excision of bursa or synovia of forearm extensor tendon sheaths with transposition of dorsal retinaculum
P1-16A37 Radical excision of bursa or synovia of extensor forearm tendon sheaths without transposition of dorsal retinaculum
P1-16A38 Radical excision of forearm extensor tendon sheaths with transposition of dorsal retinaculum
P1-16A39 Excision or curettage of benign tumor of radius with autograft
P1-16A3A Excision or curettage of benign tumor of ulna with autograft
P1-16A40 Excision or curettage of bone cyst of radius with autograft
P1-16A41 Excision or curettage of bone cyst of ulna with autograft
P1-16A42 Excision or curettage of benign tumor of radius with allograft
P1-16A43 Excision or curettage of benign tumor of ulna with allograft
P1-16A44 Excision or curettage of bone cyst of radius with allograft
P1-16A45 Excision or curettage of bone cyst of ulna with allograft
P1-16A46 Reduction of open Monteggia type of fracture dislocation at elbow with uncomplicated soft tissue closure
P1-16A47 Reduction of open radial head or neck fracture with uncomplicated soft tissue closure
P1-16A48 Reduction of open ulnar fracture, proximal end, with uncomplicated soft tissue closure
P1-16A49 Open reduction of closed or open ulnar fracture proximal end, with or without internal or external skeletal fixation
P1-16A50 Repair of flexor tendon or muscle of forearm, primary, single, each tendon or muscle
P1-16A51 Repair of flexor tendon or muscle of forearm, secondary, single, each tendon or muscle
P1-16A52 Repair of flexor tendon or muscle or forearm, secondary with free graft, each tendon or muscle
P1-16A53 Repair of extensor tendon or muscle of forearm, primary, single, each tendon or muscle
P1-16A54 Repair of extensor tendon or muscle of forearm, secondary, single, each tendon or muscle
P1-16A55 Repair of extensor tendon or muscle of forearm, secondary with tendon graft, each
P1-16A56 Lengthening of flexor or extensor tendon of forearm, single, each
P1-16A57 Shortening of flexor or extensor tendon of forearm, single, each
P1-16A58 Forearm flexor origin slide for cerebral palsy
Flexor origin slide for cerebral palsy, wrist
P1-16A59 Forearm flexor origin slide for cerebral palsy with tendon transfer
Flexor origin slide for cerebral palsy, wrist with tendon transfer
P1-16A5A Forearm flexor origin slide for Volkmann contracture
P1-16A5B Forearm flexor origin slide for Volkmann contracture with tendon transfer
P1-16A60 Multiple osteotomies of radius and ulna with realignment on intramedullary rod
P1-16A61 Multiple osteotomies of radius with realignment on intramedullary rod
P1-16A62 Multiple osteotomies of ulna with realignment on intramedullary rod
P1-16A63 Osteoplasty of radius, shortening
P1-16A64 Osteoplasty of ulna, shortening
P1-16A65 Osteoplasty of radius, lengthening with autograft
P1-16A66 Osteoplasty of ulna, lengthening with autograft

1-168-16B Shoulder and Arm: Surgical Repairs, Closures and Reconstructions — Continued

P1-16A67 Osteoplasty of radius and ulna, shortening
P1-16A68 Osteoplasty of radius and ulna, lengthening with autograft
P1-16A70 Repair of nonunion or malunion, of ulna without graft such as compression technique
P1-16A71 Repair of nonunion or malunion of radius without graft such as compression technique
P1-16A73 Repair of nonunion or malunion of radius with iliac or other autograft
P1-16A74 Repair of nonunion or malunion of ulna with iliac or other autograft
P1-16A76 Repair of nonunion or malunion of radius and ulna without graft, such as compression technique
P1-16A78 Repair of nonunion or malunion of radius and ulna with iliac or other autograft
P1-16A80 Repair of defect of radius with autograft
P1-16A81 Repair of defect of ulna with autograft
P1-16A82 Repair of defect of radius and ulna with autograft
P1-16A83 Arthroplasty of distal radius with prosthetic replacement
P1-16A84 Arthroplasty of distal ulna with prosthetic replacement
P1-16A85 Arthroplasty with prosthetic replacement of distal radius and partial or entire carpus
P1-16A90 Prophylactic treatment of radius and ulna without methyl methacrylate
P1-16A91 Prophylactic treatment of radius without methyl methacrylate
P1-16A92 Prophylactic treatment of ulna without methyl methacrylate
P1-16AA1 Arrest of bone growth of radius
P1-16AA2 Arrest of bone growth of ulna
P1-16AA3 Epiphysiodesis of distal radius
P1-16AA4 Epiphyseal arrest by stapling of distal radius
    Stapling of epiphyseal plate of radius
P1-16AA5 Epiphysiodesis of ulna
P1-16AA6 Epiphyseal arrest by stapling of ulna
    Stapling of epiphyseal plate of ulna
P1-16AB0 Epiphysiodesis of distal radius and ulna
P1-16AB1 Epiphyseal arrest by stapling of distal radius and ulna
    Epiphyseal stapling of radius and ulna
P1-16B01 Reduction of open radial shaft fracture with uncomplicated soft tissue closure
P1-16B02 Open reduction of closed radial shaft fracture
P1-16B03 Open reduction of closed radial shaft fracture with internal skeletal fixation
P1-16B04 Open reduction of closed radial shaft fracture with external skeletal fixation
P1-16B05 Open reduction of open radial shaft fracture
P1-16B06 Open reduction of open radial shaft fracture with external skeletal fixation
P1-16B07 Open reduction of open radial shaft fracture with internal skeletal fixation
P1-16B08 Reduction of open ulnar shaft fracture with uncomplicated soft tissue closure
P1-16B10 Open reduction of closed ulnar shaft fracture
P1-16B11 Open reduction of closed ulnar shaft fracture with external skeletal fixation
P1-16B12 Open reduction of closed ulnar shaft fracture with internal skeletal fixation
P1-16B13 Open reduction of open ulnar shaft fracture
P1-16B14 Open reduction of open ulnar shaft fracture with internal skeletal fixation
P1-16B15 Open reduction of open ulnar shaft fracture with external skeletal fixation
P1-16B16 Reduction of open radial and ulnar shaft fractures with uncomplicated soft tissue closure
P1-16B17 Open reduction of closed or open radial and ulnar shaft fractures
P1-16B18 Open reduction of closed or open radial and ulnar shaft fractures with external skeletal fixation
P1-16B19 Open reduction of closed or open radial and ulnar shaft fractures with internal skeletal fixation
    Open reduction of fracture of radius and ulna with internal fixation
P1-16B20 Reduction of open distal radial fracture or epiphyseal separation with fracture of ulnar styloid with uncomplicated soft tissue closure
P1-16B21 Reduction of open distal radial fracture or epiphyseal separation without fracture of ulnar styloid with uncomplicated soft tissue closure
P1-16B22 Open reduction of closed or open distal radial fracture or epiphyseal separation with fracture of ulnar styloid
P1-16B23 Open reduction of closed or open distal radial fracture or epiphyseal separation with fracture of ulnar styloid with internal or external skeletal fixation
P1-16B24 Open reduction of closed or open distal radial fracture or epiphyseal separation without fracture of ulnar styloid
P1-16B25 Open reduction of closed or open distal radial fracture or epiphyseal separation without fracture of ulnar styloid with internal or external skeletal fixation
P1-16B26 Open reduction of closed or open distal radioulnar dislocation, acute
P1-16B27 Open reduction of closed or open distal radioulnar dislocation, chronic
P1-16B31 Change in bone length of radius
P1-16B32 Change in bone length of ulna
P1-16B33 Lengthening of bone of ulna
P1-16B34 Shortening of bone of ulna
P1-16B40 Repair or plastic operation on radius and ulna, NOS
P1-16B41 Osteoplasty of radius, NOS
P1-16B42 Osteoplasty of ulna, NOS

P1-16B50 Internal fixation of radius and ulna without fracture reduction
P1-16B51 Open reduction of fracture of radius and ulna
P1-16B52 Open reduction of fracture of radius
P1-16B53 Open reduction of fracture of ulna
P1-16B54 Open reduction of fracture of radius with internal fixation
P1-16B55 Open reduction of fracture of ulna with internal fixation
P1-16B56 Open reduction of separated epiphysis of radius and ulna
P1-16B57 Reconstruction of below-elbow amputation
  Krukenberg operation
P1-16B60 Reattachment of forearm
P1-16B62 Suture of ligament of upper extremity, NOS
P1-16B63 Suture of capsule of upper extremity, NOS
  Capsulorrhaphy of upper extremity, NOS
P1-16B64 Capsulorrhaphy for recurrent anterior dislocation of upper extremity
  Magnuson operation for recurrent shoulder dislocation
  Putti-Platt operation
P1-16B65 Nicola operation for recurrent dislocation of shoulder
P1-16B66 Bankhart capsulorrhaphy for recurrent anterior dislocation of upper extremity
  Bankhart type operation
P1-16B67 Bankhart type operation with stapling
P1-16B68 Bristow operation for dislocation of shoulder
P1-16B69 Capsulorrhaphy for recurrent anterior dislocation, any type with bone block
P1-16B6A Capsulorrhaphy for recurrent anterior dislocation, any type with coracoid process transfer
P1-16B70 Capsulorrhaphy for recurrent posterior dislocation with bone block
P1-16B71 Capsulorrhaphy for recurrent posterior dislocation without bone block
P1-16B72 Capsulorrhaphy for recurrent dislocation with any type multi-directional instability
P1-16B75 Staple capsulorrhaphy of shoulder
  Dutoit and Roux operation
P1-16B80 Periosteal suture of clavicle
  Suture of periosteum of clavicle
P1-16B82 Periosteal suture of scapula
  Suture of periosteum of scapula
P1-16B84 Periosteal suture of humerus
  Suture of periosteum of humerus
P1-16B86 Periosteal suture of ulna
  Suture of periosteum of ulna
P1-16B87 Periosteal suture of radius
  Suture of periosteum of radius
P1-16B90V Imbrication of forelimb
P1-16B92V Suture of wound of forelimb

1-16C Shoulder and Arm: Destructive Procedures

P1-16C00 Destructive procedure of shoulder and arm, NOS
P1-16C01 Destruction of lesion of shoulder joint, NOS
P1-16C02 Lateral fasciotomy of elbow with stripping
P1-16C04 Medial fasciotomy of elbow with stripping
P1-16C05 Osteoclasis of clavicle
P1-16C06 Osteoclasis of scapula
P1-16C07 Osteoclasis of humerus
P1-16C20 Local destruction of lesion of elbow joint, NOS
P1-16C23 Osteoclasis of ulna
P1-16C24 Osteoclasis of radius
P1-16C25 Tenolysis of flexor tendon of forearm
P1-16C26 Tenolysis of extensor tendon of forearm
P1-16C27 Complex tenolysis of extensor tendon of dorsum of hand, including hand and forearm
P1-16C30V Cryosurgery of forelimb

1-16D Shoulder and Arm: Transplantations and Transpositions

P1-16D01 Muscle transfer, any type for paralysis of shoulder, single
P1-16D02 Muscle transfer, any type for paralysis of shoulder or upper arm, multiple
P1-16D04 Grafting of bone of clavicle
P1-16D05 Grafting of bone of scapula
P1-16D06 Muscle or tendon transfer, any type, upper arm, single
P1-16D07 Muscle transfer, any type for paralysis of upper arm, single
P1-16D08 Muscle or tendon transfer, any type, elbow, single
P1-16D10 Transplantation or transfer of flexor tendon of forearm
P1-16D11 Transplantation or transfer of extensor tendon of forearm
P1-16D12 Transplantation or transfer of flexor tendon of forearm with tendon grafts
P1-16D13 Transplantation or transfer of extensor tendon of forearm with tendon grafts
P1-16D15 Transplantation of long tendon of biceps for chronic tenosynovitis
P1-16D20 Grafting of radius and ulna
P1-16D22 Grafting of bone of radius
P1-16D24 Grafting of bone of ulna
P1-16D30 Grafting of bone of humerus

1-16E Shoulder and Arm: Manipulations

P1-16E02 Fitting of prosthetic upper limb device, NOS
P1-16E03 Fitting of prosthesis or prosthetic device of arm, NOS
P1-16E04 Fitting of prosthesis or prosthetic device of shoulder
P1-16E05 Fitting of prosthesis or prosthetic device of upper arm
P1-16E06 Fitting of prosthesis or prosthetic device of lower arm
P1-16E10 Removal or bivalving of full arm cast

1-16E Shoulder and Arm: Manipulations — Continued

P1-16E11 Removal or bivalving of shoulder spica
P1-16E12 Application of shoulder spica
P1-16E13 Strapping of shoulder, Velpeau type
P1-16E14 Strapping of elbow
P1-16E15 Reduction of closed elbow dislocation without anesthesia
P1-16E16 Strapping of wrist
P1-16E20 Closed reduction of fracture of arm, NOS
P1-16E21 Reduction of fracture of arm with internal fixation
P1-16E22 Reduction of closed sternoclavicular dislocation without manipulation
P1-16E23 Reduction of closed sternoclavicular dislocation with manipulation
P1-16E24 Reduction of closed acromioclavicular dislocation without manipulation
P1-16E25 Reduction of closed acromioclavicular dislocation with manipulation
P1-16E26 Reduction of closed shoulder dislocation with manipulation without anesthesia
P1-16E27 Reduction of closed shoulder dislocation with manipulation requiring anesthesia
P1-16E28 Reduction of closed shoulder dislocation with fracture of greater tuberosity with manipulation
P1-16E29 Reduction of closed shoulder dislocation with surgical or anatomical neck fracture with manipulation
P1-16E2A Manipulation under anesthesia of shoulder joint including application of fixation apparatus
P1-16E30 Closed reduction of dislocation of shoulder
P1-16E31 Reduction of closed clavicular fracture without manipulation
P1-16E32 Reduction of closed clavicular fracture with manipulation
P1-16E33 Reduction of closed scapular fracture without manipulation
P1-16E34 Reduction of closed scapular fracture with manipulation
P1-16E36 Reduction of closed humeral fracture without manipulation
P1-16E37 Reduction of closed humeral fracture with manipulation
P1-16E38 Reduction of closed greater tuberosity fracture without manipulation
P1-16E39 Reduction of closed greater tuberosity fracture with manipulation
P1-16E40 Reduction of closed humeral shaft fracture without manipulation
P1-16E41 Reduction of closed humeral shaft fracture with manipulation
P1-16E42 Reduction of closed humeral shaft fracture with percutaneous insertion of pin or rod
P1-16E43 Reduction of closed humeral supracondylar fracture without manipulation
P1-16E44 Reduction of closed humeral transcondylar fracture without manipulation
P1-16E45 Reduction of closed humeral supracondylar fracture without manipulation and with traction
P1-16E46 Reduction of closed humeral transcondylar fracture without manipulation and with traction
P1-16E47 Reduction of closed humeral supracondylar fracture with manipulation
P1-16E48 Reduction of closed humeral transcondylar fracture with manipulation
P1-16E49 Reduction of closed humeral supracondylar fracture with manipulation and traction
P1-16E4A Reduction of closed humeral transcondylar fracture with manipulation and traction
P1-16E50 Reduction of closed humeral supracondylar fracture with manipulation and percutaneous skeletal fixation
P1-16E51 Reduction of closed humeral transcondylar fracture with manipulation and percutaneous skeletal fixation
P1-16E52 Reduction of closed humeral lateral epicondylar fracture without manipulation
P1-16E53 Reduction of closed humeral medial epicondylar fracture without manipulation
P1-16E54 Reduction of closed humeral lateral epicondylar fracture with manipulation
P1-16E55 Reduction of closed humeral medial epicondylar fracture with manipulation
P1-16E56 Reduction of closed humeral lateral condylar fracture without manipulation
P1-16E57 Reduction of closed humeral medial condylar fracture without manipulation
P1-16E58 Reduction of closed humeral lateral condylar fracture with manipulation
P1-16E59 Reduction of closed humeral medial condylar fracture with manipulation
P1-16E5A Closed reduction of fracture of humerus, NOS
P1-16E5B Closed reduction of fracture of humerus without internal fixation
P1-16E60 Closed reduction of fracture of humerus with internal fixation
P1-16E61 Closed reduction of separated epiphysis of humerus
P1-16E63 Reduction of closed comminuted elbow fracture with traction and without manipulation
P1-16E64 Reduction of closed comminuted elbow fracture with traction and manipulation
P1-16E65 Reduction of closed ulnar shaft fracture without manipulation
P1-16E66 Closed reduction of dislocation of elbow
P1-16E67 Reduction of closed elbow dislocation requiring anesthesia
P1-16E68 Reduction of closed Monteggia type of fracture dislocation at elbow
    Reduction of closed fracture of proximal ulna with dislocation of radial head

P1-16E69 Reduction of radial head subluxation in child, nursemaid elbow with manipulation
P1-16E70 Reduction of closed radial head or neck fracture without manipulation
P1-16E71 Reduction of closed radial head or neck fracture with manipulation
P1-16E72 Reduction of closed fracture of proximal end of ulna, olecranon process without manipulation
P1-16E73 Reduction of closed fracture of proximal end of ulna with manipulation
P1-16E74 Reduction of closed radial shaft fracture without manipulation
P1-16E75 Reduction of closed radial shaft fracture with manipulation
P1-16E77 Reduction of closed ulnar shaft fracture with manipulation
P1-16E78 Reduction of closed radial and ulnar shaft fractures without manipulation
P1-16E79 Reduction of closed radial and ulnar shaft fractures with manipulation
P1-16E7A Reduction of closed distal radial fracture, Colles or Smith type, or epiphyseal separation with or without fracture of ulnar styloid without manipulation
P1-16E80 Reduction of closed distal radial fracture or epiphyseal separation without fracture of ulnar styloid without manipulation
P1-16E81 Reduction of closed distal radial fracture or epiphyseal separation with fracture of ulnar styloid with manipulation
P1-16E82 Reduction of closed distal radial fracture or epiphyseal separation without fracture of ulnar styloid with manipulation
P1-16E83 Reduction of closed complex distal radial fracture or epiphyseal separation with fracture of ulnar styloid with manipulation
P1-16E84 Treatment of closed complex distal radial fracture or epiphyseal separation without fracture of ulnar styloid with manipulation
P1-16E85 Treatment of closed complex distal radial fracture or epiphyseal separation with fracture of ulnar styloid with manipulation, percutaneous pinning or pins and plaster technique
P1-16E86 Treatment of closed complex distal radial fracture or epiphyseal separation without fracture of ulnar styloid with manipulation, percutaneous pinning or pins and plaster technique
P1-16E87 Reduction of closed distal radioulnar dislocation with manipulation
P1-16E88 Closed reduction of fracture of radius and ulna
P1-16E89 Closed reduction of fracture of ulna
P1-16E8A Closed reduction of fracture of radius
P1-16E90 Closed reduction of fracture of radius and ulna with internal fixation
P1-16E92 Reduction of fracture of radius with internal fixation
P1-16E93 Reduction of fracture of ulna with internal fixation
P1-16E94 Closed reduction of separated epiphysis of radius and ulna
P1-16E95 Reduction of closed ulnar styloid fracture
P1-16E96 Reduction of closed radiocarpal or intercarpal dislocation, one or more bones with manipulation
P1-16E97 Application of plaster figure of eight, shoulder to hand
Application of plaster figure of eight, long arm
P1-16E98 Application of plaster figure of eight, elbow to finger
Application of plaster figure of eight, short arm
P1-16E99 Application of long arm splint, shoulder to hand
P1-16EA0 Application of short arm splint, forearm to hand, static
P1-16EA2 Application of short arm splint, forearm to hand, dynamic
P1-16EA5V Manipulation of muscle of shoulder of forelimb
P1-16EA6V Manipulation of forelimb with application of splint

1-17 OPERATIVE PROCEDURES ON THE UPPER EXTREMITY: WRIST AND HAND

1-170 Wrist and Hand: General and Miscellaneous Operative Procedures

P1-17000 Operative procedure on wrist and hand, NOS
P1-17010 Operative procedure on wrist, NOS
P1-17012 Diagnostic procedure on carpals and metacarpals, NOS
P1-17014 Operation on bone injury of carpals and metacarpals, NOS
P1-17020 Operative procedure on hands, NOS
P1-17021 Operation on soft tissue of hand, NOS
P1-17022 Operation on muscle, tendon and fascia of hand, NOS
P1-17023 Operation on bursa of hand, NOS
P1-17024 Operation on fascia of hand, NOS
P1-17025 Operation on muscle of hand, NOS
P1-17026 Operation on tendon of hand, NOS
P1-17040 Operative procedure on fingers, NOS
P1-17042 Operation for bone injury of phalanges of hand, NOS
Operation on bone injury of fingers, NOS
P1-17048 Diagnostic procedure on phalanges of hand, NOS

1-171-172 Wrist and Hand: Incisions

P1-17100 Arthrotomy of wrist, NOS
Incision of joint of wrist, NOS
P1-17102 Division of cartilage of wrist
Division of joint cartilage of wrist
P1-17103 Division of joint capsule of wrist
P1-17104 Division of ligament of wrist
Division of joint ligament of wrist
P1-17105 Capsulotomy of wrist
P1-17106 Arthrotomy of wrist joint with joint exploration
P1-17108V Incision and drainage of forefoot
P1-17110 Tendon sheath incision at wrist for other stenosing tenosynovitis
P1-17111 Decompression fasciotomy of wrist
P1-17112 Decompression fasciotomy of wrist, flexor and extensor compartment
P1-17113 Open tenotomy of flexor or extensor tendon of wrist, single, each
P1-17114 Arthrotomy of mediocarpal joint for infection with exploration and drainage
P1-17115 Arthrotomy of radiocarpal joint for infection with exploration and drainage
P1-17116 Arthrotomy for infection with drainage of carpometacarpal joint
P1-17117 Arthrotomy for infection with exploration and drainage of carpometacarpal joint
P1-17118 Arthrotomy for infection with exploration of carpometacarpal joint
P1-17120 Incision and drainage of wrist for deep abscess
P1-17121 Incision and drainage of hematoma of wrist
P1-17122 Incision and drainage of infected bursa of wrist
P1-17123 Deep incision with opening of bone cortex of wrist
P1-17130 Incision of bone of carpals and metacarpals, NOS
Incision of carpals and metacarpals, NOS
P1-17132 Division of carpals and metacarpals, NOS
Osteotomy of carpals and metacarpals, NOS
P1-17135 Deep incision with opening of bone cortex of hand
P1-17140 Arthrotomy of hand, NOS
Incision of joint of hand, NOS
P1-17142 Division of cartilage of hand
Division of joint cartilage of hand
P1-17143 Division of joint capsule of hand
P1-17144 Division of ligament of hand
Division of joint ligament of hand
P1-17150 Incision of tendon of hand
Exploration of tendon of hand
P1-17151 Exploration of tendon sheath of hand
P1-17152 Drainage of tendon of hand
P1-17153 Release of tendon sheath of hand
P1-17154 Release for tenosynovitis of hand
P1-17155 Release for de Quervain's tenosynovitis of hand
P1-17156 Release for tenosynovitis of abductor pollicis longus
P1-17157 Release for tenosynovitis of external pollicis brevis
P1-17158 Decompression of tendon of hand
P1-17159 Splitting of tendon sheath of hand
P1-1715A Puncture of bursa of hand
P1-1715B Bursotomy of hand
Exploration of bursa of hand
Incision of bursa of hand
P1-1715C Drainage of bursa of hand
P1-1715D Multiple drainage of palmar bursa
P1-1715E Complicated drainage of palmar bursa
P1-17160 Incision of muscle of hand
Exploration of muscle of hand
Myotomy of hand
P1-17161 Decompression of muscle of hand
P1-17162 Drainage of palm
P1-17163 Drainage of tendon sheath, one digit and palm
P1-17165 Incision of midpalmar space
Drainage of midpalmar space
Drainage of middle palmar space
Incision and drainage of palmar space
Incision of middle palmar space
P1-17166 Decompression of hand, injection injury
P1-17167 Incision of thenar space
Drainage of thenar space
Incision and drainage of thenar space
P1-17168 Decompressive fasciotomy of hand
P1-17169 Palmar fasciotomy for Dupuytren's contracture, closed, subcutaneous
Palmar fasciotomy for release of Dupuytren's contracture
P1-1716A Palmar fasciotomy for Dupuytren's contracture, open, partial
P1-17170 Incision of fascia of hand
Exploration of fascia of hand
P1-17171 Incision of soft tissue of hand, NOS
Exploration of soft tissue of hand, NOS
P1-17172 Aspiration of soft tissue of hand, NOS
P1-17175 Aponeurotomy of hand
P1-17176 Division of tendon of hand
Incision of tendon of hand with division
Transection of tendon of hand
P1-17177 Myotenotomy of hand
P1-17178 Release of tendon of hand
P1-17179 Tenotomy of hand
P1-17180 Division of fascia of hand
Fasciotomy of hand
Incision of fascia of hand with division
P1-17182 Division of muscle of hand
Release of intrinsic muscle of hand
Incision of muscle of hand with division
Myotomy of hand with division
Release of muscle of hand
Transection of muscle of hand
P1-17183 Division of soft tissue of hand, NOS
Incision of soft tissue of hand with division

P1-17187 Subcutaneous tenotomy, single, each digit
P1-17188 Open flexor tenotomy of palm, single, each
Open flexor tenotomy of finger, single, each
P1-17189 Open extensor tenotomy of hand, single, each
Open extensor tenotomy of finger, single, each
P1-17190 Aspiration of bursa of hand
Bursocentesis of hand
Drainage of bursa of hand by aspiration
P1-17192 Aspiration of fascia of hand
P1-17193 Aspiration of muscle of hand
P1-17195 Aspiration of tendon of hand
P1-171A0 Drainage of finger abscess, simple
P1-171A1 Drainage of finger abscess, complicated
P1-171A2 Drainage of one digit
P1-171A3 Deep incision with opening of bone cortex of finger
P1-171A4 Decompression of fingers, injection injury
P1-171A5 Tendon sheath incision for trigger finger
Release of trigger finger or thumb
P1-17200 Arthrotomy for infection with drainage of metacarpophalangeal joint
Arthrotomy for infection with exploration and drainage of metacarpophalangeal joint
Arthrotomy for infection with exploration of metacarpophalangeal joint
P1-17202 Arthrotomy for infection with drainage of interphalangeal joint of finger, each
Arthrotomy for infection with exploration and drainage of interphalangeal joint of finger, each
Arthrotomy for infection with exploration of interphalangeal joint of finger, each
P1-17204 Capsulotomy for contracture of metacarpophalangeal joint, single, each
P1-17205 Capsulotomy for contracture of interphalangeal joint of finger, single, each
P1-17210 Incision of phalanges of hand, NOS
P1-17211 Osteotomy of phalanges,of hand
P1-17212 Arthrotomy of finger, NOS
P1-17214 Division of cartilage of finger
Division of joint cartilage of finger
P1-17215 Division of joint capsule of finger
P1-17216 Division of ligament of finger
Division of joint ligament of finger

1-173-174 Wrist and Hand: Excisions

P1-17302 Arthrotomy of wrist joint for biopsy
P1-17303 Arthrotomy of wrist joint with exploration and biopsy
P1-17304 Arthrotomy of wrist joint with exploration and removal of loose or foreign body
P1-17305 Arthrotomy of wrist joint for synovectomy
P1-17306 Exploration for removal of deep foreign body of wrist
P1-17307V Debridement of sesamoid bone of forefoot
P1-17310 Decompression fasciotomy of wrist with debridement of nonviable muscle and/or nerve
P1-17311 Decompression fasciotomy of wrist extensor compartment with debridement of nonviable muscle and/or nerve
P1-17312 Decompression fasciotomy of wrist flexor compartment with debridement of nonviable muscle and/or nerve
P1-17313 Decompression fasciotomy of wrist, flexor and extensor compartment, with debridement of nonviable muscle and nerve
P1-17315 Biopsy of soft tissue of wrist, superficial
P1-17316 Biopsy of soft tissue of wrist, deep
P1-17317 Excision of tumor of wrist area, deep, intramuscular
P1-17318 Excision of tumor of wrist area, deep, subfascial
P1-17319 Radical resection of tumor of soft tissue of wrist area
P1-1731A Arthrotomy for synovial biopsy of carpometacarpal joint
P1-17320 Excision of lesion of tendon sheath of wrist
P1-17322 Excision of ganglion of wrist, primary
Excision of ganglion of wrist
Ganglionectomy of tendon sheath of wrist
P1-17323 Excision of ganglion of wrist, recurrent
P1-17324 Radical excision of bursa of synovia of flexors of wrist
P1-17325 Radical excision of bursa of synovia of extensors of wrist
P1-17326 Synovectomy of extensor tendon sheath of wrist, single compartment
P1-17327 Synovectomy of extensor tendon sheath of wrist, single compartment with resection of distal ulna
P1-17328 Capsulectomy of wrist
P1-17329 Sequestrectomy of wrist
P1-17330 Disarticulation through wrist
Amputation by disarticulation of forefoot
Amputation of forefoot
P1-17331 Disarticulation through wrist, secondary closure or scar revision
P1-17332 Disarticulation through wrist, reamputation
P1-17334 Revision of arthroplasty including removal of implant of wrist joint
P1-17336 Excisional biopsy of joint structure of wrist
Biopsy of joint structure of wrist
P1-17337 Synovectomy of wrist
P1-17338 Local excision of lesion of wrist joint, NOS
Excision of lesion of wrist joint, NOS
P1-17340 Arthrectomy of wrist, NOS
Excision of wrist joint, NOS
P1-17341 Chondrectomy of wrist
P1-17342 Excision of meniscus of wrist
Meniscectomy of wrist
P1-17350 Amputation of arm through wrist
Amputation of wrist

1-173-174 Wrist and Hand: Excisions — Continued

P1-17350 (cont.) Disarticulation of wrist
P1-17352 Arthrotomy of mediocarpal joint for infection with removal of foreign body
P1-17353 Arthrotomy of radiocarpal joint for infection with removal of foreign body
P1-17354 Arthrotomy for infection with removal of foreign body of carpometacarpal joint
P1-17355 Arthrotomy for infection with removal of foreign body of metacarpophalangeal joint
P1-17356 Wedge osteotomy of carpals and metacarpals
P1-17357 Excision or curettage of benign tumor of carpal bones
P1-17358 Excision or curettage of bone cyst of carpal bones
P1-17359 Partial ostectomy of carpals or metacarpals, NOS
Carpectomy, one bone
Partial carpectomy
P1-1735A Total ostectomy of carpals and metacarpals
Carpectomy, all bones of proximal row
Total carpectomy
P1-1735B Excision of carpals and metacarpals for graft
P1-17360 Transmetacarpal amputation
Amputation of arm through carpals
Metacarpal amputation
Transcarpal amputation
P1-17361 Transmetacarpal amputation, secondary closure or scar revision
P1-17362 Transmetacarpal amputation, reamputation
P1-17363 Synovectomy of carpometacarpal joint
P1-17364 Excision or curettage of benign tumor of metacarpal bone
P1-17365 Excision or curettage of bone cyst of metacarpal bone
P1-17366 Partial excision of metacarpal bone
P1-17367 Radical resection for tumor of metacarpal bone
P1-17368 Metacarpal amputation with finger or thumb
P1-17369 Sequestrectomy of carpals or metacarpals
P1-1736A Excisional biopsy of carpals or metacarpals
P1-1736B Excision of lesion of bone, carpal or metacarpal, NOS
Local excision of lesion or tissue of carpals or metacarpals, NOS
P1-17370V Debridement of forefoot
P1-17371V Debridement of joint of forefoot
P1-17372 Debridement of open fracture, carpal or metacarpal
P1-17373V Excision of lesion of forefoot
P1-17374V Debridement of carpus region
P1-17376 Excision of tumor or vascular malformation of hand, deep, subfascial, intramuscular
P1-17377 Radical resection of tumor of soft tissue of hand
P1-17378 Palmar fasciectomy without z-plasty
P1-17379 Palmar fasciectomy without z-plasty, partial with release of single digit including proximal interphalangeal joint
P1-1737A Palmar fasciectomy without z-plasty, partial with release of each additional digit, including proximal interphalangeal joint
P1-17380 Synovectomy of flexor tendon sheath of palm, radical, single, each digit
P1-17382 Excision of flexor tendon of palm, single, each
P1-17383 Sequestrectomy of phalanges of hand
P1-17384 Excisional biopsy of phalanges of hand
P1-17385 Excision of lesion of phalanges of hand
P1-17386 Debridement of open fracture of hand, NOS
P1-17387 Excisional biopsy of joint structure of hand and finger
Biopsy of joint structure of hand and finger
P1-17388 Synovectomy of hand
P1-17389 Local excision of lesion of joint of hand, NOS
P1-17390 Arthrectomy of hand, NOS
Excision of joint of hand, NOS
P1-17391 Chondrectomy of hand
P1-17394 Removal of foreign body from tendon of hand
P1-17395 Removal of rice bodies from tendon sheaths of hand
P1-17396 Removal of foreign body from muscle of hand
P1-17397 Removal of foreign body from bursa of hand
P1-17398 Removal of calcareous deposit from bursa of hand
P1-17399 Removal of foreign body from fascia of hand
P1-1739A Removal of foreign body from soft tissue of hand
P1-17401 Curettage of tendon sheath of hand
P1-17402 Excision of ganglion of tendon sheath of hand
P1-17403 Excision of lesion of tendon sheath of hand
Excision of lesion of tendon sheath or capsule of hand
P1-17404 Excision of xanthoma of tendon sheath of hand
P1-17405 Tenectomy of tendon sheath of hand
P1-17406 Curettage of muscle of hand
P1-17407 Excision of lesion of muscle of hand
P1-17408 Excision of heterotopic bone from muscle of hand
Excision of myositis ossificans of hand
P1-1740A Curettage of bursa of hand
P1-1740B Curettage of tendon of hand
P1-17410 Excision of cyst of hand
P1-17411 Excision of lesion of fascia of hand
P1-17412 Excision of lesion of soft tissue of hand
P1-17413 Excision of lesion of tendon of hand
P1-17414 Removal of calcareous deposit of tendon of hand
P1-17415 Tenectomy of hand
Excision of tendon of hand
Resection of tendon of hand
P1-17416 Excision of tendon of hand for graft
Tenonectomy of hand for graft
P1-17417 Synovectomy of tendon sheath of hand
Tenonectomy of hand
Tenosynovectomy of hand

P1-17418 Bursectomy of hand
Excision of bursa of hand
Resection of bursa of hand
P1-1741A Aponeurectomy of hand
Excision of aponeurosis of hand
P1-17420 Excision of palmar fascia, NOS
Adams operation
Excision of fascia of hand
Fasciectomy of hand
P1-17421 Dupuytren operation fasciectomy
Dupuytren operation fasciotomy with excision
Palmar fasciectomy for release of Dupuytren's contracture
Release of Dupuytren's contracture by palmar fasciectomy
Release of Dupuytren's contracture by fasciotomy with excision
Resection of fascia of hand
P1-17422 Excision of fascia of hand for graft
Fasciectomy of hand for graft
Resection of fascia of hand for graft
P1-17425 Debridement of muscle of hand
P1-17426 Excision of muscle of hand, NOS
Myectomy of hand, NOS
Resection of muscle of hand, NOS
P1-17427 Excision of muscle of hand for graft
Myectomy of hand for graft
Resection of muscle of hand for graft
P1-17428 Excision of soft tissue of hand, NOS
Resection of soft tissue of hand, NOS
P1-17430 Amputation of hand
Amputation through hand
P1-17431 Removal of foreign body from hand, NOS
Removal of foreign body from forefoot, NOS
P1-17432 Removal of foreign body from hand without incision
P1-17440 Lateral fasciotomy with annular ligament of finger resection
P1-17441 Medial fasciotomy with annular ligament of finger resection
P1-17442 Arthrotomy for infection with removal of foreign body of interphalangeal joint of finger, each
P1-17443 Arthrotomy for synovial biopsy of metacarpophalangeal joint
P1-17444 Arthrotomy for synovial biopsy of interphalangeal joint of finger, each
P1-17445 Excision of tumor or vascular malformation of finger, deep, subfascial, intramuscular
P1-17446 Radical resection of tumor of soft tissue of finger
P1-17447 Synovectomy of flexor tendon sheath of finger, radical, single, each digit
P1-17448 Excision of lesion of tendon sheath or capsule of finger
P1-17449 Excision of flexor tendon of finger
P1-17450 Excision or curettage of benign tumor of proximal, middle or distal phalanx of finger
P1-17451 Partial excision of bone of proximal or middle phalanx of finger
P1-17452 Partial excision of bone of distal phalanx of finger
P1-17453 Radical resection for tumor of proximal or middle phalanx of finger
P1-17454 Radical resection for tumor of distal phalanx of finger
P1-17455 Capsulectomy for contracture of metacarpophalangeal joint, single, each
P1-17456 Capsulectomy for contracture of interphalangeal joint of finger, single, each
P1-17457 Amputation of finger or thumb, primary, any joint or phalanx, single, including neurectomies with direct closure
P1-17458 Amputation of finger or thumb, secondary, any joint or phalanx, single, including neurectomies with direct closure
P1-17459 Wedge osteotomy of phalanges, NOS
P1-17460 Partial phalangectomy, NOS
P1-17461 Total phalangectomy, NOS
Amputation of foredigit, NOS
P1-17462 Debridement of open fracture of phalanges of hand
P1-17463V Excision of lesion of foredigit
P1-17464 Synovectomy of finger
P1-17465 Excision of lesion of joint of finger, NOS
Local excision of lesion of joint of finger, NOS
P1-17466 Dewebbing of syndactyly of fingers
P1-17468 Arthrectomy of finger, NOS
Excision of joint of finger, NOS
P1-17469 Chondrectomy of finger
P1-17470 Amputation of finger, except thumb
Disarticulation of finger, except thumb
P1-17471 Ray amputation of finger
P1-17472 Revision of current traumatic amputation of finger
Kutler amputation
P1-17474 Amputation of thumb
Disarticulation of thumb

1-175 Wrist and Hand: Injections and Implantations

P1-17500 Injection procedure for wrist arthrography
P1-17502 Implantation of wrist joint
P1-17503 Implantation of prosthesis or prosthetic device of acetabulum of wrist joint
P1-17504 Implantation of Swanson prosthesis of wrist
P1-17506 Internal fixation of carpal or metacarpal
P1-17507 Insertion of bone growth stimulator into carpals and metacarpals
P1-17510 Removal of prosthesis of joint structures of wrist
Arthrotomy for removal of prosthesis of wrist

1-175 Wrist and Hand: Injections and Implantations — Continued

P1-17510 (cont.) Removal of wrist prosthesis
P1-17511 Removal of wrist prosthesis, complicated
P1-17512 Removal of internal fixation device from carpals and metacarpals
P1-17520 Implantation of joint of hand
P1-17522 Implantation of prosthesis or prosthetic device of acetabulum of joint of hand
P1-17523 Implantation of Swanson prosthesis of hand
P1-17525 Removal of implant from hand, NOS
P1-17526 Removal of prosthesis of joint structures of hand
 Arthrotomy for removal of prosthesis of hand
P1-17530 Injection into bursa of hand
P1-17532 Injection of therapeutic substance into bursa of hand
P1-17533 Injection into tendon of hand
P1-17534 Injection of therapeutic substance into tendon of hand
P1-17536 Injection into fascia of hand
P1-17537 Injection of therapeutic substance into fascia of hand
P1-17538 Injection into soft tissue of hand
P1-17539 Injection of therapeutic substance into soft tissue of hand
P1-17540 Irrigation of tendon of hand
P1-17542 Irrigation of muscle of hand
P1-17550 Implantation of joint of finger
P1-17552 Implantation of prosthesis or prosthetic device of acetabulum of joint of finger
P1-17554 Implantation of Swanson prosthesis of finger
P1-17555 Removal of internal fixation device from phalanges of hand
P1-17556 Removal of implant from finger, NOS
P1-17557 Removal of prosthesis of joint structures of finger
 Arthrotomy for removal of prosthesis of finger

1-177 Wrist and Hand: Endoscopy

P1-17700 Arthroscopy of wrist, NOS
 Diagnostic arthroscopy of wrist
P1-17701 Diagnostic arthroscopy of wrist with synovial biopsy
P1-17702 Arthroscopy of wrist with partial synovectomy
P1-17703 Arthroscopy of wrist with complete synovectomy
P1-17704 Arthroscopy of wrist with excision of triangular fibrocartilage
P1-17705 Arthroscopy of wrist with excision of triangular fibrocartilage and joint debridement
P1-17706 Arthroscopy of wrist with joint debridement
P1-17707 Arthroscopy of wrist with internal fixation for fracture
P1-17708 Arthroscopy of wrist for infection with lavage and drainage
P1-17709 Arthroscopy of wrist with internal fixation for instability
P1-17710 Arthroscopy of hand, NOS
P1-17720 Arthroscopy of finger, NOS

1-178-17B Wrist and Hand: Surgical Repairs, Closures and Reconstructions

P1-17800 Arthroplasty of wrist, NOS
 Repair of wrist, NOS
P1-17801 Arthroplasty of wrist with implant
 Arthroplasty of wrist with synthetic joint prosthesis
P1-17802 Arthroplasty of wrist, pseudoarthrosis type with internal fixation
P1-17804 Arthrotomy of distal radioulnar joint for repair of triangular cartilage complex
P1-17805 Radical excision of bursa or synovia of wrist extensors with transposition of dorsal retinaculum
P1-17806 Radical excision of bursa or synovia of wrist extensors without transposition of dorsal retinaculum
P1-17808 Repair of flexor tendon or muscle of wrist, primary, single, each tendon or muscle
P1-17809 Repair of flexor tendon or muscle of wrist, secondary, single, each tendon or muscle
P1-17810 Repair of flexor tendon or muscle of wrist, secondary, with free graft, including obtaining graft, each tendon or muscle
P1-17811 Repair of extensor tendon or muscle of primary, single, each tendon or muscle
P1-17812 Repair of extensor tendon or muscle of wrist, secondary, single, each tendon or muscle
P1-17813 Repair of extensor tendon or muscle of wrist, secondary, with tendon graft, each
P1-17814 Lengthening of flexor or extensor tendon of wrist, single, each
P1-17815 Shortening of flexor or extensor tendon of wrist, single, each
P1-17816 Tenodesis at wrist for flexors of fingers
P1-17817 Tenodesis at wrist for extensors of fingers
P1-17820 Centralization of wrist on ulna
P1-17821 Open reduction of closed or open radiocarpal or intercarpal dislocation, one or more bones
P1-17822 Reduction of open radiocarpal or intercarpal dislocation, one or more bones with uncomplicated soft tissue closure
P1-17823 Arthrodesis of wrist joint, NOS
 Arthrodesis of wrist, NOS
P1-17824 Arthrodesis of wrist joint with sliding graft
P1-17825 Arthrodesis of wrist joint with iliac or other autograft
P1-17826 Intercarpal fusion
P1-17827 Intercarpal fusion with autograft
P1-17828 Arthroplasty of carpometacarpal joint
P1-17829V Stapling of carpus
P1-17830 Open reduction of closed or open carpometacarpal fracture dislocation of thumb

P1-17831 Reduction of open carpometacarpal fracture dislocation of thumb with uncomplicated soft tissue closure
P1-17832 Reduction of open carpometacarpal fracture dislocation of thumb with uncomplicated soft tissue closure with skeletal fixation
P1-17833 Open reduction of closed or open carpometacarpal fracture dislocation of thumb with internal or external skeletal fixation
P1-17834 Reduction of open carpometacarpal dislocation, except Bennett fracture, single with uncomplicated soft tissue closure
P1-17835 Open reduction of closed or open carpometacarpal dislocation, except Bennett fracture, single
P1-17836 Open reduction of closed or open carpometacarpal dislocation, except Bennett fracture, single with internal or external skeletal fixation
P1-17837 Open reduction of closed or open carpometacarpal dislocation, except Bennett fracture, complex, delayed reduction
P1-17838 Open reduction of closed or open carpometacarpal dislocation, except Bennett fracture, complex, multiple reduction
P1-17839 Metacarpocarpal arthrodesis
    Metacarpocarpal fusion
P1-1783A Arthrodesis of carpometacarpal joint of thumb
P1-17840 Arthrodesis of carpometacarpal joint of thumb with internal fixation
P1-17841 Arthrodesis of carpometacarpal joint of thumb with internal fixation and autograft
P1-17842 Arthrodesis of carpometacarpal joint of thumb with autograft
P1-17843 Arthrodesis of carpometacarpal joint of digits, other than thumb
P1-17844 Arthrodesis of carpometacarpal joint of digits, other than thumb with autograft
P1-17845 Open reduction of dislocation of wrist
P1-17846 Carporadial arthrodesis
    Carporadial fusion
    Gill-Stein operation
    Smith-Peterson operation
    Bost radiocarpal fusion
    Radiocarpal fusion
P1-17850 Total wrist replacement
P1-17851 Arthroplasty of carpocarpal joint with implant
P1-17852 Arthroplasty of carpometacarpal joint with implant
P1-17853 Kessler arthroplasty of carpometacarpal joint
P1-17854 Arthroplasty of carpocarpal joint without implant
P1-17855 Arthroplasty of carpometacarpal joint without implant
P1-17859 Arthroplasty of carpals with synthetic joint prosthesis
P1-17860 Excision or curettage of benign tumor of carpal bones with autograft
P1-17861 Excision or curettage of bone cyst of carpal bones with autograft
P1-17862 Excision or curettage of benign tumor of carpal bones with allograft
P1-17863 Excision or curettage of bone cyst of carpal bones with allograft
P1-17864 Excision or curettage of benign tumor of metacarpal bone with autograft
P1-17865 Excision or curettage of bone cyst of metacarpal with autograft
P1-17866 Radical resection for tumor of metacarpal with autograft
P1-17867 Amputation of metacarpal with finger or thumb, single with interosseous transfer
P1-17868 Amputation of metacarpal with finger or thumb, single, without interosseous transfer
P1-17869 Repair of nonunion of scaphoid bone with radial styloidectomy
P1-1786A Repair of nonunion of scaphoid bone without radial styloidectomy
P1-17871 Arthroplasty with prosthetic replacement of scaphoid
P1-17872 Arthroplasty with prosthetic replacement of lunate
P1-17873 Arthroplasty with prosthetic replacement of trapezium
P1-17874 Interposition arthroplasty of carpometacarpal joints
P1-17875 Interposition arthroplasty of intercarpal joints
P1-17876 Open reduction of closed or open carpal scaphoid fracture
P1-17877 Reduction of open carpal scaphoid fracture with uncomplicated soft tissue closure
P1-17878 Open reduction of closed or open carpal scaphoid fracture with skeletal fixation
P1-17879 Open reduction of closed or open carpal fracture, each bone
P1-1787A Reduction of open carpal fracture with uncomplicated soft tissue closure, each bone
P1-17881 Open reduction of closed or open trans-scaphoperilunar type of fracture dislocation
P1-17882 Open reduction of lunate dislocation
P1-17883 Osteotomy for correction of deformity of metacarpal
P1-17884 Osteoplasty for lengthening of metacarpal or phalanx of finger
P1-17885 Open reduction of closed or open metacarpal fracture, single, each
P1-17886 Reduction of open metacarpal fracture, single with uncomplicated soft tissue closure, each
P1-17887 Open reduction of closed or open metacarpal fracture, single, with internal skeletal fixation, each
P1-17888 Open reduction of closed or open metacarpal fracture, single, with external skeletal fixation, each

1-178-17B Wrist and Hand: Surgical Repairs, Closures and Reconstructions — Continued

P1-17889 Change in bone length of carpals and metacarpals, NOS
P1-17890 Osteoplasty of carpal or metacarpal, NOS
P1-17891 Open reduction of fracture of carpals and metacarpals
P1-17892 Internal fixation of carpals and metacarpals without fracture reduction
P1-17894 Open reduction of fracture of carpals and metacarpals with internal fixation
P1-17896 Arthroplasty of carpals
P1-17897 Metacarpal lengthening and transfer of local flap
    Cocked hat procedure
P1-17898 Replantation of hand, complete amputation
P1-17899 Replantation of hand, incomplete amputation
P1-17901 Internal fixation of bone of phalanges of hand
P1-17902 Arthroplasty of hand with synthetic joint prosthesis
P1-17903 Repair of tendon sheath of hand, NOS
P1-17904 Repair of tendon of hand by suture
    Repair of tendon of hand by suture, direct, immediate, primary
P1-17906 Repair of fascia of hand by suture
    Repair of fascia of hand by suture, direct
P1-17907 Repair of muscle of hand by suture
    Repair of muscle of hand by suture, direct
P1-17910 Release of scar contracture of flexor or extensor of hand with skin grafts, rearrangement flaps or z-plasties
P1-17911 Palmar fasciectomy with z-plasty
P1-17912 Palmar fasciectomy with z-plasty, partial excision with release of single digit including proximal interphalangeal joint
P1-17913 Palmar fasciectomy with z-plasty, partial with release of each additional digit, including proximal interphalangeal joint
P1-17914 Flexor tendon repair or advancement, single, not in no man's land, primary without free graft, each tendon
P1-17915 Flexor tendon repair or advancement, single, not in no man's land, secondary without free graft, each tendon
P1-17916 Flexor tendon repair or advancement, single, not in no man's land, secondary with free graft, each tendon
P1-17917 Flexor tendon repair or advancement, single, in no man's land, primary, each tendon
P1-17918 Flexor tendon repair or advancement, single, in no man's land, secondary, each tendon
P1-17919 Flexor tendon repair or advancement, single, in no man's land, secondary with free graft, each tendon
P1-17920 Profundus tendon repair or advancement with intact sublimis, primary
P1-17921 Profundus tendon repair or advancement with intact sublimis, secondary with free graft
P1-17922 Profundus tendon repair or advancement with intact sublimis, secondary without free graft
P1-17923 Flexor tendon excision with implantation of plastic tube or rod for delayed tendon graft of hand
P1-17924 Removal of tube or rod and insertion of flexor tendon graft of hand
P1-17925 Extensor tendon repair of dorsum of hand, single, primary without free graft, each
P1-17926 Extensor tendon repair of dorsum of hand, single, secondary without free graft, each
P1-17927 Extensor tendon repair of dorsum of hand, single, primary with free graft, each
P1-17928 Extensor tendon repair of dorsum of hand, single, secondary with free graft, each
P1-17929 Extensor tendon excision with implantation of plastic tube or rod for delayed extensor tendon graft of hand
P1-1792A Removal of tube or rod and insertion of extensor tendon graft of hand
P1-17930 Extensor tendon repair by central slip repair, secondary, using local tissues
P1-17931 Extensor tendon repair by central slip repair, secondary, with free graft
P1-17932 Extensor tendon repair with distal insertion, closed, splinting with percutaneous pinning
P1-17933 Extensor tendon repair with distal insertion, closed, splinting without percutaneous pinning
P1-17934 Extensor tendon repair with distal insertion, open, primary repair without graft
P1-17935 Extensor tendon repair with distal insertion, open, secondary repair without graft
P1-17936 Extensor tendon repair with distal insertion, open, primary repair with free graft
P1-17937 Extensor tendon repair with distal insertion, open, secondary repair with free graft
P1-17938 Extensor tendon realignment of hand
P1-17939 Extensor tendon lengthening of hand, single, each
P1-1793A Extensor tendon shortening of hand, single, each
P1-1793B Flexor tendon lengthening of hand, single, each
P1-1793C Flexor tendon shortening of hand, single, each
P1-1793D Correction of claw finger, NOS
P1-17940 Reconstruction of tendon pulley of hand
    Reconstruction of tendon pulley for opponensplasty of hand
P1-17941 Hand tendon pulley reconstruction with local tissues
P1-17942 Hand tendon pulley reconstruction with tendon or fascial graft
P1-17943 Hand tendon pulley reconstruction with tendon prosthesis
P1-17944 Thenar muscle release for thumb contracture
P1-17945 Cross intrinsic transfer

P1-17951 Repair of cleft hand
P1-17952 Repair of intrinsic muscles of hand
P1-17954 Osteoplasty of phalanges of hand
P1-17956 Open reduction of fracture of hand
P1-17957 Open reduction of fracture of phalanges of hand
P1-17958 Open reduction of fracture of hand with internal fixation
P1-17959 Open reduction of fracture of phalanges of hand with internal fixation
P1-1795A Open reduction of dislocation of hand
P1-1795B Arthroplasty of hand, NOS
P1-17963 Reattachment of tendon of hand
P1-17964 Reattachment of muscle of hand
P1-17965 Change of length of muscle of hand, NOS
P1-17966 Change of length of tendon of hand, NOS
P1-17967 Lengthening of muscle of hand
P1-17968 Shortening of muscle of hand
P1-17969 Lengthening of tendon of hand
P1-1796A Plication of tendon of hand
P1-1796B Shortening of tendon of hand
P1-17974 Opponensplasty of hand
P1-17977 Plastic operation on hand, NOS
  Repair of hand, NOS
P1-17978 Plastic operation on hand with graft of fascia
  Repair of hand with graft or implant of fascia
P1-17979 Plastic operation on hand with graft of muscle
  Repair of hand with graft or implant of muscle
P1-1797A Repair of muscle of hand by graft or implant of fascia
P1-1797B Repair of tendon of hand by graft or implant
P1-1797C Repair of tendon of hand by graft or implant of fascia
P1-1797D Repair of tendon of hand by graft or implant of muscle
P1-17980 Plastic operation on hand with graft, NOS
  Plastic operation on hand with implant, NOS
  Repair of hand with graft or implant, NOS
P1-17981 Repair of fascia of hand by graft, NOS
P1-17982 Repair of fascia of hand by graft of tendon
P1-17983 Repair of muscle of hand by graft or implant of tendon
  Repair of hand with graft or implant of tendon
P1-17984 Repair of muscle of hand by graft or implant, NOS
P1-17986 Fixation of tendon of hand
  Reattachment of tendon of hand to skeletal attachment
  Tenodesis of hand
P1-17987 Fowler tenodesis of hand
P1-17989 Myotenontoplasty of hand
P1-17990 Myotenoplasty of hand
  Tenomyoplasty of hand
P1-17991 Repair of ruptured tendon of hand
  Repair of tendon of hand
  Tenoplasty of hand
P1-17992 Tenosuspension of hand
P1-17994 Fasciodesis of hand
P1-17995 Fascioplasty of hand, NOS
  Repair of fascia of hand, NOS
P1-17996 Lengthening of fascia of hand
P1-17997 Musculoplasty of hand
  Myoplasty of hand
P1-17998 Plication of fascia of hand
P1-1799B Repair of hernia of fascia of hand
P1-1799C Repair of muscle of hand
P1-17A00 Reattachment of hand at wrist
  Reattachment of wrist
P1-17A01 Replantation of digit, except thumb, includes metacarpophalangeal joint to insertion of flexor sublimis tendon, complete amputation
P1-17A02 Replantation of digit, except thumb, includes metacarpophalangeal joint to insertion of flexor sublimis tendon, incomplete amputation, devascularized extremity with soft tissue pedicle
P1-17A03 Replantation of digit, except thumb, includes distal tip to sublimis tendon insertion, complete amputation
P1-17A04 Replantation of digit, except thumb, incomplete amputation
P1-17A05 Replantation of thumb, including carpometacarpal joint to metacarpophalangeal joint, complete amputation
P1-17A06 Replantation of thumb, incomplete amputation, devascularized extremity with soft tissue pedicle
P1-17A07 Replantation of thumb including distal tip to metacarpophalangeal joint, complete amputation
P1-17A08 Replantation of thumb, including distal tip to metacarpophalangeal joint, incomplete amputation, devascularized extremity with soft tissue pedicle
P1-17A09 Arthroplasty of finger with synthetic joint prosthesis
P1-17A0A Arthroplasty of metacarpophalangeal joint with synthetic joint prosthesis
P1-17A10 Release of scar contracture of flexor or extensor of finger with skin grafts, rearrangement flaps, or z-plasties
P1-17A11 Synovectomy of proximal interphalangeal joint of finger including extensor reconstruction, each
P1-17A12 Excision or curettage of benign tumor of proximal, middle or distal phalanx of finger with autograft
P1-17A13 Excision or curettage of bone cyst of proximal, middle or distal phalanx of finger with autograft

1-178-17B Wrist and Hand: Surgical Repairs, Closures and Reconstructions — Continued

P1-17A14 Radical resection for tumor of proximal or middle phalanx of finger with autograft
P1-17A15 Excision of constricting ring of finger with multiple z-plasties
P1-17A16 Amputation of finger or thumb, primary, any joint or phalanx, single, including neurectomies with local advancement flaps
P1-17A17 Amputation of finger or thumb, secondary, any joint or phalanx, single, including neurectomies with local advancement flaps
P1-17A18 Flexor tendon excision with implantation of plastic tube or rod for delayed tendon graft of finger
P1-17A19 Removal of tube or rod and insertion of flexor tendon graft of finger
P1-17A20 Extensor tendon excision with implantation of plastic tube or rod for delayed extensor tendon graft of finger
P1-17A21 Removal of tube or rod and insertion of extensor tendon graft of finger
P1-17A22 Extensor tendon repair of dorsum of finger, single, primary without free graft, each tendon
P1-17A23 Extensor tendon repair of dorsum of finger, single, secondary without free graft, each tendon
P1-17A24 Extensor tendon repair of dorsum of finger, single, primary with free graft, each tendon
P1-17A25 Extensor tendon repair of dorsum of finger, single, secondary with free graft, each tendon
P1-17A26 Tenodesis for proximal interphalangeal finger joint stabilization
P1-17A27 Tenodesis for distal interphalangeal finger joint stabilization
P1-17A30 Extensor tendon lengthening of finger, single, each
P1-17A31 Extensor tendon shortening of finger, single, each
P1-17A32 Flexor tendon lengthening of finger, single, each
P1-17A33 Flexor tendon shortening of finger, single, each
P1-17A34 Capsulodesis for metacarpophalangeal joint stabilization, single digit
P1-17A35 Capsulodesis for metacarpophalangeal joint stabilization, two digits
P1-17A36 Capsulodesis for metacarpophalangeal joint stabilization, three or four digits
P1-17A37 Arthroplasty of metacarpophalangeal joint, single, each
    Fowler arthroplasty of metacarpophalangeal joint
    Arthroplasty of metacarpophalangeal joint
P1-17A38 Arthroplasty of metacarpophalangeal joint with prosthetic implant, single, each
P1-17A39 Arthroplasty of interphalangeal joint of finger, single, each
P1-17A3A Arthroplasty of interphalangeal joint of finger with prosthetic implant, single, each
P1-17A3B Synovectomy of metacarpophalangeal joint including intrinsic release and extensor hood reconstruction, each
P1-17A40 Primary repair of collateral ligament of metacarpophalangeal joint
P1-17A41 Primary repair of collateral ligament of metacarpophalangeal joint with tendon or fascial graft
P1-17A42 Primary repair of collateral ligament of metacarpophalangeal joint with local tissue
P1-17A43 Reconstruction of collateral ligament of interphalangeal joint of finger, single, including graft, each
P1-17A44 Repair and reconstruction of finger, volar plate of interphalangeal joint
P1-17A45 Pollicization of a digit
    Pollicization with carry over of nerves and blood supply
P1-17A46 Reconstruction of thumb with toe
P1-17A47 Positional change of other finger
P1-17A48 Osteotomy for correction of deformity of phalanx of finger
P1-17A49 Repair of bifid digit of hand
P1-17A4A Reconstruction of supernumerary digit of hand with soft tissue and bone
P1-17A4B Open reduction of dislocation of finger, NOS
P1-17A50 Open reduction of closed or open metacarpophalangeal dislocation, single
P1-17A51 Reduction of open metacarpophalangeal dislocation, single, with uncomplicated soft tissue closure
P1-17A52 Open reduction of closed or open metacarpophalangeal dislocation, single with internal skeletal fixation
P1-17A53 Open reduction of closed or open metacarpophalangeal dislocation, single with external skeletal fixation
P1-17A54 Reduction of open phalangeal shaft fracture of proximal or middle phalanx of finger or thumb with uncomplicated soft tissue closure, each
P1-17A55 Open reduction of closed or open phalangeal shaft fracture of proximal or middle phalanx of finger or thumb, each
P1-17A56 Open reduction of closed or open phalangeal shaft fracture of proximal or middle phalanx of finger or thumb with internal or external skeletal fixation, each
P1-17A57 Open reduction of closed or open articular fracture, involving metacarpophalangeal or proximal interphalangeal joint, each
P1-17A58 Reduction of open articular fracture, involving metacarpophalangeal or proximal interphalangeal joint with uncomplicated soft tissue closure, each
P1-17A59 Open reduction of closed or open distal phalangeal fracture of finger or thumb, each

P1-17A60 Reduction of open distal phalangeal fracture of finger or thumb with uncomplicated soft tissue closure, each
P1-17A61 Reduction of open interphalangeal finger joint dislocation, single, with uncomplicated soft tissue closure
P1-17A62 Open reduction of closed or open interphalangeal finger joint dislocation, single
P1-17A63 Fusion in opposition of thumb with autogenous graft
P1-17A64 Arthrodesis of metacarpophalangeal joint
P1-17A65 Arthrodesis of metacarpophalangeal joint with internal fixation
P1-17A66 Arthrodesis of metacarpophalangeal joint with internal fixation and autograft
P1-17A67 Arthrodesis of metacarpophalangeal joint with autograft
P1-17A68 Arthrodesis of interphalangeal joint of finger
  Arthrodesis of finger
  Interphalangeal arthrodesis of finger
  Interphalangeal fusion of joint of finger
  Interphalangeal fusion of finger
P1-17A69 Arthrodesis of interphalangeal joint of finger, each additional interphalangeal joint
P1-17A70 Arthrodesis of interphalangeal joint of finger with internal fixation
P1-17A71 Arthrodesis of interphalangeal joint of finger with internal fixation, each additional interphalangeal joint
P1-17A72 Arthrodesis of interphalangeal joint of finger with internal fixation with autograft
P1-17A73 Arthrodesis of interphalangeal joint of finger without internal fixation with autograft
P1-17A74 Arthrodesis of interphalangeal joint of finger with internal fixation and autograft, each additional joint
P1-17A75 Arthrodesis of interphalangeal joint of finger without internal fixation with autograft, each additional joint
P1-17A76 Arthroplasty of finger, NOS
P1-17A77 Curtis arthroplasty of interphalangeal joint of finger
P1-17A78 Carroll and Taber arthroplasty of proximal interphalangeal joint of finger
P1-17A79 Arthroplasty of metacarpophalangeal and interphalangeal joint
P1-17A7A Arthroplasty of metacarpophalangeal and interphalangeal joint with implant
P1-17A80 Lengthening of bone for reconstruction of thumb
P1-17A81 Reconstruction of thumb with bone graft and skin graft
P1-17A82 Thompson operation on thumb, apposition with bone graft
P1-17A83 Unlisted reconstruction of thumb, NOS
P1-17A84 Phalangization of fifth metacarpal
P1-17A85 Repair of macrodactyly of finger
  Repair of macrodactylia of finger
  Reduction of size of finger for macrodactyly repair
  Shortening of finger for macrodactyly repair
P1-17A86 Tsuge operation on finger for macrodactyly repair
P1-17A87 Revision of mallet finger
  Fowler operation release for mallet finger repair
  Repair of mallet finger
P1-17A88 Release of extensor tendon of hand by central slip for repair of mallet finger
P1-17A90 Repair of bifid finger
P1-17A91 Reattachment of fingers and thumb
P1-17A92 Reattachment of finger
  Reattachment of fingers, except thumb
P1-17B04 Capsulorrhaphy or reconstruction of wrist
P1-17B05 Suture of periosteum of carpal or metacarpal
P1-17B06 Suture of periosteum of phalanges of hand
P1-17B07 Suture of tendon sheath of hand, NOS
P1-17B08 Suture of tendon of hand, NOS
  Tendinosuture of hand
  Tenorrhaphy of hand
  Tenosuture of hand
P1-17B09 Suture of tendon of hand to skeletal attachment
  Tenorrhaphy to skeletal attachment of hand
  Tenosuture to skeletal attachment of hand
P1-17B10 Delayed suture of tendon of hand, NOS
P1-17B11 Suture of flexor tendon of hand, NOS
P1-17B12 Delayed suture of flexor tendons of hand
P1-17B17 Aponeurorrhaphy of hand
P1-17B20 Myorrhaphy of hand
  Myosuture of hand
  Suture of muscle of hand
P1-17B22 Suture of fascia of hand
P1-17B23 Suture of fascia to skeletal attachment of hand
P1-17B24 Suture of bursa of hand
P1-17B26 Closure of cleft hand
  Barsky operation for closure of cleft hand
  Closure of palmar cleft
P1-17B30V Suture of wound of forefoot
P1-17B50V Plastic operation on hoof of forelimb
P1-17B55V Plastic operation on claw of forelimb

1-17C Wrist and Hand: Destructive Procedures

P1-17C00 Destructive procedure of wrist and hand, NOS
P1-17C01 Local destruction of lesion of wrist joint, NOS
P1-17C02 Tenolysis of flexor tendon of wrist
P1-17C03 Tenolysis of extensor tendon of wrist
P1-17C10 Osteoclasis of carpal or metacarpal bone
P1-17C11 Osteoclasis of phalanges of hand
P1-17C12 Local destruction of lesion of joint of hand, NOS

1-17C Wrist and Hand: Destructive Procedures — Continued

P1-17C20 Lysis of adhesions of hand
P1-17C21 Lysis of adhesions of bursa of hand
P1-17C22 Lysis of adhesions of fascia of hand
P1-17C23 Lysis of adhesions of muscle of hand
  Myoclasis of hand
P1-17C25 Stripping of fascia of hand
P1-17C30 Lysis of adhesions of tendon of hand
  Tendolysis of hand
  Tenolysis of hand
P1-17C31 Simple tenolysis of flexor tendon of palm
  Simple tenolysis of flexor tendon of finger
P1-17C33 Tenolysis of extensor tendon of dorsum of hand, each
  Tenolysis of extensor tendon of dorsum of finger, each
P1-17C34 Complex tenolysis of extensor tendon of dorsum of finger including hand and forearm
P1-17C40 Local destruction of lesion of joint of finger, NOS
P1-17C50V Cauterization of forefoot
P1-17C55V Cauterization of hoof of forefoot

1-17D Wrist and Hand: Transplantations and Transpositions

P1-17D02 Grafting of carpals and metacarpals
P1-17D04 Grafting of phalanges of hand
P1-17D05 Grafting of fascia of hand
P1-17D06 Grafting of muscle of hand
P1-17D07 Grafting of skin, free thumb for pollicization
  Grafting of skin pedicle attachment to site of thumb for pollicization
P1-17D09 Grafting of bone of thumb with transfer of skin flap
P1-17D10 Tendon transplantation or transfer of flexor or extensor of wrist, single, each
P1-17D12 Tendon transplantation or transfer of flexor or extensor of wrist, single, with tendon graft, each tendon
P1-17D14 Tendon transfer or transplant of carpometacarpal area of hand, single, without free graft, each
P1-17D16 Tendon transfer or transplant of carpometacarpal area of hand, single, with free tendon graft, each
P1-17D20 Tendon transfer or transplant of carpometacarpal area of dorsum of hand, single, without free graft, each
P1-17D22 Tendon transfer or transplant of carpometacarpal area of dorsum of hand, single, with free tendon graft, each
P1-17D24 Tendon transfer or transplant of palmar area, single, without free tendon graft, each
P1-17D25 Tendon transfer or transplant of palmar area, single, with free tendon graft, each
P1-17D26 Opponensplasty by sublimis tendon transfer type
P1-17D27 Opponensplasty by tendon transfer with graft
P1-17D28 Opponensplasty by hypothenar muscle transfer
P1-17D29 Opponensplasty by other method
P1-17D30 Repair of tendon of hand by transfer or transplantation
  Bunnell operation for tendon of hand transfer
  Transfer of tendon of hand
  Transplantation of tendon of hand
P1-17D31 Advancement of tendon of hand
P1-17D32 Advancement of tendon profundus
  Wagner operation
P1-17D33 Recession of tendon of hand
P1-17D34 Zancolli operation for tendon transfer of biceps
P1-17D35 Transposition of tendon of hand, NOS
  Hand tendon transposition, NOS
P1-17D37 Hand muscle transplantation, NOS
  Hand muscle transfer, NOS
P1-17D40 Transposition of muscle of hand, NOS
  Hand muscle transposition, NOS
P1-17D41 Transfer of hand muscle origin
P1-17D45 Grafting of tendon of hand
P1-17D46 Transplantation of fascia of hand
P1-17D48 Tendon transfer to restore intrinsic function, ring and small finger
P1-17D49 Tendon transfer to restore intrinsic function, all four fingers
P1-17D50 Toe to finger transfer, first stage
P1-17D51 Transfer of toe to finger, except thumb
P1-17D53 Toe to finger transfer, each delay
P1-17D54 Toe to finger transfer, second stage
P1-17D55 Grafting of thumb for reconstruction
P1-17D56 Grafting of skin pedicle attachment to site of thumb for reconstruction
P1-17D57 Transfer of toe to thumb with amputation
P1-17D58 Transfer of digit to replace absent thumb, NOS
P1-17D59 Transplantation of finger for replacing absent thumb, same hand
  Transfer of digital finger to thumb, same hand
P1-17D60 Transfer of finger to opposite hand with amputation
  Transplant of finger to opposite hand with amputation
P1-17D65 Transfer of finger, except thumb
  Transfer of finger to finger, except thumb
P1-17D72 Bone graft of scaphoid
  Russe operation

1-17E Wrist and Hand: Manipulations

P1-17E02 Closed reduction of dislocation of wrist, NOS
P1-17E04 Reduction of carpometacarpal dislocation of thumb with manipulation
P1-17E05 Reduction of closed carpometacarpal fracture dislocation of thumb with manipulation

P1-17E06 Reduction of closed carpometacarpal fracture dislocation of thumb with manipulation and skeletal fixation
P1-17E07 Reduction of closed carpometacarpal dislocation, except Bennett fracture, single, with manipulation without anesthesia
P1-17E08 Reduction of closed carpometacarpal dislocation, except Bennett fracture, single with manipulation and anesthesia
P1-17E09 Reduction of closed carpometacarpal dislocation, except Bennett fracture, single, with manipulation and percutaneous pinning
P1-17E10 Reduction of closed carpal fracture without manipulation, each bone
P1-17E11 Reduction of closed carpal fracture with manipulation, each bone
P1-17E12 Reduction of closed carpal scaphoid fracture without manipulation
P1-17E13 Reduction of closed carpal scaphoid fracture with manipulation
P1-17E14 Reduction of closed trans-scaphoperilunar type of fracture dislocation with manipulation
P1-17E15 Reduction of lunate dislocation with manipulation
P1-17E16 Closed reduction of fracture of carpals and metacarpals
P1-17E17 Closed reduction of fracture of carpals and metacarpals with internal fixation
Reduction of fracture of carpal and metacarpal with internal fixation
P1-17E18 Reduction of closed metacarpal fracture, single without manipulation, each
P1-17E19 Reduction of closed metacarpal fracture, single with manipulation, each
P1-17E1A Reduction of closed metacarpal fracture, single with manipulation with skeletal fixation, each
P1-17E1BV Manipulation of carpal region with application of splint
P1-17E20 Fitting of prosthesis of hand
Fitting of prosthetic device of hand
P1-17E21 Application of plaster figure of eight, hand and lower forearm
Application of plaster figure of eight, gauntlet
P1-17E22 Strapping of hand
P1-17E23 Application of finger splint, static
P1-17E24 Application of finger splint, dynamic
P1-17E25 Strapping of finger
P1-17E27 Closed reduction of dislocation of hand
P1-17E30 Closed reduction of fracture of hand, NOS
P1-17E31 Reduction of fracture of hand with internal fixation
P1-17E32 Closed reduction of fracture of phalanges of hand
P1-17E33 Closed reduction of fracture of phalanges of hand with internal fixation
P1-17E34 Closed reduction of dislocation of finger
P1-17E36 Reduction of closed metacarpophalangeal dislocation, single, with manipulation and without anesthesia
P1-17E37 Reduction of closed metacarpophalangeal dislocation, single with manipulation requiring anesthesia
P1-17E38 Reduction of closed metacarpophalangeal dislocation, single, with manipulation and with percutaneous pinning
P1-17E39 Reduction of closed phalangeal shaft fracture of proximal or middle phalanx of finger or thumb without manipulation, each
P1-17E3A Reduction of closed phalangeal shaft fracture of proximal or middle phalanx of finger or thumb with manipulation, each
P1-17E40 Reduction of unstable phalangeal shaft fracture of proximal or middle phalanx of finger or thumb with manipulation requiring traction or fixation, each
P1-17E41 Reduction of closed articular fracture, involving metacarpophalangeal or proximal interphalangeal joint without manipulation, each
P1-17E42 Reduction of closed articular fracture, involving metacarpophalangeal or proximal interphalangeal joint with manipulation, each
P1-17E43 Reduction of closed distal phalangeal fracture of finger or thumb without manipulation, each
P1-17E44 Reduction of closed distal phalangeal fracture of finger or thumb with manipulation, each
P1-17E45 Reduction of closed distal phalangeal fracture of finger or thumb with percutaneous pinning, each
P1-17E46 Reduction of closed interphalangeal finger joint dislocation, single, with manipulation without anesthesia
P1-17E47 Reduction of closed interphalangeal finger joint dislocation, single with manipulation with anesthesia
P1-17E48 Reduction of closed interphalangeal finger joint dislocation, single with manipulation with percutaneous pinning

1-18-19 OPERATIVE PROCEDURES ON THE LOWER EXTREMITY

1-18 OPERATIVE PROCEDURES ON THE LOWER EXTREMITY: THIGH AND LEG

1-180 Thigh and Leg: General and Miscellaneous Operative Procedures

P1-18010 Operative procedure on femur, NOS
P1-18012 Diagnostic procedure on femur, NOS
P1-18014 Operation on bone injury of femur, NOS
P1-18020 Operative procedure on knee, NOS
P1-18022 Diagnostic procedure on patella, NOS

1-180 Thigh and Leg: General and Miscellaneous Operative Procedures — Continued

P1-18030 Operative procedure on lower leg, NOS
P1-18032 Diagnostic procedure on tibia and fibula, NOS
P1-18034 Diagnostic procedure on fibula
P1-18036 Diagnostic procedure on tibia
P1-18038 Operation on bone injury of tibia and fibula, NOS

1-181 Thigh and Leg: Incisions

P1-18100 Incision of thigh, NOS
P1-18101 Incision of leg, NOS
P1-18102 Incision of bone of femur, NOS
Deep incision with opening of bone cortex of femur, NOS
Incision of femur without division, NOS
P1-18103 Osteotomy of femur
Schanz operation
P1-18104 Osteotomy of shaft of femur
P1-18105 Supracondylar osteotomy of femur
P1-18106 Osteotomy, intertrochanteric, with external fixation and cast
P1-18107 Osteotomy, subtrochanteric, with external fixation and cast
P1-18108 Drilling of femoral head
Graber-Duvernay operation
P1-18109V Incision and drainage of hindlimb
P1-18110 Incision and drainage of deep abscess of thigh region
P1-18111 Incision and drainage of deep hematoma of thigh region
P1-18112 Incision and drainage of deep infected bursa of thigh region
P1-18113 Open iliotibial fasciotomy
P1-18114 Subcutaneous closed tenotomy of adductor or hamstring, single
P1-18115 Subcutaneous closed tenotomy of adductor or hamstring, multiple
P1-18116 Open tenotomy of hamstring, knee to hip, single
P1-18117 Open tenotomy of hamstring, knee to hip, multiple, one leg
P1-18118 Open tenotomy of hamstring, knee to hip, multiple, bilateral
P1-18119 Division of iliotibial band
P1-1811AV Tenotomy of hindlimb, NOS
Division of tendon of hindlimb, NOS
P1-18120 Incision and drainage of deep abscess of knee region
P1-18121 Incision and drainage of deep hematoma of knee region
P1-18122 Incision and drainage of deep infected bursa of knee region
P1-18123 Deep incision with opening of bone cortex of knee
P1-18126 Arthrotomy of knee for infection
P1-18127 Arthrotomy of knee for infection with drainage
P1-18128 Arthrotomy of knee for infection with exploration
P1-18129 Arthrotomy of knee for infection with removal of foreign body
P1-1812A Arthrotomy of knee with joint exploration
P1-18131 Capsulotomy of knee, posterior capsular release
P1-18132 Incision of patella
Incision of patella without division
P1-18134 Osteotomy of patella
P1-18138V Division of stifle ligament
P1-18140 Arthrotomy of knee, NOS
P1-18141 Division of cartilage of knee
Division of joint cartilage of knee
P1-18142 Division of joint capsule of knee
P1-18143 Division of ligament of knee
Division of joint ligament of knee
P1-18144 Patellar retinacula release
Eggers operation for tendon release of patella
P1-18145 Lateral retinacula release of knee
P1-18150 Decompression fasciotomy of leg, anterior compartment only
P1-18151 Decompression fasciotomy of leg, posterior compartment only
P1-18152 Decompression fasciotomy of leg, anterior and posterior compartments
P1-18153 Incision and drainage of leg for deep abscess
P1-18154 Incision and drainage of hematoma of leg
P1-18155 Incision and drainage of infected bursa of leg
P1-18170 Incision of tibia and fibula without division, NOS
Deep incision with opening of bone cortex of leg, NOS
P1-18171 Incision of fibula
P1-18172 Incision of tibia
P1-18174 Osteotomy of tibia
P1-18175 Osteotomy of fibula
P1-18176 Osteotomy of tibia and fibula, NOS
Division of tibia and fibula
Osteotomy of bone of leg, NOS

1-183-184 Thigh and Leg: Excisions

P1-18300 Amputation of leg, NOS
Amputation of lower limb, NOS
Lower limb amputation, NOS
Hind limb amputation, NOS
P1-18303V Biopsy of hindlimb
P1-18304 Biopsy of soft tissue of leg area, superficial
P1-18305 Biopsy of soft tissue of leg area, deep
P1-18306 Radical resection of tumor of soft tissue of leg area
P1-18307 Excision of tumor of leg area, deep, intramuscular
P1-18308 Excision of tumor of leg area, deep, subfascial
P1-18309 Excision of lesion of tendon sheath or capsule of leg

P1-1830A Debridement of open fracture of leg, NOS
P1-1830BV Excision of lesion of hindlimb
P1-1830CV Excision of lesion of muscle of hindlimb
P1-18310 Removal of foreign body of lower limb, except foot
  Removal of foreign body without incision from lower limb, except foot
  Removal of foreign body of hindlimb
P1-18312 Radical resection for infection of greater trochanter of femur
P1-18313 Radical resection for tumor of greater trochanter of femur
P1-18315 Excision or curettage of benign tumor of femur
P1-18316 Excision or curettage of bone cyst of femur
P1-18317 Partial excision of femur
P1-18318 Radical resection for tumor of bone of femur
P1-18319V Removal of foreign body from femur
P1-18320 Amputation of thigh through femur
P1-18321 Amputation of thigh through femur, open
P1-18322 Amputation of thigh through femur, immediate fitting technique including first cast
P1-18323 Amputation of thigh through femur, open, circular guillotine technique
P1-18324 Amputation of thigh through femur, secondary closure or scar revision
P1-18325 Amputation of thigh through femur, reamputation
P1-18326 Amputation above-knee
  AK amputation
  Amputation of leg above knee
  Amputation of leg through femur
  Amputation supracondylar, above-knee
  Kirk amputation of thigh
P1-18328 Amputation below-knee conversion into above-knee amputation
P1-18330 Excisional biopsy of femur
  Biopsy of femur
P1-18331 Excision of lesion of femur
  Local excision of lesion or tissue of femur
P1-18332 Excision of femur for graft
P1-18333 Resection of femoral head and neck of femur
  Girdlestone operation on femoral head and neck
P1-18334 Partial ostectomy of femur, NOS
P1-18335 Total ostectomy of femur, NOS
P1-18336 Debridement of open fracture of femur
P1-18337 Sequestrectomy of femur
P1-18338 Wedge osteotomy of trochanter of femur
  Gant trochanter wedge osteotomy
  Whitman trochanter wedge osteotomy
P1-18340 Biopsy of soft tissue of thigh area, superficial
P1-18341 Biopsy of soft tissue of thigh area, deep
P1-18342 Excision of tumor of thigh area, deep, intramuscular
P1-18343 Excision of tumor of thigh area, deep, subfascial
P1-18344 Radical resection of tumor of soft tissue of thigh area
P1-18345 Removal of deep foreign body from thigh region
P1-18348 Biopsy of soft tissue of knee area, superficial
P1-18349 Biopsy of soft tissue of knee area, deep
P1-18350 Excision of tumor of knee area, deep, intramuscular
P1-18351 Excision of tumor of knee area, deep, subfascial
P1-18352 Radical resection of tumor of soft tissue of knee area
P1-18353 Arthrotomy of knee with removal of foreign body
P1-18354 Excision of prepatellar bursa
P1-18355 Arthrotomy of knee for synovial biopsy only
P1-18360 Arthrotomy of knee with joint exploration and biopsy
P1-18361 Arthrotomy of knee with joint exploration, biopsy and removal of loose or foreign bodies
P1-18362 Arthrotomy of knee with joint exploration and removal of loose or foreign bodies
P1-18363 Arthrotomy of knee for excision of lateral semilunar cartilage
P1-18364 Arthrotomy of knee for excision of medial semilunar cartilage
P1-18365 Arthrotomy of knee for excision of medial and lateral semilunar cartilages
P1-18366 Arthrotomy of knee for anterior synovectomy
P1-18367 Arthrotomy of knee for posterior synovectomy
P1-18368 Arthrotomy of knee for synovectomy, anterior and posterior including popliteal area
P1-18370 Radical resection for tumor of bone of knee
P1-18371 Removal of deep foreign body from knee area
P1-18373 Wedge osteotomy of patella
P1-18374 Sequestrectomy of patella
P1-18375 Excisional biopsy of patella
  Biopsy of patella
P1-18376 Excision of lesion of patella
  Local excision of lesion or tissue of patella
P1-18377 Debridement of patella
P1-18378 Shaving of patella
P1-18379 Partial excision of patella
  Hemipatellectomy
  Partial patellectomy
  Partial removal of patella
P1-1837A Open reduction of dislocation of knee
P1-18380 Patellectomy
  Complete excision of patella
  Complete removal of patella
  Total ostectomy of patella
P1-18381 Arthrectomy of knee, NOS
  Excision of knee joint, NOS
P1-18382 Excisional biopsy of joint structure of knee
  Biopsy of joint structure of knee
P1-18383 Chondrectomy of semilunar cartilage of knee
  Arthrectomy of knee for semilunar cartilage excision

1-183-184 Thigh and Leg: Excisions — Continued

P1-18383 (cont.) Excision of semilunar cartilage of knee
P1-18384 Excision of meniscus of knee, NOS
Meniscectomy of knee, NOS
P1-18385 Synovectomy of knee
P1-18386 Excision of lesion of knee joint, NOS
P1-18387 Excision of Baker's cyst of knee
Excision of synovial cyst of popliteal space
Excision of popliteal cyst of knee
P1-18388 Knee disarticulation
Disarticulation at knee
Batch-Spittler-McFaddin amputation
Callander's amputation
Gritti-Stokes amputation
Mazet amputation
S.P. Rogers amputation
Disarticulation of knee
Amputation by disarticulation of stifle joint
P1-1838AV Open reduction of stifle ligament
P1-1838BV Excision of cartilage of stifle joint
P1-18402 Removal of foreign body of popliteal space
P1-18405 Partial excision of proximal fibula
P1-18406 Partial excision of proximal tibia
P1-18407 Excision or curettage of benign tumor of fibula
P1-18408 Excision or curettage of benign tumor of tibia
P1-18409 Excision or curettage of bone cyst of fibula
P1-1840A Excision or curettage of bone cyst of tibia
P1-18410 Osteotomy of proximal tibia including fibular excision or osteotomy before epiphyseal closure
P1-18411 Osteotomy of proximal tibia including fibular excision or osteotomy after epiphyseal closure
P1-18412 Partial excision of tibia
P1-18413 Partial excision of fibula
P1-18414 Radical resection for tumor of tibia
P1-18415 Radical resection for tumor of fibula
P1-18418 Excision of tibia and fibula for graft
P1-18420 Amputation of leg through tibia and fibula
Amputation below-knee, NOS
Amputation of leg below knee
BK amputation, NOS
P1-18421 Amputation of leg through tibia and fibula with immediate fitting technique including application of first cast
P1-18423 Amputation of leg through tibia and fibula, open, circular
Amputation of leg through tibia and fibula, open, guillotine technique
P1-18425 Amputation of leg through tibia and fibula, secondary closure or scar revision
P1-18426 Amputation of leg through tibia and fibula, reamputation
P1-18430 Sequestrectomy of tibia and fibula
P1-18431 Sequestrectomy of fibula
P1-18432 Sequestrectomy of tibia
P1-18433 Wedge osteotomy of tibia
Coventry operation
P1-18434 Wedge osteotomy of fibula
P1-18435 Excisional biopsy of fibula
P1-18436 Excisional biopsy of tibia
P1-18437 Excision of lesion of fibula
P1-18438 Excision of lesion of tibia
P1-18439 Local excision of lesion or tissue of tibia and fibula
P1-1843A Partial ostectomy of tibia and fibula, NOS
P1-1843B Total ostectomy of tibia and fibula
P1-18440 Debridement of open fracture of fibula
P1-18441 Debridement of open fracture of tibia
P1-18442 Debridement of open fracture of tibia and fibula
P1-18450V Tenectomy of hindlimb
P1-18451V Debridement of hindlimb
P1-18452V Debridement of stifle ligament

1-185 Thigh and Leg: Injections and Implantations

P1-18500 Injection of knee, NOS
Injection of stifle joint, NOS
P1-18505 Injection procedure for knee arthrography
P1-18510 Implantation of prosthetic device of leg
Insertion of prosthesis or prosthetic device of lower extremity
Insertion of prosthesis or prosthetic device of leg, bioelectric or cineplastic
P1-18511 Implantation of prosthesis or prosthetic device of acetabulum of lower extremity
Implantation of prosthesis or prosthetic device of acetabulum of leg, bioelectric or cineplastic
P1-18514 Replacement of prosthesis of lower extremity
Replacement of prosthesis of leg, bioelectric or cineplastic
P1-18516 Prophylactic treatment of femur with methyl methacrylate
P1-18517 Prophylactic treatment of femoral neck and proximal femur with methyl methacrylate
P1-18519 Insertion of bone growth stimulator into femur
P1-18520 Insertion of prosthesis or prosthetic device of femoral head
Insertion of Austin-Moore prosthesis
Insertion of Eicher prosthesis
Insertion of Thompson prosthesis
P1-18521 Insertion of prosthesis or prosthetic device of femoral head with use of methyl methacrylate
P1-18524 Removal of internal fixation device of femur
P1-18525 Replacement of prosthesis of femur
P1-18530 Insertion of bone growth stimulator into patella
P1-18532 Removal of internal fixation device from patella
P1-18540 Implantation of knee joint
P1-18542 Implantation of prosthesis or prosthetic device of acetabulum of knee joint
Implantation of prosthesis or prosthetic device of acetabulum of knee, bioelectric or cineplastic

P1-18544 Implantation of Swanson prosthesis of knee
P1-18546 Removal of knee prosthesis including total knee, methyl methacrylate and insertion of spacer
P1-18547 Arthrotomy for removal of prosthesis of knee
  Removal of prosthesis of joint structures of knee
P1-18550 Insertion of bone growth stimulator into tibia and fibula
P1-18552 Prophylactic treatment of tibia with methyl methacrylate
P1-18555 Removal of internal fixation device of fibula
P1-18556 Removal of internal fixation device of tibia

1-187 Thigh and Leg: Endoscopy

P1-18700 Arthroscopy of knee, NOS
  Diagnostic arthroscopy of knee, NOS
P1-18701 Diagnostic arthroscopy of knee with synovial biopsy
P1-18704 Arthroscopy of knee for synovectomy, limited
P1-18705 Arthroscopy of knee for synovectomy, major, two or more compartments
P1-18706 Arthroscopy of knee for shaving of articular cartilage
P1-18708 Arthroscopy of knee for debridement of articular cartilage
P1-18710 Arthroscopy of knee, surgical, for synovectomy, limited, plica or shelf resection
P1-18712 Arthroscopy of knee with medial and lateral meniscectomy
P1-18714 Arthroscopy of knee with medial meniscectomy
P1-18716 Arthroscopy of knee with lateral meniscectomy
P1-18724 Arthroscopy of knee for infection with lavage and drainage
P1-18725 Arthroscopy of knee for removal of foreign body
  Arthroscopy of knee for removal of loose body
P1-18730 Surgical arthroscopy of knee for infection with lavage and drainage
P1-18731 Arthroscopy of knee, multiple drilling
P1-18732 Arthroscopy of knee, drilling for intact osteochondritis dissecans lesion
P1-18734 Arthroscopy of knee, drilling for intact osteochondritis dissecans lesion with internal fixation
P1-18735 Arthroscopy of knee, drilling for osteochondritis dissecans lesion with bone grafting and internal fixation
P1-18736 Arthroscopy of knee with lysis of adhesions with manipulation
P1-18737 Arthroscopy of knee, drilling for osteochondritis dissecans with bone grafting without internal fixation
P1-18738 Arthroscopy of knee with lysis of adhesions without manipulation
P1-18740 Arthroscopy of knee for abrasion arthroplasty
P1-18741 Arthroscopy of knee with meniscus repair
P1-18742 Arthroscopy of knee with lateral meniscus repair
P1-18743 Arthroscopy of knee with medial meniscus repair
P1-18744 Arthroscopy of knee with medial and lateral meniscus repair
P1-18750 Arthroscopically aided anterior cruciate ligament augmentation
P1-18752 Arthroscopically aided anterior cruciate ligament reconstruction
P1-18754 Arthroscopically aided anterior cruciate ligament repair
P1-18755 Arthroscopically aided posterior cruciate ligament augmentation
P1-18756 Arthroscopically aided posterior cruciate ligament reconstruction
P1-18758 Arthroscopically aided posterior cruciate ligament repair

1-188-18B Thigh and Leg: Surgical Repairs, Closures and Reconstructions

P1-18800 Surgical repair of lower extremity, NOS
  Plastic repair of lower extremity, NOS
  Plastic repair of hindlimb, NOS
P1-18803 Reattachment of lower extremity, NOS
  Lower leg reattachment, NOS
P1-18804 Replantation of leg, complete amputation
P1-18805 Replantation of leg, incomplete amputation
P1-18806V Anastomosis of muscle of hindlimb, NOS
P1-18807 Suture of joint capsule with arthroplasty of lower extremity, NOS
P1-18808 Cineplasty or cineplastic prosthesis of lower extremity
  Cineplasty or cineplastic prosthesis of leg
P1-18809 Repair of fascial defect of leg
P1-1880AV Suture of wound of hindlimb
P1-18810 Repair or suture of flexor tendon of leg, primary without graft
P1-18811 Repair or suture of flexor tendon of leg, secondary with graft
P1-18812 Repair or suture of flexor tendon of leg, secondary without graft
P1-18813 Repair or suture of extensor tendon of leg, primary without graft
P1-18814 Repair or suture of extensor tendon of leg, secondary with graft
P1-18815 Repair or suture of extensor tendon of leg, secondary without graft
P1-18816 Lengthening of tendon of leg, single
P1-18817 Shortening of tendon of leg, single
P1-18818 Lengthening of tendon of leg, multiple, each
P1-18819 Shortening of tendon of leg, multiple, each
P1-18820 Osteotomy, multiple with realignment on intramedullary rod
P1-18821 Equalization of leg, lengthening or shortening, by bone fusion

1-188-18B Thigh and Leg: Surgical Repairs, Closures and Reconstructions — Continued

P1-18822 Reduction of open fracture of leg
P1-18823 Reduction of open fracture of leg with internal fixation
P1-18826 Intertrochanteric osteotomy with internal fixation and cast
P1-18827 Radical resection for infection of greater trochanter of femur with skin flaps
P1-18828 Subtrochanteric osteotomy with internal fixation and cast
P1-18829 Open reduction of slipped femoral epiphysis with bone graft
P1-18830 Radical resection for tumor of greater trochanter of femur with skin flaps
P1-18831 Open reduction of slipped femoral epiphysis, multiple pinning
P1-18832 Open reduction of slipped femoral epiphysis with osteoplasty of femoral neck
P1-18833 Open reduction of slipped femoral epiphysis, single pinning
P1-18834 Open reduction of slipped femoral epiphysis, closed manipulation with multiple pinning
P1-18836 Open reduction of slipped femoral epiphysis, closed manipulation with single pinning
P1-18838 Open reduction of slipped femoral epiphysis, osteotomy and internal fixation
P1-1883A Prophylactic treatment of femur
P1-1883B Prophylactic treatment without methyl methacrylate of femoral neck and proximal femur
P1-1883C Internal fixation of patella
P1-1883D Internal fixation of femur
P1-18840 Open treatment of slipped femoral epiphysis, NOS
P1-18842 Open reduction of closed or open intertrochanteric femoral fracture with internal fixation
P1-18843 Reduction of open femoral fracture, proximal end, neck, with uncomplicated soft tissue closure with manipulation
P1-18844 Reduction of open femoral fracture, proximal end, neck, in situ pinning of undisplaced or impacted fracture
P1-18845 Open reduction of closed femoral fracture, proximal end, neck, internal fixation or prosthetic replacement
P1-18846 Open reduction of open femoral fracture, proximal end, neck, with internal fixation or prosthetic replacement
P1-18847 Replacement of prosthesis of femur with use of methyl methacrylate
P1-18848 Osteotomy of femoral neck
P1-18849 Osteotomy and transfer of greater trochanter
P1-1884A Replacement of femoral head by prosthesis with use of methyl methacrylate
P1-18850 Excision or curettage of benign tumor of femur with allograft
P1-18851 Excision or curettage of bone cyst of femur with allograft
P1-18852 Excision or curettage of benign tumor of femur with autograft
P1-18853 Excision or curettage of bone cyst of femur with autograft
P1-18854 Excision or curettage of benign tumor of femur with internal fixation
P1-18855 Excision or curettage of bone cyst of femur with internal fixation
P1-18858 Intramedullary nailing of femur
P1-1885A Replacement of femoral head by prosthesis
    Moore operation
    Replacement of femoral head
P1-18860 Reduction of open intertrochanteric femoral fracture with uncomplicated soft tissue closure
P1-18861 Reduction of open pertrochanteric femoral fracture with uncomplicated soft tissue closure
P1-18863 Reduction of open subtrochanteric femoral fracture with uncomplicated soft tissue closure
P1-18864 Acetabuloplasty with use of methyl methacrylate
P1-18865 Open reduction of closed or open subtrochanteric femoral fracture with internal fixation
P1-18866 Open reduction of closed or open greater trochanteric fracture
P1-18867 Open reduction of closed or open greater trochanteric fracture with external skeletal fixation
P1-18868 Open reduction of closed or open greater trochanteric fracture with internal skeletal fixation
P1-18869 Reduction of open femoral shaft fracture with uncomplicated soft tissue closure
P1-1886A Open reduction of closed or open femoral shaft fracture
P1-18870 Open reduction of closed or open femoral shaft fracture with external skeletal fixation
P1-18871 Open reduction of closed or open femoral shaft fracture with internal skeletal fixation
P1-18872 Reduction of open femoral fracture, distal end, lateral condyle with uncomplicated soft tissue closure
P1-18873 Reduction of open femoral fracture, distal end, medial condyle with uncomplicated soft tissue closure
P1-18874 Open reduction of closed or open femoral fracture, distal end, lateral condyle
P1-18875 Open reduction of closed or open femoral fracture, distal end, lateral condyle with external skeletal fixation
P1-18876 Open reduction of closed or open femoral fracture, distal end, lateral condyle with internal skeletal fixation

P1-18877 Open reduction of closed or open femoral fracture, distal end, medial condyle
P1-18878 Open reduction of closed or open femoral fracture, distal end, medial condyle with external skeletal fixation
P1-18879 Open reduction of closed or open femoral fracture, distal end, medial condyle with internal skeletal fixation
P1-1887A Reduction of open distal femoral epiphyseal separation with uncomplicated soft tissue closure
P1-1887B Open reduction of closed or open distal femoral epiphyseal separation
P1-18880 Trochanterplasty, NOS
P1-18881 Open reduction of closed or open distal femoral epiphyseal separation with external skeletal fixation
P1-18882 Open reduction of closed or open distal femoral epiphyseal separation with internal skeletal fixation
P1-18884 Osteotomy of shaft of femur with fixation
P1-18885 Osteotomy of femur, supracondylar with fixation
P1-18886 Osteotomy, multiple, femoral shaft with realignment on intramedullary rod
P1-18887 Osteoplasty of femur, shortening
  Shortening of femur
P1-18888 Osteoplasty of femur, lengthening
  Lengthening of femur
P1-18889 Osteoplasty of femur, combined, lengthening and shortening with femoral segment transfer
  Change in bone length of femur
  Equalization of leg at femur
P1-18890 Repair of malunion, of femur, distal to head and neck
P1-18891 Repair of nonunion or malunion of femur, distal to head and neck with iliac bone graft
P1-18892 Repair of union or malunion of femur, distal to head and neck with other autogenous bone graft
P1-18895 Lengthening of gastrocnemius muscle
  Vulpius operation
P1-18896 Internal fixation of femur without fracture reduction
P1-18898 Open reduction of separated epiphysis of femur
P1-1889A Insertion of bone peg in femoral neck
  Albee Delbet operation
P1-1889B Femoral shortening with blade plate
  Blount operation
P1-188A0 Arrest of bone growth of femur, NOS
P1-188A1 Equalization of leg by epiphyseal stapling, NOS
P1-188A2 Epiphyseal arrest by epiphysiodesis or stapling of greater trochanter
P1-188A3 Hemiepiphyseal arrest of proximal leg or distal femur
P1-188A4 Femoral shortening by epiphyseal stapling
  Blount operation with epiphyseal stapling
  Equalization of leg by epiphyseal stapling of femur
  Stapling of epiphyseal plate of femur
P1-188A5 Epiphyseal arrest by epiphysiodesis or stapling of distal femur
P1-188A6 Epiphyseal arrest by epiphysiodesis, combined, proximal and distal tibia and fibula and distal femur
P1-188A7 Epiphyseal arrest by stapling, combined, proximal and distal tibia and fibula and distal femur
P1-188A8 Epiphyseal arrest by epiphysiodesis or stapling, combined distal femur, proximal tibia and fibula
P1-18900 Osteoplasty of femur, NOS
  Repair or plastic operation on femur, NOS
P1-18903 Quadricepsplasty
  Repair of quadriceps
P1-18904 Open reduction of fracture of femur
P1-18906 Open reduction of fracture of femur with internal fixation
P1-18911 Suture of quadriceps rupture, secondary reconstruction including fascial or tendon graft
P1-18915 Reattachment of extremity at thigh
P1-18920 Revision of total knee arthroplasty with allograft, one component
P1-18921 Suture of infrapatellar tendon, secondary reconstruction including fascial or tendon graft
P1-18922 Revision of total knee arthroplasty, one component
P1-18923 Revision of total knee arthroplasty with allograft, all components
P1-18924 Revision of total knee arthroplasty, all components
P1-18925 Suture of hamstring muscle rupture, secondary reconstruction including fascial or tendon graft
P1-18926 Lengthening of hamstring, NOS
P1-18927 Lengthening of hamstring tendon, single
P1-18928 Lengthening of hamstring tendon, multiple, one leg
P1-18929 Lengthening of hamstring tendon, multiple, bilateral
P1-18930 Arthrotomy with open meniscus repair
P1-18931 Primary repair of torn capsule of knee, collateral
P1-18932 Primary repair of torn ligament and capsule of knee, collateral
P1-18933 Primary repair of torn ligament of knee, collateral
P1-18934 Primary repair of torn capsule of knee, cruciate
P1-18935 Primary repair of torn ligament and capsule of knee, cruciate
P1-18936 Primary repair of torn ligament of knee, cruciate

1-188-18B Thigh and Leg: Surgical Repairs, Closures and Reconstructions — Continued

P1-18937 Primary repair of torn capsule of knee, collateral and cruciate ligaments
P1-18938 Primary repair of torn ligament and capsule of knee, collateral and cruciate ligaments
P1-18939 Primary repair of torn ligament of knee, collateral and cruciate ligaments
P1-1893A Anterior tibial tubercle plastic repair for chondromalacia patellae
    Maquet procedure
P1-18940 Arthroplasty of knee with constrained prosthesis
    Arthroplasty of knee with constrained prosthesis, Walldius type
P1-18941 Reconstruction for recurrent dislocating patella, Hauser type procedure
P1-18942 Reconstruction for recurrent dislocating patella with extensor realignment
P1-18943 Reconstruction for recurrent dislocating patella with extensor realignment and muscle advancement or release
P1-18945 Reconstruction for recurrent dislocating patella with muscle advancement or release
P1-18946 Reconstruction for recurrent dislocating patella with patellectomy
P1-18947 Ligamentous reconstruction of knee, extra-articular
P1-18948 Ligamentous reconstruction of knee, intra-articular
P1-18949 Ligamentous reconstruction of knee, intra-articular and extra-articular
P1-1894A Quadricepsplasty, Bennett type
P1-1894B Quadricepsplasty, Thompson type
P1-18950 Arthroplasty of patella
P1-18951 Arthroplasty of patella with prosthesis
P1-18952 Arthroplasty of knee, tibial plateau
P1-18953 Arthroplasty of knee, tibial plateau with debridement and partial synovectomy
P1-18954 Arthroplasty of knee, femoral condyles
P1-18955 Arthroplasty of knee, tibial plateaus
P1-18956 Arthroplasty of knee, femoral condyles with debridement and partial synovectomy
P1-18957 Arthroplasty of knee, tibial plateaus with debridement and partial synovectomy
P1-18959 Arthroplasty of knee, condyle and plateau, lateral compartment
P1-1895A Arthroplasty of knee, condyle and plateau, medial compartment
P1-18960 Arthroplasty of knee, condyle and plateau, medial and lateral compartments
P1-18961 Arthroplasty of knee, condyle and plateau, medial and lateral compartments with patella resurfacing
P1-18962 Reduction of open patellar fracture, with uncomplicated soft tissue closure
P1-18963 Open reduction of closed or open patellar fracture with excision
P1-18964 Open reduction of closed or open patellar fracture with repair
P1-18965 Open reduction of closed or open patellar fracture with repair and excision
P1-18966 Open reduction of closed or open intercondylar spine fractures of knee with internal fixation
P1-18967 Reduction of open knee dislocation with uncomplicated soft tissue closure
P1-18968 Open reduction of closed or open knee dislocation
P1-18969 Open reduction of closed or open knee dislocation with external skeletal fixation
P1-1896A Open reduction of closed or open knee dislocation with internal skeletal fixation
P1-18970 Open reduction of closed or open knee dislocation with external skeletal fixation with primary ligamentous repair
P1-18971 Open reduction of closed or open knee dislocation with internal skeletal fixation with primary ligamentous repair
P1-18972 Open reduction of closed or open knee dislocation with primary ligamentous repair
P1-18973 Reduction of open patellar dislocation with uncomplicated soft tissue closure
P1-18974 Open reduction of closed or open patellar dislocation
P1-18975 Open reduction of closed or open patellar dislocation with partial patellectomy
P1-18976 Open reduction of closed or open patellar dislocation with total patellectomy
P1-18977 Fusion of knee, NOS
    Arthrodesis of knee, NOS
    Albert operation
P1-18978 Internal fixation of patella without fracture reduction
P1-1897A Excision of patella for graft
P1-1897B Operation with graft for slipping patella
P1-18980 Revision of knee replacement
P1-18981 Patellapexy
P1-18982 Patellaplasty, NOS
    Plastic operation on patella, NOS
    Osteoplasty of patella, NOS
    Repair of patella, NOS
P1-18984 Knee arthrodesis with plate
    Charnley operation on knee
    Lucas and Murray operation
P1-18985 Total replacement of knee
    Total arthroplasty of knee, geomedic or polycentric
P1-18986 Repair of knee, five-in-one
P1-18987 Triad knee repair
    O'Donoghue operation
P1-18989 Repair of recurrent dislocation of patella
    Roux-Goldthwait operation
P1-18990 Repair of knee cruciate ligaments, NOS
P1-18991 Reconstruction of anterior cruciate ligament of knee
    Campbell operation on anterior cruciate ligament

P1-18991 (cont.) Hey-Groves operation
  Surgical repair of cranial cruciate ligament of knee
P1-18993 Repair of knee collateral ligaments, NOS
P1-18994 Arthroplasty of knee, NOS
  Repair of knee joint, NOS
P1-18995V Anastomosis of stifle ligament
P1-18996V Imbrication of stifle joint
P1-18997V Imbrication of stifle ligament
P1-18998V Plastic operation of stifle ligament
P1-18999 Bone graft with microvascular anastomosis of fibula
P1-189A0 Arrest of bone growth of fibula
P1-189A1 Arrest of bone growth of tibia
P1-189A2 Equalization of leg by epiphyseal stapling of fibula
  Stapling of epiphyseal plate of fibula
P1-189A3 Equalization of leg by epiphyseal stapling of tibia
  Stapling of epiphyseal plate of tibia
P1-189A4 Epiphyseal arrest by epiphysiodesis or stapling of proximal tibia and fibula
P1-189A5 Epiphyseal arrest by epiphysiodesis of distal tibia
P1-189A6 Epiphyseal arrest by stapling of distal tibia
P1-189A7 Epiphyseal arrest by epiphysiodesis of distal fibula
P1-189A8 Epiphyseal arrest by stapling of distal fibula
P1-189A9 Epiphyseal arrest by epiphysiodesis of distal tibia and fibula
P1-189AA Epiphyseal arrest by stapling of distal tibia and fibula
  Epiphyseal stapling of tibia and fibula
P1-189B0 Epiphyseal arrest by epiphysiodesis, combined, proximal and distal tibia and fibula
P1-189B1 Epiphyseal arrest by stapling, combined, proximal and distal tibia and fibula
P1-18A00 Internal fixation of fibula
P1-18A01 Internal fixation of tibia
P1-18A02 Intramedullary nailing of fibula
P1-18A03 Intramedullary nailing of tibia
P1-18A04 Open reduction of fracture of tibia and fibula with internal fixation
P1-18A10 Osteotomy of tibia and fibula, multiple with realignment on intramedullary rod, Sofield type procedure
P1-18A11 Excision or curettage of benign tumor of fibula with autograft
P1-18A12 Excision or curettage of benign tumor of tibia with autograft
P1-18A13 Excision or curettage of bone cyst of fibula with autograft
P1-18A14 Excision or curettage of bone cyst of tibia with autograft
P1-18A15 Excision or curettage of benign tumor of fibula with allograft
P1-18A16 Excision or curettage of benign tumor of tibia with allograft
P1-18A17 Excision or curettage of bone cyst of fibula with allograft
P1-18A18 Excision or curettage of bone cyst of tibia with allograft
P1-18A20 Reduction of open tibial fracture, proximal plateau with uncomplicated soft tissue closure
P1-18A21 Open reduction of closed or open proximal tibial fracture with external skeletal fixation
P1-18A22 Open reduction of closed or open proximal tibial fracture with internal skeletal fixation
P1-18A23 Open reduction of closed or open proximal tibial fracture without internal or external skeletal fixation
P1-18A24 Open reduction of closed or open proximal tibial fracture with external skeletal fixation with autogenous graft
P1-18A25 Open reduction of closed or open proximal tibial fracture with internal skeletal fixation with autogenous graft
P1-18A26 Open reduction of closed or open proximal tibial fracture without internal or external skeletal fixation with autogenous graft
P1-18A27 Repair for dislocating peroneal tendons
P1-18A28 Repair for dislocating peroneal tendons with fibular osteotomy
P1-18A29 Osteoplasty of tibia and fibula, lengthening
P1-18A30 Repair of malunion of tibia
P1-18A31 Repair of nonunion or malunion of tibia without graft
P1-18A33 Repair of nonunion of tibia
P1-18A34 Repair of malunion of tibia with sliding graft
P1-18A35 Repair of nonunion of tibia with sliding graft
P1-18A36 Repair of malunion of tibia with iliac autograft
P1-18A37 Repair of malunion of tibia with unlisted autograft
P1-18A38 Repair of nonunion of tibia with iliac autograft
P1-18A39 Repair of nonunion of tibia with unlisted autograft
P1-18A40 Repair of malunion of tibia by synostosis with fibula, unlisted method
P1-18A41 Repair of nonunion of tibia by synostosis with fibula, unlisted method
P1-18A42 Repair of congenital pseudoarthrosis of tibia
P1-18A4A Change in bone length of tibia
P1-18A4B Lengthening of bone of tibia
  Anderson operation
P1-18A4C Shortening of bone of tibia
P1-18A4D Change in bone length of fibula
P1-18A4E Equalization of leg by fibula
P1-18A4F Equalization of leg by tibia
P1-18A54 Prophylactic treatment of tibia without methyl methacrylate
P1-18A55 Reduction of open tibial shaft fracture with uncomplicated soft tissue closure
P1-18A56 Open reduction of closed or open tibial shaft fracture with internal skeletal fixation, simple

1-188-18B Thigh and Leg: Surgical Repairs, Closures and Reconstructions — Continued

P1-18A57 Open reduction of closed or open tibial shaft fracture with internal skeletal fixation, complicated
P1-18A58 Reduction of open distal tibial fracture with uncomplicated soft tissue closure
P1-18A59 Open reduction of closed or open distal tibial fracture with fixation
P1-18A5A Osteoplasty of tibia
P1-18A5B Osteoplasty of fibula
P1-18A5C Change in bone length of tibia and fibula, NOS
P1-18A5D Repair or plastic operation on tibia and fibula, NOS
P1-18A60 Open reduction of closed or open proximal fibula or shaft fracture
P1-18A61 Reduction of open proximal fibula or shaft fracture with uncomplicated soft tissue closure
P1-18A62 Internal fixation of tibia and fibula without fracture reduction
P1-18A63 Open reduction of closed or open proximal fibula or shaft fracture with internal skeletal fixation
P1-18A64 Open reduction of fracture of tibia and fibula
P1-18A65 Open reduction of fracture of fibula
P1-18A66 Open reduction of fracture of tibia
P1-18A67 Open reduction of closed or open proximal fibula or shaft fracture with external skeletal fixation
P1-18A68 Reduction of open distal fibular fracture with uncomplicated soft tissue closure
P1-18A69 Open reduction of closed or open distal fibular fracture with fixation
P1-18A6A Open reduction of fracture of fibula with internal fixation
P1-18A6B Reduction of open tibial and fibular shaft fractures with uncomplicated soft tissue closure
P1-18A6C Open reduction of fracture of tibia with internal fixation
P1-18A70 Open reduction of closed or open tibial and fibular shaft fractures
P1-18A71 Open reduction of closed or open tibial and fibular shaft fractures with external skeletal fixation
P1-18A72 Open reduction of separated epiphysis of tibia and fibula
P1-18A73 Open reduction of closed or open tibial and fibular shaft fractures with internal skeletal fixation
P1-18A74 Open reduction of separation of epiphysis of fibula
P1-18A75 Open reduction of separation of epiphysis of tibia
P1-18A82 Repair of peroneal tendon
  Ellis Jones operation
  Johanson operation on peroneal tendon
P1-18B00 Suture of capsule or ligament of lower extremity
P1-18B01 Capsulorrhaphy of lower extremity, NOS
P1-18B02 Suture of ligament of lower extremity, NOS
P1-18B04 Suture of periosteum of femur
  Periosteal suture of femur
P1-18B06 Suture of quadriceps rupture, primary
P1-18B07 Suture of infrapatellar tendon, primary
P1-18B08 Suture of hamstring muscle rupture, primary
P1-18B09 Suture of ligament of knee
P1-18B11 Suture of periosteum of patella
  Periosteal suture of patella
P1-18B20 Periosteal suture of tibia and fibula
P1-18B21 Suture of periosteum of fibula
P1-18B22 Suture of periosteum of tibia

1-18C Thigh and Leg: Destructive Procedures

P1-18C00 Destructive procedure of thigh and leg, NOS
P1-18C04 Osteoclasis of femur
P1-18C06 Osteoclasis of patella
P1-18C08 Tenolysis including tibia, fibula and ankle flexor, single
P1-18C09 Tenolysis including tibia, fibula and ankle flexor, multiple
P1-18C10 Tenolysis of extensor of foot, multiple
P1-18C12 Osteoclasis of fibula
P1-18C14 Osteoclasis of tibia
P1-18C16 Osteoclasis of tibia and fibula
P1-18C20 Local destruction of lesion of knee joint, NOS
P1-18C50V Cauterization of hindlimb, NOS

1-18D Thigh and Leg: Transplantations and Transpositions

P1-18D10 Transfer of single tendon of leg, superficial
  Transplant of single tendon of leg, superficial
P1-18D11 Transfer of single tendon of leg, each additional tendon
  Transplant of single tendon of leg, each additional tendon
P1-18D13 Tendon or muscle transfer, hamstring to femur
P1-18D20 Bone graft for nonunion of femoral head
P1-18D22 Bone graft for nonunion of femoral intertrochanteric area
P1-18D24 Bone graft for nonunion of femoral neck
P1-18D26 Bone graft for nonunion of femoral subtrochanteric area
P1-18D28 Bone graft of femur
P1-18D30 Transplant of hamstring tendon to patella, single
P1-18D31 Transplant of hamstring tendon to patella, multiple
P1-18D32 Bone graft of patella
P1-18D33 Transfer of tendon pes anserinus for repair of knee
  Slocum operation

P1-18D33 (cont.) Transplantation of tendon pes anserinus for repair of knee
Pes anserinus transfer
P1-18D34 Patellar stabilization by tendon transfer
Goldthwaite operation
P1-18D35 Gastrocnemius recession
Strayer procedure
P1-18D36 Transfer of single tendon, anterior tibial through interosseous space
P1-18D37 Transfer of single tendon, posterior tibial through interosseous space
P1-18D38 Grafting of tibia and fibula
P1-18D39 Grafting of fibula
P1-18D3A Grafting of tibia
P1-18D3B Sliding inlay graft of tibia
P1-18D40 Anterior tibialis tendon transfer for repair of flat foot
Young operation
P1-18D42 Transplantation of gracilis muscle
P1-18D44 Hamstring tendon transfer
Durham operation
Eggers operation
Transfer of biceps femoris tendon
P1-18D48V Transposition of muscle of hindlimb
P1-18D49V Graft of stifle ligament
P1-18D50 Transfer of bone shaft, fibula into tibia
P1-18D52 Transfer of tibialis posterior tendon
Barr operation
P1-18D54 Tibial tendon transfer
Garceau operation
P1-18D56 Soft tissue release with peroneus brevis tendon transfer
Osmond-Clark operation

1-18E Thigh and Leg: Manipulations

P1-18E00 Fitting of prosthesis of leg, NOS
Fitting of prosthesis or prosthetic device of leg, NOS
P1-18E01 Fitting of prosthesis above knee
Fitting of prosthesis or prosthetic device above knee
P1-18E02 Application of long leg cast
P1-18E03 Application of cylinder cast, thigh to ankle
P1-18E04 Application of long leg cast, walker or ambulatory type
P1-18E05 Application of long leg cast, brace type
P1-18E06 Application of short leg cast below knee to toes
P1-18E07 Application of short leg cast below knee to toes, walking or ambulatory type
P1-18E08 Adding walker to previously applied cast
P1-18E09 Application of clubfoot cast with molding or manipulation, short leg
P1-18E0A Application of clubfoot cast with molding or manipulation, long leg
P1-18E10 Application of long leg splint, thigh to ankle or toes
P1-18E11 Application of short leg splint calf to foot
P1-18E12 Removal or bivalving of full leg cast
P1-18E14 Closed reduction of fracture of leg, NOS
P1-18E15 Reduction of fracture of leg with internal fixation
P1-18E16 Application of hip spica cast, both legs
P1-18E17 Application of hip spica cast, one leg
P1-18E18 Application of hip spica cast, one and one-half spica
P1-18E19 Removal or bivalving of hip spica
P1-18E1A Strapping of hip
P1-18E20 Closed reduction of separated epiphysis of femur
P1-18E21 Treatment of slipped femoral epiphysis by traction without reduction
P1-18E22 Treatment of slipped femoral epiphysis by multiple pinning, in situ
P1-18E23 Treatment of slipped femoral epiphysis by single pinning, in situ
P1-18E24 Reduction of closed femoral fracture, proximal end, neck without manipulation
P1-18E25 Reduction of closed femoral fracture, proximal end, neck with manipulation including skeletal traction
P1-18E26 Reduction of closed femoral fracture, proximal end, neck, in situ pinning of undisplaced or impacted fracture
P1-18E27 Reduction of closed intertrochanteric femoral fracture without manipulation
P1-18E28 Reduction of closed pertrochanteric femoral fracture without manipulation
P1-18E29 Reduction of closed subtrochanteric femoral fracture without manipulation
P1-18E2A Reduction of closed intertrochanteric femoral fracture with manipulation
P1-18E30 Reduction of closed pertrochanteric femoral fracture with manipulation
Reduction of closed subtrochanteric femoral fracture with manipulation
P1-18E31 Reduction of closed greater trochanteric fracture without manipulation
P1-18E32 Reduction of closed femoral shaft fracture without manipulation
P1-18E33 Reduction of closed femoral shaft fracture with manipulation
P1-18E34 Reduction of closed femoral fracture, distal end, lateral condyle without manipulation
P1-18E35 Reduction of closed femoral fracture, distal end, medial condyle without manipulation
P1-18E36 Reduction of closed femoral fracture, distal end, lateral condyle with manipulation
P1-18E37 Reduction of closed femoral fracture, distal end, medial condyle with manipulation
P1-18E38 Fitting of prosthesis or prosthetic device of leg below knee
Fitting of prosthesis below knee
P1-18E40 Reduction of closed distal femoral epiphyseal separation without manipulation

1-18E Thigh and Leg: Manipulations — Continued

P1-18E41 Reduction of closed distal femoral epiphyseal separation with manipulation
P1-18E42 Closed reduction of fracture of femur
P1-18E43 Closed reduction of fracture of femur with internal fixation
  Reduction of fracture of femur with internal fixation
P1-18E44 Application of patellar tendon bearing, cast
P1-18E45 Strapping of knee
P1-18E46 Reduction of closed patellar fracture without manipulation
P1-18E47 Reduction of closed intercondylar spine fractures of knee
P1-18E48 Reduction of closed knee dislocation
  Closed reduction of dislocation of knee
P1-18E49 Reduction of closed knee dislocation with anesthesia
P1-18E50 Reduction of closed patellar dislocation
P1-18E51 Reduction of closed patellar dislocation with anesthesia
P1-18E52 Manipulation of knee joint under general anesthesia
P1-18E54 Reduction of closed tibial fracture, proximal without manipulation
P1-18E55 Reduction of closed tibial fracture, proximal with manipulation
P1-18E56 Reduction of closed tibial shaft fracture without manipulation
P1-18E57 Reduction of closed tibial shaft fracture with manipulation
P1-18E58 Reduction of closed distal tibial fracture without manipulation
P1-18E59 Reduction of closed distal tibial fracture with manipulation
P1-18E60 Reduction of closed proximal fibula or shaft fracture without manipulation
P1-18E61 Reduction of closed proximal fibula or shaft fracture with manipulation
P1-18E62 Reduction of closed distal fibular fracture without manipulation
P1-18E63 Reduction of closed distal fibular fracture with manipulation
P1-18E64 Reduction of closed tibial and fibular shaft fractures without manipulation
P1-18E65 Reduction of closed tibial and fibular shaft fractures with manipulation
P1-18E66 Closed reduction of fracture of tibia and fibula
P1-18E68 Closed reduction of fracture of fibula
P1-18E69 Closed reduction of fracture of tibia
P1-18E70 Closed reduction of fracture of tibia and fibula with internal fixation
P1-18E71 Reduction of fracture of fibula with internal fixation
P1-18E72 Reduction of fracture of tibia with internal fixation
P1-18E74 Closed reduction of separation of epiphysis of fibula
P1-18E75 Closed reduction of separation of epiphysis of tibia
P1-18E78 Closed reduction of separated epiphysis of tibia and fibula
P1-18E80V Manipulation of hindlimb with application of splint
P1-18E81V Manipulation of stifle joint ligament with splint

1-19 OPERATIVE PROCEDURES ON THE LOWER EXTREMITY: ANKLE AND FOOT

1-190 Ankle and Foot: General and Miscellaneous Operative Procedures

P1-19010 Operative procedure on ankle, NOS
P1-19020 Operative procedure on foot or toes, NOS
P1-19022 Diagnostic procedure on tarsals and metatarsals, NOS
P1-19028 Operation for bone injury of tarsals and metatarsals, NOS
P1-19030 Diagnostic procedure on phalanges of foot, NOS
P1-19038 Operation for bone injury on phalanges of foot, NOS

1-191 Ankle and Foot: Incisions

P1-19100 Arthrotomy of ankle, NOS
P1-19101 Arthrotomy of ankle with drainage
P1-19102 Arthrotomy of ankle for infection
P1-19103 Arthrotomy of ankle with exploration
  Arthrotomy of ankle with joint exploration
  Arthrotomy of ankle with joint exploration without biopsy
  Arthrotomy of ankle with joint exploration without removal of loose or foreign body
P1-19105 Incision and drainage of ankle for deep abscess
P1-19106 Incision and drainage of hematoma of ankle
P1-19107 Incision and drainage of infected bursa of ankle
P1-19108 Deep incision with opening of bone cortex of ankle
P1-19109V Incision and drainage of hindfoot
P1-1910A Division of cartilage of ankle
  Division of joint cartilage of ankle
P1-1910B Division of joint capsule of ankle
P1-1910C Division of ligament of ankle
  Division of joint ligament of ankle
P1-19112 Incision and drainage of infected bursa of foot
P1-19113 Deep dissection below fascia for deep infection of foot with tendon sheath involvement, single bursal space, specify
P1-19114 Deep dissection below fascia for deep infection of foot, single bursal space, specify
P1-19115 Deep dissection below fascia for deep infection of foot with tendon sheath involvement, multiple areas

P1-19116 Deep dissection below fascia for deep infection of foot, multiple areas
P1-19117 Deep incision with opening of bone cortex of foot
P1-19118 Fasciotomy of foot and toe
P1-19119 Fasciotomy of foot
P1-1911A Fasciotomy of toe
P1-19120 Subcutaneous tenotomy of toe, single
P1-19121 Subcutaneous tenotomy of toe, multiple
P1-19122 Arthrotomy with drainage of intertarsal or tarsometatarsal joint
P1-19123 Arthrotomy with drainage of tarsometatarsal joint
P1-19124 Arthrotomy with exploration of intertarsal or tarsometatarsal joint
P1-19125 Arthrotomy with exploration of tarsometatarsal joint
P1-19126 Arthrotomy with drainage of metatarsophalangeal joint
P1-19127 Arthrotomy with exploration of metatarsophalangeal joint
P1-19128 Arthrotomy with drainage of interphalangeal joint of toe
P1-19129 Arthrotomy with exploration of interphalangeal joint of toe
P1-1912A Tarsal tunnel release
P1-19130 Open tenotomy of extensor of foot
P1-19131 Open tenotomy of extensor of toe
P1-19132 Open tenotomy of flexor of foot, multiple
P1-19133 Tenotomy of abductor hallucis muscle
  Release of abductor hallucis muscle
P1-19134 Open tenotomy of flexor of foot, single
P1-19135 Division of plantar fascia and muscle
  Steindler stripping
P1-19136 Open tenotomy of flexor of toe, single
P1-19137 Capsulotomy of midfoot, medial release only
P1-19138 Capsulotomy of midtarsal region
  Heyman type procedure
P1-19139 Capsulotomy for contracture of metatarsophalangeal joint, single, each
P1-1913A Capsulotomy for contracture of metatarsophalangeal joint with tenorrhaphy, single, each
P1-1913B Capsulotomy for contracture of interphalangeal joint of toe, single, each
P1-19140 Incision of tarsals or metatarsals, NOS
P1-19141 Incision of phalanges of foot, NOS
P1-19142 Division of tarsals and metatarsals, NOS
P1-19143 Osteotomy of tarsal
P1-19144 Osteotomy of metatarsal
P1-19145 Osteotomy of phalanges of foot
P1-19146 Arthrotomy of foot and toe
P1-19147 Division of cartilage of foot and toe
  Division of joint cartilage of foot and toe
P1-19148 Division of ligament of foot and toe
  Division of joint ligament of foot and toe
P1-19149 Division of joint capsule of foot and toe
P1-19150 Achillotenotomy
  Achillotomy
  Division of Achilles tendon
  Tenotomy of Achilles tendon
  Hauser achillotenotomy
P1-19151 Tenotomy of Achilles tendon, subcutaneous with general anesthesia
P1-19152 Tenotomy of Achilles tendon, subcutaneous with local anesthesia
P1-19153 Plantar dissection
  Bost operation
P1-19156 Osteotomy of calcaneus
P1-19157 Osteotomy of calcaneus without internal fixation
P1-19158 Osteotomy of talus
P1-19159 Osteotomy of midtarsal bones, except calcaneus or talus

1-193-194 Ankle and Foot: Excisions

P1-19300 Arthrectomy of ankle, NOS
  Chondrectomy of ankle, NOS
  Excision of ankle joint, NOS
P1-19301 Biopsy of soft tissue of ankle area, superficial
P1-19302 Biopsy of soft tissue of ankle area, deep
P1-19306 Arthrotomy of ankle with removal of foreign body
P1-19308 Radical resection of tumor of soft tissue of ankle area
P1-19309 Excision of tumor of ankle area, deep, intramuscular
P1-1930A Excision of tumor of ankle area, deep, subfascial
P1-19310 Arthrotomy of ankle with joint exploration and biopsy
P1-19312 Arthrotomy of ankle with joint exploration and removal of foreign body
  Arthrotomy of ankle with joint exploration and removal of loose body
P1-19313 Arthrotomy of ankle for synovectomy
P1-19314 Arthrotomy of ankle for synovectomy including tenosynovectomy
P1-19315 Excision of lesion of tendon sheath or capsule of ankle
P1-19318 Amputation of ankle through malleoli of tibia and fibula with plastic closure and resection of nerves
  Amputation of ankle through malleoli of tibia and fibula
  Pirogoff amputation
  Syme amputation
  Burgess operation
P1-19319 Ankle disarticulation
  Amputation of ankle
  Guyon amputation
  Amputation of leg through ankle joints
  Disarticulation of ankle
  Amputation by disarticulation of hindfoot
P1-1931A Supramalleolar amputation of foot
P1-19320 Excisional biopsy of joint structure of ankle
  Biopsy of joint structure of ankle

1-193-194 Ankle and Foot: Excisions — Continued

P1-19321 Synovectomy of ankle
P1-19322 Excision of lesion of ankle joint, NOS
  Local excision of lesion of ankle joint, NOS
P1-19324 Radical resection for tumor of calcaneus
P1-19325 Radical resection for tumor of talus
P1-19326 Excision of tumor of foot, deep, intramuscular
P1-19327 Excision of tumor of foot, deep, subfascial
P1-19328 Radical resection of tumor of soft tissue of foot
P1-19332 Arthrotomy with removal of foreign body of intertarsal or tarsometatarsal joint
P1-19333 Arthrotomy with removal of foreign body of tarsometatarsal joint
P1-19335 Arthrotomy with removal of loose body of intertarsal joint
P1-19337 Arthrotomy with removal of loose body of tarsometatarsal joint
P1-19338 Arthrotomy with removal of foreign body of metatarsophalangeal joint
  Arthrotomy with removal of loose body of metatarsophalangeal joint
P1-1933A Arthrotomy with removal of foreign body of interphalangeal joint of toe
  Arthrotomy with removal of loose body of interphalangeal joint of toe
P1-19340 Arthrotomy for synovial biopsy of intertarsal joint
P1-19341 Arthrotomy for synovial biopsy of tarsometatarsal joint
P1-19342 Arthrotomy for synovial biopsy of metatarsophalangeal joint
P1-19345 Arthrotomy for synovial biopsy of interphalangeal joint of toe
P1-19347 Partial fasciectomy of plantar fascia
P1-19348 Radical fasciectomy of plantar fascia
P1-19349 Synovectomy of intertarsal joint, each
P1-1934A Synovectomy of tarsometatarsal joint, each
P1-1934B Synovectomy of metatarsophalangeal joint, each
P1-19350 Excision of interdigital Morton neuroma of foot, single, each
P1-19351 Synovectomy of flexor tendon sheath of foot
P1-19352 Synovectomy of extensor tendon sheath of foot
P1-19353 Excision of lesion of capsule of foot
  Excision of lesion of fibrous sheath of foot
P1-19355 Excision of lesion of tendon of foot
P1-19356 Excision of lesion of capsule of toes
  Excision of lesion of fibrous sheath of toes
P1-19358 Excision of lesion of tendon of toes
P1-19360 Excision or curettage of benign tumor of calcaneus
P1-19361 Excision or curettage of benign tumor of talus
P1-19362 Excision or curettage of bone cyst of calcaneus
P1-19363 Excision or curettage of bone cyst of talus
P1-19364 Excision or curettage of benign tumor of metatarsal bones, except talus or calcaneus
P1-19365 Excision or curettage of benign tumor of tarsal bones, except talus or calcaneus
P1-19366 Excision or curettage of bone cyst of metatarsal bones, except talus or calcaneus
P1-19367 Excision or curettage of bone cyst of tarsal bones, except talus or calcaneus
P1-19368 Excision or curettage of benign tumor of phalanges of foot
P1-19369 Excision or curettage of bone cyst of phalanges of foot
P1-19370 Ostectomy, partial excision of fifth metatarsal head
P1-19371 Ostectomy, complete excision of first metatarsal head
P1-19372 Ostectomy, complete excision of other metatarsal head
P1-19373 Ostectomy, complete excision of fifth metatarsal head
P1-19374 Ostectomy, complete excision of all metatarsal heads with partial proximal phalangectomy, except first metatarsal
P1-19376 Ostectomy, excision of tarsal coalition
P1-19377 Ostectomy of calcaneus, NOS
P1-19378 Ostectomy of calcaneus for spur
P1-19379 Ostectomy of calcaneus for spur with plantar fascial release
P1-19380 Partial excision of calcaneus
P1-19381 Partial excision of talus
P1-19382 Partial excision of metatarsal bone, except talus or calcaneus
P1-19383 Partial excision of tarsal bone, except talus or calcaneus
P1-19384 Partial excision of phalanx of toe
P1-19385 Condylectomy of phalangeal base of toe, single, each
P1-19386 Talectomy
P1-19387 Metatarsectomy
P1-19388 Phalangectomy of toe, single, each
P1-19389 Resection of head of phalanx of toe
P1-1938A Hemiphalangectomy of toe, single, each
P1-1938B Interphalangeal joint excision of toe, single, each
P1-1938C Astragalectomy
P1-19390 Radical resection for tumor of tarsal
P1-19391 Radical resection for tumor of metatarsal
P1-19392 Radical resection for tumor of phalanx of toe
P1-19393 Removal of foreign body of foot, deep
P1-19394 Removal of foreign body of foot, complicated
P1-19395 Condylectomy of metatarsal head, first through fifth, single, each
P1-19396 Exostectomy of metatarsal head, first through fifth, single, each
  Partial ostectomy of metatarsal head, first through fifth, each
P1-19397 Sesamoidectomy of first toe
P1-19398 Midtarsal amputation of foot
  Chopart type procedure
P1-1939A Amputation of metatarsal with toe, single

P1-1939B Amputation of toe at metatarsophalangeal joint
P1-1939C Amputation of toe at interphalangeal joint
P1-19400 Debridement of open fracture of foot, NOS
  Debridement of open fracture of tarsal and metatarsal, NOS
P1-19401 Debridement of open fracture of phalanges of foot
P1-19402 Excision of accessory navicular bone
  Kidner operation
P1-19404 Sequestrectomy of tarsals or metatarsals
P1-19405 Sequestrectomy of phalanges of foot
P1-19406 Removal of internal fixation device from tarsals and metatarsals
P1-19407 Anterior tarsal wedge osteotomy
  Cole operation
P1-19408 Wedge osteotomy of tarsal
  Elmslie-Cholmeley operation
P1-19409 Wedge osteotomy of calcaneus
  Dwyer operation
P1-1940A Excisional biopsy of tarsal and metatarsal
  Biopsy of tarsals and metatarsals
P1-1940B Wedge osteotomy of metatarsal
P1-1940C Excisional biopsy of phalanges of foot
P1-1940D Excision of tarsals and metatarsals for graft
P1-19410 Excision of bunion, NOS
  Bunionectomy, NOS
P1-19411 Radical bunionectomy
  Keller operation
  Mayo operation
  Silver operation
P1-19412 Bunionectomy with osteotomy of first metatarsal
  Bunionectomy with soft tissue correction and osteotomy of the first metatarsal
  Lapidus operation
P1-19413 Excision of bunionette
P1-19416 Dewebbing of syndactyly of toes
P1-19417 Partial ostectomy of tarsals and metatarsals, NOS
P1-19418 Resection of metatarsal heads and bases of phalanges
  Clayton operation
P1-19419 Excision of lesion of tarsal and metatarsal
P1-19420 Excisional biopsy of joint structure of foot and toe
  Biopsy of joint structure of foot and toe
P1-19421 Excision of lesion of phalanges of foot
P1-19422 Arthrectomy of foot and toe
  Chondrectomy of foot and toe
  Excision of joint of foot and toe, NOS
P1-19423 Sesamoidectomy
P1-19424 Synovectomy of foot and toe
P1-19425 Total ostectomy of tarsals and metatarsals
P1-19426 Excision of lesion of joint of foot and toe, NOS
  Local excision of lesion of joint of foot and toe, NOS
P1-19427 Talectomy for foot stabilization
  Whitman operation for foot stabilization
P1-19428 Excision of sinus tarsi
P1-19429 Proximal phalangectomy for hammer toe
  Ruiz-Mora operation
P1-1942A Wedge osteotomy of tarsals and metatarsals
P1-19430 Amputation of toe
  Amputation of hinddigit
P1-19431 Disarticulation of toe
P1-19432 Amputation of hallux
P1-19434 Amputation of foot
  Transmetatarsal amputation of foot
  Hindfoot amputation
  Hey foot amputation
  Amputation of leg through foot
  Lisfranc foot amputation
  Amputation through foot
  Transmetatarsal amputation
P1-19440 Removal of foreign body from foot
  Removal of foreign body from foot without incision
  Removal of foreign body of hindfoot
P1-19442V Excision of lesion of hindfoot
P1-19444V Excision of lesion of hinddigit
P1-19445V Debridement of sesamoid bone of hindfoot
P1-19446V Debridement of hindfoot

1-195 Ankle and Foot: Injections and Implantations

P1-19500 Injection of ankle, NOS
P1-19501 Injection of joint of ankle, NOS
P1-19502 Injection of foot, NOS
P1-19503 Injection of joint of foot, NOS
  Injection of joint of hindfoot, NOS
P1-19505 Injection procedure for ankle arthrography
P1-19510 Insertion of bone growth stimulator into tarsals and metatarsals
P1-19512 Implantation of joint of toe
P1-19513 Implantation of prosthesis or prosthetic device of acetabulum of joint of toe
  Implantation of Swanson prosthesis of toe
P1-19520 Removal of prosthesis of joint structures of ankle
  Removal of ankle implant
  Arthrotomy for removal of prosthesis of ankle
P1-19522 Removal of internal fixation device from phalanges of foot
P1-19523 Removal of prosthesis of joint structures of foot and toe
  Arthrotomy for removal of prosthesis of foot and toe

1-197 Ankle and Foot: Endoscopy

P1-19700 Arthroscopy of ankle, NOS
P1-19704 Arthroscopy of ankle for partial synovectomy
P1-19706 Arthroscopy of ankle for debridement, limited
P1-19708 Arthroscopy of ankle for debridement, extensive

1-197 Ankle and Foot: Endoscopy — Continued

P1-19710 Arthroscopy of ankle with removal of foreign body
  Arthroscopy of ankle with removal of loose body
P1-19724 Arthroscopy of foot, NOS
P1-19726 Arthroscopy of toe, NOS

1-198-19B Ankle and Foot: Surgical Repairs, Closures and Reconstructions

P1-19800 Arthroplasty of ankle, NOS
  Repair of ankle, NOS
P1-19802 Suture of joint capsule with arthroplasty of ankle
P1-19803 Arthrotomy of ankle for posterior capsular release without Achilles tendon lengthening
P1-19804 Arthrotomy of ankle for posterior capsular release with Achilles tendon lengthening
P1-19805 Open reduction of closed or open bimalleolar ankle fracture
P1-19806 Lengthening of tendon of ankle, single
P1-19807 Shortening of tendon of ankle, single
P1-19808 Lengthening of tendon of ankle, multiple
P1-19809 Shortening of tendon of ankle, multiple
P1-1980A Arthroplasty of ankle with implant
P1-1980C Arthroplasty of ankle, secondary reconstruction, total ankle
P1-19810 Reduction of open bimalleolar ankle fracture with uncomplicated soft tissue closure
P1-19811 Open reduction of closed or open bimalleolar ankle fracture with internal skeletal fixation
P1-19812 Reduction of open trimalleolar ankle fracture with uncomplicated soft tissue closure
P1-19813 Open reduction of closed or open trimalleolar ankle fracture, medial and lateral malleolus only
P1-19814 Open reduction of closed or open trimalleolar ankle fracture with external skeletal fixation, medial and lateral malleolus only
P1-19815 Open reduction of closed or open trimalleolar ankle fracture with internal skeletal fixation, medial and lateral malleolus only
P1-19816 Open reduction of closed or open trimalleolar ankle fracture, medial and lateral malleolus, including internal skeletal fixation of posterior lip
P1-19817 Open reduction of closed or open trimalleolar ankle fracture with external skeletal fixation, medial and lateral malleolus, including internal skeletal fixation of posterior lip
P1-19818 Open reduction of closed or open trimalleolar ankle fracture with internal skeletal fixation, medial and lateral malleolus, including internal skeletal fixation of posterior lip
P1-19819 Reduction of proximal tibiofibular joint dislocation
P1-19821 Reduction of proximal tibiofibular joint dislocation with anesthesia
P1-19822 Open reduction of proximal tibiofibular joint dislocation with excision
P1-19823 Open reduction of proximal tibiofibular joint dislocation with fixation
P1-19824 Reduction of ankle dislocation
P1-19825 Reduction of ankle dislocation with anesthesia
P1-19826 Reduction of open ankle dislocation with uncomplicated soft tissue closure
P1-19827 Open reduction of closed or open ankle dislocation
P1-19828 Open reduction of closed or open ankle dislocation with fixation
P1-19829 Arthrodesis of ankle, NOS
  Ankle fusion, NOS
  Fusion of joint of ankle, NOS
P1-19830 Arthrodesis of distal tibiofibular joint
P1-19831 Arthrodesis of proximal tibiofibular joint
P1-19832 Total ankle replacement
P1-19833 Open reduction of dislocation of ankle
P1-19834 Open reduction of diastasis of ankle mortise
P1-19835 Pantalar arthrodesis
  Fusion of pantalar joint
P1-19836 Tibiotalar arthrodesis
  Fusion of tibiotalar joint
P1-19837 Bone block of ankle
  Campbell operation for bone block of ankle
P1-19838 Charnley operation on ankle
P1-19839 Goldthwaite operation for ankle stabilization
P1-1983A Triple arthrodesis of ankle
  Dunn operation
  Hoke operation
  Lambrinudi operation
P1-19840 Subtalar arthrodesis
  Fusion of subtalar joint
  Grice operation
P1-19842 Watson-Jones operation for reconstruction of lateral ligaments of ankle
P1-19843 Ankle reattachment
  Reattachment of ankle
P1-19845 Replantation of foot, complete amputation
P1-19846 Replantation of foot, incomplete amputation
P1-19847 Free osteocutaneous flap with microvascular anastomosis, metatarsal
P1-19848 Free osteocutaneous flap with microvascular anastomosis, great toe with web space
P1-19849 Internal fixation of tarsal or metatarsal
P1-19850 Internal fixation of phalanges of foot
P1-19851 Reconstruction of foot and toes with synthetic joint prosthesis
P1-19852 Suture of joint capsule with arthroplasty of foot
P1-19853 Reconstruction of foot and toes with fixation device
P1-19854 Primary open repair of ruptured Achilles tendon
  Primary percutaneous repair of ruptured Achilles tendon

P1-19856 Primary open repair of ruptured Achilles tendon with graft
Primary percutaneous repair of ruptured Achilles tendon with graft
P1-19857 Secondary repair of ruptured Achilles tendon
P1-19858 Secondary repair of ruptured Achilles tendon with graft
P1-19859 Capsulotomy of midfoot with tendon lengthening
P1-1985A Capsulotomy of midfoot, extensive, including posterior talotibial capsulotomy and tendon lengthening as for resistant clubfoot deformity
P1-19860 Excision or curettage of benign tumor of calcaneus with iliac autograft
P1-19861 Excision or curettage of benign tumor of calcaneus with other autograft
P1-19862 Excision or curettage of benign tumor of talus with iliac autograft
P1-19863 Excision or curettage of benign tumor of talus with other autograft
P1-19864 Excision or curettage of bone cyst of calcaneus with iliac autograft
P1-19865 Excision or curettage of bone cyst of calcaneus with other autograft
P1-19866 Excision or curettage of bone cyst of talus with iliac autograft
P1-19867 Excision or curettage of bone cyst of talus with other autograft
P1-19868 Excision or curettage of benign tumor of calcaneus with allograft
P1-19869 Excision or curettage of benign tumor of talus with allograft
P1-1986A Excision or curettage of bone cyst of calcaneus with allograft
P1-1986B Excision or curettage of bone cyst of talus with allograft
P1-19870 Excision or curettage of benign tumor of metatarsal bones, except talus or calcaneus, with iliac autograft
P1-19871 Excision or curettage of benign tumor of metatarsal bones, except talus or calcaneus, with other autograft
P1-19872 Excision or curettage of benign tumor of tarsal bones, except talus or calcaneus, with iliac autograft
P1-19873 Excision or curettage of benign tumor of tarsal bones, except talus or calcaneus, with other autograft
P1-19874 Excision or curettage of bone cyst of metatarsal bones, except talus or calcaneus, with iliac autograft
P1-19875 Excision or curettage of bone cyst of metatarsal bones, except talus or calcaneus, with other autograft
P1-19876 Excision or curettage of bone cyst of tarsal bones, except talus or calcaneus, with iliac autograft
P1-19877 Excision or curettage of bone cyst of tarsal bones, except talus or calcaneus, with other autograft
P1-19878 Excision or curettage of benign tumor of metatarsal bones, except talus or calcaneus, with allograft
P1-19879 Excision or curettage of benign tumor of tarsal bones, except talus or calcaneus, with allograft
P1-1987A Excision or curettage of bone cyst of metatarsal bones, except talus or calcaneus, with allograft
P1-1987B Excision or curettage of bone cyst of tarsal bones, except talus or calcaneus, with allograft
P1-19881 Repair of flexor tendon of foot, single, primary
P1-19882 Repair of flexor tendon of foot, single, secondary
P1-19883 Repair of flexor tendon of foot, single, secondary, with free graft
P1-19884 Repair of extensor tendon of foot, single, primary
P1-19885 Repair of extensor tendon of foot, single, secondary
P1-19886 Repair of extensor tendon of foot, single, secondary, with free graft
P1-19887 Advancement of posterior tibial tendon with excision of accessory navicular bone
P1-19889 Lengthening of abductor hallucis muscle
P1-1988A Lengthening of tendo calcaneus by incomplete tenotomy
White operation
P1-19890 Webbing operation for soft corn
Creation of syndactylism of toes
P1-19891 Hammer toe operation, one toe
Repair of hammer toe
Correction of hammer toe
P1-19892 Repair of hallux valgus, NOS
P1-19893 Hammer toe operation for cock-up fifth toe with plastic skin closure
P1-19894 Hallux valgus correction with sesamoidectomy, simple exostectomy
P1-19895 Hallux valgus correction without sesamoidectomy, simple exostectomy
P1-19897 Hallux valgus, bunion, correction with sesamoidectomy, Keller, McBride or Mayo type procedure
P1-19898 Hallux valgus, bunion, correction without sesamoidectomy, Keller, McBride or Mayo type procedure
P1-19900 Hallux valgus correction with sesamoidectomy, resection of joint with implant
P1-19901 Hallux valgus correction without sesamoidectomy, resection of joint with implant
P1-19902 Hallux valgus correction with sesamoidectomy and tendon transplants

1-198-19B Ankle and Foot: Surgical Repairs, Closures and Reconstructions — Continued

P1-19903 Hallux valgus correction without sesamoidectomy with tendon transplants
P1-19904 Hallux valgus, bunion correction with or without sesamoidectomy with tendon transplants
  Joplin type procedure
P1-19905 Hallux valgus correction with sesamoidectomy and metatarsal osteotomy
P1-19906 Hallux valgus correction with metatarsal osteotomy without sesamoidectomy
  Mitchell operation for hallux valgus repair
  Metatarsal wedge osteotomy for hallux valgus repair
  Wilson operation
  Angulation osteotomy for hallux valgus
P1-19907 Bunionectomy with arthrodesis
P1-19908 Bunionectomy with soft tissue correction and arthrodesis
P1-19909 Hallux valgus, bunion, correction with sesamoidectomy, Lapidus type procedure
P1-1990A Hallux valgus, bunion, correction without sesamoidectomy, Lapidus type procedure
P1-19910 Bunionectomy with soft tissue correction, NOS
  McBride operation
P1-19911 Bunionectomy with adductor tendon transfer
  Hauser bunionectomy
  Joplin operation
P1-19914 Hallux valgus correction with sesamoidectomy
  Hallux valgus correction with sesamoidectomy by other methods
P1-19916 Osteotomy of calcaneus with internal fixation
P1-19917 Osteotomy of midtarsal bones, except calcaneus or talus with autograft
P1-19918 Hallux valgus correction by phalanx osteotomy
P1-19919 Osteotomy of midtarsal bones, other than calcaneus or talus with autograft
P1-1991A Osteotomy of metatarsal base or shaft, single, for shortening or angular correction, first metatarsal
P1-19920 Osteotomy of metatarsal base or shaft, single, with lengthening for shortening or angular correction, first metatarsal
P1-19921 Osteotomy of metatarsal, base or shaft, single for shortening or angular correction, first metatarsal with autograft
P1-19922 Osteotomy of metatarsal, base or shaft, single with lengthening for shortening or angular correction, first metatarsal with autograft
P1-19923 Osteotomy of metatarsal, base or shaft, single for shortening or angular correction, except first metatarsal
P1-19924 Osteotomy of metatarsal, base or shaft, single with lengthening for shortening or angular correction, except first metatarsal
P1-19925 Osteotomy of metatarsals, multiple, for cavus foot
  Swanson type procedure for cavus foot
P1-19926 Osteotomy for angular correction of proximal phalanx of first toe
P1-19927 Osteotomy for rotational correction of proximal phalanx of first toe
P1-19928 Osteotomy for shortening of proximal phalanx of first toe
P1-19929 Osteotomy for angular correction of other phalanges, any toe
P1-19930 Osteotomy for rotational correction of other phalanges, any toe
P1-19931 Osteotomy for shortening of other phalanges, any toe
P1-19932 Reconstruction of angular deformity of toe by soft tissue procedure
P1-19933 Repair of malunion of tarsal bones
P1-19934 Repair of nonunion of tarsal bones
P1-19938 Kidner operation with tendon transfer
P1-19940 Repair of malunion of metatarsal bones
P1-19941 Repair of malunion of metatarsal with bone graft
P1-19942 Repair of nonunion of metatarsal with bone graft
P1-19943 Repair of nonunion of metatarsal bones
P1-19944 Reconstruction of toe for macrodactyly by soft tissue resection
P1-19945 Reconstruction of toe for macrodactyly with bone resection
P1-19946 Reconstruction of toes for polydactyly
P1-19947 Reconstruction of cleft foot
P1-19950 Open reduction of closed or open calcaneal fracture
P1-19951 Reduction of open calcaneal fracture with uncomplicated soft tissue closure
P1-19952 Open reduction of closed or open calcaneal fracture with external skeletal fixation
P1-19953 Open reduction of closed or open calcaneal fracture with internal skeletal fixation
P1-19954 Open reduction of closed or open calcaneal fracture with external skeletal fixation with autogenous bone graft
P1-19955 Open reduction of closed or open calcaneal fracture with external skeletal fixation with primary iliac autogenous bone graft
P1-19956 Open reduction of closed or open calcaneal fracture with internal skeletal fixation with autogenous bone graft
P1-19957 Open reduction of closed or open calcaneal fracture with internal skeletal fixation with primary iliac autogenous bone graft
P1-19958 Open reduction of closed or open calcaneal fracture with autogenous bone graft
P1-19959 Open reduction of closed or open calcaneal fracture with primary iliac autogenous bone graft
P1-19960 Open reduction of closed or open talus fracture

P1-19961 Reduction of open talus fracture with uncomplicated soft tissue closure
P1-19962 Open reduction of closed or open talus fracture with internal skeletal fixation
P1-19963 Reduction of open tarsal bone fracture with uncomplicated soft tissue closure
P1-19964 Open reduction of closed or open tarsal bone fracture
P1-19965 Open reduction of closed or open tarsal bone fracture with external skeletal fixation
P1-19966 Open reduction of closed or open tarsal bone fracture with internal skeletal fixation
P1-19967 Reduction of open metatarsal fracture with uncomplicated soft tissue closure
P1-19968 Open reduction of closed or open metatarsal fracture
P1-19969 Open reduction of closed or open metatarsal fracture with external skeletal fixation
P1-1996A Open reduction of closed or open metatarsal fracture with internal skeletal fixation
P1-19970 Reduction of open fracture of great toe, phalanx or phalanges with uncomplicated soft tissue closure
P1-19971 Open reduction of closed or open fracture of great toe, phalanx or phalanges
P1-19972 Open reduction of closed or open fracture of great toe, phalanx or phalanges with external skeletal fixation
P1-19973 Open reduction of closed or open fracture of great toe, phalanx or phalanges with internal skeletal fixation
P1-19974 Reduction of open fracture of phalanx or phalanges of foot, except great toe with uncomplicated soft tissue closure
P1-19976 Open reduction of closed or open fracture of phalanx or phalanges of foot, except great toe
P1-19977 Open reduction of closed or open fracture of phalanx or phalanges of foot, except great toe with external skeletal fixation
P1-19978 Open reduction of closed or open fracture of phalanx or phalanges of,foot, except great toe with internal skeletal fixation
P1-19979 Reduction of open tarsal bone dislocation with uncomplicated soft tissue closure
P1-19980 Open reduction of closed or open tarsal bone dislocation
P1-19981 Open reduction of closed or open tarsal bone dislocation with external skeletal fixation
P1-19982 Open reduction of closed or open tarsal bone dislocation with internal skeletal fixation
P1-19983 Reduction of open talotarsal joint dislocation with uncomplicated soft tissue closure
P1-19984 Open reduction of closed or open talotarsal joint dislocation
P1-19985 Open reduction of closed or open talotarsal joint dislocation with external skeletal fixation
P1-19986 Open reduction of closed or open talotarsal joint dislocation with internal skeletal fixation
P1-19987 Reduction of open tarsometatarsal joint dislocation with uncomplicated soft tissue closure
P1-19988 Open reduction of closed or open tarsometatarsal joint dislocation
P1-19989 Open reduction of closed or open tarsometatarsal joint dislocation with external skeletal fixation
P1-19990 Open reduction of closed or open tarsometatarsal joint dislocation with internal skeletal fixation
P1-19991 Reduction of open metatarsophalangeal joint dislocation with uncomplicated soft tissue closure
P1-19992 Open reduction of closed or open metatarsophalangeal joint dislocation
P1-19993 Reduction of open interphalangeal toe joint dislocation with uncomplicated soft tissue closure
P1-19994 Open reduction of closed or open interphalangeal toe joint dislocation
P1-19998 Midtarsal arthrodesis, multiple
P1-19999 Midtarsal arthrodesis, transverse
P1-199A0 Tarsometatarsal arthrodesis, NOS
  Tarsometatarsal arthrodesis, single joint
  Tarsometatarsal fusion, NOS
P1-199A1 Tarsometatarsal arthrodesis, multiple
P1-199A2 Tarsometatarsal arthrodesis, transverse
P1-199A3 Tarsometatarsal arthrodesis, multiple, with osteotomy as for flatfoot correction
P1-199A4 Tarsometatarsal arthrodesis, transverse, with osteotomy as for flatfoot correction
P1-199B0 Midtarsal arthrodesis, NOS
  Fusion of joint of midtarsal
  Hoke operation for midtarsal fusion
  Midtarsal fusion
  Miller operation
P1-199B1 Midtarsal arthrodesis, navicular-cuneiform, with tendon lengthening and advancement
P1-199B2 Midtarsal arthrodesis, single joint
P1-199B3 Midtarsal arthrodesis, multiple, with osteotomy as for flatfoot correction
P1-199B4 Midtarsal arthrodesis, transverse, with osteotomy as for flatfoot correction
P1-19A00 Metatarsophalangeal arthrodesis
  McKeever arthrodesis
  Fusion of metatarsophalangeal joint
  Metatarsophalangeal fusion
P1-19A01 Arthrodesis of interphalangeal joint of great toe
P1-19A04 Arthrodesis of metatarsophalangeal joint of great toe
P1-19A05 Fusion of first metatarsophalangeal joint for hallux valgus repair
  Mckeever operation
P1-19A08 Arthrodesis of interphalangeal joint of great toe with extensor hallucis longus transfer to first metatarsal neck

1-198-19B Ankle and Foot: Surgical Repairs, Closures and Reconstructions — Continued

P1-19A12 Correction of bunionette
P1-19A14 Repair of claw toe
P1-19A15 Excision, fusion and repair of toes, NOS
P1-19A16 Change in bone length of tarsals and metatarsals, NOS
P1-19A18 Osteoplasty of tarsal or metatarsal, NOS
    Repair or plastic operation of tarsals and metatarsals, NOS
P1-19A19 Filleting of hammer toe
P1-19A20 Osteoplasty of phalanges of foot
P1-19A21 Internal fixation of tarsals and metatarsals without fracture reduction
P1-19A22 Open reduction of fracture of tarsals and metatarsals
P1-19A23 Open reduction of fracture of foot
P1-19A24 Open reduction of fracture of foot with internal fixation
    Open reduction of fracture of tarsals and metatarsals with internal fixation
P1-19A26 Open reduction of fracture of phalanges of foot
P1-19A27 Open reduction of fracture of phalanges of foot with internal fixation
P1-19A28 Open reduction of dislocation of foot and toe
P1-19A29 Open reduction of dislocation of foot
P1-19A2A Open reduction of dislocation of toe
P1-19A31 Correction of metatarsus varus
    Heyman-Herndon operation
P1-19A3B Arthrodesis of foot, NOS
    Fusion of joint of foot, NOS
    Fusion of tarsal joints, NOS
P1-19A40 Fusion of joint of toe, NOS
    Interphalangeal arthrodesis of toe
    Arthrodesis of toe, NOS
    Johanson operation for hammer toe
P1-19A41 Correction of overlapping toes
P1-19A44 Arthroplasty of foot with synthetic joint prosthesis
P1-19A45 Arthroplasty of toe with synthetic joint prosthesis
P1-19A46 Metatarsal arthroplasty of foot
P1-19A47 Tendon transfer and arthrodesis to correct claw toe
    Dickson-Diveley operation
P1-19A48 Transfer of extensor hallucis longus tendon
    Johanson operation for claw toe
P1-19A49 Modified Johanson operation for claw toe with arthrodesis
P1-19A4A Muscle transfer for claw toe repair
    Girdlestone operation for claw toe repair
    Girdlestone-Taylor operation
P1-19A52 Correction of clubfoot, NOS
    Goldner operation
    Turco operation
    Evans operation
    Gelman operation
    McCauley operation
    Release of clubfoot, NOS
    Clubfoot release, NOS
P1-19A53 Soft tissue release for clubfoot
    Brockman operation
    Heyman operation
P1-19A5A Replacement of joint of foot and toe, NOS
P1-19A60 Plastic achillotomy
    Plastic achillotenotomy
P1-19A62 Lengthening of Achilles tendon
    Lengthening of heel cord
    Poncet operation
P1-19A63 Shortening of Achilles tendon
    Shortening of heel cord
P1-19A70 Reattachment of extremity of foot
P1-19A72 Reattachment of extremity of toe
P1-19B00 Suture of capsule of ankle
    Capsulorrhaphy of ankle
P1-19B02 Suture of ligament of ankle
P1-19B05 Primary suture of ruptured ligament of ankle, collateral
    Primary suture of severed ligament of ankle, collateral
    Primary suture of torn ligament of ankle, collateral
P1-19B07 Primary suture of ruptured ligaments of ankle, both collateral ligaments
    Primary suture of severed ligaments of ankle, both collateral ligaments
    Primary suture of torn ligaments of ankle, both collateral ligaments
P1-19B08 Suture for secondary repair of ruptured ligament of ankle, collateral
    Suture for secondary repair of severed ligament of ankle, collateral
    Suture for secondary repair of torn ligament of ankle, collateral
P1-19B10 Suture of periosteum of tarsal or metatarsal
P1-19B12 Suture of periosteum of phalanges of foot
P1-19B20 Suture of capsule of foot
    Capsulorrhaphy of foot
P1-19B21 Suture of ligament of foot
P1-19B22 Suture of ligament of foot and toes
P1-19B24 Achillorrhaphy
P1-19B25 Delayed achillorrhaphy
P1-19B30 Suture of flexor tendon of foot, single, primary
P1-19B31 Suture of flexor tendon of foot, single, secondary, with free graft
P1-19B32 Suture of extensor tendon of foot, single, primary
P1-19B33 Suture of extensor tendon of foot, single, secondary
P1-19B34 Suture of extensor tendon of foot, single, secondary, with free graft
P1-19B50V Plastic operation on hoof of hindlimb
P1-19B55V Plastic operation on claw of hindlimb

1-19C Ankle and Foot: Destructive Procedures

P1-19C00 Destructive procedure of ankle and foot, NOS
P1-19C06 Local destruction of lesion of ankle joint, NOS
P1-19C08 Local destruction of lesion of joint of foot and toe, NOS
P1-19C10 Tenolysis of flexor of foot, single
P1-19C11 Tenolysis of flexor of foot, multiple
P1-19C12 Tenolysis of extensor of foot, single
P1-19C14 Osteoclasis of tarsal or metatarsal
P1-19C16 Osteoclasis of phalanges of foot
P1-19C50V Cauterization of hindfoot
P1-19C55V Cauterization of hoof of hindfoot

1-19D Ankle and Foot: Transplantations and Transpositions

P1-19D12 Grafting of tarsal or metatarsal
P1-19D14 Grafting of phalanges of foot
P1-19D19 Transfer of anterior tibial tendon into tarsal bone

1-19E Ankle and Foot: Manipulations

P1-19E00 Manipulation of ankle and foot, NOS
P1-19E04 Wedging of clubfoot cast
P1-19E05 Removal or bivalving of boot cast
P1-19E06 Strapping of ankle
P1-19E07 Strapping of toes
P1-19E08 Strapping of Unna boot
P1-19E10 Reduction of closed bimalleolar ankle fracture without manipulation
P1-19E11 Reduction of closed bimalleolar ankle fracture with manipulation
P1-19E12 Reduction of closed trimalleolar ankle fracture without manipulation
P1-19E13 Reduction of closed trimalleolar ankle fracture with manipulation
P1-19E14 Manipulation of ankle under general anesthesia
P1-19E15 Closed reduction of dislocation of ankle
P1-19E16 Closed reduction of diastasis of ankle mortise
P1-19E20 Closed reduction of fracture of tarsal or metatarsal
P1-19E21 Reduction of closed calcaneal fracture without manipulation
P1-19E22 Reduction of closed calcaneal fracture with manipulation including Cotton or Bohler type reduction
P1-19E23 Reduction of closed calcaneal fracture with manipulation and skeletal fixation
P1-19E25 Reduction of closed talus fracture without manipulation
P1-19E26 Reduction of closed talus fracture with manipulation
P1-19E27 Reduction of closed talus fracture with manipulation and percutaneous pinning
P1-19E28 Reduction of closed tarsal bone fracture without manipulation
P1-19E29 Reduction of closed tarsal bone fracture with manipulation
P1-19E30 Reduction of closed tarsal bone fracture with manipulation and percutaneous pinning
P1-19E31 Reduction of closed metatarsal fracture without manipulation
P1-19E32 Reduction of closed metatarsal fracture with manipulation
P1-19E33 Reduction of closed metatarsal fracture with manipulation and percutaneous pinning
P1-19E34 Reduction of closed fracture of great toe, phalanx or phalanges without manipulation
P1-19E36 Reduction of closed fracture of great toe, phalanx or phalanges with manipulation
P1-19E37 Reduction of closed fracture of great toe, phalanx or phalanges with manipulation and percutaneous pinning
P1-19E38 Reduction of closed fracture of phalanx or phalanges, except great toe, without manipulation
P1-19E39 Reduction of closed fracture of phalanx or phalanges, except great toe, with manipulation
P1-19E40 Reduction of closed sesamoid fracture
P1-19E41 Reduction of closed tarsal bone dislocation
P1-19E42 Reduction of closed tarsal bone dislocation with anesthesia
P1-19E44 Reduction of closed tarsal bone dislocation with percutaneous skeletal fixation
P1-19E45 Reduction of closed talotarsal joint dislocation
P1-19E46 Reduction of closed talotarsal joint dislocation with anesthesia
P1-19E47 Reduction of closed tarsometatarsal joint dislocation
P1-19E48 Reduction of closed tarsometatarsal joint dislocation with anesthesia
P1-19E49 Reduction of closed tarsometatarsal joint dislocation with percutaneous skeletal fixation
P1-19E50 Reduction of closed metatarsophalangeal joint dislocation
P1-19E51 Reduction of closed metatarsophalangeal joint dislocation with anesthesia
P1-19E52 Reduction of closed interphalangeal toe joint dislocation
P1-19E53 Reduction of closed interphalangeal toe joint dislocation with anesthesia
P1-19E55 Closed reduction of fracture of foot, NOS
P1-19E56 Closed reduction of fracture of tarsals and metatarsals
P1-19E57 Closed reduction of fracture of phalanges of foot
P1-19E58 Closed reduction of fracture of foot with internal fixation
    Closed reduction of fracture of tarsals and metatarsals with internal fixation
P1-19E61 Closed reduction of fracture of phalanges of foot with internal fixation
P1-19E71 Closed reduction of dislocation of foot

1-19E Ankle and Foot: Manipulations — Continued

P1-19E72 Closed reduction of dislocation of toe

P1-19E79 Closed reduction of dislocation of foot and toe

SECTION 1-2 OPERATIVE PROCEDURES ON THE RESPIRATORY TRACT

1-20 GENERAL OPERATIVE PROCEDURES ON THE RESPIRATORY TRACT

1-200 Respiratory Tract: General and Miscellaneous Operative Procedures

P1-20000 Operative procedure on respiratory tract, NOS
 Operation on respiratory tract, NOS

P1-20010 Diagnostic procedure on respiratory tract, NOS

P1-20020 Operative procedure on upper respiratory tract, NOS

P1-20022 Diagnostic procedure on upper respiratory tract, NOS

P1-20030 Operative procedure on lower respiratory tract, NOS

P1-20032 Diagnostic procedure on lower respiratory tract, NOS

1-21 OPERATIVE PROCEDURES ON THE NOSE AND NASOPHARYNX

1-210 Nose and Nasopharynx: General and Miscellaneous Operative Procedures

P1-21000 Operation on nose, NOS

P1-21010 Operation on nasopharynx, NOS

P1-21020 Control of hemorrhage of nose, NOS
 Control of epistaxis, NOS
 Control of epistaxis by unlisted technique, NOS

1-211 Nose and Nasopharynx: Incisions

P1-21100 Incision of nose, NOS
 Rhinotomy, NOS

P1-21104 Incision and exploration of nose

P1-21105 Incision and exploration of frontonasal duct

P1-21106 Nasal chondrotomy

P1-21107 Nasal septotomy

P1-21110 Conchotomy

P1-21120 Drainage of abscess of nose by internal approach

P1-21124 Drainage of abscess of nasal septum

P1-21130 Drainage of hematoma of nose by internal approach

P1-21134 Drainage of hematoma of nasal septum

1-213 Nose and Nasopharynx: Excisions

P1-21300 Intranasal biopsy, NOS

P1-21302 Excision of intranasal lesion by internal approach
 Excision of intranasal lesion of nose

P1-21304 Excision of intranasal lesion by external approach

P1-21310 Simple excision of nasal polyps
 Nasal polypectomy

P1-21314 Extensive excision of nasal polyps

P1-21320 Removal of intranasal foreign body, simple
 Removal of rhinolith
 Removal of intraluminal foreign body from nose without incision

P1-21322 Removal of foreign body from nose by incision
 Removal of intranasal foreign body by lateral rhinotomy

P1-21324 Removal of intranasal foreign body requiring general anesthesia

P1-21360 Submucous resection of nasal septum
 Submucous chondrectomy of nasal septum
 Submucous excision of cartilage of nasal septum
 Submucous nasal septectomy
 Nasal septectomy

P1-21362 Submucous resection with cartilage scoring or contouring

P1-21364 Submucous resection of nasal septum with replacement with graft

P1-21366 Partial submucous resection of turbinate

P1-21368 Complete submucous resection of turbinate

P1-21370 Turbinectomy
 Complete excision of turbinate
 Conchectomy

P1-21372 Partial excision of turbinate

P1-21376 Sequestrectomy of bone of nose

P1-21380 Control of epistaxis by excision of nasal mucosa with grafting

P1-21382 Pinsker operation for obliteration of nasoseptal telangiectasia

P1-21390 Excision of dermoid cyst of nose, superficial

P1-21392 Excision of dermoid cyst of nose, deep

P1-21399 Local excision of lesion of nose

P1-213A0 Excision of skin of nose for rhinophyma
 Surgical planing of skin of nose for rhinophyma

P1-213B0 Partial rhinectomy

P1-213B2 Total rhinectomy
 Amputation of nose

P1-21400 Excision of lesion of nasopharynx
 Biopsy of visible lesion of nasopharynx

P1-21404 Biopsy of nasopharynx, survey for unknown primary lesion

1-215 Nose and Nasopharynx: Injections and Implantations

P1-21500 Control of epistaxis by packing, NOS
P1-21502 Anterior packing of nose
  Packing of nose for anterior epistaxis
P1-21504 Packing of posterior nose
P1-21506 Control of epistaxis by packing of posterior and anterior nose
P1-21508 Replacement of nasal packing
  Replacement of pack of nose
P1-21509 Removal of nasal pack
P1-21510 Insertion of nasal septal prosthesis
P1-21514 Implant of inert material into nose
P1-21520 Displacement therapy of nose, Proetz type
P1-21530 Therapeutic injection into turbinates
P1-21534 Irrigation of nasal passages

1-217 Nose and Nasopharynx: Endoscopy

P1-21700 Endoscopy of nose
  Rhinoscopy
  Nasal endoscopy
P1-21740 Nasopharyngoscopy
P1-21750 Nasal endoscopy with nasal polypectomy
P1-21760 Nasal endoscopy with removal of foreign body

1-218-21A Nose and Nasopharynx: Surgical Repairs, Closures and Reconstructions

P1-21800 Repair of nose, NOS
P1-21802 Repair of laceration of nose
  Rhinorrhaphy
  Suture of laceration of nose
P1-21804 Rhinorrhaphy for epistaxis
  Suture of nose for epistaxis
P1-21814 Repair of nasal fistula
  Closure of oronasal fistula
P1-21818 Repair of nasopharyngeal fistula
  Closure of nasopharyngeal fistula
P1-21820 Repair of choanal atresia, intranasal
P1-21824 Repair of choanal atresia, transpalatine
P1-21830 Repair of nasolabial flaps
P1-21832 Open reduction of nasal fracture
P1-21900 Control of epistaxis by ligation of artery, NOS
P1-21902 Ligation of external carotid artery for nasal hemorrhage
P1-21903 Ligation of ethmoidal arteries for epistaxis
  Control of epistaxis by ligation of ethmoidal artery
P1-21904 Transantral ligation of internal maxillary artery for epistaxis
  Ligation of maxillary artery for nasal hemorrhage
  Control of epistaxis by transantral ligation of the maxillary artery
P1-21A00 Rhinoplasty, NOS
P1-21A02 Limited rhinoplasty, NOS
  Denonvillier operation, limited rhinoplasty
P1-21A04 Primary rhinoplasty of alar cartilages
P1-21A06 Primary rhinoplasty with elevation of nasal tip
  Nasal tip rhinoplasty
P1-21A08 Primary rhinoplasty with lateral and alar cartilages and elevation of nasal tip
P1-21A10 Complete primary rhinoplasty
P1-21A12 Primary rhinoplasty including major septal repair
  Total nasal reconstruction
P1-21A20 Secondary rhinoplasty, minor revision
P1-21A22 Secondary rhinoplasty, intermediate revision with osteotomies
P1-21A24 Secondary rhinoplasty, major revision
P1-21A30 Revision rhinoplasty
P1-21A40 Functional reconstruction of internal nose
P1-21A60 Rhinoplasty augmentation with synthetic implant
P1-21A70 Rhinoseptoplasty
  Septorhinoplasty
P1-21A80 Nasal septoplasty
  Nasal septoplasty without graft
P1-21A84 Nasal septoplasty with graft
P1-21A90 Repair of nasal septal perforation
  Closure of nasal septal perforation
P1-21AA0 Osteoplasty of nasal bones
  Repair of nasal bone
P1-21B10 Reattachment of amputated nose

1-21C Nose and Nasopharynx: Destructive Procedures

P1-21C00 Destructive procedure of nose and nasopharynx, NOS
P1-21C06 Destruction of intranasal lesion, NOS
P1-21C12 Electrocoagulation of nose for epistaxis
P1-21C14 Control of anterior nasal hemorrhage by simple cautery and packing
  Control of epistaxis by cauterization and packing
P1-21C15 Control of anterior nasal hemorrhage by complex cautery and packing
P1-21C16 Control of posterior nasal hemorrhage with cautery and packs, initial
P1-21C18 Control of secondary nasopharyngeal hemorrhage, simple, with cauterization
  Control of postadenoidectomy hemorrhage, simple
P1-21C19 Control of secondary nasopharyngeal hemorrhage, complex
  Control of postadenoidectomy hemorrhage, complex
P1-21C1A Control of nasopharyngeal hemorrhage, primary or secondary, complicated and requiring hospitalization
P1-21C1B Control of nasopharyngeal hemorrhage, primary or secondary, with secondary surgical intervention
P1-21C30 Lysis of adhesions of nose, NOS
  Lysis of intranasal synechia

1-21C Nose and Nasopharynx: Destructive Procedures — Continued

P1-21C34 Lysis of adhesions of choanae of nasopharynx
  Lysis of adhesions of nasopharynx
  Scrub of posterior nasal adhesions
P1-21C42 Crushing of nasal septum
  Adams operation for crushing of nasal septum
P1-21C60 Cauterization of turbinates, superficial
P1-21C62 Cauterization of turbinates, intramural
P1-21C64 Cryosurgery of turbinates
  Cryotherapy of nasal turbinates
  Turbinectomy by cryosurgery
P1-21C66 Diathermy of nasal turbinates
  Turbinectomy by diathermy
P1-21C70 Surgical fracture of nasal turbinates
  Therapeutic fracture of nasal turbinates
P1-21C72 Refracture of nasal bones

1-21D Nose and Nasopharynx: Transplantations and Transpositions

P1-21D00 Graft of nose, NOS
P1-21D10 Graft of nasal septum
P1-21D20 Graft of nose tip
P1-21D30 Graft of nasolabial flaps
P1-21D40 Weir operation for correction of nostrils
P1-21D50 Reconstruction of nose, total with arm flap
P1-21D60 Reconstruction of nose, total with forehead flap

1-21E Nose and Nasopharynx: Manipulations

P1-21E00 Manipulation of displaced nasal septum
P1-21E10 Closed reduction of nasal fracture
P1-21E30 Dilation of nares
P1-21E40 Dilation of sphenoid ostia
P1-21E50 Dilation of nasopharynx
  Dilation of choanae of nasopharynx
P1-21E60 Dilation of frontonasal duct

1-23 OPERATIVE PROCEDURES ON THE ACCESSORY SINUSES

1-230 Accessory Sinuses: General and Miscellaneous Operative Procedures

P1-23000 Operation on accessory sinus, NOS
  Operation on nasal sinus, NOS
P1-23010 Pterygomaxillary fossa surgery by any approach, NOS

1-231 Accessory Sinuses: Incisions

P1-23100 Sinusotomy, NOS
P1-23102 Sinusotomy by intranasal approach, NOS
  Intranasal antrotomy
P1-23103 Perinasal sinusotomy
P1-23104 Sinusotomy, multiple, NOS
P1-23105 Sinusotomy, combined, three or more sinuses
P1-23110 Aspiration of nasal sinus, NOS
P1-23112 Aspiration of nasal sinus through natural ostium
P1-23114 Aspiration of nasal sinus by puncture
  Puncture of nasal sinus
P1-23120 Maxillary sinusotomy by intranasal approach
  Maxillary antrotomy by intranasal approach
P1-23121 Maxillary antrotomy by external approach
P1-23122 Maxillary sinusotomy by Caldwell-Luc approach
P1-23124 Radical maxillary antrotomy, NOS
P1-23125 Denker operation for radical maxillary antrotomy
P1-23130 Frontal sinusotomy, NOS
  Exploration of frontal sinus
P1-23131 Frontal sinusotomy with trephine
P1-23132 Frontal sinusotomy by intranasal approach
P1-23133 Frontal sinusotomy by transorbital approach, unilateral
P1-23134 Frontal sinusotomy, obliterative without osteoplastic flap by brow incision
P1-23135 Frontal sinusotomy, obliterative without osteoplastic flap by coronal incision
P1-23136 Frontal sinusotomy, obliterative with osteoplastic flap by brow approach
P1-23137 Frontal sinusotomy, obliterative with osteoplastic flap by coronal approach
P1-23138 Frontal sinusotomy, nonobliterative with osteoplastic flap by brow approach
P1-23139 Frontal sinusotomy, nonobliterative with osteoplastic flap by coronal approach
P1-23140 Ethmoid sinusotomy
  Ethmoidotomy
  Exploration of ethmoid sinus
P1-23150 Sphenoid sinusotomy
  Exploration of sphenoid sinus
  Sphenoidotomy
P1-23154 Sphenoid sinusotomy with biopsy
P1-23156 Sphenoid sinusotomy with removal of polyp

1-233 Accessory Sinuses: Excisions

P1-23300 Nasal sinusectomy, NOS
P1-23301 Biopsy of nasal sinus, NOS
P1-23302 Core needle biopsy of nasal sinus
P1-23304 Fine needle biopsy of nasal sinus
  Fine needle aspiration biopsy of nasal sinus
P1-23306 Excision of lesion of nasal sinus, NOS
P1-23308 Removal of foreign body from nasal sinus, NOS
P1-23309 Removal of foreign body from maxillary sinus, NOS
P1-2330A Removal of foreign body from maxillary sinus by Caldwell-Luc approach
P1-23310 Excision of lesion of maxillary sinus, NOS
P1-23311 Excision of lesion of maxillary sinus by Caldwell-Luc approach
P1-23312 Caldwell-Luc operation with removal of membrane lining

P1-23313 Radical maxillary sinusotomy with removal of antrochoanal polyps
P1-23314 Maxillary sinusectomy, NOS
  Maxillectomy without orbital exenteration
P1-23316 Maxillectomy with orbital exenteration
P1-23317 Maxillary antrectomy, NOS
P1-23318 Radical maxillary antrectomy
P1-2331A Excision of tooth from nasal sinus
P1-2331B Removal of impacted tooth from maxillary sinus
P1-23320 Frontal sinusectomy, NOS
P1-23322 Excision of lesion from frontal sinus
P1-23324 Removal of foreign body from frontal sinus
P1-23330 Ethmoid sinusectomy, NOS
  Ethmoidectomy, NOS
P1-23331 Excision of lesion of ethmoid sinus
P1-23332 Anterior ethmoidectomy by intranasal approach
P1-23334 Total ethmoidectomy by intranasal approach
P1-23336 Total ethmoidectomy by extranasal approach
P1-23337 Exenteration of ethmoid air cells
P1-23338 Removal of foreign body from ethmoid sinus
P1-23340 Sphenoid sinusectomy, NOS
  Sphenoidectomy, NOS
P1-23342 Excision of lesion from sphenoid sinus
P1-23344 Removal of foreign body from sphenoid sinus

1-235 Accessory Sinuses: Injections and Implantations

P1-23500 Irrigation of nasal sinus, NOS
  Aspiration and lavage of nasal sinus, NOS
P1-23501 Cannulation of nasal sinus by puncture
P1-23502 Aspiration and lavage of nasal sinus by puncture
P1-23503 Cannulation of nasal sinus through natural ostium
P1-23504 Lavage of nasal sinus through natural ostium
P1-23510 Irrigation by cannulation of maxillary sinus
P1-23520 Irrigation by cannulation of sphenoid sinus

1-237 Accessory Sinuses: Endoscopy

P1-23700 Nasal sinus endoscopy, NOS
P1-23704 Nasal sinus endoscopy, multiple sinuses
P1-23706 Endoscopic biopsy of nasal sinus, NOS
P1-23710 Nasal endoscopy with maxillary antrostomy
P1-23712 Maxillary sinus endoscopy without biopsy
P1-23713 Maxillary sinus endoscopy with biopsy
P1-23714 Maxillary sinus endoscopy with removal of foreign body
P1-23715 Maxillary sinus endoscopy with removal of cyst
P1-23716 Maxillary sinus endoscopy with removal of mucous membrane
P1-23717 Maxillary sinus endoscopy with removal of mucous membrane and polyps
P1-23718 Maxillary sinus endoscopy with removal of polyps
P1-23719 Maxillary sinus endoscopy with removal of fungus ball
P1-23720 Nasal endoscopy with partial ethmoidectomy
P1-23724 Nasal endoscopy with total ethmoidectomy
P1-23730 Diagnostic sphenoid endoscopy
P1-23732 Sphenoid endoscopy with biopsy
P1-23734 Sphenoid endoscopy with removal of mucous membrane

1-238 Accessory Sinuses: Surgical Repairs, Closures and Reconstructions

P1-23800 Repair of nasal sinus, NOS
P1-23802 Repair of bone of accessory sinus
P1-23804 Fistulization of nasal sinus, NOS
P1-23810 Elevation of orbital bone fragments of frontal sinus
P1-23818 Reconstruction of frontonasal duct
P1-23820 Elevation of orbital bone fragments of maxillary sinus
P1-23834 Exteriorization of maxillary sinus
P1-23850 Repair of nasal sinus fistula, NOS
  Closure of nasal sinus fistula, NOS
  Closure of fistula of nasal sinus, NOS
P1-23854 Repair of oroantral fistula
  Closure of oroantral fistula
P1-23856 Repair of oromaxillary fistula
  Closure of oromaxillary fistula

1-23C Accessory Sinuses: Destructive Procedures

P1-23C10 Obliteration of maxillary sinus

1-23D Accessory Sinuses: Transplantations and Transpositions

P1-23D10 Transplantation of accessory sinus mucosa, NOS

1-23E Accessory Sinuses: Manipulations

P1-23E00 Manipulation of accessory sinus, NOS

1-25 OPERATIVE PROCEDURES ON THE LARYNX

1-250 Larynx: General and Miscellaneous Operative Procedures

P1-25010 Operation on larynx, NOS
P1-25060 Operation on vocal cord, NOS

1-251 Larynx: Incisions

P1-25100 Incision of larynx, NOS
  Laryngotomy, NOS
P1-25110 Incision and exploration of larynx
  Diagnostic laryngotomy
P1-25120 Laryngocentesis
  Puncture of larynx

1-251 Larynx: Incisions — Continued

P1-25150 Division of congenital web of larynx
P1-25160 Cordotomy of vocal cord

1-253-254 Larynx: Excisions

P1-25300 Excision of lesion of larynx, NOS
P1-25301 Incisional biopsy of larynx
P1-25302 Excisional biopsy of larynx
P1-25310 Removal of foreign body of larynx by incision
P1-25312 Core needle biopsy of larynx
P1-25313 Fine needle biopsy of larynx
  Fine needle aspiration biopsy of larynx
P1-25330V Marks procedure for laryngeal hemiplegia
P1-25332V Laryngeal ventriculectomy
P1-25340 Excision of lesion of vocal cord
P1-25342 Cordectomy of vocal cord
P1-25343 Submucous resection of vocal cord
P1-25345 Epiglottidectomy
  Excision of epiglottis
P1-25346 Ventriculocordectomy
P1-25348 Punch resection of vocal cord
P1-25350 Excision of lesion of epiglottis
P1-25360 Cricoidectomy
P1-25362 Cricothyroidectomy
  Thyrocricoidectomy
P1-25390 Arytenoidectomy by external approach
P1-25400 Laryngectomy, NOS
P1-25402 Total laryngectomy
  Total laryngectomy without radical neck dissection
P1-25404 Total laryngectomy with radical neck dissection
  Radical dissection of neck with laryngectomy
P1-25406 Hemilaryngectomy
P1-25410 Partial laryngectomy, NOS
P1-25411 Partial submucous laryngectomy
P1-25412 Partial horizontal laryngectomy
P1-25413 Partial laterovertical laryngectomy
  Partial lateral laryngectomy
P1-25414 Partial anterovertical laryngectomy
  Partial vertical laryngectomy
P1-25415 Partial antero-latero-vertical laryngectomy
P1-25416 Partial supraglottic laryngectomy
  Subtotal supraglottic laryngectomy without radical neck dissection
  Partial glottosupraglottic laryngectomy
P1-25418 Subtotal supraglottic laryngectomy with radical neck dissection
P1-25430 Laryngopharyngectomy
  Pharyngolaryngectomy
P1-25432 Total laryngectomy with partial pharyngectomy and synchronous tracheostomy
  Laryngopharyngectomy with synchronous tracheostomy
P1-25434 Radical laryngopharyngectomy with synchronous thyroidectomy
  Thyroidectomy with laryngectomy
P1-25436 Pharyngolaryngectomy with radical neck dissection without reconstruction
P1-25438 Pharyngolaryngectomy with radical neck dissection and reconstruction
P1-25439 Complete laryngectomy with radical neck dissection, synchronous thyroidectomy and synchronous tracheostomy
P1-25440 Laryngoesophagectomy
P1-25442 Laryngopharyngoesophagectomy with radical neck dissection and synchronous thyroidectomy
P1-25450 Laryngotomy with removal of laryngocele
P1-25452 Laryngotomy with removal of tumor

1-255 Larynx: Injections and Implantations

P1-25500 Injection of larynx, NOS
P1-25502 Injection of vocal cords, NOS
  Augmentation of vocal cords, NOS
P1-25530 Replacement of laryngeal stent
P1-25534 Removal of keel, tantalum plate or stent from larynx
P1-25550 Implant of larynx, NOS
  Implant of inert material into larynx
P1-25551V Teflon implant into epiglottis
P1-25552 Implant of vocal cords
  Implant of inert material into vocal cords
P1-25554 Insertion of valved tube into larynx
  Insertion of artifical pharyngeal valve
P1-25560 Insertion of oropharyngeal airway

1-257 Larynx: Endoscopy

P1-25700 Laryngoscopy, NOS
  Laryngotracheoscopy, NOS
  Endoscopic exploration of larynx, NOS
  Endoscopy of larynx, NOS
P1-25702 Endoscopy of larynx through stoma
P1-25704 Endoscopic biopsy of larynx, NOS
P1-25708 Endoscopic removal of foreign body from larynx, NOS
P1-25710 Indirect laryngoscopy, NOS
P1-25711 Indirect laryngoscopy, diagnostic
P1-25712 Indirect laryngoscopy with biopsy
P1-25714 Indirect laryngoscopy with removal of foreign body
P1-25716 Indirect laryngoscopy with removal of lesion
P1-25718 Indirect laryngoscopy with vocal cord injection
P1-25720 Direct laryngoscopy, NOS
P1-25722 Direct laryngoscopy, diagnostic, except newborn
P1-25723 Direct laryngoscopy, diagnostic, with operating microscope
P1-25724 Direct laryngoscopy, diagnostic, newborn
P1-25726 Direct laryngoscopy for aspiration
P1-25727 Direct laryngoscopy with insertion of obturator
P1-25728 Direct laryngoscopy with dilation
P1-25730 Direct laryngoscopy with foreign body removal

P1-25731 Direct laryngoscopy direct with foreign body removal with operating microscope
P1-25732 Direct laryngoscopy with biopsy
P1-25733 Direct laryngoscopy with biopsy with operating microscope
P1-25734 Direct laryngoscopy with excision of tumor
P1-25735 Direct laryngoscopy with excision of tumor with operative microscope
P1-25736 Direct laryngoscopy with stripping of vocal cords
P1-25737 Direct laryngoscopy with stripping of vocal cords with operative microscope
P1-25738 Direct laryngoscopy with stripping of epiglottis
P1-25740 Direct laryngoscopy with arytenoidectomy
P1-25741 Direct laryngoscopy with arytenoidectomy with operating microscope
P1-25744 Direct laryngoscopy with injection into vocal cord, therapeutic
P1-25745 Direct laryngoscopy with injection into vocal cord, therapeutic with operating microscope
P1-25750 Flexible fiberoptic laryngoscopy, NOS
P1-25752 Flexible fiberoptic laryngoscopy, diagnostic
P1-25754 Flexible fiberoptic laryngoscopy with biopsy
P1-25756 Flexible fiberoptic laryngoscopy with removal of foreign body
P1-25758 Flexible fiberoptic laryngoscopy with removal of lesion
P1-2575A Flexible fiberoptic laryngoscopy with stroboscopy

1-258-259 Larynx: Surgical Repairs, Closures and Reconstructions

P1-25800 Repair of larynx, NOS
P1-25802 Suture of larynx
  Laryngorrhaphy
  Repair of laceration of larynx
P1-25810 Repair of stoma of larynx
  Revision of stoma of larynx
  Repair of laryngostomy
  Laryngostomy revision
P1-25820 Closure of stoma of larynx
  Take-down of laryngostomy
  Take-down of stoma of larynx
P1-25850 Repair of fistula of larynx, NOS
  Repair of laryngeal fistula, NOS
P1-25852 Repair of laryngotracheal fistula
P1-25854 Repair of laryngotracheal cleft
P1-25860 Marsupialization of cyst of larynx
P1-25900 Laryngoplasty, NOS
P1-25910 Laryngoplasty with cricoid split
P1-25920 Laryngoplasty with open reduction of fracture
P1-25930 Laryngoplasty for laryngeal stenosis with graft
P1-25932 Laryngoplasty for laryngeal stenosis with core mold
P1-25940 Laryngoplasty for laryngeal web, two stage, with keel insertion and removal
P1-25950 Construction of artificial larynx
  Asai operation on larynx
P1-25A00 Arytenoidopexy by external approach
P1-25A10 Cordopexy of vocal cord
P1-25A20 Abduction procedure of arytenoid
P1-25A30 Arthrodesis of cricoarytenoid
P1-25A50 Repair of epiglottis, NOS
P1-25A52 Repair of fistula of vocal cord

1-25C Larynx: Destructive Procedures

P1-25C00 Destructive procedure on larynx, NOS
P1-25C02 Cauterization of larynx
P1-25C04 Cauterization of vocal cords
P1-25C10 Lysis of adhesions of larynx
P1-25C20 Stripping of vocal cords
P1-25C30 Destruction of lesion of larynx, NOS

1-25D Larynx: Transplantations and Transpositions

P1-25D00 Graft of larynx, NOS
P1-25D10 Transposition of vocal cords
P1-25D40 Laryngeal reinnervation by neuromuscular pedicle

1-25E Larynx: Manipulations

P1-25E00 Dilation of larynx
P1-25E20 Reduction of fracture of larynx, NOS
  Treatment of closed laryngeal fracture with closed manipulative reduction
P1-25E24 Treatment of closed laryngeal fracture without manipulation

1-26 OPERATIVE PROCEDURES ON THE TRACHEA AND BRONCHI

1-260 Trachea and Bronchi: General and Miscellaneous Operative Procedures

P1-26000 Operation on trachea and bronchus, NOS
P1-26010 Operation on bronchus, NOS
P1-26040 Operation on trachea, NOS

1-261 Trachea and Bronchi: Incisions

P1-26100 Incision of trachea, NOS
  Tracheostomy, NOS
  Tracheotomy, NOS
P1-26102 Incision and exploration of trachea
P1-26120 Planned tracheostomy
P1-26122 Planned tracheostomy, under two years
P1-26124 Permanent tracheostomy, NOS
  Tracheostomy, fenestration procedure with skin flaps
P1-26128 Temporary tracheostomy
P1-26130 Tracheostomy, emergency procedure by transtracheal approach
  Emergency tracheotomy for assistance in breathing
  Emergency tracheostomy for assistance in breathing

1-261 Trachea and Bronchi: Incisions — Continued

P1-26132 Tracheostomy, emergency procedure by cricothyroid membrane approach
  Thyrocricotomy for assistance in breathing
  Cricothyreotomy for assistance in breathing
P1-26138 Thyrocondrotomy
P1-26140 Mediastinal tracheostomy
P1-26180 Incision of bronchus, NOS
  Bronchostomy, NOS
  Bronchotomy, NOS
P1-26182 Incision and exploration of bronchus
P1-26190 Aspiration of trachea, percutaneous
  Tracheal puncture, percutaneous for aspiration of mucus
P1-26192 Puncture and aspiration of bronchus
P1-26194 Nasotracheal aspiration, NOS

1-263 Trachea and Bronchi: Excisions

P1-26300 Biopsy of trachea
P1-26302 Excision of lesion of trachea
P1-26304 Excision of tracheal tumor by cervical approach
P1-26306 Excision of tracheal tumor by thoracic approach
P1-26310 Removal of foreign body from trachea by incision
P1-26314 Core needle biopsy of trachea
P1-26315 Fine needle biopsy of trachea
  Fine needle aspiration biopsy of trachea
P1-26340 Resection of trachea
P1-26350 Open biopsy of bronchus
P1-26352 Excision of lesion of bronchus
P1-26354 Excision of bronchogenic cyst
P1-26360 Core needle biopsy of bronchus
P1-26362 Fine needle biopsy of bronchus
  Aspiration biopsy of bronchus
P1-26380 Excision of bronchus, wide sleeve, NOS

1-265 Trachea and Bronchi: Injections and Implantations

P1-26500 Injection of trachea, percutaneous, NOS
P1-26502 Transtracheal percutaneous injection for bronchography
P1-26504 Injection of locally acting therapeutic substance into trachea, percutaneous
P1-26510 Irrigation of trachea, NOS
  Aspiration of trachea with lavage, NOS
  Lavage of trachea, NOS
P1-26513 Nasotracheobronchial catheter aspiration
P1-26514 Tracheobronchial catheter aspiration with fiberscope, bedside
P1-26520 Insertion of endotracheal tube
  Intubation of trachea
P1-26521 Transglottic catheterization of trachea
P1-26522 Intubation of larynx
P1-26523 Laryngeal catheterization
P1-26524 Endotracheal intubation, emergency procedure
P1-26530 Percutaneous transtracheal introduction of indwelling tube for therapy
P1-26540 Replacement of tracheal stent
P1-26560 Catheterization of bronchus
  Insertion of catheter into bronchus
P1-26562 Catheterization of bronchus with lavage, NOS
  Irrigation of bronchus, NOS
  Aspiration of bronchus with lavage, NOS
  Lavage of bronchus, NOS
  Bronchoalveolar lavage
  BAL procedure
P1-26570 Catheterization for bronchography
P1-26572 Instillation of contrast material for bronchography without catheterization
P1-26580 Catheterization with bronchial brush biopsy

1-267 Trachea and Bronchi: Endoscopy

P1-26700 Endoscopy of trachea, NOS
  Tracheoscopy, NOS
P1-26702 Endoscopy of trachea through stoma
P1-26710 Endoscopic biopsy of trachea
P1-26714 Endoscopic brush biopsy of trachea
P1-26724 Endoscopic removal of intraluminal foreign body from trachea
P1-26730 Bronchoscopy, NOS
  Endoscopy of bronchus, NOS
P1-26732 Fiberoptic bronchoscopy
P1-26734 Fiberoptic bronchoscopy with biopsy of bronchus
P1-26740 Bronchoscopy with cell washing or brushing
P1-26741 Bronchoscopy with brush biopsy
P1-26742 Bronchoscopy with cell washing
P1-26750 Bronchoscopy with biopsy
  Endoscopy of bronchus with biopsy
P1-26751 Endoscopy with excision of lesion from bronchus
P1-26752 Bronchoscopy with excision of tumor
P1-26753 Removal of intraluminal foreign body bronchus
P1-26756 Bronchoscopy with closed reduction of fracture
P1-26760 Tracheobronchoscopy through established tracheostomy incision
  Bronchoscopy through tracheostomy
P1-26762 Bronchoscopy through tracheostomy with biopsy of bronchus
P1-26763 Bronchoscopy through tracheostomy with biopsy of lung
P1-26764 Bronchoscopy with destruction of tumor by laser surgery
P1-26765 Bronchoscopy for relief of stenosis with laser surgery
P1-26770 Bronchoscopy with transbronchial lung biopsy
  Fiberoptic bronchoscopy with biopsy of lung
P1-26772 Bronchoscopy with transbronchial lung biopsy, with fluoroscopic guidance

P1-26774 Bronchoscopy with transbronchial needle aspiration biopsy
P1-26780 Bronchoscopy with bronchial dilation
P1-26781 Bronchoscopy with tracheal dilation
P1-26782 Bronchoscopy with tracheal dilation and placement of tracheal stent
P1-26783 Bronchoscopy with removal of foreign body
P1-26784 Bronchoscopy with drainage of lung abscess
P1-26786 Bronchoscopy with therapeutic aspiration of tracheobronchial tree, initial
P1-26788 Bronchoscopy with therapeutic aspiration of tracheobronchial tree, subsequent
P1-26790 Bronchoscopy with injection of contrast material for segmental bronchography
P1-26799 Bronchoscopy with unlisted bronchoscopic procedure
P1-267A0 Laryngotracheobronchoscopy
P1-267A2 Laryngotracheobronchoscopy with biopsy

1-268-269 Trachea and Bronchi: Surgical Repairs, Closures and Reconstructions

P1-26800 Repair of trachea, NOS
  Tracheoplasty, NOS
P1-26802 Suture of trachea
  Tracheorrhaphy
  Suture of laceration of trachea
P1-26804 Suture of external tracheal wound or injury by cervical approach
P1-26806 Suture of external tracheal wound or injury by intrathoracic approach
P1-26812 Tracheoplasty by cervical approach
P1-26814 Tracheoplasty by intrathoracic approach
P1-26820 Closure of tracheostomy
  Closure of stoma of trachea
  Take-down of stoma of trachea
P1-26821 Revision of tracheostomy
  Revision of stoma of trachea
  Repair of stoma of trachea
P1-26822 Tracheostomy revision, simple, without flap rotation
P1-26823 Tracheostomy revision, complex with flap rotation
P1-26824 Surgical closure of tracheostomy with plastic repair
P1-26825 Surgical closure of tracheostomy without plastic repair
P1-26828 Repair of tracheal fistula
  Surgical closure of tracheal fistula without plastic repair
P1-26829 Surgical closure of tracheal fistula with plastic repair
P1-2682A Closure of external fistula of trachea
P1-2682B Repair of internal or complex fistula of trachea
P1-26850 Carinal reconstruction
P1-26860 Revision of tracheostomy scar
P1-26870 Excision of tracheal stenosis and anastomosis by cervical approach
P1-26874 Excision of tracheal stenosis and anastomosis by cervicothoracic approach
P1-26890 Construction of tracheoesophageal fistula and subsequent insertion of an alaryngeal speech prosthesis
P1-26892 Tracheoplasty with creation of tracheopharyngeal fistulization, each stage
P1-26893 Repair of tracheoesophageal fistula
P1-26900 Repair of bronchus, NOS
P1-26904 Suture of bronchus, NOS
  Bronchorrhaphy, NOS
  Repair of laceration of bronchus by suture
  Suture of laceration of bronchus
P1-26910 Repair of stoma of bronchus
  Revision of stoma of bronchus
P1-26920 Take-down of stoma of bronchus
  Bronchostomy closure
P1-26930 Bronchoplasty, NOS
P1-26934 Bronchoplasty with excision of stenosis and anastomosis
P1-26936 Bronchotracheal anastomosis
  Anastomosis of bronchus to trachea
P1-26940 Repair of bronchocutaneous fistula
P1-26942 Repair of bronchoesophageal fistula
P1-26944 Repair of bronchovisceral fistula

1-26C Trachea and Bronchi: Destructive Procedures

P1-26C00 Local destruction of lesion of trachea, NOS
P1-26C10 Lysis of adhesions of trachea
P1-26C50 Local destruction of lesion of bronchus, NOS
P1-26C60 Ligation of bronchus

1-26D Trachea and Bronchi: Transplantations and Transpositions

P1-26D00 Graft of trachea
P1-26D02 Reconstruction of trachea with graft
P1-26D40 Bronchoplasty with graft repair

1-26E Trachea and Bronchi: Manipulations

P1-26E00 Dilation of trachea
P1-26E40 Dilation of bronchus

1-28 OPERATIVE PROCEDURES ON THE LUNGS AND PLEURA

1-280 Lungs and Pleura: General and Miscellaneous Operatives Procedures

P1-28010 Operation on lung, NOS
  Pulmonary operation, NOS
P1-28040 Operation on pleural cavity, NOS
P1-28042 Control of hemorrhage of pleural cavity, NOS
P1-28044 Control of postoperative hemorrhage of pleural cavity

1-281 Lungs and Pleura: Incisions

P1-28100 Incision of lung, NOS
 Pneumonotomy, NOS
P1-28102 Incision and exploration of lung
P1-28110 Drainage of lung by incision
 Cavernostomy of lung
 Pneumonostomy with open drainage
P1-28120 Pneumocentesis
 Pneumonocentesis
 Puncture of lung for aspiration
P1-28152 Tube thoracostomy with water seal
 Closed drainage of pleura
P1-28154 Tube thoracostomy without water seal
 Tube drainage of pleural cavity
P1-28160 Thoracentesis
 Pleurocentesis
 Puncture of pleural cavity for aspiration
P1-28164 Thoracentesis with insertion of tube with water seal for pneumothorax
P1-28166 Thoracentesis with insertion of tube without water seal for pneumothorax
P1-28170 Thoracostomy with open flap drainage for empyema
P1-28172 Thoracostomy with rib resection for empyema
P1-28174 Major thoracotomy with cardiac massage
P1-28199 Incision of pleura, NOS

1-283 Lungs and Pleura: Excisions

P1-28300 Biopsy of lung, NOS
P1-28302 Limited thoracotomy for biopsy of lung, NOS
P1-28304 Excision of lesion of lung, NOS
P1-28306 Wedge resection of lung, single site
 Segmental excision of lung
P1-28308 Wedge resection of lung, multiple sites
 Segmental lobectomy of lung with resection of adjacent lobes
P1-28310 Segmental lobectomy
 Partial lobectomy of lung
P1-28311 Apicectomy lung
P1-28312 Segmental lobectomy with bronchoplasty
P1-28314 Segmental lobectomy with concomitant decortication
P1-28316 Lingulectomy of lung
P1-28320 Percutaneous core needle biopsy of lung
P1-28322 Percutaneous fine needle biopsy of lung
 Percutaneous fine needle aspiration biopsy of lung
P1-28330 Total lobectomy of lung
 Lobectomy of lung
P1-28332 Total lobectomy with bronchoplasty
P1-28334 Total lobectomy of lung with concomitant decortication
P1-28339 Excision of accessory or ectopic lung tissue
P1-28350 Pneumonectomy
 Total pneumonectomy
P1-28354 Extrapleural pneumonectomy without empyemectomy
P1-28356 Extrapleural pneumonectomy with empyemectomy
P1-28360 Major thoracotomy with exploration and biopsy of lung
P1-28361 Thoracotomy for excision of emphysematous bleb of lung
 Excision of cyst of lung
P1-28362 Major thoracotomy with cyst removal and with a pleural procedure
P1-28363 Major thoracotomy with excision or plication of bullae with a pleural procedure
P1-28364 Major thoracotomy with excision or plication of bullae
 Stapling of emphysematous blebs
 Plication of emphysematous bleb
P1-28370 Major thoracotomy with removal of intrapulmonary foreign body
 Thoracotomy for removal of foreign body from lung
P1-28374 Major thoracotomy with control of traumatic hemorrhage and repair of lung tear
P1-28375 Major thoracotomy for postoperative complications
P1-28390 Radical resection of thoracic structures
P1-28391 Resection of lung with resection of chest wall
P1-28392 Resection of lung with reconstruction of chest wall without prosthesis
P1-28393 Resection of lung with major reconstruction of chest wall with prosthesis
P1-28394 Complete excision of lung with mediastinal dissection
 Mediastinotomy with pneumonectomy
P1-28396 Excision of Pancoast tumor of lung
P1-283A0 Open biopsy of pleura
 Limited thoracotomy for biopsy of pleura
 Open pleural biopsy
P1-283A2 Percutaneous core needle biopsy of pleura
P1-283A3 Percutaneous fine needle biopsy of pleura
 Fine needle aspiration biopsy of pleura
P1-283C0 Major thoracotomy with open intrapleural pneumonolysis
P1-283C2 Major thoracotomy with removal of fibrin deposit
P1-283C4 Major thoracotomy with removal of intrapleural foreign body
P1-283D0 Pleurectomy, NOS
 Excision of pleura, NOS
P1-283D2 Parietal pleurectomy
 Total decortication of lung
P1-283D4 Partial pleurectomy
 Partial decortication of lung
P1-283D6 Decortication of lung and parietal pleurectomy
P1-283D8 Empyemectomy
P1-283D9 Empyemectomy with lobectomy

1-285 Lungs and Pleura: Injections and Implantations

P1-28500 Therapeutic pneumothorax
 Therapeutic pneumothorax with intrapleural injection of air

P1-28500 (cont.) Therapeutic collapse of lung

P1-28510 Surgical pneumoperitoneum for collapse of lung

P1-28520 Plombage of lung

P1-28522 Creation of oleothorax

P1-28540 Removal of tube from pleural cavity
  Removal of thoracotomy tube

1-287 Lungs and Pleura: Endoscopy

P1-28700 Endoscopy of lung, NOS

1-288 Lungs and Pleura: Surgical Repairs, Closures and Reconstructions

P1-28800 Repair of lung, NOS

P1-28810 Suture of lung, NOS
  Closure of laceration of lung, NOS

P1-28820 Open repair of major bronchial fistula, NOS

P1-28830 Repair of pleura, NOS
  Suture of pleura, NOS

P1-28832 Pleuropexy

P1-28840 Repair of pleural fistula, NOS

P1-28841 Repair of bronchopleural fistula

P1-28842 Repair of bronchopleurocutaneous fistula

P1-28843 Repair of bronchopleuromediastinal fistula

P1-28844 Repair of esophagopleurocutaneous fistula

P1-28845 Repair of hepatopleural fistula

P1-28846 Repair of pleurocutaneous fistula

P1-28847 Repair of pleuroperitoneal fistula

P1-28860 Repair of lung hernia through chest wall

1-28C Lungs and Pleura: Destructive Procedures

P1-28C00 Surgical collapse of lung, NOS
  Thoracolysis for collapse of lung

P1-28C02 Local destruction of lesion of lung

P1-28C08 Cauterization of lung

P1-28C10 Surgical collapse of lung by destruction of phrenic nerve
  Phrenicectomy for collapse of lung
  Phrenicotripsy for collapse of lung
  Avulsion of phrenic nerve for collapse of lung
  Phrenicoexeresis for collapse of lung
  Phrenemphraxis for collapse of lung

P1-28C20 Pneumonolysis, NOS
  Pneumonolysis for collapse of lung

P1-28C21 Pneumonolysis, extraperiosteal, including filling or packing procedures

P1-28C22 Pleurolysis
  Lysis of adhesions of pleura

P1-28C30 Pleurodesis, NOS
  Scarification of pleura
  Obliteration of pleural cavity
  Pleurosclerosis

P1-28C31 Pleural scarification for repeat pneumothorax

P1-28C32 Chemical pleurodesis, NOS
  Chemical pleurosclerosis, NOS

P1-28C33 Chemotherapy administration into pleural cavity requiring thoracentesis

P1-28C34 Pleurodesis with cancer chemotherapy substance

P1-28C36 Pleurodesis with tetracycline

P1-28C38 Pleural poudrage
  Pleural abrasion

1-28D Lungs and Pleura: Transplantations and Transpositions

P1-28D00 Transplant of lung, NOS

P1-28D10 Autotransplant of lung

P1-28D20 Reimplantation of lung

1-28E Lungs and Pleura: Manipulations

P1-28E10 Manipulation of lung, NOS

SECTION 1-3 OPERATIVE PROCEDURES ON THE CARDIOVASCULAR SYSTEM

1-30 GENERAL OPERATIVE PROCEDURES ON THE CARDIOVASCULAR SYSTEM

1-300 Cardiovascular System: General and Miscellaneous Operative Procedures

P1-30000 Cardiovascular procedure, NOS

P1-30010 Vascular surgery procedure, NOS
  Operation on vessels, NOS

P1-30022 Diagnostic procedure on blood vessel, NOS

P1-30080 Control of hemorrhage, NOS

P1-30081 Control of postoperative hemorrhage, NOS

P1-30082 Control of hemorrhage following vascular surgery, NOS

1-301 Cardiovascular System: Incisions

P1-30100 Incision of blood vessel, NOS
  Angiotomy, NOS

P1-30102 Exploration of blood vessel, NOS

P1-30104 Division of aberrant vessel, NOS

P1-30105 Division of aberrant vessel with reanastomosis

P1-30110 Incision of artery, NOS
  Arteriotomy, NOS

P1-30114 Exploration of artery, NOS

P1-30115 Transection of artery with ligation
  Division of artery with ligation

P1-30120 Puncture of artery, NOS
  Arterial puncture, NOS

P1-30122 Arterial puncture for withdrawal of blood for diagnosis

P1-30124 Percutaneous arterial cutdown

P1-30126 Arterial cutdown for prolonged infusion therapy

1-301 Cardiovascular System: Incisions — Continued

P1-30130 Aneurysmotomy, NOS

1-303 Cardiovascular System: Excisions

P1-30300 Excision of blood vessel, NOS
  Angiectomy, NOS
P1-30302 Excision of artery, NOS
  Arteriectomy, NOS
P1-30310 Biopsy of blood vessel, NOS
  Excisional biopsy of blood vessel, NOS
P1-30312 Biopsy of artery, NOS
  Excisional biopsy of artery, NOS
P1-30314 Excision of lesion of blood vessel, NOS
P1-30316 Excision of lesion of artery, NOS
P1-30320 Removal of embolus, NOS
  Embolectomy, NOS
P1-30322 Removal of thrombus, NOS
  Thrombectomy, NOS
P1-30324 Aneurysmectomy, NOS
  Dissection of aneurysm and removal, NOS
P1-30326 Excision of arteriovenous aneurysm
  Excision of arteriovenous fistula
P1-30327 Aneurysmectomy with anastomosis
P1-30328 Aneurysmectomy with graft replacement by interposition
P1-30330 Endarterectomy, NOS
  Intimectomy
P1-30331 Gas endarterectomy
P1-30332 Gas endarterectomy with patch graft
P1-30333 Thromboendarterectomy
P1-30334 Angiectomy with graft replacement by interposition
P1-30335 Arteriectomy with graft replacement by interposition
P1-30336 Angiectomy with anastomosis
P1-30337 Arteriectomy with anastomosis
P1-30340 Thrombectomy of arterial graft
P1-30341 Thrombectomy and repair of arterial graft
P1-30342 Removal of embolus of bovine graft
  Embolectomy of bovine graft
P1-30343 Removal of thrombus of bovine graft
  Thrombectomy of bovine graft
P1-30344 Removal of embolus from arteriovenous shunt or cannula
P1-30345 Removal of thrombus from arteriovenous shunt or cannula
P1-30360 Removal of vascular graft or prosthesis, NOS
P1-30362 Removal of arterial graft or prosthesis, NOS
P1-30370 Resection of vessel with anastomosis, NOS
P1-30372 Resection of vessel with replacement, NOS
P1-30380 Excision of infected graft
P1-30381 Excision of infected graft with revascularization

1-305 Cardiovascular System: Injections and Implantations

P1-30500 Injection of cardiovascular system, NOS
  Vascular injection, NOS
  Injection of blood vessel, NOS
P1-30520 Insertion of vessel-to-vessel cannula, NOS
P1-30521 Insertion of Allen-Brown cannula
P1-30522 Cannulation of artery
P1-30523 Insertion of catheter into artery
  Catheterization of artery
P1-30524 Direct arteriovenous anastomosis
  Arteriovenous cannulation
  Arteriovenous catheterization
P1-30525 Arterial catheterization or cannulation for monitoring, percutaneous
P1-30526 Arterial catheterization or cannulation for sampling, percutaneous
P1-30527 Introduction of catheter for arteriovenous shunt created for dialysis
P1-30528 Introduction of needle for arteriovenous shunt created for dialysis
P1-30529 Implantation of tissue mandril for vascular graft
  Insertion of mandril
P1-3052A Pilojection of aneurysm, Gallagher type
P1-30530 Selective embolization of artery
P1-30532 Replacement of cannula of arteriovenous shunt
P1-30534 Irrigation of vascular catheter, NOS
P1-30537 Total body perfusion
P1-30540 Insertion of cannula for hemodialysis, NOS
P1-30541 Arteriovenous shunt for renal dialysis by external cannula
  Creation of arteriovenous shunt or fistula for dialysis by external cannula
  Formation of arteriovenous fistula by external cannula for renal dialysis
P1-30542 Insertion of cannula for hemodialysis, unlisted purpose, arteriovenous, external
  Insertion of Scribner shunt
  Insertion of cannula for hemodialysis, unlisted purpose, arteriovenous, external, Scribner type
P1-30543 Insertion of cannula for hemodialysis, unlisted purpose, arteriovenous, external closure
  Insertion of cannula for hemodialysis, unlisted purpose, arteriovenous, external revision
P1-30546 Insertion of cannula for hemodialysis, unlisted purpose, arteriovenous, internal
  Insertion of cannula for hemodialysis, unlisted purpose, arteriovenous, internal, Cimino type
P1-30550 Insertion of Thomas shunt
P1-30554 Insertion of implantable intra-arterial infusion pump
P1-30555 Revision of implanted intra-arterial infusion pump

P1-30557 Cannula declotting without balloon catheter
P1-30558 Cannula declotting with balloon catheter
P1-30560 Removal of arteriovenous shunt device
P1-30561 Removal of Scribner shunt
P1-30562 Removal of implanted intra-arterial infusion pump
P1-30563 Removal of arteriovenous shunt for renal dialysis
P1-30567 Revision of vessel-to-vessel arteriovenous cannula
P1-30568 Revision of arteriovenous shunt for renal dialysis
Revision of cannula for dialysis
P1-30580 Prolonged extracorporeal circulation for cardiopulmonary bypass
P1-30581 Regional extracorporeal circulation, except hepatic
P1-30585 Cardioassist by aortic balloon pump
P1-30589 Insertion of cannula for prolonged extracorporeal circulation for cardiopulmonary insufficiency

1-307 Cardiovascular System: Endoscopy

P1-30700 Percutaneous angioscopy, NOS

1-308-309 Cardiovascular System: Surgical Repairs, Closures and Reconstructions

P1-30800 Repair of blood vessel, NOS
Angioplasty, NOS
P1-30802 Repair of great vessels, NOS
P1-30804 Repair of artery, NOS
Arterioplasty, NOS
P1-30812 Repair of aneurysm, NOS
Repair of aneurysm, false or true
P1-30814 Repair of arteriovenous fistula
Plastic repair of arteriovenous aneurysm
P1-30820 Reattachment of peripheral vessels, NOS
P1-30822 Great vessel repair with unlisted major procedure
P1-30824 Rastelli operation in repair of transposition of great vessels
P1-30830 Repair of graft-enteric fistula
P1-30832 Repair of aneurysm without graft of unspecified artery
P1-30833 Repair of ruptured aneurysm without graft of unspecified artery
P1-30834 Repair of arteriovenous fistula by division
P1-30836 Repair of arteriovenous fistula by coagulation
P1-30838 Arteriovenous fistulization
P1-30839 Repair of laceration of great vessels
P1-30840 Repair of blood vessel with patch graft, NOS
Grafting of blood vessel with patch, NOS
P1-30841 Repair of blood vessel with synthetic, dacron or teflon patch graft
Grafting of blood vessel with synthetic patch, dacron or teflon
P1-30842 Repair of blood vessel with tissue patch graft of vein, autogenous or homograft
Grafting of blood vessel with tissue patch of vein, autogenous or homograft
P1-30843 Implantation of tissue mandril with blood vessel repair
Insertion of tissue mandril, Spark type, with blood vessel repair
P1-30845 Repair of artery with patch graft
Grafting of artery with patch
P1-30846 Repair of artery with synthetic, dacron or teflon patch graft
Grafting of artery with synthetic, dacron or teflon patch
P1-30847 Repair of artery with tissue patch graft of vein, autogenous or homograft
Grafting of artery with tissue patch of vein, autogenous or homograft
P1-30848 Arterial bypass graft with vein, NOS
P1-30850 Insertion of graft of great vessels without bypass
P1-30852 Insertion of graft of great vessels with cardiopulmonary bypass
P1-30853 Repair of aneurysm with graft of unspecified artery
P1-30854 Repair of ruptured aneurysm with graft of unspecified artery
P1-30855 Creation of arteriovenous fistula by autogenous graft
P1-30856 Composite bypass graft
P1-30857 Revision of arteriovenous fistula without thrombectomy with autogenous graft
P1-30858 Revision of arteriovenous fistula without thrombectomy with nonautogenous graft
P1-30859 Revision of arteriovenous fistula with thrombectomy with autogenous graft
P1-3085A Revision of arteriovenous fistula with thrombectomy with nonautogenous graft
P1-3085B Creation of arteriovenous fistula with nonautogenous graft
P1-30862 Anastomosis of artery by suture of distal to proximal end
P1-30864 Surgical construction of arteriovenous shunt, NOS
Arteriovenous shunt, NOS
Arteriovenostomy, NOS
Formation of arteriovenous shunt
Arteriovenous anastomosis
P1-30865 Mandril anastomosis
P1-30866 Arteriovenous anastomosis for renal dialysis
Arteriovenostomy for renal dialysis
Formation of arteriovenous fistula for kidney dialysis
Arteriovenous shunt for renal dialysis
P1-30870 Creation of vascular bypass, NOS
P1-30871 Anastomosis of artery with bypass graft, NOS
Creation of arterial vascular bypass, NOS
P1-30872 Creation of arterial bypass with vein graft

1-308-309 Cardiovascular System: Surgical Repairs, Closures and Reconstructions — Continued

P1-30873 Creation of arterial bypass with mandril grown graft
P1-30874 Creation of arterial bypass with nonautogenous graft
P1-30875 Creation of arterial bypass with synthetic graft
P1-30880 Revision of vascular procedure, NOS
P1-30881 Revision of anastomosis of blood vessel, NOS
P1-30882 Revision of anastomosis of artery, NOS
P1-30890 Take-down of vascular anastomosis or bypass
  Take-down of vascular anastomosis
  Take-down of anastomosis of blood vessel
P1-30891 Take-down of arterial bypass
P1-30892 Take-down of arterial anastomosis
P1-30894 Take-down of arteriovenous shunt
P1-30895 Take-down of arteriovenous shunt with creation of new shunt
  Removal of arteriovenous shunt with creation of new shunt
P1-30900 Repair of blood vessel with suture, NOS
  Suture of blood vessel, NOS
  Angiorrhaphy, NOS
P1-30902 Repair of artery with suture
  Angiorrhaphy of artery
  Arteriorrhaphy
  Suture of artery
P1-30904 Suture of great vessel
  Repair of laceration of great vessels by suture
P1-30905 Suture of artery of great vessels
P1-30910 Repair of aneurysm by suture
  Aneurysmorrhaphy by suture
  Aneurysmorrhaphy
P1-30912 Aneurysmoplasty
  Matas operation for aneurysm
  Endoaneurysmorrhaphy
  Endoaneurysmoplasty
P1-30913 Aneurysmorrhaphy by clipping
  Repair of aneurysm by clipping
  Clipping of aneurysm
P1-30914 Aneurysmorrhaphy by electrocoagulation
  Repair of aneurysm by coagulation
  Repair of aneurysm by electrocoagulation
P1-30915 Aneurysmorrhaphy by filipuncture
  Repair of aneurysm by filipuncture
P1-30916 Aneurysmorrhaphy by wiring
  Aneurysmorrhaphy by wrapping
  Repair of aneurysm by trapping
  Repair of aneurysm by wiring
P1-30918 Aneurysmorrhaphy by methyl methacrylate
  Repair of aneurysm by methyl methacrylate
P1-30920 Suture repair of great vessels with cardiopulmonary bypass
P1-30921 Suture repair of great vessels without bypass
P1-30922 Repair of arteriovenous fistula by suture
  Suture of arteriovenous fistula
  Ligation of arteriovenous fistula
P1-30923 Division of arteriovenous fistula with ligation
  Repair of arteriovenous fistula by ligation
P1-30930 Surgical occlusion of blood vessel, NOS
P1-30931 Ligation of blood vessel, NOS
P1-30932 Ligation of artery, NOS
P1-30933 Stapling of artery, NOS
P1-30934 Repair of aneurysm by occlusion
P1-30935 Repair of aneurysm by ligation
  Ligation of aneurysm
P1-30937 Repair of arterial graft
P1-30946 Repair of arteriovenous fistula by occlusion
P1-30947 Repair of arteriovenous fistula by clipping
  Clipping of arteriovenous fistula

1-30C Cardiovascular System: Destructive Procedures

P1-30C00 Destructive procedure of blood vessel, NOS
  Angiotripsy, NOS
P1-30C10 Lysis of adhesions of blood vessel, NOS
  Lysis of adhesions of peripheral blood vessel, NOS
  Freeing of blood vessel, NOS
P1-30C12 Lysis of adhesions of artery-vein-nerve bundle
  Freeing of vascular bundle
  Freeing of artery-vein-nerve bundle
  Dissection of vascular bundle
  Dissection of artery-vein-nerve bundle
P1-30C14 Coagulation or electrocoagulation of arteriovenous fistula
P1-30C16 Embolization of arteriovenous fistula

1-30D Cardiovascular System: Transplantations and Transpositions

P1-30D00 Transplantation of blood vessel, NOS
P1-30D02 Transplantation of artery, NOS
P1-30D04 Reimplantation of artery, NOS

1-30E Cardiovascular System: Manipulations

P1-30E00 Manipulation of cardiovascular system, NOS

1-31 OPERATIVE PROCEDURES ON THE HEART

1-310 Heart: General and Miscellaneous Operative Procedures

P1-31000 Operative procedure on heart, NOS
  Cardiac surgery procedure, NOS
  Operation on heart, NOS
P1-31002 Exploration of heart
P1-31004 Open heart surgery, NOS
P1-31005 Systemic hypothermia in open heart surgery
P1-31010 Diagnostic procedure on heart, NOS
P1-31012 Diagnostic procedure on papillary muscle of heart
P1-31020 Revision of heart procedure, NOS

P1-31021 Revision of corrective procedure on heart, NOS
P1-31030 Operation on papillary muscle of heart, NOS
P1-31031 Operation on chordae tendineae, NOS
P1-31032 Operation on trabeculae carneae cordis, NOS
P1-31034 Operation on cardiac septum, NOS
P1-31080 Operation on heart and pericardium, NOS
P1-31090 Temporary cardioassist with artificial heart

1-311 Heart: Incisions

P1-31100 Incision of heart, NOS
  Cardiotomy
  Cardiac valvotomy, NOS
P1-31102 Exploratory cardiotomy
P1-31104 Incision of atrium of heart, NOS
  Atriotomy, NOS
P1-31110 Cardiocentesis
  Puncture of heart
P1-31111 Decompression of heart
P1-31120 Incision of subvalvular tissue for discrete subvalvular aortic stenosis
P1-31121 Ventriculomyotomy for idiopathic hypertrophic subaortic stenosis
P1-31124 Division of papillary muscle of heart
P1-31125 Division of chordae tendineae
P1-31126 Division of trabeculae carneae cordis
P1-31130 Atrial septostomy
  Interatrial fistulization
  Formation of interatrial fistula
  Formation of interatrial septal defect
  Creation of atrial septal defect
  Blalock-Hanlon operation
  Creation of interatrial fistula
P1-31131 Closed atrial septostomy
P1-31132 Open atrial septostomy with inflow occlusion
P1-31133 Atrial septostomy by transvenous balloon method, Rashkind type
  Rashkind operation
  Balloon atrioseptostomy
  Atrial septectomy by transvenous balloon method, Rashkind type
P1-31134 Atrial septostomy by blade method
P1-31140 Exploratory cardiotomy with removal of foreign body without bypass
P1-31142 Exploratory cardiotomy with removal of foreign body with cardiopulmonary bypass
P1-31150 Incision of endocardium, NOS
P1-31152 Incision of myocardium, NOS
  Myocardiotomy
P1-31153 Ventriculomyocardiotomy
  Ventriculotomy of heart
P1-31156 Enlargement of pre-existing atrial septal defect
P1-31157 Enlargement of pre-existing foramen ovale

1-313-314 Heart: Excisions

P1-31300 Myocardial resection, NOS
  Resection of myocardium, NOS
P1-31304 Resection of left ventricle of heart
P1-31307 Excision of trabeculae carneae cordis
P1-31310 Biopsy of heart, NOS
  Excisional biopsy of heart, NOS
P1-31312 Endomyocardial biopsy
P1-31320 Aneurysmectomy of heart, NOS
  Excision of aneurysm of heart, NOS
  Excision of aneurysm of myocardium, NOS
P1-31321 Atrial aneurysmectomy
P1-31322 Auricular aneurysmectomy
P1-31323 Aneurysmectomy of ventricle of heart
  Ventricular aneurysmectomy
P1-31325 Excision of aneurysm of sinus of Valsalva
P1-31330 Excision of intracardiac tumor with cardiopulmonary bypass
P1-31332 Resection of external cardiac tumor
P1-31333 Resection of subvalvular tissue for discrete subvalvular aortic stenosis
  Excision of aortic subvalvular ring
P1-31334 Ventriculomyectomy for idiopathic hypertrophic subaortic stenosis
P1-31335 Right ventricular resection for infundibular stenosis with commissurotomy
P1-31336 Right ventricular resection for infundibular stenosis without commissurotomy
  Infundibulectomy of heart
  Resection of infundibulum of right heart
  Resection of right ventricle of heart for infundibular stenosis
P1-31337 Infundibulectomy of ventricle in total repair of tetralogy of Fallot
P1-31339 Excision of common wall between posterior left atrium and coronary sinus with roofing of resultant defect with patch graft
P1-31340 Closed atrial septectomy
P1-31341 Open atrial septectomy with inflow occlusion
  Open atrial septectomy
P1-31342 Atrial septectomy by blade method
P1-31350 Excision of lesion of heart, NOS
  Excision of lesion of myocardium, NOS
P1-31351 Excision of lesion of ventricle of heart
P1-31352 Excision of lesion of atrium
P1-31353 Excision of cardioma
P1-31354 Excision of diverticulum of ventricle of heart
P1-31356 Myocardiectomy of infarcted area
P1-31360 Removal of foreign body from heart
P1-31400 Donor cardiectomy-pneumonectomy with preparation and maintenance of homograft
P1-31402 Heart-lung transplant with recipient cardiectomy-pneumonectomy
P1-31404 Donor cardiectomy with preparation and maintenance of homograft

1-315-316 Heart: Injections and Implantations

P1-31500 Injection of heart, NOS
  Puncture of heart for intracardiac injection, NOS

1-315-316 Heart: Injections and Implantations — Continued

P1-31502 Intracardiac injection for cardiac resuscitation
P1-31504 Injection of therapeutic substance into heart
  Introduction of therapeutic substance into heart
P1-31505 Induced cardioplegia
  Induced cardiac arrest
P1-31506 Insertion of carotid pacemaker
  Implantation of electronic stimulator into carotid sinus
P1-31510 Insertion of intracardiac pacemaker, NOS
  Insertion of cardiac pacemaker, NOS
  Insertion of electrode in heart, NOS
  Implantation of cardiac electrode, NOS
P1-31511 Insertion of permanent pacemaker with transvenous electrodes, ventricular
  Initial insertion of transvenous pacemaker electrode leads into ventricle
  Initial insertion of electrode into ventricle of heart
P1-31512 Insertion of permanent pacemaker with transvenous electrodes, AV sequential
P1-31513 Insertion of permanent transvenous electrodes
P1-31514 Replacement of permanent transvenous electrodes
  Repositioning of permanent transvenous electrodes
P1-31515 Repair of pacemaker electrodes
  Repair of cardiac pacemaker electrode, NOS
P1-31516 Repair of pacemaker with replacement of pulse generator
  Repair of cardiac pacemaker with replacement of pulse generator
P1-31520 Initial implantation of electrode into cardiac atrium and ventricle
  Initial insertion of transvenous lead electrodes into atrium and ventricle
P1-31522 Temporary insertion of pacemaker into atrium by transvenous route
  Implantation of cardiac electrode, temporary transvenous pacemaker system
  Insertion of temporary transvenous cardiac electrode and pacemaker catheter
P1-31523 Initial implantation of electrode into cardiac atrium
  Initial insertion of transvenous lead electrode into atrium
P1-31524 Insertion of permanent atrial pacemaker with transvenous electrodes
P1-31525 Implantation of electrode into cardiac epicardium by sternotomy or thoracotomy approach
  Insertion of electrode into heart epicardium by sternotomy or thoracotomy approach
  Insertion of permanent pacemaker with epicardial electrode by thoracotomy approach
  Insertion of epicardial pacemaker electrode leads
P1-31526 Insertion of permanent pacemaker with epicardial electrode by xiphoid approach
P1-31530 Removal of epicardial electrodes with replacement of epicardial lead
  Removal of cardiac pacemaker from epicardium with replacement of epicardial lead
  Replacement of epicardial pacemaker electrode leads
  Replacement of electronic heart device, epicardial electrode
P1-31532 Revision of pacemaker electrode leads
  Revision of cardiac pacemaker electrodes
  Reposition of cardiac pacemaker electrodes
P1-31534 Implantation of electrode into cardiac atrium and ventricle, replacement
  Insertion of electrode into heart atrium and ventricle, replacement
P1-31535 Implantation of electrode into cardiac atrium, replacement
  Insertion of electrode into heart atrium, replacement
P1-31536 Implantation of electrode into cardiac ventricle, replacement
  Insertion of electrode into heart ventricle, replacement
P1-31537 Removal of cardiac pacemaker electrodes with replacement
P1-31538 Removal of cardiac pacemaker from epicardium with replacement of atrial and/or ventricular leads
P1-31539 Replacement of transvenous atrial and ventricular pacemaker electrode leads
P1-3153A Replacement of transvenous atrial pacemaker electrode leads
P1-3153B Replacement of transvenous ventricular pacemaker electrode leads
P1-31540 Replacement of temporary transvenous pacemaker system
P1-31542 Reposition of cardiac pacemaker pocket
  Revision of cardiac pacemaker pocket
  Revision of skin pocket for pacemaker
P1-31543 Implantation of heart pacemaker
P1-31544 Insertion of pacemaker pulse generator
P1-31545 Insertion of unspecified permanent pacemaker, initial
P1-31546 Replacement of unspecified permanent pacemaker
P1-31547 Initial implantation of cardiac single-chamber device
  Initial insertion of single-chamber device not specified as rate-responsive
P1-31548 Implantation of rate-responsive cardiac single-chamber device
  Initial insertion of rate-responsive single-chamber device

P1-31548 (cont.) Insertion of cardiac pacemaker single-chamber rate-responsive device

P1-31549 Initial implantation of cardiac dual-chamber device
  Initial insertion of cardiac dual-chamber device
  Initial insertion of cardiac pacemaker dual-chamber device

P1-31550 Replacement of electronic heart device, transvenous electrode

P1-31553 Replacement of electronic heart device, myocardial electrode

P1-31557 Implantation of cardiac single-chamber device, replacement
  Insertion of cardiac pacemaker single-chamber device, replacement
  Removal of cardiac pacemaker with replacement, single-chamber device
  Replacement of cardiac pacemaker device, single-chamber

P1-31558 Reinsertion of cardiac pacemaker battery
  Replacement of electronic heart device battery

P1-31559 Replacement of electronic heart device, pulse generator
  Replacement of pacemaker pulse generator

P1-31560 Replacement of pacemaker device with single-chamber device, not specified as rate-responsive

P1-31561 Implantation of cardiac single-chamber device replacement, rate-responsive
  Insertion of cardiac pacemaker, single-chamber device replacement, rate-responsive

P1-31562 Removal of cardiac pacemaker with replacement by single-chamber device, rate-responsive
  Replacement of any type of pacemaker device with single-chamber device, rate-responsive
  Replacement of any type of pacemaker device with dual-chamber device

P1-31564 Implantation of cardiac dual-chamber device, replacement
  Insertion of cardiac pacemaker dual-chamber device, replacement
  Removal of cardiac pacemaker with replacement by dual-chamber device

P1-31566 Revision of permanent cardiac pacemaker device
  Revision of pacemaker device

P1-31570 Repair of cardiac pacemaker, NOS

P1-31573 Repair of cardiac pulse generator

P1-31575 Implantation of cardiac temporary transvenous pacemaker system during and immediately following cardiac surgery
  Implantation of electrode for cardiac temporary transvenous pacemaker system during and immediately following cardiac surgery
  Insertion of electrode of heart for temporary transvenous pacemaker system during and immediately following cardiac surgery
  Insertion of cardiac pacemaker during and immediately following cardiac surgery
  Insertion of cardiac temporary transvenous pacemaker system during and immediately following cardiac surgery
  Insertion of pacemaker during and immediately following cardiac surgery

P1-31576 Subcutaneous implantation of cardiac pacemaker

P1-31577 Implantation of automatic cardioverter/defibrillator, total system (AICD)

P1-31578 Implantation of cardioverter/defibrillator leads only
  Implantation of automatic implantable cardioverter/defibrillator pads with sensing electrodes

P1-31579 Implantation of automatic implantable cardioverter/defibrillator pads without sensing electrodes

P1-3157A Implantation of automatic implantable cardioverter/defibrillator pads with sensing electrodes and insertion of automatic implantable cardioverter/defibrillator pulse generator

P1-3157C Implantation of automatic cardioverter/defibrillator pulse generator only
  Insertion of automatic implantable cardioverter/defibrillator pulse generator

P1-31580 Replacement of cardioverter/defibrillator leads only

P1-31581 Replacement of automatic cardioverter/defibrillator pulse generator only
  Replacement of automatic implantable cardioverter/defibrillator pulse generator

P1-31582 Repositioning of cardioverter/defibrillator leads
  Revision of automatic implantable cardioverter/defibrillator pads and electrodes

P1-31583 Repositioning of cardioverter/defibrillator pulse generator

P1-31584 Relocation of automatic implantable cardioverter/defibrillator

P1-31585 Revision of automatic implantable cardioverter/defibrillator

P1-31586 Replacement of automatic cardioverter/defibrillator, total system
  Replacement of AICD

P1-31592 Implantation of baffle, atrial or interatrial
  Formation of pericardial baffle, interatrial

P1-315A0 Implantation of artificial heart

P1-315A1 Implantation of heart auxiliary ventricle

P1-315A2 Implantation of heart assist system
  Insertion of Kantrowitz heart pump

1-315-316 Heart: Injections and Implantations — Continued

P1-315A2 (cont.) Insertion of artificial cardioassist pump
P1-315A5 Implantation of outflow tract prosthesis in total repair of tetralogy of Fallot
  Insertion of outflow tract prosthesis in total repair of tetralogy of Fallot
P1-315B0 Removal of heart assist system with replacement
  Removal of pump assist device of heart with replacement
P1-315B2 Replacement of artificial heart
P1-315B8 Repair of heart assist system
P1-315C0 Removal of heart assist system, NOS
P1-315C1 Removal of pacemaker device, NOS
  Removal of permanent pacemaker
P1-315C2 Removal of Kantrowitz heart pump
P1-315C3 Removal of pacemaker electrode leads without replacement
P1-315C4 Removal of epicardial electrodes
  Removal of cardiac pacemaker from epicardium or myocardium
  Removal of electronic heart device, epicardial electrode
P1-315C5 Removal of transvenous electrodes
  Removal of electronic heart device, transvenous electrode
P1-315C6 Removal of electronic heart device, myocardial electrode
P1-315C7 Removal of electronic heart device, NOS
P1-315C8 Removal of electronic heart device battery
P1-315C9 Removal of electronic heart device pulse generator
  Removal of pulse generator of cardiac pacemaker
P1-315D0 Removal of cardioverter/defibrillator pulse generator without replacement
  Removal of pulse generator cardioverter/defibrillator
P1-315D1 Removal of automatic implantable cardioverter/defibrillator pads and electrodes
P1-31600 Cardiac catheterization, NOS
  Cardiac catheterization procedure, NOS
  Insertion of catheter into heart chamber, NOS
P1-31602 Catheterization of right heart
  Introduction of catheter into right heart
  Cardiac catheterization, right heart, NOS
  Right heart catheterization
P1-31604 Catheterization of left heart
  Cardiac catheterization, left heart, NOS
P1-31606 Catheterization of both left and right heart
  Cardiac catheterization, combined right and left heart, NOS
P1-31610 Cardiac catheterization, left heart, retrograde, percutaneous
P1-31611 Left heart catheterization, retrograde, from the brachial artery, axillary artery or femoral artery, percutaneous
P1-31612 Cardiac catheterization, left heart, transseptal
P1-31614 Cardiac catheterization, left heart, by left ventricular puncture
P1-31616 Cardiac catheterization, left heart, combined transseptal and retrograde
P1-31620 Cardiac catheterization, right heart and retrograde left
  Combined right heart catheterization and retrograde left heart catheterization
P1-31622 Cardiac catheterization, right heart and transseptal left
  Combined right heart catheterization and transseptal left heart catheterization through intact septum with or without retrograde left heart catheterization
P1-31624 Cardiac catheterization, right heart and left ventricular puncture
  Combined right heart catheterization with left ventricular puncture with retrograde left heart catheterization
P1-31625 Combined right heart catheterization with left ventricular puncture without retrograde left heart catheterization
P1-31626 Combined right heart catheterization and left heart catheterization through existing septal opening with retrograde left heart catheterization
P1-31627 Combined right heart catheterization and left heart catheterization through existing septal opening without retrograde left heart catheterization
P1-31628 Combined right heart catheterization and transseptal left heart catheterization through intact septum without retrograde left heart catheterization
P1-31629 Combined transseptal and retrograde left heart catheterization
P1-3162A Left heart catheterization, retrograde, from the brachial artery, axillary artery or femoral artery by left ventricular puncture
P1-3162B Left heart catheterization, retrograde, from the brachial artery, axillary artery or femoral artery by cutdown
P1-31640 Intraventricular and/or intra-atrial mapping of tachycardia site with catheter manipulation to record from multiple sites to identify origin of tachycardia
P1-31642 Injection procedure during cardiac catheterization including use of automatic power injectors

1-317 Heart: Endoscopy

P1-31700 Endoscopy of heart, NOS

1-318-319 Heart: Surgical Repairs, Closures and Reconstructions

P1-31800 Repair of heart, NOS
  Cardioplasty, NOS

P1-31802 Repair of heart and pericardium
P1-31810 Creation of cardiac pacemaker pocket new site in subcutaneous tissue
  Formation of cardiac pacemaker pocket new site in subcutaneous tissue
P1-31812 Debridement of skin or subcutaneous tissue of pacemaker pocket
P1-31813 Relocation of cardiac pacemaker pocket to new site in subcutaneous tissue
P1-31814 Repair of cardiac pacemaker pocket in skin or subcutaneous tissue
P1-31820 Repair of postinfarction ventricular septal defect with myocardial resection
P1-31821 Repair of postinfarction ventricular septal defect without myocardial resection
P1-31824 Repair of atrial septal defect, secundum, with cardiopulmonary bypass and patch
P1-31825 Repair of atrial septal defect, secundum, with cardiopulmonary bypass without patch
P1-31826 Repair of atrial septal defect and ventricular septal defect with direct closure
P1-31827 Repair of atrial septal defect and ventricular septal defect with patch closure
P1-31828 Repair of complete atrioventricular canal with prosthetic valve
P1-31829 Repair of complete atrioventricular canal without prosthetic valve
P1-31830 Repair of sinus of Valsalva fistula with cardiopulmonary bypass
P1-31831 Repair of sinus of Valsalva fistula with cardiopulmonary bypass and repair of ventricular septal defect
P1-31832 Repair of sinus of Valsalva aneurysm with cardiopulmonary bypass
P1-31835 Repair of hypoplastic left heart syndrome
P1-31836 Heart transplant with recipient cardiectomy
P1-31838 Heart transplant without recipient cardiectomy
P1-31839 Repair of papillary muscle of heart
  Reattachment of papillary muscle of heart
P1-3183A Repair of chordae tendineae
P1-31840 Repair of heart septum with prosthesis, NOS
  Repair of septal defect of heart with prosthesis, NOS
P1-31842 Closure of foramen ovale with prosthesis by open heart technique
  Repair of foramen ovale with prosthesis by open heart technique
P1-31843 Closure of foramen ovale with prosthesis by closed heart technique
  Repair of foramen ovale with prosthesis by closed heart technique
P1-31845 Repair of atrial septal defect with prosthesis by open heart technique
P1-31846 Repair of atrial septal defect with prosthesis by closed heart technique
P1-31847 Repair of ostium secundum defect with prosthesis by open heart technique
P1-31848 Repair of ostium secundum defect with prosthesis by closed heart technique
P1-31850 Repair of ventricular septal defect with prosthesis
P1-31851 Repair of supracristal defect with prosthesis
P1-31852 Repair of atrioventricular canal defect with prosthesis
P1-31853 Repair of ostium primum defect
P1-31854 Repair of ostium primum defect with prosthesis
P1-31860 Repair of heart septum with tissue graft, NOS
P1-31861 Repair of septal defect of heart with tissue graft, NOS
P1-31862 Repair of atrial septal defect with tissue graft
P1-31863 Repair of foramen ovale with tissue graft
  Closure of foramen ovale with tissue graft
P1-31864 Repair of ostium secundum defect with tissue graft
P1-31865 Repair of ostium primum defect with tissue graft
P1-31866 Repair of ventricular septal defect with tissue graft
P1-31867 Repair of supracristal defect with tissue graft
P1-31868 Repair of atrioventricular canal defect with tissue graft
P1-31869 Repair of endocardial cushion defect with tissue graft
P1-31870 Atrioplasty, NOS
P1-31871 Closure of atrial septal defect with umbrella device, King-Mills type
  Insertion of atrial septal umbrella
  Insertion of King-Mills umbrella device for closure of septal defect
P1-31872 Atrioseptoplasty
  Septal atrioplasty of heart
  Atrioseptopexy
  Closure of atrial septal defect
  Correction of atrial septal defect
  Repair of atrial septal defect
  Repair of atrial septum of heart, NOS
P1-31873 Closure of septal fenestration of heart
  Closure of septum defect of heart
P1-31874 Closure of patent foramen ovale
  Repair of patent foramen ovale
P1-31875 Repair of ostium secundum defect
P1-31876 Correction of ventricular septal defect
  Repair of ventricular septal defect
P1-31877 Repair of supracristal defect of heart
P1-31878 Ventriculoseptoplasty
  Ventriculoseptopexy
P1-31879 Repair of atrioventricular canal defect
P1-3187A Repair of endocardial cushion defect
  Closure of endocardial cushion defect
P1-3187B Repair of endocardial cushion defect with prosthesis
P1-31880 Heart revascularization, NOS
P1-31881 Implantation of blood vessels into myocardium
  Implantation of artery branches to heart muscle

1-318-319 Heart: Surgical Repairs, Closures and Reconstructions — Continued

P1-31881 (cont.) Indirect cardiac revascularization
 Sewell operation of heart
 Heart revascularization by arterial implant
P1-31883 Implantation of systemic arteries into myocardium, Vineberg type operation
 Vineberg operation
P1-31884 Implantation of mammary artery into ventricle
 Anastomosis of internal mammary artery to myocardium
 Anastomosis of thoracic artery to myocardium
P1-31885 Aorto-myocardial shunt
P1-31886 Cardiac revascularization with bypass anastomosis, NOS
P1-31890 Augmentation of outflow tract in total repair of tetralogy of Fallot
 Grafting of outflow tract in total repair of tetralogy of Fallot
P1-31891 Correction of tetralogy of Fallot, one-stage
 Repair of tetralogy of Fallot, one-stage
 Complete repair of tetralogy of Fallot
 Total repair of tetralogy of Fallot
P1-31892 Complete repair of tetralogy of Fallot with transannular patch
P1-31893 Complete repair of tetralogy of Fallot with closure of previous shunt
P1-31894 Repair of atrial heart septum in total repair of tetralogy of Fallot
P1-31895 Repair of ventricular septal defect in total repair of tetralogy of Fallot
P1-31896 Repair of ventricular septal defect with prosthesis in total repair of tetralogy of Fallot
P1-31897 Repair of pulmonary heart valve with prosthesis in total repair of tetralogy of Fallot
 Replacement of pulmonary heart valve in total repair of tetralogy of Fallot
P1-31898 Take-down of systemic-pulmonary artery anastomosis in total repair of tetralogy of Fallot
P1-31900 Repair of total anomalous pulmonary venous connection, one-stage
 Correction of total anomalous pulmonary venous connection, one-stage
 Complete repair of anomalous venous return, supracardiac type
P1-31902 Anastomosis of common pulmonary trunk and left atrium, posterior wall
P1-31904 Division of common wall between posterior left atrium and coronary sinus with roofing of resultant defect and patch graft
 Incision of common wall between posterior left atrium and coronary sinus with roofing of resultant defect with patch graft
P1-31905 Enlargement of atrial septal defect in repair of total anomalous pulmonary venous connection
P1-31906 Enlargement of foramen ovale in repair of total anomalous pulmonary venous connection
P1-31907 Repair of atrial septal defect in total repair of total anomalous pulmonary venous connection
P1-31908 Repair of ventricular septum in total repair of total anomalous pulmonary venous connection
P1-31909 Pulmonary vein to atrium shunt construction
P1-31910 Total repair of truncus arteriosus
 Total correction of truncus arteriosus
P1-31911 Total repair of truncus arteriosus, one-stage
 Correction of truncus arteriosus, one-stage
P1-31912 Total repair of truncus arteriosus, Rastelli type operation
 Creation of conduit of right ventricle and pulmonary artery in repair of truncus arteriosus
 Rastelli operation in repair of truncus arteriosus
 Shunt of right ventricle and pulmonary artery in repair of truncus arteriosus
P1-31913 Formation of conduit of right ventricle and pulmonary artery in repair of pulmonary artery atresia in truncus arteriosus
P1-31914 Reimplantation of pulmonary artery for hemitruncus repair
P1-31915 Repair of heart atrial septum in total repair of truncus arteriosus
P1-31917 Interatrial transposition of venous return
 Baffes operation
 Mustard operation
 Transposition of interatrial venous return
P1-31918 Correction of transposition of great vessels
 Senning operation
P1-31920 Creation of conduit between right ventricle and pulmonary artery
 Formation of conduit of right ventricle and distal pulmonary artery
 Creation of shunt of right ventricle and distal pulmonary artery
 Rastelli operation
P1-31921 Creation of conduit of right ventricle and pulmonary artery in repair of pulmonary artery atresia
 Formation of conduit of right ventricle and pulmonary artery in repair of pulmonary artery atresia
 Creation of shunt of right ventricle and pulmonary artery in repair of pulmonary artery atresia
P1-31922 Creation of conduit of right ventricle and pulmonary artery in repair of transposition of great vessels
 Creation of shunt of right ventricle and pulmonary artery in repair of transposition of great vessels

P1-31924 Creation of conduit between left ventricle and aorta
Formation of apicoaortic shunt
Construction of apicoaortic conduit
P1-31926 Creation of conduit of right atrium and pulmonary artery
Formation of conduit of right atrium and pulmonary artery
Creation of shunt of right atrium and pulmonary artery
Fontan operation
P1-31930 Repair of cardiac wound without bypass
P1-31931 Repair of cardiac wound with cardiopulmonary bypass
P1-31932 Direct closure of sinus venosus with anomalous pulmonary venous drainage
P1-31933 Direct closure of sinus venosus without anomalous pulmonary venous drainage
P1-31934 Patch closure of sinus venosus with anomalous pulmonary venous drainage
P1-31935 Patch closure of sinus venosus without anomalous pulmonary venous drainage
P1-31936 Patch closure of endocardial cushion defect with repair of mitral and tricuspid cleft
P1-31937 Patch closure of endocardial cushion defect with repair of mitral cleft
P1-31938 Patch closure of endocardial cushion defect with repair of tricuspid cleft
P1-31939 Patch closure of endocardial cushion defect without repair of mitral and tricuspid cleft
P1-3193A Patch closure of endocardial cushion defect without repair of mitral cleft
P1-3193B Patch closure of endocardial cushion defect without repair of tricuspid cleft
P1-31940 Closure of ventricular septal defect
P1-31941 Patch closure of endocardial cushion defect with repair of separate ventricular septal defect
P1-31942 Closure of ventricular septal defect with patch
P1-31943 Closure of ventricular septal defect without patch
P1-31944 Closure of ventricular septal defect with infundibular resection and patch
P1-31945 Closure of ventricular septal defect with infundibular resection and without patch
P1-31946 Closure of ventricular septal defect with pulmonary valvotomy and patch
P1-31947 Closure of ventricular septal defect with pulmonary valvotomy and without patch
P1-31948 Closure of ventricular septal defect with patch and removal of pulmonary artery band, with gusset
P1-31949 Closure of ventricular septal defect with patch and removal of pulmonary artery band, without gusset
P1-3194A Closure of ventricular septal defect with removal of pulmonary artery band, with gusset
P1-3194B Closure of ventricular septal defect with removal of pulmonary artery band, without gusset or patch
P1-31950 Ligation of atrium of heart
Ligation of auricle of heart
P1-31954 Resuture of cardiac septum prosthesis
P1-31960 Suture of heart, NOS
Cardiorrhaphy, NOS
P1-31962 Cardio-omentopexy
P1-31963 Cardiomyopexy
P1-31964 Cardiopericardiopexy
P1-31966 Cardiopneumopexy
P1-31968 Cardiosplenopexy
P1-31969 Plication of ventricle of heart
P1-31971 Cardiac external resuscitation by massage with open chest
Cardiac massage with open chest

1-31C Heart: Destructive Procedures

P1-31C00 Destructive procedure on heart, NOS
P1-31C01 Destruction of tissue of heart, NOS
P1-31C02 Catheter ablation of tissue of heart
P1-31C04 Destruction of lesion of heart, NOS
P1-31C05 Catheter ablation of lesion of heart
P1-31C06 Cardioschisis
P1-31C08 Cardiolysis
Brauer operation
Lysis of adhesions of heart
P1-31C10 Operative ablation of supraventricular arrhythmogenic focus or tracts and/or foci without cardiopulmonary bypass
P1-31C11 Operative ablation of supraventricular arrhythmogenic focus, tracts and/or foci with cardiopulmonary bypass
P1-31C13 Operative ablation of arrhythmogenic focus or pathway without cardiopulmonary bypass
P1-31C14 Intracardiac catheter ablation of arrhythmogenic focus or tracts including intracardiac mapping with temporary pacemaker placement
P1-31C15 Intracardiac catheter ablation of arrhythmogenic focus or tracts including intracardiac mapping without temporary pacemaker placement

1-31D Heart: Transplantations and Transpositions

P1-31D00 Transplantation of heart, NOS
Heart transplantation
P1-31D01 Grafting of heart for revascularization
Grafting of myocardium for revascularization
P1-31D02 Grafting of mediastinal fat to myocardium
P1-31D03 Grafting of omentum to myocardium

1-31E Heart: Manipulations

P1-31E00 Manual external cardiac massage with closed chest
External cardiac resuscitation by massage

1-32 OPERATIVE PROCEDURES ON THE HEART VALVES

1-320 Heart Valves: General and Miscellaneous Operative Procedures

P1-32000 Operative procedure on heart valve, NOS
P1-32010 Operation on heart valve adjacent structure, NOS

1-321 Heart Valves: Incisions

P1-32100 Incision of heart valve, NOS
  Cardiac valvulotomy, NOS
  Closed heart valvulotomy
P1-32102 Commissurotomy, NOS
P1-32103 Fenestration of cardiac valve, NOS
P1-32110 Valvulotomy of tricuspid valve, NOS
  Closed heart valvotomy of tricuspid valve
P1-32112 Valvotomy of tricuspid valve with cardiopulmonary bypass
P1-32130 Valvulotomy of pulmonary valve, NOS
  Brock operation for pulmonary valvotomy
  Pulmonary valvulotomy
P1-32131 Closed heart valvotomy of pulmonary valve
P1-32132 Closed transventricular pulmonary valve commissurotomy
  Closed valvotomy of pulmonary valve by transventricular approach
P1-32133 Pulmonary valve commissurotomy by transvenous balloon method
  Valvotomy of pulmonary valve by transvenous balloon method
P1-32134 Open pulmonary valve commissurotomy with inflow occlusion
  Open valvotomy of pulmonary valve with inflow occlusion
P1-32135 Open pulmonary valve commissurotomy with cardiopulmonary bypass
  Open valvotomy of pulmonary valve with cardiopulmonary bypass
P1-32136 Valvulotomy of pulmonary valve in total repair of tetralogy of Fallot
P1-32150 Mitral valvotomy, NOS
  Valvulotomy of mitral valve, NOS
  Mitral valvulotomy, NOS
P1-32152 Closed mitral valve commissurotomy
P1-32153 Posterior mitral commissurotomy
P1-32154 Open mitral valve commissurotomy with cardiopulmonary bypass
  Open valvotomy of mitral valve with cardiopulmonary bypass
P1-32155 Closed heart valvotomy of mitral valve
  Closed valvotomy of mitral valve
P1-32180 Aortic valvotomy, NOS
  Valvulotomy of aortic valve, NOS
P1-32182 Closed heart valvotomy of aortic valve
P1-32183 Aortic valve commissurotomy with inflow occlusion
  Valvotomy of aortic valve with inflow occlusion
P1-32184 Aortic valve commissurotomy with cardiopulmonary bypass
  Valvotomy of aortic valve with cardiopulmonary bypass

1-323 Heart Valves: Excisions

P1-32300 Excision of heart valve, NOS
P1-32302 Excision of cusp of heart valve, NOS
P1-32310 Valvectomy of tricuspid valve with cardiopulmonary bypass
P1-32312 Excision of cusp of tricuspid valve
P1-32350 Excision of cusp of mitral valve
P1-32380 Excision of cusp of aortic valve
P1-32382 Resection of aortic valve for subvalvular stenosis

1-325 Heart Valves: Injections and Implantations

P1-32500 Implantation of heart valve, NOS
P1-32502 Implantation of heart valve with tissue graft
P1-32504 Implantation of heart valve prosthesis or synthetic device
P1-32510 Implantation of tricuspid valve with tissue graft
P1-32512 Implantation of tricuspid valve prosthesis or synthetic device
P1-32531 Implantation of pulmonary valve prosthesis or synthetic device
P1-32532 Implantation of outflow tract prosthesis in pulmonary valvuloplasty
  Insertion of outflow tract prosthesis in pulmonary valvuloplasty
P1-32550 Implantation of mitral valve with tissue graft
P1-32552 Implantation of mitral valve prosthesis or synthetic device
P1-32580 Implantation of aortic valve with tissue graft
P1-32582 Implantation of aortic valve prosthesis or synthetic device

1-327 Heart Valves: Endoscopy

P1-32700 Endoscopy of heart valve, NOS

1-328-329 Heart Valves: Surgical Repairs, Closures and Reconstructions

P1-32800 Cardiac valvuloplasty, NOS
  Repair of heart valve, NOS
P1-32802 Advancement of leaflet of heart valve, NOS
P1-32803 Bicuspidization of heart valve
P1-32804 Repair of heart valve with prosthesis or tissue graft
  Replacement of heart valve with prosthesis or tissue graft
P1-32810 Valvuloplasty of tricuspid valve, NOS
  Repair of tricuspid valve without replacement
P1-32811 Open heart valvuloplasty of tricuspid valve without replacement

P1-32812 Valvuloplasty of tricuspid valve with cardiopulmonary bypass
P1-32813 Replacement of tricuspid valve, NOS
P1-32814 Replacement of tricuspid valve with cardiopulmonary bypass
P1-32815 Correction of tricuspid atresia
P1-32816 Tricuspid valve repositioning and plication for Ebstein anomaly
  Plication of tricuspid valve with repositioning
P1-32817 Replacement of tricuspid valve with tissue graft
P1-32818 Repair of tricuspid valve with tissue graft
P1-32819 Repair of tricuspid valve with prosthesis
P1-3281A Repair of tricuspid atresia
P1-32830 Valvuloplasty of pulmonary valve, NOS
P1-32831 Implantation of pulmonary valve with tissue graft
P1-32832 Replacement of pulmonary valve, NOS
P1-32833 Open heart valvuloplasty of pulmonary valve without replacement
  Repair of pulmonary valve without replacement by open heart technique
P1-32834 Valvuloplasty of pulmonary valve in total repair of tetralogy of Fallot
P1-32835 Augmentation of outflow tract of pulmonary valve
  Outflow tract augmentation of pulmonic valve without commissurotomy and infundibular resection
P1-32836 Outflow tract augmentation of pulmonic valve with commissurotomy and without infundibular resection
P1-32837 Outflow tract augmentation of pulmonic valve with commissurotomy and infundibular resection
P1-32838 Outflow tract augmentation of pulmonic valve without commissurotomy and with infundibular resection
P1-32839 Percutaneous balloon valvuloplasty of pulmonary valve
P1-32840 Repair of pulmonary valve with tissue graft
  Replacement of pulmonary valve with tissue graft
P1-32842 Repair of pulmonary valve with prosthesis
  Replacement of pulmonary valve with prosthesis
P1-32850 Repair of mitral valve without replacement
  Valvuloplasty of mitral valve
P1-32851 Valvuloplasty of mitral valve with cardiopulmonary bypass and prosthetic ring
P1-32852 Radical reconstructive valvuloplasty of mitral valve with cardiopulmonary bypass and ring
P1-32853 Radical reconstructive valvuloplasty of mitral valve with cardiopulmonary bypass and without ring
P1-32854 Repair of mitral valve with prosthesis
P1-32855 Replacement of mitral valve, NOS
  Excision and replacement of mitral valve
P1-32856 Replacement of mitral valve with prosthesis
P1-32857 Replacement of mitral valve with cardiopulmonary bypass
P1-32858 Atriocommissuropexy of mitral valve
P1-32859 Valvuloplasty of mitral valve with cardiopulmonary bypass
P1-3285A Bicuspidization of mitral valve
P1-3285B Hinging of mitral valve
  Neostrophingic mobilization of mitral valve
P1-32860 Open heart valvuloplasty of mitral valve without replacement
P1-32862 Repair of mitral valve with tissue graft
P1-32864 Replacement of mitral valve with tissue graft
P1-32880 Valvuloplasty of aortic valve
  Aortic valvuloplasty
P1-32881 Bicuspidization of aortic valve
P1-32882 Open heart valvuloplasty of aortic valve without replacement
  Repair of aortic valve without replacement
P1-32883 Percutaneous balloon valvuloplasty of aortic valve
P1-32890 Replacement of aortic valve, NOS
  Excision and replacement of aortic valve, NOS
P1-32891 Replacement of aortic valve with cardiopulmonary bypass
P1-32892 Open heart valvuloplasty of aortic valve with cardiopulmonary bypass
P1-32894 Replacement of aortic valve with aortic annulus enlargement of noncoronary cusp
P1-32895 Replacement of aortic valve with transventricular aortic annulus enlargement
P1-32896 Repair of aortic valve with tissue graft
  Replacement of aortic valve with tissue graft
P1-32897 Repair of aortic valve with prosthesis
  Replacement of aortic valve with prosthesis
P1-32900 Replacement of heart valve poppet, prosthetic
  Reinsertion of heart valve, prosthetic
P1-32901 Percutaneous balloon valvuloplasty of heart
P1-32902 Annuloplasty
  Reconstruction of cardiac valve annulus
P1-32910 Single valve replacement with commissurotomy of another valve
P1-32911 Single valve replacement with valvuloplasty of another valve
P1-32912 Single valve replacement with commissurotomy of two valves
P1-32913 Single valve replacement with valvuloplasty of two valves
P1-32914 Double valve replacement
P1-32915 Double valve replacement with commissurotomy of one valve
P1-32916 Double valve replacement with valvuloplasty of one valve
P1-32921 Replacement of unspecified heart valve
P1-32922 Triple valve replacement

1-328-329 Heart Valves: Surgical Repairs, Closures and Reconstructions — Continued

P1-32930 Open heart valvuloplasty without replacement of valve, NOS
P1-32932 Percutaneous valvuloplasty
P1-32933 Plication of annulus of heart valve
P1-32934 Resuture of heart valve prosthesis, poppet
P1-32935 Revision of prosthesis of heart valve, NOS

1-32C Heart Valves: Destructive Procedures

P1-32C00 Destructive procedure of heart valve, NOS

1-32D Heart Valves: Transplantations and Transpositions

P1-32D00 Transplantation of heart valve, NOS

1-32E Heart Valves: Manipulations

P1-32E00 Manipulation of heart valve, NOS

1-33 OPERATIVE PROCEDURES ON THE CORONARY ARTERIES

1-330 Coronary Arteries: General and Miscellaneous Operative Procedures

P1-33000 Operative procedure on coronary arteries, NOS
P1-33002 Operation on vessels of heart, NOS

1-331 Coronary Arteries: Incisions

P1-33100 Incision of coronary artery, NOS

1-333 Coronary Arteries: Excisions

P1-33300 Excision of coronary artery, NOS
P1-33310 Removal of coronary artery obstruction, NOS
P1-33311 Removal of coronary artery thrombus
P1-33314 Endarterectomy of coronary artery
  Thromboendarterectomy of coronary artery
P1-33315 Gas endarterectomy of coronary artery
P1-33320 Removal of coronary artery obstruction by percutaneous transluminal balloon, single vessel
P1-33321 Removal of coronary artery obstruction by percutaneous transluminal balloon with thrombolytic agent
P1-33322 Removal of coronary artery obstruction, percutaneous transluminal, multiple vessels
P1-33324 Thromboendarterectomy of coronary artery by open chest approach
  Endarterectomy of coronary artery by open chest approach
  Removal of coronary artery obstruction by open chest approach
P1-33326 Removal of coronary artery obstruction by direct intracoronary artery infusion
P1-33328 Excision of aneurysm of coronary artery

1-335 Coronary Arteries: Injections and Implantations

P1-33500 Injection of coronary artery, NOS
P1-33512 Injection of thrombolytic agent direct into coronary artery
  Intracoronary artery thrombolytic infusion
P1-33520 Perfusion of coronary artery, NOS
P1-33523 Selective introduction of catheter in coronary artery

1-337 Coronary Arteries: Endoscopy

P1-33700 Endoscopy of coronary artery, NOS

1-338 Coronary Arteries: Surgical Repairs, Closures and Reconstructions

P1-33800 Coronary angioplasty, NOS
  Repair of coronary artery, NOS
P1-33820 Coronary angioplasty by open chest approach
P1-33822 Graft of anomalous coronary artery with cardiopulmonary bypass
P1-33830 Repair of aneurysm of coronary artery
P1-33831 Repair of coronary arteriocardiac chamber fistula
P1-33832 Repair of coronary arteriovenous chamber fistula
P1-33834 Repair of arteriovenous fistula of coronary artery by ligation
P1-33835 Graft of anomalous coronary artery without cardiopulmonary bypass
P1-33840 Aortocoronary bypass for heart revascularization, NOS
  Aortocoronary artery bypass graft
  ACB graft
  CAB graft
  Vascular aortocoronary bypass
  Coronary bypass
  Cardiac revascularization with aortocoronary bypass anastomosis
P1-33841 Aortocoronary artery bypass graft with prosthesis
P1-33842 Aortocoronary artery bypass graft with vein graft
P1-33843 Aortocoronary artery bypass graft with saphenous vein graft
P1-33850 Coronary angioplasty with bypass
P1-33854 Coronary angioplasty with bypass combined with vascularization
P1-33855 Aortocoronary bypass of one coronary artery
  Cardiac revascularization with bypass aortocoronary anastomosis of one coronary vessel
P1-33857 Coronary artery bypass with autogenous graft, single graft
P1-33858 Coronary artery bypass with nonautogenous graft, single graft
P1-33859 Coronary artery bypass, nonautogenous cadaver graft, single graft

P1-33860 Aortocoronary bypass of two coronary arteries
Cardiac revascularization with bypass aortocoronary anastomosis of two coronary vessels
P1-33862 Coronary artery bypass with autogenous graft, two grafts
P1-33863 Coronary artery bypass, nonautogenous graft, two grafts
P1-33864 Coronary artery bypass, nonautogenous cadaver graft, two grafts
P1-33870 Aortocoronary bypass of three coronary arteries
Cardiac revascularization with bypass aortocoronary anastomosis of three coronary vessels
P1-33872 Coronary artery bypass with autogenous graft, three grafts
P1-33873 Coronary artery bypass with nonautogenous graft, three or more grafts
P1-33874 Coronary artery bypass, nonautogenous cadaver graft, three or more grafts
P1-33875 Aortocoronary bypass of four or more coronary arteries
Cardiac revascularization with bypass aortocoronary anastomosis of four coronary vessels
P1-33876 Coronary artery bypass with autogenous graft, four grafts
P1-33877 Coronary artery bypass with autogenous graft, five grafts
P1-33878 Coronary artery bypass with autogenous graft, six or more grafts
P1-33879 Aortocoronary artery bypass graft, repeated
P1-33880 Anastomosis of internal mammary artery to coronary artery, single vessel
Bypass internal mammary-coronary artery, single
Cardiac revascularization with bypass anastomosis of internal mammary to coronary artery, single vessel
Single internal mammary-coronary artery bypass
Coronary artery bypass with autogenous graft of internal mammary artery, single graft
P1-33882 Anastomosis of internal mammary artery to coronary artery, double vessel
Bypass of internal mammary-coronary artery, double vessel
Double internal mammary-coronary artery bypass
Cardiac revascularization with bypass anastomosis of internal mammary-coronary artery, double vessel
P1-33883 Coronary artery bypass with autogenous graft, internal mammary artery, two coronary grafts
P1-33884 Anastomosis of thoracic artery to coronary artery, single
Cardiac revascularization with bypass anastomosis of thoracic artery to coronary artery, single vessel
P1-33885 Anastomosis of thoracic artery to coronary artery, double
Cardiac revascularization with bypass anastomosis of thoracic artery to coronary artery, double vessel
P1-33887 Coronary artery bypass, autogenous graft, internal mammary artery, three coronary grafts
P1-33888 Coronary artery bypass, autogenous graft, internal mammary artery, four coronary grafts
P1-33889 Coronary artery bypass, autogenous graft, internal mammary artery, five coronary grafts
P1-3388A Coronary artery bypass, autogenous graft, internal mammary artery, six or more coronary grafts
P1-33890 Aorta-coronary sinus shunt
Beck operation for aorta-coronary sinus shunt
P1-33892 Ligation of anomalous coronary artery
P1-33894 Ligation of coronary sinus
P1-33896 Ligation of arteriovenous fistula of coronary artery

1-33C Coronary Arteries: Destructive Procedures

P1-33C00 Destructive procedure of coronary artery, NOS
P1-33C10 Thrombolysis of coronary artery by intravenous infusion
P1-33C12 Thrombolysis of coronary artery by intracoronary infusion, including selective coronary angiography

1-33D Coronary Arteries: Transplantations and Transpositions

P1-33D00 Transplantation of coronary artery, NOS

1-33E Coronary Arteries: Manipulations

P1-33E00 Manipulation of coronary artery, NOS

1-34 OPERATIVE PROCEDURES ON THE AORTA

1-340 Aorta: General and Miscellaneous Operative Procedures

P1-34000 Operation on aorta, NOS
P1-34020 Operation on aortic body, NOS

1-341 Aorta: Incisions

P1-34100 Incision of aorta, NOS
Aortotomy, NOS
Angiotomy of aorta , NOS
Arteriotomy of aorta, NOS
Exploration of aorta, NOS
P1-34101 Incision of ascending aorta
Angiotomy of ascending aorta

1-341 Aorta: Incisions — Continued

P1-34101 (cont.) Arteriotomy of ascending aorta
  Exploration of ascending aorta
P1-34102 Incision of aortic arch
  Angiotomy of aortic arch
  Arteriotomy of aortic arch
  Exploration or aortic arch
P1-34103 Incision of descending aorta
  Angiotomy of descending aorta
  Arteriotomy of descending aorta
  Exploration of descending aorta
P1-34110 Division of aorta
P1-34111 Division of ascending aorta
P1-34112 Division of aortic arch
P1-34113 Division of descending aorta

1-343 Aorta: Excisions

P1-34300 Excision of aorta, NOS
  Arteriectomy of aorta, NOS
P1-34301 Excision of ascending aorta
  Arteriectomy of ascending aorta
P1-34302 Excision of aortic arch
  Arteriectomy of aortic arch
P1-34303 Excision of descending aorta
  Arteriectomy of descending aorta
P1-34305 Resection of aorta with anastomosis, NOS
P1-34306 Resection of ascending aorta with anastomosis
P1-34307 Resection of aortic arch with anastomosis
P1-34308 Resection of descending aorta with anastomosis
P1-34310 Excision of lesion of aorta, NOS
P1-34311 Excision of lesion of ascending aorta
P1-34312 Excision of lesion of aortic arch
P1-34313 Excision of lesion of descending aorta
P1-34315 Aneurysmectomy of aorta, NOS
P1-34316 Aneurysmectomy of ascending aorta
P1-34317 Aneurysmectomy of aortic arch
P1-34318 Aneurysmectomy of descending aorta
P1-34319 Aneurysmectomy of sinus of Valsalva
P1-3431A Aneurysmectomy of aorta with anastomosis, NOS
P1-3431B Aneurysmectomy of ascending aorta with anastomosis
P1-3431C Aneurysmectomy of aortic arch with anastomosis
P1-3431D Aneurysmectomy of descending aorta with anastomosis
P1-34320 Embolectomy of aorta, NOS
  Removal of embolus of aorta, NOS
P1-34321 Embolectomy of ascending aorta
  Removal of embolus of ascending aorta
P1-34322 Embolectomy of aortic arch
  Removal of embolus of aortic arch
P1-34323 Embolectomy of descending aorta
  Removal of embolus of descending aorta
P1-34325 Thrombectomy of aorta, NOS
  Removal of thrombus of aorta, NOS
P1-34326 Thrombectomy of ascending aorta
  Removal of thrombus of ascending aorta
P1-34327 Thrombectomy of aortic arch
  Removal of thrombus of aortic arch
P1-34328 Thrombectomy of descending aorta
  Removal of thrombus of descending aorta
P1-34330 Endarterectomy of aorta, NOS
  Thromboendarterectomy of aorta, NOS
  Intimectomy of aorta, NOS
P1-34331 Endarterectomy of ascending aorta
  Thromboendarterectomy of ascending aorta
  Intimectomy of ascending aorta
P1-34332 Endarterectomy of aortic arch
  Thromboendarterectomy of aortic arch
  Intimectomy of aortic arch
P1-34333 Endarterectomy of descending aorta
  Thromboendarterectomy of descending aorta
  Intimectomy of descending aorta
P1-34335 Gas endarterectomy of aorta, NOS
P1-3433A Endarterectomy of aorta with patch graft
P1-34340 Excision of coarctation of aorta with end-to-end anastomosis
P1-34341 Excision of coarctation of aorta without associated patent ductus arteriosus and with direct anastomosis
P1-34342 Excision of coarctation of aorta with associated patent ductus arteriosus and direct anastomosis
P1-34343 Excision of coarctation of aorta with associated patent ductus arteriosus and graft
P1-34344 Excision of coarctation of aorta with associated patent ductus arteriosus and repair using left subclavian artery
P1-34345 Excision of coarctation of aorta with associated patent ductus arteriosus and repair using prosthetic material
P1-34346 Excision of coarctation of aorta without associated patent ductus arteriosus with repair using left subclavian artery
P1-34347 Excision of coarctation of aorta without associated patent ductus arteriosus with repair using prosthetic material
P1-34348 Excision of coarctation of aorta without associated patent ductus arteriosus with graft
P1-34350 Excision of lesion of aorta with end-to-end anastomosis, NOS
P1-34352 Excision of lesion of aorta with interposition graft replacement
P1-34360 Arteriectomy of thoracoabdominal aorta
  Resection of thoracoabdominal aorta
P1-34361 Arteriectomy of thoracic aorta
  Resection of thoracic aorta
P1-34362 Arteriectomy of abdominal aorta
  Resection of abdominal aorta
P1-34365 Arteriectomy with graft replacement of thoracic aorta
  Angiectomy with graft replacement of thoracic aorta

P1-34366 Aneurysmectomy with graft replacement of thoracic aorta
P1-34367 Arteriectomy with graft replacement of thoracoabdominal aorta
  Angiectomy with graft replacement of thoracoabdominal aorta
  Excision with graft replacement of thoracoabdominal aorta
P1-34368 Aneurysmectomy with graft replacement of thoracoabdominal aorta
P1-34369 Aneurysmectomy with graft replacement of abdominal aorta
P1-34370 Excision of lesion of thoracic aorta with end-to-end anastomosis
P1-34371 Excision of lesion of thoracoabdominal aorta with end-to-end anastomosis
P1-34372 Excision of lesion of thoracic aorta with interposition graft replacement
P1-34373 Excision of lesion of thoracoabdominal aorta with interposition graft replacement
P1-34374 Excision of lesion of abdominal aorta with end-to-end anastomosis
P1-34375 Excision of lesion of abdominal aorta with interposition graft replacement
P1-34376 Thromboendarterectomy without graft of abdominal aorta
P1-34377 Thromboendarterectomy with graft of abdominal aorta
P1-34378 Resection of abdominal aorta with replacement
  Arteriectomy with graft replacement of abdominal aorta
  Angiectomy with graft replacement of abdominal aorta
P1-34381 Embolectomy with catheter of aortoiliac artery by abdominal incision
P1-34382 Thrombectomy with catheter of aortoiliac artery by abdominal incision
P1-34383 Embolectomy without catheter of aortoiliac artery by abdominal incision
P1-34384 Thrombectomy without catheter of aortoiliac artery by abdominal incision
P1-34385 Embolectomy without catheter of aortoiliac artery by leg incision
P1-34386 Thrombectomy without catheter of aortoiliac artery by leg incision
P1-34387 Embolectomy with catheter of aortoiliac artery by leg incision
P1-34388 Thrombectomy with catheter of aortoiliac artery by leg incision
P1-34390 Aorto-iliac thromboendarterectomy, NOS
  Aorto-iliac endarterectomy, NOS
P1-34391 Thromboendarterectomy without graft, combined aortoiliac
P1-34392 Thromboendarterectomy with graft, combined aortoiliac
P1-34393 Thromboendarterectomy with graft, combined aortoiliofemoral
P1-34394 Thromboendarterectomy without graft, combined aortoiliofemoral

1-345 Aorta: Injections and Implantations

P1-34500 Injection of aorta, NOS
P1-34512 Introduction of aortic catheter by translumbar route
P1-34513 Introduction of aortic needle by translumbar route
P1-34514 Introduction of catheter into aorta, initial placement
P1-34515 Selective introduction of catheter into aorta, initial placement
P1-34518 Percutaneous insertion of intra-aortic balloon catheter
P1-34519 Insertion of intra-aortic balloon counterpulsation
  Insertion of intra-aortic balloon pump
  Insertion of pulsation-type balloon into aorta
P1-34520 Embolization of aorta, NOS

1-347 Aorta: Endoscopy

P1-34700 Endoscopy of aorta, NOS

1-348-349 Aorta: Surgical Repairs, Closures and Reconstructions

P1-34800 Aortoplasty, NOS
  Repair of aorta, NOS
P1-34810 Correction of coarctation of aorta with anastomosis
P1-34811 Correction of coarctation of aorta with graft replacement
P1-34812 Intraoperative transluminal aortic angioplasty
P1-34820 Re-entry operation of aorta
P1-34821 Fenestration of aorta
P1-34822 Fenestration of aortic aneurysm
P1-34823 Fenestration of dissecting aneurysm of thoracic aorta
  Repair of dissecting aneurysm of thoracic aorta by fenestration
P1-34826 Repair of aneurysm of sinus of Valsalva
P1-34827 Repair of fistula of sinus of Valsalva
P1-34829 Aortoplasty for supravalvular stenosis
P1-34830 Insertion of graft of aorta without bypass
P1-34831 Insertion of graft of aorta with cardiopulmonary bypass
P1-34840 Suture of aorta, NOS
P1-34841 Suture repair of aorta without bypass
P1-34842 Suture repair of aorta with cardiopulmonary bypass
P1-34850 Surgical occlusion of aorta, NOS
P1-34851 Ligation of aorta, NOS
P1-34852 Ligation of ascending aorta
P1-34853 Ligation of aortic arch
P1-34854 Ligation of descending aorta
P1-34856 Closure of aorticopulmonary fistula or fenestration
  Obliteration of aortopulmonary septal defect

1-348-349 Aorta: Surgical Repairs, Closures and Reconstructions — Continued

P1-34856 (cont.) Aorticopulmonary window operation
 Repair of aorticopulmonary window
P1-34857 Obliteration of aortopulmonary septal defect with cardiopulmonary bypass
P1-34858 Closure of aortoduodenal fistula
P1-34859 Pulmonary-aortic anastomosis
 Pott anastomosis
P1-34860 Creation of shunt of ascending aorta to pulmonary artery
 Shunt of ascending aorta to pulmonary artery by Waterston operation
 Waterston operation for aorta-right pulmonary artery anastomosis
P1-34861 Ascending aorta graft with cardiopulmonary bypass, with coronary implant, with valve suspension and without valve replacement
P1-34862 Ascending aorta graft with cardiopulmonary bypass, with coronary implant, without valve suspension or valve replacement
P1-34863 Ascending aorta graft with cardiopulmonary bypass, without coronary implant, with valve suspension, without valve replacement
P1-34864 Ascending aorta graft with cardiopulmonary bypass, without coronary implant, without valve suspension or valve replacement
P1-34865 Ascending aorta graft with cardiopulmonary bypass, with coronary implant, valve suspension and valve replacement
P1-34866 Ascending aorta graft with cardiopulmonary bypass, with coronary implant, without valve suspension, with valve replacement
P1-34867 Ascending aorta graft with cardiopulmonary bypass, without coronary implant, with valve suspension and valve replacement
P1-34868 Ascending aorta graft with cardiopulmonary bypass, without coronary implant, without valve suspension, with valve replacement
P1-34869 Creation of shunt of descending aorta to pulmonary artery
 Potts-Smith operation, descending aorta-left pulmonary artery anastomosis
 Shunt of descending aorta to pulmonary artery, Potts-Smith
 Anastomosis of descending aorta to pulmonary artery
P1-3486A Shunt of left subclavian to descending aorta by Blalock-Park operation
P1-34870 Repair of hypoplastic aortic arch using autogenous material
P1-34871 Repair of hypoplastic aortic arch using prosthetic material
P1-34872 Repair of interrupted aortic arch using autogenous material
P1-34873 Repair of interrupted aortic arch using prosthetic material
P1-34874 Transverse arch graft with cardiopulmonary bypass
P1-34876 Repair of thoracoabdominal aortic aneurysm with graft and without cardiopulmonary bypass
P1-34877 Repair of thoracoabdominal aortic aneurysm with graft and cardiopulmonary bypass
P1-34878 Descending thoracic aorta graft without bypass
P1-34879 Descending thoracic aorta graft with bypass
P1-34890 Repair of aneurysm of abdominal aorta without graft
P1-34892 Repair of aneurysm of abdominal aorta with graft
P1-34893 Direct repair of ruptured aneurysm of abdominal aorta without patch graft
P1-34894 Repair of ruptured aneurysm of abdominal aorta with graft
P1-34895 Repair of ruptured aneurysm of abdominal aorta without graft
P1-34896 Repair of aneurysm of abdominal aorta involving visceral vessels with graft
P1-34897 Repair of aneurysm of abdominal aorta involving visceral vessels without graft
P1-34898 Repair of ruptured aneurysm of abdominal aorta involving visceral vessels with graft
P1-34899 Repair of ruptured aneurysm of abdominal aorta involving visceral vessels without graft
P1-3489A Repair of aneurysm of abdominal aorta involving iliac vessels with graft
P1-3489B Repair of aneurysm of abdominal aorta involving iliac vessels without graft
P1-3489C Repair of ruptured aneurysm of abdominal aorta involving iliac vessels with graft
P1-3489D Repair of ruptured aneurysm of abdominal aorta involving iliac vessels without graft
P1-34900 Creation of aortosubclavian shunt
 Creation of vascular aortosubclavian bypass
 Anastomosis of aorta to subclavian artery
 Subclavian-aortic anastomosis
P1-34901 Aortosubclavian bypass graft with other than vein
 Aortosubclavian bypass graft with vein
P1-34902 Creation of aortocarotid shunt
 Creation of aortocarotid vascular bypass
P1-34903 Creation of aorta-subclavian-carotid vascular bypass
P1-34904 Creation of aorta-carotid-brachial vascular bypass
P1-34905 Creation of aortorenal shunt
 Creation of aortorenal vascular bypass
 Anastomosis of aorta to renal artery
 Aortorenal bypass graft with vein
P1-34906 Aortorenal bypass graft with other than vein
P1-34907 Creation of aortoiliac shunt
 Aortoiliac vascular bypass
 Aortoiliac bypass graft with vein
 Aortoiliac bypass graft with other than vein

P1-34908 Creation of aortofemoral shunt
Creation of aortofemoral vascular bypass
Aortofemoral bypass graft with vein
Aortofemoral bypass graft with other than vein

P1-34909 Aortoiliofemoral vascular bypass
Aortoiliofemoral shunt
Aorta-iliac-femoral vascular bypass
Aortoiliofemoral bypass graft with vein, unilateral
Aortoiliofemoral bypass graft with vein, bilateral

P1-3490A Abdominal aorta-iliac artery dacron bypass graft

P1-34910 Aortoiliac to popliteal vascular bypass

P1-34911 Aortofemoral to popliteal vascular bypass
Aortofemoral-popliteal bypass graft with vein
Aortofemoral-popliteal bypass graft with other than vein

P1-34912 Aortopopliteal vascular bypass

P1-34913 Creation of aortoceliac shunt
Aortoceliac vascular bypass
Aortoceliac bypass graft with vein
Aortoceliac anastomosis

P1-34914 Aortoceliac bypass graft with other than vein

P1-34915 Creation of aortomesenteric shunt
Aortomesenteric vascular bypass
Aortomesenteric bypass graft with vein
Aortomesenteric anastomosis

P1-34916 Aortomesenteric bypass graft with other than vein

P1-34918 Aortic-superior mesenteric vascular bypass

P1-34920 Removal of intra-aortic balloon with repair of aorta

P1-34921 Removal of intra-aortic balloon with repair of aorta with graft

1-34C Aorta: Destructive Procedures

P1-34C00 Destructive procedure of aorta, NOS

P1-34C10 Denervation of aortic body

1-34D Aorta: Transplantations and Transpositions

P1-34D00 Transplantation of aorta, NOS

1-34E Aorta: Manipulations

P1-34E00 Manipulation of aorta, NOS

1-35 OPERATIVE PROCEDURES ON THE ARTERIES OF THE HEAD AND NECK

1-350 Head and Neck Arteries: General and Miscellaneous Operative Procedures

P1-35000 Operative procedure on artery of head and neck, NOS

P1-35050 Operation on carotid body, NOS

1-351 Head and Neck Arteries: Incisions

P1-35100 Incision of artery of head and neck, NOS
Angiotomy of artery of head and neck, NOS
Arteriotomy of head and neck, NOS

P1-35102 Exploration of artery of head and neck, NOS

P1-35104 Division of artery of head and neck, NOS

P1-35106 Incision of intracranial artery, NOS
Intracranial angiotomy of artery, NOS
Intracranial arteriotomy, NOS

P1-35107 Exploration of intracranial artery, NOS

P1-35108 Division of intracranial artery, NOS

P1-35109 Filipuncture of cerebral aneurysm

P1-35110 Exploration for postoperative thrombosis of neck

P1-35111 Exploration for postoperative hemorrhage of neck

P1-35112 Exploration of carotid artery

1-353 Head and Neck Arteries: Excisions

P1-35300 Excision of artery of head and neck, NOS
Arteriectomy of head and neck, NOS

P1-35304 Excision of lesion of artery of head and neck, NOS

P1-35306 Aneurysmectomy of head and neck artery, NOS

P1-35310 Carotid endarterectomy, NOS
Carotid thromboendarterectomy, NOS

P1-35311 Thromboendarterectomy without graft of carotid artery by neck incision

P1-35313 Thrombectomy without catheter of carotid artery by neck incision

P1-35314 Embolectomy without catheter of carotid artery by neck incision

P1-35315 Thromboendarterectomy with graft of carotid artery by neck incision

P1-35316 Thrombectomy with catheter of carotid artery by neck incision

P1-35317 Embolectomy with catheter of carotid artery by neck incision

P1-35318V Exteriorization of carotid artery

P1-35320 Excision of carotid body, NOS
Carotid glomectomy, NOS

P1-35322 Excision of carotid body lesion, NOS

P1-35323 Excision of carotid body tumor without excision of carotid artery

P1-35324 Excision of carotid body tumor with excision of carotid artery

P1-35330 Thromboendarterectomy without graft of vertebral artery by neck incision

P1-35331 Thromboendarterectomy with graft of vertebral artery by neck incision

P1-35336 Biopsy of temporal artery

P1-35340 Removal of embolus from intracranial artery
Intracranial embolectomy

1-353 Head and Neck Arteries: Excisions — Continued

P1-35342 Removal of thrombus from intracranial artery
  Intracranial thrombectomy
P1-35344 Endarterectomy of intracranial artery
  Intracranial thromboendarterectomy
  Intracranial intimectomy
P1-35345 Intracranial gas endarterectomy
P1-35346 Intracranial arteriectomy with anastomosis
  Intracranial angiectomy of artery with anastomosis
  Resection of intracranial artery with anastomosis
P1-35350 Intracranial aneurysmectomy, NOS
P1-35351 Intracranial aneurysmectomy with anastomosis
P1-35352 Intracranial aneurysmectomy with graft replacement
P1-35354 Excision of intracranial artery, NOS
  Intracranial arteriectomy, NOS
P1-35355 Intracranial arteriectomy with graft replacement
  Intracranial angiectomy of artery with graft replacement
  Resection of intracranial artery with replacement
P1-35358 Excision of lesion of intracranial artery
P1-35360 Removal of embolus of head and neck artery
  Embolectomy of head and neck artery
P1-35361 Thrombectomy of head and neck artery
  Removal of thrombus of head and neck artery
P1-35362 Endarterectomy of head and neck artery
  Thromboendarterectomy of head and neck artery
  Intimectomy of head and neck artery
P1-35363 Gas endarterectomy of head and neck artery
P1-35364 Arteriectomy with anastomosis of head and neck artery
  Angiectomy with anastomosis of head and neck artery
  Resection of artery of head and neck with anastomosis
P1-35365 Aneurysmectomy with anastomosis of head and neck artery
P1-35366 Arteriectomy with graft replacement of head and neck artery
  Angiectomy with graft replacement of head and neck artery
  Resection of artery of head and neck with replacement
P1-35367 Aneurysmectomy with graft replacement of head and neck artery

1-355 Head and Neck Arteries: Injections and Implantations

P1-35500 Injection of artery of head and neck, NOS
P1-35510 Introduction of catheter into carotid artery
P1-35512 Introduction of catheter, each additional selective cerebral artery catheter placement
P1-35513 Introduction of needle into carotid artery
P1-35514 Perfusion of carotid artery
P1-35515 Embolization of artery of neck
P1-35516 Introduction of catheter into vertebral artery
P1-35517 Introduction of catheter into vertebral artery, each additional placement
P1-35518 Introduction of needle into vertebral artery

1-357 Head and Neck Arteries: Endoscopy

P1-35700 Endoscopy of artery of head and neck, NOS

1-358-359 Head and Neck Arteries: Surgical Repairs, Closures and Reconstructions

P1-35800 Repair of artery of head and neck, NOS
P1-35804 Coating of aneurysm of brain, NOS
P1-35810 Embolization of artery of head, NOS
  Embolization of intracranial artery, NOS
P1-35830 Direct repair of artery of neck
P1-35831 Repair of artery of neck with vein graft
P1-35832 Repair of artery of neck with graft other than vein
P1-35834 Repair of congenital arteriovenous fistula of head and neck
P1-35836 Repair of acquired or traumatic arteriovenous fistula of head and neck
P1-35840 Direct repair of aneurysm without graft of carotid artery by neck incision
P1-35841 Direct repair of aneurysm with graft of carotid artery by neck incision
P1-35843 Repair of ruptured aneurysm with graft of carotid artery by neck incision
P1-35844 Repair of ruptured aneurysm without graft of carotid artery by neck incision
P1-35848 Repair of aneurysm without graft of vertebral artery
P1-35849 Repair of aneurysm with graft of vertebral artery
P1-35850 Creation of external-internal carotid bypass, NOS
P1-35851 Creation of carotid-carotid shunt, NOS
P1-35852 Bypass graft with vein of carotid artery
  Carotid-carotid bypass graft with vein
P1-35853 Bypass graft of carotid artery with other than vein
P1-35855 Creation of carotid-subclavian shunt, NOS
  Vascular bypass of carotid to subclavian artery
P1-35856 Carotid-subclavian artery bypass graft with vein
  Subclavian-carotid artery bypass graft with vein
P1-35857 Carotid-subclavian artery bypass graft with other than vein
P1-35860 Creation of carotid-vertebral artery shunt

P1-35861 Carotid-vertebral artery bypass graft with vein
P1-35862 Carotid-vertebral artery bypass graft with other than vein
P1-35863 Bypass graft with other than vein, vertebral-carotid transposition
P1-35870 Creation of subclavian-vertebral artery shunt
P1-35871 Subclavian-vertebral artery bypass graft with vein
P1-35872 Subclavian-vertebral bypass graft with other than vein
P1-35873 Bypass graft with other than vein, vertebral-subclavian transposition
P1-35879 Anastomosis of extracranial-intracranial arteries, NOS
P1-35900 Surgical occlusion of artery of head and neck, NOS
P1-35901 Ligation of artery of head and neck, NOS
P1-35902 Ligation of major artery of neck, NOS
P1-35910 Surgical occlusion of intracranial artery, NOS
P1-35911 Ligation of intracranial artery, NOS
P1-35912 Application of clamp to cerebral aneurysm, Crutchfield or Silverstone, NOS
    Clamping of cerebral aneurysm, NOS
    Clipping of cerebral aneurysm, NOS
P1-35914 Trapping of cerebral aneurysm, NOS
P1-35920 Ligation of temporal artery
P1-35922 Ligation of thyroid artery
P1-35923 Ligation of external carotid artery
P1-35924 Ligation of common carotid artery
P1-35925 Ligation of internal carotid artery
P1-35926 Ligation of internal carotid artery with gradual occlusion by Silverstone or Crutchfield clamp
P1-35927 Ligation of common carotid artery with gradual occlusion by Silverstone or Crutchfield clamp
P1-35930 Percutaneous transluminal vertebral artery balloon angioplasty

1-35C Head and Neck Arteries: Destructive Procedures

P1-35C00 Destructive procedure on artery of head and neck, NOS
P1-35C10 Coagulation of aneurysm of cerebral vessel
    Electrocoagulation of aneurysm of cerebral artery
P1-35C12 Denervation of carotid body
P1-35C13 Stripping of carotid sinus

1-35D Head and Neck Arteries: Transplantations and Transpositions

P1-35D00 Transplantation of artery of head and neck, NOS

1-35E Head and Neck Arteries: Manipulations

P1-35E20 Stimulation of carotid sinus

1-36 OPERATIVE PROCEDURES ON THE ARTERIES OF THE THORAX AND ABDOMEN

1-360 Thoracic and Abdominal Arteries: General and Miscellaneous Operative Procedures

P1-36000 Operative procedure on the arteries of the thorax and abdomen, NOS

1-361 Thoracic and Abdominal Arteries: Incisions

P1-36100 Incision of thoracic artery, NOS
    Thoracic angiotomy of artery, NOS
    Thoracic arteriotomy, NOS
P1-36102 Exploration of thoracic artery
P1-36104 Division of thoracic artery
P1-36110 Exploration for postoperative hemorrhage of chest
P1-36112 Exploration for postoperative thrombosis of chest
P1-36120 Incision of abdominal artery
    Angiotomy of abdominal artery
    Abdominal arteriotomy
P1-36122 Division of abdominal artery
P1-36124 Exploration of abdominal artery
P1-36125 Exploration for postoperative thrombosis of abdomen
P1-36126 Exploration for postoperative hemorrhage of abdomen
P1-36130 Release of celiac artery axis
    Strong operation for unbridling of celiac artery axis
    Unbridling of celiac artery axis
P1-36132 Release of median arcuate ligament

1-363-364 Thoracic and Abdominal Arteries: Excisions

P1-36300 Excision of artery of thorax and abdomen, NOS
P1-36310 Removal of pulmonary embolus
P1-36312 Pulmonary artery embolectomy with cardiopulmonary bypass
P1-36313 Pulmonary artery embolectomy without bypass
P1-36314 Pulmonary endarterectomy with embolectomy and cardiopulmonary bypass
P1-36315 Pulmonary endarterectomy without embolectomy and with cardiopulmonary bypass
P1-36317 Thrombectomy of pulmonary artery
    Removal of thrombus of pulmonary artery
P1-36320 Embolectomy with catheter of innominate artery by neck incision
P1-36321 Thrombectomy with catheter of innominate artery by neck incision
P1-36322 Embolectomy without catheter of innominate artery by neck incision

1-363-364 Thoracic and Abdominal Arteries: Excisions — Continued

P1-36323 Thrombectomy without catheter of innominate artery by neck incision
P1-36324 Embolectomy with catheter of innominate artery by thoracic incision
P1-36325 Thrombectomy with catheter of innominate artery by thoracic incision
P1-36326 Embolectomy without catheter of innominate artery by thoracic incision
P1-36327 Thrombectomy without catheter of innominate artery by thoracic incision
P1-36328 Thromboendarterectomy without graft of innominate artery by thoracic incision
P1-36330 Embolectomy with catheter of subclavian artery by neck incision
P1-36331 Thrombectomy with catheter of subclavian artery by neck incision
P1-36332 Embolectomy without catheter of subclavian artery by neck incision
P1-36333 Thrombectomy without catheter of subclavian artery by neck incision
P1-36334 Embolectomy with catheter of subclavian artery by thoracic incision
P1-36335 Thrombectomy with catheter of subclavian artery by thoracic incision
P1-36336 Embolectomy without catheter of subclavian artery by thoracic incision
P1-36337 Thrombectomy without catheter of subclavian artery by thoracic incision
P1-36338 Thromboendarterectomy with graft of subclavian artery by neck incision
P1-36339 Thromboendarterectomy without graft of subclavian artery by neck incision
P1-3633A Thromboendarterectomy without graft of subclavian artery by thoracic incision
P1-36350 Embolectomy with catheter of celiac artery by abdominal incision
P1-36351 Thrombectomy with catheter of celiac artery by abdominal incision
P1-36352 Embolectomy without catheter of celiac artery by abdominal incision
P1-36354 Thrombectomy without catheter of celiac artery by abdominal incision
P1-36355 Thromboendarterectomy without graft of celiac artery
P1-36358 Arteriectomy with anastomosis of abdominal artery
P1-36360 Embolectomy with catheter of mesenteric artery by abdominal incision
P1-36361 Thrombectomy with catheter of mesenteric artery by abdominal incision
P1-36362 Embolectomy without catheter of mesenteric artery by abdominal incision
P1-36363 Thrombectomy without catheter of mesenteric artery by abdominal incision
P1-36364 Thromboendarterectomy without graft of mesenteric artery
P1-36370 Embolectomy with catheter of renal artery by abdominal incision
P1-36371 Thrombectomy with catheter of renal artery by abdominal incision
P1-36372 Embolectomy without catheter of renal artery by abdominal incision
P1-36373 Thrombectomy without catheter of renal artery by abdominal incision
P1-36374 Thromboendarterectomy without graft of renal artery
P1-36378 Excision of aberrant renal artery
P1-36380 Thromboendarterectomy without graft of iliac artery
P1-36382 Thromboendarterectomy without graft of iliofemoral artery
P1-36400 Removal of embolus from thoracic artery, NOS
  Embolectomy of thoracic artery, NOS
P1-36402 Removal of thrombus from thoracic artery, NOS
  Thrombectomy of thoracic artery, NOS
P1-36404 Thoracic endarterectomy
  Endarterectomy of thoracic artery
  Intimectomy of thoracic artery
P1-36405 Gas endarterectomy of thoracic artery
P1-36406 Thromboendarterectomy of thoracic artery
P1-36410 Angiectomy with anastomosis of thoracic artery
  Arteriectomy with anastomosis of thoracic artery
  Resection of thoracic artery with anastomosis
P1-36411 Thoracic aneurysmectomy, NOS
P1-36412 Aneurysmectomy with anastomosis of thoracic artery
P1-36420 Excision of thoracic artery, NOS
  Thoracic arteriectomy, NOS
P1-36421 Resection of thoracic artery with replacement
P1-36424 Excision of lesion of thoracic artery
P1-36440 Excision of abdominal artery, NOS
  Abdominal arteriectomy, NOS
P1-36442 Embolectomy of abdominal artery
  Removal of embolus from abdominal artery
P1-36443 Thrombectomy of abdominal artery
  Removal of thrombus from abdominal artery
P1-36444 Endarterectomy of abdominal artery
  Intimectomy of abdominal artery
P1-36445 Gas endarterectomy of abdominal artery
P1-36446 Thromboendarterectomy of abdominal artery
P1-36450 Excision of lesion from abdominal artery
P1-36452 Angiectomy with anastomosis of abdominal artery
  Resection of abdominal artery with anastomosis
P1-36453 Aneurysmectomy of abdominal artery
P1-36454 Aneurysmectomy with anastomosis of abdominal artery

P1-36458 Resection of abdominal artery with replacement

1-365 Thoracic and Abdominal Arteries: Injections and Implantations

P1-36500 Injection of thoracic and abdominal artery, NOS
P1-36510 Embolization of thoracic artery
P1-36512 Introduction of catheter, each additional selective thoracic artery catheter placement
P1-36520 Introduction of catheter into pulmonary artery
P1-36522 Pulmonary catheterization with Swan-Ganz catheter
Insertion and placement of flow directed catheter, Swan-Ganz, for monitoring purposes
Insertion of Swan-Ganz catheter into pulmonary artery
P1-36530 Embolization of abdominal artery
P1-36532 Transcatheter embolization for gastric bleeding
P1-36535 Introduction of catheter, each additional selective abdominal artery catheter placement

1-367 Thoracic and Abdominal Arteries: Endoscopy

P1-36700 Endoscopy of thoracic and abdominal artery, NOS

1-368-36A Thoracic and Abdominal Arteries: Surgical Repairs, Closures and Reconstructions

P1-36800 Repair of artery of thorax and abdomen, NOS
P1-36812 Repair of patent ductus arteriosus, NOS
Division of patent ductus arteriosus
P1-36813 Division of patent ductus arteriosus, up to age 18
P1-36814 Division of patent ductus arteriosus, over age 18
P1-36815 Division of patent ductus arteriosus, simultaneous procedure
P1-36816 Ligation of patent ductus arteriosus
Closure of patent ductus arteriosus
P1-36817 Ligation of patent ductus arteriosus, simultaneous procedure
P1-36820 Direct repair of intrathoracic artery without bypass
P1-36822 Direct repair of intrathoracic artery with bypass
P1-36823 Repair with vein graft of intrathoracic artery without bypass
P1-36824 Repair with vein graft of intrathoracic artery with bypass
P1-36825 Repair with graft other than vein of intrathoracic artery without bypass
P1-36827 Repair with graft other than vein of intrathoracic artery with bypass
P1-36830 Total correction of transposition of great vessels, NOS
P1-36831 Repair of transposition of the great arteries, atrial baffle procedure, Mustard or Senning type with cardiopulmonary bypass
P1-36832 Repair of transposition of the great arteries, atrial baffle procedure, Mustard or Senning type with cardiopulmonary bypass, with removal of pulmonary band
P1-36833 Repair of transposition of the great arteries, atrial baffle procedure, Mustard or Senning type with cardiopulmonary bypass, with closure of ventricular septal defect
P1-36834 Repair of transposition of the great arteries, atrial baffle procedure, Mustard or Senning type with cardiopulmonary bypass, with repair of subpulmonic obstruction
P1-36835 Repair of transposition of the great arteries, aortic pulmonary artery reconstruction, Jatene type
P1-36836 Repair of transposition of the great arteries, aortic pulmonary artery reconstruction, Jatene type, with removal of pulmonary band
P1-36837 Repair of transposition of the great arteries, aortic pulmonary artery reconstruction, Jatene type, with closure of ventricular septal defect
P1-36838 Repair of transposition of the great arteries, aortic pulmonary artery reconstruction, Jatene type, with repair of subpulmonic obstruction
P1-36840 Excision with graft replacement of thoracic artery
Angiectomy with graft replacement of thoracic artery
Arteriectomy with graft replacement of thoracic artery
P1-36841 Aneurysmectomy with graft replacement of thoracic artery
P1-36844 Surgical occlusion of thoracic artery, NOS
P1-36845 Ligation of thoracic artery
P1-36846 Ligation of major artery of chest
P1-36850 Banding of pulmonary artery
Müller operation for banding of pulmonary artery
P1-36853 Rastelli operation for repair of pulmonary artery atresia
P1-36857 Pulmonary bypass operation
P1-36858 Cardiopulmonary bypass operation
Heart lung bypass
P1-36860 Thromboendarterectomy with graft of innominate artery by thoracic incision
P1-36861 Repair of aneurysm without graft of innominate artery by thoracic incision
P1-36862 Repair of aneurysm with graft of innominate artery by thoracic incision

1-368-36A Thoracic and Abdominal Arteries: Surgical Repairs, Closures and Reconstructions — Continued

P1-36863 Repair of ruptured aneurysm without graft of innominate artery by thoracic incision
P1-36864 Repair of ruptured aneurysm with graft of innominate artery by thoracic incision
P1-36866 Bardenheurer operation for ligation of innominate artery
P1-36870 Intraoperative transluminal subclavian-axillary angioplasty
P1-36871 Thromboendarterectomy with graft of subclavian artery by thoracic incision
P1-36872 Direct repair of aneurysm without graft of subclavian artery by neck incision
P1-36873 Direct repair of aneurysm with graft of subclavian artery by neck incision
P1-36874 Repair of aneurysm without graft of subclavian artery by thoracic incision
P1-36875 Repair of aneurysm with graft of subclavian artery by thoracic incision
P1-36876 Repair of ruptured aneurysm without graft of subclavian artery by neck incision
P1-36877 Repair of ruptured aneurysm with graft of subclavian artery by neck incision
P1-36878 Repair of ruptured aneurysm without graft of subclavian artery by thoracic incision
P1-36879 Repair of ruptured aneurysm with graft of subclavian artery by thoracic incision
P1-3687A Ligation of subclavian artery
  Touroff operation for ligation of subclavian artery
P1-36880 Direct repair of intra-abdominal artery
P1-36881 Repair with vein graft of intra-abdominal artery
P1-36882 Repair with graft other than vein of intra-abdominal artery
P1-36883 Excision with graft replacement of abdominal artery
  Angiectomy with graft replacement of abdominal artery
P1-36884 Aneurysmectomy with graft replacement of abdominal artery
P1-36885 Surgical occlusion of abdominal artery, NOS
P1-36886 Ligation of abdominal artery, NOS
P1-36887 Ligation of major artery of abdomen
P1-36888 Ligation of gastric artery
  Gastric vasoligation
P1-36889 Ligation of splenic artery
P1-3688A Intraoperative transluminal angioplasty of visceral artery, NOS
P1-36890 Intraoperative transluminal angioplasty of renal artery
P1-36892 Thromboendarterectomy with graft of renal artery
P1-36893 Repair of aneurysm without graft of renal artery
P1-36894 Repair of aneurysm with graft of renal artery
P1-36895 Repair of ruptured aneurysm without graft of renal artery
P1-36896 Repair of ruptured aneurysm with graft of renal artery
P1-36899 Aortofemoral-popliteal artery in-situ vein bypass graft
P1-36901 Repair of aneurysm without graft of splenic artery
P1-36902 Repair of aneurysm with graft of splenic artery
P1-36903 Repair of ruptured aneurysm without graft of splenic artery
P1-36904 Repair of ruptured aneurysm with graft of splenic artery
P1-36910 Thromboendarterectomy with graft of celiac artery
P1-36911 Repair of aneurysm without graft of celiac artery
P1-36912 Repair of aneurysm with graft of celiac artery
P1-36913 Repair of ruptured aneurysm without graft of celiac artery
P1-36914 Repair of ruptured aneurysm with graft of celiac artery
P1-36920 Repair of aneurysm without graft of hepatic artery
P1-36921 Repair of aneurysm with graft of hepatic artery
P1-36922 Repair of ruptured aneurysm without graft of hepatic artery
P1-36923 Repair of ruptured aneurysm with graft of hepatic artery
P1-36930 Thromboendarterectomy with graft of mesenteric artery
P1-36931 Repair of aneurysm without graft of mesenteric artery
P1-36932 Repair of aneurysm with graft of mesenteric artery
P1-36933 Repair of ruptured aneurysm without graft of mesenteric artery
P1-36934 Repair of ruptured aneurysm with graft of mesenteric artery
P1-36940 Intraoperative transluminal angioplasty of iliac artery
P1-36941 Thromboendarterectomy with graft of iliac artery
P1-36942 Thromboendarterectomy with graft of iliofemoral artery
P1-36943 Repair of aneurysm without graft of iliac artery
P1-36944 Repair of aneurysm with graft of iliac artery
P1-36945 Repair of ruptured aneurysm without graft of iliac artery
P1-36946 Repair of ruptured aneurysm with graft of iliac artery
P1-36948 Central shunt with prosthetic graft
P1-36950 Creation of intrathoracic vascular shunt or bypass, NOS
P1-36951 Anastomosis of intrathoracic artery
  Intrathoracic arterial bypass

P1-36952 Creation of shunt left-to-right, systemic to pulmonary circulation
Creation of left-to-right shunt, systemic-pulmonary artery
Creation of systemic-pulmonary artery shunt
Anastomosis of systemic to pulmonary artery
P1-36953 Take-down of systemic-pulmonary artery anastomosis
P1-36957 Anastomosis of pulmonary-subclavian artery by Blalock-Taussig operation
Blalock-Taussig operation, subclavian-pulmonary anastomosis
Shunt of subclavian to pulmonary artery
Creation of subclavian-pulmonary shunt
P1-36958 Creation of pulmonary-innominate artery shunt
Blalock operation, systemic-pulmonary anastomosis
Anastomosis of pulmonary-innominate artery by Blalock operation
P1-36959 Caval-pulmonary artery anastomosis
Shunt of vena cava to pulmonary artery, Glenn type operation
Anastomosis of superior vena cava to pulmonary artery
Glenn operation for anastomosis of superior vena cava to right pulmonary artery
Shunt of vena cava to pulmonary artery
Anastomosis of pulmonary artery and superior vena cava
P1-3695A Vascular subclavian-subclavian bypass
P1-3695B Subclavian-subclavian artery bypass graft with vein
P1-3695C Subclavian-subclavian artery bypass graft with other than vein
P1-3695D Anastomosis of carotid-subclavian artery
P1-36960 Vascular subclavian-axillary bypass
P1-36961 Subclavian-axillary artery bypass graft with vein
P1-36962 Subclavian-axillary artery bypass graft with other than vein
P1-36965 Axillary-axillary artery bypass graft
P1-36966 Axillary-axillary artery bypass graft with vein
P1-36967 Axillary-axillary artery bypass graft with other than vein
P1-36970 Intra-abdominal vascular shunt or bypass, NOS
Arterial intra-abdominal bypass
P1-36972 Vascular bypass of renal artery
P1-36973 Vascular bypass of renal artery with graft
P1-36976 Ilioiliac shunt
Ilioiliac vascular bypass
P1-36977 Ilioiliac bypass graft with vein
P1-36978 Ilioiliac bypass graft with other than vein
P1-36979 Common hepatic-common iliac-renal vascular bypass
P1-36980 Iliofemoral shunt
P1-36981 Iliofemoral bypass graft with vein
P1-36982 Iliofemoral bypass graft with other than vein
P1-36990 Splenorenal bypass graft
P1-36991 Splenorenal bypass graft with vein
P1-36992 Splenorenal bypass graft with other than vein
P1-36A10 Repair of anal sphincter aneurysm, false or true
P1-36A12 Repair of congenital arteriovenous fistula of thorax and abdomen
P1-36A13 Repair of acquired or traumatic arteriovenous fistula of thorax and abdomen
P1-36A25 Ligation of adrenal artery

1-36C Thoracic and Abdominal Arteries: Destructive Procedures

P1-36C00 Destructive procedure of thoracic artery, NOS
P1-36C10 Destructive procedure of abdominal artery, NOS

1-36D Thoracic and Abdominal Arteries: Transplantations and Transpositions

P1-36D00 Transplantation of thoracic artery, NOS
P1-36D04 Reimplantation of anomalous pulmonary artery
P1-36D10 Transplantation of abdominal artery, NOS
P1-36D20 Transplantation of aberrant renal artery
Transection of aberrant renal artery with reimplantation
Reimplantation of aberrant renal artery
Reattachment of aberrant renal artery
Reposition of aberrant renal artery
Hellstom operation for transplantation of aberrant renal artery

1-36E Thoracic and Abdominal Arteries: Manipulations

P1-36E00 Manipulation of thoracic artery, NOS
P1-36E10 Manipulation of abdominal artery, NOS

1-37 OPERATIVE PROCEDURES ON THE ARTERIES OF THE EXTREMITIES

1-370 Arteries of The Extremities: General and Miscellaneous Operative Procedures

P1-37000 Operation procedure on artery of extremity, NOS

1-371 Arteries of The Extremities: Incisions

P1-37100 Incision of artery of upper limb
Angiotomy of upper limb artery
Arteriotomy of upper limb
P1-37102 Exploration of artery of upper limb
P1-37104 Division of artery of upper limb
P1-37120 Incision of artery of lower limb
Angiotomy of lower limb artery

1-371 Arteries of The Extremities: Incisions — Continued

P1-37120 (cont.) Arteriotomy of lower limb
P1-37122 Exploration of artery of lower limb
P1-37124 Division of artery of lower limb
P1-37126 Exploration of femoral artery
P1-37127 Exploration of popliteal artery
P1-37128 Exploration for postoperative hemorrhage of extremity
P1-37129 Exploration for postoperative thrombosis of extremity
P1-3712A Unbridling of artery of limb

1-373 Arteries of The Extremities: Excisions

P1-37300 Excision of artery of extremity, NOS
P1-37310 Excision of upper limb artery, NOS
Arteriectomy of upper limb, NOS
P1-37312 Excision of lesion of artery of upper limb
P1-37314 Aneurysmectomy of upper limb artery
P1-37315 Endarterectomy of upper limb artery
Intimectomy of upper limb artery
P1-37316 Gas endarterectomy of upper limb artery
P1-37317 Thromboendarterectomy of upper limb artery
P1-37318 Embolectomy of upper limb artery
P1-37321 Embolectomy without catheter of axillary artery by arm incision
P1-37322 Thrombectomy without catheter of axillary artery by arm incision
P1-37323 Embolectomy without catheter of brachial artery by arm incision
P1-37324 Thrombectomy without catheter of brachial artery by arm incision
P1-37325 Embolectomy without catheter of innominate artery by arm incision
P1-37326 Thrombectomy without catheter of innominate artery by arm incision
P1-37327 Embolectomy without catheter of subclavian artery by arm incision
P1-37328 Thrombectomy without catheter of subclavian artery by arm incision
P1-37329 Embolectomy without catheter of radial artery by arm incision
P1-3732A Thrombectomy without catheter of radial artery by arm incision
P1-3732B Embolectomy without catheter of ulnar artery by arm incision
P1-3732C Thrombectomy without catheter of ulnar artery by arm incision
P1-37330 Embolectomy with catheter of axillary artery by arm incision
P1-37333 Thrombectomy with catheter of axillary artery by arm incision
P1-37334 Embolectomy with catheter of brachial artery by arm incision
P1-37335 Thrombectomy with catheter of brachial artery by arm incision
P1-37336 Embolectomy with catheter of innominate artery by arm incision
P1-37337 Thrombectomy with catheter of innominate artery by arm incision
P1-37338 Embolectomy with catheter of subclavian artery by arm incision
P1-37339 Thrombectomy with catheter of subclavian artery by arm incision
P1-37340 Embolectomy with catheter of radial artery by arm incision
P1-37341 Thrombectomy with catheter of radial artery by arm incision
P1-37342 Embolectomy with catheter of ulnar artery by arm incision
P1-37343 Thrombectomy with catheter of ulnar artery by arm incision
P1-37345 Thromboendarterectomy without graft of axillary-brachial artery
P1-37346 Thromboendarterectomy with graft of axillary-brachial artery
P1-37350 Resection of upper limb artery with anastomosis
Angiectomy with anastomosis of upper limb artery
Arteriectomy with anastomosis of upper limb
P1-37352 Aneurysmectomy with anastomosis of upper limb artery
P1-37353 Aneurysmectomy with graft replacement of upper limb artery
P1-37354 Angiectomy with graft replacement of upper limb artery
Resection of upper limb artery with replacement by graft
Arteriectomy with graft replacement of upper limb
P1-37360 Excision of lower limb artery, NOS
Arteriectomy of lower limb, NOS
P1-37361 Resection of lower limb artery with replacement by graft
Angiectomy with graft replacement of lower limb artery
Arteriectomy with graft replacement of lower limb
P1-37362 Angiectomy with anastomosis of lower limb artery
Arteriectomy with anastomosis of lower limb
Resection of lower limb artery with anastomosis
P1-37364 Aneurysmectomy of lower limb artery
P1-37365 Aneurysmectomy with graft replacement of lower limb artery
P1-37366 Aneurysmectomy with anastomosis of lower limb artery
P1-37367 Excision of lesion of artery of lower limb
P1-37370 Endarterectomy of lower limb artery
Intimectomy of lower limb

P1-37372 Gas endarterectomy of lower limb artery
P1-37374 Embolectomy of lower limb artery
Removal of embolus of lower limb artery
P1-37375 Thrombectomy of lower limb artery
Removal of thrombus of lower limb artery
P1-37376 Thromboendarterectomy of lower limb artery
P1-37377 Femoral endarterectomy
P1-37378 Embolectomy of femoral artery
P1-37381 Embolectomy without catheter of femoropopliteal artery by leg incision
P1-37382 Thrombectomy without catheter of femoropopliteal artery by leg incision
P1-37383 Embolectomy without catheter of popliteal-tibio-peroneal artery by leg incision
P1-37384 Thrombectomy without catheter of popliteal-tibio-peroneal artery by leg incision
P1-37385 Embolectomy with catheter of femoropopliteal artery by leg incision
P1-37386 Thrombectomy with catheter of femoropopliteal artery by leg incision
P1-37387 Embolectomy with catheter of popliteal-tibio-peroneal artery by leg incision
P1-37388 Thrombectomy with catheter of popliteal-tibio-peroneal artery by leg incision
P1-37390 Thromboendarterectomy without graft of common femoral artery
Thromboendarterectomy of common femoral artery
P1-37391 Thromboendarterectomy with graft of common femoral artery
P1-37392 Thromboendarterectomy without graft of deep profunda femoral artery
P1-37393 Thromboendarterectomy with graft of deep profunda femoral artery
P1-37394 Thromboendarterectomy with graft of femoral and popliteal arteries
P1-37395 Thromboendarterectomy with graft of femoral, popliteal and tibioperoneal arteries

1-375 Arteries of The Extremities: Injections and Implantations

P1-37500 Injection of artery of extremity, NOS
P1-37502 Perfusion of limb, NOS
P1-37503 Perfusion of upper limb
P1-37504 Perfusion of lower limb
P1-37510 Embolization of artery of upper limb
P1-37512 Embolization of artery of lower limb
P1-37520 Introduction of catheter into artery of extremity
P1-37521 Arterial catheterization or cannulation for transfusion, percutaneous
P1-37522 Insertion of tissue mandril of artery of extremity
P1-37525 Introduction of needle into artery of extremity
P1-37528 Introduction of catheter, retrograde, brachial artery
P1-37529 Introduction of needle, retrograde, brachial artery

1-377 Arteries of The Extremities: Endoscopy

P1-37700 Endoscopy of artery of extremity, NOS

1-378-379 Arteries of The Extremities: Surgical Repairs, Closures and Reconstructions

P1-37800 Surgical repair of artery of extremity, NOS
P1-37810 Direct repair of artery of upper extremity
P1-37811 Direct repair of artery of hand
P1-37812 Direct repair of artery of finger
P1-37814 Repair of artery with vein graft of upper extremity
P1-37815 Repair of artery with graft other than vein of upper extremity
P1-37816 Repair of aneurysm without graft of radial artery
P1-37817 Repair of aneurysm without graft of ulnar artery
P1-37818 Repair of aneurysm without graft of axillary-brachial artery of arm by incision
P1-37820 Repair of aneurysm with graft of radial artery
P1-37821 Repair of aneurysm with graft of ulnar artery
P1-37822 Axillary-brachial artery vascular bypass
P1-37823 Repair of aneurysm with graft of axillary-brachial artery of arm by incision
P1-37824 Repair of ruptured aneurysm without graft of axillary-brachial artery of arm by incision
P1-37825 Repair of ruptured aneurysm with graft of axillary-brachial artery of arm by incision
P1-37830 Surgical occlusion of upper limb artery, NOS
P1-37832 Ligation of artery of upper limb
P1-37850 Direct repair of artery of lower extremity
P1-37851 Repair of artery with vein graft of lower extremity
P1-37852 Repair of artery with graft other than vein of lower extremity
P1-37854 Intraoperative transluminal femoral-popliteal angioplasty
P1-37856 Repair of aneurysm without graft of common femoral artery
P1-37857 Repair of aneurysm without graft of popliteal artery
P1-37858 Repair of aneurysm with graft of common femoral artery
P1-37859 Repair of aneurysm with graft of popliteal artery
P1-3785A Repair of ruptured aneurysm without graft of common femoral artery
P1-3785B Repair of ruptured aneurysm without graft of popliteal artery
P1-3785C Repair of ruptured aneurysm with graft of common femoral artery
P1-3785D Repair of ruptured aneurysm with graft of popliteal artery
P1-37860 Femoral-femoral artery vascular bypass
P1-37861 Femoral-femoral artery bypass graft with vein
P1-37862 Femoral-femoral artery bypass graft with other than vein

1-378-379 Arteries of The Extremities: Surgical Repairs, Closures and Reconstructions — Continued

P1-37863 Femoral-popliteal artery bypass graft
  Femoral-popliteal artery vascular bypass
  Creation of femoropopliteal shunt
P1-37864 Femoral-popliteal artery bypass graft with vein
  Femoral-popliteal in-situ vein bypass
P1-37865 Femoral-popliteal artery bypass graft with other than vein
P1-37867 Femoral-anterior tibial artery bypass graft with vein
  Femoral-anterior tibial artery in-situ vein bypass
P1-37868 Femoral-anterior tibial artery bypass graft with other than vein
P1-3786B Peroneal artery bypass graft with vein
  Peroneal artery in-situ vein bypass
P1-3786C Peroneal artery bypass graft with other than vein
P1-37870 Posterior tibial artery bypass graft with vein
  Posterior tibial artery in-situ vein bypass
P1-37871 Posterior tibial artery bypass graft with other than vein
P1-37874 Popliteal-peroneal artery bypass graft with vein
P1-37875 Popliteal-peroneal artery bypass graft with other than vein
P1-37877 Popliteal-tibial artery vascular bypass
P1-37878 Popliteal-tibial artery bypass graft with vein
  Popliteal-tibial artery in-situ vein bypass
P1-37879 Popliteal-tibial artery bypass graft with other than vein
P1-37880 Axillary-femoral artery bypass graft with vein
P1-37881 Axillary-femoral artery bypass graft with other than vein
P1-37882 Axillary-femoral-femoral artery bypass graft with vein
P1-37883 Axillary-femoral-femoral artery bypass graft with other than vein
P1-37885 Axillary-femoral vascular bypass
  Superficial axillofemoral vascular bypass
  Axillary-femoral shunt
P1-37887 Bifemoral bypass graft with vein
P1-37888 Bifemoral artery bypass graft with other than vein
P1-37890 Femoroperoneal vascular bypass
  Femoroperoneal shunt
P1-37891 Femorotibial vascular bypass, anterior or posterior
P1-37892 Iliofemoral vascular bypass
P1-37894 Surgical occlusion of lower limb artery, NOS
P1-37895 Ligation of artery of lower limb
P1-37896 Reattachment of artery of extremity
P1-37900 Repair of congenital arteriovenous fistula of extremity
P1-37901 Repair of acquired or traumatic arteriovenous fistula of extremity
P1-37905 Peripheral arterial bypass, NOS
  Vascular bypass of peripheral artery
  Peripheral vascular shunt or bypass
P1-37908 Ligation of major artery of extremity, NOS

1-37C Arteries of The Extremities: Destructive Procedures

P1-37C00 Destructive procedure of artery of extremity, NOS
P1-37C10 Destructive procedure of artery of upper extremity, NOS
P1-37C20 Destructive procedure of artery of lower extremity, NOS

1-37D Arteries of The Extremities: Transplantations and Transpositions

P1-37D00 Transplantation of artery of extremity, NOS
P1-37D10 Transplantation of artery of upper extremity, NOS
P1-37D20 Transplantation of artery of lower extremity, NOS

1-37E Arteries of The Extremities: Manipulations

P1-37E00 Manipulation of artery of extremity, NOS
P1-37E10 Manipulation of artery of upper extremity, NOS
P1-37E20 Manipulation of artery of lower extremity, NOS

1-38 OPERATIVE PROCEDURES ON THE VEINS

1-380 Veins: General and Miscellaneous Operative Procedures

P1-38000 Operator procedure on veins, NOS

1-381-382 Veins: Incisions

P1-38100 Incision of vein, NOS
  Phlebotomy, NOS
  Venotomy, NOS
P1-38104 Exploration of vein
P1-38108 Division of varicose vein
P1-38110 Incision of intracranial vein
  Intracranial phlebotomy
  Intracranial venotomy
P1-38114 Exploration of intracranial vein
P1-38117 Division of intracranial vein
P1-38118 Division of intracranial varicose vein
P1-38120 Incision of vein of head and neck
  Phlebotomy of head and neck vein
  Venotomy of head and neck vein
P1-38124 Exploration of vein of head and neck
P1-38127 Division of vein head and neck
P1-38128 Division of varicose vein of head and neck
P1-38130 Incision of vein of upper limb
  Phlebotomy of upper limb vein

P1-38130 (cont.) Venotomy of upper limb vein
P1-38134 Exploration of vein of upper limb
P1-38137 Division of vein of upper limb
P1-38138 Division of varicose vein of upper limb
  Varicotomy of peripheral veins of upper limb
P1-38140 Incision of thoracic vein
  Thoracic phlebotomy
  Thoracic venotomy
P1-38144 Exploration of thoracic vein
P1-38147 Division of thoracic vein
P1-38148 Division of thoracic varicose vein
P1-38150 Incision of abdominal vein
  Abdominal phlebotomy
  Abdominal venotomy
  Angiotomy of abdominal vein
P1-38154 Exploration of abdominal vein
P1-38157 Division of abdominal vein
P1-38158 Division of abdominal varicose vein
P1-38160 Incision of vein of lower limb
  Incision of peripheral veins of lower limb
  Phlebotomy of lower limb vein
  Venotomy of lower limb vein
  Angiotomy of lower limb vein
P1-38164 Exploration of vein of lower limb
  Exploration of peripheral veins of lower limb
P1-38167 Division of vein of lower limb
P1-38168 Division of varicose vein of lower limb
  Transection of varicose vein of lower limb
  Varicotomy of peripheral veins of lower limb
P1-38200 Venipuncture, NOS
  Puncture of vein, NOS
  Introduction of needle into vein
P1-38201 Venipuncture, under age 3 years
P1-38202 Venipuncture, child over age 3 years, by physician
P1-38204 Venipuncture of sagittal sinus, under age 3 years
P1-38205 Venipuncture of scalp vein, under age 3 years
P1-38206 Venipuncture of jugular vein, up to age 3 years
P1-38207 Venipuncture of femoral vein, up to age 3 years
P1-38210 Routine venipuncture for collection of specimen, NOS
P1-38220 Venous cutdown, NOS
P1-38221 Venipuncture, cutdown, up to age 1
P1-38222 Venipuncture, cutdown, over age 1

1-383-384 Veins: Excisions

P1-38300 Excision of vein, NOS
  Phlebectomy, NOS
  Venectomy, NOS
P1-38302 Excision of varicose vein
  Varicose phlebectomy
  Cockett operation for varicose vein
P1-38304 Phlebectomy with anastomosis
P1-38310 Biopsy of vein, NOS
  Excisional biopsy of vein, NOS
P1-38312 Excision of lesion of vein, NOS
P1-38314 Thrombectomy of venous graft
P1-38315 Phlebectomy with graft replacement
P1-38318 Removal of implantable intravenous infusion pump
P1-38319 Removal of implantable venous access port
P1-38320 Intracranial phlebectomy, NOS
P1-38322 Excision of lesion of intracranial vein
P1-38323 Phlebectomy of intracranial varicose vein
  Excision of intracranial varicose vein
P1-38324 Intracranial phlebectomy with anastomosis
P1-38325 Intracranial phlebectomy with graft replacement
P1-38330 Phlebectomy of head and neck vein
P1-38331 Excision of lesion of vein of head and neck
P1-38332 Phlebectomy of varicose vein of head and neck
  Excision of varicose vein of head and neck
P1-38333 Phlebectomy with anastomosis of head and neck vein
P1-38334 Phlebectomy with graft replacement of head and neck
P1-38335 Direct thrombectomy of subclavian vein by neck incision
P1-38336 Direct thrombectomy of subclavian vein by arm incision
P1-38337 Direct thrombectomy of axillary vein by arm incision
P1-38339 Thrombectomy with catheter of subclavian vein by neck incision
P1-3833A Thrombectomy with catheter of axillary vein by arm incision
P1-3833B Thrombectomy with catheter of subclavian vein by arm incision
P1-38340 Phlebectomy of upper limb vein
P1-38341 Excision of lesion of vein of upper limb
P1-38342 Excision of varicose vein of upper limb
  Extirpation of varicose vein of upper limb
  Phlebectomy of varicose vein of upper limb
  Stripping of varicose veins of upper limb
  Cockett operation of upper limb
P1-38343 Phlebectomy with anastomosis of upper limb vein
P1-38344 Phlebectomy with graft replacement of upper limb vein
P1-38350 Thoracic phlebectomy
P1-38351 Excision of lesion of thoracic vein
P1-38352 Excision of thoracic varicose vein
  Thoracic phlebectomy of varicose vein
P1-38353 Thoracic phlebectomy with anastomosis
P1-38354 Thoracic phlebectomy with graft replacement
P1-38360 Abdominal phlebectomy
  Excision of abdominal vein
P1-38361 Excision of lesion of abdominal vein

1-383-384 Veins: Excisions — Continued

P1-38362 Embolectomy of abdominal vein
  Removal of embolus of abdominal vein
P1-38363 Thrombectomy of abdominal vein
  Removal of thrombus of abdominal vein
P1-38364 Direct thrombectomy of iliac vein by abdominal incision
P1-38365 Direct thrombectomy of vena cava by abdominal incision
P1-38366 Direct thrombectomy of iliac vein by leg incision
P1-38367 Direct thrombectomy of vena cava by leg incision
P1-38368 Direct thrombectomy of iliac vein by abdominal and leg incision
P1-38369 Direct thrombectomy of vena cava by abdominal and leg incision
P1-38370 Thrombectomy with catheter of iliac vein by abdominal incision
P1-38371 Thrombectomy with catheter of vena cava by abdominal incision
P1-38372 Thrombectomy with catheter of iliac vein by leg incision
P1-38373 Thrombectomy with catheter of vena cava by leg incision
P1-38374 Thrombectomy with catheter of iliac vein by abdominal and leg incision
P1-38375 Thrombectomy with catheter of vena cava by abdominal and leg incision
P1-38376 Excision of abdominal varicose vein
  Phlebectomy of abdominal varicose vein
P1-38378 Excision of ovarian varicose vein
P1-38380 Aneurysmectomy of abdominal vein
P1-38381 Aneurysmectomy with anastomosis of abdominal vein
P1-38382 Angiectomy with anastomosis of abdominal vein
  Resection of abdominal vein with anastomosis
  Phlebectomy with anastomosis of abdominal vein
P1-38383 Aneurysmectomy with graft replacement of abdominal vein
P1-38384 Angiectomy with graft replacement of abdominal vein
  Resection of abdominal vein with replacement by graft
  Phlebectomy with graft replacement of abdominal vein
P1-38390 Phlebectomy of lower limb vein
  Excision of lower limb vein
P1-38391 Excision of lesion of lower limb vein
  Excision of lesion of vein of lower limb
P1-38392 Embolectomy of lower limb vein
  Removal of embolus of lower limb vein
P1-38393 Aneurysmectomy of lower limb vein
P1-38394 Thrombectomy of lower limb vein
  Removal of thrombus of lower limb vein
P1-38395 Direct thrombectomy of femoropopliteal vein by leg incision
P1-38396 Direct thrombectomy of femoropopliteal vein by abdominal and leg incision
P1-38397 Thrombectomy with catheter of femoropopliteal vein by leg incision
P1-38398 Thrombectomy with catheter of femoropopliteal vein by abdominal and leg incision
P1-383A0 Excision of varicose vein of lower limb
  Phlebectomy of varicose vein of lower limb
  Extirpation of varicose vein of lower limb
  Cockett operation of lower limb
  Stripping of varicose vein of lower limb
P1-383A1 Stripping of varicose saphenous vein
P1-38410 Ligation and division of long saphenous vein at distal interruptions
P1-38411 Ligation and division of long saphenous vein at saphenofemoral junction
P1-38412 Ligation and division of short saphenous vein at saphenopopliteal junction
P1-38413 Ligation, division and complete stripping of long saphenous veins
P1-38414 Ligation, division and complete stripping of short saphenous veins
P1-38415 Ligation, division and complete stripping of long and short saphenous veins
P1-38417 Ligation, division and complete stripping of long and short saphenous veins with radical excision of ulcer and skin graft
P1-38418 Complete stripping of long and short saphenous veins with interruption of communicating veins of lower leg and excision of deep fascia
P1-38419 Ligation, division and excision of recurrent or secondary varicose veins of one leg
  Excision of recurrent or secondary varicose veins of one leg
P1-38420 Angiectomy with anastomosis of lower limb vein
  Phlebectomy with anastomosis of lower limb vein
  Resection of lower limb vein with anastomosis
P1-38421 Aneurysmectomy with anastomosis of lower limb vein
P1-38422 Aneurysmectomy with graft replacement of lower limb vein
P1-38424 Angiectomy with graft replacement of lower limb vein
  Phlebectomy with graft replacement of lower limb vein
  Resection of lower limb vein with replacement by graft

1-385 Veins: Injections and Implantations

P1-38500 Injection of vein, NOS

P1-38502 Push transfusion of blood, up to age 2
P1-38510 Introduction of therapeutic substance into vein
P1-38511 Intravenous chemotherapy administration by push technique
P1-38512 Intravenous chemotherapy administration by infusion technique, up to one hour
P1-38513 Intravenous chemotherapy administration by infusion technique, one to 8 hours, each additional hour
P1-38514 Intravenous chemotherapy administration by infusion technique, initiation of prolonged infusion, more than 8 hours, requiring the use of a portable or implantable pump
P1-38520 Catheterization of vein, NOS
  Introduction of catheter into vein, NOS
  Insertion of catheter into vein, NOS
  Venous catheterization, NOS
P1-38522 Venous catheterization for selective organ blood sampling
P1-38523 Venous sampling through catheter without angiography, NOS
P1-38524 Insertion of catheter for central venous pressure monitoring
P1-38525 Placement of central venous catheter, percutaneous, up to age 2
P1-38526 Placement of central venous catheter, percutaneous, over age 2
P1-38527 Placement of central venous catheter, cutdown, up to age 2
P1-38528 Placement of central venous catheter, cutdown, over age 2
P1-38530 Insertion of implantable intravenous infusion pump
P1-38531 Insertion of implantable venous access port
P1-38532 Insertion of cannula for hemodialysis, vein to vein
P1-38534 Catheterization of inferior vena cava
P1-38536 Catheterization of umbilical vein
P1-38537 Introduction of catheter into superior vena cava
P1-38538 Insertion of antiembolic filter into vena cava
P1-38539 Implantation of umbrella into vena cava
  Insertion of Mobitz-Uddin umbrella into vena cava
P1-3853A Insertion of sieve into vena cava
  Insertion of vena cava sieve
P1-38540 Introduction of catheter into inferior vena cava
P1-38542 Catheterization of hepatic vein
P1-38543 Catheterization of renal vein
P1-38545 Venous catheterization for renal dialysis
P1-38550 Insertion of extravascular umbrella of inferior vena cava, partial
P1-38551 Insertion of extravascular umbrella of inferior vena cava, complete
P1-38553 Insertion of intravascular umbrella of inferior vena cava, partial
P1-38555 Insertion of intravascular umbrella of inferior vena cava, complete
P1-38556 Insertion of intravascular device in femoral vein, partial
P1-38557 Insertion of intravascular device in femoral vein, complete
P1-38558 Insertion of intravascular device in common iliac vein, partial
P1-38559 Insertion of intravascular device in common iliac vein, complete
P1-38560 Revision of implantable intravenous infusion pump
P1-38561 Revision of implantable venous access port

1-387 Veins: Endoscopy

P1-38700 Endoscopy of vein, NOS

1-388 Veins: Surgical Repairs, Closures and Reconstructions

P1-38800 Repair of vein, NOS
P1-38804 Anastomosis of veins, NOS
  Venovenostomy, NOS
  Phlebophlebostomy, NOS
P1-38806 Repair of venous graft
P1-38807 Thrombectomy and repair of venous graft
P1-38810 Repair of vein with suture
  Suture of vein
  Venorrhaphy
  Angiorrhaphy of vein
  Phleborrhaphy
P1-38814 Repair of laceration of large vein
P1-38815 Stapling of vein
P1-38816 Ligation of vein
P1-38817 Division of vein with ligation
  Transection of vein with ligation
P1-38818 Ligation of venous connection between anomalous vein and left innominate vein
P1-38819 Ligation of venous connection between anomalous vein and superior vena cava
P1-38824 Revision of anastomosis of vein
P1-38830 Ligation of varicose vein, NOS
  Linton operation for varicose vein
P1-38832 Stripping of varicose veins, NOS
P1-38850 Ligation of vein of head and neck, NOS
P1-38852 Ligation of intracranial vein, NOS
P1-38853 Ligation of internal jugular vein
P1-38854 Ligation of vein of thyroid
P1-38855 Ligation of varicose vein of head and neck
P1-38856 Ligation of intracranial varicose vein
P1-38858 Stripping of varicose veins of head and neck
P1-38859 Stripping of intracranial varicose veins
P1-38866 Plication of superior vena cava
P1-38867 Anastomosis of pulmonary vein and azygos vein
P1-38869 Ligation of thoracic vein
P1-3886A Ligation of thoracic varicose vein
P1-3886B Stripping of thoracic varicose veins
P1-38880 Intra-abdominal venous shunt
  Venous intra-abdominal bypass

1-388 Veins: Surgical Repairs, Closures and Reconstructions — Continued

P1-38881 Caval-mesenteric vein anastomosis
  Caval-mesenteric vein shunt
  Cannulation of caval-mesenteric vein
  Creation of mesocaval shunt
  Superior mesenteric-caval shunt
  Mesenteric-caval anastomosis
  Mesocaval anastomosis
  Anastomosis of mesenteric vein to vena cava
P1-38882 Shunt of portal vein to vena cava
  Creation of portal-systemic shunt
  Porto-caval shunt
  Portacaval anastomosis
  Anastomosis of inferior vena cava and portal vein
  Anastomosis of portal vein to inferior vena cava
P1-38883 Renoportal anastomosis
  Creation of renoportal shunt
  Renoportal cannulation
P1-38884 Anastomosis of renal vein and splenic vein
  Splenorenal anastomosis
  Anastomosis of splenic and renal vein
  Splenorenal vascular bypass
  Creation of splenorenal shunt
  Creation of lienorenal shunt
  Splenorenal cannulation
P1-38885 Proximal splenorenal anastomosis
P1-38886 Distal splenorenal anastomosis
P1-38887 Creation of porto-splenic shunt
P1-38890 Interruption of vena cava, NOS
P1-38891 Partial or complete interruption of inferior vena cava, extravascular or intravascular, umbrella type
P1-38892 Plication of inferior vena cava
P1-38893 Plication of inferior vena cava, partial
P1-38894 Plication of inferior vena cava, complete
P1-38910 Surgical occlusion of abdominal vein, NOS
  Ligation of abdominal vein
P1-38911 Ligation of inferior vena cava
P1-38912 Suture of inferior vena cava, partial
  Ligation of inferior vena cava, partial
P1-38913 Suture of inferior vena cava, complete
  Ligation of inferior vena cava, complete
P1-38914 Clipping of inferior vena cava, partial
P1-38915 Clipping of inferior vena cava, complete
P1-38919 Ligation of adrenal vein
P1-38921 Ligation of common iliac vein, partial
P1-38922 Ligation of common iliac vein, complete
P1-38924 Ligation of abdominal varicose vein
P1-38925 Stripping of abdominal varicose vein
P1-38930 Surgical occlusion of upper limb veins, NOS
P1-38931 Ligation of vein of upper limb
P1-38932 Ligation of varicose vein of upper limb
  Ligation of varices of peripheral vein of upper limb
P1-38940 Surgical occlusion of lower limb veins, NOS
P1-38941 Ligation of vein of lower limb
P1-38943 Valvuloplasty of femoral vein
P1-38944 Saphenopopliteal vein anastomosis
P1-38945 Ligature of femoral vein, complete
P1-38946 Ligature of femoral vein, partial
P1-38948 Ligation of saphenous perforators, subfascial, radical, Linton type, with skin graft
P1-38949 Ligation of saphenous perforators, subfascial, radical, Linton type, without skin graft
P1-38950 Stripping and ligation of veins of leg, NOS
P1-38951 Stripping and ligation of saphenous vein
P1-38952 Ligation of varicose vein of lower limb
P1-38954 Stripping of lower limb varicose veins
P1-38960 Construction of venous valves
P1-38962 Plication of peripheral vein

1-38C Veins: Destructive Procedures

P1-38C00 Destructive procedure of vein, NOS
P1-38C02 Venotripsy, NOS
P1-38C10 Injection of sclerosing agent in vein
  Injection of sclerosing solution, single vein
P1-38C12 Injection of sclerosing agent in varicose vein
  Injection of varicose vein with sclerosing agent
P1-38C14 Single injection of sclerosing solution for spider veins of face
P1-38C15 Multiple injections of sclerosing solution for spider veins of face
P1-38C16 Single injection of sclerosing solution for spider veins of trunk
P1-38C17 Multiple injections of sclerosing solution for spider veins of trunk
P1-38C18 Single injection of sclerosing solution for spider veins of limb
P1-38C19 Multiple injections of sclerosing solution for spider veins of limb
P1-38C1A Injection of sclerosing solution of multiple veins of same leg

1-38D Veins: Transplantations and Transpositions

P1-38D00 Grafting of vein with patch
  Repair of vein with patch graft
P1-38D01 Repair of vein with patch graft of tissue
  Grafting of vein with tissue patch
P1-38D02 Grafting of vein with synthetic patch, dacron or teflon
P1-38D03 Cross-over vein graft to venous system
P1-38D04 Venous valve transposition, any vein donor
P1-38D20 Transplantation of aberrant renal vein
  Transection of aberrant renal vein with reimplantation
P1-38D40 Transplantation of peripheral vein

1-38E Veins: Manipulations

P1-38E00 Manipulation of vein, NOS

1-39 OPERATIVE PROCEDURES ON THE PERICARDIUM

1-390 Pericardium: General and Miscellaneous Operative Procedures

P1-39000 Operation on pericardium, NOS
P1-39010 Diagnostic procedure on pericardium, NOS

1-391 Pericardium: Incisions

P1-39100 Incision of pericardium, NOS
  Pericardiotomy, NOS
P1-39102 Pericardiotomy for removal of clot
P1-39110 Pericardiostomy, NOS
  Creation of pericardial window for drainage
  Creation of pericardial window
  Formation of pericardial window
  Fenestration of pericardium
  Window operation on pericardium
P1-39112 Tube pericardiostomy
P1-39120 Pericardiocentesis, NOS
  Puncture of pericardium
P1-39121 Initial pericardiocentesis
P1-39122 Subsequent pericardiocentesis
P1-39123 Decompression of pericardium
  Drainage of pericardium
  Aspiration of pericardium

1-393 Pericardium: Excisions

P1-39300 Pericardiectomy, NOS
P1-39302 Epicardiectomy, NOS
P1-39310 Partial resection of pericardium for drainage
  Resection of pericardium for drainage
P1-39312 Subtotal pericardiectomy without cardiopulmonary bypass
P1-39313 Subtotal pericardiectomy with cardiopulmonary bypass
P1-39316 Resection of pericardium for chronic constrictive pericarditis
P1-39320 Biopsy of pericardium
  Excisional biopsy of pericardium
P1-39322 Complete pericardiectomy without cardiopulmonary bypass
P1-39323 Complete pericardiectomy with cardiopulmonary bypass
P1-39324 Decortication of pericardium
  Delorme operation pericardiectomy
  Decortication of heart
  Decortication of ventricle of heart
P1-39330 Excision of lesion of pericardium
P1-39332 Excision of cyst of pericardium
  Excision of pericardial cyst
P1-39334 Excision of pericardial tumor
P1-39336 Excision of scar of pericardium
  Resection of pericardium for removal of adhesions
  Excision of pericardial adhesions
P1-39340 Removal of foreign body from pericardium
  Pericardiotomy for removal of foreign body
P1-39350 Excision of lesion of epicardium, NOS
P1-39352 Excision of scar of epicardium

1-395 Pericardium: Injections and Implantations

P1-39500 Injection of pericardium, NOS
P1-39510 Injection of therapeutic substance into pericardium
  Introduction of therapeutic substance into pericardium

1-397 Pericardium: Endoscopy

P1-39700 Endoscopy of pericardium, NOS

1-398 Pericardium: Surgical Repairs, Closures and Reconstructions

P1-39800 Pericardioplasty, NOS
  Repair of pericardium, NOS
P1-39840 Pericardiorrhaphy, NOS
  Suture of pericardium, NOS
P1-39842 Closure of pleuropericardial fistula
  Repair of pleuropericardial fistula

1-39C Pericardium: Destructive Procedures

P1-39C00 Destructive procedure of pericardium, NOS
P1-39C10 Pericardiolysis
  Lysis of adhesions of pericardium
P1-39C20 Abrasion of epicardial surface
  Scarification of pericardium
  Formation of adhesions of pericardium
P1-39C22 Epicardial poudrage
  Beck operation
  Intrapericardial poudrage

1-39D Pericardium: Transplantations and Transpositions

P1-39D00 Grafting of pericardium, NOS

1-39E Pericardium: Manipulations

P1-39E00 Manipulation of pericardium, NOS

SECTION 1-4 OPERATIVE PROCEDURES ON THE INTEGUMENTARY SYSTEM

1-40 GENERAL OPERATIVE PROCEDURES ON THE INTEGUMENTARY SYSTEM

1-400 Integumentary System: General and Miscellaneous Operative Procedures

P1-40000 Operation on skin, NOS
P1-40010 Diagnostic procedure on skin, NOS
P1-40040 Operation on subcutaneous tissue, NOS

1-401-402 Integumentary System: Incisions

P1-40100 Incision of skin, NOS
P1-40102 Incision and exploration of skin
P1-40104 Incision and exploration of sinus tract
P1-40106 Incision or expression of comedones and milia
P1-40110 Incision and drainage of skin, NOS
P1-40111 Incision of skin abscess, NOS
P1-40112 Incision and drainage of skin abscess, simple
P1-40113 Incision and drainage of skin abscess, complicated
P1-40114 Incision and drainage of pustules and cysts
P1-40117 Incision and drainage of furuncle
P1-40119 Incision and drainage of postoperative wound infection, complex
P1-40120 Incision of sebaceous cyst, NOS
P1-40121 Incision and drainage of noninfected sebaceous cyst, one lesion
P1-40125 Incision and drainage of infected sebaceous cyst, one lesion
P1-40128 Incision and drainage of carbuncle, simple
P1-40129 Incision and drainage of carbuncle, complicated
P1-4012A Incision of sweat glands of skin
P1-40130 Incision and drainage of noninfected epithelial inclusion cyst with complete removal of sac and treatment of cavity
P1-40131 Incision and drainage of infected epithelial inclusion cyst with complete removal of sac and treatment of cavity
P1-40134 Incision and drainage of suppurative hidradenitis, simple
P1-40135 Incision and drainage of suppurative hidradenitis, complicated
P1-40140 Incision and drainage of hematoma, simple
P1-40141 Incision and drainage of hematoma, complicated
P1-40150 Aspiration of skin, NOS
P1-40151 Puncture aspiration of hematoma of skin
P1-40152 Puncture aspiration of bulla of skin
P1-40153 Puncture aspiration of cyst of skin
P1-40154 Puncture aspiration of abscess of skin
P1-40160 Relaxation of scar contracture of skin
    Release of scar tissue of skin
P1-40161 Release of web contracture of skin
    Relaxation of web contracture of skin
P1-40162 Escharotomy
P1-40164 Undercutting of hair follicles
    Incision of hair follicles
P1-40200 Incision of subcutaneous tissue, NOS
P1-40202 Panniculotomy
P1-40210 Incision and exploration of subcutaneous tissue
P1-40211 Incision and drainage of subcutaneous tissue
P1-40212 Incision and drainage of abscess of subcutaneous tissue
P1-40214 Aspiration of subcutaneous tissue
P1-40216 Incision of hematoma of subcutaneous tissue

1-403-404 Integumentary System: Excisions

P1-40300 Local excision of skin
    Reduction of size of skin
P1-40301 Wedge resection of skin
P1-40303 Punch biopsy of skin
P1-40305 Excision of lesion of skin
P1-40306 Elliptical excision of skin lesion
P1-40307 Partial excision of skin lesion
P1-40308 Curettage of skin lesion
P1-40309 Curettage of skin lesion under local anesthesia
P1-40310 Biopsy of skin, one lesion
P1-40312 Radical excision of skin lesion
P1-40313 Radical excision of lesion of skin involving underlying or adjacent structure
P1-40314 Excision of scar of skin
    Escharectomy
    Excision of cicatrix of skin
P1-40315 Excision of keloid
P1-40316 Excision of tattoo of skin
P1-40317 Excision of lesion of sweat gland
    Excision of lesion of apocrine gland
P1-40320V Excision of scent gland
P1-40322V Biopsy of scent gland
P1-40330 Excision of skin tags, up to 15 lesions
P1-40332 Enucleation of cyst of skin
P1-40336 Removal of sutures under anesthesia
P1-40340 Removal of foreign body from skin without incision
P1-40342 Removal of foreign body from skin with incision
P1-40360 Debridement of skin and subcutaneous tissue
P1-40361 Debridement of skin, partial thickness
P1-40362 Debridement of skin, full thickness
P1-40364 Debridement of wound of skin
    Surgical toilet of skin wound
P1-40365 Debridement of infection of skin
P1-40366 Debridement of eczematous or infected skin, up to 10% of body surface
P1-40369 Acne surgery, NOS
P1-40370 Curettement of benign lesion without chemical cauterization
P1-40375 Curettement of benign lesion with chemical cauterization
P1-40380 Shaving of benign lesion without chemical cauterization
    Paring of benign lesion without chemical cauterization
P1-40385 Shaving of benign lesion with chemical cauterization
    Paring of benign lesion with chemical cauterization
P1-40390 Excision of pressure ulcer, NOS
    Excision of unlisted pressure ulcer, NOS
P1-40391 Excision of unlisted pressure ulcer with primary suture, NOS

P1-40392 Excision of unlisted pressure ulcer with skin flap closure
P1-40393 Excision of unlisted pressure ulcer with local skin flap closure and with ostectomy
P1-40394 Excision of unlisted pressure ulcer with muscle or myocutaneous flap closure
P1-40395 Excision of unlisted pressure ulcer with muscle or myocutaneous flap closure with ostectomy
P1-403A0 Initial local treatment of first degree burn
P1-403A1 Excisional debridement of burn, NOS
P1-403A2 Nonexcisional debridement of burn
Removal of skin necrosis or slough
P1-403A3 Dressings and debridement of small burn without anesthesia
P1-403A4 Dressings and debridement of medium burn without anesthesia
P1-403A6 Dressings and debridement of small burn with anesthesia
P1-403A7 Dressings and debridement of medium burn with anesthesia
P1-403A9 Dressings and debridement of major burn with anesthesia
P1-403AA Dressings and debridement of major burn without anesthesia
P1-403AB Nonexcisional debridement of wound or infection of integumentary system
P1-403C0 Rhytidectomy, NOS
P1-403C2 Rhytidectomy of subcutaneous and musculoaponeurotic system
SMAS flap, rhytidectomy
P1-403D0 Biopsy of mucous membrane
P1-40400 Biopsy of subcutaneous tissue, NOS
P1-40402 Excision of lesion of subcutaneous tissue
P1-40403 Punch biopsy of subcutaneous tissue
P1-40404 Enucleation of cyst of subcutaneous tissue
P1-40420 Debridement of subcutaneous tissue
P1-40430 Removal of foreign body of subcutaneous tissue, NOS
P1-40431 Removal of foreign body of subcutaneous tissue by incision, simple
P1-40432 Removal of foreign body of subcutaneous tissue, complicated
P1-40440 Panniculectomy
Excision of fat pad, NOS
Adipectomy
Cutaneolipectomy
Lipectomy
P1-40444 Local excision of skin and subcutaneous tissue, NOS
P1-40445 Excision of excessive skin and subcutaneous tissue, NOS
P1-40448 Fistulectomy of skin and subcutaneous tissue
P1-40460 Mohs' chemosurgery, NOS
Mohs' operation, chemosurgical excision of skin
P1-40462 Mohs' chemosurgery, fixed tissue technique
P1-40464 Mohs' chemosurgery, fresh tissue technique
P1-40470 Chemosurgery by Mohs' technique, first stage, NOS
Chemosurgery by Mohs' technique, first stage, including the removal of all gross tumor and delineation of margins
Chemosurgery, first stage, including the removal of all gross tumor and delineation of margins
P1-40472 Chemosurgery by Mohs' technique, second stage, NOS
Chemosurgery, second stage, including the removal of all gross tumor and delineation of margins
P1-40474 Chemosurgery by Mohs' technique, third stage, NOS
Chemosurgery by Mohs' technique, third stage, including the removal of all gross tumor and delineation of margins

1-405 Integumentary System: Injections and Implantations

P1-40500 Injection of skin, NOS
P1-40510 Insertion of filling material under skin for filling of defect
Insertion of tissue expander of skin
P1-40512 Implant of silicone under skin for filling of defect
P1-40514 Implant of silicone under skin for augmentation, NOS
P1-40515 Subcutaneous injection of filling material
P1-40520 Tattooing of skin, NOS
Pigmenting of skin
P1-40521 Tattooing of skin lesion
Tattooing of skin defect
P1-40522 Tattooing to correct color defects of skin
P1-40531 Intralesional injection of skin
P1-40536 Intravenous injection of agent to test blood flow in flap or graft
P1-40560 Irrigation of wound catheter of integument
P1-40561 Replacement of wound catheter of integument
P1-40562 Replacement of wound drain of integument
P1-40563 Replacement of wound packing of integument
P1-40565 Removal of tissue expander of skin without insertion of prosthesis
Removal of skin tissue expander
P1-40566 Replacement of tissue expander of skin with permanent prosthesis
P1-40568 Removal of intraluminal foreign body from artificial stoma without incision
P1-40570 Insertion of infusion pump beneath skin
Implantation of infusion pump beneath skin
P1-40580V Insertion of metal device into subcutaneous tissue

1-407 Integumentary System: Endoscopy

P1-40710 Endoscopy of integument, NOS

1-408-409 Integumentary System: Surgical Repairs, Closures and Reconstructions

P1-40800 Dermatoplasty, NOS
P1-40810 Closure of skin by suture, NOS
  Repair of skin wound without graft
  Suture of skin laceration
  Suture of skin without graft
P1-40812 Suture of subcutaneous tissue without skin graft
  Repair of subcutaneous tissue laceration by suture
P1-40813 Resuture of wound of skin, NOS
P1-40814 Resuture of wound of skin and subcutaneous tissue without graft
P1-40816 Complicated surgical repair of skin wound, over 7.5 cm
P1-40818 Suture of ulcer of skin
  Closure of ulcer of skin
P1-40819 Closure of skin wound by tape
P1-40820 Treatment of superficial wound dehiscence by simple closure
P1-40821 Treatment of superficial wound dehiscence with packing
P1-40822 Secondary closure of surgical dehiscence, complicated
  Secondary closure of extensive surgical wound or dehiscence
P1-40850 V-Y operation of skin and subcutaneous tissue without skin graft
  Closure of skin V-Y type
P1-40851 Z-plasty of skin, NOS
P1-40852 Z-plasty of skin with excision of lesion
P1-40854 Revision of scar of skin
P1-40855 Revision of scar of skin with excision
P1-40858 Dermodesis
P1-40860 Reconstruction of subcutaneous tissue without skin graft
P1-40880 Ligation of dermal appendage, NOS
P1-40881 Ligation of wart
P1-40890 Repair of syndactyly, NOS
  Correction of syndactyly, NOS
P1-40892 Repair of syndactyly, each web space, with skin flaps
P1-40894 Repair of syndactyly, each web space, with skin flaps and grafts
P1-40896 Repair of syndactyly, each web space, complex
P1-40899 Syndactylization
  Webbing of digits
P1-40900V Plastic repair of exoskeleton
P1-40910V Repair of shell

1-40C Integumentary System: Destructive Procedures

P1-40C00 Destruction of lesion of skin, NOS
P1-40C10 Destruction of benign skin lesions, other than face, one lesion
P1-40C14 Destruction of benign skin lesions, other than face, complicated lesions
P1-40C15 Destruction of milia, up to 15 lesions
P1-40C16 Destruction of molluscum contagiosum, up to 15 lesions
P1-40C17 Destruction of flat warts, up to 15 lesions
P1-40C18 Destruction of premalignant skin lesion
P1-40C1B Destruction of premalignant skin lesions, complicated lesions
P1-40C1D Destruction of lesion of subcutaneous tissue, NOS
P1-40C1E Avulsion of subcutaneous tissue
P1-40C20 Dermabrasion, NOS
  Removal of superficial layer of skin by dermabrasion
  Abrasion of skin
  Sandpapering of skin
  Planing of skin
P1-40C21 Partial dermabrasion
  Superficial dermabrasion
P1-40C22 Complete dermabrasion
P1-40C23 Excision of tattoo by dermabrasion
  Tattoo removal by abrasion
P1-40C24 Abrasion of single lesion of skin
P1-40C26 Regional dermabrasion, other than face
P1-40C30 Salabrasion of 20 sq cm or less of skin
P1-40C32 Salabrasion of over 20 sq cm of skin
P1-40C36 Fulguration of skin
P1-40C37 Cauterization of skin
  Fulguration of subcutaneous tissue, NOS
P1-40C38 Chemical cauterization of wound
P1-40C39 Cauterization of subcutaneous tissue
P1-40C40 Cryotherapy of skin, NOS
P1-40C41 Cryotherapy of skin lesion with carbon dioxide
P1-40C42 Cryotherapy of skin lesion with liquid nitrogen
P1-40C44 Cryotherapy of warts
P1-40C48 Cryotherapy of subcutaneous tissue
P1-40C50 Epilation of skin, NOS
  Depilation of skin, NOS
P1-40C51 Epilation by electrolysis
P1-40C52 Electrolysis of skin, NOS
P1-40C53 Electrolysis of hair follicles
P1-40C54 Electrosurgical destruction of fibrocutaneous tags
P1-40C58 Electrolysis of subcutaneous tissue
P1-40C60 Chemexfoliation of skin, NOS
  Chemical peel of skin, NOS
  Chemopeel of skin, NOS
P1-40C61 Phenopeel of skin
  Acidpeel of skin
P1-40C62 Regional chemexfoliation, NOS
P1-40C70V Hot iron branding of animal
  Branding of animal

P1-40C70V (cont.) Branding of livestock

1-40D Integumentary System: Transplantations and Transpositions

P1-40D00 Skin grafting, NOS
P1-40D02 Graft of skin and mucous membrane, NOS
P1-40D04 Excision of skin for graft
P1-40D10 Free skin graft, NOS
P1-40D11 Autogenous skin free graft, NOS
P1-40D12 Full-thickness skin graft, NOS
P1-40D14 Partial-thickness skin graft
  Split-thickness skin graft
P1-40D16 Pinch graft, single
P1-40D17 Pinch graft, multiple
P1-40D18 Punch graft for hair transplant
P1-40D20 Pedicle graft, NOS
  Formation of island pedicle flap graft, NOS
P1-40D21 Double pedicle flap graft, NOS
P1-40D22 Formation of neurovascular pedicle flap graft
  Skin pedicle graft preparation
  Cutting and preparation of pedicle grafts
  Skin pedicle graft design and raising
  Raising of pedicle graft
P1-40D23 Flap graft, NOS
P1-40D24 Advancement of pedicle graft, NOS
  Transection of pedicle graft
P1-40D25 Advancement of flap graft, NOS
P1-40D26 Attachment of pedicle or flap graft
  Transfer of pedicle or flap graft
P1-40D27 Rotation flap graft of skin
P1-40D28 Delaying of pedicle graft
  Delay of skin pedicle graft
P1-40D29 Intermediate transfer of pedicle flap
  Transfer of "walking" tube graft
P1-40D30 Formation of free flap graft by microvascular technique
  Free transplantation of skin flap by microsurgical technique
P1-40D50 Preparation or creation of recipient site for skin graft
P1-40D52 Graft to hair-bearing skin
P1-40D70 Adjacent integumentary tissue transfer or rearrangement, complicated, any area
P1-40D80 Revision of skin graft
P1-40D82 Debridement of skin graft
  Defatting of graft
P1-40D90 Dermal-fat skin graft
P1-40D91 Dermal-fat-fascia graft
P1-40D92 Composite graft
P1-40DA0 Homograft of skin, NOS
  Application of skin allograft
P1-40DA4 Graft of amnionic membrane to skin
P1-40DB0 Xenograft of skin
  Application of xenograft to skin
  Heterograft of skin
P1-40DB1 Pigskin graft, NOS
  Porcine skin graft, NOS

1-40E Integumentary System: Manipulations

P1-40E10 Manipulation of skin, NOS
P1-40E20 Enlargement of sinus tract of skin, NOS
P1-40E30 Manual expression of sebaceous gland, NOS

1-41 OPERATIVE PROCEDURES ON THE SKIN OF THE HEAD AND NECK

1-410 Skin of Head and Neck: General and Miscellaneous Operative Procedures

P1-41010 Operation on skin of head, NOS
P1-41040 Operation on skin of neck, NOS

1-411 Skin of Head and Neck: Incisions

P1-41110 Incision of face, NOS
P1-41114 Incision of cheek
P1-41120 Submaxillary incision
P1-41122 Submaxillary incision with drainage
P1-41150 Incision of supraclavicular fossa
P1-41152 Incision of supraclavicular fossa with drainage
  Drainage of supraclavicular fossa
P1-41170 Incision of neck, NOS

1-413-414 Skin of Head and Neck: Excisions

P1-41300 Excision of skin of head and neck, NOS
P1-41320 Excision of benign lesion of face and ears, NOS
P1-41321 Excision of benign lesion of face and ears, lesion diameter 0.5 cm or less
P1-41322 Excision of benign lesion of face and ears, lesion diameter 0.6 to 1.0 cm
P1-41323 Excision of benign lesion of face and ears, lesion diameter 1.1 to 2.0 cm
P1-41324 Excision of benign lesion of face and ears, lesion diameter 2.1 to 3.0 cm
P1-41325 Excision of benign lesion of face and ears, lesion diameter 3.1 to 4.0 cm
P1-41326 Excision of benign lesion of face and ears, lesion diameter over 4.0 cm
P1-41330 Excision of benign lesion of scalp and neck, NOS
P1-41331 Excision of benign lesion of scalp and neck, lesion diameter 0.5 cm or less
P1-41332 Excision of benign lesion of scalp and neck, lesion diameter 0.6 to 1.0 cm
P1-41333 Excision of benign lesion of scalp and neck, lesion diameter 1.1 to 2.0 cm
P1-41334 Excision of benign lesion of scalp and neck, lesion diameter 2.1 to 3.0 cm
P1-41335 Excision of benign lesion of scalp and neck, lesion diameter 3.1 to 4.0 cm
P1-41336 Excision of benign lesion of scalp and neck, lesion diameter over 4.0 cm
P1-41350 Excision of malignant lesion of face and ears, NOS

1-413-414 Skin of Head and Neck: Excisions — Continued

P1-41351 Excision of malignant lesion of face and ears, lesion diameter 0.5 cm or less
P1-41352 Excision of malignant lesion of face and ears, lesion diameter 0.6 to 1.0 cm
P1-41353 Excision of malignant lesion of face and ears, lesion diameter 1.1 to 2.0 cm
P1-41354 Excision of malignant lesion of face and ears, lesion diameter 2.1 to 3.0 cm
P1-41355 Excision of malignant lesion of face and ears, lesion diameter 3.1 to 4.0 cm
P1-41356 Excision of malignant lesion of face and ears, lesion diameter over 4.0 cm
P1-41360 Excision of malignant lesion of scalp and neck, NOS
P1-41361 Excision of malignant lesion of scalp and neck, lesion diameter 0.5 cm or less
P1-41362 Excision of malignant lesion of scalp and neck, lesion diameter 0.6 to 1.0 cm
P1-41363 Excision of malignant lesion of scalp and neck, lesion diameter 1.1 to 2.0 cm
P1-41364 Excision of malignant lesion of scalp and neck, lesion diameter 2.1 to 3.0 cm
P1-41365 Excision of malignant lesion of scalp and neck, lesion diameter 3.1 to 4.0 cm
P1-41366 Excision of malignant lesion of scalp and neck, lesion diameter over 4.0 cm
P1-41380 Removal of suture of skin of head and neck
P1-41382 Debridement of forehead lacerations
P1-41384 Removal of foreign body from supraclavicular fossa by incision
P1-41386 Suction assisted lipectomy of head and neck
P1-41398 Excision of excessive skin and subcutaneous tissue of submental fat pad
P1-41410V Excision of scent gland of head
P1-41414V Biopsy of muzzle
P1-41416V Transection of horn
  Dehorn
P1-41417V Amputation of cornual process
P1-41420V Biopsy of snout

1-415 Skin of Head and Neck: Injections and Implantations

P1-41510 Injection into skin of head, NOS
P1-41512V Ear tattooing
P1-41514V Tattooing of skin of nose
P1-41520 Injection into skin of neck, NOS
P1-41540 Implantation into skin of head, NOS
P1-41550 Implantation into skin of neck, NOS

1-417 Skin of Head and Neck: Endoscopy

P1-41710 Endoscopy of skin of head
P1-41740 Endoscopy of skin of neck

1-418 Skin of Head and Neck: Surgical Repairs, Closures and Reconstructions

P1-41800 Facial rhytidoplasty
  Face lift
  Facial rhytidectomy, NOS
P1-41801 Rhytidectomy of forehead
P1-41802 Rhytidectomy of glabellar frown lines
P1-41803 Rhytidectomy of cheek, chin, or neck
P1-41804 Rhytidectomy of neck with platysmal tightening
P1-41812 Fascial sling for facial weakness
  Facial meloplasty
P1-41814 Fascial sling of mouth
P1-41816 Z-plasty of eyelid
P1-41818 Revision of scars of face
P1-41830 Simple repair of superficial wounds of scalp and neck, NOS
P1-41837 Simple repair of wounds of face and ears, NOS
P1-41840 Layer closure of wounds of scalp and neck, NOS
P1-41850 Layer closure of wounds of face and ears, NOS
P1-41860 Complex surgical repair of forehead, cheeks, chin, mouth, and neck
P1-41865 Complex surgical repair of eyelids, nose, ears and lips
P1-4186A Galeaplasty, NOS
P1-4186B Complex surgical repair of scalp

1-41C Skin of Head and Neck: Destructive Procedures

P1-41C10 Destruction of benign facial lesions, first lesion
P1-41C18 Destruction of complicated benign facial lesions
P1-41C30 Dermabrasion of face, NOS
P1-41C32 Segmental dermabrasion of face
P1-41C34 Dermabrasion of facial scars
P1-41C40 Chemexfoliation of face, NOS
  Chemical peel of face
P1-41C42 Regional chemexfoliation of face
P1-41C44 Chemical exfoliation for acne
P1-41C50V Cauterization of horn

1-41D Skin of Head and Neck: Transplantations and Transpositions

P1-41D00 Graft of head and neck, NOS
P1-41D02 Fasciocutaneous flap of head and neck
P1-41D04 Muscle flap of head and neck
P1-41D06 Myocutaneous flap of head and neck
P1-41D10 Split-thickness graft of scalp, 100 sq cm or less
P1-41D14 Split-thickness graft of face, eyelids, mouth, neck, ears, orbits, 100 sq cm or less
P1-41D20 Full thickness free graft including closure of donor site of scalp, 20 sq cm or less

P1-41D23 Full thickness free graft including closure of donor site of forehead, cheeks, chin, mouth, neck, 20 sq cm or less

P1-41D25 Full thickness free graft, including closure of donor site of nose, ears, eyelids, and lips, 20 sq cm or less

P1-41D40 Formation of tubed pedicle graft, head and neck, NOS

P1-41D42 Formation of large flap graft, head and neck, NOS

P1-41D50 Primary attachment of pedicle flap graft to recipient site requiring minimal preparation, scalp

P1-41D52 Primary attachment of pedicle flap graft to recipient site requiring minimal preparation, forehead, cheeks, chin, mouth or neck

P1-41D53 Primary attachment of pedicle flap graft to recipient site requiring minimal preparation, eyelids, nose, ears or lips

P1-41D60 Intermediate delay of small flap at scalp

P1-41D61 Intermediate delay of small flap at forehead, cheeks, chin or neck

P1-41D62 Intermediate delay of small flap at eyelids, nose, ears or lips

P1-41D63 Intermediate delay of any flap, primary delay of small flap, or sectioning pedicle of tubed or direct flap at scalp

P1-41D64 Intermediate delay of any flap, primary delay of small flap, or sectioning pedicle of tubed or direct flap at forehead, cheeks, chin or neck

P1-41D65 Intermediate delay of any flap, primary delay of small flap, or sectioning pedicle of tubed or direct flap at eyelids, nose, ears or lips

P1-41D66 Excisional preparation of recipient site and attachment of direct or tubed pedicle flap at scalp

P1-41D67 Excisional preparation of recipient site and attachment of direct or tubed pedicle flap at forehead, cheeks, chin, mouth or neck

P1-41D68 Excisional preparation of recipient site and attachment of direct or tubed pedicle flap at eyelids, nose, ears or lips

P1-41D70 Adjacent tissue transfer or rearrangement of skin of eyelids, nose, ears and lips, defect 10 sq cm or less

P1-41D72 Adjacent tissue transfer or rearrangement on scalp of defect 10 sq cm or less

P1-41D74 Adjacent tissue transfer or rearrangement of skin of forehead, cheeks, chin, mouth and neck, defect 10.1 sq cm to 30.0 sq cm

P1-41D76 Intermediate sectioning pedicle of tubed or direct flap at scalp

P1-41D77 Intermediate sectioning pedicle of tubed or direct flap at forehead, cheeks, chin or neck

P1-41D78 Intermediate sectioning pedicle of tubed or direct flap at eyelids, nose, ears or lips

P1-41D80 Ear pedicle graft preparation

P1-41D84 Graft for facial nerve paralysis with free fascia graft

P1-41D90 Replantation of skin of scalp
  Replantation of scalp

P1-41D92 Hair transplant

P1-41D94 Transplant of hair follicles to scalp

1-41E Skin of Head and Neck: Manipulations

P1-41E10 Manipulation of skin of head, NOS

P1-41E40 Manipulation of skin of neck, NOS

1-43 OPERATIVE PROCEDURES ON THE SKIN OF THE TRUNK

1-430 Skin of Trunk: General and Miscellaneous Operative Procedures

P1-43010 Operation on skin of trunk, NOS

1-431 Skin of Trunk: Incisions

P1-43100 Incision of skin of trunk, NOS

P1-43110 Incision and drainage of pilonidal cyst, simple
  Incision and exploration of pilonidal sinus

P1-43114 Incision and drainage of pilonidal cyst, complicated

P1-43130 Incision and exploration of skin of groin

P1-43134 Incision of gluteal skin

1-433 Skin of Trunk: Excisions

P1-43310 Excision of benign lesion of trunk, NOS

P1-43320 Excision of malignant lesion of trunk, NOS

P1-43340 Excision of sacral pressure ulcer with primary suture

P1-43342 Excision of sacral pressure ulcer with primary suture with ostectomy

P1-43344 Excision of sacral pressure ulcer with local skin flap closure

P1-43346 Excision of sacral pressure ulcer with local skin flap closure with ostectomy

P1-43348 Excision of coccygeal pressure ulcer with coccygectomy with primary suture

P1-43349 Excision of coccygeal pressure ulcer with coccygectomy with skin flap closure

P1-43350 Excision of ischial pressure ulcer with primary suture

P1-43351 Excision of ischial pressure ulcer with primary suture with ischiectomy

P1-43352 Excision of ischial pressure ulcer with skin flap closure

P1-43354 Excision of ischial pressure ulcer with skin flap closure and with ostectomy

P1-43356 Excision of ischial pressure ulcer with ostectomy, with muscle flap or myocutaneous flap closure

P1-43360 Excision of pilonidal cyst or sinus, NOS
  Excision of pilonidal cyst or sinus, simple

P1-43362 Excision of pilonidal cyst or sinus, extensive

P1-43364 Excision of pilonidal cyst or sinus, complicated

1-433 Skin of Trunk: Excisions — Continued

P1-43370 Excision of skin and subcutaneous tissue for hidradenitis, inguinal with primary suture
P1-43371 Excision of skin and subcutaneous tissue for hidradenitis, inguinal with other closure
P1-43373 Excision of skin and subcutaneous tissue for hidradenitis, perianal with primary closure
P1-43374 Excision of skin and subcutaneous tissue for hidradenitis, umbilical with primary closure
P1-43375 Excision of skin and subcutaneous tissue for hidradenitis, umbilical with other closure
P1-43380 Excision of lesion of skin of groin region
P1-43381 Excision of lesion of subcutaneous tissue of groin
P1-43382 Excision of excessive skin and subcutaneous tissue of abdomen
P1-43383 Excision of excessive skin and subcutaneous tissue of buttock
P1-43384 Suction assisted lipectomy of trunk

1-435 Skin of Trunk: Injections and Implantations

P1-43510 Injection into skin of trunk, NOS
P1-43540 Implantation into skin of trunk, NOS

1-437 Skin of Trunk: Endoscopy

P1-43700 Endoscopy of skin of trunk, NOS

1-438 Skin of Trunk: Surgical Repairs, Closures and Reconstructions

P1-43810 Simple repair of wounds of trunk, NOS
P1-43820 Layer closure of wounds of trunk, NOS
P1-43830 Complex surgical repair of wounds of trunk, NOS
P1-43840 Marsupialization of pilonidal cyst or sinus
Exteriorization of pilonidal cyst or sinus
P1-43860 Reduction of size of abdominal wall
P1-43862 Reduction of buttocks
P1-43864 Augmentation of buttock
Fanny-lift operation

1-43C Skin of Trunk: Destructive Procedures

P1-43C10 Destructive procedure of lesion on skin of trunk

1-43D Skin of Trunk: Transplantations and Transpositions

P1-43D00 Skin graft to trunk, NOS
P1-43D02 Myocutaneous flap of trunk
P1-43D03 Muscle flap of trunk
P1-43D04 Fasciocutaneous flap of trunk
P1-43D10 Split-thickness graft to trunk, 100 sq cm or less, adult
P1-43D16 Full thickness graft to trunk including closure of donor site, 20 sq cm or less
P1-43D20 Adjacent tissue transfer or rearrangement to trunk, defect 10 sq cm or less
P1-43D24 Adjacent tissue transfer or rearrangement to trunk, complicated
P1-43D26 Delay of flap or sectioning of pedicle or direct flap of trunk

1-43E Skin of Trunk: Manipulations

P1-43E10 Manipulation of skin of trunk, NOS

1-45 OPERATIVE PROCEDURES ON THE SKIN OF THE EXTREMITIES

1-450 Skin of Extremities: General and Miscellaneous Operative Procedures

P1-45010 Operation on skin of upper extremity, NOS
P1-45020 Operation on fingernail
P1-45060 Operation on skin of lower extremity, NOS
P1-45070 Operation on toenail

1-451 Skin of Extremities: Incisions

P1-45110 Onychotomy, NOS
Incision of nailbed or nailfold
P1-45111 Incision and drainage of onychia, simple
Onychotomy with drainage
P1-45112 Incision and drainage of onychia, complicated
P1-45113 Incision and drainage of paronychia, simple
Incision of paronychia
P1-45114 Incision and drainage of paronychia, complicated
P1-45115 Piercing of nail
P1-45116 Aspiration of nail
Evacuation of subungual hematoma
P1-45118 Incision of ingrown nail
P1-45130 Incision of axilla
P1-45132 Incision and exploration of axilla
P1-45133 Incision of hematoma of axilla
P1-45134 Incision and drainage of axilla
P1-45136 Incision of antecubital fossa
P1-45137 Incision and drainage of antecubital fossa
P1-45150 Incision of popliteal space
P1-45152 Incision and exploration of popliteal space
P1-45154 Incision of hematoma of popliteal space
P1-45156 Incision and drainage of popliteal space
P1-45160V Incision and drainage of skin of forelimb
P1-45162V Incision and drainage of skin of hindlimb

1-453 Skin of Extremities: Excisions

P1-45310 Removal of nail, NOS
Onychectomy, NOS
Avulsion of nail
Excision of nail
Declawing, NOS
Onychectomy of claw, NOS

P1-45311 Partial excision of nail and nail matrix
  Partial excision of claw
P1-45312 Complete excision of nail and nail matrix
P1-45313 Partial excision of nail and nail matrix for permanent removal with amputation of tuft of distal phalanx
P1-45314 Complete excision of nail and nail matrix for permanent removal with amputation of tuft of distal phalanx
P1-45315 Wedge excision of skin of nail fold
P1-45316V Excision of nail fold
P1-45317 Debridement of skin or subcutaneous tissue of nail, nail bed, or nail fold
  Debridement of nail
  Debridement of infected nail bed or fold
  Debridement of nail bed
  Debridement of nail fold
P1-45318 Debridement of multiple nails, nail beds or nail folds
P1-45319V Debridement of beak
P1-45320V Excision of hoof
  Amputation of hoof
P1-45321V Partial excision of hoof
P1-45322V Excision of lesion of hoof
P1-45324V Excision of lesion of claw
P1-45325V Resection of pad of forefoot
  Amputation of pad of forefoot
P1-45326V Resection of pad of hindfoot
  Amputation of pad of hindfoot
P1-45327 Biopsy of nail
  Biopsy of nail bed
P1-45328V Biopsy of claw
  Biopsy of claw bed
P1-45329V Biopsy of hoof
  Biopsy of hoof bed
P1-4532A Excision of lesion of skin of extremity, NOS
P1-4532B Excision of lesion of skin of upper extremity, NOS
  Excision of lesion of skin of forelimb
P1-4532C Excision of lesion of skin of lower extremity, NOS
  Excision of lesion of skin of hindlimb
P1-45330 Excision of benign lesion of skin of extremities, NOS
P1-45340 Excision of malignant lesion of skin of extremities, NOS
P1-45350 Excision of subcutaneous tumor of extremities
P1-45351 Excision of subcutaneous vascular malformation of extremity, NOS
P1-45352 Excision of subcutaneous tumor of shoulder area
P1-45354 Excision of skin and subcutaneous tissue for hidradenitis, axillary with primary suture
P1-45355 Excision of skin and subcutaneous tissue for hidradenitis, axillary with other closure
P1-45360 Excision of excessive skin and subcutaneous tissue of leg
P1-45361 Excision of excessive skin and subcutaneous tissue of hip
P1-45362 Excision of excessive skin and subcutaneous tissue of thigh
P1-45364 Excision of excessive skin and subcutaneous tissue of arm
P1-45365 Excision of knee fat pad
P1-45366 Excision of trochanteric lipomatosis
P1-45368 Suction assisted lipectomy of upper extremity
P1-45369 Suction assisted lipectomy of lower extremity
P1-45370 Removal of supernumerary digit, NOS
P1-45371 Removal of supernumerary toe
P1-45372 Removal of supernumerary finger
P1-45375 Removal of subcutaneous foreign body from foot
P1-45376 Removal of foreign body from popliteal space
P1-45377 Removal of subcutaneous foreign body from upper extremity
P1-45378 Removal of subcutaneous foreign body from shoulder
P1-45379 Removal of foreign body from skin of axilla
P1-45386 Excision of trochanteric pressure ulcer with primary suture
P1-45387 Excision of trochanteric pressure ulcer with primary suture with ostectomy
P1-45388 Excision of trochanteric pressure ulcer with skin flap closure
P1-45389 Excision of trochanteric pressure ulcer with muscle or myocutaneous flap closure
P1-4538A Excision of trochanteric pressure ulcer with muscle or myocutaneous flap closure with ostectomy
P1-4538B Excision of trochanteric pressure ulcer with bipedicle flap closure
P1-4538C Excision of trochanteric pressure ulcer with bipedicle flap closure with ostectomy
P1-4538D Excision of trochanteric pressure ulcer with local rotation skin flap closure with ostectomy
P1-45390 Excision of leg pressure ulcer with primary suture
P1-45391 Excision of leg pressure ulcer with primary suture with ostectomy
P1-45393 Excision of leg pressure ulcer with local skin flap
P1-45394 Excision of leg pressure ulcer with local skin flap with ostectomy
P1-45396 Excision of leg pressure ulcer with muscle or myocutaneous flap closure with ostectomy
P1-45398V Biopsy of skin of forefoot
P1-45399V Biopsy of skin of hindfoot

1-455 Skin of Extremities: Injections and Implantations

P1-45510 Injection of skin of extremities, NOS
P1-45540 Implantation of skin of extremities, NOS

1-457 Skin of Extremities: Endoscopy

P1-45710 Endoscopy of skin of extremities, NOS

1-458 Skin of Extremities: Surgical Repairs, Closures and Reconstructions

P1-45808V Plastic operation of hoof
P1-45809V Plastic operation of claw
P1-45810 Simple repair of wounds of extremities, NOS
P1-45820 Layer closure of wounds of extremities, NOS
P1-45830 Complex surgical repair of skin of extremities, NOS
P1-45860 Ligation of supernumerary digit, NOS
P1-45861 Ligation of supernumerary toes
P1-45862 Ligation of supernumerary fingers
P1-45865 Onychoplasty, NOS
  Repair of ingrown toenail, NOS
P1-45870 Creation of syndactyly, NOS
P1-45872 Formation of syndactyly of toe
  Reconstruction of toes, syndactyly, each web
P1-45874 Reconstruction of toes, syndactyly with skin graft, each web
P1-45876 Creation syndactyly of finger
  Formation of syndactyly of finger
P1-45879 Reduction of batwing arms
P1-45890V Suture of skin wound of limb, NOS
P1-45891V Suture of skin wound of forelimb, NOS
P1-45892V Suture of skin wound of forefoot, NOS
P1-45895V Suture of skin wound of hindlimb, NOS
P1-45896V Suture of skin wound of hindfoot, NOS

1-45C Skin of Extremities: Destructive Procedures

P1-45C20 Avulsion of nail, NOS
P1-45C22 Partial avulsion of nail
  Partial avulsion of single nail plate
P1-45C24 Complete avulsion of nail
  Complete avulsion of single nail plate
P1-45C30 Debridement of nails by electric grinder, five or less
P1-45C40 Chemexfoliation of skin of extremities, NOS
P1-45C50V Cauterization of hoof

1-45D Skin of Extremities: Transplantations and Transpositions

P1-45D10 Skin graft to extremity, NOS
P1-45D11 Attachment of pedicle graft to extremity
P1-45D12 Attachment of flap graft to extremity
P1-45D16 Myocutaneous flap to extremity
P1-45D17 Muscle flap to extremity
P1-45D18 Fasciocutaneous flap to extremity
P1-45D20 Full thickness graft to extremity, including closure of donor site, 20 sq cm or less
P1-45D26 Split-thickness graft to extremities, 100 sq cm or less, adult
P1-45D30 Delay of flap or sectioning of pedicle or direct flap of extremities
P1-45D32 Adjacent tissue transfer or rearrangement of skin of extremity, defect 10 sq cm or less
P1-45D36 Adjacent tissue transfer or rearrangement of skin of extremity, complicated
P1-45D37 Filleting of toe flap including preparation of recipient site
P1-45D38 Filleting of finger flap including preparation of recipient site
P1-45D39 Graft of skin pedicle attachment to thumb

1-45E Skin of Extremities: Manipulations

P1-45E00 Manipulation of skin of extremity, NOS
P1-45E10 Manipulation of skin of upper extremity, NOS
P1-45E20 Manipulation of skin of lower extremity, NOS

1-48 OPERATIVE PROCEDURES ON THE BREAST

1-480 Breast: General and Miscellaneous Operative Procedures

P1-48000 Operation on breast, NOS
P1-48010 Diagnostic procedure on breast, NOS
P1-48040 Operation on nipple, NOS
P1-48050 Diagnostic procedure on nipple, NOS
P1-48090 Breast procedure, NOS

1-481 Breast: Incisions

P1-48100 Mammotomy, NOS
  Mastotomy, NOS
P1-48102 Incision of skin of breast
P1-48112 Incision and exploration of breast
P1-48114 Incision and deep exploration of breast
  Mastotomy with deep exploration
P1-48118 Mastotomy with drainage of deep abscess
P1-48120 Periprosthetic capsulotomy of breast
P1-48140 Aspiration of breast
  Evacuation of cyst of breast
  Aspiration of cyst of breast
P1-48180 Incision and exploration of nipple

1-483 Breast: Excisions

P1-48300 Excision of breast tissue, NOS
P1-48301 Incisional biopsy of breast mass, NOS
P1-48302 Excisional biopsy of breast mass, NOS
  Local excision of lump in breast
P1-48303 Periprosthetic capsulectomy of breast
P1-48304 Core needle biopsy of breast
P1-48305 Fine needle biopsy of breast
  Fine needle aspiration biopsy of breast
P1-48306 Blind biopsy of breast, NOS
P1-48307 Wedge excision of breast, NOS
P1-48309 Excision of lesion of skin of breast
P1-4830A Excision of lesion of subcutaneous tissue of breast
P1-48310 Excision of benign tumor of breast, NOS

P1-48311 Excision of fibroadenoma of breast
P1-48312 Excision of hamartoma of breast
P1-48317 Excision of cyst of breast
P1-48319 Excision of malignant tumor of breast, NOS
P1-48320 Excision of nipple, NOS
  Amputation of teat, NOS
P1-48321 Excision of accessory nipple
P1-48322 Excision of nipple lesion
P1-48324 Nipple exploration with excision of lactiferous duct
P1-48326 Excision of lactiferous duct fistula of breast
  Excision of lesion of mammary duct
  Excision of lesion of breast ducts
P1-48327 Excision of intraductal papilloma of breast
P1-48328 Removal of foreign body from breast
P1-48329V Removal of foreign body from teat
P1-48340 Partial mastectomy, NOS
  Subtotal mastectomy
P1-48344 Segmental excision of breast
  Resection of quadrant of breast
  Segmental resection of breast
  Tylectomy of breast
P1-48345 Excision of accessory breast
  Excision of supernumerary breast
P1-48346 Excision of aberrant tissue of breast
  Excision of ectopic tissue of breast
P1-48350 Mastectomy, NOS
  Mammectomy, NOS
P1-48351 Unilateral mastectomy, NOS
P1-48352 Bilateral mastectomy, NOS
P1-48353 Unilateral simple mastectomy, NOS
P1-48354 Bilateral simple mastectomy
P1-48355 Unilateral mastectomy extended simple
P1-48356 Bilateral mastectomy extended simple
P1-48359 Mastectomy for gynecomastia
P1-48360 Radical mastectomy, NOS
  Halsted mastectomy
  Urban operation, extended radical mastectomy
  Radical mastectomy including pectoral muscles and axillary lymph nodes
P1-48361 Unilateral radical mastectomy
P1-48362 Bilateral radical mastectomy
  Mastectomy extended radical bilateral
P1-48363 Radical mastectomy, including pectoral muscles, axillary and internal mammary lymph nodes
P1-48364 Modified radical mastectomy, NOS
P1-48365 Modified radical mastectomy, including axillary lymph nodes and pectoralis minor muscle
P1-48366 Modified radical mastectomy, unilateral
P1-48367 Modified radical mastectomy, bilateral
P1-48370 Mastectomy with excision of regional lymph nodes, NOS
  Unilateral simple mastectomy with regional lymphadenectomy
P1-48371 Partial mastectomy with axillary lymphadenectomy
P1-48373 Bilateral mastectomy with excision of bilateral regional lymph nodes
P1-48390 Subcutaneous mastectomy, NOS
  Unilateral mastectomy with preservation of skin and nipple
  Unilateral subcutaneous mammectomy
P1-48394 Bilateral subcutaneous mammectomy
  Bilateral subcutaneous mastectomy
  Bilateral mastectomy with preservation of skin and nipple
P1-48395 Mastectomy with preservation of skin and nipple with synchronous implant
  Unilateral subcutaneous mastectomy with synchronous implant
  Unilateral subcutaneous mammectomy with synchronous implant
P1-48396 Bilateral subcutaneous mammectomy with synchronous implant
  Bilateral mastectomy with preservation of skin and nipple with synchronous implant

1-485 Breast: Injections and Implantations

P1-48500 Injection of breast, NOS
P1-48504V Infusion of mammary gland, NOS
P1-48510 Insertion of prosthetic device into breast, NOS
  Insertion of tissue expander into breast
  Insertion of breast implants, NOS
P1-48512 Bilateral breast implants
  Bilateral insertion of prosthesis into breast
P1-48513 Unilateral breast implant
P1-48514 Mammoplasty with injection into one breast
P1-48515 Mammoplasty with injection into both breasts
P1-48516 Unilateral implant of silicone into breast
P1-48517 Bilateral implant of silicone into breast
  Unilateral injection of prosthesis into breast
P1-48518 Immediate insertion of breast prosthesis
P1-48519 Delayed insertion of breast prosthesis
P1-48520 Removal of breast implant, NOS
  Removal of mammary implant material
P1-48521 Removal of intact mammary implant
P1-48530 Injection procedure for mammary ductogram
  Injection procedure only for mammary galactogram
P1-48540 Injection of therapeutic agent into breast

1-487 Breast: Endoscopy

P1-48700 Endoscopy of breast, NOS

1-488 Breast: Surgical Repairs, Closures and Reconstructions

P1-48810 Suture of skin of breast
  Mastorrhaphy
  Suture of laceration of breast
P1-48814 Fixation of pendulous breast
  Mastopexy

1-488 Breast: Surgical Repairs, Closures and Reconstructions — Continued

P1-48820 Mammoplasty, NOS
  Mastoplasty, NOS
  Breast reconstruction, NOS
  Mammaplasty, NOS
P1-48824 Mammoplasty revision
P1-48826 Revision of breast implant
  Revision of breast prosthesis
P1-48828 Revision of reconstructed breast
P1-48830 Reduction mammaplasty
  Reduction mammoplasty
  McKissock operation, breast reduction
P1-48832 Reduction mammoplasty, unilateral
  Breast reduction, unilateral
  Biesenberger operation, reduction mammoplasty, unilateral
P1-48834 Reduction mammoplasty, bilateral
  Breast reduction, bilateral
  Biesenberger operation, reduction mammoplasty, bilateral
P1-48840 Augmentation mammoplasty, NOS
  Augmentation mammaplasty without prosthetic implant
P1-48880 Repair of nipple, NOS
  Nipple and areola reconstruction
  Reconstruction of nipple, NOS
  Theleplasty, NOS
  Mammilliplasty, NOS
  Plastic operation of teat
P1-48882V Suture of wound of teat
P1-48884 Correction of inverted nipples
P1-48885V Closure of teat fistula

1-48C Breast: Destructive Procedures

P1-48C00 Destruction of tissue of breast, NOS
P1-48C10 Destruction of lesion of breast, NOS
P1-48C50V Cauterization of mammary gland, NOS
P1-48C54V Teat cryosurgery, NOS

1-48D Breast: Transplantations and Transpositions

P1-48D10 Grafting of breast, NOS
P1-48D20 Mammoplasty with pedicle graft
  Pedicle graft to breast
  Skin pedicle graft to breast
P1-48D30 Mammoplasty with split-thickness graft
  Split-thickness graft to breast
P1-48D32 Mammoplasty with full-thickness graft
  Full-thickness graft to breast
P1-48D34 Grafting of skin and dermal-fat for breast augmentation
P1-48D40 Mammoplasty with muscle flap
  Muscle flap graft to breast
  Breast reconstruction with muscle or myocutaneous flap
P1-48D50 Breast reconstruction with free flap
P1-48D80 Transposition of nipple
  Graft of nipple

1-48E Breast: Manipulations

P1-48E10 Preparation of moulage for custom breast implant
P1-48E50V Manipulation of teat
P1-48E52V Dilation of teat

SECTION 1-5 OPERATIVE PROCEDURES ON THE DIGESTIVE SYSTEM

1-50 GENERAL OPERATIVE PROCEDURES ON THE DIGESTIVE SYSTEM

1-500 Digestive System: General and Miscellaneous Procedures

P1-50000 Operation on digestive tract, NOS
P1-50020 Operation on digestive organ, NOS

1-51-58 OPERATIVE PROCEDURES ON THE DIGESTIVE TRACT

1-51 OPERATIVE PROCEDURES ON THE MOUTH AND LIPS

1-510 Mouth and Lips: General and Miscellaneous Operative Procedures

P1-51005 Operation on face, NOS
P1-51010 Operation on mouth, NOS
  Operation on oral cavity, NOS
P1-51020 Operation on lip, NOS
P1-51030 Operation on palate, NOS
P1-51040 Operation on uvula, NOS

1-511 Mouth and Lips: Incisions

P1-51110 Incision of lip, NOS
  Cheilotomy
P1-51111 Incision of abscess of lip
P1-51112 Incision and drainage of vestibule of mouth, simple
P1-51113 Incision and drainage of vestibule of mouth, complicated
P1-51114 Incision of labial frenum
  Labial frenotomy
P1-51120 Incision of mouth, NOS
P1-51122 Incision of buccal space
P1-51124 Incision and drainage of buccal space
P1-51130 Incision of floor of mouth, NOS
  Incision of sublingual space
P1-51131 Incision and drainage of sublingual space, NOS
P1-51132 Incision and drainage of sublingual space by intraoral approach
P1-51133 Incision and drainage of sublingual space by extraoral approach
P1-51134 Incision and drainage of supramylohyoid space by intraoral approach

P1-51135 Incision and drainage of supramylohyoid space by extraoral approach
P1-51136 Incision and drainage of submental space by intraoral approach
P1-51137 Incision and drainage of submental space by extraoral approach
P1-51138 Incision and drainage of submandibular space by intraoral approach
P1-51139 Incision and drainage of submandibular space by extraoral approach
P1-5113A Incision and drainage of masticator space by intraoral approach
P1-5113B Incision and drainage of masticator space by extraoral approach
P1-51140 Incision and drainage of Ludwig's angina
P1-51150 Incision of palate
 Fenestration of palate
P1-51152 Drainage of abscess of palate
P1-51160 Incision of uvula
 Transection of uvula
 Uvulotomy
P1-51162 Drainage of abscess of uvula

1-513 Mouth and Lips: Excisions

P1-51300 Biopsy of lip, NOS
P1-51301 Excision of lesion of lip
P1-51302 Excision of lesion of lip by wide excision
P1-51303 Lip shave
P1-51306 Wedge resection of lip
 Transverse wedge excision of lip with primary closure
P1-51307 Resection of more than one-fourth of lip
P1-51308 Vermilionectomy, NOS
 Vermilionectomy with mucosal advancement
P1-51309 Excision of labial frenulum
 Frenectomy of lip
P1-5130A V-excision of lip with primary direct linear closure
P1-51310 Biopsy of vestibule of mouth
P1-51311 Excision of buccal mucosa
P1-51312 Excision of lesion of vestibule of mouth without repair
P1-51314 Excision of lesion of vestibule of mouth with simple repair
P1-51316 Excision of lesion of vestibule of mouth with complex repair
P1-51318 Excision of lesion of vestibule of mouth, complex, with excision of underlying muscle
P1-51319 Excision of nasolabial cyst
P1-51320 Removal of embedded foreign body from vestibule of mouth, simple
P1-51321 Removal of embedded foreign body from vestibule of mouth, complicated
P1-51330 Excision of lesion of mouth, NOS
P1-51332 Removal of foreign body from mouth by incision
 Removal of foreign body from oral cavity by incision
P1-51333 Removal of foreign body from gum
P1-51340 Biopsy of floor of mouth
P1-51342 Excision of lesion from floor of mouth
P1-51346 Radical excision of floor of mouth
P1-51360 Biopsy of palate, NOS
P1-51361 Excision of lesion of palate without closure
 Local excision of lesion of palate
P1-51363 Resection of lesion of palate, extensive
 Excision of lesion of palate by wide excision
P1-51364 Excision of nasopalatine cyst
P1-51365 Excision of nasopalatine cyst by wide excision
P1-51366 Resection of palate
P1-51367 Resection of alveolar process and palate, en bloc
P1-51368 Removal of foreign body from palate by incision
 Removal of penetrating foreign body from palate
P1-51369 Excision of lesion of palate with simple primary closure
P1-5136A Excision of lesion of palate with local flap closure
P1-51381 Excision of lesion of uvula without closure
P1-51382 Excision of lesion of soft palate
P1-51384 Resection of soft palate
P1-51390 Excision of uvula
 Uvulectomy
P1-51391 Biopsy of uvula
P1-51392 Clipping of tip of uvula
P1-51394 Excision of lesion of uvula with simple primary closure
P1-51395 Excision of lesion of uvula with local flap closure
P1-51399 Biopsy of uvula and soft palate

1-515 Mouth and Lips: Injections and Implantations

P1-51510 Injection of mouth, NOS
P1-51560 Injection of lips, NOS
P1-51580 Insertion of pin-retained palatal prosthesis

1-517 Mouth and Lips: Endoscopy

P1-51710 Endoscopy of mouth, NOS

1-518-519 Mouth and Lips: Surgical Repairs, Closures and Reconstructions

P1-51800 Plastic repair of mouth, NOS
 Repair of mouth, NOS
 Stomatoplasty, NOS
P1-51802 Repair of lip, NOS
 Cheiloplasty
P1-51804 Cheilostomatoplasty
P1-51805 Rhinocheiloplasty
P1-51810 Suture of mouth
 Stomatorrhaphy
P1-51812 Repair of mouth laceration, NOS

1-518-519 Mouth and Lips: Surgical Repairs, Closures and Reconstructions — Continued

P1-51813 Repair of laceration of floor of mouth, up to 2.5 cm
P1-51814 Repair of laceration of floor of mouth, over 2.5 cm
P1-51815 Repair of laceration of floor of mouth, complex
P1-51820 Vestibuloplasty, NOS
P1-51821 Anterior vestibuloplasty
P1-51822 Posterior vestibuloplasty, unilateral
P1-51823 Posterior vestibuloplasty, bilateral
P1-51824 Vestibuloplasty of entire arch
P1-51825 Complex vestibuloplasty
P1-51831 Suture of lip
  Cheilorrhaphy
P1-51832 Repair of notched lip
P1-51834 V-Y operation of lip
P1-51835 Full-thickness repair of lip, vermilion only
P1-51836 Full-thickness repair of lip, up to half vertical height
P1-51837 Full-thickness repair of lip, over one half vertical height
P1-51838 Full thickness repair of lip, complex
P1-51840 Closure of laceration of vestibule of mouth, 2.5 cm or less
P1-51842 Closure of laceration of vestibule of mouth, over 2.5 cm
P1-51844 Closure of laceration of vestibule of mouth, complex
P1-51850 Repair of fistula of mouth, NOS
  Closure of fistula of mouth, NOS
  Fistulectomy of mouth, NOS
P1-51854 Repair of nasolabial fistula
  Closure of nasolabial fistula
P1-51880 Palatoplasty, NOS
  Repair of palate, NOS
  Plastic repair of palate, NOS
P1-51882 Suture of palate
  Palatorrhaphy
P1-51883 Suture of laceration of palate, NOS
  Repair of laceration of palate, up to 2 cm
P1-51884 Repair of laceration of palate, over 2 cm
P1-51885 Repair of laceration of palate, complex
P1-51890 Repair of uvula
P1-51892 Suture of uvula
P1-51900 Repair of cleft lip, NOS
  Harelip operation
  Reconstruction of cleft lip, NOS
P1-51901 Full thickness excision of lip, reconstruction with local flap
  Estlander operation, lip reconstruction
P1-51902 Primary repair of cleft lip, unilateral, partial
P1-51903 Primary repair of cleft lip, unilateral, complete
P1-51904 Primary repair of cleft lip, bilateral, single stage procedure
P1-51905 Primary repair of cleft lip, bilateral, one of two stages
P1-51906 Primary repair of cleft lip, secondary by recreation of defect and reclosure
P1-51907 Primary repair of cleft lip with cross lip pedicle flap including sectioning and insertion of pedicle
P1-51908 Full thickness excision of lip by reconstruction with cross lip flap
  Abbe-Estlander operation, cross lip flap
P1-51909 Lemesurier operation, cleft lip repair
P1-51910 Millard operation, cleft lip repair
P1-51911 Thompson operation, cleft lip repair
P1-51912 Rhinocheiloplasty repair for cleft lip
P1-51934 Repair of uvula with synchronous cleft palate repair
P1-51936 Uvulopalatopharyngoplasty
P1-51938 Uvulopharyngoplasty
P1-51950 Repair of cleft palate, NOS
  Uranorrhaphy for cleft palate repair
  Suture of cleft palate
  Palatorrhaphy for cleft palate
  Uranoplasty for cleft palate repair
  Palatoplasty for cleft palate
  Correction of cleft palate
P1-51952 Palatoplasty for cleft palate, soft palate
P1-51953 Palatoplasty for cleft palate, hard palate
P1-51955 Repair of anterior palate including vomer flap
P1-51956 Palatoplasty for cleft palate, soft and hard palate
  Uranostaphylorrhaphy
P1-51960 Pharyngeal flap operation, cleft palate repair
  Pharyngorrhaphy for cleft palate
  Palatoplasty for cleft palate, attachment of pharyngeal flap
  Graft of palate for cleft palate repair
  Palatopharyngoplasty
  Pharyngoplasty for cleft palate
P1-51961 Palatoplasty for lengthening of palate with pharyngeal flap
P1-51963 Palatoplasty for lengthening of palate with island flap
P1-51964 Palatoplasty for cleft palate by secondary lengthening procedure
  Lengthening of palate, subsequent procedure
P1-51965 Dorrance operation, push-back operation for cleft palate
P1-51966 Langenbeck operation, cleft palate repair
P1-51967 Palatoplasty for cleft palate with closure of alveolar ridge, soft tissue only
P1-51968 Wardill operation, cleft palate repair
P1-51969 Palatoplasty for cleft palate with closure of alveolar ridge with bone graft to alveolar ridge
P1-51970 Revision of cleft palate repair
  Palatoplasty for cleft palate, major revision

1-51C Mouth and Lips: Destructive Procedures

P1-51C00 Destructive procedure on mouth and lips, NOS

P1-51C10 Cryocauterization for destruction of lesion of vestibule of mouth
P1-51C12 Thermocauterization for destruction of lesion of vestibule of mouth
P1-51C14 Chemical cauterization for destruction of lesion of vestibule of mouth
P1-51C16 Laser beam destruction of lesion of vestibule of mouth
P1-51C20 Local destruction of lesion of bony palate
P1-51C21 Wide destruction of lesion of bony palate
P1-51C24 Cryotherapy of palate
  Cryosurgery for destruction of lesion of palate
P1-51C26 Cauterization of palate
P1-51C27 Thermocauterization for destruction of lesion of palate
P1-51C28 Chemocauterization of palate
  Chemical cauterization for destruction of lesion of palate
P1-51C40 Cryosurgery for destruction of lesion of uvula
P1-51C42 Thermocauterization for destruction of lesion of uvula
P1-51C44 Chemical cauterization for destruction of lesion of uvula

1-51D Mouth and Lips: Transplantations and Transpositions

P1-51D04 Excision of mucosa of vestibule of mouth as donor graft
P1-51D10 Graft of mouth, except palate, NOS
P1-51D12 Full-thickness graft of mouth, except palate
P1-51D14 Full-thickness graft to lip and mouth
P1-51D16 Attachment of pedicle or flap graft to lip and mouth
P1-51D17 Graft to buccal sulcus
P1-51D19 Skin graft to lip and mouth, NOS
P1-51D20 Graft of lip
P1-51D22 Full-thickness graft of lip
P1-51D24 Graft of vermilion border of lip
P1-51D26 Attachment of pedicle graft to lip
P1-51D50 Graft of palate

1-51E Mouth and Lips: Manipulations

P1-51E10 Manipulation of tissue of mouth, NOS
P1-51E16 Removal of intraluminal foreign body from oral cavity
  Removal of intraluminal foreign body from mouth without incision
P1-51E40 Manipulation of tissue of lips, NOS

1-52 OPERATIVE PROCEDURES ON THE TONGUE

1-520 Tongue: General and Miscellaneous Operative Procedures

P1-52010 Operation on tongue, NOS

1-521 Tongue: Incisions

P1-52100 Incision of tongue, NOS
  Glossotomy
P1-52120 Incision and drainage of lesion of tongue
P1-52140 Incision of lingual frenum
  Division of frenulum of tongue
  Tongue tie operation
  Lingual frenotomy

1-523 Tongue: Excisions

P1-52300 Biopsy of tongue, NOS
  Excision of tissue of tongue
P1-52302 Excision of lesion of tongue
  Excisional biopsy of tongue
P1-52306 Excision of lesion of tongue without closure
P1-52310 Core needle biopsy of tongue
P1-52312 Fine needle biopsy of tongue
  Fine needle aspiration biopsy of tongue
P1-52316 Excision of lingual frenum
  Lingual frenectomy
  Frenectomy of tongue
P1-52320 Biopsy of anterior two-thirds of tongue
P1-52322 Biopsy of posterior one-third of tongue
P1-52324 Excision of lesion of tongue with closure, anterior two-thirds
P1-52326 Excision of lesion of tongue with closure, posterior one-third
P1-52328 Excision of lesion of tongue with closure with local tongue flap
P1-52340 Glossectomy, NOS
  Resection of tongue, NOS
P1-52342 Wedge resection of tongue
P1-52344 Partial glossectomy
  Partial excision of tongue
  Glossectomy, less than one-half of tongue
P1-52346 Hemiglossectomy
P1-52348 Total excision of tongue
  Complete glossectomy
  Total glossectomy
  Radical excision of tongue
  Radical glossectomy
  Whitehead operation, radical glossectomy
P1-52350 Partial glossectomy with unilateral radical neck dissection
P1-52352 Complete glossectomy with tracheostomy with unilateral radical neck dissection
P1-52354 Complete glossectomy without tracheostomy with unilateral radical neck dissection
P1-52356 Glossectomy with resection of floor of mouth with suprahyoid neck dissection
P1-52357 Glossectomy with resection of floor of mouth and mandibular resection without radical neck dissection
P1-52358 Glossectomy with resection of floor of mouth with mandibular resection and radical neck dissection
  Commando operation, radical glossectomy
P1-52360 Complete glossectomy with tracheostomy without radical neck dissection

1-525 Tongue: Injections and Implantations

P1-52510 Injection of tongue, NOS
P1-52540 Implantation of tongue, NOS

1-527 Tongue: Endoscopy

P1-52710 Endoscopy of tongue, NOS

1-528 Tongue: Surgical Repairs, Closures and Reconstructions

P1-52800 Glossoplasty, NOS
Repair of tongue, NOS
P1-52808 Frenoplasty
Lingual frenoplasty
P1-52812 Fascial sling of tongue
P1-52820 Suture of tongue
Glossorrhaphy
Suture of laceration of tongue
P1-52822 Repair of laceration of anterior two-thirds of tongue, up to 2.5 cm
P1-52824 Repair of laceration of posterior one-third of tongue, up to 2.5 cm
P1-52826 Repair of laceration of tongue, over 2.5 cm
P1-52827 Repair of laceration of tongue, complex
P1-52860 Suture of tongue to lip for micrognathia
Fusion of lip to tongue
Douglas operation, suture of tongue to lip for micrognathia
P1-52880 Fixation of tongue
Glossopexy
P1-52882 Fixation of tongue with mechanical K wire

1-52C Tongue: Destructive Procedures

P1-52C00 Destruction of tissue of tongue, NOS
P1-52C10 Destruction of lesion of tongue
P1-52C20 Lysis of adhesions of tongue

1-52D Tongue: Transplantations and Transpositions

P1-52D10 Transplant of tissue of tongue, NOS
Tongue graft, NOS
P1-52D40 Transposition of tissue of tongue, NOS

1-52E Tongue: Manipulations

P1-52E10 Manipulation of tongue, NOS

1-53 OPERATIVE PROCEDURES ON THE PHARYNX

1-530 Pharynx: General and Miscellaneous Operative Procedures

P1-53000 Operation on pharynx, NOS
P1-53006 Operation on hypopharynx, NOS
P1-53010 Operation on oropharynx, NOS
P1-53020 Operation on pyriform sinus, NOS
P1-53030 Control of oropharyngeal hemorrhage, NOS
P1-53032 Control of oropharyngeal hemorrhage, simple
P1-53034 Control of oropharyngeal hemorrhage, complicated
P1-53036 Control of oropharyngeal hemorrhage with secondary surgical intervention

1-531 Pharynx: Incisions

P1-53100 Pharyngotomy, NOS
Incision of pharynx, NOS
P1-53120 Incision and drainage of lateral pharyngeal space
P1-53121 Incision and drainage of parapharyngeal abscess by intraoral approach
P1-53122 Incision and drainage of parapharyngeal abscess by external approach
P1-53125 Incision and drainage of retropharyngeal tissue
P1-53126 Incision and drainage of retropharyngeal abscess by intraoral approach
P1-53128 Incision and drainage of retropharyngeal abscess by external approach
P1-53130 Division of congenital web of pharynx
P1-53140 Aspiration of diverticulum of pharynx
P1-53160 Cricopharyngeal myotomy

1-533 Pharynx: Excisions

P1-53300 Excision of tissue of pharynx, NOS
P1-53301 Pharyngeal biopsy, NOS
P1-53302 Biopsy of oropharynx
P1-53303 Biopsy of supraglottic mass
P1-53310 Excision of lesion of pharynx
P1-53311 Excision of pharyngeal bands
P1-53314 Biopsy of hypopharynx
P1-53320 Removal of foreign body from pharynx, NOS
P1-53321 Removal of intraluminal foreign body from pharynx without incision
P1-53322 Removal of foreign body from pharynx by pharyngotomy
P1-53325 Removal of calculus of pharynx
P1-53330 Pharyngectomy
P1-53332 Partial pharyngectomy
Limited pharyngectomy
P1-53333 Resection of lateral pharyngeal wall with direct closure by advancement of lateral and posterior pharyngeal walls
Resection of lateral pyriform sinus with direct closure by advancement of lateral and posterior pharyngeal walls
P1-53334 Resection of pharyngeal wall requiring closure with myocutaneous flap
P1-53340 Pharyngeal diverticulectomy by cricopharyngeal myotomy
Pharyngoesophageal diverticulectomy by cricopharyngeal myotomy
Hypopharyngeal diverticulectomy by cricopharyngeal myotomy
P1-53342 Diverticulectomy of hypopharynx with myotomy by cervical approach
Diverticulectomy of hypopharynx by cervical approach

P1-53360 Excision of branchial cleft vestige, NOS
P1-53361 Excision of branchial cleft cyst confined to skin and subcutaneous tissues
P1-53362 Excision of branchial cleft cyst or fistula extending beneath subcutaneous tissues into pharynx

1-535 Pharynx: Injections and Implantations

P1-53510 Injection of pharynx, NOS
P1-53540 Implantation of pharynx, NOS

1-537 Pharynx: Endoscopy

P1-53700 Endoscopy of pharynx, NOS
  Pharyngoscopy, NOS

1-538 Pharynx: Surgical Repairs, Closures and Reconstructions

P1-53800 Repair of pharynx, NOS
  Pharyngoplasty, NOS
P1-53804 Pharyngoesophageal repair
P1-53812 Z-plasty of hypopharynx
P1-53814 Pharyngoplasty with silastic implant
P1-53815 Construction of artificial pharyngeal valve
P1-53820 Reconstruction of pharynx, NOS
P1-53830 Repair of pharyngeal fistula, NOS
  Closure of pharyngeal fistula, NOS
P1-53832 Repair of pharyngoesophageal fistula
  Closure of pharyngoesophageal fistula
P1-53834 Repair of branchial cleft fistula or cyst
  Fistulectomy of branchial cleft fistula or cyst
  Closure of branchial cleft fistula or cyst
P1-53840 Suture of pharynx
  Pharyngorrhaphy
P1-53842 Suture of laceration of pharynx
P1-53850 Diverticulopexy of hypopharynx
  Suspension of diverticulum of pharynx
P1-53852 Diverticulopexy of hypopharynx with myotomy
P1-53860 Repair of nasopharyngeal atresia
  Correction of nasopharyngeal atresia
P1-53880 Pharyngostomy

1-53C Pharynx: Destructive Procedures

P1-53C00 Destruction of tissue of pharynx, NOS
P1-53C02 Lysis of adhesions of pharynx
P1-53C10 Electrocoagulation of lesion of pharynx
P1-53C12 Cauterization of pharynx, NOS

1-53D Pharynx: Transplantations and Transpositions

P1-53D10 Transplantation of pharyngeal tissue, NOS
P1-53D40 Transposition of pharyngeal tissue, NOS

1-53E Pharynx: Manipulations

P1-53E10 Dilation of pharynx

1-54 OPERATIVE PROCEDURE ON THE ESOPHAGUS

1-540 Esophagus: General and Miscellaneous Operative Procedures

P1-54000 Operation on esophagus, NOS

1-541 Esophagus: Incisions

P1-54100 Incision of esophagus, NOS
  Esophagotomy, NOS
P1-54102 Esophagotomy by cervical approach
P1-54104 Esophagotomy by thoracic approach
P1-54106 Incision and exploration of esophagus
P1-54110 Incision of esophageal web
  Dewebbing of esophagus
P1-54130 Esophagomyotomy, NOS
  Heller operation, esophagomyotomy
  Cardiomyotomy of esophagus
  Myotomy of esophagus
  Esophagogastromyotomy
P1-54131 Esophagomyotomy without hiatal hernia repair by abdominal approach
P1-54132 Esophagomyotomy without hiatal hernia repair by thoracic approach

1-543 Esophagus: Excisions

P1-54300 Biopsy of esophagus, NOS
  Open biopsy of esophagus
P1-54302 Incisional biopsy of esophagus
P1-54304 Open excisional biopsy of esophagus
  Excision of lesion of esophagus
P1-54305 Excision of local lesion of esophagus with primary repair by cervical approach
P1-54306 Excision of local lesion of esophagus with primary repair by thoracic approach
P1-54310 Diverticulectomy of esophagus, NOS
  Dahlman operation, excision of esophageal diverticulum
  Excision of diverticulum of esophagus
P1-54311 Diverticulectomy of esophagus with myotomy
P1-54312 Diverticulectomy of esophagus by cervical approach
P1-54313 Diverticulectomy of esophagus with myotomy by cervical approach
P1-54314 Diverticulectomy of esophagus by thoracic approach
P1-54315 Diverticulectomy of esophagus with myotomy by thoracic approach
P1-54330 Wide excision of malignant lesion of cervical esophagus
P1-54332 Excision of malignant lesion of cervical esophagus with laryngectomy
P1-54334 Excision of malignant lesion of cervical esophagus with radical neck dissection
P1-54336 Excision of malignant lesion of cervical esophagus with laryngectomy and radical neck dissection
P1-54337 Wooky operation, excision of esophagus with radical neck dissection

1-543 Esophagus: Excisions — Continued

P1-54340 Removal of foreign body from esophagus by incision
P1-54341 Esophagotomy with removal of foreign body by cervical approach
P1-54342 Esophagotomy with removal of foreign body by thoracic approach
P1-54360 Esophagectomy, NOS
P1-54362 Total esophagectomy
P1-54364 Subtotal resection of esophagus
  Partial esophagectomy
P1-54370 Esophagectomy of upper two-thirds level with segment replacement, one stage
P1-54371 Esophagectomy of upper two-thirds level with segment replacement, two stages
P1-54372 Esophagectomy of upper two-thirds level with gastric anastomosis and vagotomy
P1-54373 Esophagectomy of upper two-thirds level with gastric anastomosis, vagotomy and pyloroplasty
P1-54374 Esophagectomy of upper two-thirds level with gastric anastomosis, vagotomy and second stage pyloroplasty
P1-54380 Total esophagectomy with gastropharyngostomy
P1-54390 Esophagogastrectomy, NOS
P1-54392 Esophagogastrectomy of lower third wuth vagotomy by combined thoracicoabdominal approach
P1-54394 Esophagogastrectomy of lower third with vagotomy by combined thoracicoabdominal approach with pyloroplasty

1-545 Esophagus: Injections and Implantations

P1-54510V Irrigation of crop
P1-54520 Insertion of catheter into esophagus, permanent tube type
P1-54524 Replacement of esophagostomy tube

1-547 Esophagus: Endoscopy

P1-54700 Endoscopy of esophagus, NOS
  Esophagoscopy, NOS
P1-54702 Diagnostic flexible fiberoptic esophagoscopy
P1-54704 Diagnostic rigid esophagoscopy
P1-54706 Esophagoscopy by intraoperative incision
P1-54708 Esophagoscopy through artificial stoma
P1-54710 Esophagoscopy for biopsy
  Endoscopic biopsy of esophagus
P1-54712 Endoscopic excision of lesion of esophagus
P1-54714 Esophagoscopy for removal of polypoid lesion
P1-54716 Esophagoscopy for biopsy and collection of specimen by brushing or washing
P1-54718 Esophagoscopy for removal of foreign body
  Endoscopic removal of intraluminal foreign body from esophagus without incision
P1-54720 Esophagoscopy for destruction of lesion or tumor
  Endoscopic destruction of lesion or tumor of esophagus, NOS
P1-54729 Esophagoscopy for control of hemorrhage
P1-54730 Esophagoscopy for insertion of plastic tube or stent
P1-54740 Esophagoscopy for injection of esophageal varices
  Injection of sclerosing agent into esophageal varices by endoscopy
  Endoscopic injection of esophageal varices
  Injection of esophageal varices by endoscopy
  Injection of varicose veins of esophagus by endoscopy
P1-54750 Esophagoscopy for direct dilation
P1-54752 Esophagoscopy for insertion of wire to guide dilation

1-548-549 Esophagus: Surgical Repairs, Closures and Reconstructions

P1-54800 Repair of esophagus, NOS
  Esophagoplasty, NOS
P1-54802 Esophagoplasty by cervical approach
P1-54803 Esophagoplasty by thoracic approach
P1-54806 Anastomosis of esophagus by intrathoracic approach, NOS
P1-54808 Anastomosis of esophagus, antethoracic, NOS
  Esophagoesophageal anastomosis, antesternal or antethoracic
P1-54810 Repair of esophageal stricture
  Thal operation, repair of esophageal stricture
P1-54812 Correction of esophageal atresia
P1-54820 Suture of esophagus
  Suture of laceration of esophagus
  Esophagorrhaphy
P1-54821 Suture of esophageal wound or injury by cervical approach
P1-54822 Suture of esophageal wound or injury by thoracic approach
P1-54828 Closure of perforation of esophagus
P1-54840 Transection of esophagus with repair for esophageal varices
P1-54842 Ligation of esophageal varices
P1-54850 Intrathoracic esophageal anastomosis with interposition of colon
P1-54859 Intrathoracic esophageal anastomosis with other interposition, NOS
P1-54860 Esophagostomy, NOS
  External fistulization of esophagus, NOS
P1-54862 Cervical esophagostomy
  Fistulization of esophagus by cervical approach
P1-54864 Thoracic esophagostomy
  Fistulization of esophagus by thoracic approach
P1-54866 Abdominal esophagostomy
  Fistulization of esophagus by abdominal approach

P1-54868 Exteriorization of esophageal pouch
P1-54870 Repair of esophageal fistula, NOS
  Closure of esophageal fistula, NOS
P1-54871 Closure of esophageal fistula by cervical approach
P1-54872 Closure of esophageal fistula by thoracic approach
P1-54873 Repair of tracheoesophageal fistula by cervical approach
P1-54874 Repair of tracheoesophageal fistula by thoracic approach
P1-54876 Repair of esophagocutaneous fistula
  Closure of esophagocutaneous fistula
P1-54878 Closure of gastroesophageal fistula
P1-54879 Repair of stoma of esophagus
P1-54890 Esophageal hiatus hernia repair, NOS
P1-54891 Esophagomyotomy with hiatal hernia repair by abdominal approach
P1-54892 Esophagomyotomy with hiatal hernia repair by thoracic approach
P1-548A0 Take-down of esophagostomy
  Closure of stoma of esophagus
  Closure of esophagostomy
  Take-down of stoma of esophagus
P1-548A1 Closure of esophagostomy by cervical approach
P1-548A2 Closure of esophagostomy by thoracic approach
P1-548A5 Revision of esophagostomy
P1-54900 Esophagoesophagostomy
  Intrathoracic esophagoesophageal anastomosis
P1-54910 Esophagogastrostomy, NOS
P1-54912 Esophagogastrostomy by thoracic approach
  Intrathoracic esophagogastric anastomosis, NOS
P1-54914 Esophagogastrostomy with vagotomy and pyloroplasty by thoracic approach
P1-54916 Esophagogastrostomy by abdominal approach
P1-54918 Esophagogastrostomy with vagotomy and pyloroplasty by abdominal approach
P1-54920 Anastomosis of esophagus to intestinal segment, NOS
  Esophagoenterostomy, NOS
  Anastomosis of esophagus to small bowel, NOS
P1-54921 Esophagoenteric anastomosis, intrathoracic, NOS
P1-54922 Intrathoracic esophageal anastomosis with interposition of small bowel, NOS
P1-54924 Esophagoduodenostomy, NOS
  Esophagoduodenal anastomosis, NOS
P1-54926 Esophagoduodenal anastomosis with interposition of small bowel
  Esophagoduodenostomy with interposition of small bowel
P1-54930 Esophagojejunostomy, NOS
P1-54931 Esophagojejunostomy with interposition of small bowel
P1-54932 Esophagojejunostomy by thoracic approach
P1-54933 Esophagojejunostomy by abdominal approach
P1-54940 Intrathoracic esophagoileostomy, NOS
P1-54941 Esophagoileostomy with interposition of small bowel
P1-54950 Intrathoracic esophagocolostomy
  Intrathoracic esophagocologastrostomy
P1-54960 Esophagogastrostomy, antesternal or antethoracic
  Formation of reversed gastric tube, antesternal or antethoracic
  Esophagogastric anastomosis, antesternal or antethoracic
  Gastric bypass operation, NOS
P1-54968 Creation of subcutaneous tunnel with esophageal anastomosis
P1-54969 Construction of subcutaneous tunnel without esophageal anastomosis
P1-54970 Esophagoenteric anastomosis, antesternal or antethoracic, NOS
  Anastomosis of esophagus to intestinal segment, antesternal or antethoracic, NOS
  Anastomosis of esophagus, antesternal or antethoracic, with interposition of small bowel
P1-54980 Esophagoileostomy, antesternal or antethoracic, with interposition of small bowel
  Esophagoileostomy, antesternal or antethoracic, NOS
P1-54986 Anastomosis of esophagus, antesternal or antethoracic, with interposition of jejunal loop
  Roux-Herzen-Judine operation, jejunal loop interposition
  Esophagojejunostomy antesternal or antethoracic, with interposition of small bowel
  Esophagojejunostomy antesternal or antethoracic, NOS
P1-54990 Esophagocolic anastomosis, antesternal or antethoracic, NOS
  Esophagocolostomy, antesternal or antethoracic, NOS
  Esophagus to colon anastomosis, antesternal or antethoracic
  Anastomosis of esophagus, antesternal or antethoracic with interposition of colon
P1-549A0 Anastomosis of esophagus, antesternal or antethoracic with insertion of prosthesis, NOS
P1-549A2 Anastomosis of esophagus, antesternal or antethoracic with insertion of rubber tube

1-54C Esophagus: Destructive Procedures

P1-54C00 Destruction of lesion of esophagus, NOS
P1-54C10 Cryotherapy of lesion of esophagus
P1-54C20 Cauterization of lesion of esophagus
P1-54C24 Electrocautery of lesion of esophagus

1-54C Esophagus: Destructive Procedures — Continued

P1-54C26 Fulguration of lesion of esophagus
P1-54C30 Chemosurgery of lesion of esophagus

1-54D Esophagus: Transplantations and Transpositions

P1-54D10 Transplantation of tissue of esophagus
P1-54D40 Transposition of tissue of esophagus

1-54E Esophagus: Manipulations

P1-54E00 Dilation of esophagus, NOS
 Bougienage of esophagus, NOS
P1-54E10 Dilation of esophagus by unguided sound or bougie with single or multiple passes
P1-54E20 Dilation of esophagus over guide wire or string
P1-54E30 Dilation of esophagus by balloon or Starck dilator
P1-54E34 Dilation of esophagus by balloon or Starck dilator, retrograde
P1-54E40 Dilation of cardiac sphincter of esophagus
 Dilation of achalasia
P1-54E50 Esophagogastric tamponade with balloon

1-55 OPERATIVE PROCEDURES ON THE STOMACH

1-550 Stomach: General and Miscellaneous Operative Procedures

P1-55000 Operation on stomach, NOS
 Gastric operation, NOS
P1-55020 Control of hemorrhage of stomach, NOS

1-551 Stomach: Incisions

P1-55100 Incision of stomach
 Gastrotomy
 Labbe operation, gastrotomy
 Gastromyotomy
 Gastrocentesis
P1-55102 Incision and exploration of stomach
P1-55106 Gastrotomy with esophageal dilation and insertion of plastic tubes
P1-55107V Puncture by trocar of rumen of stomach
P1-55108V Incision of rumen of stomach
P1-55109V Incision and exploration of rumen of stomach
P1-55110 Pyloromyotomy, NOS
 Pyloric sphincterotomy
 Pyloroduodenotomy
P1-55112 Ramstedt operation, pyloromyotomy with wedge resection
 Fredet-Ramstedt operation, pyloromyotomy with wedge resection
P1-55114 Gastric cardiotomy
P1-55151 Truncal vagotomy
 Subdiaphragmatic vagotomy
P1-55152 Transection of vagus nerve by abdominal approach
P1-55153 Transection of vagus nerve by transthoracic approach
P1-55154 Selective vagotomy
P1-55155 Highly selective vagotomy
 Transection of vagi limited to proximal stomach
 Parietal cell vagotomy
P1-55160 Truncal vagotomy with pyloroplasty
P1-55161 Truncal vagotomy with pyloroplasty and gastrostomy
P1-55163 Selective vagotomy with pyloroplasty
P1-55164 Selective vagotomy with pyloroplasty and gastrostomy
P1-55166 Highly selective vagotomy with pyloroplasty
 Parietal cell vagotomy with pyloroplasty
P1-55167 Parietal cell vagotomy with pyloroplasty and gastrostomy

1-553 Stomach: Excisions

P1-55300 Biopsy of stomach, NOS
P1-55302 Open biopsy of stomach
 Biopsy of stomach by laparotomy
P1-55303 Excision of lesion of stomach, NOS
P1-55304 Gastric polypectomy
P1-55305 Wedge resection of stomach
P1-55306 Core needle biopsy of stomach
P1-55307 Fine needle biopsy of stomach
 Fine needle aspiration biopsy of stomach
P1-55308 Removal of foreign body from stomach by incision
 Gastrotomy with foreign body removal
P1-55310 Excision of ulcer of stomach
P1-55312 Excision of stomach diverticulum
 Diverticulectomy of stomach
P1-55314 Excision of tumor of stomach
P1-55330 Gastrectomy, NOS
P1-55331 Subtotal gastrectomy
 Partial gastrectomy
P1-55332 Hemigastrectomy
P1-55333 Hemigastrectomy by abdominal approach
P1-55334 Hemigastrectomy by thoracic approach
P1-55335 Hemigastrectomy with vagotomy
P1-55336 Resection of stomach fundus
 Gastric fundusectomy
 Gastric fundectomy
P1-55337 Proximal subtotal gastrectomy by abdominal approach
P1-55338 Proximal subtotal gastrectomy by thoracic approach
P1-55339 Pyloric antrectomy
 Pylorectomy
 Gastropylorectomy
P1-5533A Sleeve resection of stomach
P1-55350 Total gastrectomy
 Schlatter operation, total gastrectomy
 Complete gastrectomy
P1-55354 Distal subtotal gastrectomy
 Gastrectomy with anastomosis to duodenum

P1-55354 (cont.) Billroth I operation
Resection of stomach with gastroduodenal anastomosis
P1-55356 Distal subtotal gastrectomy with vagotomy
P1-55358 Esophagoduodenostomy with complete gastrectomy
P1-55359 Esophagojejunostomy with complete gastrectomy
P1-55360 Resection of stomach with gastrojejunal anastomosis
Billroth II operation
P1-55361 Hofmeister operation, gastrectomy
P1-55362 Polya operation, gastrectomy
P1-55370 Total gastrectomy with intestinal interposition, NOS
Complete gastrectomy with intestinal interposition, NOS
Total gastrectomy with repair by intestinal transplant
P1-55372 Partial gastrectomy with jejunal transposition
Gastrectomy with jejunal transposition
Henley operation, jejunal transposition
P1-55380V Removal of foreign body from rumen of stomach
P1-55385V Abomasectomy

1-555 Stomach: Injections and Implantations

P1-55500 Intubation of stomach, NOS
P1-55501 Intubation for gastric decompression, NOS
P1-55502 Insertion of nasogastric tube for intestinal decompression
P1-55506 Replacement of nasogastric tube
P1-55510 Irrigation of stomach
Nasogastric irrigation
Gastric lavage
P1-55512 Irrigation of gastrostomy
P1-55520 Nasogastric intubation for enteral infusion of concentrated nutritional substances
Gastric gavage
P1-55540 Insertion of gastric balloon
Insertion of balloon into stomach
P1-55542 Removal of gastric balloon
P1-55549 Removal of device from digestive system, NOS
P1-55560 Percutaneous placement of gastrostomy tube
P1-55561 Change of gastrostomy tube
Replacement of gastrostomy tube
P1-55562 Removal of gastrostomy tube
P1-55570V Insertion of magnet into rumen of stomach
P1-55572V Removal of magnet from rumen of stomach

1-557 Stomach: Endoscopy

P1-55700 Endoscopy of stomach, NOS
Gastroscopy, NOS
P1-55702 Esophagogastroscopy
P1-55704 Upper gastrointestinal endoscopy for directed placement of percutaneous gastrostomy tube
P1-55710 Transabdominal gastroscopy
Operative endoscopy of stomach
P1-55712 Gastroscopy through artificial stoma
Percutaneous endoscopy through gastrostomy
Endoscopy of stomach through stoma
P1-55714 Esophagogastroscopy through stoma
P1-55720 Operative esophagogastroscopy
P1-55730 Endoscopic biopsy of stomach
P1-55731 Endoscopic brush biopsy of stomach
Gastroesophageal brush biopsy
P1-55740 Upper gastrointestinal endoscopy for dilation of gastric outlet obstruction
P1-55741 Endoscopic dilation of pylorus
Endoscopic dilation of pyloric sphincter
P1-55742 Endoscopic dilation of sphincter of pylorus by incision
P1-55744 Endoscopic dilation of gastrojejunostomy site
P1-55750 Endoscopic destruction of lesion of stomach
P1-55752 Endoscopic excision of lesion of stomach
P1-55760 Upper gastrointestinal endoscopy for injection and sclerosis of gastric varices
P1-55762 Endoscopic control of gastric bleeding
P1-55770 Endoscopic removal of foreign body from stomach
Endoscopic removal of intraluminal foreign body from stomach and small intestine without incision

1-558-55A Stomach: Surgical Repairs, Closures and Reconstructions

P1-55810 Repair of stomach, NOS
P1-55830 Gastroplasty, NOS
P1-55832 Cardioplasty of stomach
P1-55833 Cardioplasty of stomach and esophagus
Esophagogastroplasty
P1-55834 Belsey operation, esophagogastric sphincter
P1-55836 Creation of esophagogastric sphincteric competence, NOS
Restoration of cardioesophageal angle
P1-55838 Pyloroplasty, NOS
Gastric pyloroplasty
Heineke-Mikulicz operation, pyloroplasty
Finney operation, pyloroplasty
P1-55839 Revision of pyloroplasty
P1-55840V Plastic operation on rumen of stomach
P1-55842V Fistulization of rumen of stomach
P1-55844V Fixation of rumen of stomach
P1-55846V Abomasopexy
P1-55847V Abomasopexy by flank approach
P1-55860 Devascularization of stomach
Tanner operation, devascularization of stomach
P1-55870 Reduction of volvulus of stomach
P1-55880 Plication of stomach
Gastroplication
P1-55882 Fundoplication
Nissen operation, fundoplication of stomach

1-558-55A Stomach: Surgical Repairs, Closures and Reconstructions — Continued

P1-55886 Esophagogastric fundoplasty, NOS
P1-55887 Esophagogastric fundoplasty with fundic patch
P1-55910 Inversion of diverticulum of stomach
 Invagination of diverticulum of stomach
P1-55920 Esophagogastropexy
P1-55922 Gastropexy
P1-55924 Anterior gastropexy for hiatal hernia
P1-55930 Gastrostomy, NOS
P1-55931 Pylorostomy
P1-55932 Temporary gastrostomy
P1-55933 Brunschwig operation, temporary gastrostomy
P1-55934 Kader operation, temporary gastrostomy
P1-55935 Witzel operation, temporary gastrostomy
P1-55936 Temporary neonatal gastrostomy for feeding
P1-55940 Permanent gastrostomy
P1-55942 Beck-Jianu operation, permanent gastrostomy
P1-55943 Frank operation, permanent gastrostomy
P1-55944 Janeway operation, permanent gastrostomy
P1-55945 Spivack operation, permanent gastrostomy
P1-55946 Ssabanejew-Frank operation, permanent gastrostomy
P1-55948 Permanent gastrostomy with construction of gastric tube
P1-55960 Gastric bypass for morbid obesity
 Gastroplasty for morbid obesity, NOS
 Gastrointestinal bypass shunt for obesity
 Bypass gastrogastrostomy
P1-55963 Printen and Mason operation, high gastric bypass
 High gastric bypass
P1-55965 Biliopancreatic bypass to ileum with partial gastrectomy
 Scopinaro operation for morbid obesity
P1-55966 Bypass gastroenterostomy
 Gastric bypass with Roux-en-Y gastroenterostomy for morbid obesity
P1-55967 Jaboulay operation, gastroduodenostomy
 Gastroduodenostomy
P1-55968 Bypass gastrojejunostomy
 Gastrojejunostomy
P1-55969 Gastrojejunostomy with vagotomy
P1-5596A Gastric stapling for obesity
P1-5596B Jejunocecostomy for obesity
P1-5596C Jejunocolostomy for obesity
P1-5596D Scott operation, intestinal bypass for obesity
P1-55970 Repair of stoma of stomach
 Revision of gastrostomy
 Revision of stoma of stomach
P1-55971 Revision of gastric anastomosis with jejunal interposition
P1-55972 Pantaloon operation, revision of gastric anastomosis
P1-55973 Steinberg operation, revision of gastric anastomosis
P1-55974 Revision of gastroduodenostomy with jejunal interposition
P1-55975 Revision of gastroduodenal anastomosis with reconstruction
P1-55976 Revision of gastroduodenal anastomosis with reconstruction and vagotomy
P1-55980 Revision of gastrojejunostomy
P1-55982 Revision of gastrojejunal anastomosis with reconstruction with partial gastrectomy
P1-55984 Revision of gastrojejunal anastomosis with reconstruction with bowel resection
P1-55986 Revision of gastrojejunal anastomosis with reconstruction with partial gastrectomy and vagotomy
P1-55988 Revision of gastrojejunal anastomosis with reconstruction with bowel resection and vagotomy
P1-55989 Take-down of gastric anastomosis
 Take-down of anastomosis of stomach
P1-55A10 Closure of gastrostomy
 Surgical closure of gastrostomy
 Closure of stoma of stomach
 Take-down of stoma of stomach
P1-55A20 Closure of gastroduodenostomy
 Take-down of gastroduodenostomy
P1-55A22 Closure of gastrojejunostomy
 Take-down of gastrojejunostomy
P1-55A30 Repair of stomach fistula, NOS
 Repair of gastric fistula, NOS
 Closure of stomach fistula, NOS
 Closure of gastric fistula, NOS
P1-55A32 Repair of gastrojejunal fistula
 Closure of gastrojejunal fistula
P1-55A34 Repair of gastroenterocolic fistula
 Closure of gastroenterocolic fistula
P1-55A36 Repair of gastrojejunocolic fistula
 Closure of gastrojejunocolic fistula
P1-55A38 Repair of gastrocolic fistula
 Closure of gastrocolic fistula
P1-55A40 Closure of stomach ulcer
 Closure of gastric ulcer
P1-55A60 Suture of stomach, NOS
 Gastrorrhaphy, NOS
P1-55A62 Repair of stomach laceration by suture
 Gastrorrhaphy for suture of wound
P1-55A64 Gastrotomy with suture repair of esophagogastric laceration
P1-55A65 Gastrotomy with suture repair of bleeding ulcer
P1-55A66 Suture of gastric ulcer
 Gastrorrhaphy for perforated gastric ulcer
 Oversewing of ulcer crater of stomach
 Oversewing of peptic ulcer crater
P1-55A67 Ligation of gastric ulcer
P1-55A70 Ligation of gastric varices
 Ligation of varicose veins of stomach
P1-55A71 Stapling of gastric varices

1-55C Stomach: Destructive Procedures

P1-55C10 Destruction of lesion of stomach, NOS
P1-55C12 Fulguration of stomach lesion
P1-55C14 Chemosurgery of stomach lesion
P1-55C20 Gastric freezing
  Gastric cooling
  Cryotherapy of stomach

1-55D Stomach: Transplantations and Transpositions

P1-55D10 Transplantation of tissue of stomach
P1-55D20V Rumen transfer
P1-55D40 Transposition of tissue of stomach

1-55E Stomach: Manipulations

P1-55E10 Manipulation of stomach, NOS
P1-55E20V Manipulation of rumen of stomach

1-56 OPERATIVE PROCEDURES ON THE SMALL INTESTINE

1-560 Small Intestine: General and Miscellaneous Operative Procedures

P1-56010 Operation on intestine, NOS
P1-56050 Operation on duodenum, NOS
P1-56052 Operation on jejunum, NOS
P1-56054 Operation on ileum, NOS
P1-56055 Procedure on Meckel's diverticulum, NOS

1-561 Small Intestine: Incisions

P1-56100 Incision of intestine, NOS
  Enterotomy, NOS
P1-56102 Incision and exploration of intestine, NOS
P1-56104 Myotomy of intestine, NOS
P1-56112 Enterolithotomy
P1-56114 Enterocentesis of intestine, NOS
P1-56120 Incision of duodenum
  Duodenotomy
P1-56122 Incision and exploration of duodenum
P1-56123 Incision and drainage of duodenum
P1-56126 Enterocentesis of duodenum
P1-56128 Ileoduodenotomy
P1-56130 Incision of small intestine
  Enterotomy of small intestine
P1-56132 Incision and exploration of small intestine
  Enterotomy of small bowel for exploration
P1-56134 Enterotomy of small bowel for decompression
  Decompression of intestine by incision
P1-56136 Enterocentesis of small intestine
P1-56140 Jejunotomy
P1-56142 Incision and exploration of jejunum
P1-56144 Ileotomy
P1-56146 Incision and exploration of ileum
P1-56148 Ileocolotomy
P1-56191 Reduction of intussusception by laparotomy
P1-56192 Reduction of volvulus by laparotomy, NOS
P1-56194 Correction of midgut volvulus, NOS
  Ladd procedure for correction of volvulus

1-563 Small Intestine: Excisions

P1-56300 Biopsy of intestine, NOS
P1-56302 Partial resection of intestine with anastomosis, NOS
  Enterectomy with anastomosis
P1-56303 Enterectomy with double-barrel enterostomy
P1-56304 Removal of foreign body from intestine by incision
P1-56305 Removal of gallstones from intestine
P1-56306 Removal of intraluminal foreign body from artifical stoma
P1-56308 Core needle biopsy of small intestine
P1-56309 Fine needle biopsy of small intestine
  Fine needle aspiration biopsy of small intestine
P1-5630A Resection of intestine for interposition, NOS
  Excision of intestine for interposition, NOS
P1-56310 Open biopsy of small intestine
  Enterotomy of small bowel for biopsy
P1-56312 Excision of lesion of small intestine
P1-56313 Excision of one or more lesions of small bowel by single enterotomy
P1-56314 Excision of one or more lesions of small bowel by multiple enterotomies
P1-56318 Excision of diverticulum of small intestine
  Diverticulectomy of small intestine
P1-56320 Partial excision of small intestine
  Segmental resection of small intestine
P1-56322 Multiple segmental resections of small intestine
P1-56324 Total excision of small intestine
  Total resection of small intestine
P1-56326 Excision of small intestine for interposition
  Resection of small intestine for interposition
P1-56327 Resection of exteriorized segment of small intestine
P1-56328 Enterotomy of small bowel for foreign body removal
  Removal of intraluminal foreign body from small intestine
P1-56329 Removal of gallstones from small intestine
P1-56340 Open biopsy of duodenum
  Duodenotomy for biopsy
P1-56342 Excision of lesion of duodenum
P1-56344 Diverticulectomy of duodenum
  Excision of diverticulum of duodenum
P1-56346 Excision of ulcer of duodenum
P1-56347 Duodenectomy
P1-56348 Excision of redundant mucosa from duodenostomy
P1-56349 Duodenotomy for foreign body removal
  Removal of foreign body from duodenum by incision
P1-5634A Removal of gallstones from duodenum
P1-56350 Open biopsy of jejunum
P1-56357 Jejunectomy
P1-56358 Excision of redundant mucosa from jejunostomy

1-563 Small Intestine: Excisions — Continued

P1-56360 Open biopsy of ileum
P1-56362 Excision of Meckel's diverticulum
  Meckel's diverticulectomy
P1-56366 Partial ileectomy
P1-56367 Total ileectomy
P1-56368 Excision of redundant mucosa from ileostomy
P1-56369 Isolation of ileal loop

1-565 Small Intestine: Injections and Implantations

P1-56510 Intubation of small intestine
P1-56511 Intubation of intestine for decompression
  Decompression of intestine by tube
P1-56512 Insertion of Miller-Abbott tube for intestinal decompression
P1-56520 Irrigation of enterostomy
P1-56522 Perfusion of small intestine
P1-56526 Perfusion of large intestine
P1-56530 Removal of tube from small intestine
P1-56531 Replacement of small intestine tube
P1-56532 Replacement of tube or enterostomy device of small intestine
P1-56540 Tube drainage of duodenum
P1-56542V Cannulation of duodenum

1-567 Small Intestine: Endoscopy

P1-56700 Endoscopy of intestine, NOS
P1-56710 Upper gastrointestinal endoscopy, simple primary examination
P1-56711 Esophagogastroduodenoscopy
P1-56712 Operative esophagogastroduodenoscopy
P1-56713 Esophagogastroduodenoscopy through stoma
  Duodenoscopy through artifical stoma
  Gastroduodenoscopy through artificial stoma
P1-56714 Gastroduodenoscopy
P1-56715 Duodenoscopy, NOS
P1-56716 Operative duodenoscopy
P1-56717 Endoscopic excision of lesion of duodenum
P1-56718 Endoscopic control of duodenal bleeding
P1-56719 Endoscopic destruction of lesion of duodenum
P1-56721 Upper gastrointestinal endoscopy for removal of foreign body
P1-56722 Upper gastrointestinal endoscopy for removal of polypoid lesion
P1-56724 Upper gastrointestinal endoscopy for control of hemorrhage by electrocoagulation
P1-56725 Upper gastrointestinal endoscopy for control of hemorrhage by laser photocoagulation
P1-56726 Upper gastrointestinal endoscopy for ablation of mucosal lesion or tumor by electrocoagulation
P1-56727 Upper gastrointestinal endoscopy for ablation of mucosal lesion or tumor by hot biopsy and fulguration
P1-56728 Upper gastrointestinal endoscopy for ablation of mucosal lesion or tumor by laser photocoagulation
P1-56730 Upper gastrointestinal endoscopy including esophagus, stomach and small bowel for collection of specimen by brushing or washing
P1-56731 Endoscopic brush biopsy of small intestine
P1-56732 Endoscopic brush biopsy of duodenum
P1-56733 Endoscopic brush biopsy of ileum
P1-56734 Endoscopic brush biopsy of jejunum
P1-56735 Upper gastrointestinal endoscopy including esophagus, stomach and small bowel for biopsy
  Esophagogastroduodenoscopy with biopsy
P1-56736 Endoscopic biopsy of small intestine
P1-56737 Endoscopic biopsy of duodenum
P1-56738 Endoscopic biopsy of jejunum
P1-56739 Endoscopic biopsy of ileum
P1-5673A Upper gastrointestinal endoscopy including esophagus, stomach and small bowel for biopsy and collection of specimen by brushing or washing
P1-5673B Upper gastrointestinal endoscopy including esophagus, stomach, duodenum and jejunum, complex diagnostic
P1-5673C Upper gastrointestinal endoscopy including esophagus, stomach and small bowel with transendoscopic tube or catheter placement
P1-56740 Endoscopy of small intestine, NOS
  Small intestinal endoscopy, diagnostic
P1-56741 Endoscopy of small intestine through artificial stoma
P1-56742 Operative endoscopy of small intestine
P1-56744 Small intestinal endoscopy with biopsy
P1-56745 Small intestinal endoscopy for removal of foreign body
P1-56746 Small intestinal endoscopy for removal of polypoid lesion
P1-56748 Small intestinal endoscopy for control of hemorrhage by electrocoagulation
P1-56749 Small intestinal endoscopy for control of hemorrhage by laser photocoagulation
P1-5674A Small intestinal endoscopy for ablation of mucosal lesion or tumor by hot biopsy and fulguration
P1-5674B Small intestinal endoscopy for ablation of mucosal lesion or tumor by laser
P1-56750 Endoscopy of jejunum
P1-56751 Operative endoscopy of jejunum
P1-56752 Endoscopy of jejunum through artificial stoma
  Percutaneous endoscopy through jejunostomy
P1-56754 Fiberoptic evaluation of small intestinal or pelvic pouch, NOS
P1-56755 Fiberoptic evaluation of small intestinal or pelvic pouch with biopsy
P1-56756 Fiberoptic evaluation of small intestinal pouch with collection of specimen by brushing or washing
P1-56757 Small intestinal endoscopy for placement of percutaneous jejunostomy tube

P1-56758 Small intestinal endoscopy for conversion of percutaneous gastrostomy tube to percutaneous jejunostomy tube
P1-56760 Endoscopy of ileum
  Ileoscopy
P1-56761 Operative endoscopy of ileum
  Operative ileoscopy
P1-56762 Endoscopy of ileum through artificial stoma
  Ileoscopy through artificial stoma
P1-56763 Fiberoptic ileoscopy through stoma
P1-56764 Fiberoptic ileoscopy through stoma with biopsy

1-568-569 Small Intestine: Surgical Repairs, Closures and Reconstructions

P1-56800 Repair of intestine, NOS
  Enteroplasty, NOS
P1-56805V Fistulization for ileus
P1-56806 Fixation of intestine
  Enteropexy
  Fixation of intestine to abdominal wall
P1-56807 Intestinal plication
P1-56810 Exteriorization of intestine, NOS
  Rankin operation, exteriorization of intestine
  Mikulicz operation, exteriorization of intestine, first stage
P1-56820 Anastomosis of intestine, NOS
  Anastomosis of bowel, NOS
  Enteroenterostomy
P1-56823 Enlargement of intestinal stoma
P1-56824 Take-down of anastomosis of intestine
P1-56829 Intestinal bypass for morbid obesity
  Enteroenterostomy, anastomosis of intestine for morbid obesity
P1-56830 Enterostomy, NOS
  Exteriorization of small intestine
P1-56831 Feeding enterostomy
  Feeding jejunostomy
  Feeding enterostomy of jejunum
P1-56832 Repair of enterostomy
  Repair of stoma of intestine
  Revision of enterostomy
P1-56833 Enterostomy, delayed opening
P1-56834 Ileostomy, delayed opening
P1-56836 Closure of enterostomy
  Take-down of intestinal stoma
  Closure of stoma of intestine
  Take-down of enterostomy
  Closure of artificial opening of intestine
P1-56840 Repair of intestinal fistula, NOS
  Closure of intestinal fistula, NOS
P1-56841 Repair of small intestine fistula, NOS
  Closure of small intestine fistula, NOS
P1-56842 Closure of intestinal cutaneous fistula
  Closure of enterocutaneous fistula
P1-56843 Closure of enterocolic fistula
P1-56844 Closure of enteroenteric fistula
P1-56845 Closure of enterovesical fistula
P1-56846 Closure of enterovesical fistula with bowel resection
P1-56847 Closure of enterovesical fistula with bladder resection
P1-56848 Closure of enterovesical fistula with bowel and bladder resection
P1-56849 Closure of fecal fistula, NOS
P1-5684A Repair of ileorectal fistula
P1-56850 Suture of intestine
  Enterorrhaphy
P1-56852 Closure of perforated ulcer of intestine
  Suture of intestinal ulcer
P1-56900 Surgical repair of small bowel, NOS
P1-56902 Plication of small intestine, NOS
P1-56904 Plication of jejunum
  Noble operation, plication of small intestine
P1-56906 Inversion of diverticulum of small intestine
P1-56910 Fixation of small intestine
  Fixation of small intestine to abdominal wall
P1-56912 Fixation of duodenum
  Fixation of duodenum to abdominal wall
P1-56914 Fixation of jejunum
  Fixation of jejunum to abdominal wall
  Jejunopexy
P1-56916 Fixation of ileum
  Ileopexy
  Fixation of ileum to abdominal wall
P1-56920 Anastomosis of small intestine to small intestine
  Enteroanastomosis small-to-small intestine
  Enteroenterostomy small-to-small intestine
  Bypass shunt small-to-small intestine
P1-56921 Duodenojejunostomy
P1-56922 Duodenoileostomy
P1-56923 Anastomosis of small-to-large intestine
  Enteroanastomosis small-to-large intestine
  Bypass shunt small-to-large intestine
  Enteroenterostomy small-to-large intestine
P1-56924 Anastomosis of small intestine to rectal stump
  Hampton operation, anastomosis of small intestine to rectal stump
  Anastomosis of rectum to small intestine
P1-56925 Duodenoduodenostomy
P1-56926 Revision of anastomosis of small intestine
P1-56927 Jejunojejunostomy
P1-56928 Jejunoileostomy
P1-56929 Ileoileostomy
P1-5692B Ileocolostomy
  Terminal ileum bypass
P1-5692C Ileotransversostomy
P1-5692D Ileosigmoidostomy
P1-5692E Ileorectostomy
  Ileorectal anastomosis
  Ileoproctostomy

1-568-569 Small Intestine: Surgical Repairs, Closures and Reconstructions — Continued

P1-5692F Ileoanal anastomosis
Anastomosis of small intestine-to-anus
P1-56930 Duodenostomy
Enterostomy of duodenum
P1-56931 Closure of duodenostomy
Take-down of duodenostomy
P1-56932 Jejunostomy
Surmay operation, jejunostomy
P1-56934 Ileostomy, NOS
Enterostomy of ileum, Brooke-Dragstedt type
Loop ileostomy
P1-56936 Closure of stoma of small intestine
P1-56945 Closure of duodenal fistula
P1-56946 Closure of jejunal fistula
P1-56947 Closure of ileal fistula
P1-56948 Closure of ileosigmoidal fistula
P1-56949 Closure of ileorectal fistula
P1-56950 Suture of small intestine, NOS
Suture of small intestine, single site
Enterorrhaphy of small intestine
P1-56951 Suture of duodenum
Suture of laceration of duodenum
Duodenorrhaphy
P1-56952 Suture of ulcer of duodenum
Closure of ulcer of duodenum
Oversewing of ulcer crater of duodenum
P1-56954 Suture of small intestine with colostomy
P1-56956 Suture of jejunum
Jejunorrhaphy
P1-56958 Suture of ileum
Ileorrhaphy
P1-56960 Ileojejunal bypass
Jejunoileostomy bypass shunt for obesity
P1-56961 Take-down of jejunoileal bypass
P1-56962 Revision of jejunoileal bypass
P1-56963 Suture of small intestine, multiple sites
P1-56969 Revision of stoma of small intestine
Enlargement of stoma of small intestine
P1-5696A Closure of artificial opening of small intestine
Closure of enterostomy of small intestine
P1-5696B Closure of enterostomy of small intestine with resection and anastomosis
P1-56970 Revision of ileostomy
Repair of ileostomy
Revision of ileostomy, simple
P1-56971 Revision of ileostomy, complicated
P1-56972 Closure of ileostomy
Take-down of ileostomy
P1-56973 Temporary ileostomy
Paul operation, temporary ileostomy
Temporary tangential ileostomy
Hendon operation, temporary ileostomy
P1-56974 Temporary tube ileostomy
P1-56975 Repair of jejunostomy
Revision of jejunostomy
P1-56976 Jejunostomy, delayed opening
P1-56977 Closure of jejunostomy
Take-down of jejunostomy
P1-56980 Permanent ileostomy
Continent ileostomy
Permanent continent ileostomy
P1-56985 Creation of endorectal ileal J-pouch with anastomosis to anus
P1-56986 Creation of endorectal ileal H-pouch with anastomosis to anus
P1-56987 Creation of endorectal ileal S-pouch with anastomosis to anus

1-56C Small Intestine: Destructive Procedures

P1-56C10 Destructive procedure of small intestine, NOS
P1-56C12 Enterolysis for acute bowel obstruction
P1-56C20 Destruction of lesion of small intestine, NOS
P1-56C21 Fulguration of lesion of small intestine, NOS
P1-56C26 Destruction of lesion of duodenum, NOS
P1-56C27 Fulguration of lesion of duodenum
P1-56C30 Correction of malrotation by lysis of duodenal bands
P1-56C32 Correction of malrotation by lysis of duodenal bands with reduction of midgut volvulus
P1-56C40V Crushing of contents of intestine

1-56D Small Intestine: Transplantations and Transpositions

P1-56D10 Transplantation of small intestine, NOS
P1-56D12 Ileostomy transplantation to new site
Transplant of ileal stoma to new site
P1-56D40 Transposition of small intestine, NOS
Transposition of intestine

1-56E Small Intestine: Manipulations

P1-56E10 Intra-abdominal manipulation of intestine, NOS
P1-56E12 Intra-abdominal manipulation of small intestine
P1-56E20 Manual reduction of torsion of intestine, NOS
Detorsion of volvulus
Reduction of volvulus of intestine
P1-56E22 Reduction of torsion of small intestine
Reduction of volvulus of small intestine
P1-56E30 Reduction of intussusception of intestine, NOS
P1-56E34 Reduction of intussusception of small intestine
P1-56E40 Enteroentectropy, NOS
P1-56E42 Ileoentectropy
P1-56E50 Manual reduction of prolapsed enterostomy, NOS
P1-56E51 Manual reduction of prolapsed ileostomy
P1-56E60 Dilation of intestinal stoma, NOS
Dilation and manipulation of enterostomy stoma, NOS

P1-56E62 Dilation of ileostomy stoma
P1-56E64 Dilation of colostomy stoma
P1-56E68 Dilation of colon, NOS

1-57 OPERATIVE PROCEDURES ON THE LARGE INTESTINE

1-570 Large Intestine: General and Miscellaneous Operative Procedures

P1-57000 Operative procedure on large intestine, NOS
P1-57060 Operation on colon, NOS
P1-57061 Operation on cecum, NOS
P1-57062 Operation on appendix, NOS
P1-57064 Operation on sigmoid, NOS

1-571 Large Intestine: Incisions

P1-57100 Incision of large intestine, NOS
  Enterotomy of large intestine, NOS
P1-57101 Incision and exploration of large intestine
P1-57102 Enterocentesis of large intestine
P1-57130 Colotomy, NOS
P1-57134 Incision and exploration of colon
P1-57135 Colocentesis
P1-57136 Myotomy of colon, NOS
P1-57170 Cecotomy
P1-57179 Sigmoidotomy
P1-57180 Incision of appendix
  Appendicotomy
P1-57185 Incision and drainage of abscess of appendix, NOS
P1-57186 Incision and drainage of appendiceal abscess by transabdominal approach

1-573-574 Large Intestine: Excisions

P1-57300 Total resection of large intestine, NOS
  Total excision of large intestine, NOS
P1-57302 Partial excision of large intestine
  Partial resection of large intestine
P1-57304 Mikulicz operation, resection of large intestine, second stage
  Resection of exteriorized segment of large intestine
P1-57306 Multiple segmental resections of large intestine
P1-57308 Excision of large intestine for interposition
  Resection of large intestine for interposition
P1-57310 Open biopsy of large intestine, NOS
P1-57312 Core needle biopsy of large intestine
P1-57313 Fine needle biopsy of large intestine
  Fine needle aspiration biopsy of large intestine
P1-57320 Excision of lesion of large intestine
P1-57321 Excision of one or more lesions of large bowel by single enterotomy
P1-57322 Excision of one or more lesions of large bowel by multiple enterotomies
P1-57323 Excision of diverticulum from large intestine
  Diverticulectomy of large intestine
P1-57324 Removal of foreign body from large intestine by incision
P1-57325 Removal of gallstones from large intestine
P1-57330 Colectomy, NOS
P1-57331 Partial resection of colon
  Segmental colectomy
P1-57332 Partial colectomy with anastomosis
P1-57333 Partial colectomy by abdominal approach
P1-57334 Partial colectomy by transanal approach
P1-57336 Partial colectomy with skin level colostomy
P1-57338 Partial colectomy with end colostomy and closure of distal segment
P1-57340 Partial colectomy with ileostomy and creation of mucofistula
P1-57342 Partial colectomy with colostomy and creation of mucofistula
P1-57344 Partial colectomy with coloproctostomy
P1-57346 Partial colectomy with coloproctostomy and colostomy
P1-57348 Excision of redundant mucosa from colostomy
P1-57349 Resection of colon for interposition
P1-57350 Right colectomy
  Enterocolectomy, NOS
  Resection of ascending colon, cecum and terminal ileum
  Right hemicolectomy
P1-57351 Cecectomy
  Resection of cecum and terminal ileum
P1-57353 Transverse colectomy
  Resection of transverse colon
P1-57354 Resection of splenic flexure of colon
P1-57355 Left colectomy
  Resection of descending colon
  Left hemicolectomy
  Resection of left hemicolon
P1-57356 Sigmoid colectomy
  Sigmoidectomy
P1-57360 Biopsy of colon, NOS
P1-57361 Open biopsy of colon
  Colotomy for biopsy
P1-57362 Excision of lesion of colon, NOS
P1-57365 Colotomy for foreign body removal
P1-57400 Total colectomy, NOS
  Complete resection of colon
P1-57403 Total abdominal colectomy with ileostomy
P1-57404 Total abdominal colectomy with ileoproctostomy
P1-57405 Total abdominal colectomy without proctectomy with continent ileostomy
P1-57407 Total abdominal colectomy with proctectomy and continent ileostomy
P1-57408 Total abdominal colectomy with rectal mucosectomy and ileoanal anastomosis
P1-57409 Total abdominal colectomy with rectal mucosectomy and ileoanal anastomosis with loop ileostomy

1-573-574 Large Intestine: Excisions — Continued

P1-57411 Total abdominal colectomy with rectal mucosectomy and ileoanal anastomosis with creation of ileal reservoir
P1-57412 Total abdominal colectomy with rectal mucosectomy and ileoanal anastomosis with creation of ileal reservoir with loop ileostomy
P1-57414 Total abdominal colectomy with proctectomy and ileostomy
P1-57416 Ileocolectomy, NOS
P1-57450 Appendectomy, NOS
 Excision of appendix, NOS
 Primary appendectomy
 Appendicectomy, NOS
P1-57451 Incidental appendectomy
 Secondary appendectomy
P1-57452 Appendectomy with drainage
 Appendicectomy with drainage
P1-57454 Appendectomy for ruptured appendix with abscess or generalized peritonitis
P1-57455 Excision of appendiceal stump
P1-57457 Biopsy of appendix

1-575 Large Intestine: Injections and Implantations

P1-57510 Removal of tube from large intestine
P1-57514 Replacement of tube or enterostomy device of large intestine

1-577 Large Intestine: Endoscopy

P1-57700 Endoscopy of large intestine, NOS
P1-57701 Endoscopic biopsy of large intestine
P1-57702 Endoscopic brush biopsy of large intestine
P1-57703 Endoscopic excision of lesion of large intestine
P1-57704 Endoscopic polypectomy of large intestine
P1-57705 Endoscopic destruction of lesion of large intestine
P1-57706 Removal of intraluminal foreign body from large intestine without incision
P1-57707 Endoscopy of large intestine through artificial stoma
P1-57710 Colonoscopy, NOS
 Endoscopy of colon, NOS
P1-57712 Intraoperative colonoscopy
 Operative endoscopy of colon
P1-57714 Colonoscopy with rigid sigmoidoscope through colotomy
P1-57720 Fiberoptic colonoscopy, NOS
P1-57721 Fiberoptic colonoscopy with biopsy
P1-57722 Fiberoptic colonoscopy for removal of polypoid lesion
P1-57723 Fiberoptic colonoscopy for ablation of mucosal lesion or tumor by electrocoagulation
P1-57724 Fiberoptic colonoscopy for ablation of mucosal lesion or tumor by laser photocoagulation
P1-57725 Fiberoptic colonoscopy for ablation of mucosal lesion by hot biopsy and fulguration
P1-57726 Fiberoptic colonoscopy for removal of foreign body
P1-57727 Fiberoptic colonoscopy for control of hemorrhage by electrocoagulation
P1-57728 Fiberoptic colonoscopy for control of hemorrhage by laser photocoagulation
P1-57730 Fiberoptic colonoscopy through colostomy
 Endoscopy of colon through artificial stoma
 Colonoscopy through artificial stoma
P1-57731 Fiberoptic colonoscopy through colostomy for removal of foreign body
P1-57732 Fiberoptic colonoscopy through colostomy for control of hemorrhage by electrocoagulation
P1-57733 Fiberoptic colonoscopy through colostomy for control of hemorrhage by laser photocoagulation
P1-57734 Fiberoptic colonoscopy through colostomy for biopsy
P1-57735 Fiberoptic colonoscopy through colostomy for removal of polypoid lesion
P1-57736 Fiberoptic colonoscopy through colostomy for ablation of mucosal lesion or tumor by laser
P1-57737 Fiberoptic colonoscopy through colostomy for ablation of mucosal lesion or tumor by hot biopsy and fulguration
P1-577A0 Sigmoidoscopy, NOS
P1-577A1 Flexible fiberoptic sigmoidoscopy
 Flexible sigmoidoscopy
P1-577A2 Intraoperative sigmoidoscopy
P1-577A3 Sigmoidoscopy through artificial stoma
P1-577A4 Sigmoidoscopy with biopsy
 Endoscopic biopsy of sigmoid colon
 Flexible fiberoptic sigmoidoscopy with biopsy
P1-577A5 Flexible fiberoptic sigmoidoscopy for removal of polypoid lesions
P1-577A6 Flexible fiberoptic sigmoidoscopy for control of hemorrhage by electrocoagulation
P1-577A7 Flexible fiberoptic sigmoidoscopy for control of hemorrhage by laser photocoagulation
P1-577A8 Flexible fiberoptic sigmoidoscopy for ablation of tumor by photocoagulation
P1-577A9 Flexible fiberoptic sigmoidoscopy for ablation of mucosal lesion or tumor by hot biopsy and fulguration
P1-577AA Flexible fiberoptic sigmoidoscopy for ablation of mucosal lesion or tumor by electrocoagulation
P1-577AB Flexible fiberoptic sigmoidoscopy for removal of foreign body
P1-577AC Flexible fiberoptic sigmoidoscopy for decompression of volvulus
P1-577B0 Rigid proctosigmoidoscopy
P1-577B1 Proctosigmoidoscopy by transabdominal approach
P1-577B2 Proctosigmoidoscopy through artificial stoma
P1-577B3 Proctosigmoidoscopy with biopsy
P1-577B4 Proctosigmoidoscopy for removal of single polyp or papilloma

P1-577B5 Proctosigmoidoscopy for removal of multiple polyps or papillomata
P1-577B6 Proctosigmoidoscopy for collection of specimen by brushing or washing
P1-577B7 Proctosigmoidoscopy for dilation
P1-577B8 Proctosigmoidoscopy for removal of foreign body
P1-577B9 Proctosigmoidoscopy for decompression of volvulus
P1-577BA Proctosigmoidoscopy for ablation of tumor by electrocoagulation
P1-577BB Proctosigmoidoscopy for ablation of tumor by hot biopsy and fulguration
P1-577BC Proctosigmoidoscopy for ablation of tumor by photocoagulation
P1-577BE Proctosigmoidoscopy for control of hemorrhage by electrocoagulation
P1-577BF Proctosigmoidoscopy for control of hemorrhage by laser photocoagulation

1-578-579 Large Intestine: Surgical Repairs, Closures and Reconstructions

P1-57800 Repair of large intestine, NOS
  Repair of large bowel, NOS
P1-57801 Fixation of large intestine to abdominal wall
P1-57802 Repair of colon
P1-57803 Colopexy
  Colofixation
P1-57804 Cecopexy
  Cecofixation
P1-57805 Cecocoloplicopexy
P1-57806 Sigmoidopexy
  Moschowitz sigmoidopexy
P1-57807 Cecoplication
P1-57808 Coloplication
P1-57809 Inversion of diverticulum of large intestine
P1-57810 Exteriorization of large intestine
P1-57816 Fistulization of appendix
  Appendicostomy
  Weir operation, appendicostomy
P1-57817 Appendicocecostomy
P1-57820 Enteroanastomosis large-to-large intestine
  Anastomosis of intestine, large-to-large
  Bypass shunt, large-to-large intestine
P1-57821 Anastomosis of intestine, large-to-rectum
P1-57822 Anastomosis of intestine, large-to-anus
P1-57823 Colocolostomy
P1-57824 Coloproctostomy
P1-57826 Revision of anastomosis of large intestine
P1-57827 Closure of enterostomy of large intestine with resection and anastomosis
P1-57828 Surgical reanastomosis of colon, NOS
P1-57830 Colostomy, NOS
P1-57831 Cecostomy, NOS
P1-57832 Transverse colostomy
P1-57833 Sigmoidostomy
  Colostomy of sigmoid
P1-57834 Colostomy with multiple biopsies
P1-57835 Tube cecostomy
P1-57836 Loop colostomy
P1-57837 Tube cecostomy with other procedure
P1-57838 Skin level cecostomy
P1-57839 Skin level cecostomy with multiple biopsies
P1-5783A Formation of mucous fistula
P1-5783B Temporary colostomy
P1-5783C Repair of stoma of large intestine
  Revision of stoma of large intestine
P1-5783D Permanent colostomy
P1-5783E Permanent magnetic colostomy
P1-5783F Perineal colostomy
P1-57900 Closure of large intestine fistula, NOS
  Repair of fistula of large intestine
P1-57901 Suture of large intestine, NOS
  Suture of large intestine, single site
  Enterorrhaphy of large intestine
P1-57902 Suture of large intestine, multiple sites
P1-57904 Suture of large intestine with colostomy
P1-57906 Take-down of stoma of large intestine
  Closure of stoma of large intestine
P1-57910 Closure of colon fistula, NOS
P1-57912 Closure of cecosigmoidal fistula
P1-57914 Closure of appendiceal fistula
  Repair of appendiceal fistula
  Closure of appendicostomy
P1-57915 Closure of intestinocolonic fistula
P1-57916 Repair of perineosigmoidal fistula
  Closure of perineosigmoidal fistula
P1-57920 Suture of colon
  Colorrhaphy
P1-57922 Suture of cecum
  Cecorrhaphy
P1-57924 Suture of sigmoid
  Sigmoidorrhaphy
P1-57930 Revision of colostomy, NOS
  Repair of colostomy
  Revision of colostomy, simple
P1-57932 Revision of colostomy, complicated
P1-57933 Delayed opening colostomy
P1-57934 Revision of colostomy with repair of paracolostomy hernia
  Repair of hernia of colostomy
  Repair of hernia of pericolostomy
P1-57936 Closure of colostomy
  Take-down of colostomy
P1-57937 Closure of cecostomy
  Take-down of cecostomy
P1-57938 Closure of sigmoidostomy
  Take-down of sigmoidostomy

1-57C Large Intestine: Destructive Procedures

P1-57C00 Destructive procedure of large intestine, NOS
  Destructive procedure of large bowel, NOS
P1-57C10 Destruction of lesion of large intestine
P1-57C12 Fulguration of lesion of large intestine

1-57D Large Intestine: Transplantations and Transpositions

P1-57D00 Transplantation of large intestine, NOS
P1-57D40 Transposition of large intestine, NOS

1-57E Large Intestine: Manipulations

P1-57E10 Intra-abdominal manipulation of large intestine
P1-57E12 Reduction of volvulus of large intestine
  Reduction of torsion of large intestine
P1-57E14 Reduction of intussusception of large intestine
P1-57E20 Inversion of appendix
P1-57E30 Manual reduction of prolapsed colostomy

1-58 OPERATIVE PROCEDURES ON THE RECTUM AND ANUS

1-580 Rectum and Anus: General and Miscellaneous Operative Procedures

P1-58010 Operation on rectum, NOS
P1-58020 Operation on perirectal tissue, NOS
P1-58024 Operation on rectum and perirectal tissue, NOS
P1-58060 Operation on anus, NOS
P1-58070 Control of hemorrhage from anus, NOS

1-581 Rectum and Anus: Incisions

P1-58100 Incision of rectum, NOS
  Proctotomy
P1-58102 Linear proctotomy
  Panas operation, linear proctotomy
P1-58104 Incision of rectal stricture
  Division of stricture of rectum
P1-58105 Incision of perirectal tissue
P1-58106 Incision of ischiorectal tissue
P1-58107 Incision of rectovaginal septum
P1-58108 Incision of pelvirectal tissue
P1-58110 Incision and exploration of rectum
P1-58130 Incision and drainage of rectal abscess, NOS
P1-58131 Incision and drainage of submucosal abscess of rectum
P1-58132 Incision and drainage of perirectal abscess
P1-58134 Incision and drainage of ischiorectal abscess
P1-58135 Incision and drainage of ischiorectal abscess with submuscular fistulectomy
P1-58136 Incision and drainage of deep retrorectal abscess
P1-58137 Incision and drainage of deep supralevator abscess
P1-58139 Incision and drainage of deep pelvirectal abscess
  Transrectal drainage of pelvic abscess
P1-58160 Incision of anus, NOS
P1-58161 Decompression of imperforate anus
  Decompression of rectum
P1-58162 Incision of septum of anus
  Incision of anal septum of infant
P1-58164 Anal sphincterotomy, NOS
P1-58165 Left lateral anal sphincterotomy
P1-58166 Posterior anal sphincterotomy
P1-58170 Anal pectenotomy
P1-58172 Cryptotomy of anus
P1-58175V Incision and drainage of anal sac
P1-58180 Incision of anal fistula
  Anal fistulotomy
P1-58181 Incision and drainage of perianal abscess, NOS
  Incision and drainage of perianal abscess, superficial
P1-58182 Incision and drainage of submucosal anal abscess by transanal approach under anesthesia
P1-58183 Incision and drainage of intramural anal abscess by transanal approach under anesthesia
P1-58184 Incision and drainage of intramural anal abscess with submuscular fistulectomy
P1-58185 Incision of thrombosed hemorrhoid
  Evacuation of thrombosed hemorrhoids
P1-58190 Incision of perianal tissue
  Undercutting of perianal tissue
  Ball operation, undercutting of perianal tissue

1-583-584 Rectum and Anus: Excisions

P1-58300 Biopsy of rectum, NOS
P1-58301 Incisional biopsy of rectum
P1-58302 Excision of lesion of rectum
P1-58304 Biopsy of anorectal wall by anal approach
P1-58306 Core needle biopsy of rectum
P1-58307 Fine needle biopsy of rectum
  Fine needle aspiration biopsy of rectum
P1-58308 Anorectal myomectomy
  Rectal myectomy
P1-58309 Excision of rectal mucosa
  Excision of redundant mucosa of rectum
P1-58310 Excision of benign tumor of rectum by transanal approach
P1-58312 Excision of malignant tumor of rectum by transanal approach
P1-58314 Proctotomy for excision of rectal tumor by transcoccygeal or transsacral approach
P1-58316 Removal of foreign body of rectum by incision
P1-58320 Resection of rectum, NOS
  Proctectomy, NOS
P1-58322 Rectosigmoidectomy
  Resection of rectosigmoid
  Proctosigmoidectomy
  Sigmoidoproctectomy
P1-58324 Partial proctectomy
  Partial resection of rectum
P1-58325 Partial proctectomy with anastomosis by abdominal and transsacral approach, one stage

P1-58326 Partial proctectomy with anastomosis by abdominal and transsacral approach, two stages
P1-58327 Partial proctectomy with anastomosis by transsacral approach only
P1-58330 Abdominoperineal pull-through procedure, NOS
 Resection of rectum by abdominoperineal pull-through, NOS
P1-58331 Endorectal resection
 Endorectal pull-through procedure
 Soave operation, endorectal pull-through
 Soave submucosal resection of rectum
P1-58332 Altemeier operation, perineal rectal pull-through
P1-58333 Swenson operation, proctectomy
P1-58340 Abdominoperineal resection
 Abdominoperineal proctectomy
 Complete proctectomy
P1-58341 Lloyd-Davies operation, abdominoperineal resection
P1-58342 Sauer-Bacon operation, abdominoperineal resection
P1-58343 Rankin operation, complete proctectomy
P1-58344 Miles operation, complete proctectomy
P1-58345 Duhamel operation, abdominoperineal pull-through
P1-58346 Proctectomy by abdominoperineal resection with colostomy, one stage
P1-58347 Proctectomy by abdominoperineal resection with colostomy, two stages
P1-58348 Complete proctectomy with subtotal or total colectomy with multiple biopsies
P1-58349 Proctectomy by combined abdominoperineal pull-through procedure, two stage
P1-58350 Transsacral rectosigmoidectomy
P1-58352 Anterior resection of rectum
P1-58353 Anterior resection of rectum with colostomy
P1-58354 Posterior resection of rectum
P1-58355 Von Kraske operation, proctectomy
P1-58356 Hartmann operation, rectal resection
P1-58358 Resection of rectum with pelvic exenteration
P1-58360V Excision of anal sac
P1-58362V Excision of lesion of anal sac
P1-58364V Excision of lesion of perianal gland
P1-58366V Biopsy of cloaca
P1-58370 Excision of rectal procidentia with anastomosis by abdominal and perineal approach
P1-58372 Excision of rectal procidentia with anastomosis by perineal approach
P1-58374 Excision of lesion of perirectal tissue
 Excision of perirectal tissue
P1-58375 Excision of lesion of pelvirectal tissue
 Excision of pelvirectal tissue
P1-58376 Excision of lesion of rectovaginal septum
P1-58377 Removal of intraluminal foreign body from rectum
P1-58378 Removal of foreign body from rectum under anesthesia
P1-58379 Excision of rectal fistula
 Fistulectomy of rectum
 Perirectal fistulectomy
P1-58380 Hemorrhoidectomy, NOS
P1-58381 Hemorrhoidectomy by simple ligature
 Hemorrhoidectomy by ligation
 Ligation of hemorrhoids
P1-58382 Ligation of internal hemorrhoids, single procedure
P1-58383 Ligation of internal hemorrhoids, multiple procedures
P1-58384 Complete external hemorrhoidectomy
P1-58385 Excision of external thrombotic hemorrhoid
P1-58387 Internal hemorrhoidectomy
P1-58388 Internal and external hemorrhoidectomy, simple
P1-58389 Internal and external hemorrhoidectomy, complex
 Lord operation, hemorrhoidectomy
 Whitehead operation, hemorrhoidectomy
P1-5838A Internal and external hemorrhoidectomy, simple, with fissurectomy
P1-5838B Internal and external hemorrhoidectomy, complex, with fissurectomy
P1-5838C Internal and external hemorrhoidectomy, simple, with fistulectomy and fissurectomy
P1-5838D Internal and external hemorrhoidectomy, complex, with fistulectomy and fissurectomy
P1-5838E Hemorrhoidectomy with anoplasty
P1-5838F Excision of external hemorrhoidal tags and papillae
P1-58400 Biopsy of anus
P1-58401 Biopsy of perianal tissue
P1-58402 Excision of perianal tissue
P1-58410 Excision of lesion of anus, NOS
P1-58412 Excision of lesion of anus, extensive, NOS
P1-58414 Curettage of anus
P1-58415 Curettage of anal fissure including dilation of anal sphincter, initial
P1-58420 Anal cryptectomy, NOS
P1-58421 Anal cryptectomy, single
P1-58422 Anal cryptectomy, multiple
P1-58426 Excision of diverticulum of anus
P1-58430 Anal fistulectomy, NOS
 Excision of anal fistula, NOS
P1-58431 Anal fistulectomy, subcutaneous
P1-58432 Anal fistulectomy, submuscular
P1-58433 Anal fistulectomy, complex
P1-58434 Anal fistulectomy, multiple
P1-58435 Anal fistulectomy, second stage
P1-58436 Anal fissurectomy
 Excision of fissure of anus
P1-58437 Fissurectomy with sphincterotomy
P1-58440 Excision of anal papilla, NOS
 Anal papillectomy
 Papillectomy of single anal tag

1-583-584 Rectum and Anus: Excisions — Continued

P1-58441 Excision of multiple anal papillae
  Excision of perianal skin tags
P1-58450 Anal sphincterectomy, NOS
P1-58460 Complete excision of anus, NOS
P1-58461 Partial excision of anus, NOS
P1-58470 Removal of Thiersch wire or suture from anal canal
P1-58471 Removal of intraluminal foreign body from anus
P1-58472 Incision and removal of foreign body from anus

1-585 Rectum and Anus: Injections and Implantations

P1-58500 Injection of rectum and anus, NOS
P1-58504V Injection of anal sac
P1-58510 Rectal irrigation
  Proctoclysis
P1-58520 Insertion of tube into rectum
P1-58522 Replacement of rectal tube
P1-58530 Insertion of pack into rectum
  Rectal packing
P1-58532 Removal of packing from rectum
P1-58540 Implant of electronic stimulator to anus
  Insertion of subcutaneous electrical anal stimulator
P1-58550 Hemorrhoidectomy by injection
  Injection of sclerosing solution into hemorrhoids
P1-58554 Perirectal injection of sclerosing solution for prolapse
P1-58560 Removal of anal seton or unlisted marker

1-587 Rectum and Anus: Endoscopy

P1-58700 Proctoscopy
  Endoscopy of rectum
P1-58702 Operative endoscopy of rectum
  Proctoscopy by transabdominal approach
P1-58704 Proctoscopy through stoma
  Endoscopy of rectum through stoma
P1-58706 Proctoscopy with biopsy
  Endoscopic biopsy of rectum
P1-58707 Endoscopic brush biopsy of rectum
P1-58710 Anoscopy, NOS
  Endoscopy of anus
P1-58712 Anoscopy for dilation, direct
P1-58714 Anoscopy for collection of specimen by brushing or washing
P1-58716 Anoscopy with coagulation for control of hemorrhage of mucosal lesion
P1-58720 Anoscopy with biopsy
P1-58722 Endoscopic excision of lesion of anus
P1-58724 Anoscopy for removal of polyp
P1-58725 Anoscopy for removal of multiple polyps
P1-58727 Endoscopic destruction of lesion of anus
P1-58728 Anoscopy for removal of foreign body

1-588-589 Rectum and Anus: Surgical Repairs, Closures and Reconstructions

P1-58800 Repair of rectum, NOS
  Rectoplasty, NOS
  Proctoplasty, NOS
P1-58802 Proctoplasty for stenosis
P1-58803 Correction of atresia of rectum
P1-58806 Anastomosis of rectum, NOS
  Rectorectostomy
P1-58807 Saucerization of rectum
P1-58810 Repair of rectal prolapse, NOS
  Proctoplasty for prolapse of mucous membrane
P1-58811 Repair of rectal prolapse by abdominal approach
  Proctopexy for prolapse by abdominal approach
P1-58813 Proctopexy for prolapse by perineal approach
P1-58815 Proctopexy
  Rectopexy
P1-58816 Puborectalis sling operation
  Sling fixation of rectum
P1-58817 Delorme operation, proctopexy
P1-58818 Pemberton operation, rectal prolapse repair
P1-58819 Ripstein operation, repair of prolapsed rectum
P1-5881A Frickman operation, abdominal proctopexy
P1-58820 Proctosigmoidopexy
P1-58822 Proctopexy combined with sigmoid resection by abdominal approach
P1-58830 Proctostomy
  Rectostomy
P1-58832 Repair of stoma of rectum
  Revision of stoma of rectum
P1-58833 Take-down of stoma of rectum
  Closure of proctostomy
  Closure of stoma of rectum
  Closure of rectostomy
P1-58840 Suture of rectum
  Rectorrhaphy
  Proctorrhaphy
P1-58842 Repair of rectal laceration
  Suture of laceration of rectum
P1-58850 Repair of rectal fistula, NOS
  Closure of rectal fistula, NOS
P1-58851 Repair of perirectal fistula
  Closure of perirectal fistula
P1-58852 Repair of vulvorectal fistula
  Closure of vulvorectal fistula
  Closure of rectovulvar fistula
  Repair of rectolabial fistula
  Closure of rectolabial fistula
P1-58853 Repair of perineorectal fistula
  Closure of perineorectal fistula
P1-58855 Repair of anal fistula
  Closure of anal fistula

P1-58856 Repair of anorectal fistula
Closure of anorectal fistula
P1-58857 Repair of rectourethral fistula
Closure of rectourethral fistula
Closure of urethrorectal fistula
P1-58859 Repair of rectovesical fistula
Closure of rectovesical fistula
Closure of vesicorectal fistula
P1-58860 Repair of rectovesical fistula with colostomy
Closure of rectovesical fistula with colostomy
P1-58861 Repair of rectourethral fistula with colostomy
Closure of rectourethral fistula with colostomy
P1-58862 Repair of congenital anovaginal fistula, NOS
P1-58863 Repair of congenital anovaginal fistula with cut-back type procedure
P1-58900 Repair of anus
Anoplasty
P1-58901 Stone operation, anoplasty
P1-58902 Construction of anus for congenital absence by perineal approach
P1-58903 Construction of anus for congenital absence by sacrococcygeal approach
P1-58904 Construction of anus for congenital absence by combined abdominal and perineal approach
P1-58906 Construction of anus for congenital absence with repair of urinary fistula
P1-58920 Suture of anus
Suture of laceration of anus
P1-58921V Temporary suture of anus
P1-58922V Suture of cloaca
P1-58924 Suture of old anal obstetric laceration
P1-58926 Anal cerclage
P1-58930 Repair of anal sphincter
Anal sphincteroplasty
P1-58932 Suture of anal sphincter
Anal sphincterorrhaphy
P1-58934 Anoplasty for stricture, infant
P1-58935 Anoplasty for stricture, adult
P1-58936 Anal sphincteroplasty for prolapse, child
P1-58937 Anal sphincteroplasty for prolapse, adult
P1-58938 Anal sphincteroplasty for incontinence, child
P1-58939 Anal sphincteroplasty for incontinence, adult
P1-58940 Anal sphincteroplasty for incontinence, adult, with muscle transplant
Transplant of gracilis muscle for anal incontinence
P1-58941 Anal sphincteroplasty for incontinence, adult, with levator muscle imbrication
P1-58942 Anal sphincteroplasty for incontinence, adult, with implantation of artificial sphincter
P1-58943 Park operation, posterior anal repair
P1-58944 Formation of artificial anus

1-58C Rectum and Anus: Destructive Procedures

P1-58C00 Destruction of lesion of rectum, NOS
Destruction of lesion of rectum, simple
P1-58C02 Destruction of lesion of rectum by any method, extensive
P1-58C06 Proctolysis
P1-58C07 Lysis of perirectal adhesions
P1-58C09V Crushing of contents of rectum
P1-58C10 Destruction of lesion of rectum by cryosurgery, NOS
P1-58C12 Cryosurgery for benign rectal tumor
P1-58C14 Cryosurgery for malignant rectal tumor
P1-58C20 Destruction of lesion of rectum by chemicals
P1-58C30 Fulguration of anus, NOS
Destruction of lesion of rectum by fulguration
P1-58C40 Destruction of lesion of rectum by electrocoagulation
P1-58C50 Destruction of lesion of rectum by cauterization
Cauterization of rectum
P1-58C51 Cauterization of anus, NOS
P1-58C52V Cauterization of anal sac
P1-58C54 Cauterization of anal fissure including dilation of anal sphincter, initial
P1-58C60 Destruction of lesion of rectum by laser
P1-58C70 Destruction of lesion of rectum by electrodesiccation
P1-58C72 Electrodesiccation of malignant tumor of rectum by transanal approach
P1-58C90 Destruction of hemorrhoids, NOS
P1-58C91 Destruction of hemorrhoids, external
P1-58C92 Destruction of hemorrhoids, internal
P1-58C93 Destruction of hemorrhoids, internal and external
P1-58C94 Destruction of hemorrhoids by cryotherapy
Cryotherapy of hemorrhoids
P1-58C95 Cauterization of hemorrhoids
Clamp and cautery of hemorrhoids
Hemorrhoidectomy by cauterization
P1-58C96 Destruction of hemorrhoids by sclerotherapy
Sclerotherapy of hemorrhoids
P1-58C97 Crushing of hemorrhoids
Hemorrhoidectomy by crushing

1-58D Rectum and Anus: Transplantations and Transpositions

P1-58D10 Transplantation of tissue of rectum
P1-58D15 Graft for rectal prolapse
P1-58D20 Transplant of tissue of anus
Thiersch operation, anus
P1-58D22 Graft for rectal incontinence
P1-58D24 Graft for rectal incontinence and prolapse
P1-58D30 Transposition of tissue of rectum
P1-58D32V Conversion of rectal position
P1-58D40 Transposition of tissue of anus

1-58D Rectum and Anus: Transplantations and Transpositions — Continued

P1-58D50 Perineal transplant for anovaginal fistula

1-58E Rectum and Anus: Manipulations

P1-58E00 Manipulation of rectum
P1-58E04V Manipulation of cloaca
P1-58E10 Dilation of rectum
  Proctectasis
P1-58E11 Dilation of anus
P1-58E12 Dilation of rectal stricture under nonlocal anesthesia
P1-58E14 Dilation of anal sphincter under nonlocal anesthesia
P1-58E20 Rectal massage for levator spasm
P1-58E30 Manual reduction of hemorrhoids
P1-58E32 Manual reduction of prolapsed rectum
P1-58E34 Reduction of prolapsed rectum under anesthesia
P1-58E35 Operative reduction of prolapse of anus
P1-58E40V Expression of anal sac

1-5A-5E OPERATIVE PROCEDURES ON THE DIGESTIVE ORGANS

1-5A OPERATIVE PROCEDURES ON THE SALIVARY GLANDS

1-5A0 Salivary Glands: General and Miscellaneous Operative Procedures

P1-5A010 Operation on salivary gland, NOS
P1-5A012 Operation on parotid gland, NOS
P1-5A014 Operation on sublingual gland, NOS
P1-5A016 Operation on submaxillary gland, NOS
P1-5A040 Operation on salivary duct, NOS
P1-5A042 Operation on parotid duct, NOS
P1-5A044 Operation on sublingual duct, NOS
P1-5A046 Operation on submaxillary duct, NOS

1-5A1 Salivary Glands: Incisions

P1-5A100 Incision of salivary gland, NOS
  Sialoadenotomy
P1-5A104 Incision and exploration of salivary gland
P1-5A110 Incision and drainage of parotid abscess, simple
  Incision and drainage of parotid space
P1-5A112 Incision and drainage of parotid abscess, complicated
P1-5A114 Incision and drainage of sublingual abscess, intraoral
P1-5A116 Incision and drainage of submaxillary abscess, intraoral
P1-5A117 Incision and drainage of submaxillary abscess, extraoral
P1-5A150 Incision of salivary duct
  Incision and probing of salivary duct
P1-5A160 Sialolithotomy, NOS
  Ptyalolithotomy, NOS
  Duct sialolithotomy, NOS
  Sialoadenolithotomy, NOS
P1-5A163 Intraoral sialolithotomy of sublingual gland, uncomplicated
P1-5A166 Intraoral sialolithotomy of submandibular gland, uncomplicated
P1-5A168 Intraoral sialolithotomy of submandibular gland, complicated
P1-5A170 Extraoral sialolithotomy of parotid gland
P1-5A172 Intraoral sialolithotomy of parotid gland, uncomplicated
P1-5A174 Intraoral sialolithotomy of parotid gland, complicated
P1-5A180V Transection of venom duct

1-5A3 Salivary Glands: Excisions

P1-5A300 Biopsy of salivary gland, NOS
P1-5A302 Incisional biopsy of salivary gland
P1-5A304 Excisional biopsy of salivary gland
  Excision of lesion of salivary gland, NOS
P1-5A305 Excision of lesion of salivary gland, en bloc
P1-5A306 Core needle biopsy of salivary gland
P1-5A307 Fine needle biopsy of salivary duct
  Fine needle aspiration biopsy of salivary gland, NOS
P1-5A308 Enucleation of cyst of salivary gland
P1-5A309 Excision of lesion of salivary duct, NOS
P1-5A320 Excision of salivary gland, NOS
  Sialoadenectomy, NOS
  Amputation of salivary gland duct, NOS
P1-5A321 Partial excision of salivary gland
  Partial sialoadenectomy
P1-5A322 Complete sialoadenectomy
  Complete excision of salivary gland
P1-5A340 Excision of sublingual gland
P1-5A342 Excision of ranula of sublingual gland, NOS
  Excision of sublingual salivary gland cyst
P1-5A350 Excision of submandibular gland
  Submandibular sialoadenectomy
  Excision of submaxillary gland
P1-5A360 Parotidectomy, NOS
  Excision of parotid gland, NOS
P1-5A361 Complete parotidectomy, NOS
P1-5A362 Partial parotidectomy
P1-5A363 Excision of lesion of parotid gland, NOS
  Excision of lesion of parotid duct, NOS
P1-5A364 Excision of lateral lobe of parotid gland without nerve dissection
P1-5A365 Excision of parotid gland tumor of lateral lobe without nerve dissection
P1-5A366 Excision of parotid gland tumor of lateral lobe with dissection and preservation of facial nerve
P1-5A367 Excision of lateral lobe of parotid gland with dissection and preservation of facial nerve
P1-5A368 Total excision of parotid gland with dissection and preservation of facial nerve
  Total excision of parotid gland tumor with dissection and preservation of facial nerve

P1-5A369 Total excision of parotid gland with en bloc removal and sacrifice of facial nerve
    Total excision of parotid gland tumor with en bloc removal and sacrifice of facial nerve
P1-5A36A Total excision of parotid gland with unilateral radical neck dissection
    Total excision of parotid gland tumor with unilateral radical neck dissection
P1-5A36B Enucleation of parotid gland cyst

1-5A5 Salivary Glands: Injections and Implantations

P1-5A500 Injection of salivary gland, NOS
P1-5A502 Injection of salivary duct, NOS
P1-5A510 Dilation and catheterization of salivary duct with injection
P1-5A512 Injection procedure for sialography

1-5A7 Salivary Glands: Endoscopy

P1-5A700 Endoscopy of salivary gland, NOS

1-5A8 Salivary Glands: Surgical Repairs, Closures and Reconstructions

P1-5A800 Repair of salivary gland, NOS
P1-5A810 Sialodochoplasty, NOS
    Repair of salivary duct, NOS
P1-5A812 Primary sialodochoplasty
P1-5A813 Secondary sialodochoplasty
P1-5A814 Simple sialodochoplasty
P1-5A815 Complicated sialodochoplasty
P1-5A840 Fistulization of salivary gland, NOS
P1-5A841 Destruction of lesion of salivary gland by marsupialization
    Marsupialization of cyst of salivary gland
P1-5A842 Fistulization of ranula, NOS
    Marsupialization of ranula of salivary gland
P1-5A843 Fistulization of ranula with prosthesis
P1-5A860 Suture of salivary gland
P1-5A862 Suture of laceration of salivary gland
P1-5A870 Repair of salivary gland fistula
    Closure of salivary fistula
P1-5A880 Ligation of salivary duct, intraoral
P1-5A882V Ligation of parotid duct
P1-5A884V Ligation of venom duct

1-5AC Salivary Glands: Destructive Procedures

P1-5AC00 Destructive procedure of salivary gland, NOS
P1-5AC10 Destruction of lesion of salivary gland, NOS

1-5AD Salivary Glands: Transplantations and Transpositions

P1-5AD30 Transplantation of salivary gland duct
P1-5AD32V Parotid duct transposition
    Transplantation of parotid gland duct
P1-5AD40 Bilateral parotid duct diversion
    Wilke type procedure, parotid duct diversion
P1-5AD41 Bilateral parotid duct diversion with excision of one submandibular gland
P1-5AD42 Bilateral parotid duct diversion with excision of both submandibular glands
P1-5AD43 Bilateral parotid duct diversion with ligation of both submandibular ducts
P1-5AD50 Transplant of salivary duct opening, NOS

1-5AE Salivary Glands: Manipulations

P1-5AE00 Dilation of salivary duct, NOS
    Ptyalectasis
P1-5AE02 Dilation and catheterization of salivary duct without injection
P1-5AE10 Dilation of Stenson's duct
    Dilation of parotid duct
P1-5AE20 Dilation of Wharton's duct
    Dilation of submandibular duct
P1-5AE30 Manipulation of salivary duct
P1-5AE50 Probing of salivary duct, NOS
P1-5AE52 Probing of salivary duct for removal of calculus
    Removal of calculus of salivary gland by probe

1-5B OPERATIVE PROCEDURES ON THE LIVER

1-5B0 Liver: General and Miscellaneous Operative Procedures

P1-5B010 Operation on liver, NOS
P1-5B012 Diagnostic procedure on liver
P1-5B020 Extracorporeal circulation for hepatic assistance

1-5B1 Liver: Incisions

P1-5B100 Incision of liver
    Hepatotomy
P1-5B101 Stromeyer-Little operation hepatotomy
P1-5B102 Incision and exploration of liver
P1-5B106 Hepatotomy with packing
P1-5B110 Hepatotomy with drainage, NOS
P1-5B112 Hepatotomy for drainage of cyst or abscess, one stage
P1-5B114 Hepatotomy for drainage of cyst or abscess, two stages
P1-5B116 Drainage of liver by aspiration
    Percutaneous aspiration of liver
P1-5B117 Evacuation of cyst of liver
P1-5B120 Hepatolithotomy of liver

1-5B3 Liver: Excisions

P1-5B300 Biopsy of liver, NOS
P1-5B302 Open biopsy of liver
P1-5B303 Wedge biopsy of liver

1-5B3 Liver: Excisions — Continued

P1-5B311 Open core needle biopsy of liver
P1-5B315 Open fine needle biopsy of liver
 Open fine needle aspiration biopsy of liver
P1-5B316 Percutaneous core needle biopsy of liver
P1-5B317 Percutaneous fine needle biopsy of liver
 Percutaneous fine needle aspiration biopsy of liver
P1-5B320 Excision of lesion of liver, NOS
P1-5B322 Excision of hydatid cyst of liver
P1-5B324 Enucleation of cyst of liver
P1-5B350 Hepatectomy, NOS
P1-5B352 Total hepatectomy
 Total resection of liver
P1-5B354 Partial hepatectomy
 Partial excision of liver
 Subtotal hepatectomy
P1-5B355 Lobectomy of liver
 Total resection of lobe of liver
P1-5B356 Hepatectomy, total left lobectomy
P1-5B357 Hepatectomy, total right lobectomy
P1-5B358 Lobectomy of liver with partial excision of adjacent lobes
P1-5B359 Hepatectomy, trisegmentectomy
P1-5B370 Removal of foreign body from liver
P1-5B372 Hepaticotomy with removal of calculus
 Hepaticostomy with removal of calculus
P1-5B373 Removal of gallstones from liver

1-5B5 Liver: Injections and Implantations

P1-5B510 Injection into liver, NOS
P1-5B512 Injection of therapeutic substance into liver, NOS
P1-5B520 Perfusion of liver
P1-5B570 Removal of liver tube

1-5B7 Liver: Endoscopy

P1-5B700 Endoscopy of liver, NOS
 Endoscopic procedure of liver, NOS

1-5B8 Liver: Surgical Repairs, Closures and Reconstructions

P1-5B800 Repair of liver, NOS
P1-5B806 Marsupialization of cyst or abscess of liver
P1-5B810 Hepatorrhaphy
 Suture of liver
 Simple hepatorrhaphy
 Repair of liver laceration
P1-5B812 Complex hepatorrhaphy
P1-5B814 Complex hepatorrhaphy with hepatic artery ligation
P1-5B816 Hepatorrhaphy with common duct or gallbladder drainage
P1-5B830 Hepatopexy
P1-5B831 Binnie operation, hepatopexy
P1-5B832 Kehr operation, hepatopexy
P1-5B850 Hepatic portoenterostomy, NOS
 Hepaticoenterostomy
P1-5B852 U-tube hepaticoenterostomy
P1-5B854 Hepatoduodenostomy
 Hepaticoduodenostomy
P1-5B856 Hepatogastrostomy
 Hepaticogastrostomy
P1-5B858 Hepatojejunostomy

1-5BC Liver: Destructive Procedures

P1-5BC00 Destructive procedure of liver, NOS
P1-5BC10 Destruction of lesion of liver
P1-5BC20 Cauterization of liver

1-5BD Liver: Transplantations and Transpositions

P1-5BD10 Transplantation of liver, NOS
P1-5BD14 Liver transplant with recipient hepatectomy
P1-5BD16 Liver transplant without recipient hepatectomy
P1-5BD20 Donor hepatectomy with preparation and maintenance of homograft

1-5BE Liver: Manipulations

P1-5BE10 Manipulation of liver, NOS

1-5C OPERATIVE PROCEDURES ON THE GALLBLADDER AND THE BILIARY TRACT

1-5C0 Gallbladder and Biliary Tract: General and Miscellaneous Operative Procedures

P1-5C010 Operation on gallbladder, NOS
P1-5C040 Operation on biliary tract, NOS

1-5C1 Gallbladder and Biliary Tract: Incisions

P1-5C100 Incision of gallbladder
 Cholecystotomy
P1-5C102 Incision and exploration of gallbladder
 Cholecystotomy with exploration
P1-5C110 Incision and drainage of gallbladder
P1-5C114 Percutaneous aspiration of gallbladder for drainage
 Percutaneous cholecystotomy
P1-5C116 Trocar cholecystotomy
P1-5C120 Cholelithotomy
 Cholecystostomy with removal of calculus
 Lithotomy of gallbladder
 Removal of calculus from gallbladder
 Removal of gallstones from gallbladder
 Bobb operation, cholelithotomy
P1-5C121 Incision and removal of foreign body from gallbladder
P1-5C160 Incision of common bile duct
 Choledochostomy, NOS
 Choledochotomy, NOS
P1-5C163 Exploration of common bile duct
 Choledochotomy with exploration

P1-5C164 Incision and exploration of common bile duct for relief of obstruction
Decompression of common bile duct
P1-5C166 Choledochostomy with transduodenal sphincteroplasty
P1-5C167 Choledochostomy with cholecystotomy
P1-5C168 Incision of bile duct with T or Y tube insertion, NOS
P1-5C170 Choledocholithotomy
Choledochostomy with removal of calculus
Lithotomy of common bile duct
P1-5C171 Percutaneous lithotomy of common duct
P1-5C172 Duodenocholedochotomy with transduodenal choledocholithotomy
P1-5C174 Choledochotomy with removal of calculus with transduodenal sphincterotomy or sphincteroplasty
P1-5C176 Choledochotomy with removal of calculus with cholecystotomy
P1-5C180 Incision of hepatic ducts, NOS
Hepaticostomy, NOS
Cholangiotomy, NOS
Cholangiostomy
Hepaticodochotomy
Hepaticotomy
P1-5C181 Hepaticotomy with drainage
P1-5C182 Incision and exploration of hepatic ducts
Incision of bile duct, except common
P1-5C184 Hepaticolithotomy
Lithotomy of hepatic ducts
P1-5C187 Exploration for congenital atresia of bile ducts without repair
P1-5C188 Exploration for congenital atresia of bile ducts with liver biopsy and cholangiography
P1-5C190 Incision of sphincter of Oddi, NOS
Choledochal sphincterotomy
P1-5C191 Transduodenal sphincterotomy

1-5C3 Gallbladder and Biliary Tract: Excisions

P1-5C300 Biopsy of gallbladder, NOS
P1-5C301 Open biopsy of gallbladder
P1-5C302 Excision of lesion of gallbladder
P1-5C304 Core needle biopsy of gallbladder
P1-5C305 Fine needle biopsy of gallbladder
Fine needle aspiration biopsy of gallbladder
P1-5C308 Percutaneous extraction of common duct stones
Removal of gallstones from hepatic ducts
Biliary duct stone extraction, percutaneous via t-tube tract with snare or basket
P1-5C330 Cholecystectomy
P1-5C331 Partial cholecystectomy
Thoreck operation, partial cholecystectomy
P1-5C332 Cholecystectomy with exploration of common duct
P1-5C333 Cholecystectomy with exploration of common duct with cholangiography
P1-5C334 Cholecystectomy with exploration of common duct with choledochoenterostomy
P1-5C335 Cholecystectomy with exploration of common duct with transduodenal sphincteroplasty without cholangiography
P1-5C336 Cholecystectomy with exploration of common duct with transduodenal sphincterotomy, with cholangiography
P1-5C360 Excision of common bile duct
Choledochectomy
P1-5C361 Biopsy of bile ducts
Open biopsy of bile ducts
P1-5C362 Excision of choledochal cyst
P1-5C363 Excision of lesion of bile ducts
Excision of lesion of hepatic ducts
P1-5C364 Excision of bile duct tumor with repair
P1-5C366 Excision of cystic duct remnant
P1-5C368 Resection of hepatic ducts
P1-5C370 Excision of ampulla of Vater, simple
P1-5C372 Excision ampulla of Vater with reimplantation of common duct
P1-5C374 Excision of diverticulum of ampulla of Vater
P1-5C376 Excision of lesion of ampulla of Vater
P1-5C378 Resection of sphincter of Oddi

1-5C5 Gallbladder and Biliary Tract: Injections and Implantations

P1-5C500 Insertion of prosthetic device into biliary tract
P1-5C504 Introduction of percutaneous transhepatic catheter for biliary drainage
P1-5C510 Insertion of catheter into common bile duct
Intubation of common bile duct
P1-5C511 Insertion of choledochohepatic tube for decompression
P1-5C512 Cannulation of ampulla of Vater
P1-5C513 Placement of choledochal stent
P1-5C515 Reinsertion of transhepatic T-tube
P1-5C516 Replacement of prosthesis in biliary tract
Replacement of stent in biliary tree
Change of percutaneous biliary drainage catheter
P1-5C517 Removal of prosthesis of bile duct
Removal of prosthetic device from bile duct
P1-5C518 Removal of T-tube from bile duct
P1-5C519 Removal of tube cholecystostomy
Removal of cholecystostomy tube
P1-5C51C Intubation of common bile duct for decompression
P1-5C520 Irrigation cholecystostomy
P1-5C521 Irrigation of biliary tube
P1-5C530 Injection procedure for percutaneous transhepatic cholangiography

1-5C7 Gallbladder and Biliary Tract: Endoscopy

P1-5C700 Endoscopic retrograde cholangiography
ERC, NOS

1-5C7 Gallbladder and Biliary Tract: Endoscopy — Continued

P1-5C710 Endoscopic retrograde cholangiopancreatography, NOS
  ERCP, NOS
P1-5C712 Endoscopic retrograde cholangiopancreatography with biopsy
P1-5C714 Endoscopic retrograde cholangiopancreatography for sphincterotomy or papillotomy
P1-5C716 Endoscopic retrograde cholangiopancreatography for pressure measurement of sphincter of Oddi
P1-5C718 Endoscopic retrograde cholangiopancreatography for removal of stone from biliary and pancreatic ducts
  Removal of calculus of bile duct by ERCP
  Removal calculus of common duct by ERCP
P1-5C720 Endoscopic retrograde cholangiopancreatography for destruction by lithotripsy of stones
P1-5C722 Endoscopic retrograde cholangiopancreatography for insertion of nasobiliary or nasopancreatic drainage tube
P1-5C724 Endoscopic retrograde cholangiopancreatography for insertion of tube or stent into bile or pancreatic duct
  Insertion of nasobiliary tube by ERCP
P1-5C726 Endoscopic retrograde cholangiopancreatography for removal or change of tube or stent
P1-5C728 Endoscopic retrograde cholangiopancreatography for removal of foreign body
P1-5C729 Sphincterotomy of sphincter of Oddi by ERCP
P1-5C730 Endoscopic retrograde cholangiopancreatography for balloon dilation of ampulla, biliary or pancreatic duct
  Dilation of biliary duct by ERCP
  Dilation of ampulla of Vater by ERCP
  Dilation of sphincter of Oddi by ERCP
P1-5C732 Endoscopic retrograde cholangiopancreatography for ablation of mucosal lesion or tumor by fulguration
  Ablation of biliary tract lesion by ERCP
P1-5C738 Endoscopic retrograde cholangiopancreatography for ablation of mucosal lesion or tumor by laser
P1-5C739 Insertion of biliary stent by ERCP
P1-5C760 Operative endoscopy of biliary tract
  Choledochoscopy
  Intraoperative endoscopy of biliary tract
P1-5C770 Percutaneous biliary endoscopy via T-tube or other tract, NOS
P1-5C772 Percutaneous biliary endoscopy via T-tube or other tract with biopsy
P1-5C774 Percutaneous biliary endoscopy via T-tube or other tract for removal of stone
P1-5C776 Percutaneous biliary endoscopy via T-tube or other tract for dilation of biliary duct stricture
P1-5C780 Endoscopic biopsy of sphincter of Oddi, NOS
P1-5C781 Endoscopic excision of lesion of sphincter of Oddi
P1-5C782 Endoscopic destruction of lesion of sphincter of Oddi
P1-5C790 Laparoscopy with guided transhepatic cholangiography
P1-5C792 Laparoscopy with guided transhepatic cholangiography and biopsy

1-5C8-5C9 Gallbladder and Biliary Tract: Surgical Repairs, Closures and Reconstructions

P1-5C805 Anastomosis of gallbladder to hepatic ducts
P1-5C810 Anastomosis of hepatic duct to gastrointestinal tract, NOS
P1-5C811 Direct anastomosis of intrahepatic ducts and gastrointestinal tract
P1-5C812 Portoenterostomy
  Anastomosis of intrahepatic duct to jejunum
P1-5C813 Roux-en-y anastomosis of extrahepatic biliary ducts and gastrointestinal tract
P1-5C820 Anastomosis of bile ducts, NOS
P1-5C821 Longmire operation, bile duct anastomosis
P1-5C822 Cholangiocholangiostomy
P1-5C823 Anastomosis of common bile duct
P1-5C824 Anastomosis of cystic duct
P1-5C826 Anastomosis of hepatic ducts
  Intrahepatic anastomosis
P1-5C828 Anastomosis of pancreatic duct
P1-5C829 Choledochopancreatostomy
P1-5C830 Revision of anastomosis of biliary tract
P1-5C840 Gallbladder to intestine anastomosis, NOS
  Winiwarter operation, cholecystoenterostomy
  Direct cholecystoenterostomy
P1-5C841 Roux-en-y cholecystoenterostomy
P1-5C842 Cholecystogastrostomy
  Gallbladder to stomach anastomosis
P1-5C844 Cholecystopancreatostomy
  Gallbladder to pancreas anastomosis
P1-5C845 Cholecystocecostomy
P1-5C846 Cholecystoduodenostomy
P1-5C848 Cholecystojejunostomy
P1-5C849 Roux-en-Y cholecystojejunostomy with jejunojejunostomy
P1-5C84A Cholecystoileostomy
P1-5C84B Cholecystocolostomy
P1-5C84D Cholecystoenterostomy with gastroenterostomy
P1-5C851 Hepaticocystoduodenostomy
P1-5C852 Hepatocholangiocystoduodenostomy
P1-5C853 Hepaticocholangiojejunostomy
P1-5C860 Choledochoenterostomy
P1-5C865 Choledochoduodenostomy
  Duodenocholedochotomy

P1-5C867 Choledochojejunostomy
P1-5C870 Repair of gallbladder
P1-5C871 Repair of laceration of gallbladder
  Cholecystorrhaphy
  Suture of gallbladder
P1-5C872 Repair of stoma of gallbladder
  Revision of cholecystostomy
P1-5C874 Take-down of stoma of gallbladder
  Closure of stoma of gallbladder
  Closure of cholecystostomy
P1-5C876 Repair of stoma of common duct
P1-5C877 Take-down of stoma of common duct
P1-5C890 Choledochoplasty
P1-5C892 Repair of common bile duct laceration
  Suture of common duct
  Choledochorrhaphy
P1-5C894 Repair of choledochoduodenal fistula
P1-5C895 Repair of bile ducts
  Suture of bile duct
P1-5C896 Repair of hepatic duct
  Suture of hepatic duct
P1-5C897 Repair of bile duct laceration, NOS
P1-5C898 Anastomosis of choledochal cyst without excision
P1-5C89A Cholecystopexy
P1-5C900 Repair of biliary tract fistula, NOS
  Closure of biliary tract fistula, NOS
P1-5C902 Repair of gallbladder fistula
  Closure of gallbladder fistula
P1-5C904 Repair of common duct fistula
  Closure of common duct fistula
P1-5C906 Repair of hepatic duct fistula
  Closure of hepatic duct fistula
P1-5C908 Repair of cholecystoenteric fistula
  Closure of cholecystoenteric fistula
P1-5C910 Repair of cholecystogastroenteric fistula
  Closure of cholecystogastroenteric fistula
P1-5C912 Repair of cholecystoduodenal fistula
  Closure of cholecystoduodenal fistula
P1-5C914 Repair of cholecystogastric fistula
  Closure of cholecystogastric fistula
P1-5C916 Repair of cholecystojejunal fistula
  Closure of cholecystojejunal fistula
P1-5C918 Repair of cholecystocolic fistula
  Closure of cholecystocolic fistula

1-5CC Gallbladder and Biliary Tract: Destructive Procedures

P1-5CC10 Crushing of bile calculus, NOS
P1-5CC12 Choledocholithotripsy
P1-5CC20 Extracorporeal shockwave lithotripsy of the bile duct
P1-5CC24 Extracorporeal shockwave lithotripsy of the gallbladder
P1-5CC28 Extracorporeal shockwave lithotripsy of the gallbladder and bile duct

1-5CD Gallbladder and Biliary Tract: Transplantations and Transpositions

P1-5CD20 Transposition of biliary fistulous tract into intestine
P1-5CD22 Transposition of biliary fistulous tract into stomach

1-5CE Gallbladder and Biliary Tract: Manipulations

P1-5CE10 Dilation of sphincter of Oddi
  Dilation of pancreatic sphincter
  Dilation of ampulla of Vater

1-5E OPERATIVE PROCEDURES ON THE PANCREAS

1-5E0 Pancreas: General and Miscellaneous Operative Procedures

P1-5E010 Operation on pancreas, NOS

1-5E1 Pancreas: Incisions

P1-5E100 Incision of pancreas
  Pancreatotomy
P1-5E104 Incision and exploration of pancreas
P1-5E120 Drainage of cyst of pancreas, NOS
P1-5E122 Internal drainage of pancreatic cyst
P1-5E126 Incision and drainage of pseudocyst of pancreas
P1-5E128 External drainage of pseudocyst of pancreas
P1-5E180 Filleting of pancreas
P1-5E200 Pancreatolithotomy
  Incision and removal of pancreatic calculus
  Pancreolithotomy
P1-5E202 Removal of foreign body from pancreas

1-5E3 Pancreas: Excisions

P1-5E300 Biopsy of pancreas, NOS
P1-5E301 Open biopsy of pancreas
P1-5E302 Incisional biopsy of pancreas
P1-5E307 Core needle biopsy of pancreas
P1-5E308 Fine needle biopsy of pancreas
  Fine needle aspiration biopsy of pancreas
P1-5E310 Excision of lesion of pancreas
P1-5E330 Pancreatectomy, NOS
P1-5E332 Total pancreatectomy
P1-5E334 Total pancreaticoduodenectomy
  Total pancreatectomy with synchronous duodenectomy
  Total pancreatoduodenectomy
P1-5E340 Distal subtotal pancreatectomy
P1-5E342 Distal subtotal pancreatectomy with splenectomy
P1-5E344 Distal subtotal pancreatectomy with pancreaticojejunostomy
P1-5E345 Radical subtotal resection of pancreas
P1-5E346 Distal subtotal pancreatectomy with splenectomy and pancreaticojejunostomy

1-5E3 Pancreas: Excisions — Continued

P1-5E347 Child operation, radical subtotal pancreatectomy
P1-5E348 Rodney Smith operation, radical subtotal pancreatectomy
P1-5E349 Near-total pancreatectomy with preservation of duodenum
P1-5E350 Proximal subtotal pancreatectomy with pancreaticoduodenectomy and pancreatic jejunostomy
  Whipple operation, proximal pancreatectomy
  Proximal pancreatectomy

1-5E5 Pancreas: Injections and Implantations

P1-5E500 Injection of pancreas, NOS
P1-5E510 Catheterization of pancreatic cyst
P1-5E520 Irrigation of pancreatic tube
P1-5E540 Removal of pancreatic drain
P1-5E544 Replacement of stent in pancreatic duct

1-5E7 Pancreas: Endoscopy

P1-5E700 Endoscopy of pancreas, NOS
  Endoscopic retrograde pancreatography
  ERP
P1-5E702 Endoscopic biopsy of pancreatic duct
P1-5E704 Endoscopic excision of lesion of pancreatic duct
P1-5E706 Endoscopic destruction of lesion of pancreatic duct
P1-5E710 Endoscopic catheterization of pancreatic duct system
P1-5E711 Endoscopic dilation of pancreatic duct
  Dilation of pancreatic duct by ERCP
P1-5E714 Endoscopic insertion of nasopancreatic drainage tube
P1-5E726 Endoscopic insertion of stent into pancreatic duct
  Insertion of pancreatic stent by ERCP
P1-5E730 Endoscopic removal of stones from pancreatic duct

1-5E8 Pancreas: Surgical Repairs, Closures and Reconstructions

P1-5E800 Repair of pancreas, NOS
P1-5E804 Repair of Wirsung's duct
P1-5E806 Repair of pancreatic fistula
  Closure of pancreatic fistula
P1-5E810 Anastomosis of pancreas, NOS
P1-5E820 Pancreas to intestine anastomosis
  Pancreaticoenterostomy
  Drainage of pancreas by anastomosis
  Enteropancreatostomy
P1-5E822 Pancreas to stomach anastomosis
  Pancreaticogastrostomy
P1-5E823 Pancreaticoduodenostomy
P1-5E824 Pancreas to jejunum anastomosis
  Roux-en-Y operation, pancreaticojejunostomy
  Pancreaticojejunostomy
  Pancreaticojejunostomy, side-to-side anastomosis
  Puestow operation, pancreaticojejunostomy
P1-5E826 Ileopancreatostomy
  Pancreaticoileostomy
P1-5E840 Internal anastomosis of pancreatic cyst to gastrointestinal tract, direct
P1-5E842 Internal anastomosis of pancreatic cyst to gastrointestinal tract, Roux-en-Y
P1-5E844 Drainage of pseudocyst of pancreas by anastomosis
  Marsupialization of cyst of pancreas
P1-5E850 Pancreaticocystoenterostomy
P1-5E852 Pancreaticocystogastrostomy
P1-5E854 Pancreaticocystoduodenostomy
P1-5E856 Pancreaticocystojejunostomy

1-5EC Pancreas: Destructive Procedures

P1-5EC10 Destructive procedure on pancreas, NOS

1-5ED Pancreas: Transplantations and Transpositions

P1-5ED10 Transplantation of pancreas, NOS
P1-5ED12 Homotransplant of pancreas
P1-5ED14 Heterotransplant of pancreas
P1-5ED20 Autotransplantation of pancreatic tissue
  Reimplantation of pancreatic tissue
P1-5ED30 Total pancreatectomy with transplantation

SECTION 1-6 OPERATIVE PROCEDURES ON THE ENDOCRINE AND HEMATOPOIETIC SYSTEMS

1-60-61 OPERATIVE PROCEDURES ON THE ENDOCRINE SYSTEM

1-60 OPERATIVE PROCEDURES ON THE ENDOCRINE SYSTEM, EXCEPT THYROID GLAND

1-600 Endocrine System: General and Miscellaneous Operative Procedures

P1-60000 Operative procedure on endocrine system, NOS
P1-60010 Operative procedure on parathyroid gland, NOS
P1-60020 Operative procedure on adrenal gland, NOS
P1-60030 Operative procedure on pituitary gland, NOS
  Operative procedure on hypophysis, NOS
P1-60040 Operative procedure on pineal gland, NOS
P1-60050 Operative procedure on carotid body, NOS

1-601 Endocrine System: Incisions

P1-60100 Exploration of parathyroid gland, NOS

P1-60101 Exploration of parathyroid with mediastinal exploration by sternal split approach
P1-60102 Exploration of parathyroid with mediastinal exploration by transthoracic approach
P1-60103 Reexploration of parathyroid gland
P1-60110 Incision of adrenal gland, NOS
Adrenalotomy, NOS
P1-60112 Incision and exploration of adrenal, NOS
P1-60113 Unilateral exploration of adrenal, NOS
P1-60114 Bilateral exploration of adrenal, NOS
P1-60115 Exploration of adrenal gland without biopsy by dorsal approach
P1-60117 Exploration of adrenal gland without biopsy by transabdominal approach
P1-60130 Incision of pituitary gland, NOS
Incision of hypophysis, NOS
P1-60131 Incision and exploration of pituitary gland
Incision and exploration of pituitary fossa
Incision and exploration of hypophysis
P1-60132 Puncture and drainage of pituitary gland
Puncture and drainage of hypophysis
P1-60134 Puncture and drainage of craniopharyngioma
P1-60136 Division of hypophyseal stalk
Section of hypophyseal stalk
P1-60150 Incision of Rathke's pouch
P1-60152 Puncture and drainage of Rathke's pouch
P1-60160 Incision of pineal gland
Pinealotomy
P1-60162 Incision and exploration of pineal gland
P1-60170 Incision of carotid body
P1-60172 Incision and exploration of carotid body

1-603-604 Endocrine System: Excisions

P1-60300 Biopsy of parathyroid gland
P1-60301 Excision of lesion of parathyroid glands
P1-60310 Parathyroidectomy, NOS
P1-60311 Complete parathyroidectomy
Global parathyroidectomy
Total parathyroidectomy
P1-60312 Subtotal parathyroidectomy
Partial excision of parathyroid glands
P1-60316 Ectopic parathyroidectomy
P1-60320 Parathyroidectomy with mediastinal exploration by cervical approach
P1-60321 Parathyroidectomy with mediastinal exploration by sternal split approach
P1-60322 Parathyroidectomy with mediastinal exploration by transthoracic approach
P1-60330 Excision of lesion of adrenal gland
P1-60332 Fine needle biopsy of adrenal gland
Fine needle aspiration biopsy of adrenal gland
P1-60340 Adrenalectomy, NOS
Excision of adrenal gland, NOS
P1-60341 Unilateral adrenalectomy
P1-60342 Total adrenalectomy, NOS
Bilateral adrenalectomy
Complete adrenalectomy
P1-60343 Partial adrenalectomy, NOS
Subtotal adrenalectomy, NOS
P1-60344 Partial bilateral adrenalectomy
Subtotal bilateral adrenalectomy
P1-60350 Complete adrenalectomy by dorsal approach
P1-60352 Complete adrenalectomy by transabdominal approach
P1-60353 Partial adrenalectomy by dorsal approach
P1-60355 Partial adrenalectomy by transabdominal approach
P1-60360 Adrenalectomy by dorsal approach with excision of adjacent retroperitoneal tumor
P1-60362 Adrenalectomy by transabdominal approach with excision of adjacent retroperitoneal tumor
P1-60368 Adrenalectomy of remaining gland
P1-60370 Exploration of adrenal gland with biopsy by dorsal approach
P1-60372 Exploration of adrenal gland with biopsy by transabdominal approach
P1-60373 Exploration of adrenal gland by dorsal approach with excision of adjacent retroperitoneal tumor
P1-60374 Exploration of adrenal gland by transabdominal approach with excision of adjacent retroperitoneal tumor
P1-60400 Excision of lesion of pituitary gland, NOS
Excisional biopsy of hypophysis
P1-60401 Excisional biopsy of pituitary gland by transfrontal approach
P1-60402 Excisional biopsy of pituitary gland by transsphenoidal approach
P1-60404 Fine needle aspiration biopsy of hypophysis
Fine needle aspiration biopsy of pituitary gland
P1-60405 Fine needle aspiration biopsy of Rathke's pouch
P1-60406 Fine needle aspiration biopsy of craniopharyngioma
P1-60407 Hypophyseal infundibulectomy
P1-60410 Partial hypophysectomy, NOS
Subtotal hypophysectomy, NOS
P1-60411 Partial excision of pituitary gland by transfrontal approach
Subtotal hypophysectomy by transfrontal approach
Partial hypophysectomy by transfrontal approach
P1-60412 Partial excision of pituitary gland by transsphenoidal approach
Partial hypophysectomy by transsphenoidal approach
P1-60418 Partial excision of pituitary gland by unspecified approach
P1-60420 Total hypophysectomy
Total excision of pituitary gland
Ablation of pituitary gland

1-603-604 Endocrine System: Excisions — Continued

P1-60420 (cont.) Total pituitectomy

P1-60421 Total excision of pituitary gland by transfrontal approach
  Ablation of pituitary gland by transfrontal approach

P1-60422 Total excision of pituitary gland by transsphenoidal approach
  Ablation of pituitary gland by transsphenoidal approach

P1-60428 Hypophysectomy by other specified approach

P1-60440 Excisional biopsy of pineal gland

P1-60441 Excision of lesion of pineal gland

P1-60442 Excision of chemodectoma of pineal gland

P1-60450 Partial excision of pineal gland
  Partial pinealectomy

P1-60452 Pinealectomy
  Complete pinealectomy
  Complete excision of pineal gland

1-605 Endocrine System: Injections and Implantations

P1-60510 Insertion of pack into sella turcica
  Packing of sella turcica

1-607 Endocrine System: Endoscopy

P1-60710 Endoscopy of parathyroid gland, NOS

P1-60720 Endoscopy of adrenal gland, NOS

P1-60740 Endoscopy of pituitary gland, NOS

P1-60760 Endoscopy of carotid body, NOS

1-608 Endocrine Sytem: Surgical Repairs, Closures and Reconstructions

P1-60800 Repair of parathyroid gland, NOS

P1-60820 Repair of adrenal gland, NOS

P1-60840 Repair of pituitary gland, NOS

P1-60860 Repair of carotid body, NOS

1-60C Endocrine System: Destructive Procedures

P1-60C00 Destructive procedure on parathyroid, NOS

P1-60C20 Destructive procedure on adrenal gland, NOS

P1-60C40 Destructive procedure on pituitary gland, NOS

P1-60C50 Destructive procedure on pineal gland, NOS

P1-60C60 Destructive procedure on carotid body, NOS

1-60D Endocrine System: Transplantations and Transpositions

P1-60D00 Transplantation of parathyroid

P1-60D20 Transplantation of adrenal gland

P1-60D22 Transplantation of adrenal gland tissue to cerebral ventricle

P1-60D40 Transplantation of pituitary gland

P1-60D50 Transplantation of pineal gland

P1-60D60 Transplantation of carotid body

1-60E Endocrine System: Manipulations

P1-60E00 Manipulation of parathyroid gland, NOS

P1-60E20 Manipulation of adrenal gland, NOS

P1-60E40 Manipulation of pituitary gland, NOS

P1-60E50 Manipulation of pineal gland, NOS

P1-60E60 Manipulation of carotid body, NOS

1-61 OPERATIVE PROCEDURES ON THE THYROID GLAND

1-610 Thyroid Gland: General and Miscellaneous Operative Procedures

P1-61010 Operative procedure on the thyroid gland, NOS

1-611 Thyroid Gland: Incisions

P1-61100 Incision of thyroid, NOS
  Thyrotomy, NOS
  Thyroidotomy, NOS

P1-61102 Incision and exploration of thyroid
  Exploration of thyroid

P1-61103 Incision and drainage of thyroid

P1-61105 Postoperative thyroidotomy
  Reopening of thyroid field wound
  Postoperative examination of thyroid field
  Postoperative drainage of thyroid
  Postoperative exploration of thyroid

P1-61114 Needle aspiration for drainage of thyroid, NOS

P1-61116 Postoperative needle aspiration for drainage of thyroid

P1-61120 Transection of isthmus of thyroid
  Division of isthmus of thyroid

P1-61140 Incision and drainage of thyroglossal tract

P1-61142 Needle aspiration for drainage of thyroglossal tract

1-613 Thyroid Gland: Excisions

P1-61300 Biopsy of thyroid, NOS

P1-61301 Excision of lesion of thyroid
  Excisional biopsy of thyroid gland

P1-61302 Excision of cyst of thyroid

P1-61304 Excision of adenoma of thyroid

P1-61310 Incisional biopsy of thyroid

P1-61311 Core needle biopsy of thyroid
  Trucut needle biopsy of thyroid

P1-61312 Fine needle biopsy of thyroid
  Fine needle aspiration biopsy of thyroid

P1-61320 Thyroidectomy, NOS

P1-61321 Total thyroidectomy, NOS
  Complete thyroidectomy

P1-61322 Secondary thyroidectomy

P1-61324 Subtotal thyroidectomy
  Partial thyroidectomy

P1-61326 Unilateral thyroid lobectomy
  Hemithyroidectomy
P1-61328 Partial lobectomy of thyroid
  Subtotal lobectomy of thyroid
P1-61330 Substernal thyroidectomy, NOS
P1-61331 Complete substernal thyroidectomy
  Total substernal thyroidectomy
P1-61332 Partial substernal thyroidectomy
P1-61333 Substernal thyroidectomy by sternal split approach
P1-61334 Substernal thyroidectomy by transthoracic approach
P1-61335 Substernal thyroidectomy by cervical approach
P1-61342 Subtotal thyroidectomy for malignancy with limited neck dissection
P1-61343 Total thyroidectomy for malignancy with limited neck dissection
P1-61344 Subtotal thyroidectomy for malignancy with radical neck dissection
P1-61345 Total thyroidectomy for malignancy with radical neck dissection
P1-61350 Unilateral thyroid lobectomy with contralateral subtotal lobectomy including isthmus
  Hemithyroidectomy with removal of isthmus and removal of portion of remaining lobe
  Unilateral thyroidectomy with removal of isthmus and removal of portion of other lobe
P1-61352 Thyroid isthmectomy
P1-61356 Excision of lingual thyroid, NOS
P1-61357 Lingual thyroidectomy by submental route
P1-61358 Lingual thyroidectomy by transoral route
P1-61359 Thyroidectomy of remaining tissue
P1-61370 Removal of foreign body of thyroid
P1-61380 Excision of thyroglossal duct cyst
  Sistrunk operation on thyroglossal duct
  Excision of thyroglossal duct sinus
P1-61382 Excision of recurrent thyroglossal duct cyst
P1-61386 Excision of thyroglossal cyst with resection of hyoid bone

1-615 Thyroid Gland: Injections and Implantations

P1-61500 Injection of thyroid, NOS

1-617 Thyroid Gland: Endoscopy

P1-61700 Endoscopy of thyroid, NOS

1-618 Thyroid Gland: Surgical Repairs, Closures and Reconstructions

P1-61800 Thyroidorrhaphy
  Suture of thyroid gland

1-61C Thyroid Gland: Destructive Procedures

P1-61C00 Destructive procedure on thyroid gland, NOS

1-61D Thyroid Gland: Transplantations and Transpositions

P1-61D00 Transplantation of thyroid tissue, NOS
P1-61D02 Autotransplantation of thyroid tissue
  Reposition of thyroid tissue
  Reimplantation of thyroid tissue

1-61E Thyroid Gland: Manipulations

P1-61E00 Manipulation of thyroid gland, NOS

1-65-67 OPERATIVE PROCEDURES ON THE HEMATOPOIETIC SYSTEM

1-65 OPERATIVE PROCEDURES ON THE LYMPHATIC SYSTEM

1-650 Lymphatic System: General and Miscellaneous Operative Procedures

P1-65000 Operation on lymphatic structure, NOS
P1-65010 Operation on lymph node, NOS
P1-65020 Operation on thoracic duct, NOS

1-651 Lymphatic System: Incisions

P1-65100 Incision of lymphoid tissue, NOS
P1-65101 Incision of lymph node, NOS
  Lymphadenotomy, NOS
P1-65102 Incision and exploration of lymphatic structure
P1-65110 Simple drainage of lymph node abscess
P1-65112 Extensive drainage of lymph node abscess
P1-65120 Lymphangiotomy, NOS
P1-65122 Incision of lymphangioma
P1-65124 Incision of cystic hygroma

1-653 Lympatic System: Excisions

P1-65300 Excision of lymph node, NOS
  Lymphadenectomy, nos
  Simple lymphadenectomy
P1-65301 Biopsy of lymph node, NOS
P1-65302 Biopsy of lymphatic structure, NOS
P1-65303 Excision of superficial lymph node
P1-65304 Excision of deep lymph node
P1-65305 Excision of lesion of lymph structure, NOS
P1-65306 Core needle biopsy of lymph node
P1-65307 Fine needle biopsy of lymph node
  Fine needle aspiration biopsy of lymph node
P1-65308 Lymphangiectomy, NOS
P1-65309 Excision of lymphangioma
  Excision of lymphocele
P1-6530A Simple excision of cystic hygroma
P1-6530B Complex excision of cystic hygroma

1-653 Lympatic System: Excisions — Continued

P1-65310 Excision of regional lymph nodes
  Block dissection of lymph nodes
P1-65312 Radical excision of lymph nodes, NOS
  Radical lymphangiectomy
P1-65320 Excision of cervical lymph nodes, NOS
P1-65321 Excision of superficial cervical lymph nodes
P1-65322 Excision of deep cervical lymph nodes
  Deep cervical lymphadenectomy
  Excision of regional cervical lymph nodes
P1-65324 Biopsy of deep cervical lymph nodes with excision scalene fat pad
  Clearance of prescalene fat pad
  Excision of scalene fat pad
P1-65326 Excision of deep jugular nodes
P1-65327 Suprahyoid lymphadenectomy
P1-65330 Radical lymph node dissection of neck region, NOS
  Complete cervical lymphadenectomy
P1-65331 Unilateral radical neck dissection
P1-65332 Bilateral radical neck dissection
P1-65333 Modified radical neck dissection
P1-65334 Unilateral modified radical neck dissection
P1-65335 Bilateral modified radical neck dissection
P1-65340 Excision of axillary lymph nodes, NOS
  Superficial axillary lymphadenectomy
P1-65341 Deep axillary lymphadenectomy
P1-65342 Bilateral axillary lymphadenectomy
P1-65344 Complete axillary lymphadenectomy
  Radical excision of axillary lymph nodes
P1-65350 Excision of internal mammary lymph nodes
P1-65352 Excision of mediastinal lymph nodes
P1-65354 Excision of bronchial lymph nodes
P1-65360 Excision of periaortic lymph nodes
P1-65362 Excision of regional periaortic lymph nodes
P1-65363 Limited retroperitoneal lymphadenectomy for staging
P1-65364 Radical excision of periaortic lymph nodes
P1-65366 Excision of iliac lymph nodes
P1-65368 Regional excision of iliac lymph nodes
P1-65369 Radical excision of iliac lymph nodes
P1-65370 Pelvic and para-aortic limited lymphadenectomy for staging
P1-65372 Extensive retroperitoneal transabdominal lymphadenectomy
P1-65376 Pelvic lymphadenectomy
P1-65380 Excision of inguinal lymph nodes
  Excision of groin lymph nodes
P1-65382 Regional excision of groin lymph nodes
  Regional excision of inguinal lymph nodes
P1-65384 Superficial inguinofemoral lymphadenectomy including Cloquet's node
P1-65386 Superficial inguinofemoral lymphadenectomy in continuity with pelvic lymphadenectomy
P1-65388 Radical dissection of groin

1-655 Lymphatic System: Injections and Implantations

P1-65500 Injection procedure for lymphangiography, NOS
P1-65520 Cannulation of thoracic duct
P1-65524 Cannulation of cisterna chyli

1-657 Lymphatic System: Endoscopy

P1-65700 Endoscopy of lymphoid structure, NOS

1-658 Lymphatic System: Surgical Repairs, Closures and Reconstructions

P1-65800 Repair of lymphoid structure, NOS
  Lymphangioplasty, NOS
P1-65802 Lymphangiorrhaphy
P1-65803 Repair of thoracic duct, NOS
  Suture of thoracic duct, NOS
P1-65804 Suture of thoracic duct by cervical approach
P1-65805 Suture of thoracic duct by thoracic approach
P1-65806 Suture of thoracic duct by abdominal approach
P1-65810 Fistulization of thoracic duct
  Lymphaticostomy of thoracic duct
P1-65811 Closure of fistula of thoracic duct
P1-65812 Repair of cisterna chyli
P1-65814 Repair of fistula of cisterna chyli
P1-65820 Ligation of lymphatic, NOS
P1-65822 Ligation of thoracic duct
P1-65824 Ligation of cisterna chyli
P1-65826 Fistulization of cisterna chyli
  Lymphaticostomy of cisterna chyli
P1-65830 Anastomosis of lymphatic, NOS
P1-65832 Correction of lymphedema, NOS

1-65C Lymphatic System: Destructive Procedures

P1-65C00 Obliteration of lymphatic structure, NOS

1-65D Lymphatic System: Tranplantations and Transpositions

P1-65D00 Graft of lymphatic structure, NOS
P1-65D10 Transplant of lymphatic structure, NOS
  Reconstruction of lymphatic by transplantation
P1-65D50 Correction of lymphedema by transplantation of autogenous lymphatics graft
P1-65D54 Charles operation for correction of lymphedema
P1-65D56 Thompson operation for correction of lymphedema

1-65E Lymphatic System: Manipulations

P1-65E10 Dilation of lymphatic structure, NOS

1-66 OPERATIVE PROCEDURES ON THE TONSILS AND ADENOIDS

1-660 Tonsils and Adenoids: General and Miscellaneous Operative Procedures

P1-66000 Operation on tonsils, NOS
P1-66010 Operation on adenoids, NOS
P1-66020 Control of hemorrhage after tonsillectomy and adenoidectomy
P1-66022 Postoperative control of hemorrhage of tonsils
P1-66024 Postoperative control of hemorrhage of adenoids

1-661 Tonsils and Adenoids: Incisions

P1-66100 Incision of tonsil, NOS
  Tonsillotomy, NOS
P1-66110 Drainage of tonsil
P1-66111 Drainage of abscess of tonsil
P1-66120 Incision and drainage of tonsil and peritonsillar structures
P1-66130 Drainage of peritonsillar tissues
P1-66132 Incision and drainage of peritonsillar abscess
  Drainage of abscess of peritonsillar tissues

1-663 Tonsils and Adenoids: Excisions

P1-66300 Biopsy of tonsil
P1-66301 Excision of lesion of tonsil
P1-66302 Removal of foreign body of tonsil by incision
P1-66304 Excision of tonsil tags
P1-66306 Excision of lingual tonsil
  Lingual tonsillectomy
P1-66310 Tonsillectomy, NOS
  Sluder operation of tonsillectomy
  Excision of tonsil, NOS
P1-66312 Primary tonsillectomy, up to age 12
P1-66314 Primary tonsillectomy, age 12 or over
P1-66316 Secondary tonsillectomy, up to age 12
P1-66318 Secondary tonsillectomy, age 12 or over
P1-66320 Radical resection of tonsil and tonsillar pillars without closure
P1-66322 Radical resection of tonsil, tonsillar pillars and retromolar trigone without closure
P1-66324 Radical resection of tonsil, tonsillar pillars and retromolar trigone with closure by local flap
P1-66326 Radical resection of tonsil, tonsillar pillars and retromolar trigone with closure by nonlocal flap
P1-66350 Biopsy of adenoids
P1-66351 Excision of lesion of adenoids
P1-66352 Curettage of adenoids
P1-66353 Removal of foreign body of adenoid by incision
P1-66358 Excision adenoidal tags
P1-66360 Adenoidectomy, NOS
  Adenoidectomy without tonsillectomy
P1-66362 Primary adenoidectomy, up to age 12
P1-66364 Primary adenoidectomy, age 12 or over
P1-66366 Secondary adenoidectomy, up to age 12
P1-66368 Secondary adenoidectomy, age 12 or over
P1-66370 Tonsillectomy with adenoidectomy, NOS
P1-66371 Tonsillectomy and adenoidectomy, up to age 12
P1-66372 Tonsillectomy and adenoidectomy, age 12 or over

1-665 Tonsils and Adenoids: Injections and Implantations

P1-66510 Injection of tonsil, NOS
P1-66540 Injection of adenoid, NOS

1-667 Tonsils and Adenoids: Endoscopy

P1-66710 Endoscopy of tonsil, NOS
P1-66740 Endoscopy of adenoid, NOS

1-668 Tonsils and Adenoids: Surgical Repairs, Closures and Reconstructions

P1-66810 Suture of adenoid fossa
P1-66850 Suture of tonsillar fossa

1-66C Tonsils and Adenoids: Destructive Procedures

P1-66C10 Cauterization of tonsillar fossa
P1-66C14 Fulguration of tonsillar fossa
P1-66C20 Cauterization of adenoid fossa
P1-66C24 Fulguration of adenoid fossa

1-66D Tonsils and Adenoids: Transplantations and Transpositions

P1-66D00 Transplantation of tonsil and adenoid, NOS

1-66E Tonsils and Adenoids: Manipulations

P1-66E10 Manipulation of tonsil, NOS
P1-66E40 Manipulation of adenoid, NOS

1-67 OPERATIVE PROCEDURES ON THE SPLEEN, THYMUS AND BONE MARROW

1-670 Spleen, Thymus and Bone Marrow: General and Miscellaneous Operative Procedures

P1-67010 Operation on spleen, NOS
P1-67020 Operation on thymus, NOS
P1-67040 Operation on bone marrow, NOS

1-671 Spleen, Thymus and Bone Marrow: Incisions

P1-67100 Incision of spleen
  Splenotomy

1-671 Spleen, Thymus and Bone Marrow: Incisions — Continued

P1-67104 Incision and exploration of spleen
P1-67110 Puncture and drainage of spleen
P1-67112 Drainage of spleen by marsupialization
P1-67130 Incision of thymus
P1-67132 Incision and exploration of thymus field

1-673 Spleen, Thymus and Bone Marrow: Excisions

P1-67300 Biopsy of spleen, NOS
 Open biopsy of spleen
P1-67304 Excision of lesion of spleen
P1-67305 Excision of cyst of spleen
P1-67310 Splenectomy
 Total splenectomy
P1-67312 Partial splenectomy
P1-67320 Excision of accessory spleen
 Excision of ectopic spleen
P1-67330 Core needle biopsy of spleen
P1-67332 Fine needle aspiration biopsy of spleen
P1-67350 Biopsy of thymus
P1-67352 Excision of lesion of thymus
P1-67360 Total thymectomy
 Excision of thymus
P1-67362 Partial thymectomy
P1-67370 Core needle biopsy of thymus
P1-67372 Fine needle biopsy of thymus
 Fine needle aspiration biopsy of thymus
P1-67380 Bone marrow aspiration procedure, NOS
P1-67381 Bone marrow aspiration procedure, posterior iliac crest
P1-67382 Bone marrow aspiration procedure, anterior iliac crest
P1-67383 Bone marrow aspiration procedure, tibia
P1-67384 Bone marrow aspiration procedure, spine
P1-67385 Bone marrow aspiration procedure, sternum
P1-67388 Bone marrow aspiration procedure, other
P1-67390 Bone marrow biopsy, needle or trocar
P1-67394 Aspiration of bone marrow from donor for transplant

1-675 Spleen, Thymus and Bone Marrow: Injections and Implantations

P1-67510 Injection procedure for splenoportography
P1-67520 Injection into bone marrow

1-677 Spleen, Thymus and Bone Marrow: Endoscopy

P1-67710 Endoscopic procedure on spleen
P1-67740 Endoscopic procedure on thymus

1-678 Spleen, Thymus and Bone Marrow: Surgical Repairs, Closures and Reconstructions

P1-67800 Repair of spleen
 Splenoplasty
P1-67804 Suture of spleen
 Splenorrhaphy
P1-67806 Splenorrhaphy with partial splenectomy
P1-67810 Splenopexy
 Fixation of spleen
P1-67820 Marsupialization of splenic cyst
P1-67830 Repair of splenocolic fistula
 Closure of splenocolic fistula
P1-67840 Repair of thymus, NOS
P1-67842 Suture of thymus
P1-67844 Thymopexy

1-67C Spleen, Thymus and Bone Marrow: Destructive Procedures

P1-67C10 Destruction of lesion of spleen, NOS

1-67D Spleen, Thymus and Bone Marrow: Transplantations and Transpositions

P1-67D10 Transplantation of spleen
P1-67D20 Transplantation of thymus
P1-67D40 Transplantation of bone marrow, NOS
P1-67D50 Allogeneic bone marrow transplantation
P1-67D60 Autologous bone marrow transplant
P1-67D62 Autologous bone marrow transplant with purging
P1-67D64 Autologous bone marrow transplant without purging

1-67E Spleen, Thymus and Bone Marrow: Manipulations

P1-67E10 Manipulation of spleen, NOS
P1-67E20 Manipulation of thymus, NOS

SECTION 1-7 OPERATIVE PROCEDURES ON THE URINARY AND MALE GENITAL SYSTEMS

1-70-75 OPERATIVE PROCEDURES ON THE URINARY SYSTEM

1-70 GENERAL OPERATIVE PROCEDURES ON THE URINARY SYSTEM

1-700 Urinary System: General and Miscellaneous Operative Procedures

P1-70010 Operation on urinary system, NOS
P1-70020 Removal of urinary system device, NOS
P1-70022 Removal of urinary drainage device, NOS
 Removal of urinary catheter
P1-70030 Genitourinary instillation, NOS

1-71 OPERATIVE PROCEDURES ON THE KIDNEY

1-710 Kidney: General and Miscellaneous Operative Procedures

P1-71010 Operation on kidney, NOS
  Renal operation, NOS
P1-71040 Perirenal operation, NOS

1-711 Kidney: Incisions

P1-71100 Incision of kidney, NOS
  Nephrotomy, NOS
P1-71104 Incision and exploration of kidney
  Nephrotomy with exploration
  Renal exploration
P1-71105 Nephrostomy
P1-71106 Nephrostomy with tube drainage
  Nephrotomy with tube drainage
  Drainage of kidney by incision
P1-71107 Drainage of renal abscess
P1-71108 Percutaneous nephrostomy
P1-71110 Percutaneous aspiration of kidney
  Percutaneous puncture of kidney
P1-71111 Percutaneous aspiration of renal pelvis
P1-71112 Evacuation of kidney cyst
P1-71120 Symphysiotomy for horseshoe kidney
  Division of isthmus of horseshoe kidney
P1-71130 Incision of kidney pelvis
  Renal pyelotomy
  Renal pelviotomy
  Incision of renal pelvis
P1-71132 Renal calicotomy
P1-71134 Incision and exploration of kidney pelvis
  Pyelotomy with exploration of kidney
P1-71136 Complicated pyelotomy
P1-71140 Renal pyelostomy
  Renal pelviostomy
P1-71142 Pyelotomy with tube drainage
  Drainage of kidney pelvis by incision
P1-71160 Incision and exploration of perirenal tissue
  Incision and exploration of perinephric area
P1-71166 Drainage of perirenal abscess
P1-71170 Transection of aberrant renal vessels

1-713 Kidney: Excisions

P1-71300 Kidney biopsy, NOS
  Renal biopsy, NOS
P1-71302 Open biopsy of kidney
  Open renal biopsy
P1-71303 Core needle biopsy of kidney
  Core needle renal biopsy
P1-71304 Fine needle biopsy of kidney
  Fine needle aspiration biopsy of kidney
P1-71310 Excision of lesion of kidney
P1-71312 Excision of cyst of kidney
  Unroofing of cyst of kidney
P1-71314 Diverticulectomy of kidney
P1-71320 Biopsy of perirenal tissue
P1-71322 Excision of perinephric cyst
P1-71324 Excision of lesion of perirenal tissue
P1-71340 Nephrectomy, NOS
P1-71342 Unilateral nephrectomy
P1-71343 Bilateral nephrectomy
P1-71344 Nephrectomy of remaining kidney
  Nephrectomy of remaining or solitary kidney
P1-71346 Partial nephrectomy
  Segmental resection of kidney
P1-71347 Excision of lesion of kidney with partial nephrectomy
P1-71348 Heminephrectomy
P1-71349 Capsulectomy of kidney
  Decapsulation of kidney
  Decortication of kidney
  Renal capsulectomy
P1-71350 Partial pelvectomy of kidney
P1-71352 Renal calicectomy
P1-71353 Renal papillectomy
P1-71360 Nephrectomy including partial ureterectomy by any approach including rib resection
P1-71362 Nephrectomy including partial ureterectomy by any approach including rib resection, radical, with regional lymphadenectomy
P1-71364 Nephrectomy including partial ureterectomy by any approach including rib resection, complicated due to prior surgery on same kidney
P1-71366 Nephrectomy with total ureterectomy and bladder cuff by same incision
  Nephroureterectomy with bladder cuff
P1-71368 Nephrectomy with total ureterectomy and bladder cuff by separate incisions
P1-71369 Nephroureterocystectomy
P1-71370 Nephrolithotomy for removal of calculus
  Removal of calculus of kidney by incision
P1-71371 Nephrolithotomy for removal of staghorn calculus
P1-71372 Nephrolithotomy complicated by congenital renal abnormality
P1-71374 Pyelolithotomy
  Pyelotomy for removal of calculus
  Removal of calculus from renal pelvis by incision
  Pelviolithotomy
P1-71375 Removal of blood clot from kidney by incision
  Pyelolithotomy for removal of coagulum
P1-71377 Nephrolithotomy by secondary operation
P1-71380 Removal of calculus of renal pelvis through percutaneous nephrostomy, NOS
  Percutaneous removal of kidney calculus
  Percutaneous extraction of kidney stone
P1-71381 Percutaneous pyelostolithotomy, up to 2 cm
  Percutaneous nephrostolithotomy, up to 2 cm
P1-71382 Percutaneous pyelostolithotomy, over 2 cm
  Percutaneous nephrostolithotomy, over 2 cm

1-713 Kidney: Excisions — Continued

P1-71383 Percutaneous extraction of kidney stone with fragmentation procedure
  Percutaneous removal of kidney calculus with ultrasound fragmentation
P1-71388 Removal of calculus of perirenal tissue
P1-71389 Removal of foreign body of perirenal tissue
P1-71390 Removal of foreign body of kidney by incision
P1-71396 Removal of foreign body of renal pelvis by incision

1-715 Kidney: Injections and Implantations

P1-71510 Percutaneous injection of renal cyst
P1-71512 Percutaneous injection of renal pelvis
P1-71514 Percutaneous injection of therapeutic substance into kidney
P1-71520 Injection procedure for pyelography through indwelling ureteral catheter by nephrostomy or pyelostomy tube
P1-71540 Irrigation of nephrostomy
P1-71542 Irrigation of renal pyelostomy
P1-71550 Insertion of drainage tube into kidney
P1-71552 Insertion of drainage tube into kidney pelvis
  Introduction of catheter or stent into renal pelvis for drainage
  Insertion of drainage tube into renal pelvis
P1-71554 Introduction of catheter or stent into renal pelvis for percutaneous injection
P1-71556 Percutaneous introduction of ureteral catheter into ureter through renal pelvis for drainage
P1-71558 Percutaneous introduction of ureteral catheter into ureter through renal pelvis for injection
P1-71560 Percutaneous introduction of guide into renal pelvis or ureter with dilation to establish nephrostomy tract
P1-71580 Removal of nephrostomy tube
P1-71581 Replacement of nephrostomy tube
  Reinsertion of nephrostomy tube or catheter
  Change of nephrostomy catheter
  Change of nephrostomy tube
P1-71582 Removal of pyelostomy tube
P1-71583 Replacement of pyelostomy tube
  Reinsertion of pyelostomy tube or catheter
  Change of pyelostomy catheter
  Change of pyelostomy tube
P1-71584 Removal of pyelostomy and nephrostomy tubes
P1-71590 Implant of mechanical kidney
P1-71592 Replacement of mechanical kidney
P1-71596 Local perfusion of kidney

1-717 Kidney: Endoscopy

P1-71700 Endoscopy of kidney, NOS
  Nephroscopy, NOS
P1-71702 Endoscopy of renal pelvis, NOS
  Renal pyeloscopy, NOS
P1-71710 Renal endoscopy through established nephrostomy or pyelostomy
P1-71711 Renal endoscopy through established nephrostomy or pyelostomy with biopsy
P1-71712 Renal endoscopy through established nephrostomy or pyelostomy with fulguration
P1-71713 Renal endoscopy through established nephrostomy or pyelostomy with fulguration and biopsy
P1-71714 Renal endoscopy through established nephrostomy or pyelostomy with ureteral catheterization
P1-71715 Renal endoscopy through established nephrostomy or pyelostomy with ureteral catheterization and dilation of ureter
P1-71716 Renal endoscopy through established nephrostomy or pyelostomy with insertion of radioactive substance
P1-71717 Renal endoscopy through established nephrostomy or pyelostomy with insertion of radioactive substance and biopsy
P1-71718 Renal endoscopy through established nephrostomy or pyelostomy with insertion of radioactive substance and fulguration
P1-71719 Renal endoscopy through established nephrostomy or pyelostomy with removal of calculus
P1-7171A Renal endoscopy through established nephrostomy or pyelostomy with removal of foreign body
P1-71720 Renal endoscopy through nephrotomy or pyelostomy
P1-71721 Renal endoscopy through nephrotomy or pyelostomy with biopsy
P1-71722 Renal endoscopy through nephrotomy or pyelostomy with fulguration
P1-71723 Renal endoscopy through nephrotomy or pyelostomy with fulguration and biopsy
P1-71724 Renal endoscopy through nephrotomy or pyelostomy with ureteral catheterization
P1-71725 Renal endoscopy through nephrotomy or pyelostomy with ureteral catheterization and dilation of ureter
P1-71726 Renal endoscopy through nephrotomy or pyelostomy with insertion of radioactive substance
P1-71727 Renal endoscopy through nephrotomy or pyelostomy with insertion of radioactive substance and biopsy
P1-71728 Renal endoscopy through nephrotomy or pyelostomy with insertion of radioactive substance and fulguration

1-718 Kidney: Surgical Repairs, Closures and Reconstructions

P1-71800 Repair of kidney, NOS
  Nephroplasty

P1-71802 Suture of kidney
Nephrorrhaphy
P1-71804 Nephropexy
Suspension of kidney
Fixation of kidney
P1-71805 Nephrocolopexy
P1-71820 Pyeloplasty, NOS
Nephropyeloplasty
Pelvi-ureteroplasty
Foley operation for pyeloplasty
Correction of ureteropelvic junction
Pyeloureteroplasty
Reconstruction of ureteropelvic junction
Pelvioplasty of kidney
P1-71821 Pyelorrhaphy
P1-71822 Simple pyeloplasty
Simple pyeloplasty with plastic operation on ureter, nephropexy, nephrostomy, pyelostomy, or ureteral splinting
P1-71826 Complicated pyeloplasty
Complicated pyeloplasty due to associated renal abnormality, solitary kidney or calicoplasty
P1-71832 Stewart operation, renal plication with pyeloplasty
P1-71834 Culp-Deweerd operation, spiral flap pyeloplasty
P1-71836 Culp-Scardino operation, ureteral flap pyeloplasty
P1-71840 Revision of nephrostomy
Repair of stoma of kidney
Revision of stoma of kidney
P1-71842 Revision of pyelostomy
P1-71850 Anastomosis of renal pelvis, NOS
Anastomosis of kidney pelvis, NOS
P1-71851 Ureteropyelostomy
P1-71852 Pyeloureterovesical anastomosis
P1-71854 Ureterocaliceal anastomosis
Ureterocalicostomy
P1-71856 Nephrocystanastomosis
P1-71858 Calico-ileoneocystostomy
P1-71859 Nephropyeloureterostomy
P1-7185A Revision of pyelointestinal anastomosis
P1-71870 Closure of fistula of kidney
Closure of renal fistula
P1-71871 Closure of nephrocutaneous fistula
P1-71872 Closure of pyelocutaneous fistula
P1-71874 Closure of reno-intestinal fistula
P1-71876 Closure of nephrovisceral fistula including visceral repair by abdominal approach
P1-71877 Closure of nephrovisceral fistula including visceral repair by thoracic approach
P1-71880 Closure of nephrostomy
Closure of artificial opening of kidney
Closure of stoma of kidney
Take-down of stoma of kidney
P1-71882 Closure of renal pyelostomy
Closure of renal pelviostomy
P1-71890 Marsupialization of cyst of kidney

1-71C Kidney: Destructive Procedures

P1-71C00 Local destruction of renal tissue, NOS
P1-71C01 Destruction of lesion of kidney, NOS
P1-71C02 Lysis of adhesions of kidney
Nephrolysis
P1-71C04 Perirenal lysis of adhesions
P1-71C06 Obliteration of caliceal diverticulum
P1-71C10 Lithotripsy of kidney, NOS
Litholapaxy of kidney
P1-71C20 Extracorporeal shockwave lithotripsy of the kidney
Ultrasonic fragmentation of urinary stone, NOS
ESWL of kidney
P1-71C22 Ultrasonic fragmentation of urinary stone through percutaneous nephrostomy
Percutaneous nephrostomy with fragmentation of kidney stone

1-71D Kidney: Transplantations and Transpositions

P1-71D00 Transplant of kidney, NOS
Kidney transplantation, NOS
Renal transplant, NOS
P1-71D10 Renal autotransplantation
Renal autotransplantation or reimplantation of kidney
Autotransplant kidney
Reimplantation of kidney
P1-71D20 Renal homotransplantation excluding donor and recipient nephrectomy
P1-71D22 Renal homotransplantation with unilateral recipient nephrectomy
P1-71D30 Donor nephrectomy
P1-71D32 Donor nephrectomy with preparation and maintenance of homograft, from living donor
P1-71D34 Donor nephrectomy with preparation and maintenance of homograft, from cadaver donor
P1-71D40 Recipient nephrectomy
P1-71D50 Removal of rejected kidney
Removal of transplanted kidney
P1-71D60 Extracorporeal bench surgery of kidney, NOS
P1-71D70 Removal of mechanical kidney
P1-71D80 Repositioning of aberrant renal vessels

1-71E Kidney: Manipulations

P1-71E10 Detorsion of kidney
Release of torsion of kidney pedicle
Reduction of torsion of kidney pedicle

1-73 OPERATIVE PROCEDURES ON THE URETER

1-730 Ureter: General and Miscellaneous Operative Procedures

P1-73010 Operation on ureter, NOS

1-731 Ureter: Incisions

P1-73100 Incision of ureter, NOS
  Ureterotomy, NOS
P1-73102 Davis operation for ureterotomy
P1-73104 Incision and exploration of ureter
P1-73110 Open ureteral meatotomy
  Cutting of ureterovesical orifice, open
P1-73120 Ureterotomy with drainage
  Drainage of ureter by incision
P1-73140 Ureterocentesis
P1-73160 Incision of periureteral tissue

1-733 Ureter: Excisions

P1-73300 Excisional biopsy of ureter, NOS
  Excision of lesion of ureter
  Open excisional biopsy of ureter
P1-73310 Excision of segment of ureter for ureteral stricture
P1-73320 Excision of ureterocele
  Ureterocelectomy
P1-73330 Core needle biopsy of ureter
P1-73332 Fine needle biopsy of ureter
  Fine needle aspiration biopsy of ureter
P1-73350 Ureterectomy, NOS
  Excision of ureter, NOS
P1-73351 Total ureterectomy
  Total excision of ureter
  Total resection of ureter
P1-73352 Partial ureterectomy
P1-73354 Ureterectomy with bladder cuff
P1-73359 Total ureterectomy of ectopic ureter by combined approach
P1-73360 Ureterolithotomy, NOS
  Removal of calculus of ureter by incision
P1-73364 Ureterolithotomy, lower one-third of ureter
P1-73365 Ureterolithotomy, middle one-third of ureter
P1-73366 Ureterolithotomy, upper one-third of ureter
P1-73368 Removal of blood clot from ureter by incision
P1-73369 Removal of foreign body of ureter by incision
P1-7336A Transvesical ureterolithotomy

1-735 Ureter: Injections and Implantations

P1-73500 Catheterization of ureter, NOS
  Ureteral catheterization, NOS
P1-73510 Irrigation of ureterostomy
P1-73512 Irrigation of ureteral catheter
P1-73514 Irrigation of ureterostomy and ureteral catheter
P1-73520 Injection procedure for ureterography through ureterostomy
P1-73522 Injection procedure for ureterography through indwelling ureteral catheter
P1-73524 Injection procedure for ureteropyelography through ureterostomy
P1-73526 Injection procedure for ureteropyelography through indwelling ureteral catheter
P1-73530 Injection procedure for visualization of ileal conduit
P1-73532 Injection procedure for ureteropyelography, NOS
P1-73534 Injection procedure for visualization of ileal conduit and ureteropyelography
P1-73550 Insertion of ureteral stent with ureterotomy
  Ureterotomy for insertion of indwelling stent, all types
P1-73552 Reinsertion of ureteral stent with ureterotomy
P1-73553 Reinsertion of ureteral stent by transurethral approach
P1-73556 Percutaneous introduction of guide into ureter with dilation to establish nephrostomy tract
P1-73558 Reinsertion of ureterostomy tube
  Replacement of ureterostomy tube
  Change of ureterostomy catheter or tube
P1-73570 Implantation of electronic stimulator to ureter
P1-73571 Removal of electronic ureteral stimulator
P1-73572 Replacement of electronic ureteral stimulator
P1-73580 Removal of ureteral splint
  Removal of ureteral stent
P1-73586 Removal of ureteral catheter
P1-73588 Removal of ureterostomy tube
P1-73589 Removal of ureterostomy tube and ureteral catheter
P1-73590 Removal of ligature of ureter
  Deligation of ureter

1-737 Ureter: Endoscopy

P1-73700 Ureteroscopy, NOS
  Endoscopy of ureter, NOS
P1-73701 Cystourethroscopy with ureteroscopy and pyeloscopy, NOS
P1-73702 Ureteroscopy with biopsy
  Endoscopic biopsy of ureter
  Cystourethroscopy with biopsy of ureter
  Transurethral excisional biopsy of ureter
P1-73703 Cystourethroscopy with insertion of ureteral guide wire through kidney to establish a percutaneous nephrostomy
P1-73704 Cystourethroscopy with unilateral ureteral meatotomy
P1-73705 Cystourethroscopy with bilateral ureteral meatotomy
P1-73706 Cystourethroscopy with ureteroscopy or pyeloscopy with biopsy and fulguration of lesion
P1-73707 Cystourethroscopy with ureteral catheterization
P1-73708 Cystourethroscopy with resection of ureterocele

P1-73709 Cystourethroscopy with ureteral catheterization and brush biopsy

P1-7370A Transurethral removal of obstruction from ureter and renal pelvis

P1-7370B Cystourethroscopy with ureteral catheterization and removal of ureteral calculus
- Transurethral removal of foreign body from ureter
- Clearance of obstruction of ureter by transurethral approach
- Removal of calculus of ureter by transurethral approach
- Cystourethroscopy with ureteroscopy or pyeloscopy for removal or manipulation of calculus

P1-7370C Cystourethroscopy with ureteral catheterization and manipulation without removal of ureteral calculus

P1-7370D Cystourethroscopy with ureteral catheterization and fragmentation and removal of ureteral calculus
- Cystourethroscopy with ureteroscopy or pyeloscopy with lithotripsy

P1-7370E Cystourethroscopy with insertion of indwelling ureteral stent
- Transurethral insertion of ureteral stent

P1-73710 Ureteral endoscopy through established ureterostomy, NOS

P1-73712 Ureteral endoscopy through established ureterostomy with ureteral catheterization

P1-73714 Ureteral endoscopy through established ureterostomy with ureteral catheterization and dilation of ureter

P1-73716 Ureteral endoscopy through established ureterostomy with biopsy

P1-73718 Ureteral endoscopy through established ureterostomy with fulguration and biopsy of lesion

P1-73720 Ureteral endoscopy through established ureterostomy with insertion of radioactive substance

P1-73722 Ureteral endoscopy through established ureterostomy with insertion of radioactive substance and biopsy

P1-73724 Ureteral endoscopy through established ureterostomy with insertion of radioactive substance and fulguration

P1-73726 Ureteral endoscopy through established ureterostomy with removal of calculus

P1-73728 Ureteral endoscopy through established ureterostomy with removal of foreign body

P1-73740 Ureteral endoscopy through ureterotomy, NOS

P1-73741 Ureteral endoscopy through ureterotomy with ureteral catheterization

P1-73742 Ureteral endoscopy through ureterotomy with irrigation

P1-73743 Ureteral endoscopy through ureterotomy with ureteropyelography

P1-73744 Ureteral endoscopy through ureterotomy with ureteral catheterization and dilation of ureter

P1-73746 Ureteral endoscopy through ureterotomy with biopsy

P1-73748 Ureteral endoscopy through ureterotomy with fulguration of lesion

P1-73750 Ureteral endoscopy through ureterotomy with insertion of radioactive substance

P1-73752 Ureteral endoscopy through ureterotomy with insertion of radioactive substance and biopsy

P1-73754 Ureteral endoscopy through ureterotomy with insertion of radioactive substance and fulguration

P1-73756 Ureteral endoscopy through ureterotomy with removal of calculus

P1-73758 Ureteral endoscopy through ureterotomy with removal of foreign body

P1-73760 Endoscopy of ileal conduit
- Cystoscopy of ileal conduit
- Looposcopy of ileal conduit

1-738 Ureter: Surgical Repairs, Closures and Reconstructions

P1-73800 Repair of ureter, NOS
- Ureteroplasty

P1-73804 Ureterorrhaphy
- Suture of ureter

P1-73806 Ligation of ureter

P1-73808 Repair of ureterocele, NOS
- Urinary cystotomy for repair of ureterocele

P1-73810 Ureteroplication
- Plication of ureter

P1-73812 Ureteropexy

P1-73840 Anastomosis of ureter, NOS
- Drainage of ureter by anastomosis, NOS

P1-73842 Ureteroureterostomy
- Ureter resection with end-to-end anastomosis
- Spatulated ureteroureterostomy

P1-73844 Transureteroureterostomy
- Crossed ureteroureterostomy

P1-73850 Ureterocystostomy
- Ureteroneocystostomy
- Ureterovesical anastomosis
- Ureter to bladder anastomosis
- Reimplantation of ureter into bladder
- Implantation of ureter into bladder

P1-73851 Ureteroneocystostomy, anastomosis of ureter to bladder for correction of vesicoureteral reflux

P1-73852 Leadbetter-Politano operation, ureteroneocystostomy

P1-73853 Hutch operation, ureteroneocystostomy

P1-73854 Bischoff operation, ureteroneocystostomy

P1-73855 Paquin operation, ureteroneocystostomy

P1-73856 Ureteroneocystostomy with bladder flap
- Replacement of ureter bladder flap

1-738 Ureter: Surgical Repairs, Closures and Reconstructions — Continued

P1-73856 (cont.) Boari operation with bladder flap
P1-73880 Ureterostomy, NOS
P1-73882 Formation of cutaneous ureterostomy
 Implantation of ureter to skin
 Ureter to skin ureterostomy
 Ureter to skin anastomosis
P1-73886 Repair of stoma of ureter
 Revision of stoma of ureter
P1-73889 Closure of stoma of ureter
 Take-down of stoma of ureter
 Closure of ureterostomy
P1-73890 Closure of ureteral fistula, NOS
P1-73892 Closure of uteroureteric fistula
P1-73893 Closure of ureterorectal fistula
P1-73894 Closure of ureterosigmoidal fistula
P1-73895 Closure of ureterovisceral fistula
 Closure of intestinoureteral fistula
P1-73896 Closure of ureterovesical fistula
P1-73897 Closure of ureterovaginal fistula
P1-73898 Closure of ureterocervical fistula
P1-73899 Closure of ureterovesicovaginal fistula
P1-7389A Closure of ureterocutaneous fistula
P1-738A0 Revision of urinary conduit, NOS
P1-73900 Ureteroenterostomy, NOS
 Urinary continent diversion including bowel anastomosis, NOS
 Transplant of ureter to intestine
 Anastomosis of ureter to intestine
 Ureteroenterostomy, direct anastomosis of ureter to intestine
P1-73912 Ureteroileostomy, NOS
 Bricker's operation, ureteroileostomy
 Ureteroileal conduit with ileal bladder including bowel anastomosis
 Ileal ureterostomy
 Ileoureterostomy with ileal bladder
 Construction of cutaneous ureteroileostomy
 Construction of ileal conduit
P1-73914 Pyeloileocutaneous anastomosis, NOS
 Pyeloileostomy
P1-73919 Revision of cutaneous ureteroileostomy
P1-73920 Ureterocolostomy
 Ureterocolic anastomosis
 Ureter to colon anastomosis
 Ureterocolon conduit including bowel anastomosis
P1-73922 Ureterocecostomy
P1-73924 Ureterosigmoidostomy
P1-73926 Ureterosigmoidostomy with creation of abdominal or perineal colostomy
 Ureteroproctostomy
P1-73929 Revision of ureterointestinal anastomosis
 Revision of ileal conduit
P1-73930 Transplantation of ureter to ileum, internal diversion only
 Ureteroileostomy for internal diversion
P1-73932 Replacement of ureter by bowel segment including bowel anastomosis
P1-73950 Urinary undiversion of ureteral anastomosis
 Take-down of ureteral anastomosis

1-73C Ureter: Destructive Procedures

P1-73C00 Ureterolysis
 Lysis of adhesions of ureter
P1-73C02 Ureterolysis with freeing and repositioning of ureter
 Lysis of adhesions of ureter with freeing and repositioning of ureter
P1-73C04 Ureterolysis with repositioning of ureter due to retroperitoneal fibrosis
P1-73C06 Ureterolysis for ovarian vein syndrome
P1-73C08 Ureterolysis for retrocaval ureter
P1-73C10 Lysis of adhesions of ureter, intraluminal
P1-73C20 Lysis of periureteral adhesions
P1-73C30 Urinary cystotomy with fragmentation of ureteral calculus
 Urinary cystotomy with extraction and fragmentation of ureteral calculus
P1-73C40 Extracorporeal shockwave lithotripsy of ureter

1-73D Ureter: Transplantations and Transpositions

P1-73D10 Transplantation of ureter, NOS
P1-73D60 Transposition of ureter, NOS

1-73E Ureter: Manipulations

P1-73E00 Dilation of ureter
 Dilation and stretching of ureter
P1-73E02 Dilation of ureterovesical orifice
 Dilation of ureteral meatus
P1-73E04 Cystostomy with insertion of ureteral catheter
P1-73E10 Splinting of ureter
P1-73E40 Manipulation of ureteral calculus by catheter

1-74 OPERATIVE PROCEDURES ON THE BLADDER

1-740 Bladder: General and Miscellaneous Operative Procedures

P1-74010 Operation on bladder, NOS
P1-74012 Operation for correction of male urinary incontinence, NOS
P1-74030 Operation on perivesical tissue, NOS
P1-74040 Control of postoperative hemorrhage of bladder, NOS
P1-74050 Operation on urachus, NOS

1-741 Bladder: Incisions

P1-74100 Incision of bladder, NOS
 Percutaneous urinary cystostomy
 Urinary cystotomy
 Urinary vesicostomy
 Cutaneous urinary vesicostomy

P1-74100 (cont.) Suprapubic cystostomy
P1-74101 Franco operation for suprapubic cystotomy
P1-74104 Incision and exploration of bladder
P1-74106 Paracentesis of bladder
Needle puncture of bladder
P1-74108 Urinary cystotomy with drainage
P1-74109 Urinary cystotomy for incision of ureterocele
P1-74110 Division of bladder neck
P1-74150 Incision of perivesical tissue
P1-74152 Incision and exploration of perivesical tissue
Exploration of retropubic space
P1-74153 Drainage of perivesical space abscess
P1-74155 Incision of space of Retzius
P1-74157 Incision of hematoma of space of Retzius

1-743 Bladder: Excisions

P1-74300 Biopsy of bladder, NOS
P1-74301 Open excisional biopsy of bladder
P1-74302 Incisional biopsy of bladder
P1-74304 Core needle biopsy of bladder
P1-74305 Fine needle biopsy of bladder
Fine needle aspiration biopsy of bladder
P1-74306 Endometrectomy of urinary bladder
P1-74309 Open curettage of bladder, NOS
P1-74310 Resection of lesion of bladder, NOS
P1-74312 Urinary cystotomy for simple excision of vesical neck
Open resection of vesical neck
Open resection of bladder neck
P1-74313 Urinary cystotomy for excision of bladder tumor
P1-74314 Urinary cystotomy for excision of bladder diverticulum
Excision of bladder diverticulum
P1-74315 Suprapubic diverticulectomy of bladder
P1-74317 Removal of blood clot from bladder by incision
P1-74319 Removal of foreign body from bladder by incision
P1-74330 Urinary cystolithotomy
Removal of calculus from bladder by incision
Lithotomy of urinary bladder
Suprapubic vesicolithotomy
P1-74334 Cystoureterolithotomy
P1-74336 Urinary cystotomy for excision of ureterocele
P1-74340 Cystectomy, NOS
P1-74342 Partial cystectomy
Partial cystectomy, simple
P1-74343 Partial cystectomy with reimplantation of ureter into bladder
P1-74344 Partial cystectomy, complicated
P1-74346 Hemicystectomy
P1-74348 Trigonectomy
P1-74350 Complete cystectomy
Total resection of bladder
P1-74351 Complete cystectomy with continent diversion by any technique, NOS
P1-74353 Complete cystectomy with ureterocutaneous transplantations
P1-74354 Complete cystectomy with bilateral pelvic lymphadenectomy
P1-74355 Complete cystectomy with ureterocutaneous transplantations with bilateral pelvic lymphadenectomy
P1-74356 Complete cystectomy with ureterosigmoidostomy with bilateral pelvic lymphadenectomy
P1-74357 Complete cystectomy with ureteroileal or sigmoid bladder, including bowel anastomosis with bilateral pelvic lymphadenectomy
P1-74360 Complete cystectomy with ureteroileal conduit including bowel anastomosis
P1-74362 Complete cystectomy with sigmoid bladder including bowel anastomosis
P1-74364 Complete cystectomy with ureterosigmoidostomy
P1-74370 Radical cystectomy
P1-74374 Radical cystoprostatectomy
P1-74390 Excision of perivesical tissue
P1-74392 Excision of lesion of perivesical tissue
Excisional biopsy of perivesical tissue
P1-74394 Removal of foreign body from perivesical tissue

1-745 Bladder: Injections and Implantations

P1-74500 Catheterization of bladder, NOS
Simple catheterization of bladder
Indwelling catheterization of bladder
P1-74502 Complicated catheterization of bladder
P1-74504 Catheterization of bladder by indwelling suprapubic catheter
Aspiration of bladder with insertion of suprapubic catheter
Drainage of bladder by indwelling suprapubic catheter
P1-74505 Change of cystostomy tube, NOS
Change of cystostomy tube, simple
P1-74506 Change of cystostomy tube, complicated
P1-74508 Removal of cystostomy tube
P1-74509 Removal of bladder catheter
P1-74510 Irrigation of urinary bladder
Simple bladder irrigation
P1-74512 Transurethral clearance of bladder
P1-74514 Irrigation of cystostomy
P1-74516 Irrigation of indwelling urinary catheter
P1-74530 Replacement of bladder catheter
P1-74540 Implantation of electronic stimulator into bladder
P1-74541 Replacement of electronic stimulator into bladder
P1-74542 Implantation of artificial bladder sphincter
Implantation of artificial urinary sphincter
P1-74543 Replacement of artificial bladder sphincter
Removal of artificial bladder sphincter with replacement

1-745 Bladder: Injections and Implantations — Continued

P1-74543 (cont.) Replacement or repair of inflatable bladder sphincter
P1-74544 Removal of artificial bladder sphincter
  Removal of artificial prosthesis from urinary sphincter
P1-74546 Removal of electronic bladder stimulator
P1-74552 Introduction of prosthesis for correction of male urinary incontinence
P1-74553 Operation for correction of urinary incontinence with placement of inflatable prosthesis in urethra or bladder
P1-74554 Surgical correction of hydraulic abnormality of inflatable sphincter device
P1-74556 Removal of perineal prosthesis introduced for male continence
P1-74557 Removal of inflatable bladder sphincter including pump, reservoir or cuff
P1-74580 Instillation of bladder, NOS
P1-74581 Injection procedure for urinary cystography
P1-74582 Injection procedure for contrast urethrocystography
P1-74584 Bladder instillation of anticarcinogenic agent
P1-74585 Urinary cystotomy for insertion of radioactive material

1-747 Bladder: Endoscopy

P1-74700 Endoscopy of bladder, NOS
  Cystoscopy, NOS
P1-74702 Transurethral cystoscopy
  Cystourethroscopy
P1-74704 Endoscopy of bladder through artificial stoma
P1-74710 Cystourethroscopy with biopsy of bladder, NOS
  Transurethral biopsy of bladder
  Cystourethroscopy with biopsy
  Transurethral excision of lesion of bladder
  Cystoscopy with biopsy
P1-74712 Cystourethroscopy with incision or resection of orifice of bladder diverticulum, single
  Diverticulectomy of bladder by transurethral approach
  Transurethral excision of bladder diverticulum
P1-74713 Cystourethroscopy with incision or resection of orifice of bladder diverticulum, multiple
P1-74715 Cystourethroscopy with resection of bladder neck
  Transurethral incision of bladder neck
  Transurethral sphincterotomy of bladder neck
  Transurethral resection of vesical neck
  Transurethral resection of bladder neck
P1-74716 Transurethral resection of postoperative bladder neck contracture
P1-74717 Transurethral electroresection of bladder neck
  Transurethral electrocoagulation of urethrovesical junction
P1-74718 Transurethral curettage of bladder
P1-74719 Transurethral destruction of lesion of bladder
P1-74720 Transurethral removal of calculus from bladder without incision
P1-74722 Transurethral removal of foreign body from bladder
  Cystourethroscopy with removal of foreign body from urethra or bladder, simple
P1-74723 Cystourethroscopy with removal of foreign body from urethra or bladder, complicated
P1-74724 Transurethral removal of blood clot from bladder
  Cystoscopy for control of hemorrhage of bladder
P1-74740 Cystourethroscopy with resection of minor bladder tumors, less than 0.5 cm
  Cystourethroscopy with resection of small bladder tumors, 0.5 to 2.0 cm
P1-74742 Cystourethroscopy with resection of medium bladder tumors, 2.0 to 5.0 cm
P1-74743 Cystourethroscopy with resection of large bladder tumors
P1-74750 Cystourethroscopy with fulguration of minor bladder tumors, less than 0.5 cm
  Cystourethroscopy with fulguration of small bladder tumors, 0.5 to 2.0 cm
P1-74752 Cystourethroscopy with fulguration of medium bladder tumors, 2.0 to 5.0 cm
P1-74753 Cystourethroscopy with fulguration of large bladder tumors
P1-74757 Cystourethroscopy with fulguration of ureterocele
P1-74758 Cystourethroscopy with fulguration of bladder or prostatic fossa
P1-74760 Cystourethroscopy with insertion of radioactive substance
P1-74762 Cystourethroscopy with insertion of radioactive substance with biopsy or fulguration
P1-74764 Cystourethroscopy with steroid injection into stricture
P1-74766 Cystourethroscopy with ejaculatory duct catheterization
P1-74770 Cystourethroscopy with dilation of bladder for interstitial cystitis, local anesthesia
P1-74771 Cystourethroscopy with dilation of bladder for interstitial cystitis, spinal anesthesia
P1-74772 Cystourethroscopy with dilation of bladder for interstitial cystitis, general anesthesia
P1-74780 Transurethral lysis of adhesions of bladder
P1-74782 Transurethral fulguration of bladder

1-748 Bladder: Surgical Repairs, Closures and Reconstructions

P1-74800 Repair of bladder, NOS
  Cystoplasty, NOS
P1-74802 Suture of bladder
  Simple cystorrhaphy

P1-74802 (cont.) Repair of laceration of bladder
Cystorrhaphy
P1-74804 Complicated cystorrhaphy
P1-74806 Repair of stoma of bladder
Revision of stoma of bladder
Revision of vesicostomy
Revision of cystostomy
P1-74808 Repair of old obstetric laceration of bladder
P1-74810 Cystourethroplasty
Repair of bladder neck
Vesicourethroplasty
Cystourethroplasty and plastic repair of bladder neck
V-Y operation of bladder neck
Plication of sphincter of urinary bladder
Sphincteroplasty of bladder neck
P1-74811 Cystourethroplasty with unilateral ureteroneocystostomy
P1-74812 Cystourethroplasty with bilateral ureteroneocystostomy
P1-74830 Repair of fistula of bladder, NOS
Closure of fistula of bladder, NOS
Repair of bladder fistula by abdominal approach
P1-74831 Repair of fistula involving bladder and intestine, NOS
Repair of enterovesical fistula
Repair of intestinovesical fistula
Repair of vesicoenteric fistula
P1-74832 Repair of ileovesical fistula
P1-74834 Repair of rectovesicovaginal fistula
P1-74835 Repair of vesicocolic fistula
P1-74836 Repair of vesicometrorectal fistula
P1-74837 Repair of vesicosigmoidal fistula
P1-74838 Repair of vesicosigmoidovaginal fistula
P1-74839 Repair of vesicourethrorectal fistula
P1-74840 Repair of cervicovesical fistula
P1-74841 Repair of urethroperineovesical fistula
P1-74842 Repair of urethrovesical fistula
Repair of vesicourethral fistula
P1-74843 Repair of urethrovesicovaginal fistula
P1-74844 Repair of vesicouterine fistula
Repair of uterovesical fistula
P1-74845 Repair of vaginovesical fistula
Repair of vesicovaginal fistula
P1-74846 Repair of vesicocervicovaginal fistula
P1-74847 Repair of vesicocutaneous fistula
P1-74848 Repair of vesicoperineal fistula
P1-74849 Closure of vesicouterine fistula with hysterectomy
P1-74850 Cystopexy, NOS
Suspension of bladder, NOS
P1-74851 Vesicourethropexy, NOS
Urethrocystopexy, NOS
Cystourethropexy, NOS
P1-74852 Repair of stress incontinence by suprapubic sling
Repair of stress incontinence by urethrovesical suspension
Urethrocystopexy by suprapubic suspension
Cystourethropexy by suprapubic suspension
P1-74853 Marshall-Marchetti repair, simple
Anterior vesicourethropexy or urethropexy, Marshall-Marchetti-Krantz type, simple
Anterior urethropexy
Anterior urethropexy, simple
P1-74854 Marshall-Marchetti repair, complicated
Anterior vesicourethropexy or urethropexy, Marshall-Marchetti-Krantz type, complicated
Anterior urethropexy, complicated
Marshall-Marchetti-Krantz operation, retropubic urethral suspension
Cystourethropexy by retropubic suspension
Urethrocystopexy by retropubic suspension
Retropubic sling operation
Repair of stress incontinence by retropubic urethral suspension
P1-74855 Goebel-Frangenheim-Stoeckel operation for urethrovesical suspension
P1-74856 Sling operation for stress incontinence with fascia or synthetic material
P1-74857 Miller operation, urethrovesical suspension
P1-74858 Oxford operation for urinary incontinence
P1-74859 Millin-Read operation for urethrovesical suspension
P1-7485A Abdomino-vaginal vesical neck suspension, Stamey, Raz, or modified Pereyra type
P1-74860 Urethrocystopexy by levator muscle sling
Levator muscle operation for urethrovesical suspension
Cystourethropexy by levator muscle sling
Repair of stress incontinence by pubococcygeal sling
P1-74862 Repair of stress incontinence by urethrovesical suspension with gracilis muscle transplant
Urethrovesical suspension with gracilis muscle transplant
P1-74870 Anastomosis of bladder, NOS
P1-74871 Enterocystoplasty
Bladder to intestine anastomosis
Enterocystoplasty including bowel anastomosis
P1-74872 Colocystoplasty
Cystocolostomy
Cystocolic anastomosis
P1-74873 Ileocystoplasty
Replacement of bladder with ileal loop
Reconstruction of bladder with ileum
Bladder to ileum anastomosis
P1-74874 Cystoproctostomy
P1-74875 Construction of sigmoid bladder
Reconstruction of bladder with sigmoid
Replacement of bladder with sigmoid
P1-74878 Reconstruction of urinary bladder, NOS
P1-74879 Augmentation of bladder, NOS

1-748 Bladder: Surgical Repairs, Closures and Reconstructions — Continued

P1-74880 Closure of cystostomy
  Take-down of stoma of bladder
  Closure of stoma of bladder
  Closure of vesicostomy
P1-74885 Repair of bladder exstrophy

1-74C Bladder: Destructive Procedures

P1-74C00 Destruction of lesion of bladder, NOS
  Open destruction of lesion of bladder
P1-74C02 Urinary cystotomy with lysis of intraluminal adhesions
P1-74C04 Lysis of perivesical adhesions
P1-74C06 Cryotherapy of bladder
  Cystostomy with cryosurgical destruction of intravesical lesion
P1-74C08 Fulguration of bladder by suprapubic approach
P1-74C20 Crushing of calculus of urinary bladder, NOS
  Lithotripsy of bladder calculus
  Cystolitholapaxy
  Litholapaxy of bladder calculus
  Crushing of contents of bladder, NOS
P1-74C21 Bigelow operation, litholapaxy
P1-74C22 Lithotripsy of bladder calculus with ultrasonic fragmentation
P1-74C23 Extracorporeal shockwave lithotripsy of bladder
P1-74C30 Litholapaxy of bladder, simple stone, less than 2.5 cm
P1-74C32 Litholapaxy of bladder, complicated stone, over 2.5 cm

1-74D Bladder: Transplantations and Transpositions

P1-74D10 Transplantation of bladder tissue
P1-74D60 Transposition of bladder tissue

1-74E Bladder: Manipulations

P1-74E00 Manipulation of bladder, NOS
P1-74E10 Dilation of bladder
  Therapeutic overdistension of bladder
P1-74E20 Dilation of bladder neck
  Dilation and stretching of bladder neck
  Dilation of vesical neck
P1-74E30V Expression of bladder by manipulation

1-75 OPERATIVE PROCEDURES ON THE URETHRA

1-750 Urethra: General and Miscellaneous Operative Procedures

P1-75010 Operation on urethra, NOS
P1-75020 Operation for anti-incontinence, NOS
P1-75030 Operation on periurethral tissue, NOS

1-751 Urethra: Incisions

P1-75100 Incision of urethra
  Urethrotomy
P1-75102 Incision and exploration of urethra
P1-75104 Release of urethral stricture
P1-75106 Incision of periurethral tissue
  Incision of bulbourethral glands
  Incision of Cowper's glands
P1-75108 Drainage of Skene's gland cyst
P1-75114 Drainage of deep periurethral abscess
P1-75120 Drainage of perineal urinary extravasation, simple
P1-75122 Drainage of perineal urinary extravasation, complicated
P1-75130 Meatotomy of urethra, NOS
  Meatotomy of urethra, except infant
  Urethral meatotomy
P1-75132 Meatotomy of infant
P1-75140 Urethrostomy
P1-75142 External urethrotomy for pendulous urethra
  Syme operation for external urethrotomy
P1-75144 External urethrotomy for perineal urethra
  Poncet operation for perineal urethrostomy

1-753 Urethra: Excisions

P1-75300 Biopsy of urethra
  Excision of urethral tissue
P1-75302 Excision of lesion of urethra
P1-75304 Excision of urethral caruncle
P1-75306 Excision of urethral diverticulum, NOS
P1-75307 Excision of female urethral diverticulum
P1-75308 Excision of urethral polyps
P1-75309 Excision of urethral prolapse
P1-75310 Excision of carcinoma of urethra
P1-75312 Excision of urethral stricture
P1-75314 Excision of urethral septum
  Excision of congenital urethral valve
P1-75330 Biopsy of periurethral tissue
  Excision of periurethral tissue
P1-75332 Excision of Skene's glands
P1-75333 Excision of bulbourethral gland
  Excision of Cowper's gland
P1-75340 Urethrectomy, NOS
  Excision of urethra, NOS
P1-75342 Partial urethrectomy
P1-75344 Total urethrectomy
P1-75346 Total urethrectomy including cystostomy in female
P1-75348 Total urethrectomy including cystostomy in male
P1-75360 Urethrolithotomy, NOS
P1-75362 Removal of calculus of urethra without incision
P1-75364 Removal of calculus of urethra with incision
P1-75366 Removal of foreign body from urethra without incision
P1-75368 Removal of foreign body from urethra with incision

1-755 Urethra: Injections and Implantations

P1-75500 Injection of urethra, NOS
P1-75510 Injection procedure for voiding urethrocystography
P1-75520 Passage of filiform and follower for acute vesical retention in male
P1-75550 Implantation of inert material into urethra
P1-75560 Removal of urethral catheter
P1-75567 Removal of urethral stent
P1-75570V Retropropulsion of urethra
  Irrigation of urethra

1-757 Urethra: Endoscopy

P1-75700 Endoscopy of urethra, NOS
  Urethroscopy, NOS
  Endoscopic exploration of urethra, NOS
P1-75710 Cystourethroscopy with dilation of urethral stricture
P1-75720 Cystourethroscopy with direct vision of internal urethrotomy
P1-75722 Cystourethroscopy with internal male urethrotomy
P1-75724 Cystourethroscopy with internal female urethrotomy
P1-75730 Cystourethroscopy with resection of posterior urethra
P1-75732 Cystourethroscopy with resection of external sphincter of bladder
P1-75734 Cystourethroscopy for treatment of the female urethral syndrome, NOS
P1-75740 Perineal urethroscopy
P1-75750 Transurethral fulguration of urethra for postoperative bleeding

1-758-759 Urethra: Surgical Repairs, Closures and Reconstructions

P1-75800 Repair of urethra, NOS
P1-75802 Suture of urethra, NOS
  Urethrorrhaphy, NOS
  Suture of laceration of urethra
P1-75803 Female urethrorrhaphy
P1-75805 Perineal urethrorrhaphy
P1-75806 Prostatomembranous urethrorrhaphy
P1-75808 Penile urethrorrhaphy
P1-75809 Repair of old obstetric urethral laceration
P1-75810 Closure of urethrostomy
  Take-down of stoma of urethra
  Closure of male urethrostomy
  Closure of stoma of urethra
P1-75812 Marsupialization of male or female urethral diverticulum
P1-75820 Repair of urethral fistula
P1-75822 Repair of urethroperineal fistula
P1-75823 Repair of urethroscrotal fistula
P1-75824 Repair of urethrovaginal fistula
P1-75825 Repair of male urethrocutaneous fistula
P1-75826 Repair of perineourethroscrotal fistula
P1-75828 Formation of urethrovaginal fistula
  Urethrovaginal fistulization
P1-75830 Urethroplasty, NOS
  Reconstruction of urethra, NOS
P1-75831 Urethroplasty for reconstruction of female urethra
P1-75832 Plastic repair of urethrocele in female
P1-75833 Urethroplasty, one-stage for reconstruction of male anterior urethra
P1-75834 Perineal urethroplasty, one stage, for repair of membranous urethra
P1-75836 Urethroplasty, first stage
  Johannson urethral reconstruction
P1-75838 Urethroplasty, second stage, with formation of urethra including urinary diversion
P1-75839 Urethroplasty, repair of membranous urethra, first stage
P1-7583A Urethroplasty, repair of membranous urethra, second stage
P1-75840 Urethroplasty with tubularization of posterior urethra or lower bladder for incontinence
P1-75841 Leadbetter urethral reconstruction
P1-75842 Swinney urethral reconstruction
P1-75843 Cecil urethral reconstruction
P1-75845 Meatoplasty of urethra
P1-75846 Urethromeatoplasty with partial excision of distal urethral segment
  Richardson urethroplasty
P1-75847 Urethromeatoplasty with mucosal advancement
P1-75848 Benenenti operation for rotation of bulbous urethra
P1-7584B Transpubic urethroplasty, one stage, for repair of membranous urethra
P1-75850 Plication of urethra, NOS
P1-75852 Plication of urethrovesical junction
P1-75854 Plastic operation on urethral sphincter by vaginal approach
  Kelly-Stoeckel operation for urethrovesical plication
  Repair of stress incontinence by plication of urethrovesical junction
P1-75862 Kaufman operation for urinary stress incontinence
P1-75864 Urethral augmentation
P1-75870 Anastomosis of urethra, end-to-end
  Reanastomosis of urethra
P1-75880 Repair of stoma of urethra
  Revision of stoma of urethra
  Revision of urethrostomy
P1-75900 Urethropexy, NOS
P1-75905 Tudor rabbit ear operation for anterior urethropexy
P1-75910 Repair of urinary stress incontinence, NOS
P1-75930 Periurethral suspension, NOS
  Repair of stress incontinence by paraurethral suspension

1-758-759 Urethra: Surgical Repairs, Closures and Reconstructions — Continued

P1-75932 Pereyra operation for paraurethral suspension

1-75C Urethra: Destructive Procedures

P1-75C00 Destruction of urethral tissue, NOS
P1-75C01 Destruction of lesion of urethra, NOS
P1-75C02 Lysis of adhesions of urethra
  Urethrolysis
P1-75C10 Cauterization of urethra, NOS
P1-75C12 Fulguration of urethra, NOS
P1-75C14 Fulguration of urethral polyps
P1-75C16 Fulguration of urethral caruncle
P1-75C18 Fulguration of Skene's glands
P1-75C20 Fulguration of carcinoma of urethra

1-75D Urethra: Transplantations and Transpositions

P1-75D10 Transplantation of urethral tissue
P1-75D40 Transposition of urethral tissue

1-75E Urethra: Manipulations

P1-75E00 Manipulation of urethra, NOS
P1-75E01 Dilation of urethra, NOS
  Dilation and stretching of urethra
P1-75E02 Dilation of urethrovesical junction
P1-75E10 Passage of urethral sound, NOS
  Bougienage of urethra, NOS
P1-75E11 Initial dilation of male urethral stricture by passage of sound or urethral dilator
P1-75E16 Dilation of male urethral stricture by passage of sound or urethral dilator with anesthesia
P1-75E40 Initial dilation of male urethral stricture by passage of filiform and follower
P1-75E50 Initial dilation of female urethra
P1-75E54 Dilation of female urethra with anesthesia

1-76-7A OPERATIVE PROCEDURES ON THE MALE GENITAL SYSTEM

1-76 GENERAL OPERATIVE PROCEDURES ON THE MALE GENITAL SYSTEM

1-760 Male Genital System: General and Miscellaneous Operative Procedures

P1-76000 Operation on male genital system, NOS
P1-76004 Intersex surgery, NOS
  Operation for sex transformation, NOS
P1-76005 Intersex surgery, male to female, NOS
P1-76007 Intersex surgery, female to male, NOS
P1-76010V Surgical sexing, male

1-77 OPERATIVE PROCEDURES ON THE PENIS

1-770 Penis: General and Miscellaneous Operative Procedures

P1-77000 Operation on penis, NOS

1-771 Penis: Incisions

P1-77100 Incision of penis, NOS
P1-77101 Incision and exploration of penis, NOS
P1-77104 Slitting of prepuce, NOS
  Preputiotomy
  Prepucotomy
  Slitting of prepuce, except newborn
P1-77105 Slitting of prepuce on newborn
P1-77110 Incision and drainage of penis, NOS
P1-77112 Superficial incision and drainage of penis
P1-77114 Deep incision and drainage of penis

1-773 Penis: Excisions

P1-77300 Circumcision, NOS
  Prepucectomy, NOS
P1-77301 Circumcision by surgical excision on newborn
P1-77302 Circumcision by clamp procedure on newborn
P1-77303 Circumcision by surgical excision, except newborn
P1-77304 Circumcision by clamp procedure, except newborn
P1-77306V Excision of lesion of penis sheath
P1-77310 Excision of lesion on penis
  Cutaneous biopsy of penis
  Simple excisional biopsy of penis
P1-77311 Biopsy of deep structures of penis
P1-77312 Core needle biopsy of penis
P1-77313 Fine needle biopsy of penis
  Fine needle aspiration biopsy of penis
P1-77314 Excision of penile plaque for Peyronie disease
P1-77315 Excision of penile plaque for Peyronie disease, with graft to 5 cm in length
P1-77316 Excision of penile plaque for Peyronie disease with graft greater than 5 cm in length
P1-77320 Removal of foreign body of penis, NOS
P1-77321 Removal of foreign body of penis without incision
P1-77322 Removal of foreign body of penis by incision
P1-77326 Removal of foreign body from deep penile tissue
P1-77338 Amputation of glans penis
P1-77340 Amputation of penis, NOS
  Penectomy, NOS
  Resection of penis, NOS
P1-77341 Partial amputation of penis
P1-77342 Complete amputation of penis
  Radical amputation of penis
P1-77346 Radical amputation of penis with bilateral inguinofemoral lymphadenectomy
P1-77348 Radical amputation of penis with bilateral pelvic lymphadenectomy

1-775 Penis: Injections and Implantations

P1-77500 Insertion of penile prosthesis, NOS
P1-77501 Insertion of inflatable penile prosthesis
Implant of inflatable penile prosthesis
P1-77502 Insertion of non-inflatable penile prosthesis
Implant of non-inflatable penile prosthesis
P1-77503 Insertion of inflatable penile prosthesis, with placement of pump, cylinders, and reservoir
P1-77507 Fitting of external prosthetic device on penis
Application of support for penis
P1-77510 Replacement of inflatable penile prosthesis
P1-77512 Replacement of non-inflatable penile prosthesis
P1-77513 Replacement of inflatable penile prosthesis, with pump, reservoir and cylinders
P1-77515 Removal of penile prosthesis, NOS
P1-77516 Removal of internal penile prosthesis
P1-77517 Removal of inflatable penile prosthesis
P1-77518 Removal of non-inflatable penile prosthesis
P1-77519 Removal of inflatable penile prosthesis, with pump, reservoir and cylinders
P1-77520 Injection procedure for corpora cavernosography
P1-77522 Injection of corpora cavernosa with pharmacologic agent
P1-77524 Injection procedure for Peyronie disease
P1-77528 Injection procedure for Peyronie disease with surgical exposure of plaque
P1-77530 Irrigation of corpora cavernosa for priapism
P1-77540 Repair of penile prosthesis, NOS
P1-77541 Repair of inflatable penile prosthesis
P1-77542 Repair of non-inflatable penile prosthesis
P1-77543 Repair of inflatable penile prosthesis, with pump, reservoir and cylinders
P1-77544 Surgical correction of hydraulic abnormality of inflatable penile prosthesis with pump, reservoir and cylinders

1-777 Penis: Endoscopy

P1-77700 Endoscopy of penis, NOS

1-778 Penis: Surgical Repairs, Closures and Reconstructions

P1-77800 Repair of penis, NOS
Balanoplasty
P1-77801 Plastic operation of penis for injury
P1-77802 Suture of laceration of penis
P1-77810 Construction of corpora cavernosa-corpus spongiosum shunt
P1-77812 Construction of corpora cavernosa-saphenous vein shunt
P1-77814 Construction of corpora cavernosa-glans penis fistulization for priapism
P1-77820 Reconstruction of penis, NOS
P1-77822 Reconstruction of penis with graft
P1-77824 Graft of penis
P1-77825 Plastic operation on penis to correct angulation
P1-77828 Replantation of penis
Reattachment of amputated penis
P1-77840 Correction of chordee without mobilization of urethra
P1-77841 Correction of chordee with mobilization of urethra
P1-77842 Plastic operation on penis for correction of chordee for first stage hypospadias repair with transplantation of prepuce or skin flap
P1-77843 Plastic operation on penis for correction of chordee for first stage hypospadias repair without transplantation of prepuce or skin flap
P1-77844 Simple one stage distal hypospadias repair with meatal advancement
P1-77845 One stage distal hypospadias repair with urethroplasty by local skin flaps
P1-77846 One stage distal hypospadias repair with urethroplasty by local skin flaps and mobilization of urethra
P1-77847 One stage distal hypospadias repair with extensive dissection to correct chordee and urethroplasty with skin graft patch
P1-77848 One stage proximal penile or penoscrotal hypospadias repair requiring extensive dissection with graft
P1-77849 One stage perineal hypospadias repair requiring extensive dissection to correct chordee and urethroplasty with graft
P1-77851 Urethroplasty for second stage hypospadias repair, including urinary diversion, less than 3 cm
P1-77852 Urethroplasty for second stage hypospadias repair, including urinary diversion, greater than 3 cm
P1-77853 Urethroplasty for second stage hypospadias repair, including urinary diversion, with free skin graft
P1-77854 Urethroplasty for third stage hypospadias repair to release penis from scrotum
Cecil repair, third stage
P1-77860 Simple repair of hypospadias complications
P1-77862 Repair of hypospadias complications with mobilization of skin flaps and urethroplasty with graft
P1-77864 Repair of hypospadias complications with extensive dissection and urethroplasty with graft
P1-77868 Repair of hypospadias cripple with extensive dissection and excision of previously constructed structures and grafts
P1-77870 Plastic operation on penis for epispadias distal to external sphincter
P1-77872 Plastic operation on penis for epispadias distal to external sphincter with incontinence
P1-77874 Plastic operation on penis for epispadias distal to external sphincter with exstrophy of bladder

1-77C Penis: Destructive Procedures

P1-77C00 Destruction of lesion of penis, NOS
P1-77C01 Simple chemical destruction of lesion of penis
P1-77C02 Simple electrodesiccation of lesion of penis
P1-77C03 Simple cryosurgical destruction of lesion of penis
P1-77C04 Simple laser surgery for destruction of lesion of penis
P1-77C05 Extensive destruction of lesion of penis by any method
P1-77C10 Lysis of penile adhesions
Division of penile adhesions
P1-77C12 Foreskin manipulation including lysis of preputial adhesions and stretching

1-77D Penis: Transplantations and Transpositions

P1-77D10 Transplantation of penis, NOS
P1-77D40 Transposition of penis, NOS

1-77E Penis: Manipulations

P1-77E01 Dilation of foreskin, except newborn
Stretching of foreskin, except newborn
P1-77E04 Dilation of foreskin in newborn
P1-77E10V Manual withdrawal of penis

1-78 OPERATIVE PROCEDURES ON THE PROSTATE

1-780 Prostate: General and Miscellaneous Operative Procedures

P1-78000 Operation on prostate, NOS

1-781 Prostate: Incisions

P1-78100 Incision of prostate, NOS
Prostatotomy, NOS
P1-78101 Incision and exploration of prostate
P1-78102 Prostatotomy by transurethral approach
P1-78103 Prostatotomy by perineal approach
P1-78104 Prostatocystotomy
P1-78105 Prostatolithotomy
P1-78110 Transurethral drainage of prostatic abscess
P1-78112 Simple prostatotomy with external drainage of prostatic abscess
P1-78114 Complicated prostatotomy with external drainage of prostatic abscess
P1-78120 Incision of periprostatic tissue
P1-78122 Incision and exploration of periprostatic tissue

1-783 Prostate: Excisions

P1-78300 Biopsy of prostate, NOS
P1-78301 Excision of lesion of prostate
P1-78310 Core needle biopsy of prostate
P1-78312 Fine needle biopsy of prostate
Fine needle aspiration biopsy of prostate
P1-78314 Transrectal biopsy of prostate
P1-78320 Prostatectomy, NOS
P1-78322 Subtotal prostatectomy, NOS
P1-78324 Radical prostatectomy, NOS
Prostatovesiculectomy
P1-78330 Transurethral prostatectomy, NOS
TUR of prostate, NOS
Loop prostatectomy
P1-78331 Excision of median bar of prostate by transurethral approach
P1-78334 Transurethral resection of prostate, first stage of two stages
P1-78335 Transurethral resection of prostate, second stage of two stages
P1-78336 Complete transurethral resection of prostate, including control of postoperative bleeding
P1-78337 Transurethral resection of residual obstructive tissue of prostate after 90 days postoperative
P1-78338 Transurethral resection of regrowth of obstructive tissue of prostate longer than one year postoperative
P1-78339 Transurethral cryosurgical removal of prostate
P1-78340 Perineal prostatectomy, NOS
Alexander operation
P1-78341 Subtotal perineal prostatectomy
P1-78342 Radical perineal prostatectomy
P1-78343 Radical perineal prostatectomy with lymph node biopsy
P1-78344 Radical perineal prostatectomy with bilateral pelvic lymphadenectomy
P1-78350 Retropubic prostatectomy, NOS
P1-78351 Subtotal retropubic prostatectomy
P1-78352 Radical retropubic prostatectomy
P1-78353 Radical retropubic prostatectomy with lymph node biopsy
P1-78354 Radical retropubic prostatectomy with bilateral pelvic lymphadenectomy
P1-78360 Suprapubic prostatectomy, NOS
P1-78361 One stage subtotal suprapubic prostatectomy
P1-78362 Two stage subtotal suprapubic prostatectomy
P1-78380 Excision of periprostatic tissue
Excisional periprostatic biopsy
P1-78382 Excision of lesion of periprostatic tissue
P1-78390 Removal of calculus of prostate

1-785 Prostate: Injections and Implantations

P1-78500 Injection of prostate, NOS
P1-78510 Exposure of prostate for insertion of radioactive substance
P1-78512 Exposure of prostate for insertion of radioactive substance with lymph node biopsy
P1-78513 Exposure of prostate for insertion of radioactive substance with bilateral pelvic lymphadenectomy

1-787 Prostate: Endoscopy

P1-78700 Endoscopy of prostate, NOS

1-788 Prostate: Surgical Repairs, Closures and Reconstructions

P1-78800 Repair of prostate, NOS
P1-78810V Marsupialization of prostate

1-78C Prostate: Destructive Prodecures

P1-78C00 Transurethral fulguration of prostate, NOS
P1-78C01 Transurethral fulguration of prostate for postoperative bleeding
P1-78C10 Electrocoagulation of prostatic bed

1-78D Prostate: Transplantations and Transpositions

P1-78D10 Transplantation of prostatic tissue, NOS
P1-78D30 Transposition of prostatic tissue, NOS

1-78E Prostate: Manipulations

P1-78E00 Prostatic massage

1-79 OPERATIVE PROCEDURES ON THE TESTIS AND EPIDIDYMIS

1-790 Testis and Epididymis: General and Miscellaneous Operative Procedures

P1-79000 Operation on testis, NOS
P1-79002 Operation on epididymis, NOS

1-791 Testis and Epididymis: Incisions

P1-79100 Incision of testis, NOS
Orchidotomy, NOS
P1-79101 Incision and exploration of testis
P1-79102 Incision and drainage of testis
P1-79110 Incision and exploration for undescended testis of inguinal or scrotal area
P1-79112 Incision and exploration for undescended testis with abdominal exploration
P1-79140 Incision of epididymis, NOS
Epididymotomy, NOS
Hagner operation on epididymis
P1-79141 Incision and exploration of epididymis
P1-79142 Incision and drainage of epididymis
P1-79145 Aspiration of spermatocele

1-793 Testis and Epididymis: Excisions

P1-79300 Excisional biopsy of testis
P1-79301 Incisional biopsy of testis
P1-79302 Trucut needle biopsy of testis
P1-79303 Fine needle biopsy of testis
Fine needle aspiration biopsy of testis
P1-79307 Removal of foreign body of testis
P1-79310 Orchidectomy, NOS
Male gonadectomy, NOS
Orchiectomy, NOS
P1-79311 Unilateral orchidectomy
Unilateral removal of testis
P1-79312 Bilateral orchidectomy
Bilateral removal of testes
Male castration
P1-79313 Radical unilateral orchiectomy
Unilateral excision of testis and spermatic cord
P1-79314 Radical bilateral orchiectomy
Bilateral excision of testes and spermatic cords
P1-79316 Orchiectomy of remaining testis
Removal of remaining testis
P1-79317 Unilateral cryptorchiectomy
P1-79318 Bilateral cryptorchiectomy
P1-79320 Unilateral removal of ovo-testis
P1-79322 Bilateral removal of ovo-testis
P1-79330 Radical orchiectomy for tumor by inguinal approach
P1-79332 Radical orchiectomy for tumor by inguinal approach with abdominal exploration
P1-79336 Simple orchiectomy with placement of testicular prosthesis by scrotal approach
P1-79350 Biopsy of epididymis
Exploration of epididymis with biopsy
P1-79352 Core needle biopsy of epididymis
P1-79353 Fine needle biopsy of epididymis
Fine needle aspiration biopsy of epididymis
P1-79354 Excision of lesion of epididymis
P1-79356 Excision of appendix of epididymis
P1-79358 Removal of foreign body of epididymis
P1-79360 Epididymectomy, NOS
Excision of epididymis
P1-79361 Unilateral epididymectomy
P1-79362 Bilateral epididymectomy
P1-79370 Excision of hydatid of Morgagni in male
Excision of appendix of testis
P1-79372 Excision of spermatocele
Excision of spermatocele without epididymectomy
Spermatocelectomy
Spermatocystectomy
P1-79374 Excision of spermatocele with epididymectomy

1-795 Testis and Epididymis: Injections and Implantations

P1-79500 Injection of testis, NOS
P1-79502 Injection of therapeutic substance into testis
P1-79510 Insertion of testicular prosthesis
Implantation of testicular prosthesis
P1-79512 Removal of testicular prosthesis
P1-79520V Electroejaculation procedure

1-797 Testis and Epididymis: Endoscopy

P1-79710 Endoscopy of testis, NOS
P1-79740 Endoscopy of epididymis, NOS

1-798 Testis and Epididymis: Surgical Repairs, Closures and Reconstructions

P1-79800 Repair of testis, NOS
  Orchidoplasty, NOS
  Orchioplasty, NOS
  Repair of testicular injury, NOS
P1-79802 Suture of laceration of testis
  Orchidorrhaphy
  Suture of testis
P1-79810 Orchidopexy
  Orchiopexy
P1-79812 Surgical reduction of torsion of testis
  Surgical release of torsion of testis
  Surgical detorsion of testis
P1-79813 Surgical reduction of torsion of testis with orchiopexy
P1-79814 Surgical reduction of torsion of testis with fixation of contralateral testis
P1-79815 Lord operation orchiopexy
P1-79816 Looposcopy orchiopexy
P1-79821 Orchiopexy, any type, second stage
  Torek operation for orchiopexy
P1-79824 Orchiopexy, any type, with hernia repair
P1-79826 Orchiopexy, any type, with hernia repair, second stage
P1-79831 Fixation of contralateral testis
P1-79832 Mobilization of testis in scrotum
P1-79850 Epididymoplasty, NOS
  Repair of epididymis
P1-79852 Repair of epididymis and spermatic cord, NOS
P1-79853 Epididymovasostomy, NOS
  Repair of epididymis and vas deferens
  Repair of vas deferens by anastomosis to epididymis
  Anastomosis of epididymis to vas deferens
P1-79854 Unilateral epididymovasostomy with anastomosis of epididymis to vas deferens
P1-79855 Bilateral epididymovasostomy with anastomosis of epididymis to vas deferens
P1-79860 Epididymorrhaphy, NOS
  Suture of laceration of epididymis
P1-79862 Suture of laceration of epididymis and spermatic cord

1-79C Testis and Epididymis: Destructive Procedures

P1-79C00 Destruction of lesion of testis, NOS

1-79D Testis and Epididymis: Transplantations and Transpositions

P1-79D00 Transplantation of testis, NOS
  Graft of testis, NOS
P1-79D02 Transplantation of testis to thigh
P1-79D10 Transplantation of testis to scrotum
  Reimplantation of testis in scrotum
  Replacement of testis in scrotum

1-79E Testis and Epididymis: Manipulations

P1-79E10 Manipulation of testis, NOS
P1-79E20 Manipulation of epididymis, NOS

1-7A OPERATIVE PROCEDURES ON THE SCROTUM, VAS DEFERENS AND SEMINAL VESICLE

1-7A0 Scrotum, Vas Deferens and Seminal Vesicle: General and Miscellaneous Operative Procedures

P1-7A000 Operation on scrotum, NOS
P1-7A010 Operation on vas deferens, NOS
P1-7A020 Operation on spermatic cord, NOS
P1-7A030 Operation on seminal vesicle, NOS

1-7A1 Scrotum, Vas Deferens and Seminal Vesicle: Incisions

P1-7A100 Incision of scrotum, NOS
  Scrototomy
P1-7A101 Incision and exploration of scrotum
P1-7A102 Drainage of scrotal wall abscess
P1-7A120 Incision of vas deferens, NOS
  Vasotomy
P1-7A122 Unilateral vasotomy
P1-7A124 Bilateral vasotomy
P1-7A125 Incision and exploration of vas deferens
P1-7A128 Vasotomy for vasograms, vesiculograms or epididymograms
P1-7A130 Incision of abscess of vas deferens
P1-7A150 Incision of spermatic cord, NOS
P1-7A151 Incision and exploration of spermatic cord
P1-7A160 Incision of tunica vaginalis, NOS
P1-7A161 Incision and exploration of tunica vaginalis
P1-7A162 Incision and drainage of tunica vaginalis
P1-7A164 Aspiration of hydrocele of tunica vaginalis
P1-7A165 Puncture aspiration of hydrocele of tunica vaginalis with injection of medication
P1-7A180 Incision of seminal vesicle, NOS
  Seminal vesiculotomy
P1-7A184 Complicated seminal vesiculotomy
P1-7A190 Percutaneous aspiration of seminal vesicle
P1-7A192 Spermatocystotomy

1-7A3 Scrotum, Vas Deferens and Seminal Vesicle: Excisions

P1-7A300 Excisional biopsy of scrotum
P1-7A302 Excision of lesion of scrotum
P1-7A310 Scrotectomy, NOS
  Resection of scrotum
P1-7A312 Partial scrotectomy
  Excision of tissue of scrotum
  Reduction of elephantiasis of scrotum
P1-7A314 Removal of foreign body of scrotum

P1-7A320 Biopsy of vas deferens
P1-7A322 Unilateral segmental vasectomy
P1-7A324 Bilateral segmental vasectomy and ligation
P1-7A326 Bilateral vasectomy including postoperative semen examination
P1-7A330 Removal of ligature of vas deferens
P1-7A332 Removal of valve of vas deferens
P1-7A334 Removal of foreign body of vas deferens
P1-7A340 Biopsy of tunica vaginalis
P1-7A341 Excision of lesion of tunica vaginalis
P1-7A342 Excision of hematocele of tunica vaginalis
P1-7A350 Hydrocelectomy, NOS
  Excision of hydrocele of tunica vaginalis
  Hydrocelectomy of tunica vaginalis
P1-7A351 Unilateral excision of hydrocele
P1-7A352 Bilateral excision of hydrocele
P1-7A357 Removal of foreign body of tunica vaginalis
P1-7A358 Hydrocelectomy of male canal of Nuck
P1-7A370 Biopsy of spermatic cord
P1-7A371 Excision of lesion of spermatic cord
P1-7A372 Excision of hydrocele of spermatic cord
  Hydrocelectomy of spermatic cord
P1-7A376 Excision of varicocele
P1-7A377 Excision of varicocele by abdominal approach
P1-7A378 Excision of varicocele with hernia repair
P1-7A379 Removal of foreign body of spermatic cord
P1-7A390 Biopsy of seminal vesicle
P1-7A391 Core needle biopsy of seminal vesicle
P1-7A392 Fine needle biopsy of seminal vesicle
  Fine needle aspiration biopsy of seminal vesicle
P1-7A394 Seminal vesiculectomy
  Seminal vesiculectomy by any approach
  Excision of seminal vesicle
P1-7A398 Excision of cyst of Müllerian duct in male

1-7A5 Scrotum, Vas Deferens and Seminal Vesicle: Injections and Implantations

P1-7A500 Injection of scrotum, NOS
P1-7A510 Insertion of valve in vas deferens

1-7A7 Scrotum, Vas Deferens and Seminal Vesicle: Endoscopy

P1-7A700 Endoscopy of scrotum, NOS

1-7A8 Scrotum, Vas Deferens and Seminal Vesicle: Surgical Repairs, Closures and Reconstructions

P1-7A800 Repair of scrotum, NOS
P1-7A801 Simple scrotoplasty
P1-7A802 Complicated scrotoplasty
P1-7A810 Suture of scrotum
  Scrotorrhaphy
  Suture of laceration of scrotum
P1-7A812 Repair of fistula of scrotum
  Closure of fistula of scrotum
P1-7A814 Reconstruction of scrotum with graft
  Graft of scrotum
P1-7A820 Repair of vas deferens, NOS
P1-7A824 Surgical reanastomosis of vas deferens
  Vasovasostomy
  Reestablishment of continuity of vas deferens
  Reconstruction of surgically divided vas deferens
  Repair of vas deferens by reconstruction
  Vasovasorrhaphy
P1-7A830 Vasorrhaphy, NOS
P1-7A832 Suture of laceration of vas deferens
P1-7A850 Repair of spermatic cord, NOS
P1-7A852 Suture of spermatic cord
  Repair of spermatic cord laceration
P1-7A856 Reduction of torsion of spermatic cord
  Detorsion of spermatic cord
P1-7A858 Repair of varicocele
P1-7A870 Repair of tunica vaginalis
P1-7A872 Suture of tunica vaginalis
  Repair of tunica vaginalis laceration
P1-7A874 Inversion of tunica vaginalis

1-7AC Scrotum, Vas Deferens and Seminal Vesicle: Destructive Procedures

P1-7AC00 Destruction of lesion of scrotum, NOS
P1-7AC10 Fulguration of scrotum
P1-7AC20 Ligation of vas deferens
  Vasoligation
P1-7AC22 Crushing of vas deferens
P1-7AC24 Division of vas deferens
  Transection of vas deferens
P1-7AC30 Ligation of spermatic cord
P1-7AC34 Lysis of adhesions of spermatic cord
P1-7AC40 Ligation of varicocele
  Vidal operation for varicocele
  High ligation of spermatic vein
P1-7AC42 Ligation of spermatic veins for varicocele by abdominal approach
P1-7AC44 Ligation of spermatic veins for varicocele with hernia repair

1-7AD Scrotum, Vas Deferens and Seminal Vesicle: Transplantations and Transpositions

P1-7AD10 Transplantation of scrotal tissue, NOS
P1-7AD20 Transplantation of vas deferens, NOS
P1-7AD30 Transplantation of seminal vesicle, NOS
P1-7AD50 Transposition of scrotal tissue, NOS
P1-7AD60 Transposition of vas deferens, NOS
P1-7AD70 Transposition of seminal vesicle, NOS

1-7AE Scrotum, Vas Deferens and Seminal Vesicle: Manipulations

P1-7AE10 Manipulation of scrotal tissue, NOS
P1-7AE20 Manipulation of vas deferens, NOS
P1-7AE30 Manipulation of seminal vesicle, NOS

SECTION 1-8 OPERATIVE PROCEDURES ON THE FEMALE GENITAL SYSTEM INCLUDING OBSTETRICS

1-80 GENERAL OPERATIVE PROCEDURES ON THE FEMALE GENITAL SYSTEM

1-800 Female Genital System: General and Miscellaneous Operative Procedures

P1-80000 Operation on female genital organs, NOS
P1-80020 Removal of device from female genital tract, NOS
P1-80030V Surgical sexing, female
P1-80034V Estrus synchronization with implants

1-81 OPERATIVE PROCEDURES ON THE VULVA

1-810 Vulva: General and Miscellaneous Operative Procedures

P1-81010 Operation on vulva, NOS
  Operation on labia, NOS
P1-81020 Operation on clitoris, NOS
P1-81030 Operation on Bartholin's gland, NOS

1-811 Vulva: Incisions

P1-81100 Incision of vulva
  Incision of labia
P1-81110 Incision and exploration of vulva
  Incision and exploration of labia
P1-81120 Incision and drainage of vulva
P1-81124 Evacuation of hematoma of vulva
P1-81130 Clitoridotomy
  Female circumcision
P1-81140 Incision of Skene's duct or gland
  Division of Skene's gland
P1-81142 Incision of Bartholin's cyst
P1-81144 Incision and drainage of Bartholin's gland abscess
P1-81150 Aspiration of Bartholin's cyst

1-813 Vulva: Excisions

P1-81300 Biopsy of vulva
  Biopsy of labia
P1-81302 Excision of lesion of vulva
  Excision of lesion of labia
  Local excision of lesion of vulva
P1-81303 Excision of cyst of vulva
  Excision of cyst of labia
P1-81310 Removal of foreign body from vulva
  Removal of foreign body from labia
P1-81311 Removal of foreign body from vulva by incision
  Removal of foreign body from labia by incision
P1-81314 Excision of redundant mucosa of vulva
P1-81320 Vulvectomy, NOS
P1-81322 Unilateral vulvectomy
  Unilateral labiectomy
P1-81324 Partial unilateral vulvectomy
P1-81326 Partial vulvectomy, less than 80% of vulvar area
P1-81328 Bilateral vulvectomy
  Complete bilateral vulvectomy
  Block dissection of vulva
  Bilateral labiectomy
  Bilateral excision of vulva
P1-81330 Radical vulvectomy without skin graft
P1-81332 Radical vulvectomy with inguinofemoral lymphadenectomy
P1-81334 Bassett operation for vulvectomy with inguinal lymph node dissection
P1-81336 Radical vulvectomy with inguinofemoral, iliac and pelvic lymphadenectomy
P1-81350 Biopsy of clitoris
P1-81352 Clitoridectomy
  Simple clitoridectomy
  Resection of clitoris
  Amputation of clitoris
P1-81354 Extensive clitoridectomy
P1-81360 Excision of Bartholin's cyst
P1-81362 Excision of hydrocele of canal of Nuck in female
  Hydrocelectomy of canal of Nuck in female
  Excision of canal of Nuck
P1-81364 Excision of Skene's gland

1-815 Vulva: Injections and Implantations

P1-81500 Injection of vulva, NOS
P1-81520 Replacement of drain of vulva
P1-81522 Removal of packing of vulva
P1-81524 Replacement of packing of vulva

1-817 Vulva: Endoscopy

P1-81700 Endoscopic procedure on vulva, NOS

1-818 Vulva: Surgical Repairs, Closures and Reconstructions

P1-81800 Repair of vulva, NOS
P1-81802 Repair of laceration of vulva
  Suture of labia
  Suture of vulva
P1-81803V Caslick operation
P1-81804 Repair of old obstetrical laceration of vulva
  Suture of old obstetrical laceration of vulva
P1-81806 Suture of clitoris
P1-81810 Repair of fistula of vulva
  Closure of fistula of vulva
P1-81830 Episiorrhaphy
  Episioplasty
P1-81832 Episioperineorrhaphy
  Episioperineoplasty

1-81C Vulva: Destructive Procedures

P1-81C11 Simple destruction of lesion of vulva
  Local destruction of lesion of vulva
P1-81C14 Extensive destruction of lesion of vulva
P1-81C20 Lysis of adhesions of vulva
P1-81C30 Cryotherapy of genital warts
P1-81C32 Cauterization of vulva
P1-81C34 Fulguration of vulva
P1-81C35 Electrocoagulation of vulva
P1-81C40 Destruction of Bartholin's gland or cyst
P1-81C41 Destruction of lesion of Bartholin's gland, NOS
P1-81C42 Destruction of lesion of Bartholin's gland by aspiration
P1-81C44 Destruction of lesion of Bartholin's gland by incision
P1-81C46 Destruction of lesion of Bartholin's gland by marsupialization
  Marsupialization of Bartholin's gland cyst
P1-81C47 Cauterization of Bartholin's gland
P1-81C50 Obliteration of Skene's gland
  Fulguration of Skene's gland

1-81D Vulva: Transplantations and Transpositions

P1-81D10 Transplantation of vulvar tissue, NOS
P1-81D20 Transposition of vulvar tissue, NOS

1-81E Vulva: Manipulations

P1-81E10 Manipulation of tissue of vulva, NOS

1-82 OPERATIVE PROCEDURES ON THE VAGINA

1-820 Vagina: General and Miscellaneous Operative Procedures

P1-82010 Operation on vagina, NOS
P1-82014 Operation on cul-de-sac, NOS
P1-82040 Operation on hymen, NOS

1-821 Vagina: Incisions

P1-82100 Incision of vagina
  Colpotomy
  Vaginotomy
P1-82102 Incision and exploration of vagina
  Colpotomy with exploration
P1-82103 Incision and exploration of cul-de-sac
P1-82106 Division of vaginal septum
P1-82108 Incision of hematoma of vagina
  Evacuation of hematoma of vagina
P1-82110 Nonobstetrical episiotomy
  Vaginoperineotomy
P1-82130 Incision of cul-de-sac
  Culdotomy
  Incision of pouch of Douglas
P1-82132 Colpoceliocentesis
  Culdocentesis
  Colpocentesis
  Drainage of cul-de-sac by aspiration
  Vaginotomy for culdocentesis
P1-82134 Evacuation of pelvic blood clot by culdocentesis
P1-82140 Colpotomy for pelvic peritoneal drainage
  Drainage of female pelvic peritoneum by incision
  Incision and drainage of cul-de-sac
P1-82142 Colpotomy with drainage of pelvic abscess
  Vaginotomy for pelvic abscess
  Incision of vagina for pelvic abscess
  Aspiration of cul-de-sac abscess
P1-82150 Incision of hymen
  Hymenotomy
  Surgical defloration

1-823 Vagina: Excisions

P1-82300 Vaginal biopsy
  Simple biopsy of vaginal mucosa
P1-82302 Extensive biopsy of vaginal mucosa requiring suture
P1-82304 Excision of lesion of vagina
P1-82305 Excision of vaginal cyst
P1-82306 Excision of vaginal tumor
P1-82307 Excision of cyst of Gartner's duct
P1-82308 Vaginal enterocelectomy
P1-82310 Excision of vaginal septum, NOS
P1-82312 Excision of urethrovaginal septum
P1-82314 Excision of vesicovaginal septum
P1-82320 Removal of foreign body from vagina by incision
P1-82350 Vaginectomy, NOS
  Colpectomy, NOS
P1-82352 Partial colpectomy
P1-82354 Complete excision of vagina
  Obliteration and total excision of vagina
  Complete colpectomy
P1-82360 Hymenectomy
P1-82362 Excision of hymenal tag
P1-82364 Excision of hymeno-urethral fusion
P1-82370 Biopsy of cul-de-sac
P1-82372 Excision of lesion of cul-de-sac
  Excision of lesion of pouch of Douglas
P1-82374 Excision of vaginal cul-de-sac
P1-82376 Endometrectomy of cul-de-sac

1-825 Vagina: Injections and Implantations

P1-82510 Insertion of diaphragm into vagina
P1-82511 Replacement of diaphragm into vagina
P1-82512 Removal of diaphragm from vagina
P1-82514 Insertion of pessary into vagina
P1-82515 Replacement of pessary in vagina
P1-82516 Removal of pessary from vagina
P1-82517 Insertion of drain into vagina
P1-82518 Replacement of drain of vagina
P1-82519 Removal of drain from vagina

1-825 Vagina: Injections and Implantations — Continued

P1-82520 Nonobstetrical insertion of pack into vagina
Tamponade of vagina
Insertion of tampon into vagina
Packing of vagina
P1-82521 Replacement of vaginal packing
Replacement of pack of vagina
P1-82522 Introduction of packing for spontaneous or traumatic nonobstetrical vaginal hemorrhage
P1-82523 Introduction of hemostatic agent for spontaneous or traumatic nonobstetrical vaginal hemorrhage
P1-82524 Removal of packing from vagina
P1-82525 Removal of intraluminal foreign body from vagina without incision
P1-82526 Insertion of mold into vagina
P1-82530 Insertion of suppository into vagina
P1-82534 Insertion of laminaria into vagina
P1-82540 Vaginal implantation of radium
P1-82550 Douche of vagina
P1-82552 Irrigation of vagina and application of medicament for treatment of bacterial disease
P1-82553 Irrigation of vagina and application of medicament for treatment of fungal disease
P1-82554 Irrigation of vagina and application of medicament for treatment of parasitic disease

1-827 Vagina: Endoscopy

P1-82700 Endoscopy of vagina
Colposcopy
Vaginoscopy
Endoscopic exploration of vagina
P1-82704 Vaginoscopy with biopsy of vagina
P1-82706 Vaginoscopy with biopsy of cervix
P1-82710 Endoscopy of cul-de-sac
Culdoscopy
Endoscopic exploration of cul-de-sac
P1-82714 Diagnostic culdoscopy with biopsy
P1-82716 Diagnostic culdoscopy with lysis of adhesions
P1-82717 Diagnostic culdoscopy with biopsy and lysis of adhesions
P1-82718 Diagnostic culdoscopy with tubal sterilization
P1-82719 Culdoscopy with removal of foreign body
P1-8271A Evacuation of pelvic blood clot by culdoscopy

1-828-829 Vagina: Surgical Repairs, Closures and Reconstructions

P1-82800 Repair of vagina, NOS
Vaginoplasty, NOS
Colpoplasty, NOS
P1-82802 Suture of vagina
Colporrhaphy
Vaginorrhaphy
Suture of laceration of vagina
Repair of laceration of vagina
P1-82803 Suture of old obstetrical laceration of vagina
Repair of old obstetrical pelvic floor laceration
P1-82806 Culdoplasty
Repair of of hernia cul-de-sac
Obliteration of cul-de-sac
Repair of pouch of Douglas
P1-82807 Partial obliteration of vagina
Partial colpocleisis
P1-82808 Total obliteration of vagina
Obliteration of vaginal vault
Closure of vagina
Complete colpocleisis
P1-82809 Colpocleisis, Le Fort type
Le Fort operation on vagina
P1-8280A Goodal-Power operation on vagina
P1-8280B Latzko operation on vagina
P1-82810 Plastic repair of introitus
P1-82812 Vaginal construction, NOS
Colpopoiesis, NOS
Reconstruction of vagina
P1-82820 Construction of artificial vagina, NOS
Construction of artificial vagina without graft
P1-82824 Construction of artificial vagina with graft
P1-82825 Abbe operation for construction of vagina
P1-82826 McIndoe operation for construction of vagina
P1-82827 Williams-Richardson operation for construction of vagina
P1-82830 Vaginopexy, NOS
Suspension of vagina
Vaginal suspension and fixation
Colpopexy, NOS
Fixation of vagina, NOS
P1-82831 Colpopexy by abdominal approach
P1-82832 Urethrovaginal fixation
P1-82833 Harrison-Richardson operation on vagina
P1-82834 Norman Miller operation on vagina
P1-82836 Sacrospinous ligament fixation to vagina for prolapse
P1-82840 Repair of vaginal fistula, NOS
Closure of fistula of vagina, NOS
P1-82842 Repair of intestinovaginal fistula, NOS
Closure of enterovaginal fistula
Repair of vaginoenteric fistula, NOS
Repair of enterovaginal fistula
Closure of intestinovaginal fistula
P1-82843 Repair of vaginoileal fistula
Closure of vaginoileal fistula
P1-82844 Repair of colovaginal fistula
Closure of colovaginal fistula
P1-82845 Repair of sigmoidovaginal fistula
Closure of sigmoidovaginal fistula
P1-82850 Repair of rectovaginal fistula, NOS
Closure of rectovaginal fistula, NOS
P1-82852 Closure of rectovaginal fistula by abdominal approach

P1-82854 Closure of rectovaginal fistula by abdominal approach with concomitant colostomy
P1-82856 Closure of rectovaginal fistula by transanal approach
P1-82858 Closure of rectovaginal fistula by vaginal approach
P1-82860 Repair of vaginocutaneous fistula
Closure of vaginocutaneous fistula
P1-82862 Repair of vaginoperineal fistula
Closure of vaginoperineal fistula
P1-82864 Closure of urethrovaginal fistula
P1-82866 Closure of urethrovaginal fistula with bulbocavernosus transplant
P1-82868 Closure of vesicovaginal fistula by transvesical and vaginal approach
P1-82869 Closure of vesicovaginal fistula by vaginal approach
P1-82870 Colpoepisiorrhaphy
Colpoperineoplasty
Colpoperineorrhaphy
P1-82900 Anterior colporrhaphy
Anterior repair of vagina
P1-82902 Colporrhaphy for repair of cystocele
Repair of cystocele
Anterior colporrhaphy for repair of cystocele without repair of urethrocele
P1-82904 Colporrhaphy for repair of urethrocele
Repair of urethrocele
P1-82905 Colpoperineoplasty with repair of urethrocele
P1-82908 Anterior colporrhaphy for repair of cystocele with repair of urethrocele
P1-82909 Pereyra procedure including anterior colporrhaphy
P1-82920 Posterior repair of vagina
Posterior colporrhaphy
Repair of rectocele
Posterior colporrhaphy for repair of rectocele without perineorrhaphy
Colporrhaphy for repair of rectocele
P1-82922 Posterior colporrhaphy for repair of rectocele with perineorrhaphy
P1-82930 Combined anteroposterior colporrhaphy
Anterior and posterior repair of vagina
Colporrhaphy for repair of cystocele and rectocele
Repair of cystocele and rectocele
P1-82932 Combined anteroposterior colporrhaphy with enterocele repair
P1-82934 Colporrhaphy for repair of enterocele
Repair of enterocele by colporrhaphy
Suture of enterocele by colporrhaphy
P1-82935 Repair of enterocele by abdominal approach
P1-82936 Repair of enterocele by vaginal approach
P1-82938 McCall culdoplasty
P1-82939 Moschowitz enterocele repair
P1-82950 Repair of hymen
Hymenorrhaphy
Plastic revision of hymen
Suture of hymen
Hymenoplasty

1-82C Vagina: Destructive Procedures

P1-82C00 Destruction of lesion of vagina, NOS
P1-82C02 Extensive destruction of lesion of vagina
P1-82C04 Cauterization of lesion of vagina
P1-82C06 Electrocoagulation of lesion of vagina
P1-82C10 Lysis of adhesions of vagina
P1-82C20 Destruction of lesion of cul-de-sac

1-82D Vagina: Transplantations and Transpositions

P1-82D10 Transplantation of vaginal tissue, NOS
P1-82D20 Transposition of vaginal tissue, NOS

1-82E Vagina: Manipulations

P1-82E00 Manipulation of vagina, NOS
P1-82E10 Dilation of vagina, NOS
Enlargement of introitus of vagina
P1-82E14 Dilation of vagina under anesthesia

1-83 OPERATIVE PROCEDURES ON THE UTERUS AND CERVIX

1-830 Uterus and Cervix: General and Miscellaneous Operative Procedures

P1-83010 Operation on uterus, NOS
P1-83030 Operation on cervix, NOS
P1-83060 Operation on uterus supporting structures, NOS
P1-83061 Operation on uterine ligament, NOS
P1-83062 Operation on round ligament, NOS
P1-83064 Operation on broad ligament, NOS

1-831 Uterus and Cervix: Incisions

P1-83100 Incision of uterus, NOS
Hysterotomy, NOS
P1-83102 Colpohysterotomy
P1-83110 Abdominouterotomy
P1-83120 Incision and exploration of uterus
P1-83122 Incision of congenital septum of uterus
P1-83130 Uterocentesis
P1-83140 Incision of hematoma of broad ligament
P1-83142 Division of uterosacral ligament
Detachment of uterosacral ligament
P1-83150 Incision of uterine cervix
Nonobstetric trachelotomy
Incision of cervix
Hysterotrachelotomy

1-833-834 Uterus and Cervix: Excisions

P1-83300 Excision of uterus and supporting structures, NOS
P1-83301 Open biopsy of uterus
Incisional biopsy of uterus

1-833-834 Uterus and Cervix: Excisions — Continued

P1-83304 Core needle biopsy of uterus
P1-83305 Fine needle biopsy of uterus
  Fine needle aspiration biopsy of uterus
P1-83306 Excision of lesion of uterus
P1-83307 Removal of intraluminal foreign body from uterus without incision
P1-83308 Hysterotomy with removal of foreign body
P1-83310 Dilation and curettage, NOS
  Curettage of uterus
  Uterine endometrectomy
  Biopsy of endometrium with dilation and curettage
P1-83311 Diagnostic dilation and curettage of uterus
P1-83312 Therapeutic dilation and curettage of uterus
P1-83313 Office endometrial curettage
P1-83314 Diagnostic aspiration curettage of uterus
  Aspiration curettage of endometrium
  Endometrial biopsy by suction
P1-83320 Open biopsy of endometrium
P1-83321 Open excision of lesion of endometrium
P1-83322 Excision of septum of uterus
  Excision of congenital septum of uterus
P1-83324 Excision of endometrial synechiae
P1-83342 Hysterotomy with removal of hydatidiform mole
P1-83350 Hysterectomy, NOS
  Bonney operation hysterectomy
  Total abdominal hysterectomy, NOS
  Total hysterectomy without removal of tube or ovary
  Richardson operation hysterectomy
  Abdominohysterectomy
  Abdominal panhysterectomy
P1-83351 Repair of intestinouterine fistula
P1-83352 Partial or subtotal hysterectomy
  Subtotal abdominal hysterectomy
  Bell-Beuttner operation for subtotal abdominal hysterectomy
  Uterine fundectomy
  Supracervical hysterectomy without removal of tube or ovary
P1-83353 Total hysterectomy with removal of both tubes and ovaries
  Bilateral hysterosalpingo-ovariectomy
P1-83356 Total hysterectomy with unilateral removal of tube and ovary
P1-83357 Total hysterectomy with unilateral removal of ovary
P1-83358 Total hysterectomy with unilateral removal of tube
P1-83360 Vaginal hysterectomy
  Vaginal panhysterectomy
  Colpohysterectomy
  Mayo operation for vaginal hysterectomy
  Tuffier operation for vaginal hysterectomy
  Ward-Mayo operation for vaginal hysterectomy
  Heaney operation for vaginal hysterectomy
P1-83362 Supracervical hysterectomy with unilateral removal of tube and ovary
P1-83364 Supracervical hysterectomy with removal of both tubes and ovaries
P1-83365 Supracervical hysterectomy without removal of tubes with removal of ovary
P1-83366 Vaginal hysterectomy with partial colpectomy
P1-83367 Vaginal hysterectomy with total colpectomy
P1-83369 Radical vaginal hysterocolpectomy
  Radical vaginal hysterectomy, Schauta type operation
P1-8336A Vaginal hysterectomy with repair of enterocele
P1-8336B Vaginal hysterectomy with partial colpectomy and repair of enterocele
P1-8336C Vaginal hysterectomy with total colpectomy and repair of enterocele
P1-8336D Vaginal hysterectomy with colpo-urethrocystopexy, Marshall-Marchetti-Krantz type
P1-8336E Vaginal hysterectomy with colpo-urethrocystopexy, Pereyra type
P1-83380 Radical abdominal hysterectomy
  Wertheim operation
  Abdominal hysterocolpectomy
P1-83384 Abdominal hysterectomy with colpo-urethrocystopexy, Marshall-Marchetti-Krantz type
P1-83386 Total hysterectomy including partial vaginectomy with limited para-aortic and pelvic lymph node biopsy
P1-83388 Radical hysterectomy with bilateral total pelvic and limited para-aortic lymphadenectomy
P1-83390 Uterine myomectomy, NOS
  Uterine fibroidectomy
  Hysteromyomectomy
P1-83392 Myomectomy of uterus, single, by abdominal approach
P1-83393 Myomectomy of uterus, single, by vaginal approach
P1-83394 Myomectomy of uterus, multiple, by abdominal approach
P1-83395 Myomectomy of uterus, multiple, by vaginal approach
P1-83400 Cervical biopsy, NOS
P1-83401 Excision of lesion of cervix, NOS
P1-83402 Biopsy of cervix with fulguration
  Local excision of single lesion of cervix with fulguration
P1-83403 Biopsy of cervix, multiple
  Local excision of multiple lesions of cervix
P1-83404 Biopsy of cervix, multiple, with fulguration
  Local excision of multiple lesions of cervix with fulguration
P1-83405 Excision of myoma of cervix
  Schroeder operation for cervical myomectomy

P1-83409 Dilation and curettage of cervical stump
P1-8340A Excision of uterosacral ligament
P1-8340B Excision of Müllerian duct
Excision of paramesonephric duct
P1-8340D Excision of Wolffian duct
Excision of mesonephric duct
P1-83420 Cone biopsy of cervix, NOS
Conization of uterine cervix
Cone biopsy of cervix without dilation and curettage, without repair
P1-83421 Excision of cervix by cryoconization
Cold knife cone biopsy of cervix
P1-83422 Excision of cervix by electroconization
P1-83423 LOOP electro excision of cervix
LEEP procedure of cervix
P1-83425 Punch biopsy of cervix
P1-83426 Cone biopsy of cervix with dilation, curettage and with repair
P1-83428 Cone biopsy of cervix without dilation and curettage, with Sturmdorf type repair
Sturmdorf operation
P1-83440 Amputation of cervix
Cervicectomy
Trachelectomy
Excision of cervical stump
Hysterotrachelectomy
P1-83441 Excision of cervical stump by abdominal approach
P1-83442 Excision of cervical stump by vaginal approach
P1-83443 Excision of cervical stump by abdominal approach with pelvic floor repair
P1-83444 Excision of cervical stump by vaginal approach with anterior repair
P1-83445 Excision of cervical stump by vaginal approach with posterior repair
P1-83446 Excision of cervical stump by vaginal approach with repair of enterocele
P1-83447 Excision of cervical stump by vaginal approach with anterior and posterior repair
P1-83448 Cervicectomy with synchronous colporrhaphy
P1-83450 Removal of penetrating foreign body from cervix
P1-83452 Removal of cerclage material from cervix
Removal of Shirodkar suture from cervix
P1-83456 Removal of intraluminal foreign body from cervix
P1-83460 Endocervical biopsy
P1-83462 Endocervical curettage
P1-83480 Biopsy of uterine ligaments, NOS
P1-83481 Incisional biopsy of uterine ligaments, NOS
Open biopsy of uterine ligaments, NOS
P1-83482 Core needle biopsy of uterine ligament
P1-83484 Fine needle biopsy of uterine ligament
Fine needle aspiration biopsy of uterine ligament
P1-83486 Excision of lesion of uterine ligament
Excision of lesion of broad ligament
P1-83490 Excision of lesion of round ligament
P1-83491 Excision of lesion of uterosacral ligament
P1-83492 Excision of cyst of broad ligament
Enucleation of cyst of broad ligament
P1-83493 Excision of cyst of mesonephric duct
P1-83494 Excision of parovarian cyst
P1-83495 Myomectomy of broad ligament
P1-83496 Excision of hydrocele of round ligament
Hydrocelectomy of round ligament
P1-83497 Excision of uterine ligament
Resection of uterine ligament
P1-83498 Excision of round ligament
Resection of round ligament
P1-83499 Excision of broad ligament
Resection of broad ligament

1-835 Uterus and Cervix: Injections and Implantations

P1-83500 Injection of uterus, NOS
P1-83510 Insertion of intrauterine contraceptive device, NOS
Insertion of intrauterine device
Insertion of IUD
P1-83511 Removal of intrauterine device, NOS
Removal of intrauterine contraceptive device
P1-83512 Replacement of IUD
P1-83520 Insertion of therapeutic device into uterus, NOS
P1-83522 Nonobstetric insertion of intrauterine tamponade
Insertion of tampon into uterus
Nonobstetric intrauterine tamponade
P1-83523 Removal of intrauterine pack
P1-83530 Insertion of pessary into cervix
P1-83534 Nonobstetrical insertion of bougie into cervix
P1-83540 Insertion of laminaria into cervix
P1-83541 Removal of laminaria from uterus

1-837 Uterus and Cervix: Endoscopy

P1-83700 Hysteroscopy, NOS
Endoscopy of uterus
Endoscopic examination of uterus
P1-83702 Diagnostic hysteroscopy
P1-83712 Laparoscopic biopsy of uterus
P1-83714 Laparoscopic biopsy of uterine ligaments
P1-83720 Hysteroscopy with biopsy
P1-83722 Hysteroscopy with lysis of intrauterine adhesions
P1-83724 Hysteroscopy with removal of submucous leiomyomata
P1-83726 Hysteroscopy with resection of intrauterine septum

1-838-839 Uterus and Cervix: Surgical Repairs, Closures and Reconstructions

P1-83800 Repair of uterus, NOS
 Hysteroplasty
 Metroplasty
P1-83801 Repair of uterus and supporting structures, NOS
P1-83802 Suture of uterus
 Suture of laceration of uterus
 Nonobstetrical hysterorrhaphy for repair of ruptured uterus
 Hysterorrhaphy
P1-83803 Suture of old obstetrical laceration of uterus
P1-83804 Hysterotrachelorrhaphy
P1-83806 Hysterotracheloplasty
P1-83810 Hysteroplasty for repair of uterine anomaly, Strassman type
 Strassman operation for uterine anomaly
P1-83820 Repair of inverted uterus, NOS
P1-83824 Repair of inverted uterus by vaginal approach
P1-83830 Surgical repair of prolapsed uterus
 Hysteropexy
 Suspension of uterus
 Uteropexy
 Uterine suspension without shortening of round ligaments or sacrouterine ligaments
P1-83831 Uterine suspension with shortening of round ligaments and sacrouterine ligaments
P1-83832 Ventrohysteropexy
 Ventrosuspension of uterus
 Ventrofixation of uterus
P1-83833 Fothergill operation on uterus
P1-83834 Fothergill-Donald operation on uterus
P1-83835 Manchester operation on uterus
P1-83836 Manchester-Donald operation on uterus
P1-83837 Manchester-Fothergill operation on uterus
P1-83838 Baldy-Webster operation on uterus
P1-83839 Coffey operation on uterus
P1-83840 Gilliam operation on uterus
P1-83841 Olshausen operation on uterus
P1-83842 Spaulding-Richardson operation on uterus
P1-83843 Duhrssen's operation on uterus
P1-83844 Watkins-Wertheim operation on uterus
P1-83845 Tomkins operation on uterus
P1-83846 Interposition operation for uterine suspension
P1-83847 Uterine suspension with presacral sympathectomy
P1-83850 Closure of fistula of uterus, NOS
P1-83851 Repair of uteroenteric fistula
 Repair of enterouterine fistula
 Repair of uterointestinal fistula
P1-83852 Repair of uterorectal fistula
 Repair of rectouterine fistula
P1-83853 Repair of abdominouterine fistula
P1-83854 Repair of uterovaginal fistula
P1-83860 Repair of cervix
 Cervicoplasty
 Uterine stomatoplasty
 Tracheloplasty
P1-83861 Repair of internal os of cervix
P1-83862 Suture of cervix
 Trachelorrhaphy by vaginal approach
 Suture of laceration of cervix
 Trachelorrhaphy
 Trachelorrhaphy, Emmet type
P1-83863 Repair of old obstetrical laceration of cervix
P1-83864 Repair of fistula of cervix
 Closure of fistula of cervix
P1-83865 Repair of cervicosigmoidal fistula
 Closure of cervicosigmoidal fistula
P1-83866 Marsupialization of nabothian cyst
P1-83868 Trachelopexy
P1-83910 Repair of uterine ligaments, NOS
 Suture of uterine ligaments, NOS
P1-83912 Repair of broad ligament of uterus
 Suture of broad ligament of uterus
P1-83914 Repair of round ligament of uterus
P1-83916 Shortening of round ligament of uterus
 Alexander operation for shortening of round ligaments
P1-83918 Shortening of endopelvic fascia
P1-83920 Advancement of round ligament
P1-83921 Shortening of uterosacral ligament
P1-83922 Adams operation on uterine ligaments
P1-83924 Alexander-Adams operation on uterine ligaments
P1-83926 Doleris operation on uterine ligaments
P1-83930 Repair of uterine ligaments by plication
P1-83931 Plication of broad ligament
P1-83932 Plication of round ligament
P1-83933 Plication of uterosacral ligament
 Suture of uterosacral ligament
 Suture of sacrouterine ligament
P1-83935 Fixation of cardinal ligament
P1-83936 Frommel operation on uterine ligaments
P1-83937 Reattachment of uterosacral ligament
P1-83940 Repair of uterine ligaments by interposition

1-83C Uterus and Cervix: Destructive Procedures

P1-83C00 Destructive procedure on uterus and supporting structures, NOS
P1-83C10 Hysterolysis, NOS
 Lysis of adhesions of uterus
P1-83C12 Intraluminal hysterolysis
 Division of endometrial synechiae
 Endometrial synechiotomy
 Lysis of uterine intraluminal adhesions
P1-83C16 Cauterization of uterus
 Coagulation of uterus
P1-83C18 Electrocoagulation of uterus
P1-83C20 Destruction of lesion of uterus, NOS
P1-83C50 Destruction of lesion of cervix
P1-83C60 Cryosurgery of lesion of cervix
 Initial cryocautery of cervix

P1-83C60 (cont.) Cryotherapy of cervix
P1-83C70 Cauterization of lesion of cervix
P1-83C72 Cauterization of cervix by laser surgery
P1-83C74 Electrocautery of cervix
Electrocoagulation of cervix
Electrocauterization of cervix
P1-83C76 Thermocauterization of cervix
P1-83C80 Cauterization of broad ligament
P1-83C82 Cauterization of round ligament
P1-83C84 Cauterization of uterosacral ligament
Electrocoagulation of broad ligament
P1-83C86 Electrocoagulation of round ligament
P1-83C88 Electrocoagulation of uterosacral ligament

1-83D Uterus and Cervix: Transplantations and Transpositions

P1-83D10 Transplantation of uterine tissue, NOS
P1-83D20 Transposition of uterine tissue, NOS

1-83E Uterus and Cervix: Manipulations

P1-83E10 Manual replacement of nonobstetric inverted uterus
Manual nonobstetric repair of inverted uterus
P1-83E20 Reduction of prolapse of uterus by pessary
P1-83E24 Reduction of retroversion of uterus by pessary
P1-83E30 Dilation of cervical canal

1-84 OPERATIVE PROCEDURES ON THE OVARIES AND FALLOPIAN TUBES

1-840 Ovaries and Fallopian Tubes: General and Miscellaneous Operative Procedures

P1-84000 Operation on ovary, NOS
P1-84010 Diagnostic procedure on ovary, NOS
P1-84050 Operation on fallopian tube, NOS
P1-84090 Female sterilization, NOS

1-841 Ovaries and Fallopian Tubes: Incisions

P1-84100 Incision of ovary, NOS
Oophorotomy, NOS
P1-84102 Salpingo-oophorotomy
P1-84110 Drainage of ovary by incision, NOS
P1-84112 Drainage of ovarian abscess by abdominal approach
P1-84114 Drainage of ovarian abscess by vaginal approach
P1-84116 Drainage of ovarian cyst by abdominal approach
P1-84118 Drainage of ovarian cyst by vaginal approach
P1-84120 Unilateral bisection of ovary
P1-84122 Bilateral bisection of ovary
P1-84130 Aspiration of ovary
P1-84150 Incision of fallopian tube
Salpingotomy
P1-84152 Incision and exploration of fallopian tube
P1-84160 Aspiration of fallopian tube
Puncture of fallopian tube with aspiration
P1-84180 Transection of fallopian tube by abdominal approach
P1-84182 Transection of fallopian tube by vaginal approach
P1-84184 Postpartum transection of fallopian tube by abdominal approach
P1-84185 Postpartum transection of fallopian tube by vaginal approach
P1-84186 Incidental transection of fallopian tube

1-843 Ovaries and Fallopian Tubes: Excisions

P1-84300 Biopsy of ovary
P1-84305 Core needle biopsy of ovary
P1-84306 Fine needle biopsy of ovary
Fine needle aspiration biopsy of ovary
P1-84310 Excision of lesion of ovary
P1-84312 Excision of cyst of ovary
Oophorocystectomy
Enucleation of ovarian cyst
Ovarian cystectomy
P1-84320 Local excision of ovary, NOS
P1-84321 Partial oophorectomy
Partial excision of ovary
P1-84322 Unilateral wedge resection of ovary
P1-84324 Bilateral wedge resection of ovary
P1-84326 Decortication of ovary
Capsulectomy of ovary
P1-84328V Removal of foreign body from ovary
P1-84330 Oophorectomy, NOS
P1-84331 Unilateral oophorectomy
P1-84332 Bilateral oophorectomy
Female castration
Spay operation
P1-84336 Unilateral salpingo-oophorectomy
Unilateral oophorectomy with salpingectomy
P1-84338 Bilateral salpingectomy with oophorectomy
Complete salpingo-oophorectomy
Bilateral salpingo-oophorectomy
P1-84339 Partial salpingo-oophorectomy
P1-84340 Oophorectomy of remaining ovary
Removal of remaining ovary
P1-84342 Oophorectomy of remaining ovary with tube
Salpingectomy of remaining tube with ovary
P1-84348V Ovariohysterectomy
P1-84350 Resection of ovarian malignancy with bilateral salpingo-oophorectomy and omentectomy
P1-84352 Resection of ovarian malignancy with bilateral salpingo-oophorectomy and omentectomy with radical node dissection

1-843 Ovaries and Fallopian Tubes: Excisions — Continued

P1-84354 Resection of ovarian malignancy with bilateral salpingo-oophorectomy and omentectomy with total abdominal hysterectomy and pelvic and limited para-aortic lymphadenectomy
P1-84356 Resection for ovarian malignancy with salpingo-oophorectomy, para-aortic and pelvic lymph node biopsies, peritoneal washings, peritoneal biopsies and diaphragmatic assessment
P1-84360 Biopsy of fallopian tube
P1-84362 Excision of lesion of fallopian tube
P1-84364 Excision of cyst of fallopian tube
  Excision of hydatid of Morgagni
P1-84370 Salpingectomy, NOS
P1-84371 Unilateral salpingectomy
P1-84372 Bilateral complete salpingectomy
  Removal of both fallopian tubes
P1-84374 Partial salpingectomy, NOS
P1-84375 Fimbriectomy of fallopian tube
P1-84376 Unilateral partial salpingectomy
  Unilateral resection of cornua of fallopian tube
P1-84377 Bilateral resection of cornua of fallopian tubes
P1-84378 Bilateral partial salpingectomy
P1-84379 Partial bilateral salpingectomy for sterilization
P1-8437A Salpingectomy of remaining fallopian tube
P1-84380 Removal of ligature from fallopian tube
P1-84384 Removal of foreign body from fallopian tube

1-845 Ovaries and Fallopian Tubes: Injections and Implantations

P1-84500 Injection of ovary, NOS
P1-84504 Injection of fallopian tube, NOS
P1-84510 Injection procedure for hysterosalpingography
P1-84520 Inflation of fallopian tube
  Rubin test on fallopian tube
  Insufflation of fallopian tube
P1-84521 Hydrotubation of oviduct
P1-84524 Inflation of fallopian tube with injection of therapeutic agent
P1-84550 Implantation of prosthesis into fallopian tube, NOS
  Insertion of prosthesis into fallopian tube, NOS
P1-84551 Replacement of prosthesis of fallopian tube
P1-84552 Implantation of Mulligan hood on fallopian tube
P1-84553 Replacement of Mulligan hood of fallopian tube
P1-84554 Replacement of stent of fallopian tube
P1-84560 Removal of prosthesis from fallopian tube
P1-84561 Removal of Mulligan hood from fallopian tube
P1-84562 Removal of silastic tubes from fallopian tube

1-847 Ovaries and Fallopian Tubes: Endoscopy

P1-84700 Endoscopy of ovary and fallopian tube, NOS
P1-84703 Bilateral endoscopic occlusion of fallopian tubes, NOS
P1-84704 Bilateral endoscopic destruction of fallopian tubes, NOS
P1-84710 Partial bilateral salpingectomy for sterilization by endoscopy
P1-84712 Bilateral segmental tubal excision and ligation by endoscopy
  Pomeroy procedure by endoscopy
P1-84713 Uchida fimbriectomy with tubal ligation by endoscopy
  Uchida operation on fallopian tube
P1-84714 Irving operation on fallopian tube
P1-84720 Ligation of fallopian tubes with division by endoscopy
  Transection of fallopian tubes by endoscopy
P1-84730 Laparoscopy with fulguration of oviducts
  Cauterization of fallopian tube by endoscopy
P1-84732 Bilateral endoscopic ligation and crushing of fallopian tubes
P1-84734 Bilateral endoscopic ligation and division of fallopian tubes
P1-84736 Laparoscopy with occlusion of oviducts by device
  Ligation of fallopian tubes with Falope ring by endoscopy
P1-84750 Laparoscopy with fulguration or excision of lesions of the ovary
P1-84760 Laparoscopy with removal of adnexal structures

1-848 Ovaries and Fallopian Tubes: Surgical Repairs, Closures and Reconstructions

P1-84800 Repair of ovary
  Oophoroplasty
P1-84802 Salpingo-oophoroplasty
P1-84803 Salpingo-oophorostomy
P1-84804 Oophoropexy
  Suspension of ovary
P1-84806 Detorsion of ovary
  Release of torsion of ovary
P1-84808 Marsupialization of ovarian cyst
P1-84809 Oophorostomy
P1-84810 Suture of ovary
  Oophororrhaphy
P1-84812 Salpingo-oophororrhaphy
P1-84820 Tubotubal anastomosis
  Salpingosalpingostomy
  Surgical reanastomosis of fallopian tube
  Reconstruction of fallopian tube
  Reestablishment of continuity of fallopian tube

P1-84822 Repair of fallopian tube, NOS
Salpingoplasty
P1-84823 Salpingostomy
P1-84824 Repair of fallopian tube by reimplantation into uterus
Tubouterine implantation
Hysterosalpingostomy
Salpingohysterostomy
P1-84826 Repair of fallopian tube with prosthesis
P1-84827 Burying of fimbriae of fallopian tube into uterine wall
P1-84828 Fimbrioplasty
P1-84830 Suture of fallopian tube
Salpingorrhaphy
P1-84860 Bilateral occlusion of fallopian tubes, NOS
P1-84862 Ligation of fallopian tube, NOS
P1-84863 Ligation of fallopian tubes by abdominal approach
P1-84864 Ligation of fallopian tubes by vaginal approach
P1-84865 Postpartum ligation of fallopian tubes
P1-84866 Incidental ligation of fallopian tubes
P1-84868 Unilateral ligation of fallopian tube
P1-84869 Ligation of fallopian tube with crushing
Madlener operation on fallopian tube
P1-84870 Bilateral ligation and division of fallopian tubes, NOS
P1-84872 Bilateral ligation and crushing of fallopian tubes
P1-84880 Occlusion of fallopian tubes by band, clip or Falope ring by suprapubic approach
P1-84882 Occlusion of fallopian tubes by band, clip or Falope ring by vaginal approach

1-84C Ovaries and Fallopian Tubes: Destructive Procedures

P1-84C00 Destructive procedure on ovaries and fallopian tubes, NOS
P1-84C02 Local destruction of ovary, NOS
P1-84C10 Lysis of adhesions of ovary
Ovariolysis
P1-84C12 Tubo-ovarian lysis of adhesions
Lysis of adhesions of ovary and fallopian tube
P1-84C20 Cauterization of ovary
P1-84C24 Electrocoagulation of ovary
P1-84C30 Ovarian denervation
P1-84C32 Denervation of uterosacral nerves
Denervation of paracervical uterine nerves
Doyle operation for paracervical uterine denervation
P1-84C50 Destruction of lesion of fallopian tube
P1-84C54 Lysis of adhesions of fallopian tube
P1-84C56 Cauterization of fallopian tube
P1-84C58 Electrocoagulation of fallopian tube
P1-84C59 Cauterization of uterotubal ostia
P1-84C60 Unilateral destruction of fallopian tube
P1-84C62 Bilateral destruction of fallopian tubes

1-84D Ovaries and Fallopian Tubes: Transplantations and Transpositions

P1-84D10 Transplant of ovary, NOS
P1-84D16 Autotransplantation of ovary
Estes operation on ovary
P1-84D20 Transposition of ovary
Reimplantation of ovary
P1-84D26 Implantation of ovary into uterine cavity
P1-84D60 Graft of fallopian tube

1-84E Ovaries and Fallopian Tubes: Manipulations

P1-84E00 Manipulation of ovary, NOS
P1-84E10 Manual rupture of ovarian cyst
P1-84E60 Dilation of fallopian tube

1-86 OBSTETRICAL OPERATIVE PROCEDURES

1-860 Obstetrics: General and Miscellaneous Operative Procedures

P1-86000 Routine obstetric care including antepartum care, vaginal delivery, and postpartum care
P1-86010 Routine obstetric care including antepartum care, cesarean delivery, and postpartum care
P1-86020 Obstetric operation, NOS
Operation to assist delivery, NOS

1-861 Obstetrics: Incisions

P1-86100 Amniocentesis, NOS
Incision and drainage of amnion
P1-86110 Amniotomy to induce labor
Surgical induction of labor by stripping of membranes
Surgical induction of labor
Induction of labor by artificial rupture of membranes
Induction of labor by rupture of membranes
P1-86120 Amniotomy at delivery, NOS
Artificial rupture of membranes at delivery, NOS
P1-86130 Episiotomy, NOS
P1-86132 Episioproctotomy
P1-86134 Episiotomy with subsequent episiorrhaphy
P1-86140 Incision of cervix to assist delivery
Obstetrical trachelotomy
Duhrssen's incisions of cervix to assist delivery
P1-86150 Pubiotomy to assist delivery
Pelviotomy to assist delivery
Symphysiotomy to assist delivery
P1-86160 Obstetrical hysterotomy
Obstetrical abdominouterotomy
P1-86170 Incision of hematoma in episiotomy site
Evacuation of hematoma in obstetric incision

1-861 Obstetrics: Incisions — Continued

P1-86172 Aspiration of hematoma in obstetric incision
P1-86180 Intrauterine cordocentesis

1-863-864 Obstetrics: Excisions

P1-86310 Cesarean section, NOS
P1-86311 Classical cesarean section
  Fundal cesarean section
  Corporeal cesarean section
  Classical transperitoneal cesarean section
P1-86312 Low cervical cesarean section
  Low cervical transperitoneal cesarean section
  Lower uterine segment cesarean section
  Laparotrachelotomy
  Cesarean section by laparotrachelotomy
P1-86314 Extraperitoneal cesarean section
  Cesarean section by peritoneal exclusion
  Norton cesarean operation
  Supravesical cesarean section
P1-86316 Vaginal cesarean section
P1-86320 Cesarean hysterectomy
  Total hysterectomy after cesarean delivery
P1-86321 Subtotal hysterectomy after cesarean delivery
P1-86322 Cesarean delivery only including postpartum care
P1-86330 Salpingectomy for tubal ectopic pregnancy by abdominal approach
P1-86331 Salpingectomy for tubal ectopic pregnancy by vaginal approach
P1-86332 Oophorectomy for ovarian ectopic pregnancy by abdominal approach
P1-86333 Oophorectomy for ovarian ectopic pregnancy by vaginal approach
P1-86340 Removal of ectopic fetus from ovary without oophorectomy
P1-86341 Removal of ectopic fetus from fallopian tube without salpingectomy
P1-86350 Removal of ectopic fetus from abdominal cavity
  Removal of extrauterine ectopic fetus
  Removal of intraperitoneal embryo
  Excision of ectopic abdominal fetus
  Removal of peritoneal ectopic fetus
P1-86360 Removal of ectopic interstitial uterine pregnancy requiring total hysterectomy
P1-86361 Removal of ectopic interstitial uterine pregnancy with partial resection of uterus
P1-86362 Removal of ectopic cervical pregnancy by evacuation
P1-86365 Removal of intraligamentous ectopic pregnancy
  Removal of ectopic intraligamentous fetus
P1-86370 Dilation and curettage of uterus after delivery
  Postpartum curettage
  Evacuation of retained placenta by curettage
  Removal of retained placenta by curettage
  Removal of secundines by curettage
P1-86371 Aspiration curettage of uterus after delivery
  Removal of retained placenta by aspiration curettage
  Removal of secundines by aspiration curettage
P1-86376 Delivery of placenta following delivery of infant outside of hospital
P1-86400 Therapeutic abortion procedure, NOS
P1-86401 Dilation and curettage for termination of pregnancy
  Induction of abortion by dilation and curettage
P1-86402 Aspiration curettage of uterus for termination of pregnancy
  Therapeutic abortion by aspiration curettage
  Suction curettage of uterus for termination of pregnancy
P1-86410 Therapeutic abortion by insertion of laminaria
P1-86412 Therapeutic abortion by hysterotomy
  Obstetrical hysterotomy for termination of pregnancy
  Incision of uterus for termination of pregnancy
P1-86414 Induced abortion following intra-amniotic injection with hysterotomy
P1-86420 Surgical treatment of spontaneous abortion of any trimester
P1-86421 Surgical treatment of missed abortion of first trimester
P1-86422 Surgical treatment of missed abortion of second trimester
P1-86423 Surgical treatment of missed abortion of third trimester
P1-86428 Surgical treatment of septic abortion
P1-86430 Dilation and curettage of uterus after abortion
P1-86432 Aspiration curettage of uterus after abortion
P1-86440 Removal of hydatidiform mole
  Uterine evacuation and curettage of hydatidiform mole
P1-86442 Hysterectomy for removal of hydatidiform mole
P1-86460 Intrauterine biopsy of fetus
P1-86462 Removal of fetal structures
P1-86465V Extraction of retained egg

1-865 Obstetrics: Injections and Implantations

P1-86510 Obstetric injection, NOS
P1-86550 Obstetric implantation, NOS

1-867 Obstetrics: Endoscopy

P1-86700 Amnioscopy
P1-86702 Laparoamnioscopy
P1-86710 Laparoscopic treatment of ectopic pregnancy without salpingectomy or oophorectomy

P1-86711 Laparoscopic treatment of ectopic pregnancy with oophorectomy
P1-86712 Laparoscopic treatment of ectopic pregnancy with salpingectomy
P1-86730 Fetoscopy

1-868 Obstetrics: Surgical Repairs, Closures and Reconstructions

P1-86800 Repair of obstetric laceration
  Episiorrhaphy for obstetrical laceration
P1-86801 Repair of obstetric laceration by other than attending physician
  Episiotomy repair by other than attending physician
P1-86802 Delayed repair of episiotomy
P1-86805 Repair of current obstetric laceration of rectum and sphincter ani
  Anal sphincteroplasty for current obstetrical laceration
  Repair of obstetric laceration of anal sphincter
  Anal sphincterorrhaphy for obstetrical laceration
  Repair of obstetric laceration of anus
P1-86808 Repair of obstetrical laceration of perineum
  Perineorrhaphy for obstetrical laceration
  Episioperineorrhaphy for obstetrical laceration
P1-86809 Repair of obstetric laceration of vulva
P1-86811 Suture of obstetric laceration of vagina
  Obstetrical vaginorrhaphy
P1-86813 Colpoperineorrhaphy following delivery
P1-86814 Repair of obstetric laceration of cervix
  Obstetrical trachelorrhaphy
P1-86815 Repair of obstetric laceration of bladder and urethra
P1-86816 Repair of obstetric laceration of urethra
P1-86817 Repair of obstetric laceration of bladder
P1-86818 Repair of obstetric laceration of pelvic floor
P1-86830 Repair of current obstetric laceration of uterus, NOS
  Suture of obstetric laceration of corpus uteri
  Hysterorrhaphy of ruptured uterus
P1-86832 Surgical correction of inverted pregnant uterus
  Incision of cervix to replace inverted uterus
  Spinelli operation for correction of inverted uterus
P1-86840 Cerclage of uterine cervix
  Suture of internal os of cervix by encirclement
  Banding of uterine cervix
  McDonald operation for encirclement suture of cervix
  Shirodkar operation on cervix
  Lash operation on cervix
  Marckwald operation on cervix
P1-86841 Cerclage of cervix during pregnancy by vaginal approach
P1-86842 Cerclage of cervix during pregnancy by abdominal approach
P1-86860 Intrauterine correction of fetal defect, NOS

1-86C Obstetrics: Destructive Procedures

P1-86C00 Destructive procedure on fetus to facilitate delivery, NOS
P1-86C10 Fetal cranioclasis
  Fetal craniotomy
  Cephalotomy of fetus
  Fetal basiotripsy
P1-86C12 Fetal decapitation
P1-86C20 Needling of hydrocephalic head
  Drainage of fetal hydrocephalic head
P1-86C22 Transabdominal encephalocentesis of fetal head
P1-86C30 Embryotomy
  Fetal Danforth operation
  Destruction of fetus
P1-86C40 Fetal clavicotomy
  Fetal cleidorrhexis
  Fetal cleidotomy

1-86D Obstetrics: Transplantations and Transpositions

P1-86D10 Obstetric transplantation, NOS
P1-86D20 Transplantation of embryo
P1-86D60 Obstetric transposition, NOS

1-86E Obstetrics: Manipulations

P1-86E00 Delivery, NOS
  Spontaneous unassisted delivery
P1-86E08 Vaginal delivery without forceps including postpartum care
P1-86E10 Manually assisted spontaneous delivery
  Assisted spontaneous delivery
P1-86E11 Delivery of cephalic presentation
  Delivery of vertex presentation
P1-86E12 Delivery of brow presentation
P1-86E13 Delivery of face presentation
P1-86E14 Delivery of shoulder presentation
P1-86E16 Delivery of transverse presentation
P1-86E21 Manual rotation of fetal head
P1-86E22 Crede maneuver
  Delivery by Crede maneuver
P1-86E24 Delivery by Ritgen maneuver
P1-86E31 Complete breech delivery
  Total breech extraction
  Total breech delivery
P1-86E32 Partial breech delivery
  Partial breech extraction
P1-86E33 Frank breech delivery
P1-86E34 Footling breech delivery
P1-86E38 Partial breech delivery with forceps to aftercoming head

1-86E Obstetrics: Manipulations — Continued

P1-86E39 Total breech delivery with forceps to aftercoming head
P1-86E41 Bracht maneuver
P1-86E42 Prague maneuver
P1-86E43 Van Hoorn maneuver
P1-86E44 Wigand-Martin maneuver
P1-86E45 Kristeller maneuver
P1-86E46 Pinard maneuver
P1-86E50 Instrumental delivery, NOS
  Forceps delivery, NOS
  Application of and delivery by forceps, NOS
P1-86E51 Vaginal delivery with forceps including postpartum care
P1-86E52 Failed forceps delivery
P1-86E53 Trial forceps delivery
P1-86E55 Delivery by double application of forceps
P1-86E56 Forceps application to aftercoming head
  Piper forceps delivery by application to aftercoming head
P1-86E60 Low forceps delivery
  Application of or delivery by low forceps
  Low forceps operation
P1-86E61 Low forceps delivery with episiotomy
P1-86E63 Mid forceps delivery
  Application of or delivery by mid forceps
  Mid forceps operation
P1-86E64 Mid forceps delivery with episiotomy
P1-86E65 High forceps delivery
  High forceps operation
  Application of or delivery by high forceps
P1-86E66 High forceps delivery with episiotomy
P1-86E68 Forceps delivery with rotation of fetal head
P1-86E70 Obstetrical version, NOS
P1-86E71 External obstetrical version
  Manual conversion of position
  External version to assist delivery
P1-86E72 Instrumental conversion of position
P1-86E73 Delivery by Scanzoni maneuver
P1-86E74 Wigand's obstetrical version
P1-86E75 External cephalic version without tocolysis
P1-86E76 External cephalic version with tocolysis
P1-86E77 Delivery by De Lee maneuver
P1-86E78 Delivery by Kielland rotation
P1-86E79 Barton's forceps delivery
P1-86E80 Internal obstetrical version
P1-86E82 Combined obstetrical version
P1-86E83 Internal and combined version without extraction
P1-86E84 Internal and combined version with extraction
  Obstetrical version with extraction
P1-86E85 Braxton Hicks obstetrical version
P1-86E86 Braxton Hicks obstetrical version with extraction
P1-86E87 Potter's obstetrical version
P1-86E88 Potter's obstetrical version with extraction
P1-86E89 Wright's obstetrical version
P1-86E8A Wright's obstetrical version with extraction
P1-86EA0 Delivery by vacuum extraction
  Vacuum extraction of fetus
P1-86EA2 Delivery by vacuum extraction with episiotomy
  Vacuum extraction of fetal head with episiotomy
P1-86EA4 Delivery by Malstrom's extraction
P1-86EA5 Delivery by Malstrom's extraction with episiotomy
P1-86EA6 Manual removal of retained placenta
  Manual removal of decidua
  Manual removal secundines
  Manual evacuation of retained placenta
  Manual removal of placenta
P1-86EA7 Manual postpartum exploration of uterus
  Manual postpartum exploration of uterine cavity
P1-86EA8 Manual replacement of obstetrical inverted uterus
  Manual repair of obstetrical inverted uterus
P1-86EA9 Replacement of prolapsed umbilical cord
P1-86EAA Extraction of fetus, NOS

SECTION 1-9 OPERATIVE PROCEDURES ON THE NERVOUS SYSTEM

1-90 GENERAL OPERATIVE PROCEDURES ON THE NERVOUS SYSTEM

1-900 Nervous System: General and Miscellaneous Operative Procedures

P1-90000 Operative procedure on nervous system, NOS
  Operation on nervous system, NOS
P1-90002 Neuromuscular diagnostic procedure, NOS
  Neurological diagnostic procedure, NOS

1-901 Nervous System: Incisions

P1-90100 Incision of nervous system, NOS
P1-90110 Tractotomy, NOS
P1-90120V General durotomy
  Exploratory durotomy
P1-90122V Exploration of epidural space

1-91 OPERATIVE PROCEDURES ON THE BRAIN

1-910 Brain: General and Miscellaneous Operative Procedures

P1-91002 Operative procedure on head, NOS
P1-91004 Operation on bone of skull, NOS
P1-91006 Diagnostic procedure on skull, NOS
P1-91010 Operation on brain, NOS
P1-91012 Diagnostic procedure on brain, NOS
P1-91014 Operation on cerebral meninges, NOS
P1-91016 Diagnostic procedure on cerebral meninges, NOS
P1-91020 Stereotactic operation on thalamus

P1-91022 Diagnostic procedure on thalamus
P1-91024 Operation on globus pallidus, NOS
P1-91026 Diagnostic procedure on globus pallidus
P1-91050 Operation to establish drainage of ventricle, NOS

1-911-912 Brain: Incisions

P1-91100 Craniotomy, NOS
  Incision of bone of skull, NOS
P1-91104 Trephination of cranium, NOS
  Burr holes, NOS
P1-91106 Burr holes or trephine, infratentorial
P1-91107 Exploratory burr holes or trephine, supratentorial, single procedure
P1-91110 Exploration of cranium, NOS
P1-91112 Exploratory craniotomy, infratentorial
  Exploratory craniectomy, infratentorial
P1-91114 Exploratory craniotomy, supratentorial
  Exploratory craniectomy, supratentorial
P1-91116 Reopening of craniotomy site
  Reopening of craniectomy site
P1-91118 Opening of cranial suture
  Linear craniectomy with opening of cranial suture
  Strip craniectomy with opening of cranial suture
  Stripping of cranial suture
P1-91119 Craniotomy for decompression of skull fracture
P1-91120 Incision of brain, NOS
  Intracerebral incision
P1-91121 Incision of cerebrum
P1-91122 Amygdalohippocampotomy
P1-91124 Amygdalotomy
P1-91125 Incision of cortical adhesions of brain
P1-91126 Incision of epidural or extradural space of brain
P1-91130 Lobotomy, NOS
  Lobotomy of brain, NOS
P1-91132 Leukotomy, NOS
  Leucotomy, NOS
  Incision of white matter of frontal lobe of brain
P1-91133 Cryoleucotomy
P1-91134 Prefrontal lobotomy
  Prefrontal leukotomy
P1-91135 Transorbital leukotomy
  Transorbital lobotomy
P1-91140 Tractotomy of brain, NOS
P1-91142 Tractotomy of medulla oblongata
  Suboccipital craniectomy for medullary tractotomy
P1-91144 Tractotomy of mesencephalon
  Suboccipital craniectomy for mesencephalic tractotomy
P1-91146 Lobotomy and tractotomy
P1-91148 Craniotomy for lobotomy including cingulotomy
P1-91149 Cingulumotomy of brain by percutaneous radiofrequency
P1-9114A Suboccipital craniectomy for mesencephalic pedunculotomy
P1-91150 Craniotomy with treatment of penetrating wound of brain
P1-91152 Exploration of brain, NOS
P1-91154 Suboccipital craniectomy for exploration of cranial nerves
P1-91156 Decompression of brain
  Intracranial decompression
  Cranial decompression
P1-91160 Suboccipital craniectomy with cervical laminectomy for decompression of medulla and spinal cord with dural graft
P1-91161 Suboccipital craniectomy with cervical laminectomy for decompression of medulla and spinal cord without dural graft
P1-91162 Suboccipital craniectomy for decompression of cranial nerves
P1-91163 Subtemporal craniectomy for compression of sensory root of gasserian ganglion
P1-91164 Subtemporal craniectomy for decompression of sensory root of gasserian ganglion
P1-91165 Decompression of lesion of brain stem or upper spinal cord by transoral approach to skull base with splitting of tongue and/or mandible
P1-91166 Decompression of lesion of brain stem or upper spinal cord by transoral approach to skull base
P1-91168 Cranial decompression, posterior fossa
P1-91169 Cranial decompression, subtemporal, supratentorial
P1-91170 Drainage of cerebrum, NOS
P1-91171 Drainage of cerebrum by aspiration through previously implanted catheter
  Aspiration of intracranial space through previously implanted catheter or reservoir, Ommaya or Rickham
P1-91172 Burr holes or trephine with drainage of brain cyst
P1-91174 Burr holes or trephine with drainage of brain abscess
P1-91175 Craniectomy for drainage of intracranial abscess, infratentorial
  Craniotomy for drainage of intracranial abscess, infratentorial
P1-91176 Craniectomy for drainage of intracranial abscess, supratentorial
  Craniotomy for drainage of intracranial abscess, supratentorial
P1-91180 Bone flap craniotomy for transection of corpus callosum
P1-91181 Trephination for transection of corpus callosum
P1-91182 Suboccipital craniectomy for section of one or more cranial nerves

1-911-912 Brain: Incisions — Continued

P1-91183 Subtemporal craniectomy for section of sensory root of gasserian ganglion
P1-91184 Craniotomy for section of tentorium cerebelli
P1-91185 Division of brain tissue, NOS
P1-91186 Division of brain tissue for cortical adhesions
P1-91188 Division of cerebral tracts
P1-91189 Division of cerebral nerve tracts
P1-91190 Encephalocentesis
  Encephalopuncture
  Cranial puncture
  Cranial tap
P1-91192 Puncture of anterior fontanel
P1-91194 Burr holes or trephine with subsequent aspiration of intracranial abscess
P1-91195 Burr holes or trephine with subsequent aspiration of intracranial cyst
P1-91200 Incision of cerebral meninges
P1-91202 Division of cerebral meninges
P1-91204 Incision of cerebral epidural space
  Incision of cerebral extradural space
P1-91205 Drainage of cerebral epidural space by incision or trephination
  Drainage of cerebral extradural space by incision or trephination
P1-91206 Drainage of intracranial space by aspiration
  Aspiration of intracranial space
P1-91207 Drainage of cerebral epidural space by aspiration
  Drainage of cerebral extradural space by aspiration
P1-91210 Burr holes with evacuation and drainage of extradural hematoma
P1-91212 Craniectomy for evacuation of extradural hematoma, infratentorial
  Craniotomy for evacuation of extradural hematoma, infratentorial
P1-91213 Craniectomy for evacuation of extradural hematoma, supratentorial
  Craniotomy for evacuation of extradural hematoma, supratentorial
P1-91215 Drainage of intracranial space, subarachnoid or subdural by incision or trephination
  Drainage of cerebral subarachnoid space by incision or trephination
P1-91216 Drainage of cerebral subarachnoid space by aspiration
  Aspiration of cerebral subarachnoid space
P1-91217 Drainage of cerebral subdural space by aspiration
P1-91220 Craniectomy for evacuation of intracerebellar hematoma, infratentorial
  Craniotomy for evacuation of intracerebellar hematoma, infratentorial
P1-91222 Craniectomy for evacuation of intracerebral hematoma, supratentorial
  Craniotomy for evacuation of intracerebral hematoma, supratentorial
P1-91224 Burr holes with aspiration of intracerebral hematoma
P1-91225 Burr holes with aspiration of intracerebral cyst
P1-91230 Incision of cerebral subarachnoid space
P1-91232 Fistulization of cerebral subarachnoid space
P1-91235 Incision of cerebral subdural space
P1-91236 Drainage of cerebral subdural space by incision or trephination
P1-91238 Burr holes with evacuation and drainage of subdural hematoma
P1-91239 Craniotomy for evacuation of subdural hematoma, supratentorial
  Craniectomy for evacuation of subdural hematoma, supratentorial
P1-91240 Craniotomy for evacuation of subdural hematoma, infratentorial
  Craniectomy for evacuation of subdural hematoma, infratentorial
P1-91242 Subdural tap through fontanel
P1-91243 Subdural tap through fontanel, infant, initial
  Subdural tap through suture, infant, initial
P1-91245 Subdural tap through suture, infant, bilateral, initial
P1-91250 Twist drill hole for subdural puncture, single procedure
P1-91251 Twist drill hole for subdural puncture followed by other surgery
P1-91252 Twist drill hole for ventricular puncture for evacuation and drainage of subdural hematoma
P1-91253 Twist drill hole for subdural puncture for evacuation and drainage of subdural hematoma
P1-91260 Cerebral ventriculotomy, NOS
P1-91261 Drainage of cerebral ventricle by incision, NOS
P1-91262 Drainage of ventricle by aspiration
P1-91263 Drainage of ventricle through previously implanted catheter
P1-91264 Fistulization of cerebral ventricle
P1-91270 Cisternal tap
  Cisternal puncture
  Cisternal puncture without injection
P1-91272 Ventriculopuncture
  Ventricular puncture through fontanel without injection
  Ventricular puncture through suture without injection
P1-91273 Ventricular puncture through implanted ventricular catheter or reservoir without injection
  Ventriculopuncture through previously implanted catheter or reservoir, Ommaya or Rickham
P1-91274 Ventricular puncture through previous burr hole without injection
P1-91280 Puncture of ventricular shunt tubing, NOS

P1-91281 Puncture of ventricular shunt tubing or reservoir for aspiration
P1-91282 Puncture of ventricular shunt tubing or reservoir for injection procedure
P1-91283 Twist drill hole for ventricular puncture, single procedure
P1-91285 Twist drill hole for ventricular puncture, single procedure followed by other surgery
P1-91286 Burr hole for ventricular puncture, single procedure
P1-91287 Burr hole for ventricular puncture followed by other surgery
P1-91290 Incision of cranial sinus, NOS
P1-91292 Incision and drainage of cranial sinus
P1-91293 Drainage of cranial sinus by trephination
P1-91294 Drainage of cranial sinus by aspiration
P1-91296 Pallidoansotomy
P1-91297 Pallidotomy
P1-91298 Thalamotomy
P1-91299 Pallidoamygdalotomy

1-913-914 Brain: Excisions

P1-91300 Craniectomy, NOS
P1-91310 Biopsy of skull, NOS
  Excisional biopsy of skull, NOS
P1-91312 Excision of lesion of cranium
  Excision of lesion of skull
P1-91314 Debridement of skull
  Removal of bone fragment of skull
P1-91315 Sequestrectomy of bone of skull
P1-91320 Craniectomy for craniostenosis, single suture
P1-91321 Craniectomy for craniostenosis, each stage
P1-91322 Craniectomy for craniostenosis, multiple sutures, one stage
P1-91323 Craniectomy for osteomyelitis
P1-91324 Craniectomy with excision of bone lesion of skull, NOS
P1-91325 Removal of granulation tissue of skull
P1-91326 Debridement of compound fracture of skull
  Removal of bone fragment of skull with debridement of compound fracture
P1-91327 Removal of bone flap of skull
P1-91328 Replacement of bone flap of skull
P1-91338 Removal of foreign body from head, NOS
  Removal of foreign body from head without incision, NOS
P1-91339 Removal of foreign body from skull, NOS
P1-91340 Excisional biopsy of brain, NOS
P1-91341 Open excisional biopsy of brain
  Incisional biopsy of brain
P1-91342 Closed excisional biopsy of brain
P1-91343 Excisional biopsy of brain, percutaneous, needle
  Needle biopsy of brain
P1-91346 Stereotactic excisional biopsy of intracranial lesion
P1-91347 Stereotactic excisional biopsy of intracranial lesion with computerized axial tomography
P1-91348 Stereotactic biopsy by aspiration of intracranial lesion
P1-91349 Stereotactic biopsy by aspiration of intracranial lesion with computerized axial tomography
P1-91350 Burr holes or trephine with biopsy of brain
P1-91351 Burr holes or trephine with biopsy of intracranial lesion
P1-91354 Biopsy of brain stem or upper spinal cord by transoral approach to skull base
P1-91355 Biopsy of brain stem or upper spinal cord by transoral approach to skull base with splitting of tongue and/or mandible
P1-91356 Craniectomy with excision of tumor, NOS
P1-91357 Craniectomy for excision of brain tumor, infratentorial or posterior fossa
P1-91358 Bone flap craniotomy, supratentorial, for excision of brain tumor, except meningioma
P1-91359 Craniectomy for excision of brain tumor, supratentorial, except meningioma
P1-9135A Trephination for excision of brain tumor, supratentorial, except meningioma
P1-91362 Craniectomy for excision of meningioma, infratentorial
P1-91363 Craniectomy for excision of brain tumor, infratentorial for midline tumor at base of skull
P1-91364 Craniectomy for excision of cerebellopontine angle tumor
P1-91365 Bone flap craniotomy, transtemporal for excision of cerebellopontine angle tumor
P1-91366 Bone flap craniotomy, transtemporal for excision of cerebellopontine angle tumor combined with middle or posterior fossa craniotomy or craniectomy
P1-91367 Craniectomy by transtemporal mastoid approach for excision of cerebellopontine angle tumor with middle or posterior fossa craniotomy or craniectomy
P1-91369 Bone flap craniotomy for excision of craniopharyngioma
P1-9136A Craniectomy for excision of craniopharyngioma
P1-9136B Trephination for excision of craniopharyngioma
P1-91370 Excision of lesion of brain stem or upper spinal cord by transoral approach to skull base
P1-91371 Excision of lesion of brain stem or upper spinal cord by transoral approach to skull base with splitting of tongue and/or mandible
P1-91372 Bone flap craniotomy for excision of cerebral epileptogenic focus with electrocorticography during surgery
P1-91373 Craniectomy for excision of cerebral epileptogenic focus with electrocorticography during surgery
P1-91374 Trephination for excision of cerebral epileptogenic focus with electrocorticography during surgery

1-913-914 Brain: Excisions — Continued

P1-91375 Bone flap craniotomy for excision of cerebral epileptogenic focus without electrocorticography during surgery
P1-91376 Craniectomy for excision of cerebral epileptogenic focus without electrocorticography during surgery
P1-91377 Trephination for excision of cerebral epileptogenic focus without electrocorticography during surgery
P1-91378 Bone flap craniotomy, supratentorial, for excision of brain abscess
P1-91379 Craniectomy for excision of brain abscess, supratentorial
P1-9137A Trephination for excision of brain abscess, supratentorial
P1-9137B Craniectomy, infratentorial or posterior fossa, for excision of brain abscess
P1-9137C Bone flap craniotomy, supratentorial, for excision or fenestration of cyst
P1-9137D Craniectomy for excision or fenestration of cyst, supratentorial
P1-9137E Trephination for excision or fenestration of cyst, supratentorial
P1-91383 Craniectomy, infratentorial, for excision or fenestration of cyst
P1-91384 Curettage of brain
P1-91385 Debridement of brain
P1-91386 Excision of intracranial lesion, NOS
P1-91387 Excision of lesion of brain by transtemporal approach, NOS
P1-91388 Excision of lesion of cerebral cortex, NOS
P1-91389 Excision of brain
  Resection of brain
  Excision of tissue of brain
P1-9138A Lobectomy of brain
  Excision of brain lobe
  Resection of brain lobe
P1-9138B Partial lobectomy of brain
P1-9138C Excision of part of frontal cortex
  Topectomy
P1-9138D Craniectomy with treatment of penetrating wound of brain
P1-91390 Bone flap craniotomy for lobectomy with electrocorticography during surgery, other than temporal lobe, partial or total
P1-91391 Craniectomy, trephination, bone flap craniotomy for lobectomy with electrocorticography during surgery, except temporal lobe, partial
P1-91392 Craniectomy, trephination, bone flap craniotomy for lobectomy with electrocorticography during surgery, except temporal lobe, total
P1-91393 Bone flap craniotomy for lobectomy with electrocorticography during surgery, temporal lobe
P1-91394 Craniectomy or trephination for lobectomy with electrocorticography during surgery, temporal lobe
P1-91395 Excision of basal ganglion
P1-91396 Cerebral hemispherectomy
  Excision of brain hemisphere
  Resection of brain hemisphere
P1-91397 Craniectomy, trephination, bone flap craniotomy for total hemispherectomy
P1-91398 Bone flap craniotomy for total hemispherectomy
P1-91399 Bone flap craniotomy for partial or subtotal hemispherectomy
P1-9139A Craniectomy, trephination, bone flap craniotomy for partial hemispherectomy
P1-913A0 Decortication of brain
P1-913A1 Intracranial microdissection
P1-91420 Removal of foreign body from brain, NOS
P1-91421 Removal of foreign body from brain without incision into brain
P1-91422 Removal of foreign body from brain with incision into brain
P1-91424 Craniotomy for excision of foreign body from brain
  Craniectomy for excision of foreign body from brain
P1-91430 Excisional biopsy of cerebral meninges, NOS
P1-91431 Closed excisional biopsy of cerebral meninges
P1-91432 Open excisional biopsy of meninges
P1-91433 Needle biopsy of cerebral meninges
  Excisional biopsy of cerebral meninges, percutaneous, needle
P1-91434 Incisional biopsy of cerebral meninges, NOS
P1-91440 Excision of lesion of cerebral meninges
P1-91441 Debridement of cerebral meninges
P1-91442 Curettage of cerebral meninges
P1-91443 Decortication of cerebral meninges
P1-91446 Bone flap craniotomy, supratentorial, for excision of meningioma
P1-91447 Craniectomy, trephination, bone flap craniotomy for excision of meningioma, supratentorial
P1-91449 Resection of cerebral meninges
  Excision of tissue of cerebral meninges
P1-91458 Removal of foreign body from cerebral meninges
P1-91460 Hypophysectomy, NOS
P1-91461 Craniotomy for hypophysectomy by intracranial approach
  Craniotomy for excision of pituitary tumor by intracranial approach
P1-91462 Excision of pituitary tumor by transnasal approach, nonstereotactic
  Hypophysectomy for pituitary tumor by transnasal approach, nonstereotactic
P1-91463 Excision of pituitary tumor by transseptal approach, nonstereotactic
  Hypophysectomy for pituitary tumor by transseptal approach, nonstereotactic
P1-91466 Excision of choroid plexus
  Choroid plexectomy

P1-91467 Excision of lesion of choroid plexus
P1-91468 Trephination for excision or coagulation of choroid plexus
P1-91469 Bone flap craniotomy for excision or coagulation of choroid plexus
P1-9146A Craniectomy, trephination, bone flap craniotomy for excision of choroid plexus
P1-91470 Pallidectomy
P1-91472 Chemopallidectomy
P1-91473 Thalamectomy
P1-91474 Chemothalamectomy
P1-91475 Cryothalamectomy

1-915-916 Brain: Injections and Implantations

P1-91500 Injection of brain, NOS
P1-91510 Cisternal puncture with injection
P1-91511 Ventricular puncture through fontanel with injection
  Ventricular puncture through suture with injection
P1-91512 Ventricular puncture through implanted ventricular catheter or reservoir with injection
P1-91513 Ventricular puncture through previous burr hole with injection
P1-91514 Injection of contrast substance or neurolytic solution, subarachnoid
P1-91515 Injection procedure for myelography, posterior fossa
P1-91516 Injection procedure for computerized axial tomography, posterior fossa
P1-91518 Irrigation by subarachnoid/subdural catheter
P1-91520 Insertion of tongs of skull with synchronous skeletal traction
P1-91521 Insertion of Barton tongs of skull with synchronous skeletal traction
P1-91522 Insertion of caliper tongs of skull with synchronous skeletal traction
P1-91523 Insertion of Gardner Wells tongs with synchronous skeletal traction
P1-91524 Insertion of Vinke tongs of skull with synchronous skeletal traction
P1-91525 Application of Crutchfield tongs of skull with synchronous skeletal traction
P1-91526 Insertion of halo device of skull with synchronous skeletal traction
P1-91527 Insertion of skull plate
P1-91530 Replacement of skull tongs
  Removal of skull tongs with synchronous replacement
P1-91531 Replacement of Barton tongs of skull
  Removal of Barton tongs with synchronous replacement
P1-91532 Replacement of caliper tongs of skull
  Removal of caliper tongs with synchronous replacement
P1-91533 Replacement of Crutchfield tongs of skull
  Removal of Crutchfield tongs with synchronous replacement
P1-91534 Replacement of Vinke tongs of skull
  Removal of Vinke tongs with synchronous replacement
P1-91535 Replacement of Gardner Wells tongs of skull
  Removal of Gardner Wells tongs with synchronous replacement
P1-91536 Replacement of halo traction device of skull
  Removal of halo traction device with synchronous replacement
P1-91537 Replacement of prosthetic plate of skull
  Replacement of skull plate
  Removal of plate of skull with synchronous replacement
P1-91540 Implantation of electrode into brain
  Intracranial implantation of electrode
  Insertion of electrode into brain
P1-91542 Craniectomy for insertion of epidural electrode array
P1-91543 Bone flap craniotomy for insertion of epidural electrode array
P1-91544 Trephination for insertion of epidural electrode array
P1-91545 Craniectomy for implantation of neurostimulator electrodes, cerebellar, cortical
P1-91546 Craniectomy for implantation of neurostimulator electrodes, cerebellar, subcortical
P1-91547 Craniectomy for implantation of neurostimulator electrodes, cerebral, cortical
  Craniotomy for implantation of neurostimulator electrodes, cerebral, cortical
P1-91548 Craniectomy for implantation of neurostimulator electrodes, cerebral, subcortical
  Craniotomy for implantation of neurostimulator electrodes, cerebral, subcortical
P1-91549 Twist drill hole for implantation of neurostimulator electrodes, cortical
  Burr holes for implantation of neurostimulator electrodes, cortical
P1-9154A Twist drill hole for implantation of neurostimulator electrodes, subcortical
  Burr holes for implantation of neurostimulator electrodes, subcortical
P1-91550 Insertion by physician of sphenoidal electrodes for electroencephalographic recording
P1-91551 Stereotactic localization, any method, for introduction of subcortical electrodes
P1-91552 Revision of intracranial neurostimulator electrodes
P1-91553 Removal of electrodes of brain with synchronous replacement
  Removal of intracranial electrodes with synchronous replacement

1-915-916 Brain: Injections and Implantations — Continued

P1-91554 Burr holes for implantation of pressure recording device
P1-91555 Twist drill hole for subdural puncture for implanting pressure recording device
P1-91556 Twist drill hole for ventricular puncture for implanting pressure recording device
P1-91557 Irrigation of ventricular shunt
P1-91558 Irrigation of ventricular catheter
P1-91560 Burr holes for implanting ventricular catheter or reservoir
P1-91561 Twist drill hole for subdural puncture for implanting ventricular catheter
P1-91562 Twist drill hole for ventricular puncture for implanting ventricular catheter
P1-91563 Implantation of Ommaya reservoir
  Insertion of Ommaya reservoir
P1-91564 Implantation of Rickham reservoir
  Insertion of Rickham reservoir
P1-91565 Insertion of Holter valve
  Insertion of Spitz-Holter valve
P1-91566 Insertion of subcutaneous continuous infusion system for connection to ventricular catheter
  Insertion of subcutaneous pump for connection to ventricular catheter
  Insertion of subcutaneous reservoir for connection to ventricular catheter
P1-91567 Insertion of subarachnoid catheter with reservoir and/or pump for drug infusion without laminectomy
P1-91568 Insertion of epidural catheter with reservoir and/or pump for drug infusion without laminectomy
P1-91569 Insertion of subarachnoid catheter with reservoir and/or pump for continuous infusion of drug, including laminectomy
P1-9156A Insertion of subarachnoid catheter with reservoir and/or pump for intermittent infusion of drug, including laminectomy
P1-91570 Stereotactic localization, any method, with insertion of catheter for brachytherapy
P1-91572 Reinsertion of holter valve
P1-91573 Reinsertion of cerebral ventricular valve
P1-91574 Ventriculocisternal intubation
P1-91575 Replacement of ventricular shunt
P1-91576 Replacement of ventricular catheter
P1-91577 Replacement of cerebral ventricular valve
P1-91578 Replacement of cerebral ventricular tube
P1-91579 Replacement of subarachnoid/subdural catheter
P1-91580 Replacement or revision of CSF shunt
P1-91581 Replacement of distal catheter in shunt system
P1-91582 Replacement of obstructed valve in shunt system
P1-91583 Revision of obstructed valve in shunt system
P1-91584 Revision of distal catheter in shunt system
P1-91585 Removal of ventricular catheter with synchronous replacement
P1-91586 Removal of ventricular reservoir with synchronous replacement
P1-91587 Removal of complete CSF shunt system with replacement by similar or other shunt at same operation
P1-91590 Implantation of electroencephalographic receiver in brain
  Implantation of intracranial electroencephalographic receiver
P1-91591 Replacement of electroencephalographic receiver in brain
  Removal of electroencephalographic receiver from brain with synchronous replacement
P1-91592 Implantation of electronic stimulator in brain
  Implantation of intracranial electronic stimulator
  Implantation of neuropacemaker in brain
  Implantation of intracranial neuropacemaker
  Implantation of neurostimulator in brain
  Implantation of pacemaker in brain
  Insertion of pacemaker in brain
  Insertion of intracranial pacemaker
  Implantation of stimoceiver in brain
  Implantation of intracranial stimoceiver
P1-91598 Revision of intracranial neurostimulator receiver
P1-915A0 Replacement of pacemaker in brain
  Replacement of intracranial pacemaker
  Replacement of neural brain pacemaker
  Removal of pacemaker of brain with synchronous replacement
  Removal of intracranial pacemaker with synchronous replacement
  Removal of electronic stimulator of brain with synchronous replacement
  Removal of intracranial electronic stimulator with synchronous replacement
  Removal of neuropacemaker of brain with synchronous replacement
  Removal of intracranial neuropacemaker with synchronous replacement
  Removal of neurostimulator of brain with synchronous replacement
  Removal of intracranial neurostimulator with synchronous replacement
  Removal of stimoceiver with synchronous replacement
P1-915B1 Incision for subcutaneous placement of brain neurostimulator receiver, direct coupling
P1-915B2 Incision for subcutaneous placement of brain neurostimulator receiver, inductive coupling
P1-91610 Removal of skull plate
  Removal of prosthetic plate of skull
P1-91614 Removal of skull tongs, NOS

P1-91615 Removal of caliper tongs from skull
P1-91616 Removal of Barton's tongs from skull
P1-91617 Removal of Crutchfield tongs from skull
P1-91618 Removal of Vinke tongs from skull
P1-91619 Removal of Gardner Wells tongs from skull
P1-91620 Removal of halo traction device from skull
P1-91630 Removal of electrodes from brain
Removal of intracranial electrodes
P1-91631 Removal of electroencephalographic receiver from brain
P1-91632 Removal of neuropacemaker of brain
Removal of intracranial electronic stimulator
Removal of neurostimulator of brain
Removal of intracranial neuropacemaker
Removal of intracranial neurostimulator
P1-91635 Removal of intracranial neurostimulator electrodes
P1-91637 Removal of intracranial neurostimulator receiver
P1-91639 Removal of complete CSF shunt system without replacement
P1-91640 Removal of cerebral ventricular catheter
P1-91641 Removal of cerebral ventricular valve
P1-91642 Removal of cerebral ventricular shunt
P1-91644 Removal of cerebral ventricular reservoir, Ommaya or Rickham
P1-91650 Bone flap craniotomy for removal of epidural electrode array without excision of cerebral tissue
P1-91651 Craniectomy for removal of epidural electrode array without excision of cerebral tissue
P1-91652 Trephination for removal of epidural electrode array without excision of cerebral tissue

1-917 Brain: Endoscopy

P1-91700 Intracranial endoscopy, NOS
P1-91702 Endoscopy of brain, NOS

1-918-919 Brain: Surgical Repairs, Closures and Reconstructions

P1-91800 Cranioplasty, NOS
Osteoplasty of cranium, NOS
Osteoplasty of skull, NOS
Repair of bone of cranium, NOS
Repair of bone of skull, NOS
P1-91802 Cranioplasty for skull defect, up to 5 cm diameter
P1-91804 Cranioplasty for skull defect, larger than 5 cm diameter
P1-91805 Osteoplasty of cranium with flap of bone
Repair of cranium with bone flap
P1-91806 Reconstruction of skull by multiple bone flaps
P1-91809 Revision of bone flap of skull
P1-91810 Elevation of skull fracture fragments
P1-91812 Elevation of depressed skull fracture, simple, extradural
P1-91813 Elevation of depressed skull fracture, comminuted, extradural
Elevation of depressed skull fracture, compound, extradural
P1-91814 Elevation of depressed skull fracture with debridement of brain
P1-91815 Reconstruction of skull by orbital advancement with suturotomy or craniotomy
P1-91816 Elevation of bone fragments of orbit of skull with debridement
P1-91820 Repair of brain, NOS
P1-91822 Cranioplasty with synchronous repair of encephalocele
Repair of cerebral encephalocele
Closure of encephalocele
P1-91824 Cranioplasty for skull defect with reparative brain surgery
P1-91825 Repair of carotid-cavernous fistula by balloon catheter
P1-91826 Repair of carotid-cavernous fistula by injection procedure
P1-91827 Repair of carotid-cavernous fistula by intra-arterial embolization
P1-91828 Repair of carotid-cavernous fistula by intracranial electrothrombosis
P1-91830 Repair of cerebral aneurysm by balloon catheter
P1-91831 Repair of cerebral aneurysm by injection procedure
P1-91832 Repair of cerebral aneurysm by intra-arterial embolization
P1-91835 Repair of cerebral aneurysm by intracranial electrothrombosis
P1-91836 Repair of intracranial aneurysm by cervical approach with application of occluding clamp to cervical carotid artery
P1-91837 Repair of intracranial aneurysm of carotid circulation by intracranial approach
P1-91838 Repair of intracranial aneurysm of vertebral-basilar circulation by intracranial approach
P1-91839 Repair of intracranial arteriovenous malformation, dural, simple
P1-9183A Repair of intracranial arteriovenous malformation, dural, complex
P1-91840 Repair of intracranial arteriovenous malformation, infratentorial, simple
P1-91841 Repair of intracranial arteriovenous malformation, infratentorial, complex
P1-91842 Repair of intracranial arteriovenous malformation, supratentorial, simple
P1-91844 Repair of intracranial arteriovenous malformation, supratentorial, complex
P1-91845 Repair of intracranial vascular malformation by injection procedure
Repair of cerebral vascular malformation by injection procedure
P1-91846 Repair of intracranial vascular malformation by intra-arterial embolization
Repair of cerebral vascular malformation by intra-arterial embolization
P1-91847 Repair of intracranial vascular malformation by electrothrombosis

1-918-919 Brain: Surgical Repairs, Closures and Reconstructions — Continued

P1-91848 Repair of cerebral vascular malformation by balloon catheter
P1-91849 Repair of intracranial aneurysm by intracranial and cervical occlusion of carotid artery
P1-9184A Repair of intracranial vascular malformation by intracranial and cervical occlusion of carotid artery
P1-9184B Repair of carotid-cavernous fistula by intracranial and cervical occlusion of carotid artery
P1-91850 Marsupialization of lesion of brain
Marsupialization of cerebral lesion
P1-91852 Marsupialization of cyst of brain
P1-91854 Closure of fistula of cerebrospinal fluid
Obliteration of cerebrospinal fistula
P1-91860 Repair of cerebral meninges, NOS
P1-91861 Cerebral duraplasty
P1-91862 Subdural patch of brain
P1-91864 Repair of cranial meningocele
Closure of cerebral meningocele
P1-91865 Craniotomy for repair of dural/CSF leak
P1-91866 Craniotomy for repair of dural/CSF leak with surgery for otorrhea
P1-91868 Elevation of depressed skull fracture with repair of dura
P1-91869 Elevation of depressed skull fracture with repair of dura and debridement of brain
P1-91870 Cerebral meningeorrhaphy
Suture of cerebral meninges
P1-91872 Suture of cerebral dura mater
Simple suture of dura mater of brain
P1-91875 Ligation of middle meningeal artery
P1-91876 Ligation of superior longitudinal sinus
P1-91878 Ventriculostomy
Anastomosis of cerebral ventricle
P1-91879 Ventriculocisternostomy
Ventriculocisternal shunt with valve
Torkildsen operation
P1-91880 Ventriculocisternostomy, third ventricle
P1-91881 Ventriculocisternostomy, third ventricle, stereotactic method
P1-91882 Ventricular shunt to intracerebral site, NOS
P1-91884 Ventricular shunt to cervical subarachnoid space
P1-91885 Ventricular shunt to cisterna magna
P1-91886 Ventricular shunt to head or neck structure
P1-91887 Ventricular shunt to nasopharynx
P1-91888 Ventricular shunt to mastoid
Ventriculomastoid anastomosis with valve
P1-91890 Ventricular shunt to circulatory system, NOS
P1-91891 Ventricular shunt to venous system
Cerebral ventriculovenostomy
P1-91892 Ventriculoatrial shunt with valve
Ventriculoatrial anastomosis with valve
Atrioventriculostomy
P1-91894 Ventriculocaval shunt with valve
Ventriculocaval anastomosis with valve
P1-91896 Creation of subarachnoid/subdural-atrial shunt
P1-91897 Creation of subarachnoid/subdural-auricular shunt
P1-91898 Creation of subarachnoid/subdural-jugular shunt
P1-91899 Creation of ventriculo-atrial shunt
P1-9189A Creation of ventriculo-auricular shunt
P1-9189B Creation of ventriculo-jugular shunt
Ventriculojugulovenostomy
Ventriculojugular shunt
P1-91910 Cerebral ventricular to thoracic cavity shunt
P1-91912 Ventriculopleural shunt with valve
Creation of ventriculo-pleural shunt
Ventriculopleural anastomosis with valve
P1-91913 Creation of subarachnoid/subdural-pleural shunt
P1-91915 Shunt from cerebral ventricle to abdominal cavity or organ, NOS
P1-91916 Ventriculoperitoneal shunt
Creation of ventriculo-peritoneal shunt
Ventriculoperitoneostomy
P1-91918 Ventriculocholecystostomy
Shunt of cerebral ventricle to gallbladder
P1-91920 Subdural-peritoneal shunt with valve
P1-91921 Creation of subarachnoid/subdural-peritoneal shunt
P1-91930 Ventricular shunt to urinary system, NOS
P1-91932 Ventricular shunt to ureter
Ventriculoureterostomy
P1-91936 Shunt of cerebral ventricle to lumbar site
Ventriculolumbar shunt with valve
P1-91938 Ventricular shunt to bone marrow
P1-91944 Shunt of cerebral ventricle to extracranial site, NOS
P1-91946 Creation of subarachnoid/subdural-other terminus shunt
P1-91948 Creation of ventriculo-other terminus shunt
P1-91950 Revision of Holter valve
P1-91952 Revision of cerebral ventricular shunt
P1-91958 Take-down of cerebral ventricular shunt

1-91C Brain: Destructive Procedures

P1-91C00 Destructive procedure on brain, NOS
Destruction of tissue of brain, NOS
P1-91C10 Destruction of cerebral lesion
P1-91C12 Lysis of cortical adhesions of brain
P1-91C14 Cryotherapy of brain
P1-91C15 Coagulation or electrocoagulation of brain tissue
P1-91C16 Creation of lesion by stereotactic method, single, subcortical structures except globus pallidus or thalamus
P1-91C17 Creation of lesion by stereotactic method, multiple stages, subcortical structures except globus pallidus or thalamus

P1-91C20 Destruction of lesion of cerebral meninges
P1-91C22 Lysis of adhesions of cortical meninges
P1-91C23 Stripping of cerebral meninges
P1-91C24 Stripping of cerebral subdural membrane
P1-91C25 Cauterization of choroid plexus
P1-91C30 Craniectomy, trephination, bone flap craniotomy for coagulation of choroid plexus
P1-91C31 Creation of lesion by stereotactic method, single, globus pallidus
P1-91C32 Creation of lesion by stereotactic method, single, thalamus
P1-91C33 Creation of lesion by stereotactic method, multiple stages, globus pallidus
P1-91C34 Creation of lesion by stereotactic method, multiple stages, thalamus
P1-91C50 Destruction of gasserian ganglion by radiofrequency
P1-91C52 Creation of lesion by stereotactic method, percutaneous, by neurolytic agent, gasserian ganglion
P1-91C53 Creation of lesion by stereotactic method, percutaneous, by neurolytic agent, trigeminal medullary tract

1-91D Brain: Transplantations and Transpositions

P1-91D10 Grafting of cerebral meninges, NOS
P1-91D12 Transplantation of dura, NOS
  Grafting of dura, NOS
P1-91D20 Osteoplasty of cranium with bone graft
  Repair of skull with graft of bone
  Repair of cranium with bone graft
  Grafting of bone of skull
  Grafting of pericranial bone
  Bone graft to skull

1-91E Brain: Manipulations

P1-91E00 Reduction of fracture of skull, NOS
P1-91E02 Reduction of closed skull fracture without operation, NOS

1-93 OPERATIVE PROCEDURES ON THE SPINAL CORD

1-930 Spinal Cord: General and Miscellaneous Operative Procedures

P1-93000 Operation on spinal cord, NOS
P1-93002 Diagnostic procedure on spinal cord, NOS
P1-93010 Operation on spinal meninges, NOS
P1-93012 Diagnostic procedure on spinal meninges, NOS
P1-93020 Operative procedure on spinal structures, NOS

1-931-932 Spinal Cord: Incisions

P1-93100 Spinal cordotomy, NOS
  Bishoff operation
  Tractotomy of spinal cord, NOS
  Division of nerve tracts of spinal cord
  Division of spinal cord tracts
  Splitting of spinal cord tracts
  Transection of nerve tracts in spinal cord
  Spinal chordotomy, NOS
  Myelotomy, NOS
P1-93102 Bilateral spinal cordotomy
P1-93103 Anterior spinal cordotomy
P1-93104 Posterior spinal cordotomy
P1-93105 Anterolateral cordotomy
  Spinothalamic cordotomy
P1-93106 One stage myelotomy
  One stage tractotomy of spinal cord
P1-93107 Two stage myelotomy
  Two stage tractotomy of spinal cord
P1-93110 Spinal percutaneous cordotomy
  Percutaneous cordotomy
  Percutaneous tractotomy
  Division of nerve tracts of spinal cord, percutaneous
  Division of spinal cord tracts, percutaneous
  Splitting of spinal cord tracts, percutaneous
P1-93111 Stereotactic cordotomy
P1-93114 Incision of spinal cord meninges, NOS
  Incision of spinal meninges, NOS
  Opening of spinal dura, NOS
P1-93116V Incision and drainage of spinal cord
P1-93120 Incision of vertebral column, NOS
P1-93122 Laminotomy, NOS
  Rachitomy, NOS
  Spondylotomy, NOS
  Laminectomy, NOS
  Rachiotomy, NOS
P1-93124 Foraminotomy, NOS
P1-93126 Exploration of disc space, NOS
P1-93128 Exploration of spinal nerve root
P1-93130 Decompression of spinal cord, NOS
P1-93134 Laminotomy for decompression and exploration
  Decompression laminectomy
  Laminectomy for decompression and exploration
  Gill operation
P1-93135 Laminotomy for decompression of nerve root including partial facetectomy, foraminotomy and excision of herniated intervertebral disc, one interspace, cervical
P1-93137 Laminotomy for decompression of nerve root including partial facetectomy, foraminotomy and excision of herniated intervertebral disc, reexploration, cervical
P1-93138 Costovertebral approach for decompression of spinal cord or nerve root, thoracic, single segment
P1-9313A Transpedicular approach for decompression of spinal cord or nerve root, single segment, thoracic
P1-93140 Laminotomy for decompression of nerve root including partial facetectomy, foraminotomy and excision of herniated intervertebral disc, one interspace, lumbar

1-931-932 Spinal Cord: Incisions — Continued

P1-93142 Transpedicular approach for decompression of spinal cord, cauda equina and/or nerve root, single segment, lumbar
P1-93144 Laminotomy for decompression of nerve root including partial facetectomy, foraminotomy and excision of herniated intervertebral disc, reexploration, lumbar
P1-93148 Reopening of laminectomy or laminotomy site
P1-93150 Incision of spinal nerve root, NOS
  Spinal radicotomy
  Spinal radiculotomy
  Spinal rhizotomy
  Transection of spinal nerve root
  Cutting of spinal nerve root
  Division of spinal nerve root
P1-93152 Posterior spinal rhizotomy
  Dana operation
  Section of posterior spinal nerve root
P1-93154 Anterior spinal rhizotomy
P1-93156 Laminectomy for cordotomy with section of one spinothalamic tract, one stage, cervical
P1-93157 Laminectomy for cordotomy with section of one spinothalamic tract, one stage, thoracic
P1-93158 Laminectomy for cordotomy with section of both spinothalamic tracts, one stage, cervical
P1-93159 Laminectomy for cordotomy with section of both spinothalamic tracts, one stage, thoracic
P1-9315A Laminectomy for cordotomy with section of both spinothalamic tracts, two stages within 14 days, cervical
P1-9315B Laminectomy for cordotomy with section of both spinothalamic tracts, two stages within 14 days, thoracic
P1-93160 Laminectomy for rhizotomy, one or two segments
P1-93162 Laminectomy for rhizotomy, more than two segments
P1-93163 Laminectomy for myelotomy, Bischof or Drez type, cervical, thoracic or thoracolumbar
P1-93164 Hemilaminectomy for decompression and exploration
P1-93165 Laminectomy for exploration or decompression of cauda equina, one or two segments, lumbar for spondylolisthesis, Gill type operation
P1-93166 Laminectomy for exploration or decompression of spinal cord, one or two segments, lumbar for spondylolisthesis, Gill type operation
P1-93167 Laminectomy for exploration or decompression of spinal cord, one or two segments, cervical
P1-93168 Laminectomy for exploration or decompression of spinal cord, one or two segments, thoracic
P1-93169 Laminectomy for exploration or decompression of spinal cord, one or two segments, lumbar, except for spondylolisthesis
P1-9316A Laminectomy for exploration or decompression of spinal cord, one or two segments, sacral
P1-93170 Laminectomy for exploration or decompression of spinal cord, more than two segments, cervical
P1-93171 Laminectomy for exploration or decompression of spinal cord, more than two segments, thoracic
P1-93172 Laminectomy for exploration or decompression of spinal cord, more than two segments, lumbar
P1-93173 Laminectomy, including unilateral or bilateral complete foraminotomy for decompression of spinal cord and/or nerve roots, single segment, cervical
P1-93174 Laminectomy, including unilateral or bilateral complete foraminotomy for decompression of spinal cord and/or nerve roots, single segment, thoracic
P1-93175 Laminectomy, including unilateral or bilateral complete foraminotomy for decompression of spinal cord, cauda equina and/or nerve roots, single segment, lumbar
P1-93179 Laminectomy, including unilateral or bilateral complete facetectomy for decompression of spinal cord and/or nerve roots, single segment, cervical
P1-93180 Laminectomy, including unilateral or bilateral complete facetectomy for decompression of spinal cord and/or nerve roots, single segment, thoracic
P1-93181 Laminectomy, including unilateral or bilateral complete facetectomy for decompression of spinal cord, cauda equina and/or nerve roots, single segment, lumbar
P1-93185 Laminectomy for drainage of intramedullary cyst or syrinx to peritoneal space
P1-93186 Laminectomy for drainage of intramedullary cyst or syrinx to subarachnoid space
P1-93187 Laminectomy and section of dentate ligaments without dural graft, cervical, one or two segments
P1-93188 Laminectomy and section of dentate ligaments without dural graft, cervical, more than two segments
P1-93189 Laminectomy for release of tethered spinal cord, lumbar
P1-93190 Anterior discectomy for decompression of spinal cord and/or nerve roots, including osteophytectomy, cervical, single interspace
P1-93192 Anterior discectomy for decompression of spinal cord and/or nerve roots, including osteophytectomy, thoracic, single interspace
P1-93194 Vertebral corpectomy, partial, anterior approach for decompression of spinal cord and/or nerve roots, cervical, single segment
P1-93196 Vertebral corpectomy, partial, transthoracic approach for decompression of spinal cord and/or nerve roots, thoracic, single segment

P1-93198 Vertebral corpectomy, partial, transperitoneal approach for decompression of spinal cord, cauda equina or nerve roots, lumbar, or sacral, single segment

P1-9319A Vertebral corpectomy, partial, retroperitoneal approach for decompression of spinal cord, cauda equina or nerve roots, lumbar, or sacral, single segment

P1-931A2 Vertebral corpectomy, partial, combined thoracolumbar approach for decompression of spinal cord, cauda equina or nerve roots, lumbar, single segment

P1-931A4 Vertebral corpectomy, complete, anterior approach for decompression of spinal cord and/or nerve roots, cervical, single segment

P1-931A6 Vertebral corpectomy, complete, transthoracic approach for decompression of spinal cord and/or nerve roots, thoracic, single segment

P1-931A8 Vertebral corpectomy, complete, transperitoneal approach for decompression of spinal cord, cauda equina or nerve roots, lumbar, or sacral, single segment

P1-931B0 Vertebral corpectomy, complete, retroperitoneal approach for decompression of spinal cord, cauda equina or nerve roots, lumbar, or sacral, single segment

P1-931B2 Vertebral corpectomy, complete, combined thoracolumbar approach for decompression of spinal cord, cauda equina or nerve roots, lumbar, single segment

P1-93200 Drainage of vertebral column, NOS
  Drainage of spinal cord

P1-93210 Microdissection, spinal procedure

P1-93220 Spinal tap
  Diagnostic spinal tap
  Spinal puncture and aspiration
  Spinal puncture
  Rachicentesis

P1-93222 Diagnostic lumbar spinal puncture
  Diagnostic lumbar tap
  Diagnostic lumbar puncture

P1-93224 Therapeutic spinal puncture, NOS

P1-93230 Lateral cervical puncture without injection

P1-93232 Percutaneous aspiration of spinal cord cyst
  Percutaneous aspiration of spinal cord syrinx

1-933-934 Spinal Cord: Excisions

P1-93300 Biopsy of spinal cord, NOS
  Excisional biopsy of spinal cord, NOS

P1-93304 Biopsy of spinal meninges, NOS
  Excisional biopsy of spinal meninges, NOS

P1-93305 Percutaneous needle biopsy of spinal cord, NOS

P1-93306 Stereotactic biopsy of lesion of spinal cord

P1-93310 Excision of lesion of spinal cord
  Excision of intraspinal lesion
  Laminectomy with excision of intraspinal lesion, NOS

P1-93312 Excision of lesion of spinal meninges

P1-93320 Resection of spinal cord

P1-93322 Resection of spinal meninges

P1-93324 Debridement of spinal cord

P1-93326 Curettage of spinal cord

P1-93327 Curettage of spinal meninges

P1-93328 Debridement of spinal meninges

P1-93329 Aspiration of lesion of spinal cord

P1-9332A Radiculectomy

P1-93330 Laminectomy for biopsy of intraspinal neoplasm, extradural, cervical

P1-93331 Laminectomy for biopsy of intraspinal neoplasm, extradural, thoracic

P1-93332 Laminectomy for biopsy of intraspinal neoplasm, extradural, lumbar

P1-93334 Laminectomy for biopsy of intraspinal neoplasm, extradural, sacral

P1-93335 Laminectomy for biopsy of intraspinal neoplasm, intradural, extramedullary, cervical

P1-93336 Laminectomy for biopsy of intraspinal neoplasm, intradural, extramedullary, thoracic

P1-93337 Laminectomy for biopsy of intraspinal neoplasm, intradural, extramedullary, lumbar

P1-93338 Laminectomy for biopsy of intraspinal neoplasm, intradural, intramedullary, cervical

P1-93339 Laminectomy for biopsy of intraspinal neoplasm, intradural, intramedullary, thoracic

P1-93340 Laminectomy for biopsy of intraspinal neoplasm, intradural, intramedullary, thoracolumbar

P1-93341 Laminectomy for biopsy of intraspinal neoplasm, intradural, sacral

P1-93342 Laminectomy for biopsy of intraspinal neoplasm, combined extradural-intradural lesion, any level

P1-93346 Laminectomy for excision of intraspinal neoplasm, extradural, cervical

P1-93347 Laminectomy for excision of intraspinal neoplasm, extradural, thoracic

P1-93348 Laminectomy for excision of intraspinal neoplasm, extradural, lumbar

P1-93349 Laminectomy for excision of intraspinal neoplasm, extradural, sacral

P1-93350 Laminectomy for excision of intraspinal neoplasm, intradural, extramedullary, cervical

P1-93351 Laminectomy for excision of intraspinal neoplasm, intradural, extramedullary, thoracic

P1-93352 Laminectomy for excision of intraspinal neoplasm, intradural, extramedullary, lumbar

P1-93353 Laminectomy for excision of intraspinal neoplasm, intradural, intramedullary, cervical

P1-93354 Laminectomy for excision of intraspinal neoplasm, intradural, intramedullary, thoracic

P1-93355 Laminectomy for excision of intraspinal neoplasm, intradural, intramedullary, thoracolumbar

1-933-934 Spinal Cord: Excisions — Continued

P1-93356 Laminectomy for excision of intraspinal neoplasm, intradural, sacral
P1-93357 Laminectomy for excision of intraspinal neoplasm, combined extradural-intradural lesion
P1-93358 Laminectomy for excision of intraspinal lesion other than neoplasm, extradural, cervical
P1-93359 Laminectomy for excision of intraspinal lesion other than neoplasm, extradural, thoracic
P1-9335A Laminectomy for excision of intraspinal lesion other than neoplasm, extradural, lumbar
P1-9335B Laminectomy for excision of intraspinal lesion other than neoplasm, extradural, sacral
P1-93360 Laminectomy for excision of intraspinal lesion other than neoplasm, intradural, cervical
P1-93361 Laminectomy for excision of intraspinal lesion other than neoplasm, intradural, thoracic
P1-93362 Laminectomy for excision of intraspinal lesion other than neoplasm, intradural, lumbar
P1-93363 Laminectomy for excision of intraspinal lesion other than neoplasm, intradural, sacral
P1-93364 Laminectomy for excision of arteriovenous malformation of spinal cord, cervical
P1-93365 Laminectomy for excision of arteriovenous malformation of spinal cord, thoracic
P1-93366 Laminectomy for excision of arteriovenous malformation of spinal cord, thoracolumbar
P1-93370 Vertebral corpectomy, partial, for excision of intraspinal lesion, single segment, extradural, cervical
P1-93371 Vertebral corpectomy, partial, for excision of intraspinal lesion, single segment, extradural, thoracic by thoracolumbar approach
P1-93372 Vertebral corpectomy, partial, for excision of intraspinal lesion, single segment, extradural, thoracic by transthoracic approach
P1-93373 Vertebral corpectomy, partial, for excision of intraspinal lesion, single segment, extradural, lumbar or sacral by retroperitoneal approach
P1-93374 Vertebral corpectomy, partial, for excision of intraspinal lesion, single segment, extradural, lumbar or sacral by transperitoneal approach
P1-93375 Vertebral corpectomy, partial, for excision of intraspinal lesion, single segment, intradural, cervical
P1-93376 Vertebral corpectomy, partial, for excision of intraspinal lesion, single segment, intradural, thoracic by transthoracic approach
P1-93377 Vertebral corpectomy, partial, for excision of intraspinal lesion, single segment, intradural, thoracic by thoracolumbar approach
P1-93378 Vertebral corpectomy, partial, for excision of intraspinal lesion, single segment, intradural, lumbar or sacral by retroperitoneal approach
P1-93379 Vertebral corpectomy, partial, for excision of intraspinal lesion, single segment, intradural, lumbar or sacral by transperitoneal approach
P1-9337A Vertebral corpectomy, partial, for excision of intraspinal lesion, single segment, each additional segment
P1-93380 Vertebral corpectomy, complete, for excision of intraspinal lesion, single segment, extradural, cervical
P1-93382 Vertebral corpectomy, complete, for excision of intraspinal lesion, single segment, extradural, thoracic by transthoracic approach
P1-93383 Vertebral corpectomy, complete, for excision of intraspinal lesion, single segment, extradural, thoracic by thoracolumbar approach
P1-93384 Vertebral corpectomy, complete, for excision of intraspinal lesion, single segment, extradural, lumbar or sacral by retroperitoneal approach
P1-93385 Vertebral corpectomy, complete, for excision of intraspinal lesion, single segment, extradural, lumbar or sacral by transperitoneal approach
P1-93386 Vertebral corpectomy, complete, for excision of intraspinal lesion, single segment, intradural, cervical
P1-93387 Vertebral corpectomy, complete, for excision of intraspinal lesion, single segment, intradural, thoracic by transthoracic approach
P1-93388 Vertebral corpectomy, complete, for excision of intraspinal lesion, single segment, intradural, thoracic by thoracolumbar approach
P1-93389 Vertebral corpectomy, complete, for excision of intraspinal lesion, single segment, intradural, lumbar or sacral by retroperitoneal approach
P1-9338A Vertebral corpectomy, complete, for excision of intraspinal lesion, single segment, intradural, lumbar or sacral by transperitoneal approach
P1-93420 Removal of foreign body from spinal canal
P1-93421 Removal of foreign body from spinal cord
P1-93422 Removal of foreign body from spinal meninges
P1-93426 Removal of foreign body from nerve root, NOS
P1-93427 Removal of bony spicules from spinal canal
P1-93430 Diagnostic spinal drainage, NOS
P1-93431 Removal of dye from spinal canal
  Lumbar puncture for removal of dye
P1-93432 Removal of pantopaque dye from spinal canal

1-935-936 Spinal Cord: Injections and Implantations

P1-93500 Injection of spinal canal, NOS
  Injection of agent into spinal canal, NOS
P1-93502 Injection of spinal saline
P1-93504 Injection of spinal steroid
P1-93505 Epidural lumbar injection of blood patch

P1-93508 Irrigation of lumbosubarachnoid shunt
P1-93509V Injection of spinal epidural space
P1-93510 Injection of spinal anesthetic agent for analgesia
P1-93511 Epidural injection of anesthetic substance, diagnostic, caudal, single
P1-93512 Epidural injection of anesthetic substance, diagnostic, lumbar, single
P1-93513 Injection of anesthetic substance, diagnostic, subarachnoid, single
P1-93514 Injection of anesthetic substance, diagnostic, subdural, single
P1-93515 Epidural injection of anesthetic substance, diagnostic, caudal, continuous
P1-93516 Epidural injection of anesthetic substance, diagnostic, lumbar, continuous
P1-93517 Injection of anesthetic substance, diagnostic, subarachnoid , continuous
P1-93518 Injection of anesthetic substance, diagnostic, subdural, continuous
P1-93519 Injection of anesthetic substance, diagnostic, subarachnoid, differential
P1-9351A Injection of anesthetic substance, diagnostic, subdural, differential
P1-93520 Epidural injection of anesthetic substance, therapeutic, caudal, single
P1-93521 Epidural injection of anesthetic substance, therapeutic, lumbar, single
P1-93522 Injection of anesthetic substance, therapeutic, subarachnoid, single
P1-93523 Injection of anesthetic substance, therapeutic, subdural, single
P1-93524 Epidural injection of anesthetic substance, therapeutic, caudal, continuous
P1-93525 Epidural injection of anesthetic substance, therapeutic, lumbar, continuous
P1-93526 Injection of anesthetic substance, therapeutic, subarachnoid, continuous
P1-93527 Injection of anesthetic substance, therapeutic, subdural, continuous
P1-93528 Injection of anesthetic substance, therapeutic, subarachnoid, differential
P1-93529 Injection of anesthetic substance, therapeutic, subdural, differential
P1-93530 Epidural injection of contrast substance, caudal
P1-93532 Epidural injection of contrast substance, lumbar
P1-93533 Injection procedure for computerized axial tomography, spinal
P1-93534 Injection procedure for discography, single, cervical
P1-93535 Injection procedure for discography, single, lumbar
P1-93536 Injection procedure for discography, multiple levels, cervical
P1-93537 Injection procedure for discography, multiple levels, lumbar
P1-93538 Injection procedure for myelography, spinal
P1-93540 Injection procedure for myelography and computerized axial tomography, spinal
P1-93542 Lateral cervical puncture with injection
P1-93544 Subarachnoid perfusion of spinal cord with refrigerated saline
P1-93550 Implantation of spine, NOS
P1-93551 Implantation of electronic stimulator of spine
P1-93552 Implantation of stimoceiver in spine
P1-93553 Implantation of electrode in spine
Insertion of electrode in spine
P1-93554 Implantation of neuropacemaker in spine
Insertion of neural pacemaker in spine
P1-93555 Implantation of neurostimulator in spine
Insertion of spinal neurostimulator
P1-93557 Incision for subcutaneous placement of spinal neurostimulator receiver, direct coupling
P1-93558 Incision for subcutaneous placement of spinal neurostimulator receiver, inductive coupling
P1-93560 Laminectomy for implantation of neurostimulator electrodes, endodural
P1-93561 Laminectomy for implantation of neurostimulator electrodes, epidural
P1-93562 Laminectomy for implantation of neurostimulator electrodes, subdural
P1-93563 Laminectomy for implantation of neurostimulator electrodes, spinal cord
P1-93570 Insertion of catheter in spinal canal space, epidural, subarachnoid or subdural, for infusion of therapeutic or palliative substances
P1-93572 Insertion of catheter into spinal canal for infusion of palliative substances
P1-93574 Insertion of catheter into spinal canal for infusion of therapeutic substances
P1-93580 Percutaneous implantation of neurostimulator electrodes, epidural
P1-93581 Stereotactic stimulation of spinal cord, percutaneous, single procedure
P1-93582 Percutaneous implantation of neurostimulator electrodes, intradural
P1-93591 Revision of spinal neurostimulator electrodes
P1-93592 Revision of spinal neurostimulator receiver
P1-93593 Removal of spinal electrodes with synchronous replacement
P1-93594 Removal of spinal electronic stimulator with synchronous replacement
Replacement of spinal neurostimulator
Removal of spinal neurostimulator with synchronous replacement
P1-93595 Removal of spinal pacemaker with synchronous replacement
Removal of spinal neuropacemaker with synchronous replacement
P1-93610 Removal of spinal pacemaker
Removal of spinal neuropacemaker
P1-93611 Removal of spinal neurostimulator
Removal of spinal electronic stimulator

1-935-936 Spinal Cord: Injections and Implantations — Continued

P1-93612 Removal of spinal electrodes
 Removal of spinal neurostimulator electrodes
P1-93614 Removal of spinal neurostimulator receiver
P1-93620 Removal of entire lumbosubarachnoid shunt system without replacement
P1-93622 Removal of spinal thecal shunt
P1-93623 Removal of pleurothecal shunt
P1-93624 Removal of subarachnoid-peritoneal shunt
P1-93625 Removal of subarachnoid-ureteral shunt
P1-93626 Removal of lumbosubarachnoid shunt
P1-93627 Removal of salpingothecal shunt

1-937 Spinal Cord: Endoscopy

P1-93700 Endoscopy of spinal canal, NOS

1-938 Spinal Cord: Surgical Repairs, Closures and Reconstructions

P1-93800 Repair of spinal cord, NOS
P1-93802 Repair of spinal meninges, NOS
P1-93810 Repair of meninges of spinal meningocele
 Repair of spinal meningocele
 Gardner operation
 Closure of spinal meningocele
 Meningeorrhaphy for spinal meningocele
P1-93811 Repair of spinal meningocele, less than 5 cm diameter
P1-93812 Repair of spinal meningocele, larger than 5 cm diameter
P1-93814 Repair of spina bifida, NOS
P1-93815 Repair of vertebral arch defect in spina bifida
P1-93816 Repair of spinal pseudomeningocele with laminectomy
P1-93817 Obliteration of sacral meningocele
P1-93818 Obliteration of lumbar pseudomeningocele
P1-93820 Repair of myelomeningocele
 Repair of spinal myelomeningocele
 Repair of meninges in spinal myelomeningocele
 Closure of myelomeningocele
 Meningeorrhaphy for myelomeningocele
P1-93821 Repair of myelomeningocele, less than 5 cm diameter
P1-93822 Repair of myelomeningocele, larger than 5 cm diameter
P1-93826 Repair of dural/CSF leak without laminectomy
P1-93828 Repair of dural/CSF leak with laminectomy
P1-93830 Creation of lumbar shunt including laminectomy
P1-93832 Creation of spinal shunt with valve, NOS
P1-93833 Creation of lumbosubarachnoid shunt with valve, NOS
P1-93834 Spinal pleurothecal shunt with valve
 Spinal pleurothecal anastomosis with valve
P1-93835 Spinal salpingothecal shunt with valve
 Spinal salpingothecal anastomosis with valve
P1-93836 Subarachnoid-peritoneal spinal shunt
 Subarachnoid-peritoneal spinal shunt with valve
 Subarachnoid-peritoneal spinal anastomosis with valve
P1-93838 Creation of lumbar subarachnoid-peritoneal shunt with laminectomy
P1-9383B Subarachnoid-ureteral spinal shunt
 Subarachnoid-ureteral spinal shunt with valve
 Subarachnoid-ureteral spinal anastomosis with valve
P1-9383C Creation of lumbar subarachnoid shunt with laminectomy
P1-9383D Creation of lumbar subarachnoid-pleural shunt with laminectomy
P1-93840 Revision of spinal thecal shunt, NOS
P1-93843 Revision of spinal pleurothecal shunt
 Revision of spinal pleurothecal anastomosis
P1-93845 Revision of spinal salpingothecal shunt
 Revision of spinal salpingothecal anastomosis
P1-93846 Revision of spinal subarachnoid-peritoneal shunt
 Revision of spinal subarachnoid-peritoneal anastomosis
P1-93847 Revision of spinal subarachnoid-ureteral shunt
 Revision of spinal subarachnoid-ureteral anastomosis
P1-93848 Revision of lumbosubarachnoid shunt
P1-93851 Replacement of lumbosubarachnoid shunt
P1-93862 Repair of diastematomyelia
P1-93864 Marsupialization of spinal cyst
P1-93866 Suture of spinal meninges
 Spinal meningeorrhaphy
P1-93868 Suture of spinal dura mater

1-93C Spinal Cord: Destructive Procedures

P1-93C00 Spinal injection of destructive agent, NOS
 Injection of destructive agent into spinal canal
P1-93C10 Injection of spinal neurolytic agent, NOS
P1-93C11 Epidural injection of neurolytic solution, caudal
P1-93C12 Epidural injection of neurolytic solution, lumbar
P1-93C13 Epidural injection of neurolytic substance, caudal
P1-93C14 Epidural injection of neurolytic substance, lumbar
P1-93C15 Injection of neurolytic substance, subarachnoid
P1-93C16 Spinal injection of alcohol

P1-93C17 Spinal injection of phenol
P1-93C20 Injection procedure for chemonucleolysis, including discography, intervertebral disc, multiple levels, lumbar
P1-93C21 Injection procedure for chemonucleolysis, including discography, intervertebral disc, single, lumbar
P1-93C22 Spinal arterial injection procedure for occlusion of arteriovenous malformation
P1-93C30 Destruction of lesion of spinal cord
P1-93C31 Destruction of lesion of spinal meninges
P1-93C32 Lysis of adhesions of spinal cord
P1-93C33 Lysis of adhesions of spinal meninges
P1-93C34 Lysis of adhesions of spinal nerve roots
Neurolysis of spinal nerve roots
P1-93C35 Lysis of adhesions of spinal cord and nerve roots
P1-93C36 Chemolysis of spinal canal structure
P1-93C40 Stripping of spinal meninges
P1-93C41 Stripping of spinal subdural membrane
P1-93C50 Coagulation or electrocoagulation of spinal cord lesion
P1-93C52 Percutaneous denervation of facet
P1-93C55 Creation of lesion of spinal cord by any modality
P1-93C56 Creation of lesion of spinal cord by percutaneous method
P1-93C57 Creation of lesion of spinal cord by stereotactic method
P1-93C60 Laminectomy for occlusion of arteriovenous malformation of spinal cord, cervical
P1-93C61 Laminectomy for occlusion of arteriovenous malformation of spinal cord, thoracic
P1-93C62 Laminectomy for occlusion of arteriovenous malformation of spinal cord, thoracolumbar

1-93D Spinal Cord: Transplantations and Transpositions

P1-93D10 Spinal dural graft
P1-93D12 Laminectomy and section of dentate ligaments, with dural graft, cervical, one or two segments
P1-93D14 Laminectomy and section of dentate ligaments, with dural graft, cervical, more than two segments

1-93E Spinal Cord: Manipulations

P1-93E00 Manipulation of spinal cord, NOS
P1-93E04 Manipulation of spinal meninges, NOS

1-95 OPERATIVE PROCEDURES ON THE NERVES

1-950 Nerves: General and Miscellaneous Operative Procedures

P1-95000 Operative procedure on nerve, NOS
P1-95001 Operative procedure on cranial nerve
P1-95002 Operative procedure on peripheral nerve
P1-95007 Diagnostic procedure on nerve, NOS
P1-95008 Diagnostic procedure on cranial nerve
P1-95009 Diagnostic procedure on peripheral nerve
P1-95010 Operation on sympathetic nerve, NOS
P1-95012 Diagnostic procedure on sympathetic nerve
P1-95018 Operation on adrenal nerve, NOS
P1-95020 Operation on nerve ganglion, NOS
P1-95022 Operation on sympathetic ganglion
P1-95025 Diagnostic procedure on nerve ganglion, NOS
P1-95026 Diagnostic procedure on cranial nerve ganglion
P1-95027 Diagnostic procedure on peripheral nerve ganglion
P1-95028 Diagnostic procedure on sympathetic ganglion

1-951 Nerves: Incisions

P1-95100 Incision of nerve, NOS
Neurotomy, NOS
P1-95102 Incision of cranial nerve, NOS
Cranial neurotomy, NOS
P1-95104 Incision of peripheral nerve, NOS
Peripheral neurotomy, NOS
P1-95105 Incision of cranial and peripheral nerves, NOS
P1-95106 Exploration of nerve, NOS
P1-95107 Exploration of cranial nerve, NOS
P1-95108 Exploration of peripheral nerve, NOS
P1-95110 Transection of nerve, NOS
Cutting of nerve, NOS
Section of nerve, NOS
Division of nerve, NOS
P1-95112 Transection of cranial nerve, NOS
Cutting of cranial nerve, NOS
Section of cranial nerve, NOS
Division of cranial nerve, NOS
P1-95114 Transection of peripheral nerve, NOS
Cutting of peripheral nerve, NOS
Section of peripheral nerve, NOS
Division of peripheral nerve, NOS
P1-95116 Extradural transection of cranial nerve
P1-95117 Extradural transection of spinal nerve, NOS
P1-95119 Microdissection of nerve
P1-95120 Decompression of nerve, NOS
P1-95122 Decompression of cranial nerve, NOS
Release of cranial nerve, NOS
P1-95124 Decompression of peripheral nerve, NOS
Release of peripheral nerve, NOS
P1-95127 Exploration of carpal tunnel
P1-95128 Exploration of tarsal tunnel
P1-95130 Decompression of median nerve
Release of carpal tunnel for nerve decompression
Release of carpal tunnel for median nerve decompression
Release of transverse carpal ligament for nerve decompression
Retinaculotomy of carpal tunnel
P1-95132 Decompression of tarsal tunnel
Release of tarsal tunnel

1-951 Nerves: Incisions — Continued

P1-95132 (cont.) Release of tarsal tunnel for tibial nerve decompression
P1-95134 Decompression of plantar digital nerve
P1-95140 Phrenicotomy
  Division of phrenic nerve
  Transection of phrenic nerve
P1-95142 Transection of greater occipital nerve
P1-95143 Transection of obturator nerve, extrapelvic, without adductor tenotomy
P1-95144 Transection of obturator nerve, extrapelvic, with adductor tenotomy
P1-95145 Transection of obturator nerve, intrapelvic, without adductor tenotomy
P1-95146 Transection of obturator nerve, intrapelvic, with adductor tenotomy
P1-95147 Transection of pudendal nerve
P1-95148 Trigeminal rhizotomy
  Frazier operation
  Subtemporal trigeminal rhizotomy
P1-95149 Division of trigeminal nerve at foramen ovale
  Pancoast operation
  Transection of trigeminal nerve
  Division of trigeminal nerve
  Cutting of trigeminal nerve
P1-9514A Retrogasserian neurotomy
P1-9514B Decompression of trigeminal nerve root
  Taarnhoj operation
P1-9514C Release of trigeminal nerve
P1-95150 Transection of inferior alveolar nerve by osteotomy
P1-95152 Transection of infraorbital nerve
P1-95154 Transection of supraorbital nerve
P1-95155 Transection of lingual nerve
P1-95156 Transection of mental nerve
P1-95160 Total facial nerve decompression
P1-95161 Decompression of facial nerve, intratemporal, lateral to geniculate ganglion
P1-95162 Decompression of facial nerve, intratemporal, lateral and medial to geniculate ganglion
P1-95163 Neurotomy of lacrimal branch nerve
  Division of lacrimal branch nerve
P1-95164 Transection of facial nerve, differential
P1-95165 Transection of facial nerve, complete
P1-95168 Decompression of auditory nerve
P1-9516A Acoustic neurotomy
  Section of acoustic nerve
  Transection of acoustic nerve
  Division of acoustic nerve
  Cutting of acoustic nerve
P1-9516B Acoustic rhizotomy
P1-9516C Exploration of auditory nerve
P1-95170 Vestibular nerve section by transcranial approach
P1-95171 Vestibular nerve section by translabyrinthine approach
P1-95172 Glossopharyngeal neurotomy
  Division of glossopharyngeal nerve
P1-95175 Division of laryngeal nerve, NOS
P1-95176 Division of inferior laryngeal nerve
P1-95177 Division of recurrent laryngeal nerve
P1-95178 Division of superior laryngeal nerve
P1-95179 Laminectomy for section of spinal accessory nerve
P1-95180 Sympathetic neurotomy
  Transection of sympathetic nerve
  Section of sympathetic nerve
  Division of sympathetic nerve
  Cutting of sympathetic nerve
  Krause operation
P1-95182 Division of sympathetic ganglion
  Section of sympathetic ganglion
P1-95184 Splanchnicotomy
P1-95185 Division of nerve of adrenal gland
P1-95186 Vagotomy, NOS
P1-95190 Division of nerve ganglion, NOS
P1-95191 Nerve ganglion decompression
P1-95192 Decompression of cranial ganglion, NOS

1-953-954 Nerves: Excisions

P1-95300 Biopsy of nerve, NOS
  Excisional biopsy of nerve, NOS
P1-95302 Open excisional biopsy of nerve
P1-95304 Closed excisional biopsy of nerve
P1-95306 Percutaneous needle biopsy of nerve
P1-95308 Incisional biopsy of cranial nerve
P1-95309 Incisional biopsy of peripheral nerve
P1-95310 Needle biopsy of cranial nerve
P1-95312 Needle biopsy of peripheral nerve
P1-95315 Biopsy of sympathetic nerve
  Excisional biopsy of sympathetic nerve
P1-95320 Excision of lesion of nerve, NOS
P1-95321 Excision of lesion of cranial nerve
P1-95322 Excision of lesion of peripheral nerve
P1-95324 Excision of Morton's neuroma of peripheral nerve
P1-95325 Excision of neuroma of cutaneous nerve
P1-95326 Excision of neuroma of digital nerve, one or both, same digit
P1-95327 Excision of neuroma of digital nerve, each additional digit
P1-95328 Excision of neuroma of hand, except digital nerve
P1-95329 Excision of neuroma of hand, each additional nerve, except same digit
P1-9532A Excision of neuroma of foot, except digital nerve
P1-9532B Excision of neuroma of foot, each additional nerve, except same digit
P1-95331 Excision of neuroma of sciatic nerve
P1-95332 Excision of neuroma of major peripheral nerve, except sciatic
P1-95333 Excision of neurofibroma of cutaneous nerve
P1-95334 Excision of neurofibroma, extensive
P1-95335 Excision of neurofibroma of major peripheral nerve

P1-95336 Excision of neurolemmoma of major peripheral nerve
P1-95337 Excision of neurolemmoma of cutaneous nerve
P1-95338 Excision of neurolemmoma, extensive
P1-95340 Debridement of peripheral nerve
P1-95341 Curettage of peripheral nerve
P1-95344 Neurectomy, NOS
  Excision of nerve, NOS
  Resection of nerve, NOS
P1-95345 Excision of cranial nerve
  Resection of cranial nerve
P1-95346 Excision of peripheral nerve
  Resection of peripheral nerve
P1-95347 Retrogasserian neurectomy
P1-95348 Trigeminal neurectomy
P1-95350 Inferior maxillary neurectomy
  Sonneberg operation
P1-95352 Phrenicectomy
  Resection of phrenic nerve
P1-95353 Popliteal neurectomy
P1-95354 Neurectomy of intrinsic musculature of foot
P1-95356 Excision of lesion of sympathetic nerve, NOS
P1-95357 Excision of neuroma of sympathetic nerve
P1-95360 Sympathectomy, NOS
  Excision of sympathetic nerve
  Resection of sympathetic nerve
  Smithwick operation
P1-95361 Curettage of sympathetic nerve
P1-95362 Cervical sympathectomy
P1-95364 Paracervical neurectomy
P1-95365 Cervicothoracic sympathectomy
P1-95366 Lumbar sympathectomy
P1-95367 Thoracolumbar sympathectomy
P1-95368 Presacral sympathectomy
  Presacral neurectomy
P1-95369 Renal sympathectomy
P1-95370 Vidianectomy
P1-95372 Hypogastric plexectomy
P1-95374 Splanchnicectomy
  Resection of splanchnic nerve
  Peet operation
P1-95378 Periarterial sympathectomy
P1-95380 Biopsy of nerve ganglion, NOS
  Excisional biopsy of nerve ganglion, NOS
P1-95381 Excisional biopsy of cranial nerve ganglion
P1-95382 Excisional biopsy of peripheral nerve ganglion
P1-95384 Open excisional biopsy of nerve ganglion
  Incisional biopsy of nerve ganglion
P1-95385 Closed excisional biopsy of nerve ganglion
P1-95386 Needle biopsy of nerve ganglion
  Percutaneous excisional biopsy of nerve ganglion
P1-95387 Excisional biopsy of sympathetic nerve ganglion
P1-95390 Ganglionectomy of nerve, NOS
P1-95391 Ganglionectomy of cranial nerve
P1-95392 Ganglionectomy of peripheral nerve
P1-95393 Ganglionectomy of sympathetic nerve
P1-95394 Gasserian ganglionectomy
  Excision of gasserian ganglion
  Excision of ganglion of trigeminal nerve
  Trigeminal ganglionectomy
P1-95396 Meckel's ganglionectomy
  Sphenopalatine ganglionectomy
P1-95397 Lumbar sympathetic ganglionectomy
P1-95398 Spinal ganglionectomy
P1-95410 Removal of foreign body from nerve, NOS
P1-95412 Removal of foreign body from cranial nerve
P1-95414 Removal of foreign body from peripheral nerve

1-955-956 Nerves: Injections and Implantations

P1-95500 Injection of nerve, NOS
P1-95502 Injection of cranial nerve
P1-95504 Injection of peripheral nerve
P1-95505 Injection of optic nerve
P1-95506 Injection of sympathetic nerve
P1-95507 Injection of laryngeal nerve, NOS
P1-95508 Injection of inferior laryngeal nerve
P1-95509 Injection of recurrent laryngeal nerve
P1-9550A Injection of superior laryngeal nerve
P1-95510 Injection into nerve ganglion, NOS
P1-95511 Injection of sympathetic ganglion
P1-95520 Injection of nerve agent, NOS
P1-95521 Nerve block, NOS
P1-95523 Injection of anesthetic agent into peripheral nerve for analgesia
  Peripheral nerve block
P1-95524 Injection of anesthetic agent into axillary nerve
P1-95525 Injection of anesthetic agent into brachial plexus
P1-95526 Injection of anesthetic agent into carotid sinus
P1-95527 Injection of anesthetic agent into celiac plexus with radiologic monitoring
P1-95528 Injection of anesthetic agent into celiac plexus without radiologic monitoring
P1-95529 Injection of anesthetic agent into cervical plexus
P1-95530 Injection of anesthetic agent into facial nerve
P1-95531 Injection of anesthetic agent into greater occipital nerve
P1-95532 Injection of anesthetic agent into ilioinguinal or iliohypogastric nerves
P1-95533 Injection of anesthetic agent into intercostal nerve, single
  Intercostal nerve block
P1-95534 Injection of anesthetic agent into intercostal nerves, multiple, regional block
P1-95535 Injection of anesthetic agent into lumbar region
P1-95536 Injection of anesthetic agent into paravertebral facet joint nerve, lumbar, single level

1-955-956 Nerves: Injections and Implantations — Continued

P1-95537 Injection of anesthetic agent into paravertebral facet joint nerve, lumbar, each additional level
P1-95538 Injection of anesthetic agent into paravertebral nerve, single vertebral level
P1-95539 Injection of anesthetic agent into paravertebral nerves, multiple levels
P1-95540 Injection of anesthetic agent into phrenic nerve
P1-95541 Injection of anesthetic agent into pudendal nerve
P1-95542 Injection of anesthetic agent into sciatic nerve
P1-95543 Injection of anesthetic agent into sphenopalatine ganglion
P1-95544 Injection of anesthetic agent into spinal accessory nerve
P1-95545 Injection of anesthetic agent into stellate ganglion
  Paravertebral stellate ganglion block
P1-95546 Injection of anesthetic agent into suprascapular nerve
P1-95547 Injection of anesthetic agent into thoracic nerve
P1-95548 Injection of anesthetic agent into trigeminal nerve
  Trigeminal nerve block
P1-95549 Injection of anesthetic agent into uterine paracervical nerve
P1-95550 Injection of anesthetic agent into vagus nerve
P1-95551 Injection of anesthetic agent into sympathetic nerve for analgesia
  Sympathetic nerve block
P1-95552 Gasserian ganglion block
P1-95554 Injection of neurolytic nerve agent, NOS
P1-95555 Injection of phenol into nerve
P1-95556 Injection of alcohol into nerve
P1-95557 Injection of neurolytic agent into sympathetic nerve
P1-95558 Injection of phenol into sympathetic nerve
P1-95559 Injection of alcohol into sympathetic nerve
P1-95561 Implantation of electrode into peripheral nerve
  Insertion of electrode into peripheral nerve
P1-95563 Insertion of pacemaker into peripheral nerve
  Insertion of neural pacemaker into peripheral nerve
  Implantation of neuropacemaker into peripheral nerve
  Implantation of neurostimulator into peripheral nerve
  Implantation of electronic stimulator into peripheral nerve
P1-95564 Implantation of stimoceiver into peripheral nerve
P1-95568 Implantation of electronic stimulator into phrenic nerve
P1-95570 Application of surface transcutaneous neurostimulator
P1-95572 Percutaneous implantation of neurostimulator electrodes into neuromuscular component, NOS
P1-95573 Percutaneous implantation of neurostimulator electrodes into autonomic nerve
P1-95574 Percutaneous implantation of neurostimulator electrodes into cranial nerve
P1-95576 Percutaneous implantation of neurostimulator electrodes into peripheral nerve
P1-95580 Removal of electrodes from peripheral nerve with synchronous replacement
P1-95582 Revision of peripheral neurostimulator electrodes
P1-95583 Revision of peripheral neurostimulator receiver
P1-95584 Removal of electronic stimulator from peripheral nerve with synchronous replacement
P1-95585 Removal of neuropacemaker from peripheral nerve with synchronous replacement
P1-95586 Replacement of neural pacemaker from peripheral nerve
  Removal of neural pacemaker from peripheral nerve with synchronous replacement
P1-95587 Removal of neurostimulator from peripheral nerve with synchronous replacement
  Replacement of neurostimulator from peripheral nerve
P1-95590 Implantation of nerve, NOS
P1-95591 Implantation of cranial nerve
P1-95592 Implantation of peripheral nerve
P1-95594 Implantation of nerve end into bone
P1-95595 Implantation of nerve end into muscle
P1-95610 Incision for implantation of neurostimulator electrodes into peripheral nerve
P1-95612 Incision for implantation of neurostimulator electrodes into cranial nerve
P1-95614 Incision for implantation of neurostimulator electrodes into autonomic nerve
P1-95615 Incision for implantation of neurostimulator electrodes into neuromuscular component, NOS
P1-95616 Incision for subcutaneous placement of nerve neurostimulator receiver, direct coupling
P1-95618 Incision for subcutaneous placement of nerve neurostimulator receiver, inductive coupling
P1-95620 Removal of electrodes from peripheral nerve
  Removal of peripheral neurostimulator electrodes
P1-95622 Removal of electronic stimulator of peripheral nerve
  Removal of neurostimulator of peripheral nerve
P1-95623 Removal of neuropacemaker of peripheral nerve

P1-95625 Removal of peripheral neurostimulator receiver

1-957 Nerves: Endoscopy

P1-95700 Endoscopic procedure of nerve, NOS

1-958-959 Nerves: Surgical Repairs, Closures and Reconstructions

P1-95800 Neuroplasty, NOS
  Repair of nerve, NOS
P1-95801 Cranial neuroplasty
  Repair of cranial nerve
P1-95802 Peripheral neuroplasty
  Repair of peripheral nerve
P1-95805 Microdissection and microrepair of nerve
  Microrepair of nerve
P1-95807 Neuroplasty of old injury, NOS
  Repair of old injury of nerve, NOS
P1-95808 Repair of old traumatic injury of cranial nerve
P1-95809 Repair of old traumatic injury of peripheral nerve
P1-9580A Reattachment of nerve, NOS
P1-95810 Phrenoplasty
P1-95812 Total facial nerve repair
P1-95813 Neuroplasty of nerve of foot
P1-95814 Neuroplasty of nerve of hand
P1-95815 Neuroplasty of major peripheral nerve of arm
P1-95816 Neuroplasty of median nerve at carpal tunnel
P1-95817 Neuroplasty of ulnar nerve at elbow
P1-95818 Neuroplasty of ulnar nerve at wrist
P1-9581A Neuroplasty of major peripheral nerve of leg
P1-95820 Neuroplasty of major peripheral nerve of brachial plexus
P1-95821 Neuroplasty of major peripheral nerve of lumbar plexus
P1-95822 Neuroplasty of major peripheral nerve branch of sciatic nerve
P1-95824 Digital neuroplasty, one or both, same digit
P1-95825 Repair of sympathetic nerve
P1-95830 Revision neuroplasty, NOS
P1-95831 Revision of previous repair of cranial nerve
P1-95832 Revision of previous repair of peripheral nerve
P1-95834 Repair of ganglion
P1-95840 Neuroanastomosis, NOS
  Anastomosis of nerve, NOS
P1-95841 Cranial neuroanastomosis
  Anastomosis of cranial nerve
P1-95842 Peripheral neuroanastomosis
  Anastomosis of peripheral nerve
P1-95844 Facial-phrenic anastomosis
P1-95845 Facial-spinal accessory anastomosis
P1-95846 Facial-accessory nerve anastomosis
  Accessory-facial nerve anastomosis
  Neuroanastomosis of accessory and facial nerve
P1-95847 Accessory-hypoglossal nerve anastomosis
  Hypoglossal-accessory nerve anastomosis
  Neuroanastomosis of accessory and hypoglossal nerve
P1-95848 Facial-hypoglossal nerve anastomosis
  Anastomosis of hypoglossal and facial nerve
  Neuroanastomosis of hypoglossal and facial nerve
P1-9584C Paracervical uterine denervation
P1-95900 Neurorrhaphy, NOS
  Suture of nerve, NOS
P1-95901 Cranial neurorrhaphy
  Suture of cranial nerve
P1-95902 Peripheral neurorrhaphy
  Suture of peripheral nerve
P1-95910 Suture of nerve requiring extensive mobilization or transposition of nerve
P1-95912 Suture of nerve requiring secondary or delayed suture
P1-95913 Suture of nerve requiring shortening of bone of extremity
P1-95914 Suture of facial nerve, extracranial
P1-95915 Suture of facial nerve, intratemporal, without grafting
P1-95916 Suture of facial nerve, intratemporal, with grafting
P1-95917 Suture of facial nerve, intratemporal, without graft, lateral to geniculate ganglion
P1-95918 Suture of facial nerve, intratemporal, without graft, lateral and medial to geniculate ganglion
P1-95919 Suture of facial nerve, intratemporal, with graft, lateral to geniculate ganglion
P1-95920 Suture of facial nerve, intratemporal, with graft, lateral and medial to geniculate ganglion
P1-95921 Suture of facial nerve, intratemporal, without decompression, lateral to geniculate ganglion
P1-95922 Suture of facial nerve, intratemporal, without decompression, lateral and medial to geniculate ganglion
P1-95923 Suture of facial nerve, intratemporal, with decompression, lateral to geniculate ganglion
P1-95924 Suture of facial nerve, intratemporal, with decompression, lateral and medial to geniculate ganglion
P1-95926 Suture of digital nerve of hand, one nerve
P1-95927 Suture of digital nerve of hand, each additional digital nerve
P1-95928 Suture of one nerve of hand, common sensory nerve
P1-95929 Suture of one nerve of hand, median motor thenar nerve
P1-95930 Suture of one nerve of hand, ulnar motor nerve
P1-95931 Suture of each additional nerve of hand
P1-95932 Suture of major peripheral nerve of arm without transposition
P1-95933 Suture of major peripheral nerve of arm including transposition

1-958-959 Nerves: Surgical Repairs, Closures and Reconstructions — Continued

P1-95934 Suture of digital nerve of foot, one nerve
P1-95941 Suture of digital nerve of foot, each additional digital nerve
P1-95942 Suture of one nerve of foot, common sensory nerve
P1-95945 Suture of each additional nerve of foot
P1-95946 Suture of major peripheral nerve of leg, except sciatic, without transposition
P1-95947 Suture of major peripheral nerve of leg, except sciatic, including transposition
P1-95950 Suture of each additional major peripheral nerve
P1-95952 Suture of posterior tibial nerve
P1-95953 Suture of sciatic nerve
P1-95954 Suture of brachial plexus
P1-95955 Suture of lumbar plexus
P1-95957 Suture of sympathetic nerve
P1-95958 Suture of sympathetic ganglion

1-95C Nerves: Destructive Procedures

P1-95C00 Destructive procedure of nerve, NOS
P1-95C01 Destruction of cranial nerve
P1-95C02 Destruction of peripheral nerve
P1-95C10 Avulsion of nerve, NOS
  Neurexeresis, NOS
P1-95C11 Avulsion of cranial nerve
P1-95C12 Avulsion of peripheral nerve
P1-95C13 Avulsion of cranial nerve, extradural
P1-95C14 Avulsion of facial nerve, differential
P1-95C15 Avulsion of facial nerve, complete
P1-95C16 Avulsion of supraorbital nerve
P1-95C17 Avulsion of infraorbital nerve
P1-95C18 Avulsion of inferior alveolar nerve by osteotomy
P1-95C19 Avulsion of mental nerve
P1-95C1A Avulsion of lingual nerve
P1-95C20 Transthoracic avulsion of vagus nerve
P1-95C21 Avulsion of abdominal vagus nerve
P1-95C22 Avulsion of vagus limited to proximal stomach
P1-95C24 Avulsion of sympathetic nerve
P1-95C25 Avulsion of greater occipital nerve
P1-95C26 Avulsion of phrenic nerve
  Phrenicoexeresis
P1-95C30 Destruction of lesion of nerve, NOS
P1-95C31 Destruction of lesion of cranial nerve
P1-95C32 Destruction of lesion of peripheral nerve
P1-95C34 Destruction of lesion of sympathetic nerve
P1-95C36 Avulsion of obturator nerve, extrapelvic, without adductor tenotomy
P1-95C37 Avulsion of obturator nerve, extrapelvic, with adductor tenotomy
P1-95C38 Avulsion of obturator nerve, intrapelvic, without adductor tenotomy
P1-95C39 Avulsion of obturator nerve, intrapelvic, with adductor tenotomy
P1-95C3A Avulsion of pudendal nerve
P1-95C3B Avulsion of spinal nerve, extradural
P1-95C40 Neurolysis, NOS
P1-95C41 Neurolysis of cranial nerve
  Lysis of adhesions of cranial nerve
P1-95C42 Neurolysis of peripheral nerve
  Lysis of adhesions of peripheral nerve
P1-95C43 Neurolysis of trigeminal nerve
  Lysis of adhesions of trigeminal nerve
P1-95C45 Neurolysis of carpal tunnel
P1-95C46 Neurolysis of tarsal tunnel
P1-95C47 Lysis of adhesions of nerve ganglion, NOS
P1-95C48 Lysis of adhesions of cranial nerve ganglion
P1-95C49 Lysis of adhesions of peripheral nerve ganglion
P1-95C50 Crushing of nerve, NOS
  Neurotripsy, NOS
P1-95C51 Crushing of cranial nerve
P1-95C52 Crushing of peripheral nerve
P1-95C54 Crushing of acoustic nerve
P1-95C55 Trigeminal neurotripsy
  Crushing of trigeminal nerve
  Compression of trigeminal nerve
P1-95C56 Crushing of sympathetic nerve
  Sympatheticotripsy
P1-95C57 Crushing of phrenic nerve
  Phrenicotripsy
  Phrenemphraxis
P1-95C60 Destruction by neurolytic agent of peripheral nerve or branch
P1-95C61 Destruction by neurolytic agent of trigeminal nerve, inferior alveolar branch
P1-95C62 Destruction by neurolytic agent of trigeminal nerve, infraorbital
P1-95C63 Destruction by neurolytic agent of trigeminal nerve, mental
P1-95C64 Destruction by neurolytic agent of trigeminal nerve, supraorbital
P1-95C65 Destruction by neurolytic agent of trigeminal nerve, second and third division branches at foramen ovale
P1-95C66 Destruction by neurolytic agent of trigeminal nerve, second and third division branches at foramen ovale under radiologic monitoring
P1-95C67 Destruction by neurolytic agent of intercostal nerve
P1-95C68 Destruction of sympathetic nerve by injection of neurolytic agent
P1-95C69 Destruction by neurolytic agent of celiac plexus without radiologic monitoring
P1-95C70 Destruction by neurolytic agent of celiac plexus with radiologic monitoring
P1-95C71 Destruction by neurolytic agent of paravertebral facet joint nerve, lumbar region, single level
P1-95C72 Destruction by neurolytic agent of paravertebral facet joint nerve, lumbar region, each additional level

P1-95C73 Destruction by neurolytic agent of pudendal nerve
P1-95C74 Internal neurolysis with operating microscope
P1-95C75 Coagulation or electrocoagulation of gasserian ganglion

1-95D Nerves: Transplantations and Transpositions

P1-95D00 Grafting of nerve, NOS
P1-95D01 Cranial nerve graft
P1-95D02 Peripheral nerve graft
P1-95D10 Nerve graft, single strand, hand, up to 4 cm length
P1-95D11 Nerve graft, single strand, hand, more than 4 cm length
P1-95D12 Nerve graft, single strand, arm, up to 4 cm length
P1-95D13 Nerve graft, single strand, arm, more than 4 cm length
P1-95D14 Nerve graft, single strand, foot, up to 4 cm length
P1-95D15 Nerve graft, single strand, foot, more than 4 cm length
P1-95D16 Nerve graft, single strand, leg, up to 4 cm length
P1-95D17 Nerve graft, single strand, leg, more than 4 cm length
P1-95D18 Nerve graft, each additional nerve, single strand
P1-95D19 Nerve graft, multiple strands, hand, up to 4 cm length
P1-95D20 Nerve graft, multiple strands, hand, more than 4 cm length
P1-95D21 Nerve graft, multiple strands, arm, up to 4 cm length
P1-95D22 Nerve graft, multiple strands, arm, more than 4 cm length
P1-95D23 Nerve graft, multiple strands, foot, up to 4 cm length
P1-95D24 Nerve graft, multiple strands, foot, more than 4 cm length
P1-95D25 Nerve graft, multiple strands, leg, up to 4 cm length
P1-95D26 Nerve graft, multiple strands, leg, more than 4 cm length
P1-95D30 Transplantation of nerve, NOS
P1-95D31 Transplantation of cranial nerve
  Cranial nerve transposition
  Neuroplasty and transposition of cranial nerve
P1-95D32 Transplantation of peripheral nerve
P1-95D34 Transposition of cranial and peripheral nerves
P1-95D36 Transposition of median nerve at carpal tunnel
  Neuroplasty and transposition of median nerve at carpal tunnel
P1-95D37 Transposition of ulnar nerve at elbow
  Neuroplasty and transposition of ulnar nerve at elbow
P1-95D38 Transposition of ulnar nerve at wrist
  Neuroplasty and transposition of ulnar nerve at wrist
P1-95D41 Nerve pedicle transfer, first stage
P1-95D42 Nerve pedicle transfer, second stage

1-95E Nerves: Manipulations

P1-95E10 Neurectasis, NOS
  Stretching of nerve, NOS
P1-95E11 Neurectasis of cranial nerve
  Stretching of cranial nerve
P1-95E12 Neurectasis of peripheral nerve
  Stretching of peripheral nerve

SECTION 1-A OPERATIVE PROCEDURES ON THE EYE, EAR AND RELATED STRUCTURES

1-A0-A9 OPERATIVE PROCEDURES ON THE EYE AND RELATED STRUCTURES

1-A1 OPERATIVE PROCEDURES ON THE ORBIT AND EYEBALL

1-A10 Orbit and Eyeball: General and Miscellaneous Operative Procedures

P1-A1000 Operative procedure on the orbit and eyeball, NOS
P1-A1010 Operation on orbit, NOS
P1-A1012 Diagnostic procedure on orbit, NOS
P1-A1020 Operation on eyeball, NOS
  Ocular operation, NOS
  Ophthalmologic operation, NOS
P1-A1022 Diagnostic procedure on eye, NOS
  Diagnostic procedure on eyeball, NOS
P1-A1030 Secondary procedure after removal of eyeball, NOS

1-A11 Orbit and Eyeball: Incisions

P1-A1100 Orbitotomy, NOS
  Incision of orbit, NOS
P1-A1104 Lateral orbitotomy
  Kroenlein operation
P1-A1106 Orbitotomy with bone flap
P1-A1108 Orbital fasciotomy
P1-A1110 Exploration of orbit, NOS
P1-A1113 Orbitotomy with bone flap by lateral approach, Kroenlein, for exploration, without biopsy
P1-A1115 Orbitotomy without bone flap by frontal approach for exploration without biopsy
P1-A1120 Decompression of orbit, NOS
P1-A1122 Decompression of orbit only by transcranial approach
P1-A1124 Orbitotomy with bone flap by lateral approach, Kroenlein, with decompression
P1-A1126 Orbitotomy with bone flap by lateral approach, Kroenlein, with drainage

1-A11 Orbit and Eyeball: Incisions — Continued

P1-A1128 Orbitotomy without bone flap by frontal approach with drainage only
P1-A1130 Dissection of orbital fibrous bands
P1-A1132 Fistulization of orbit
P1-A1140 Incision and drainage of eyeball

1-A13 Orbit and Eyeball: Excisions

P1-A1300 Biopsy of eyeball and orbit, NOS
P1-A1302 Transconjunctival biopsy of orbit
P1-A1304 Excisional biopsy of orbit
P1-A1306 Excisional biopsy of orbit by aspiration
  Diagnostic aspiration of orbit
  Aspirational biopsy of orbit
P1-A1308 Excision of lesion of orbit
P1-A1310 Excisional biopsy of eye
P1-A1312 Excision of lesion of eyeball
P1-A1320 Orbitotomy without bone flap by frontal approach with removal of lesion
P1-A1322 Exploration of orbit by transcranial approach with removal of lesion
P1-A1324 Orbitotomy with bone flap by lateral approach, Kroenlein, with removal of lesion
P1-A1325 Exploration of orbit by transcranial approach with biopsy
P1-A1326 Orbitotomy with bone flap by lateral approach, Kroenlein, for exploration with biopsy
P1-A1327 Orbitotomy without bone flap by frontal approach for exploration with biopsy
P1-A1330 Evisceration of eyeball
  Evisceration of ocular contents
  Evisceration of ocular contents without implant
P1-A1332 Evisceration of ocular contents with implant into scleral shell
  Evisceration of eyeball with implant into scleral shell
  Removal of ocular contents with synchronous implant into scleral shell
P1-A1334 Evisceration of orbit
  Excision of orbital contents
  Orbitectomy
  Exenteration of orbit
  Removal of orbital contents only
P1-A1336 Exenteration of orbit with temporalis muscle transplant
  Grafting of temporalis muscle to orbit with exenteration of orbit
  Exenteration of orbit without skin graft, with temporalis muscle transplant
P1-A1337 Exenteration of orbit with therapeutic removal of orbital bone
  Exenteration of orbit without skin graft, with therapeutic removal of bone
P1-A1338 Exenteration of orbit with removal of adjacent structures
P1-A1339 Radical orbitomaxillectomy
  Radical orbitomaxillary discission
  Radical orbitomaxillary resection
P1-A1340 Excision of eye, NOS
  Ophthalmectomy, NOS
  Enucleation of eye, NOS
  Enucleation of eye without implant, NOS
  Enucleation of eyeball, NOS
  Removal of eyeball, NOS
P1-A1342 Excision of eye with implant into Tenon's capsule
  Ophthalmectomy with implant into Tenon's capsule
  Enucleation of eye with implant, muscles not attached to implant
  Enucleation of eyeball with implant into Tenon's capsule
  Removal of eyeball with implant
  Insertion of ocular implant with synchronous evisceration
  Insertion of ocular implant with synchronous enucleation
  Implantation of inert material in Tenon's capsule with enucleation of eyeball
  Insertion of ocular prosthesis or prosthetic device with orbital exenteration
P1-A1344 Excision of eye with implant and attachment of muscles
  Ophthalmectomy with implant and attachment of muscles
  Enucleation of eyeball with implant and attachment of muscles
  Removal of eyeball with implant and attachment of muscles
  Enucleation of eye with implant and muscles attached to implant
  Enucleation of eyeball with synchronous implant into Tenon's capsule with attachment of muscles
  Insertion of ocular implant with synchronous enucleation and muscle attachment to implant
P1-A1360 Removal of foreign body from eye, NOS
P1-A1362 Removal of superficial foreign body from eye without incision
P1-A1364 Removal of penetrating foreign body from eye, NOS
P1-A1365 Removal of foreign body of orbit by incision
P1-A1366 Exploration of orbit by transcranial approach with removal of foreign body
P1-A1367 Orbitotomy with bone flap by lateral approach, Kroenlein, with removal of foreign body
P1-A1368 Orbitotomy without bone flap by frontal approach with removal of foreign body

1-A15 Orbit and Eyeball: Injections and Implantations

P1-A1510 Injection of orbit, NOS
P1-A1511 Injection of eye, NOS

P1-A1512 Retrobulbar injection of therapeutic agent
Retrobulbar injection of medication
P1-A1514 Retrobulbar injection of alcohol
P1-A1516 Injection of therapeutic agent into Tenon's capsule
P1-A1520 Irrigation of eye, NOS
P1-A1530 Implantation of eye, Iowa type
P1-A1532 Insertion of ocular implant following or secondary to enucleation
Insertion of ocular implant following or secondary to evisceration
Insertion of ocular prosthesis or prosthetic device, secondary
Secondary insertion of ocular implant
P1-A1533 Insertion of ocular implant, secondary, after evisceration, in scleral shell
P1-A1534 Insertion of ocular implant secondary, after enucleation, muscles attached to implant
P1-A1535 Insertion of ocular implant secondary, after enucleation, muscles not attached to implant
P1-A1550 Orbitotomy with insertion of implant
P1-A1552 Implantation of orbit
Implantation of inert material in orbit
Insertion of orbital implant outside muscle cone
P1-A1557 Revision of orbital implant outside muscle cone
P1-A1560 Insertion of globe into eye socket
P1-A1562 Reinsertion of implant of eyeball with conjunctival graft
Reinsertion of ocular implant with conjunctival graft
P1-A1564 Reinsertion of ocular implant with attachment of muscles to implant
P1-A1565 Reinsertion of ocular implant with use of foreign material for reinforcement
P1-A1566 Reinsertion of ocular implant without conjunctival graft
P1-A1567 Implantation of inert material in scleral shell, reinsertion
Implantation of inert material in Tenon's capsule, reinsertion
P1-A1569 Implantation of inert material in orbit, reinsertion
P1-A1570 Removal of ocular implant
P1-A1571 Removal of eye prosthesis
P1-A1572 Removal of orbital implant
Removal of orbital implant outside muscle cone
P1-A1580 Revision of ocular implant
P1-A1581 Revision of orbital implant
P1-A1584 Revision and reinsertion of ocular implant

1-A18 Orbit and Eyeball: Surgical Repairs, Closures and Reconstructions

P1-A1800 Repair of eye, NOS
Repair of eyeball, NOS
P1-A1802 Repair of injury of eyeball
P1-A1804 Suture of eyeball, NOS
P1-A1810 Repair of eye, multiple structures
Repair of eyeball, multiple structures
P1-A1812 Repair of eye for eyeball rupture
P1-A1814 Repair of orbit, NOS
P1-A1815 Repair of orbit wound, NOS
Repair of injury of orbit, NOS
P1-A1820 Repair of eyeball socket
P1-A1821 Enlargement of eye socket
Enlargement of orbit of eye
P1-A1822 Reconstruction of eye socket
Restoration of eye socket
P1-A1830 Repair of eyeball socket with graft
Reconstruction of eye socket with graft
Revision of enucleation of socket with graft
Restoration of eye socket with graft
Grafting of eye socket
Grafting of orbit
P1-A1832 Revision of exenteration of eye cavity with secondary graft
Secondary graft after exenteration of eye cavity
P1-A1835 Revision of enucleation of socket, NOS
P1-A1836 Revision of exenteration of cavity of orbit, NOS

1-A1C Orbit and Eyeball: Destructive Procedures

P1-A1C00 Destructive procedure of orbit, NOS
P1-A1C02 Destructive procedure of eyeball, NOS
P1-A1C10 Photocoagulation of eye
Photocoagulation of eyeball
P1-A1C20 Destruction of lesion of eye, NOS
P1-A1C22 Photocoagulation of orbital lesion

1-A1D Orbit and Eyeball: Transplantations and Transpositions

P1-A1D10 Grafting of temporalis muscle to orbit

1-A1E Orbit and Eyeball: Manipulations

P1-A1E00 Manipulation of eyeball, NOS

1-A2 OPERATIVE PROCEDURES ON THE EYELID AND LACRIMAL APPARATUS

1-A20 Eyelid and Lacrimal Apparatus: General and Miscellaneous Operative Procedures

P1-A2000 Operation on eyelid, NOS
P1-A2002 Diagnostic procedure on eyelid, NOS
P1-A2010 Operation on canthus, NOS
P1-A2012 Diagnostic procedure on canthus, NOS
P1-A2014 Operation on tarsus, NOS
P1-A2016 Diagnostic procedure on tarsus, NOS

1-A20 Eyelid and Lacrimal Apparatus: General and Miscellaneous Operative Procedures — Continued

P1-A2020 Operation on lacrimal system, NOS
P1-A2022 Diagnostic procedure on lacrimal system, NOS
P1-A2024 Operation on lacrimal gland, NOS
P1-A2050 Operation on conjunctiva, NOS
P1-A2052 Diagnostic procedure on conjunctiva, NOS
P1-A2060V Operation on nictitating membrane, NOS
 Operation on third eyelid, NOS

1-A21-A22 Eyelid and Lacrimal Apparatus: Incisions

P1-A2100 Blepharotomy, NOS
 Incision of eyelid, NOS
P1-A2104 Incision of eyelid margin
 Incision of eyelid margin for trichiasis
P1-A2110 Incision of tarsal gland
 Incision of meibomian gland
P1-A2112 Incision of chalazion
P1-A2114 Incision of hordeolum
 Incision of stye
P1-A2116 Incision of zeisian gland
P1-A2118 Incision of eyebrow
P1-A2120 Exploration of eyelid, NOS
P1-A2122 Blepharotomy with drainage of abscess of eyelid
 Drainage of abscess of eyelid
P1-A2123 Division of symblepharon without insertion of conformer or contact lens
P1-A2130 Reopening of blepharorrhaphy
 Severing of blepharorrhaphy
 Severing of tarsorrhaphy
 Reopening of tarsorrhaphy
 Division of blepharorrhaphy
 Division of tarsorrhaphy
P1-A2132 Reopening of cilia base
P1-A2140 Canthotomy
P1-A2142 Reopening of canthorrhaphy
 Severing of canthorrhaphy
 Division of canthorrhaphy
P1-A2145 Division of palpebral ligament
P1-A2146 Division of canthal ligament
P1-A2150 Incision of conjunctiva
P1-A2152 Peritomy
P1-A2154 Incision of conjunctiva with drainage of cyst
P1-A2156 Incision and expression of conjunctival follicles
P1-A2200 Dacryoadenotomy
 Incision of lacrimal gland
P1-A2202 Incision and drainage of lacrimal gland
P1-A2204 Exploration of lacrimal gland
P1-A2210 Dacryocystotomy
 Incision of lacrimal sac
 Dacryocystostomy
 Ammon's operation
P1-A2214 Incision of lacrimal canaliculus
P1-A2216 Incision of nasolacrimal duct for stricture
 Division of nasolacrimal duct for stricture with drainage
P1-A2218 Incision of lacrimal punctum
 Snip incision of lacrimal punctum
 Slitting of lacrimal papilla
P1-A2220 Incision of lacrimal passage, NOS
P1-A2222 Exploration of lacrimal sac
P1-A2224 Incision and drainage of lacrimal sac
P1-A2226 Division of lacrimal canaliculus
 Division of lacrimal ductules
 Slitting of lacrimal canaliculus
P1-A2227 Slitting of lacrimal canaliculus for removal of streptothrix
 Evacuation of streptothrix from lacrimal duct
P1-A2228 Slitting of lacrimal canaliculus for passage of tube
P1-A2230V Division of nictitating membrane
 Splitting of third eyelid

1-A23-A24 Eyelid and Lacrimal Apparatus: Excisions

P1-A2300 Biopsy of eyelid, NOS
 Excisional biopsy of eyelid, NOS
P1-A2302 Resection of orbicularis oculi muscle
P1-A2304 Excision of lesion of eyelid, NOS
 Removal of lesion of eyelid, NOS
P1-A2306 Excision of lesion of eyelid, except chalazion, without closure
P1-A2308 Excision of lesion of eyelid, except chalazion, with simple direct closure
P1-A2310 Excision of lesion of eyelid by halving procedure
 Wheeler operation
P1-A2312 Excision of lesion of eyelid by wedge resection
P1-A2314 Excision of lesion of eyelid, minor
P1-A2315 Excision of lesion of eyelid, major, partial-thickness
P1-A2316 Excision of lesion of eyelid, major, full-thickness
P1-A2320 Excision of chalazion, single
P1-A2321 Excision of chalazion, multiple, same lid
P1-A2322 Excision of chalazion, multiple, different lids
P1-A2323 Excision of chalazion with general anesthesia, complicated, single
P1-A2324 Excision of chalazion with general anesthesia, complicated, multiple
P1-A2325 Excision of verucca of eyelid
 Excision of wart of eyelid
P1-A2328 Curettage of eyelid
P1-A2329 Curettage of chalazion
P1-A2330 Blepharectomy
 Excision of eyelid
P1-A2332 Tarsectomy of eyelid
 Excision of tarsal plate of eyelid
P1-A2333 Excision of tarsal plate by wedge resection
P1-A2334 Ciliectomy of eyelid margin
 Cyclectomy of eyelid margin
 Excision of cilia base

P1-A2335 Excision of meibomian gland
P1-A2336 Excision of fascia of eyelid
P1-A2337 Epilation of eyelid
P1-A2338 Excision of lesion of eyebrow
P1-A2340 Blepharorhytidectomy, NOS
  Removal of redundant skin of eyelid
P1-A2341 Rhytidectomy of lower eyelid
P1-A2342 Rhytidectomy of upper eyelid
P1-A2344 Removal of foreign body of eyelid by incision
  Removal of embedded foreign body of eyelid
P1-A2345 Removal of foreign body of canthus by incision
P1-A2360 Biopsy of conjunctiva
  Excisional biopsy of conjunctiva
P1-A2362 Excision of lesion of conjunctiva
P1-A2363 Excision of lesion of conjunctiva, up to 1 cm
P1-A2364 Excision of lesion of conjunctiva, over 1 cm
P1-A2365 Excision of lesion of conjunctiva with adjacent sclera
P1-A2367 Simple excision of pterygium
  Excision of pterygium without graft
  Removal of pterygium
  Resection of pterygium
P1-A2368 Curettage of conjunctiva for trachoma follicles
  Removal of trachoma follicles from conjunctiva
P1-A2370 Grattage of conjunctiva, NOS
P1-A2371 Excision of ring of conjunctiva around cornea
  Excision of conjunctival ring
  Peridectomy
  Peritectomy
P1-A2374 Removal of superficial foreign body from conjunctiva
P1-A2375 Removal of embedded foreign body from conjunctiva
  Removal of subconjunctival foreign body
  Removal of embedded foreign body from conjunctiva by incision
P1-A2410 Biopsy of lacrimal gland
  Excisional biopsy of lacrimal gland
P1-A2412 Biopsy of lacrimal sac
  Excisional biopsy of lacrimal sac
P1-A2414 Excision of lesion of lacrimal gland by frontal approach
P1-A2415 Excision of lacrimal gland tumor by frontal approach
P1-A2416 Excision of lacrimal gland tumor involving osteotomy
P1-A2418 Excision of fistula of lacrimal gland
  Fistulectomy of lacrimal gland
P1-A2420 Dacryoadenectomy, NOS
  Excision of lacrimal gland, NOS
P1-A2421 Partial excision of lacrimal gland
  Partial dacryoadenectomy
  Partial excision of lacrimal gland, except for tumor
P1-A2422 Total excision of lacrimal gland
  Total dacryoadenectomy
  Total excision of lacrimal gland, except for tumor
P1-A2424 Removal of foreign body of lacrimal gland, NOS
P1-A2425 Removal of foreign body of lacrimal gland by incision
P1-A2426 Removal of foreign body of lacrimal canaliculi, NOS
P1-A2427 Removal of foreign body of lacrimal canaliculi by incision
P1-A2428 Removal of calculus of lacrimal gland, NOS
P1-A2429 Removal of calculus of lacrimal gland by incision
P1-A242A Removal of calculus of lacrimal canaliculi, NOS
P1-A242B Removal of calculus of lacrimal canaliculi by incision
P1-A2430 Dacryocystectomy, NOS
  Excision of lacrimal sac
  Extirpation of lacrimal sac
P1-A2431 Complete dacryocystectomy
P1-A2432 Partial dacryocystectomy
P1-A2434 Excision of nasolacrimal duct
P1-A2440 Excision of lesion of lacrimal sac
P1-A2442 Excision of fistula of lacrimal sac
  Fistulectomy of lacrimal sac
P1-A2450 Removal of foreign body of lacrimal passage, NOS
P1-A2451 Removal of foreign body of lacrimal sac
P1-A2452 Removal of foreign body of lacrimal punctum
P1-A2453 Removal of calculus of lacrimal passage, NOS
P1-A2454 Removal of calculus of lacrimal sac
P1-A2455 Removal of calculus of nasolacrimal duct
  Removal of dacryolith of nasolacrimal duct
P1-A2456 Removal of calculus of lacrimal punctum
P1-A2460 Removal of foreign body of lacrimal passage by incision
P1-A2462 Removal of foreign body of lacrimal punctum by incision
P1-A2464 Removal of foreign body of lacrimal sac by incision
P1-A2465 Removal of calculus of lacrimal sac by incision
P1-A2466 Removal of calculus of lacrimal passage by incision
P1-A2467 Removal of calculus of lacrimal punctum by incision
P1-A2480V Excision of nictitating membrane, NOS
P1-A2482V Partial excision of nictitating membrane
P1-A2484V Excision of lesion of nictitating membrane
P1-A2486V Debridement of nictitating membrane

1-A25 Eyelid and Lacrimal Apparatus: Injections and Implantations

P1-A2510 Subconjunctival injection

1-A25 Eyelid and Lacrimal Apparatus: Injections and Implantations — Continued

P1-A2512 Injection of contrast medium for dacryocystography
P1-A2513 Probing of lacrimal punctum
P1-A2514 Irrigation of lacrimal punctum
  Probing of lacrimal punctum with irrigation
P1-A2516 Irrigation of lacrimal canaliculus
  Irrigation of lacrimal canaliculi
P1-A2517 Probing of lacrimal canaliculi
  Probing of lacrimal canaliculi without irrigation
P1-A2518 Probing of lacrimal canaliculi with irrigation
P1-A2520 Cannulation of lacrimal apparatus, NOS
P1-A2521 Lacrimal apparatus intubation for dilation, NOS
P1-A2522 Syringing of nasolacrimal duct, NOS
  Irrigation of nasolacrimal duct, NOS
P1-A2523 Syringing of lacrimal duct or sac, NOS
P1-A2526 Probing of nasolacrimal duct with irrigation
P1-A2527 Probing of nasolacrimal duct without irrigation and with general anesthesia
P1-A2528 Probing of nasolacrimal duct with irrigation and with general anesthesia
P1-A2529 Catheterization of lacrimonasal duct, NOS
  Catheterization of nasolacrimal duct, NOS
  Insertion of nasolacrimal tube or stent, NOS
P1-A2530 Intubation of nasolacrimal duct with irrigation
  Irrigation of nasolacrimal duct with insertion of tube or stent
  Syringing of nasolacrimal duct with insertion of tube or stent
P1-A2532 Probing of nasolacrimal duct with insertion of tube or stent
  Probing of nasolacrimal duct without irrigation with insertion of tube or stent
P1-A2534 Probing of nasolacrimal duct with irrigation and insertion of tube or stent
P1-A2536 Dilation of nasolacrimal duct with insertion of tube or stent
P1-A2538 Intranasal intubation of lacrimal apparatus for tear drainage

1-A28-A2A Eyelid and Lacrimal Apparatus: Surgical Repairs, Closures and Reconstructions

P1-A2800 Repair of lacrimal system, NOS
P1-A2810 Repair of punctum of lacrimal system
P1-A2811 Repair of punctum of lacrimal system for eversion
  Repair of punctum of lacrimal system for correction of eversion
  Correction of everted lacrimal punctum
P1-A2814 Repair of canaliculus of lacrimal system
  Repair of lacrimal canaliculus
  Plastic repair of lacrimal canaliculi
  Lacrimal canaliculoplasty
P1-A2816 Nasolacrimal anastomosis
  Fistulization of lacrimal sac into nasal cavity
  Canaliculorhinostomy
  Canaliculodacryocystorhinostomy
  Dacryocystorhinostomy
  Johanson operation
  Jones operation
  Summerskill operation
  Toti operation
  West operation
P1-A2820 Anastomosis of lacrimal sac to conjunctival sac
  Conjunctivodacryocystorhinostomy
  Conjunctivocystorhinostomy
  Stallard operation
  Conjunctivodacryocystostomy
P1-A2822 Conjunctivorhinostomy
  Conjunctivorhinostomy without tube
  Canthocystostomy
P1-A2823 Conjunctivorhinostomy with insertion of stent
  Conjunctivorhinostomy with insertion of tube
  Conjunctivodacryocystostomy with insertion of tube
  Conjunctivodacryocystostomy with insertion of stent
  Stallard operation with insertion of tube or stent
  Conjunctivodacryocystorhinostomy with insertion of tube or stent
P1-A2824 Suture of lacrimal canaliculus, NOS
P1-A2826 Closure of lacrimal punctum
P1-A2827 Ligation for closure of lacrimal punctum
P1-A2828 Closure of lacrimal fistula
P1-A2830 Repair of eyebrow, NOS
P1-A2840 Blepharoplasty, NOS
  Repair of eyelid, NOS
  Tarsoplasty
P1-A2841 Blepharoplasty of lower eyelid
P1-A2842 Blepharoplasty of lower eyelid with extensive herniated fat pad
P1-A2844 Blepharoplasty of upper eyelid
P1-A2845 Blepharoplasty of upper eyelid with excessive skin weighting down lid
P1-A2848 Extensive blepharoplasty, NOS
P1-A2850 Repair of eyelid laceration, NOS
P1-A2851 Linear repair of laceration of eyelid
P1-A2852 Linear repair of laceration of eyebrow
P1-A2853 Repair of eyelid, partial-thickness
  Repair of eyelid laceration, partial-thickness
P1-A2855 Repair of eyelid, partial-thickness involving lid margin
  Repair of eyelid laceration, partial-thickness involving lid margin
P1-A2857 Repair of eyelid, full-thickness
  Repair of eyelid laceration, full-thickness

P1-A2859 Repair of eyelid, full-thickness involving lid margin
  Repair of eyelid laceration, full-thickness involving lid margin
P1-A2860 Repair of eyelid retraction
  Correction of lid retraction
  Correction of eyelid retraction
P1-A2870 Advancement of eyelid muscle
P1-A2871 Enlargement of palpebral fissure
P1-A2872 Narrowing of palpebral fissure
P1-A2875 Shortening of eyelid margin
P1-A2877 Reposition of cilia base
P1-A2878 Rhytidoplasty of eyelid
P1-A2880 Excision and repair of eyelid, including lid margin, tarsus, conjunctiva, canthus, over one-fourth of lid margin
P1-A2882 Excision and repair of eyelid, including lid margin, tarsus, conjunctiva, canthus, up to one-fourth of lid margin
P1-A2884 Suture of eyelid
  Suture of skin of eyelid
P1-A2885 Suture of eyebrow
  Suture of skin of eyebrow
P1-A2886 Suture of recent wound of eyelid, direct closure, partial-thickness
P1-A2887 Suture of recent wound of eyelid, direct closure, full-thickness
P1-A2890 Blepharorrhaphy, NOS
  Suture of palpebral fissure, NOS
  Tarsorrhaphy, NOS
P1-A2894 Reconstruction of lateral canthus
  Revision of lateral canthus
P1-A2895 Tensing of orbicularis oculi muscle
P1-A2896 Adjustment of lid position, NOS
P1-A2897 Lateral canthopexy
P1-A28A0 Repair of epicanthus
P1-A28A1 Z-plasty of epicanthus
P1-A28A2 Repair of telecanthus
P1-A28A3 Canthoplasty, NOS
P1-A28A4 Medial canthoplasty
P1-A28B0 Construction of canthorrhaphy, NOS
  Canthorrhaphy, NOS
P1-A28B1 Construction of canthorrhaphy with transposition of tarsal plate
P1-A28B2 Construction of intermarginal adhesions
P1-A28B3 Construction of intermarginal adhesions with transposition of tarsal plate
P1-A28B4 Construction of median tarsorrhaphy
P1-A28B5 Construction of median tarsorrhaphy with transposition of tarsal plate
P1-A2900 Repair of conjunctiva, NOS
  Conjunctivoplasty, NOS
P1-A2910 Repair of laceration of conjunctiva
P1-A2911 Repair of laceration of conjunctiva by mobilization and rearrangement without hospitalization
P1-A2912 Repair of laceration of conjunctiva by mobilization and rearrangement with hospitalization
P1-A2914 Repair of conjunctiva for late effect of trachoma
P1-A2915 Conjunctivoplasty with conjunctival graft
P1-A2916 Conjunctivoplasty with extensive rearrangement
P1-A2917 Conjunctivoplasty with buccal mucous membrane graft
P1-A2918 Conjunctivoplasty with reconstruction of cul-de-sac and conjunctival graft
P1-A2919 Conjunctivoplasty with reconstruction of cul-de-sac and extensive rearrangement
P1-A291A Conjunctivoplasty with reconstruction of cul-de-sac and buccal mucous membrane graft
P1-A2920 Conjunctival flap, partial
P1-A2921 Conjunctival flap, bridge
P1-A2922 Conjunctival flap, total
P1-A2923 Conjunctival flap, total, Gunderson thin flap or purse string flap
P1-A2924 Operation on pterygium, NOS
P1-A2925 Transposition of pterygium
  McReynolds operation
  Dissection of pterygium with reposition
P1-A2926 Transposition of pterygium without graft
P1-A2927 Transposition of pterygium with graft
P1-A2928 Excision of pterygium with graft
P1-A2930 Repair of symblepharon, NOS
P1-A2931 Repair of symblepharon without graft
P1-A2932 Repair of symblepharon by division with insertion of conformer
  Division of symblepharon with insertion of conformer or contact lens
P1-A2935 Suture of conjunctiva, NOS
P1-A2936 Direct closure of laceration of conjunctiva
P1-A2937 Direct closure of laceration of conjunctiva with nonperforating scleral laceration
P1-A2940 Repair of blepharoptosis, NOS
  Correction of blepharoptosis, NOS
  Correction of eyelid ptosis, NOS
P1-A2941 Repair of blepharoptosis by resection or advancement of levator muscle or aponeurosis
  Berke operation
  Sling operation on eyelid levator muscle
  Resection of levator palpebrae muscle
  Blascovic operation
  Myectomy of levator palpebrae
  Shortening of levator palpebrae muscle
  Tenectomy of levator palpebrae
P1-A2942 Lengthening of levator palpebrae muscle
  Recession of levator palpebrae superioris muscle
  Myotomy of levator palpebrae
  Tenotomy of levator palpebrae
P1-A2950 Repair of blepharoptosis by frontalis muscle suture technique
P1-A2952 Repair of blepharoptosis by frontalis muscle technique with fascial sling
  Crawford operation

1-A28-A2A Eyelid and Lacrimal Apparatus: Surgical Repairs, Closures and Reconstructions — Continued

P1-A2952 (cont.) Tarso-frontalis sling of eyelid

P1-A2954 Repair of blepharoptosis by levator muscle technique
  Plication of levator for blepharoptosis
  Tucking of levator palpebrae for blepharoptosis

P1-A2955 Repair of blepharoptosis by other levator muscle technique

P1-A2957 Sling operation on tarsus muscle of eyelid

P1-A2958 Repair of blepharoptosis by conjunctivo-tarso-levator resection, Fasanella-Servat type

P1-A2959 Resection of extraocular tarsal muscle for blepharoptosis
  Müller resection of extraocular muscle for blepharoptosis

P1-A295A Repair of blepharoptosis by tarsolevator resection, external approach

P1-A295B Repair of blepharoptosis by tarsolevator resection, internal approach

P1-A2960 Repair of blepharoptosis by tarsal technique, NOS

P1-A2961 de Grandmont operation
  de Grandmont tarsectomy

P1-A2962 Repair of blepharoptosis by orbicularis oculi muscle sling

P1-A2963 Attachment of orbicularis oculi to eyebrow

P1-A2964 Palpebral ligament sling operation
  Eyelid fascia lata sling operation

P1-A2967 Fixation of palpebral ligament

P1-A2970 Repair of blepharoptosis by superior rectus tendon transplant

P1-A2971 Repair of blepharoptosis by superior rectus technique with fascial sling

P1-A2972 Reduction of overcorrection of ptosis
  Revision of ptosis overcorrection

P1-A2980 Repair of blepharophimosis

P1-A2982 Repair of ectropion, NOS

P1-A2983 Repair of entropion, NOS

P1-A2984 Repair of entropion by thermocauterization

P1-A2985 Repair of ectropion by thermocauterization

P1-A2986 Repair of ectropion by suture
  Suture repair of ectropion
  Suture of eyelid with ectropion repair

P1-A2987 Repair of entropion by suture
  Suture repair of entropion
  Suture of eyelid with entropion repair

P1-A2988 Repair of entropion with wedge resection
  Fox operation
  Excision of tarsal wedge for repair of entropion

P1-A2990 Repair of entropion, extensive

P1-A2991 Repair of ectropion by blepharoplasty and excision of tarsal wedge
  Repair of ectropion with wedge resection

P1-A2992 Repair of ectropion by blepharoplasty
  Repair of ectropion with lid reconstruction
  V-Y operation for ectropion
  Kuhnt-Szymanowski operation

P1-A2994 Repair of entropion with lid reconstruction
  Wheeler operation for repair of entropion

P1-A2995 Reconstruction of eyelid, NOS

P1-A2996 Reconstruction of eyelid with graft
  Reconstruction of eyelid with flap

P1-A2997 Reconstruction of eyelid, partial-thickness

P1-A2998 Reconstruction of eyelid, partial-thickness, involving lid margin

P1-A2999 Reconstruction of eyelid, full-thickness

P1-A299A Reconstruction of eyelid, full-thickness, involving lid margin

P1-A299B Reconstruction of eyelid with skin flap
  Reconstruction of eyelid with skin graft

P1-A29A0 Reconstruction of eyebrow
  Restoration of eyebrow

P1-A29A1 Restoration of eyebrow with graft

P1-A2A11 Reconstruction of eyelid with mucous membrane flap
  Reconstruction of eyelid with mucous membrane graft

P1-A2A12 Reconstruction of eyelid with hair follicle graft
  Reconstruction of eyelid with graft or flap bearing hair follicles

P1-A2A20 Reconstruction of eyelid with tarsoconjunctival flap

P1-A2A22 Reconstruction of eyelid with tarsoconjunctival flap from opposing lid

P1-A2A23 Reconstruction of eyelid, full-thickness, by transfer of tarsoconjunctival flap from opposing eyelid, up to two-thirds of eyelid, first stage

P1-A2A24 Reconstruction of eyelid, full-thickness, by transfer of tarsoconjunctival flap from opposing eyelid, total eyelid, lower, first stage

P1-A2A25 Reconstruction of eyelid, full-thickness, by transfer of tarsoconjunctival flap from opposing eyelid, total eyelid, upper, first stage

P1-A2A26 Reconstruction of eyelid, full-thickness, by transfer of tarsoconjunctival flap from opposing eyelid, second stage

P1-A2A30 Correction of trichiasis by incision of lid margin

P1-A2A31 Correction of trichiasis by incision of lid margin with free mucous membrane graft

P1-A2A34 Reconstruction of conjunctival cul-de-sac

P1-A2A35 Reconstruction of conjunctival cul-de-sac with graft

P1-A2A43 Repair of symblepharon with free graft
  Grafting for symblepharon repair

P1-A2A45 Repair of symblepharon with free graft of buccal mucous membrane

P1-A2A46 Repair of symblepharon with free graft of conjunctiva

P1-A2A50V Fixation of nictitating membrane
P1-A2A51V Temporary joining of sclera and nictitating membrane

1-A2C Eyelid and Lacrimal Apparatus: Destructive Procedures

P1-A2C00 Destructive procedure of eyelid, NOS
P1-A2C02 Destructive procedure of lacrimal apparatus, NOS
P1-A2C10 Cauterization of lacrimal canaliculi, NOS
P1-A2C11 Obliteration of lacrimal canaliculi, NOS
P1-A2C12 Cauterization of lacrimal punctum
P1-A2C13 Cauterization of lacrimal punctum for eversion
P1-A2C14 Obliteration of lacrimal punctum, NOS
P1-A2C15 Laser photocoagulation for closure of lacrimal punctum
P1-A2C16 Thermocauterization for closure of lacrimal punctum
P1-A2C17 Destruction of lacrimal sac, NOS
Gifford operation
P1-A2C18 Destruction of lesion of lacrimal sac, NOS
P1-A2C20 Cauterization of lacrimal sac
P1-A2C22 Cauterization of lacrimal gland
P1-A2C30 Destruction of lesion of eyelid, NOS
P1-A2C32 Destruction of lesion of lid margin, up to 1 cm
P1-A2C34 Lysis of adhesions of eyelid
P1-A2C36 Cryotherapy of eyelid
P1-A2C40 Cauterization of eyelid
P1-A2C41 Cauterization of chalazion of eyelid
P1-A2C42 Cauterization of eyelid for entropion
P1-A2C43 Cauterization of eyelid for ectropion
P1-A2C44 Cauterization of meibomian gland
P1-A2C50 Epilation of eyelid by forceps, NOS
P1-A2C51 Cryosurgical epilation of eyelid
P1-A2C52 Electrosurgical epilation of eyelid
P1-A2C54 Destruction of lesion of eyebrow
P1-A2C55 Epilation of eyebrow by forceps
P1-A2C56 Cryosurgical epilation of eyebrow
P1-A2C57 Electrosurgical epilation of eyebrow
P1-A2C58 Correction of trichiasis by epilation with forceps
P1-A2C59 Correction of trichiasis by epilation with electrosurgery
P1-A2C5A Correction of trichiasis by epilation with cryotherapy
P1-A2C60 Destruction of lesion of conjunctiva
P1-A2C61 Lysis of adhesions of conjunctiva
P1-A2C62 Cauterization of conjunctiva
P1-A2C63 Cauterization of conjunctival lesion
P1-A2C64 Rolling of conjunctiva
P1-A2C65 Scarification of conjunctiva
P1-A2C68 Scraping of trachoma follicles

1-A2D Eyelid and Lacrimal Apparatus: Transplantations and Transpositions

P1-A2D00 Free graft to conjunctiva, NOS
P1-A2D10 Transplantation of conjunctiva for pterygium
P1-A2D12 Transplantation of superior rectus tendon for blepharoptosis
P1-A2D14 Transplantation of hair follicles of eyelid
P1-A2D16 Transplantation of hair follicles of eyebrow
P1-A2D18 Transposition of eyelash flaps
P1-A2D20 Grafting of fascia of eyelid
P1-A2D22 Grafting of fascia to tarsal cartilage
P1-A2D30V Nictitating membrane flap

1-A2E Eyelid and Lacrimal Apparatus: Manipulations

P1-A2E00 Manipulation of eyelid, NOS
P1-A2E02 Stretching of eyelid
P1-A2E10 Manipulation of lacrimal apparatus, NOS
P1-A2E12 Manipulation of lacrimal passage, NOS
P1-A2E13 Dilation of lacrimal punctum
Dilation of lacrimal punctum without irrigation
P1-A2E14 Dilation of lacrimal punctum with irrigation
P1-A2E16 Dilation of lacrimal duct
Anel operation
P1-A2E20 Probing of nasolacrimal duct, NOS
Probing of nasolacrimal duct without irrigation
P1-A2E22 Dilation of nasolacrimal duct, retrograde
P1-A2E25 Expression of conjunctival follicles

1-A3 OPERATIVE PROCEDURES ON THE CORNEA

1-A30 Cornea: General and Miscellaneous Operative Procedures

P1-A3000 Operative procedure on cornea, NOS
Operation on cornea, NOS
P1-A3010 Diagnostic procedure on cornea, NOS

1-A31 Cornea: Incisions

P1-A3100 Incision of cornea, NOS
Keratotomy, NOS
P1-A3102 Radial keratotomy
P1-A3104 Delimiting keratotomy
Gifford keratotomy
Saemisch operation
P1-A3110 Division of blood vessels of cornea

1-A33 Cornea: Excisions

P1-A3300 Keratectomy, NOS
Excision of cornea, NOS
P1-A3310 Removal of corneal epithelium, NOS
P1-A3312 Mechanical removal of corneal epithelium
Curettage of corneal epithelium
Abrasion of corneal epithelium
Scraping of corneal epithelium

1-A33 Cornea: Excisions — Continued

P1-A3312 (cont.) Shaving of corneal epithelium
Curettage of corneal epithelium without chemocauterization
Abrasion of corneal epithelium without chemocauterization
P1-A3313 Curettage of corneal epithelium with chemocauterization
Abrasion of corneal epithelium with chemocauterization
P1-A3314 Removal of corneal epithelium with application of chelating agent
P1-A3316 Scraping of cornea, diagnostic, for smear and culture
Removal of corneal epithelium for smear or culture
Curettage of corneal epithelium for smear or culture
Abrasion of corneal epithelium for smear or culture
Scraping of corneal epithelium for smear or culture
P1-A3317 Scraping of cornea, diagnostic, for smear
P1-A3318 Scraping of cornea, diagnostic, for culture
P1-A3320 Biopsy of cornea
Excisional biopsy of cornea
P1-A3322 Abscission of cornea
Excision of prominence of cornea in staphyloma
P1-A3328 Corneal wedge resection for correction of surgically induced astigmatism
P1-A3330 Excision of lesion of cornea, NOS
P1-A3332 Excision of lesion of cornea by partial keratectomy
P1-A3334 Fistulectomy of cornea
P1-A3336 Keratectomy for pterygium
P1-A3350 Removal of implant of cornea
Removal of artificial implant from cornea
P1-A3360 Magnet extraction of foreign body from cornea
Removal of foreign body of cornea by magnet
P1-A3362 Removal of foreign body of cornea by incision
P1-A3364 Removal of foreign body of eye without slit lamp
P1-A3366 Removal of foreign body of cornea with slit lamp

1-A35 Cornea: Injections and Implantations

P1-A3510 Keratocentesis, NOS
Paracentesis of cornea, NOS
P1-A3520 Tattooing of cornea, NOS
P1-A3521 Chemical tattooing of cornea
P1-A3522 Mechanical tattooing of cornea
P1-A3530 Implantation of cornea, NOS
P1-A3531 Implantation of epikeratoprosthesis
P1-A3532 Insertion of keratoprosthesis

1-A38 Cornea: Surgical Repairs, Closures and Reconstructions

P1-A3800 Keratoplasty, NOS
Repair of cornea, NOS
P1-A3802 Reconstruction of cornea, NOS
Reconstructive surgery on cornea, NOS
P1-A3808 Radial keratoplasty
P1-A3810 Lamellar keratoplasty, NOS
P1-A3812 Lamellar keratoplasty with autograft
P1-A3814 Closure of fistula of cornea with lamellar autograft
P1-A3816 Closure of fistula of cornea with lamellar homograft
P1-A3820 Penetrating keratoplasty, NOS
Penetrating keratoplasty, except in aphakia
P1-A3821 Penetrating keratoplasty with homograft
P1-A3822 Penetrating keratoplasty with autograft
P1-A3826 Penetrating keratoplasty in aphakia
P1-A3828 Penetrating keratoplasty in pseudophakia
P1-A3830 Refractive keratoplasty
Keratomeleusis
P1-A3834 Epikeratophakia
P1-A3836 Keratophakia
P1-A3838 Corneal relaxing incision for correction of surgically induced astigmatism
P1-A3840 Operation on pterygium with corneal graft
Keratectomy for pterygium with corneal graft
Excision of pterygium with corneal graft
Ombrain operation
P1-A3842 Repair of cornea with conjunctival flap
Suture of cornea with conjunctival flap
Corneoconjunctivoplasty
P1-A3843 Repair of corneal laceration with conjunctival flap
Repair of corneal wound with conjunctival flap
P1-A3844 Repair of postoperative wound dehiscence of cornea
Repair of corneal wound postcataract dehiscence
P1-A3850 Suture of cornea, NOS
P1-A3851 Suture of corneal laceration
P1-A3854 Corneoscleral suture
P1-A3855 Corneoscleral suture with conjunctival flap
P1-A3857 Closure of fistula of cornea
P1-A3870 Thermokeratoplasty
TKP operation
P1-A3872 Repair of filtering bleb by corneal graft
P1-A3873 Repair of filtering bleb by suture
P1-A3874 Repair of filtering bleb by suture with conjunctival flap
P1-A3880 Repair of nonperforating laceration of cornea without removal of foreign body
P1-A3881 Repair of nonperforating laceration of cornea with removal of foreign body

P1-A3882 Repair of perforating laceration of cornea not involving uveal tissue
P1-A3884 Repair of perforating laceration of cornea with reposition or resection of uveal tissue
P1-A3886 Repair of laceration of cornea with application of tissue glue
P1-A3888 Repair of laceration of cornea and sclera with application of tissue glue

1-A3C Cornea: Destructive Procedures

P1-A3C00 Destructive procedure of cornea, NOS
P1-A3C10 Destruction of lesion of cornea, NOS
P1-A3C12 Destruction of lesion of cornea by cryotherapy
  Cryotherapy of corneal lesion
P1-A3C14 Cryotherapy of corneal lesion to reshape cornea
P1-A3C20 Destruction of lesion of cornea by electrocauterization
  Electrocautery of corneal lesion
P1-A3C21 Cauterization of fistula of cornea
P1-A3C22 Cauterization of ulcer of cornea
P1-A3C23 Cauterization of superficial pannus
P1-A3C30 Thermocauterization for destruction of lesion of cornea
P1-A3C32 Photocoagulation for destruction of lesion of cornea
P1-A3C36 Chemocauterization of corneal epithelium

1-A3D Cornea: Transplantations and Transpositions

P1-A3D00 Corneal transplant, NOS
  Grafting of cornea, NOS
P1-A3D10 Donor keratectomy
  Excision of cornea from donor

1-A4 OPERATIVE PROCEDURES ON THE ANTERIOR SEGMENT OF THE EYE

1-A40 Anterior Segment of Eye: General and Miscellaneous Operative Procedures

P1-A4000 Operative procedure on anterior segment of eye, NOS
P1-A4002 Diagnostic procedure on anterior segment of eye, NOS
P1-A4010 Operative procedure on anterior chamber of eye, NOS
P1-A4012 Diagnostic procedure on anterior chamber of eye
P1-A4018 Operation for glaucoma, NOS
  Intraocular release of pressure, NOS
P1-A4020 Operative procedure on iris, NOS
  Operation on iris, NOS
P1-A4022 Diagnostic procedure on iris, NOS
P1-A4030 Operative procedure on ciliary body, NOS
  Operation on ciliary body, NOS
P1-A4032 Diagnostic procedure on ciliary body
P1-A4040 Operative procedure on sclera, NOS
  Operation on sclera, NOS
P1-A4042 Diagnostic procedure on sclera, NOS

1-A41 Anterior Segment of Eye: Incisions

P1-A4100 Iridotomy, NOS
  Sphincterotomy of iris, NOS
  Discission of iris, NOS
  Puncture of iris, NOS
P1-A4102 Iridotomy by stab incision except transfixion
P1-A4104 Iridotomy by stab incision with transfixion for iris bombé
  Iridotomy for iris bombé
  Iridotomy with transfixion
  Transfixion of iris bombé
P1-A4106 Iridotomy by photocoagulation, NOS
P1-A4107 Iridotomy by photocoagulation, one or more sessions for glaucoma
P1-A4110 Pupillotomy
P1-A4112 Iridosclerotomy
P1-A4120 Division of goniosynechiae
P1-A4121 Division of anterior synechiae iris
P1-A4122 Division of posterior synechiae of iris
P1-A4125 Severing of adhesions of anterior segment of eye, incisional technique for goniosynechiae
P1-A4126 Severing of adhesions of anterior segment of eye, incisional technique for anterior synechiae, except goniosynechiae
P1-A4127 Severing of adhesions of anterior segment of eye, incisional technique for posterior synechiae
P1-A4128 Severing of adhesions of anterior segment of eye, incisional technique for corneovitreal adhesions
P1-A4140 Paracentesis of anterior chamber of eye, NOS
P1-A4141 Paracentesis of anterior chamber of eye with diagnostic aspiration of aqueous
  Diagnostic aspiration of aqueous of eye
  Diagnostic aspiration of anterior chamber of eye
P1-A4142 Paracentesis of anterior chamber of eye with therapeutic release of aqueous
  Therapeutic aspiration of anterior chamber of eye
  Therapeutic evacuation of anterior chamber of eye
P1-A4144 Paracentesis of anterior chamber of eye with discission of anterior hyaloid membrane without air injection
P1-A4145 Paracentesis of anterior chamber of eye with discission of anterior hyaloid membrane and air injection
P1-A4146 Paracentesis of anterior chamber of eye with removal of vitreous without air injection
P1-A4147 Paracentesis of anterior chamber of eye with removal of vitreous by air injection

1-A41 Anterior Segment of Eye: Incisions — Continued

P1-A4148 Paracentesis of anterior chamber of eye with removal of vitreous by discission of anterior hyaloid membrane without air injection
P1-A4149 Paracentesis of anterior chamber of eye with removal of vitreous by discission of anterior hyaloid membrane with air injection
P1-A4150 Paracentesis of anterior chamber of eye with removal of blood without irrigation or air injection
Aspiration of hyphema
Keratocentesis for hyphema
Evacuation of anterior chamber of eye for hyphema
P1-A4152 Paracentesis of anterior chamber of eye with removal of blood by air injection
P1-A4153 Paracentesis of anterior chamber of eye with removal of blood by irrigation
P1-A4154 Paracentesis of anterior chamber of eye with removal of blood by irrigation and air injection
P1-A4160 Cyclotomy, NOS
Cyclicotomy, NOS
Ciliarotomy, NOS
P1-A4162 Exploration of ciliary body
P1-A4168 Cyclodialysis, NOS
Heine operation
P1-A4170 Goniotomy, NOS
Barkan operation
Goniotomy without goniopuncture
P1-A4172 Goniotomy with goniopuncture
Barkan operation with goniopuncture
P1-A4174 Goniopuncture
Goniopuncture without goniotomy
P1-A4180 Exploratory sclerotomy, NOS
Exploration of sclera by incision, NOS
Incision of sclera, NOS
P1-A4181 Anterior sclerotomy
P1-A4182 Posterior sclerotomy
P1-A4183 Incision of abscess of sclera
P1-A4184 Sclerostomy, NOS
Scheie sclerostomy
P1-A4186 Corneoscleral trephination
P1-A4190 Trabeculotomy, NOS
P1-A4191 Trabeculotomy ab externo
P1-A4192 Trabeculodialysis
P1-A4194 Phlebogoniostomy
P1-A4195 Goniospasis
P1-A4196 Scleral fistulizing procedure, NOS
Fistulization of sclera, NOS
P1-A4197 Fistulization of sclera by trephination
P1-A4198 Facilitation of intraocular circulation, NOS

1-A43 Anterior Segment of Eye: Excisions

P1-A4300 Excision of lesion of anterior segment of eye, NOS
Removal of lesion of anterior segment of eye, NOS
P1-A4302 Excision of lesion of anterior chamber of eye, NOS
P1-A4304 Removal of epithelial downgrowth of anterior chamber of eye
P1-A4310 Biopsy of iris
Excisional biopsy of iris
P1-A4312 Excision of lesion of iris
P1-A4314 Excision of prolapsed iris
P1-A4320 Ciliectomy of ciliary body
Cyclectomy of ciliary body
P1-A4322 Excision of lesion of ciliary body
P1-A4324 Excision of prolapsed ciliary body
P1-A4328 Iridocyclectomy
P1-A4330 Excision of lesion of sclera
P1-A4332 Curettage of sclera
P1-A4340 Iridectomy, NOS
Corectomy, NOS
Ziegler operation, NOS
P1-A4342 Formation of pupil by iridectomy
P1-A4344 Iridocystectomy
P1-A4346 Sclerectomy, NOS
Resection of sclera, NOS
Holth punch operation on sclera
P1-A4347 Trephine sclerectomy
P1-A4348 Iridosclerectomy
Lagrange operation
P1-A4349 Posterior sclerotomy with iridectomy
P1-A434A Anterior sclerotomy with iridectomy
P1-A4350 Iridectomy with scleral trephination
Elliot operation
Trephination of sclera with iridectomy
P1-A4352 Iridectomy with scleral fistulization
Fistulization of sclera with iridectomy
P1-A4353 Iridectomy with filtering operation for glaucoma
P1-A4355 Fistulization of sclera for glaucoma by trephination with iridectomy
P1-A4357 Iridectomy with scleral thermocauterization
Scheie operation
P1-A4360 Iridectomy for removal of lesion with corneal section
P1-A4361 Iridectomy for removal of lesion with corneoscleral section
P1-A4362 Iridectomy with corneal section, peripheral, for glaucoma
P1-A4363 Iridectomy with corneoscleral section, peripheral, for glaucoma
P1-A4364 Iridectomy with corneal section, sector, for glaucoma
P1-A4365 Iridectomy with corneoscleral section, sector, for glaucoma
P1-A4366 Iridectomy with corneal section and cyclectomy
P1-A4367 Iridectomy with corneoscleral section and cyclectomy
P1-A4368 Iridectomy with corneal section, optical
P1-A4369 Iridectomy with corneoscleral section, optical
P1-A4370 Resection of uveal tissue

P1-A4372 Ocular trabeculectomy
P1-A4374 Trabeculectomy ab externo
P1-A4377 Opticociliary neurectomy
P1-A4381 Removal of blood clot from anterior segment of eye
P1-A4382 Removal of intraocular foreign body from anterior segment of eye, NOS
P1-A4383 Removal of foreign body of iris by incision
P1-A4384 Removal of foreign body of sclera by incision
P1-A4385 Removal of foreign body of anterior chamber of eye by incision
P1-A4387 Removal of foreign body of ciliary body by incision
P1-A4388 Removal of foreign body of anterior segment of eye without use of magnet
P1-A4390 Removal of foreign body from anterior chamber of eye without use of magnet
  Nonmagnetic extraction of foreign body from anterior chamber of eye
P1-A4391 Removal of foreign body of iris without use of magnet
P1-A4392 Removal of foreign body of sclera without use of magnet
P1-A4393 Removal of foreign body of ciliary body without use of magnet
P1-A4394 Removal of of foreign body of external eye, scleral nonperforating
P1-A4395 Removal of intraocular foreign body from anterior segment of eye with use of magnet, NOS
P1-A4396 Magnet extraction of foreign body from iris
  Removal of foreign body of iris with use of magnet
P1-A4397 Magnet extraction of foreign body from sclera
  Removal of foreign body of sclera with use of magnet
P1-A4398 Magnet extraction of foreign body from ciliary body
  Removal of foreign body of ciliary body with use of magnet
P1-A4399 Magnet extraction of intraocular foreign body from anterior chamber of eye
P1-A43A0 Removal of foreign body of anterior chamber of eye by incision with use of magnet

1-A45 Anterior Segment of Eye: Injections and Implantations

P1-A4500 Injection of anterior segment of eye, NOS
P1-A4510 Injection of anterior chamber of eye, NOS
P1-A4512 Injection of liquid in anterior chamber of eye
P1-A4514 Injection of air in anterior chamber of eye
P1-A4516 Injection of medication in anterior chamber of eye
P1-A4520 Injection of sympathetic ciliary ganglion
P1-A4530 Irrigation of anterior chamber of eye
P1-A4534 Insertion of catheter in anterior chamber of eye for permanent drainage in glaucoma
P1-A4535 Removal of implanted material from anterior segment of eye

1-A47 Anterior Segment of Eye: Endoscopy

P1-A4700 Gonioscopy, NOS

1-A48 Anterior Segment of Eye: Surgical Repairs, Closures and Reconstructions

P1-A4810 Iridoplasty, NOS
  Repair of iris, NOS
  Formation of pupil, NOS
P1-A4811 Repair of ciliary body, NOS
P1-A4812 Coreoplasty
  Needling of pupillary membrane
P1-A4813 Reposition of iris
P1-A4815 Repair of uveal hernia
  Reposition of uveal tissue
P1-A4817 Reopening of iris in anterior chamber of eye
P1-A4818 Suture of iris and ciliary body with retrieval of suture through small incision
P1-A4820 Iridesis
  Iridodesis
P1-A4822 Iridencleisis
  Holth iridencleisis
P1-A4824 Iridotasis
  Borthen operation
P1-A4826 Iridencleisis and iridotasis
P1-A4830 Scleroplasty, NOS
  Repair of sclera, NOS
P1-A4832 Repair of scleral fistula
P1-A4834 Repair of scleral staphyloma
P1-A4835 Repair of scleral staphyloma with graft
P1-A4841 Suture of laceration of sclera
P1-A4842 Repair of laceration of sclera by application of tissue glue
P1-A4843 Repair of perforating laceration of sclera not involving uveal tissue
P1-A4844 Repair of laceration of sclera with synchronous repair of conjunctiva
P1-A4845 Repair of perforating laceration of sclera with reposition or resection of uveal tissue
P1-A4846 Postoperative revision of scleral fistulization procedure, NOS
  Revision of scleral fistulization procedure, NOS
P1-A4850 Surgical construction of filtration bleb
P1-A4851 Repair of filtering bleb
P1-A4852 Repair of filtering bleb by scleroplasty
P1-A4853 Revision of filtering bleb
P1-A4854 Closure of filtering bleb
P1-A4860 Repair of operative wound of anterior segment of eye, any type, minor procedure
P1-A4862 Repair of operative wound of anterior segment of eye, any type, major procedure
P1-A4864 Revision of operative wound of anterior segment of eye, NOS
P1-A4865 Revision of operative wound of anterior segment of eye, any type, minor procedure
P1-A4866 Revision of operative wound of anterior segment of eye, any type, major procedure

1-A48 Anterior Segment of Eye: Surgical Repairs, Closures and Reconstructions — Continued

P1-A4870 Reduction of ciliary body
  Diminution of ciliary body
P1-A4880 Reformation of chamber of eye
P1-A4890 Trabeculoplasty by laser surgery, one or more sessions

1-A4C Anterior Segment of Eye: Destructive Procedures

P1-A4C00 Destructive procedure of anterior segment of eye, NOS
P1-A4C10 Destruction of lesion of iris
  Nonexcisional destruction of lesion of iris
P1-A4C12 Destruction of cyst of iris
P1-A4C15 Lysis of goniosynechiae, NOS
P1-A4C16 Freeing of goniosynechiae with injection of air or liquid
  Lysis of goniosynechiae with injection of air or liquid
P1-A4C18 Lysis of anterior adhesions of iris, NOS
  Synechiotomy of anterior iris, NOS
P1-A4C19 Freeing of anterior synechiae with injection of air or liquid
  Lysis of anterior synechiae with injection of air or liquid
P1-A4C1A Lysis of posterior adhesions of iris
  Freeing of posterior synechiae
  Lysis of posterior synechiae
  Synechiotomy of posterior iris
P1-A4C30 Lysis of corneovitreal adhesions
P1-A4C34 Corelysis
P1-A4C35 Cryotherapy of iris
P1-A4C36 Cauterization of iris
P1-A4C37 Photocoagulation of iris
P1-A4C38 Coreoplasty by photocoagulation, one or more sessions for improvement of vision
P1-A4C40 Destruction of lesion of sclera
P1-A4C42 Cauterization of sclera
P1-A4C43 Cauterization of sclera with iridectomy
P1-A4C44 Thermosclerectomy
P1-A4C45 Thermocauterization of sclera with iridectomy
P1-A4C50 Nonexcisional destruction of lesion of ciliary body, NOS
P1-A4C51 Nonexcisional destruction of cyst of ciliary body
P1-A4C52 Electrolysis of ciliary body, NOS
  Cycloelectrolysis, NOS
  Cyclodiathermy, NOS
P1-A4C56 Cryotherapy of ciliary body
  Cyclocryotherapy, NOS
P1-A4C60 Photocoagulation of ciliary body
  Cyclophotocoagulation
P1-A4C62 Cycloanemization
P1-A4C66 Destruction of epithelial downgrowth of anterior chamber of eye

1-A5 OPERATIVE PROCEDURES ON THE OCULAR LENS

1-A50 Lens: General and Miscellaneous Operative Procedures

P1-A5000 Operative procedure on ocular lens, NOS
  Operation on lens, NOS

1-A51 Lens: Incisions

P1-A5100 Capsulotomy of lens, NOS
P1-A5101 Incisional discission of lens capsule, initial
  Capsulotomy of lens with discission of lens
  Slitting of lens
P1-A5102 Incisional discission of lens capsule, subsequent
P1-A5103 Incisional discission of anterior hyaloid
P1-A5110 Discission of membranous cataract, primary
P1-A5112 Discission of membranous cataract, secondary
  Discission of after cataract
P1-A5114 Incisional discission of secondary membranous cataract and anterior hyaloid
P1-A5116 Discission of congenital cataract
P1-A5117 Needling of lens capsule
P1-A5118 Needling of secondary cataract
P1-A5130 Laser surgery for discission of lens capsule, one or more stages
P1-A5132 Laser surgery for discission of anterior hyaloid, one or more stages
P1-A5134 Laser surgery for discission of secondary membranous cataract, one or more stages
P1-A5136 Laser surgery for discission of secondary membranous cataract and anterior hyaloid, one or more stages

1-A53 Lens: Excisions

P1-A5300 Extraction of lens of eye, NOS
P1-A5302 Aspiration of lens, NOS
P1-A5304 Excision and prosthetic replacement of lens, NOS
P1-A5306 Expression of lens, linear, one or more stages
P1-A5308 Curette evacuation of lens
P1-A5320 Extraction of cataract, NOS
  Excision of cataract, NOS
  Cataract extraction, NOS
P1-A5321 Extraction of primary membranous cataract by excision
P1-A5322 Extraction of primary membranous cataract by discission
P1-A5323 Extraction of primary membranous cataract by needling
P1-A5324 Extraction of primary membranous cataract by mechanical fragmentation
  Extraction of primary membranous cataract by phacofragmentation
P1-A5326 Excision of secondary membrane
  Extraction of after cataract by excision
  Extraction of secondary membrane by excision

P1-A5326 (cont.) Excision of after cataract

P1-A5327 Extraction of secondary membrane by discission
  Extraction of after cataract by discission

P1-A5328 Extraction of secondary membrane by needling
  Extraction of after cataract by needling

P1-A5329 Extraction of after cataract with capsulotomy

P1-A532A Removal of secondary membranous cataract with iridectomy

P1-A532B Extraction of secondary membrane with capsulectomy
  Extraction of after cataract with capsulectomy

P1-A532C Extraction of after cataract with iridocapsulectomy
  Extraction of secondary membrane with iridocapsulectomy

P1-A5330 Extraction of secondary membrane by mechanical fragmentation
  Extraction of secondary membrane by phacofragmentation
  Extraction of after cataract by mechanical fragmentation
  Extraction of after cataract by phacofragmentation

P1-A5332 Removal of secondary membranous cataract, after cataract, with corneoscleral section and without iridectomy

P1-A5333 Removal of secondary membranous cataract, after cataract, with corneoscleral section, with iridectomy and iridocapsulotomy

P1-A5334 Aspiration of cataract, NOS
  Aspiration of lens material, one or more stages

P1-A5335 Aspiration of cataract by phacoemulsification
  Extraction of cataract by emulsification and aspiration

P1-A5336 Aspiration of cataract by phacofragmentation
  Extraction of cataract by phacofragmentation with aspiration
  Extraction of cataract by ultrasonic phacofragmentation
  Ultrasonic fragmentation of cataract with aspiration

P1-A5339 Mechanical fragmentation of cataract with extraction by posterior route
  Extraction of cataract by phacofragmentation with aspiration by posterior route

P1-A5340 Extraction of cataract by rotoextraction with aspiration

P1-A5341 Extraction of cataract by rotoextraction with aspiration by posterior route

P1-A5343 Cryoextraction of cataract by intracapsular approach

P1-A5344 Erysiphake extraction of cataract by intracapsular approach

P1-A5345 Zonulolysis with lens extraction

P1-A5350 Intracapsular extraction of lens, NOS
  ICCE
  Intracapsular extraction of lens without iridectomy and without enzymes

P1-A5352 Intracapsular extraction of lens without iridectomy and with enzymes

P1-A5353 Intracapsular extraction of lens without iridectomy for dislocated lens

P1-A5355 Intracapsular extraction of lens with iridectomy and without enzymes

P1-A5356 Intracapsular extraction of lens with iridectomy and enzymes

P1-A5357 Intracapsular extraction of lens with iridectomy for dislocated lens

P1-A5360 Intracapsular extraction of lens by inferior temporal route

P1-A5361 Cryoextraction of cataract by inferior temporal route

P1-A5362 Erysiphake extraction of cataract by inferior temporal route

P1-A5370 Extracapsular extraction of lens, NOS

P1-A5372 Extracapsular extraction of lens by aspiration and irrigation technique

P1-A5373 Extracapsular extraction of cataract by curette evacuation

P1-A5374 Extracapsular extraction of lens by linear extraction technique

P1-A5375 Extracapsular extraction of cataract by emulsification with aspiration
  Extracapsular extraction of cataract by phacoemulsification with aspiration

P1-A5376 Extracapsular extraction of cataract by mechanical fragmentation with aspiration by posterior route
  Extracapsular extraction of cataract by phacofragmentation with aspiration by posterior route

P1-A5377 Extracapsular extraction of cataract by rotoextraction with aspiration

P1-A5378 Extracapsular extraction of cataract by rotoextraction with aspiration by posterior route

P1-A5379 Extracapsular extraction of cataract by mechanical fragmentation with aspiration
  Extracapsular extraction of cataract by phacofragmentation with aspiration

P1-A5380 Extracapsular extraction of lens with iridectomy, NOS

P1-A5385 Extracapsular extraction of lens by inferior temporal route

P1-A5386 Extracapsular extraction of cataract by inferior temporal route

P1-A5390 Capsulectomy of lens

P1-A5391 Capsulectomy with extraction of lens

P1-A5392 Iridocapsulectomy

P1-A5394 Removal of foreign body from lens, NOS

P1-A5395 Nonmagnetic extraction of foreign body from lens without extraction of lens
  Removal of foreign body from lens without use of magnet

1-A53 Lens: Excisions — Continued

P1-A5396 Magnet extraction of foreign body from lens
  Removal of foreign body from lens with use of magnet
  Magnet extraction of foreign body from lens without extraction of lens

P1-A5397 Capsulotomy of lens with removal of foreign body
  Removal of foreign body of lens by incision

P1-A5398 Capsulotomy of lens with removal of foreign body by magnet extraction
  Removal of foreign body of lens by incision with use of magnet

1-A55 Lens: Injections and Implantations

P1-A5500 Injection of lens, NOS

P1-A5510 Irrigation of traumatic cataract, NOS

P1-A5520 Insertion of prosthetic intraocular lens
  Insertion of pseudophakos, NOS

P1-A5524 Insertion of prosthetic lens subsequent to cataract extraction
  Secondary insertion of intraocular lens prosthesis

P1-A5535 Intracapsular cataract extraction with insertion of intraocular lens prosthesis, one stage procedure
  Insertion of prosthetic lens with cataract extraction, one-stage

P1-A5537 Extracapsular cataract removal, manual, with insertion of intraocular lens prosthesis, one stage procedure

P1-A5538 Extracapsular cataract removal by phacoemulsification with insertion of intraocular lens prosthesis, one stage procedure

P1-A5540 Removal of implant of lens
  Removal of prosthesis of lens
  Removal of pseudophakos

1-A58 Lens: Surgical Repairs, Closures and Reconstructions

P1-A5800 Repair of ocular lens, NOS

P1-A5810 Repair of postcataract wound dehiscence with conjunctival flap

P1-A5820V Lens couching procedure
  Surgical displacement of lens of eye

1-A5C Lens: Destructive Procedures

P1-A5C00 Destructive procedure of lens, NOS

P1-A5C10 Mechanical fragmentation of primary membranous cataract, NOS

P1-A5C20 Mechanical fragmentation of secondary membrane, NOS
  Mechanical fragmentation of after cataract, NOS

1-A6 OPERATIVE PROCEDURES ON THE POSTERIOR SEGMENT OF THE EYE

1-A60 Posterior Segment of Eye: General and Miscellaneous Operative Procedures

P1-A6000 Operative procedure on posterior segment of eye, NOS

P1-A6010 Operation on posterior chamber of eye, NOS

P1-A6012 Diagnostic procedure on posterior chamber of eye, NOS

P1-A6020 Operation on choroid, NOS

P1-A6022 Diagnostic procedure on choroid, NOS

P1-A6030 Operation on retina, NOS

P1-A6032 Diagnostic procedure on retina, NOS

P1-A6040 Operation on vitreous, NOS

P1-A6042 Diagnostic procedure on vitreous, NOS

1-A61 Posterior Segment of Eye: Incisions

P1-A6100 Incision of posterior segment of eye, NOS

P1-A6110 Release of encircling material of posterior segment of eye

P1-A6120 Exploration of choroid, NOS

P1-A6130 Discission of vitreous strands by anterior approach

P1-A6132 Discission of vitreous strands by posterior approach

P1-A6134 Division of vitreous cicatricial bands by anterior approach

P1-A6136 Division of vitreous cicatricial bands by posterior approach

P1-A6138 Discission of vitreous strands without removal by pars plana approach

1-A63 Posterior Segment of Eye: Excisions

P1-A6300 Vitrectomy, NOS
  Excision of vitreous opacity, NOS

P1-A6310 Diagnostic aspiration of vitreous

P1-A6312 Aspiration of vitreous with replacement
  Extraction of vitreous with replacement
  Removal of vitreous with replacement

P1-A6314 Anterior sclerotomy with removal of vitreous
  Removal of vitreous by anterior approach
  Vitrectomy by anterior approach
  Excision of vitreous opacity by anterior approach

P1-A6315 Partial removal of vitreous by anterior approach

P1-A6316 Partial removal of vitreous by anterior approach, limbal incision

P1-A6317 Partial removal of vitreous by anterior approach, open sky technique

P1-A6318 Subtotal removal of vitreous by anterior approach with mechanical vitrectomy

P1-A6324 Mechanical vitrectomy, NOS

P1-A6325 Mechanical vitrectomy by anterior approach

P1-A6326 Posterior sclerotomy with removal of vitreous
P1-A6327 Mechanical vitrectomy by posterior approach
P1-A6328 Mechanical vitrectomy by pars plana approach
P1-A6329 Mechanical vitrectomy by pars plana approach with endolaser panretinal photocoagulation
P1-A632A Mechanical vitrectomy by pars plana approach with epiretinal membrane stripping
P1-A6330 Aspiration or release of choroidal fluid by pars plana approach
P1-A6331 Aspiration or release of subretinal fluid by pars plana approach
P1-A6332 Aspiration or release of vitreous fluid by pars plana approach
P1-A6333 Removal of encircling tube of eye
  Removal of scleral buckle
P1-A6340 Removal of foreign body from posterior segment of eye, NOS
P1-A6342 Removal of foreign body from retina by incision
P1-A6343 Removal of foreign body from choroid by incision
P1-A6344 Removal of foreign body from vitreous by incision
P1-A6350 Magnet extraction of foreign body from posterior segment of eye, NOS
  Removal of foreign body from posterior segment of eye with use of magnet, NOS
P1-A6351 Magnet extraction of foreign body from retina
  Removal of foreign body from retina with use of magnet
P1-A6352 Magnet extraction of foreign body from choroid
  Removal of foreign body from choroid with use of magnet
P1-A6353 Magnet extraction of foreign body from vitreous
  Removal of foreign body from vitreous with use of magnet
P1-A6354 Magnet extraction of foreign body from posterior segment of eye by anterior route
P1-A6355 Magnet extraction of foreign body from posterior segment of eye by posterior route
P1-A6360 Removal of foreign body from posterior segment of eye without use or magnet
  Nonmagnetic extraction of intraocular foreign body from posterior segment of eye
P1-A6361 Removal of foreign body from retina without use of magnet
P1-A6362 Removal of foreign body from choroid without use of magnet
P1-A6363 Removal of foreign body from vitreous without use of magnet

1-A65 Posterior Segment of Eye: Injections and Implantations

P1-A6500 Injection of posterior segment of eye, NOS
P1-A6501 Injection of vitreous substitute, NOS
P1-A6502 Injection of vitreous substitute, pars plana approach
P1-A6503 Injection of vitreous substitute for reattachment of retina
  Replacement of vitreous for retinal reattachment
P1-A6520 Implantation of custodis eye
P1-A6522 Implantation of retinal attachment
P1-A6523 Implantation of retinal attachment with buckling
P1-A6524 Implantation of vitreous, NOS
P1-A6525 Implantation of vitreous for retinal reattachment
P1-A6526 Implantation of vitreous for retinal reattachment with buckling
P1-A6530 Removal of surgically implanted material from posterior segment of eye
P1-A6531 Removal of implanted material from posterior segment of eye, extraocular
P1-A6532 Removal of implanted material from posterior segment of eye, intraocular
P1-A6538 Removal of retinal implant

1-A68 Posterior Segment of Eye: Surgical Repairs, Closures and Reconstructions

P1-A6800 Surgical repair of posterior segment of eye, NOS
P1-A6810 Repair of choroid, NOS
P1-A6812 Reattachment of choroid and retina, NOS
P1-A6814 Reinforcement of sclera, NOS
P1-A6815 Scleral reinforcement without graft, NOS
P1-A6816 Scleral reinforcement with graft, NOS
P1-A6820 Repair of retina for retinal tear or defect
P1-A6822 Repair of retina for retinal detachment
  Reattachment of retina
P1-A6823 Shortening of sclera for repair of retinal detachment
P1-A6826 Suture of retina for reattachment
P1-A6830 Repair of retinal detachment, one or more stages
P1-A6832 Repair of retinal detachment, more than one stage, subsequent operation
P1-A6834 Repair of retinal detachment, any method, with vitrectomy and removal of lens by same technique, with air tamponade, one or more stages
P1-A6840 Scleral buckling
  Buckling procedure of sclera
P1-A6842 Constriction of globe for scleral buckling
P1-A6843 Encircling procedure of sclera for buckling
  Cerclage of sclera
  Cinching for scleral buckling
P1-A6844 Indentation of sclera for buckling
P1-A6845 Infolding of sclera for buckling
P1-A6846 Outfolding of sclera for buckling
P1-A6847 Overlapping of sclera for buckling

1-A68 Posterior Segment of Eye: Surgical Repairs, Closures and Reconstructions — Continued

P1-A6848 Pleating of sclera for buckling
P1-A6850 Resection of sclera with scleral buckling
P1-A6851 Lamellar resection of sclera for retinal reattachment
P1-A6852 Shortening of sclera by scleral buckling
P1-A6854 Scleral buckling for repair of retinal detachment, one or more stages, without implant
P1-A6855 Scleral buckling with implant
  Encircling procedure of sclera for buckling with implant
P1-A6856 Scleral buckling for repair of retinal detachment, one or more stages, with implant
  Repair of retina for retinal detachment by scleral buckling
P1-A6857 Scleral buckling with vitreous implant
P1-A6859 Lamellar resection of sclera with implant
P1-A6860 Scleral buckling with vitrectomy
P1-A6861 Scleral buckling with air tamponade
P1-A6862 Cerclage for retinal reattachment
P1-A6863 Sclerectomy for retinal reattachment
P1-A6864 Trephine sclerectomy with implant
P1-A6870 Repair of retina for retinal tear or defect by diathermy
P1-A6871 Diathermy for repair of retinal detachment, one or more stages, without drainage of subretinal fluid
P1-A6872 Diathermy for repair of retinal detachment, one or more stages, with drainage of subretinal fluid
P1-A6873 Diathermy for prophylaxis of retinal detachment without drainage, one or more stages
P1-A6874 Reattachment of retina by diathermy
  Repair of retina for retinal detachment by diathermy
P1-A6875 Reattachment of retina by electrocoagulation
P1-A6876 Electrocoagulation of retina for repair of tear
P1-A6878 Reattachment of choroid and retina by diathermy
P1-A6879 Reattachment of choroid and retina by electrocoagulation
P1-A6880 Repair of retina for retinal tear or defect by cryotherapy
  Cryotherapy of retina for repair of tear or defect
  Cryoretinopexy for repair of tear or defect
P1-A6882 Repair of retina for retinal detachment by cryotherapy
  Reattachment of retina by cryotherapy
  Cryoretinopexy reattachment
P1-A6883 Cryotherapy for repair of retinal detachment, one or more stages, with drainage of subretinal fluid
P1-A6884 Cryotherapy for repair of retinal detachment, one or more stages, without drainage of subretinal fluid
P1-A6885 Cryotherapy for prophylaxis of retinal detachment without drainage, one or more stages
P1-A6888 Reattachment of choroid and retina by cryotherapy
P1-A6890 Repair of retina for retinal tear or defect by photocoagulation
P1-A6891 Repair of retina for retinal detachment by photocoagulation
P1-A6892 Photocoagulation for repair of retinal detachment, one or more stages, without drainage of subretinal fluid
P1-A6893 Photocoagulation for repair of retinal detachment, one or more stages, with drainage of subretinal fluid
P1-A6894 Photocoagulation for prophylaxis of retinal detachment without drainage, one or more stages
P1-A6895 Reattachment of retina by photocoagulation
P1-A6896 Reattachment of choroid and retina by photocoagulation
P1-A68A0 Repair of retina for retinal tear or defect by laser photocoagulation
  Laser photocoagulation of retina for repair of tear or defect
P1-A68A1 Repair of retina for retinal tear or defect by xenon arc photocoagulation
  Repair of retinal tear by xenon arc photocoagulation
P1-A68A2 Repair of retinal detachment by laser photocoagulation
  Reattachment of retina by laser photocoagulation
P1-A68A3 Repair of retinal detachment with xenon arc photocoagulation
  Reattachment of retina by xenon arc photocoagulation
P1-A68A6 Reattachment of choroid and retina by laser photocoagulation
P1-A68A8 Reattachment of choroid and retina by xenon arc photocoagulation

1-A6C Posterior Segment of Eye: Destructive Procedures

P1-A6C00 Destructive procedure on posterior segment of eye, NOS
P1-A6C10 Destruction of lesion of retina, NOS
P1-A6C11 Destruction of lesion of choroid, NOS
P1-A6C12 Destruction of chorioretinopathy
  Destruction of chorioretinal lesion
P1-A6C14 Lysis of adhesions of vitreous by anterior approach
P1-A6C16 Lysis of adhesions of vitreous by posterior approach
P1-A6C20 Destruction of lesion of retina by diathermy
P1-A6C21 Destruction of lesion of choroid by diathermy
P1-A6C22 Destruction of chorioretinal lesion by diathermy

P1-A6C23 Diathermy for destruction of lesion of retina, one or more stages
P1-A6C24 Diathermy for destruction of extensive or progressive retinopathy, one or more stages
P1-A6C25 Fulguration of retina
P1-A6C26 Fulguration of choroid
P1-A6C28 Electrocoagulation of retina for destruction of lesion
P1-A6C30 Destruction of lesion of retina by cryotherapy
P1-A6C31 Cryotherapy for destruction of lesion of retina, one or more stages
P1-A6C32 Cryotherapy for destruction of extensive or progressive retinopathy, one or more stages
P1-A6C34 Destruction of lesion of choroid by cryotherapy
P1-A6C36 Destruction of chorioretinal lesion by cryotherapy
P1-A6C40 Destruction of lesion of retina by photocoagulation
P1-A6C41 Photocoagulation for destruction of lesion of retina, one or more stages
P1-A6C42 Photocoagulation for destruction of extensive or progressive retinopathy, one or more stages
P1-A6C43 Destruction of lesion of choroid by photocoagulation
P1-A6C44 Destruction of chorioretinal lesion by photocoagulation, NOS
P1-A6C45 Destruction of lesion of retina by xenon arc photocoagulation
P1-A6C46 Destruction of lesion of choroid by xenon arc photocoagulation
P1-A6C47 Destruction of chorioretinal lesion by xenon arc photocoagulation
P1-A6C48 Destruction of lesion of retina by laser photocoagulation
P1-A6C49 Destruction of lesion of choroid by laser photocoagulation
P1-A6C4A Destruction of chorioretinal lesion by laser photocoagulation
P1-A6C50 Destruction of lesion of retina by radiation therapy
P1-A6C51 Destruction of lesion of choroid by radiation therapy
P1-A6C52 Destruction of chorioretinal lesion by radiation therapy
P1-A6C53 Destruction of lesion of retina by implantation of radiation source
P1-A6C54 Radiation by implantation for destruction of localized lesion of retina, one or more stages
P1-A6C55 Destruction of lesion of choroid by implantation of radiation source
P1-A6C58 Destruction of chorioretinal lesion by implantation of radiation source
P1-A6C60 Laser surgery for severing of vitreous face adhesions, one or more stages
  Laser surgery for severing of vitreous membranes, one or more stages
  Laser surgery for severing of vitreous opacities, one or more stages
  Laser surgery for severing of vitreous sheets, one or more stages
  Laser surgery for severing of vitreous strands, one or more stages

1-A6D Posterior Segment of Eye: Transplantations and Transpositions

P1-A6D10 Transplantation of vitreous, NOS
P1-A6D12 Transplantation of vitreous by anterior approach

1-A9 OPERATIVE PROCEDURES ON THE EXTRAOCULAR MUSCLES

1-A90 Extraocular Muscles: General and Miscellaneous Operative Procedures

P1-A9000 Operation on extraocular muscle, NOS
  Surgical procedure on ocular muscle, NOS
P1-A9001 Operation on single extraocular muscle
P1-A9002 Operation on single extraocular muscle with temporary detachment from globe
P1-A9004 Operation on multiple extraocular muscles
P1-A9005 Operation on two or more extraocular muscles, one or both eyes
P1-A9006 Operation on multiple extraocular muscles with temporary detachment from globe
P1-A9007 Operation on two or more extraocular muscles involving temporary detachment from globe, one or both eyes
P1-A9010 Diagnostic procedure on extraocular muscle, NOS
P1-A9020 Operation on tendon of extraocular muscle, NOS
P1-A9024 Diagnostic procedure on tendon of extraocular muscle
P1-A9030 Operation on extraocular muscle and tendon, NOS
P1-A9034 Diagnostic procedure on extraocular muscle and tendon with temporary detachment from globe

1-A91 Extraocular Muscles: Incisions

P1-A9100 Incision of extraocular muscle, NOS
P1-A9102 Myotomy of oblique or rectus muscle of eye, NOS
P1-A9104 Multiple myotomies of eye, two or more muscles
P1-A9110 Tenotomy of eye
P1-A9114 Multiple tenotomies of eye, two or more tendons
P1-A9120 Transection of muscle of eye
P1-A9124 Multiple transections of muscles of eye, two or more muscles

1-A93 Extraocular Muscles: Excisions

P1-A9300 Excision of extraocular muscle, NOS
  Myectomy of eye muscle, NOS
  Resection of eye muscle, NOS
  Resection of extraocular muscle, NOS
  Resection of one extraocular muscle, NOS
P1-A9302 Resection of extraocular muscle with suture of original insertion
P1-A9304 Myectomy of eye muscle, multiple
P1-A9306 Tenectomy of eye
P1-A9308 Tenectomy of eye, multiple, two or more tendons
P1-A9320 Excisional biopsy of extraocular muscle or tendon
P1-A9322 Biopsy of extraocular muscle
  Excisional biopsy of eye muscle
P1-A9324 Biopsy of extraocular tendon
P1-A9330 Excision of lesion of extraocular muscle
P1-A9334 Excision of lesion of ocular tendon

1-A98 Extraocular Muscles: Surgical Repairs, Closures and Reconstructions

P1-A9800 Surgical repair of extraocular muscle, NOS
P1-A9810 Advancement of eye muscle, NOS
  Advancement of extraocular muscle, NOS
P1-A9812 Advancement of eye muscle, multiple, with resection or recession
  Advancement of extraocular muscle, multiple, with resection or recession
P1-A9814 Recession of eye muscle
  Recession of extraocular muscle
  Recession of one extraocular muscle
P1-A9816 Recession of extraocular muscles, multiple, with advancement or resection
P1-A9820 Lengthening of extraocular muscle, NOS
  Lengthening procedure on one extraocular muscle, NOS
P1-A9822 Lengthening of extraocular muscles, two or more muscles
P1-A9824 Shortening of extraocular muscle, NOS
  Shortening procedure on one extraocular muscle, NOS
P1-A9826 Shortening of eye muscles, multiple, two or more muscles, with lengthening
P1-A9828 Plication of eye muscle, oblique or rectus
  Cinching of ocular muscle, oblique or rectus
  Folding of eye muscle
  Tucking of eye muscle
  Pleating of eye muscle
P1-A9829 Plication of eye muscles, two or more muscles
  Cinching of ocular muscles, two or more muscles
  Folding of eye muscles, two or more muscles
  Pleating of eye muscles, two or more muscles
  Tucking of eye muscles, two or more muscles
P1-A9830 Resection of extraocular muscle with advancement or recession of other eye muscle
P1-A9840 Strabismus surgery, NOS
  Strabismus operation, NOS
P1-A9841 Strabismus surgery, initial, any technique for one muscle
P1-A9842 Strabismus surgery, initial, any procedure for two muscles, one eye
P1-A9843 Strabismus surgery, initial, any procedure for two muscles, both eyes
P1-A9844 Strabismus surgery, initial, any procedure for three or more muscles, one eye
P1-A9845 Strabismus surgery, initial, any procedure for three or more muscles, both eyes
P1-A9846 Strabismus surgery, subsequent, without reoperation of muscles
P1-A9847 Strabismus surgery, subsequent, with reoperation of muscles
P1-A9848 Adjustable suture technique during strabismus surgery
P1-A9850 Repair of wound of extraocular muscle, tendon and Tenon's capsule
P1-A9851 Repair of wound of extraocular muscle
P1-A9852 Repair of wound of extraocular tendon
P1-A9853 Repair of wound of Tenon's capsule
P1-A9860 Suture of extraocular muscle, NOS
P1-A9862 Suture of ocular tendon
P1-A9864 Suture of Tenon's capsule
P1-A9866 Attachment of rectus eye muscle to frontalis
P1-A9868 Freeing of entrapped extraocular muscle
P1-A9870 Revision of extraocular muscle surgery, NOS

1-A9C Extraocular Muscles: Destructive Procedures

P1-A9C00 Destructive procedure on extraocular muscle, NOS
P1-A9C10 Lysis of adhesions of eye muscle, NOS
  Lysis of adhesions of extraocular muscle, NOS
P1-A9C20 Chemodenervation of extraocular muscle

1-A9D Extraocular Muscles: Transplantations and Transpositions

P1-A9D00 Transposition of eye muscle
  Transposition of extraocular muscle
P1-A9D10 Transposition of extraocular muscle, one or more stages, one or more muscles, with displacement of plane of action more than 5 mm

1-AB-AD OPERATIVE PROCEDURES ON THE EAR

1-AB OPERATIVE PROCEDURES ON THE EXTERNAL EAR

1-AB0 External Ear: General and Miscellaneous Operative Procedures

P1-AB000 Operation on the ear, NOS

P1-AB010 Operation on external ear, NOS
  Surgical procedure on external ear, NOS

P1-AB012 Diagnostic procedure on external ear, NOS

1-AB1 External Ear: Incisions

P1-AB100 Incision of external ear, NOS

P1-AB102 Incision of skin of ear

P1-AB104 Incision of auricle of ear

P1-AB110 Incision of hematoma of external ear

P1-AB130 Drainage of external ear, NOS

P1-AB132 Drainage of external ear abscess, simple

P1-AB134 Drainage of external ear abscess, complicated

P1-AB136 Drainage of external ear hematoma, simple

P1-AB138 Drainage of external ear hematoma, complicated

P1-AB140 Piercing of external ear
  Piercing of ear lobe
  Piercing of pinna

P1-AB150 Exploration of external auditory canal

P1-AB152 Incision of external auditory canal
  Incision of external auditory meatus

P1-AB154 Drainage of external auditory canal abscess

P1-AB160 Unroofing of external ear, NOS

P1-AB162 Unroofing of external auditory canal, NOS

1-AB3-AB4 External Ear: Excisions

P1-AB300 Biopsy of external ear
  Excisional biopsy of external ear

P1-AB302 Excision of lesion of external ear, NOS

P1-AB303 Excision of lesion of auricle of ear, NOS
  Excision of lesion of pinna, NOS

P1-AB320 Biopsy of external auditory canal

P1-AB321 Excision of lesion of external auditory canal
  Excision of lesion of external auditory meatus

P1-AB322 Excision of soft tissue lesion from external auditory canal

P1-AB324 Excision of exostosis from external auditory canal

P1-AB330 Partial excision of external ear

P1-AB332 Partial excision of external ear, simple repair

P1-AB340 Curettage of external ear

P1-AB350 Excision of preauricular lesion of ear

P1-AB352 Excision of preauricular sinus of ear, radical

P1-AB354 Excision of preauricular appendage, remnant
  Excision of periauricular skin tags

P1-AB356 Excision of congenital preauricular cyst, fistula or sinus

P1-AB360 Excision of lesion of external ear, radical

P1-AB361 Radical excision of lesion of external auditory canal or meatus, NOS

P1-AB362 Radical excision of external auditory canal lesion without neck dissection

P1-AB364 Radical excision of external auditory canal lesion with neck dissection

P1-AB370 Excision of lesion of auricle of ear, radical
  Excision of lesion of pinna, radical

P1-AB380 Excision of external ear, complete amputation
  Amputation of external ear
  Complete excision of external ear
  Auriculectomy

P1-AB400 Removal of impacted ear wax from one or both ears
  Removal of impacted cerumen from one or both ears

P1-AB404V Removal of hair from external auditory canal

P1-AB410 Removal of foreign body from external auditory canal, NOS
  Removal of intraluminal foreign body from ear without incision, NOS

P1-AB412 Removal of foreign body from external auditory canal without general anesthesia

P1-AB414 Removal of foreign body from external auditory canal with general anesthesia

P1-AB418 Removal of foreign body from ear with incision

1-AB5 External Ear: Injections and Implantations

P1-AB500 Irrigation of ear
  Syringing of ear

P1-AB510 Packing of external auditory canal

P1-AB520 Application of prosthesis for missing ear
  Prosthetic replacement of ear

1-AB7 External Ear: Endoscopy

P1-AB700 Endoscopy of ear
  Otoscopy

1-AB8-AB9 External Ear: Surgical Repairs, Closures and Reconstructions

P1-AB800 Repair of external ear, NOS
  Otoplasty of external ear, NOS

P1-AB802 Repair of auricle of ear, NOS
  Otoplasty of auricle, NOS
  Repair of pinna, NOS

P1-AB820 Repair of ear cartilage, NOS
  Otoplasty of cartilage of ear, NOS

P1-AB830 Repair of lop ear
  Repair of bat ear

P1-AB850 Repair of prominent or protruding ear
  Correction of prominent ear
  Otoplasty of prominent or protruding ear
  Reconstruction of prominent or protruding ear

P1-AB852 Otoplasty of protruding ear without size reduction

P1-AB854 Otoplasty of protruding ear with size reduction

1-AB8-AB9 External Ear: Surgical Repairs, Closures and Reconstructions — Continued

P1-AB856 Setback of ear
  Pinning of ear
P1-AB860 Repair of auditory canal or meatus of ear
  Meatoplasty of ear
  Otoplasty of auditory canal or meatus
  Canaloplasty of external auditory meatus
  Reconstruction of external auditory canal
P1-AB862 Pattee operation on auditory canal
P1-AB864 Construction of ear meatus, osseous, skin-lined
  Reconstruction of meatus of ear, osseous, skin-lined
P1-AB870 Correction of atresia of external meatus of ear
  Construction of patent meatus of ear
  Reconstruction of external auditory canal for congenital atresia, single stage
P1-AB900 Closure of cervicoaural fistula
P1-AB910 Suture of external ear
  Suture of skin of ear
  Repair of ear laceration by suture

1-ABC External Ear: Destructive Procedures

P1-ABC00 Destructive procedure of external ear, NOS
P1-ABC04 Destruction of lesion of external ear, NOS
P1-ABC10 Cryotherapy of external ear
P1-ABC20 Cauterization of external ear
P1-ABC30 Coagulation or electrocoagulation of external ear

1-ABD External Ear: Transplantations and Transpositions

P1-ABD10 Grafting of auricle of ear
P1-ABD20 Grafting of external auditory meatus of ear
  Grafting of skin of auditory meatus of ear
P1-ABD30 Reconstruction of external ear with graft or implant
  Construction of ear auricle with graft or with implant
P1-ABD40 Reconstruction otoplasty of cartilage of ear
P1-ABD42 Graft of ear cartilage to ear
P1-ABD44 Autogenous graft of rib cartilage to ear
P1-ABD50 Postauricular grafting
  Postauricular grafting of skin of ear
  Wolff procedure for postauricular grafting
P1-ABD60 Reattachment of amputated ear
  Otopexy

1-AC OPERATIVE PROCEDURES ON THE MIDDLE EAR

1-AC0 Middle Ear: General and Miscellaneous Operative Procedures

P1-AC000 Operative procedure on middle ear, NOS
  Operation on the middle ear, NOS
P1-AC010 Operation on ossicular chain of middle ear, NOS
P1-AC050 Operation on eustachian tube, NOS

1-AC1-AC2 Middle Ear: Incisions

P1-AC100 Incision of middle ear, NOS
P1-AC102 Middle ear exploration through ear canal incision
P1-AC104 Middle ear exploration through postauricular incision
P1-AC110 Division of otosclerotic process of middle ear
P1-AC120 Hypotympanotomy
P1-AC130 Exploration of tympanum
P1-AC132 Exploration of tympanum by transtympanic route
  Transtympanic exploration of middle ear
P1-AC140 Division of tympanum
P1-AC142 Plicotomy of tympanum
P1-AC160 Atticotomy of ear
P1-AC162 Atticoantrostomy of ear
  Atticoantrotomy of ear
P1-AC170 Ossiculotomy, NOS
P1-AC172 Stapes mobilization
P1-AC174 Tenotomy of stapedius
P1-AC175 Tenotomy of tensor tympani
P1-AC177 Perforation of footplate
  Cody tack operation
  Fick operation
P1-AC180 Stapedotomy with reestablishment of ossicular continuity, without use of foreign material
P1-AC182 Stapedotomy with reestablishment of ossicular continuity, with use of foreign material
P1-AC184 Stapedotomy with reestablishment of ossicular continuity, without use of foreign material and with footplate drill out
P1-AC186 Stapedotomy with reestablishment of ossicular continuity, with use of foreign material and footplate drill out
P1-AC1A0 Tympanotomy
  Tympanostomy
  Myringostomy
  Paracentesis of tympanum
  Aspiration of middle ear
  Tympanocentesis
P1-AC1B0 Tympanotomy with intubation
  Myringotomy with aspiration and drainage
  Drainage of middle ear by myringotomy
  Myringotomy with insertion of tube
  Myringotomy with insertion of tube or drainage device, button or grommet
  Drainage of middle ear with intubation
  Tube myringotomy
  Paracentesis of tympanum with intubation
  Aspiration of middle ear with intubation
P1-AC1B2 Tympanostomy with local or topical anesthesia

P1-AC1B3 Tympanostomy with general anesthesia
P1-AC1B5 Myringotomy including aspiration with general anesthesia
P1-AC1B7 Myringotomy including aspiration and eustachian tube inflation
P1-AC1B8 Myringotomy including aspiration and eustachian tube inflation with general anesthesia
P1-AC200 Mastoidotomy, NOS
Incision of mastoid, NOS
P1-AC201 Exploration of mastoid
P1-AC202 Mastoid antrotomy
Transmastoid antrotomy
P1-AC210 Incision of petrous pyramid
Exploration of petrous pyramid air cells
P1-AC212 Intrapetrosal drainage
Frenckner operation
Ramadier operation
P1-AC214 Extrapetrosal drainage
Almoor operation
Eagleton operation

1-AC3-AC4 Middle Ear: Excisions

P1-AC300 Excision of middle ear structure, NOS
P1-AC301 Ossiculectomy of middle ear, NOS
P1-AC303 Biopsy of middle ear, NOS
Excisional biopsy of middle ear, NOS
P1-AC308 Excision of lesion of middle ear, NOS
P1-AC310 Debridement of mastoidectomy cavity, simple
P1-AC312 Debridement of mastoidectomy cavity, complex
P1-AC320 Tympanectomy
Myringectomy
Myringodectomy
P1-AC322 Removal of outer attic wall of middle ear
P1-AC324 Excision of petrous apex cells
Exenteration of petrous pyramid air cells
Apicectomy of petrous pyramid
P1-AC326 Petrous apicectomy including radical mastoidectomy
P1-AC330 Removal of tumor of temporal bone
P1-AC331 Resection of temporal bone by external approach
P1-AC332 Excision of scar of mastoid
P1-AC335 Tympanosympathectomy
Sympathectomy of tympanum
Tympanic neurectomy
P1-AC340 Stapedectomy, NOS
P1-AC341 Stapedectomy with incus replacement
Stapedectomy with incus replacement by homograft or prosthesis
P1-AC342 Stapedectomy with reestablishment of ossicular continuity without use of foreign material
P1-AC343 Stapedectomy with reestablishment of ossicular continuity without use of foreign material, with footplate drill out
P1-AC344 Stapedectomy with reestablishment of ossicular continuity with use of foreign material
P1-AC346 Stapedectomy with reestablishment of ossicular continuity with use of foreign material and footplate drill out
P1-AC350 Remobilization of stapes
P1-AC352 Transcrural mobilization of stapes
P1-AC354 Bisection of stapes footplate
P1-AC355 Bisection of stapes footplate with incus replacement
P1-AC356 Ossiculectomy with stapedectomy
P1-AC357 Ossiculectomy with stapes mobilization
P1-AC360 Revision of stapedectomy, NOS
P1-AC370 Mastoidectomy, NOS
Excision of mastoid, NOS
P1-AC371 Excision of lesion of mastoid bone
P1-AC372 Mastoidectomy, cortical, conservative
P1-AC373 Simple mastoidectomy, complete
Schwartze operation
Stacke operation
P1-AC374 Antrectomy of mastoid
P1-AC376 Radical mastoidectomy
P1-AC377 Radical mastoidectomy, modified
P1-AC378 Tympanomastoidectomy
P1-AC380 Revision of mastoidectomy
P1-AC381 Revision of mastoidectomy with apicectomy
P1-AC382 Revision of mastoidectomy resulting in tympanoplasty
P1-AC383 Revision of mastoidectomy resulting in complete mastoidectomy
P1-AC384 Revision of mastoidectomy resulting in radical mastoidectomy
P1-AC385 Revision of mastoidectomy resulting in modified radical mastoidectomy
P1-AC390 Incudectomy, NOS
P1-AC392 Incudectomy with stapedectomy
P1-AC420 Excision of glomus jugulare tumor
Glomectomy jugulare
P1-AC422 Excision of aural glomus tumor, transcanal
P1-AC423 Excision of aural glomus tumor, transmastoid
P1-AC424 Excision of aural glomus tumor, extended, extratemporal
P1-AC425 Excision of aural polyp

1-AC5 Middle Ear: Injections and Implantations

P1-AC500 Injection of middle ear, NOS
P1-AC504 Catheterization of eustachian tube
Intubation of eustachian tube
Cannulation of eustachian tube
P1-AC506 Transtympanic eustachian tube catheterization
P1-AC508 Politzerization of eustachian tube
P1-AC510 Injection of eustachian tube with inert material
P1-AC512 Insufflation of eustachian tube
Inflation of eustachian tube
P1-AC513 Transnasal eustachian tube inflation without catheterization
P1-AC514 Transnasal eustachian tube inflation with catheterization

1-AC5 Middle Ear: Injections and Implantations — Continued

P1-AC520 Injection of tympanum
P1-AC522 Insertion of myringotomy device with intubation
P1-AC530 Focal application of phase control substance of middle ear, baffle technique
P1-AC540 Implantation of electromagnetic bone conduction hearing device in temporal bone
P1-AC550 Removal of implant of middle ear, NOS
P1-AC551 Removal of implant of tympanum
P1-AC552 Removal of catheter from middle ear
  Removal of tube from tympanostomy
  Removal of tube from tympanum
  Removal of myringotomy device or tube
P1-AC555 Removal of silastic tubes from ear
P1-AC556 Removal of Shepard's tube from ear
P1-AC557 Ventilating tube removal by another physician
P1-AC560 Removal of electromagnetic bone conduction hearing device in temporal bone

1-AC8-AC9 Middle Ear: Surgical Repairs, Closures and Reconstructions

P1-AC800 Repair of middle ear, NOS
  Middle ear otoplasty, NOS
P1-AC804 Eustachian tuboplasty, NOS
P1-AC810 Repair of mastoid antrum or cavity, NOS
P1-AC812 Mastoid myoplasty
P1-AC820 Myringoplasty, NOS
P1-AC821 Tympanic membrane repair without perforation
P1-AC822 Tympanic membrane repair without site preparation
P1-AC823 Tympanic membrane repair with site preparation
P1-AC824 Tympanic membrane repair with perforation, closure without patch
P1-AC825 Tympanic membrane repair with perforation, closure with patch
P1-AC826 Myringoplasty epitympanic, type I
  Tympanoplasty, type I with graft
  Derlacki operation
P1-AC830 Tympanoplasty type II with graft against incus or malleus
  Tympanoplasty with incudostapediopexy
  Myringomalleolabyrinthopexy
P1-AC834 Tympanoplasty type III with graft against mobile and intact stapes
  Myringostapediopexy
P1-AC836 Ossiculectomy with tympanoplasty
P1-AC838 Reconstruction of ossicles with tympanoplasty
P1-AC840 Tympanoplasty type IV with air pocket over round window
P1-AC842 Tympanoplasty type V with fenestra in semicircular canal
P1-AC850 Tympanoplasty with antrotomy, without ossicular chain reconstruction
P1-AC851 Tympanoplasty with antrotomy, with ossicular chain reconstruction
P1-AC852 Tympanoplasty with antrotomy, with ossicular chain reconstruction and synthetic prosthesis
P1-AC854 Tympanoplasty with mastoidotomy, without ossicular chain reconstruction
P1-AC855 Tympanoplasty with mastoidotomy, with ossicular chain reconstruction
P1-AC856 Tympanoplasty with mastoidotomy, with ossicular chain reconstruction and synthetic prosthesis
P1-AC857 Tympanoplasty without mastoidectomy, initial, without ossicular chain reconstruction
P1-AC858 Tympanoplasty without mastoidectomy, initial, with ossicular chain reconstruction
P1-AC859 Tympanoplasty without mastoidectomy, initial, with ossicular chain reconstruction and synthetic prosthesis
P1-AC860 Tympanoplasty with mastoidectomy, without ossicular chain reconstruction
P1-AC861 Tympanoplasty without mastoidectomy, revision, without ossicular chain reconstruction
P1-AC862 Tympanoplasty without mastoidectomy, revision, with ossicular chain reconstruction
P1-AC863 Tympanoplasty without mastoidectomy, revision, with ossicular chain reconstruction and synthetic prosthesis
P1-AC864 Tympanoplasty with mastoidectomy, with ossicular chain reconstruction
P1-AC865 Tympanoplasty with mastoidectomy, with intact or reconstructed canal wall, without ossicular chain reconstruction
P1-AC866 Tympanoplasty with mastoidectomy, radical, without ossicular chain reconstruction
P1-AC867 Tympanoplasty with mastoidectomy, with intact or reconstructed canal wall, with ossicular chain reconstruction
P1-AC868 Tympanoplasty with mastoidectomy, radical, with ossicular chain reconstruction
P1-AC870 Myringoplasty revision, NOS
  Tympanoplasty revision, NOS
P1-AC872 Ossiculectomy with tympanoplasty revision
P1-AC874 Revision of mastoid antrum
P1-AC875 Reconstruction of mastoid cavity
P1-AC876 Reconstruction of ossicles with stapedectomy
P1-AC877 Revision stapedectomy with incus replacement by homograft or prosthesis
P1-AC878 Reconstruction of ossicles by graft or prosthesis, NOS
P1-AC900 Closure of fistula of middle ear, NOS
P1-AC902 Closure of fistula of ear drum
  Closure of fistula of tympanic membrane
  Closure of perforation of ear drum
  Closure of perforation of tympanic membrane
P1-AC910 Closure of fistula of mastoid antrum
P1-AC912 Closure of postauricular fistula of mastoid

P1-AC922 Incudopexy
P1-AC924 Incudostapediopexy
P1-AC925 Malleostapediopexy
P1-AC926 Incudostapediopexy with incus replacement
P1-AC928 Malleostapediopexy with incus replacement
P1-AC930 Fenestration of tympanic membrane
P1-AC932 Fenestration of stapes footplate with vein graft
P1-AC934 Fenestration of stapes footplate with incus replacement
P1-AC935 Revision of fenestration operation, NOS

1-ACC Middle Ear: Destructive Procedures

P1-ACC00 Destructive procedure on middle ear, NOS
P1-ACC10 Lysis of adhesions of middle ear
  Adhesiolysis of middle ear
P1-ACC12 Transcanal tympanolysis
P1-ACC14 Stapediolysis
P1-ACC20 Coagulation or electrocoagulation of middle ear
P1-ACC30 Obliteration of tympanomastoid cavity
P1-ACC32 Mastoid obliteration

1-AD OPERATIVE PROCEDURES ON THE INNER EAR

1-AD0 Inner Ear: General and Miscellaneous Operative Procedures

P1-AD000 Operation on the inner ear, NOS

1-AD1 Inner Ear: Incisions

P1-AD100 Incision of inner ear, NOS
P1-AD104 Drainage of inner ear
P1-AD110 Sacculotomy of inner ear
  Tack operation
P1-AD120 Decompression of internal auditory canal
P1-AD130 Vestibulotomy, NOS
P1-AD140 Labyrinthotomy, transtympanic
P1-AD142 Labyrinthotomy, membranous
P1-AD144 Labyrinthotomy, osseous
  Opening of bony labyrinth of ear
P1-AD150 Labyrinthotomy without cryosurgery, transcanal
P1-AD151 Labyrinthotomy without cryosurgery, with mastoidectomy
P1-AD152 Labyrinthotomy without tack procedure, transcanal
P1-AD154 Labyrinthotomy without tack procedure, with mastoidectomy
P1-AD160 Decompression of labyrinth
P1-AD162 Fistulization of labyrinth for decompression
P1-AD170 Incision of endolymphatic sac
P1-AD180 Decompression of endolymphatic sac
P1-AD182 Fistulization of endolymphatic sac for decompression
P1-AD190 Endolymphatic sac operation without shunt
P1-AD196 Perilymphatic tap

1-AD3 Inner Ear: Excisions

P1-AD300 Excision of inner ear, NOS
  Endaural resection, NOS
P1-AD304 Biopsy of inner ear, NOS
  Excisional biopsy of inner ear, NOS
P1-AD310 Otonecrectomy of inner ear
P1-AD320 Labyrinthectomy, transtympanic
P1-AD322 Labyrinthectomy, membranous
P1-AD324 Labyrinthectomy, osseous
P1-AD325 Labyrinthectomy, transcanal
P1-AD326 Labyrinthectomy with mastoidectomy
P1-AD330 Removal of utricle of labyrinth

1-AD5 Inner Ear: Injections and Implantations

P1-AD500 Injection into inner ear, NOS
P1-AD510 Implantation of cochlear prosthetic device, NOS
  Implantation of cochlear prosthetic device, electrode and receiver
P1-AD512 Implantation of electromagnetic hearing aid
  Implantation of electromagnetic hearing device
P1-AD513 Implantation of cochlear prosthetic device, single channel
  Implantation of cochlear electronic stimulator, single channel
P1-AD514 Implantation of cochlear prosthetic device, multiple channels
  Implantation of cochlear electronic stimulator, multiple channels
P1-AD515 Implantation of cochlear electrode
  Implantation of cochlear electronic stimulator
P1-AD524 Implantation of cochlear prosthetic device, internal coil only
P1-AD525 Cochlear device implantation without mastoidectomy
P1-AD526 Cochlear device implantation with mastoidectomy
P1-AD533 Replacement of cochlear prosthesis
P1-AD534 Replacement of cochlear prosthesis, single channel
P1-AD535 Replacement of cochlear prosthesis, multiple channels
P1-AD536 Replacement of electromagnetic bone conduction hearing device in temporal bone
P1-AD538 Repair of electromagnetic bone conduction hearing device in temporal bone
  Repair of cochlear prosthetic device
P1-AD540 Removal of cochlear implant or prosthetic device

1-AD8 Inner Ear: Surgical Repairs, Closures and Reconstructions

P1-AD800 Surgical repair of inner ear, NOS
P1-AD810 Repair of oval and round windows
P1-AD812 Repair of oval window fistula
  Closure of fistula of oval window of ear

1-AD8 Inner Ear: Surgical Repairs, Closures and Reconstructions — Continued

P1-AD814 Repair of round window fistula
  Closure of fistula of round window of ear
P1-AD830 Fenestration of inner ear, initial
  Arslan operation
P1-AD832 Fenestration of inner ear with graft
P1-AD835 Fenestration of labyrinth with graft
P1-AD836 Fenestration of semicircular canals with graft
P1-AD837 Fenestration of vestibule with graft
P1-AD838 Fenestration of oval window, ear canal
P1-AD839 Lempert's fenestration
P1-AD840 Revision of fenestration of inner ear
P1-AD842 Revision of tack operation of inner ear
P1-AD850 Endolymph-perilymph shunt
P1-AD852 Endolymphatic sac operation with shunt
P1-AD854 Endolymphatic-subarachnoid shunt
P1-AD855 Semicircular-subarachnoid shunt
P1-AD864 Closure of perilymph fistula

1-ADC Inner Ear: Destructive Procedures

P1-ADC00 Destructive procedure of inner ear, NOS
  Osteoclasis of inner ear, NOS
P1-ADC01 Injection of inner ear for destruction, NOS
  Ablation of inner ear by injection of substance, NOS
  Destruction of inner ear by injection, NOS
P1-ADC02 Injection of vestibule for destruction
  Destruction of vestibule by injection
P1-ADC04 Injection of semicircular canals for destruction
  Destruction of semicircular canals by injection
P1-ADC08 Injection of inner ear with alcohol
P1-ADC10 Ablation of inner ear by cryosurgery, NOS
P1-ADC11 Ablation of inner ear by ultrasound
P1-ADC15 Labyrinthotomy with cryosurgery, transcanal
P1-ADC16 Labyrinthotomy with cryosurgery, with mastoidectomy
P1-ADC20 Coagulation or electrocoagulation of inner ear, NOS
P1-ADC22 Coagulation or electrocoagulation of semicircular canals
P1-ADC30 Labyrinthotomy with tack procedure, transcanal
P1-ADC32 Labyrinthotomy with tack procedure and mastoidectomy

1-ADD Inner Ear: Transplantations and Transpositions

P1-ADD00 Grafting of inner ear, NOS

SECTION 1-B OPERATIVE PROCEDURES ON TOPOGRAPHIC REGIONS

1-B0 GENERAL OPERATIVE PROCEDURES ON TOPOGRAPHIC REGIONS

1-B00 Topographic Regions: General and Miscellaneous Operative Procedures

P1-B0000 Operative procedure on unspecified topographic region

1-B1 OPERATIVE PROCEDURES ON THE THORAX AND CHEST WALL

1-B10 Thorax and Chest Wall: General and Miscellaneous Operative Procedures

P1-B1010 Operation on thorax, NOS
  Operation on chest wall, NOS

1-B11 Thorax and Chest Wall: Incisions

P1-B1100 Incision of thorax, NOS
  Thoracotomy, NOS
  Thoracostomy, NOS

1-B13 Thorax and Chest Wall: Excisions

P1-B1300 Biopsy of thorax, NOS
  Biopsy of chest wall, NOS
P1-B1302 Excision of lesion of thorax
  Excision of lesion of chest wall
P1-B1304 Excision of scar of thorax
P1-B1305 Removal of suture of thorax
P1-B1307 Removal of foreign body from thorax
P1-B1320 Excision of chest wall tumor including ribs
P1-B1322 Excision of chest wall tumor involving ribs with plastic reconstruction
P1-B1324 Excision of chest wall tumor involving ribs with plastic reconstruction and mediastinal lymphadenectomy
P1-B1340 Removal of Abrams bar from chest wall
P1-B1350 Resection of chest wall
  Thoracoplasty
  Thoracectomy for lung collapse
  Thoracectomy, NOS
  Resection of thorax, NOS
P1-B1352 Extrapleural resection of ribs, all stages
  Extrapleural thoracoplasty, all stages
P1-B1355 Schede type thoracoplasty, all stages
P1-B1356 Extrapleural thoracoplasty, all stages, with closure of bronchopleural fistula
P1-B1359 Delorme operation, thoracoplasty
P1-B135A Eloesser operation, thoracoplasty
P1-B135B Estlander operation, thoracoplasty
P1-B135C Fowler operation, thoracoplasty
P1-B135D Wilms operation, thoracoplasty

1-B15 Thorax and Chest Wall: Injections and Implantations

P1-B1510 Injection into chest wall, NOS
P1-B1520 Implantation into chest wall, NOS
P1-B1530 Removal of device from thorax, NOS
P1-B1532 Removal of pectus deformity implant device

1-B17 Thorax and Chest Wall: Endoscopy

P1-B1700 Thoracoscopy, NOS
  Transpleural thoracoscopy, NOS
  Cavernoscopy of thorax, NOS
P1-B1710 Thoracoscopy with biopsy

1-B18 Thorax and Chest Wall: Surgical Repairs, Closures and Reconstructions

P1-B1800 Repair of chest wall, NOS
P1-B1804 Suture of laceration of chest wall
P1-B1810 Repair of stoma of thorax
  Revision of stoma of thorax
P1-B1820 Closure of stoma of thorax
  Closure of thoracostomy
P1-B1824 Closure of chest wall following open flap drainage for empyema
  Clagett operation, chest wall closure
P1-B1840 Repair of fistula of thorax, NOS
P1-B1842 Repair of abdominothoracic fistula
  Repair of thoracoabdominal fistula
P1-B1845 Repair of thoracogastric fistula
P1-B1846 Repair of thoracointestinal fistula
P1-B1847 Repair of hepatothoracic fistula
P1-B1900 Major reconstruction of chest wall, NOS
P1-B1920 Reconstruction of chest wall with implant, NOS
  Repair of chest wall with implant, NOS
P1-B1940 Costosternoplasty for pectus excavatum repair
  Chondrosternoplasty for pectus excavatum repair
P1-B1944 Repair of pectus excavatum deformity with implant
  Repair of funnel chest with implant
P1-B1950 Repair of pectus carinatum deformity with implant

1-B1C Thorax and Chest Wall: Destructive Procedures

P1-B1C10 Destruction of lesion of chest wall, NOS
P1-B1C20 Lysis of adhesions of thorax

1-B1D Thorax and Chest Wall: Transplantations and Transpositions

P1-B1D10 Transplantation of tissue of chest wall
P1-B1D40 Transposition of tissue of chest wall

1-B1E Thorax and Chest Wall: Manipulations

P1-B1E10 Manipulation of tissue of chest wall, NOS

1-B2 OPERATIVE PROCEDURES ON THE MEDIASTINUM

1-B20 Mediastinum: General and Miscellaneous Operative Procedures

P1-B2010 Operation on mediastinum, NOS

1-B21 Mediastinum: Incisions

P1-B2100 Incision of mediastinum
  Mediastinotomy
P1-B2110 Incision and exploration mediastinum, NOS
  Mediastinotomy with exploration, NOS
P1-B2111 Mediastinotomy with exploration by cervical approach
P1-B2112 Mediastinotomy with exploration by sternal split approach
P1-B2113 Mediastinotomy with exploration by transthoracic approach
P1-B2116 Mediastinotomy with drainage by cervical approach
P1-B2117 Mediastinotomy with drainage by sternal split approach
P1-B2118 Mediastinotomy with drainage by transthoracic approach

1-B23 Mediastinum: Excisions

P1-B2300 Excision of tissue of mediastinum
  Open biopsy of mediastinum
P1-B2302 Excision of lesion of mediastinum
P1-B2304 Excision of mediastinal cyst
P1-B2306 Excision of mediastinal tumor
P1-B2308 Removal of foreign body from mediastinum
P1-B2310 Percutaneous core needle biopsy of mediastinum
P1-B2312 Fine needle biopsy of mediastinum
  Fine needle aspiration biopsy of mediastinum

1-B25 Mediastinum: Injections and Implantations

P1-B2540 Removal of mediastinal drain
P1-B2542 Removal of tube from mediastinum

1-B27 Mediastinum: Endoscopy

P1-B2700 Mediastinoscopy, NOS
  Mediastinoscopy without biopsy
  Endoscopic exploration of mediastinum
P1-B2710 Mediastinoscopy with biopsy

1-B28 Mediastinum: Surgical Repairs, Closures and Reconstructions

P1-B2810 Repair of fistula of mediastinum, NOS
P1-B2812 Repair of bronchomediastinal fistula

1-B28 Mediastinum: Surgical Repairs, Closures and Reconstructions — Continued

P1-B2814 Repair of mediastinocutaneous fistula

1-B2C Mediastinum: Destructive Procedures

P1-B2C00 Destruction of tissue of mediastinum, NOS
P1-B2C10 Destruction of lesion of mediastinum, NOS
P1-B2C20 Lysis of adhesions of mediastinum

1-B2D Mediastinum: Transplantations and Transpositions

P1-B2D10 Transplantation of tissue of mediastinum, NOS
P1-B2D60 Transposition of tissue of mediastinum, NOS

1-B2E Mediastinum: Manipulations

P1-B2E10 Manipulation of tissue of mediastinum, NOS

1-B3 OPERATIVE PROCEDURES ON THE DIAPHRAGM

1-B30 Diaphragm: General and Miscellaneous Operative Procedures

P1-B3010 Operation on diaphragm, NOS

1-B31 Diaphragm: Incisions

P1-B3110 Incision of diaphragm, NOS

1-B33 Diaphragm: Excisions

P1-B3300 Biopsy of diaphragm
  Excision of tissue of diaphragm
P1-B3310 Excision of lesion of diaphragm
P1-B3350 Resection of diaphragm, NOS

1-B35 Diaphragm: Injections and Implantations

P1-B3510 Injection of diaphragm, NOS
P1-B3540 Implantation of diaphragm, NOS
P1-B3542 Implantation of diaphragmatic pacemaker

1-B38 Diaphragm: Surgical Repairs, Closures and Reconstructions

P1-B3800 Repair of diaphragm, NOS
P1-B3804 Suture of laceration of diaphragm
P1-B3806 Repair of fistula of diaphragm, NOS
  Closure of fistula of diaphragm, NOS
P1-B3810 Plication of diaphragm
P1-B3812 Imbrication of diaphragm, NOS
P1-B3814 Imbrication of diaphragm for eventration, paralytic
P1-B3816 Imbrication of diaphragm for eventration, nonparalytic
P1-B3850 Repair of diaphragmatic hernia, NOS
P1-B3851 Repair of diaphragmatic hiatal hernia
  Repair of parahiatal diaphragmatic hernia
  Repair of paraesophageal diaphragmatic hernia
P1-B3852 Repair of paraesophageal hiatus hernia, transabdominal, with fundoplasty, vagotomy and pyloroplasty, except neonatal
P1-B3854 Hill-Allison operation, diaphragmatic hernia repair
P1-B3856 Repair of diaphragmatic hiatal hernia by thoracoabdominal approach
P1-B3857 Repair of neonatal diaphragmatic hernia
P1-B3858 Repair of diaphragmatic hernia by abdominal approach
  Repair of esophageal hiatal hernia by abdominal approach
P1-B3859 Repair of diaphragmatic hernia by thoracic approach
  Repair of diaphragmatic hernia by transpleural approach
  Repair of diaphragmatic hernia by transthoracic approach
P1-B3860 Repair of esophageal hiatal hernia by combined thoracoabdominal approach with dilation of stricture
P1-B3862 Repair of esophageal hiatal hernia by combined thoracoabdominal approach with dilation of stricture with gastroplasty
P1-B3864 Plication of diaphragm for hernia repair by thoracoabdominal approach
P1-B3867 Collis-Nissen operation for hiatal hernia repair with esophagogastroplasty
P1-B3870 Repair of traumatic diaphragmatic hernia, acute
P1-B3872 Repair of traumatic diaphragmatic hernia, chronic
P1-B3880 Repair of parasternal diaphragmatic hernia
P1-B3890 Reconstruction of diaphragm, NOS

1-B3C Diaphragm: Destructive Procedures

P1-B3C10 Destruction of tissue of diaphragm, NOS

1-B3D Diaphragm: Transplantations and Transpositions

P1-B3D10 Transplantation of tissue of diaphragm, NOS
P1-B3D60 Transposition of tissue of diaphragm, NOS

1-B3E Diaphragm: Manipulations

P1-B3E10 Manipulation of tissue of diaphragm, NOS

1-B6 OPERATIVE PROCEDURES ON THE ABDOMEN

1-B60 Abdomen: General and Miscellaneous Operative Procedures

P1-B6010 Operation on abdominal region, NOS
P1-B6020 Operation on umbilicus, NOS
P1-B6030 Control of hemorrhage of abdominal cavity, NOS

P1-B6032 Control of hemorrhage of laparotomy site, NOS

P1-B6040 Laparotomy for staging of Hodgkin's disease or lymphoma
Staging celiotomy for Hodgkin's disease or lymphoma

P1-B6042 Laparotomy for staging of ovarian cancer
Staging celiotomy for ovarian cancer

1-B61 Abdomen: Incisions

P1-B6100 Incision of abdominal wall
P1-B6104 Incision and exploration of abdominal wall
P1-B6110 Incision of epigastric region
P1-B6112 Incision of flank
P1-B6120 Incision of umbilicus
P1-B6122 Incision of urachal cyst or sinus
P1-B6130 Laparotomy, NOS
Celiotomy, NOS
P1-B6140 Exploratory laparotomy
Exploratory celiotomy
Exploration of abdomen
P1-B6142 Reopening of laparotomy site
Exploration of laparotomy site
P1-B6150 Reopening of recent laparotomy incision for removal of hematoma or control of bleeding
P1-B6160 Abdominal paracentesis
Abdominal tap
Abdominocentesis
Percutaneous abdominal paracentesis
Peritoneocentesis
Celiocentesis
Peritoneocentesis, initial
Aspiration of ascites
Drainage of abdomen
P1-B6170 Incision and drainage of abdomen for pancreatitis

1-B63 Abdomen: Excisions

P1-B6300 Biopsy of abdominal wall
P1-B6304 Excision of lesion of abdominal wall
P1-B6306 Excision of subfascial abdominal wall tumor
Excision of desmoid tumor of abdomen
P1-B6307 Debridement of abdominal wall
P1-B6308 Removal of foreign body from abdominal wall
P1-B6309 Removal of foreign body from abdominal cavity
P1-B630A Removal of suture from abdominal wall
P1-B6310 Biopsy of umbilicus
P1-B6312 Excision of umbilicus
Umbilectomy
Omphalectomy
P1-B6315 Excision of urachal cyst or sinus
Excision of urachal cyst
Excision of urachal sinus
P1-B6316 Excision of urachal cyst with umbilical hernia repair
P1-B6318 Excision of omphalomesenteric duct
P1-B6319 Exploratory laparotomy with biopsy
P1-B6320 Excision of intra-abdominal mass, NOS
Excision of intra-abdominal tumor, simple
P1-B6321 Excision of intra-abdominal tumor, extensive
P1-B6322 Excision of intra-abdominal cysts, simple
P1-B6323 Excision of intra-abdominal cysts, extensive
P1-B6324 Excision of intra-abdominal endometriomas, simple
P1-B6325 Excision of intra-abdominal endometriomas, extensive
P1-B6340 Core needle biopsy of abdominal wall mass
P1-B6342 Fine needle biopsy of abdominal wall mass
Fine needle aspiration biopsy of abdominal wall mass
P1-B6344 Core needle biopsy of intra-abdominal mass
P1-B6346 Fine needle aspiration biopsy of intra-abdominal mass
Fine needle biopsy of intra-abdominal mass

1-B65 Abdomen: Injections and Implantations

P1-B6500 Peritoneal lavage
Irrigation of peritoneal cavity
Peritoneal lavage, initial
P1-B6501 Peritoneal lavage, subsequent
P1-B6510 Injection of locally-acting therapeutic substance into peritoneal cavity, NOS
P1-B6514 Chemotherapy administration into peritoneal cavity requiring paracentesis
P1-B6530 Insertion of intraperitoneal cannula or catheter for dialysis
P1-B6531 Insertion of intraperitoneal cannula or catheter for drainage
P1-B6535 Insertion of cordis cannula into abdomen
P1-B6536 Insertion of Crosby-Cooney button into abdomen
P1-B6537 Insertion of Davidson button into abdomen
P1-B6540 Removal of device from abdomen, NOS
P1-B6542 Removal of peritoneal drainage device
Removal of tube from peritoneum
P1-B6544 Removal of tube from retroperitoneum
Removal of retroperitoneal drainage device

1-B67 Abdomen: Endoscopy

P1-B6700 Laparoscopy, NOS
Endoscopy of abdomen
Celioscopy
Peritoneoscopy
P1-B6702 Laparoscopy with biopsy
Peritoneoscopy with biopsy
P1-B6706 Laparoscopy with excision of lesion
P1-B6710 Laparoscopy with aspiration
P1-B6720 Laparoscopy with lysis of adhesions
P1-B6730 Laparoscopy with fulguration of lesion

1-B68 Abdomen: Surgical Repairs, Closures and Reconstructions

P1-B6800 Repair of abdominal wall, NOS
Abdominoplasty

1-B68 Abdomen: Surgical Repairs, Closures and Reconstructions — Continued

P1-B6801 Suture of abdominal wall, NOS
  Laparorrhaphy
P1-B6802 Repair of wound of abdominal wall, NOS
P1-B6804 Delayed closure of abdominal wall
  Secondary closure of abdominal wall
  Delayed closure of granulating abdominal wound
P1-B6806 Tertiary closure of abdominal wall
P1-B6810 Closure of abdominal wall dehiscence
  Reclosure of postoperative disruption of abdominal wall
  Closure of abdominal wall evisceration
  Repair of abdominal wall dehiscence
P1-B6900 Repair of hernia of abdominal wall, NOS
  Abdominal herniorrhaphy, NOS
P1-B6901 Repair of ventral hernia
  Repair of incisional hernia
  Ventral herniorrhaphy
P1-B6902 Repair of ventral hernia with prosthesis or graft
  Repair of incisional hernia with prosthesis or graft
P1-B6906 Repair of recurrent ventral hernia
P1-B6910 Repair of hypogastric hernia
P1-B6912V Hypochondrial hernioplasty
  Subchondral hernioplasty
P1-B6914 Repair of hypogastric hernia with prosthesis or graft
P1-B6920 Repair of epigastric hernia, NOS
  Repair of epigastric hernia, simple
P1-B6922 Repair of epigastric hernia, complex
P1-B6924 Repair of epigastric hernia with prosthesis or graft
P1-B6930 Repair of spigelian hernia
P1-B6934 Repair of spigelian hernia with prosthesis or graft
P1-B6940 Repair of omental hernia
P1-B6950 Repair of retroperitoneal hernia
P1-B6960 Repair of lumbar hernia
P1-B6970 Repair of umbilical hernia, NOS
  Umbilical herniorrhaphy
P1-B6971 Repair of umbilical hernia, up to age 5 years
P1-B6972 Repair of umbilical hernia, age 5 and greater
P1-B6973 Repair of umbilical hernia with prosthesis
P1-B6976 Repair of paraumbilical hernia
P1-B6977 Repair of paraumbilical hernia with prosthesis
P1-B6978 Reconstruction of umbilicus
P1-B6980 Repair of gastroschisis, NOS
P1-B6982 Repair of gastroschisis with prosthesis or graft
P1-B6990 Repair of omphalocele, NOS
P1-B6992 Repair of small omphalocele with primary closure
P1-B6993 Repair of large omphalocele without prosthesis
P1-B6994 Repair of large omphalocele with prosthesis
  Repair of omphalocele with prosthesis
P1-B6996 Gross operation repair of omphalocele, first stage
P1-B6997 Gross operation repair of omphalocele, second stage
P1-B6999 Repair of omphalocele with staged closure of prosthesis
P1-B6A00 Creation of peritoneal-venous shunt
  Creation of peritoneovascular shunt
  Formation of abdominovenous shunt
P1-B6A02 Formation of peritoneojugular shunt
  Formation of LeVeen shunt
P1-B6A04 Revision of peritoneal-venous shunt

1-B6C Abdomen: Destructive Procedures

P1-B6C10 Destruction of lesion of abdominal wall or umbilicus
P1-B6C12V Cauterization of navel
P1-B6C20 Lysis of adhesions of abdomen, NOS

1-B6D Abdomen: Transplantations and Transpositions

P1-B6D10 Transplantation of abdominal tissue
P1-B6D40 Transposition of abdominal tissue

1-B6E Abdomen: Manipulations

P1-B6E10 Manipulation of abdominal tissue, NOS

1-B7 OPERATIVE PROCEDURES ON THE PERITONEUM, RETROPERITONEUM AND MESENTERY

1-B70 Peritoneum, Retroperitoneum and Mesentery: General and Miscellaneous Operative Procedures

P1-B7010 Operation on peritoneum, NOS
P1-B7040 Operation on retroperitoneum, NOS
P1-B7080 Operation on omentum, NOS
P1-B7090 Operation on mesentery, NOS

1-B71 Peritoneum, Retroperitoneum and Mesentery: Incisions

P1-B7100 Incision of peritoneum
  Peritoneotomy
P1-B7102 Ladd operation, mobilization of intestine
P1-B7104 Incision and exploration of subdiaphragmatic space
P1-B7110 Drainage of peritoneal abscess, transabdominal
  Drainage of localized peritonitis, transabdominal
P1-B7112 Incision and drainage of subdiaphragmatic abscess
  Incision and drainage of subphrenic space
  Incision and drainage of subphrenic abscess

P1-B7113 Incision and drainage of subhepatic space
P1-B7114 Incision and drainage of perigastric space
P1-B7116 Incision and drainage of perisplenic space
P1-B7119 Intraperitoneal drainage for hematoma
P1-B7140 Incision of retroperitoneum
P1-B7142 Incision and exploration of retroperitoneum
P1-B7150 Incision and drainage of retroperitoneal abscess
P1-B7154 Incision and drainage of extraperitoneal abscess
P1-B7180 Incision of omentum
Omentotomy
P1-B7182 Incision and drainage of omental abscess

1-B73 Peritoneum, Retroperitoneum and Mesentery: Excisions

P1-B7300 Biopsy of peritoneum
Excision of peritoneal tissue
P1-B7304 Excision of lesion of peritoneum
P1-B7306 Removal of foreign body from retroperitoneum
P1-B7320 Biopsy of omentum
P1-B7322 Excision of lesion of omentum
P1-B7324 Omentectomy
Resection of omentum
Omentumectomy
P1-B7330 Epiploectomy
Excision of appendices epiploicae
P1-B7340 Excision of falciform ligament
P1-B7342 Excision of gastrocolic ligament
P1-B7360 Excision of lesion of retroperitoneum
Exploration of retroperitoneal area with biopsy
P1-B7362 Excision of retroperitoneal cysts, simple
P1-B7363 Excision of retroperitoneal cysts, extensive
P1-B7364 Excision of retroperitoneal endometriomas, simple
P1-B7365 Excision of retroperitoneal endometriomas, extensive
P1-B7366 Excision of retroperitoneal mass, simple
P1-B7367 Excision of retroperitoneal mass, extensive
P1-B7370 Core needle biopsy of retroperitoneal mass
P1-B7372 Fine needle biopsy of retroperitoneal mass
Fine needle aspiration biopsy of retroperitoneal tumor
P1-B7390 Biopsy of mesentery
P1-B7392 Excision of lesion of mesentery
P1-B7394 Resection of mesentery
Mesenterectomy

1-B75 Peritoneum, Retroperitoneum and Mesentery: Injections and Implantations

P1-B7510 Injection into peritoneum, NOS
P1-B7520 Surgical pneumoperitoneum, NOS
Injection of air into peritoneal cavity, NOS
Surgical pneumoperitoneum, initial
P1-B7530 Injection into retroperitoneum, NOS
P1-B7540 Injection into mesentery, NOS

1-B77 Peritoneum, Retroperitoneum and Mesentery: Endoscopy

P1-B7710 Endoscopy of retroperitoneum, NOS

1-B78 Peritoneum, Retroperitoneum and Mesentery: Surgical Repairs, Closures and Reconstructions

P1-B7810 Repair of peritoneum, NOS
P1-B7812 Suture of peritoneum
P1-B7820 Repair of retroperitoneal tissue
P1-B7840 Repair of omentum, NOS
Omentoplasty
P1-B7842 Suture of omentum
Omentorrhaphy
P1-B7844 Omentopexy
P1-B7845 Talma-Morison operation, omentopexy
P1-B7860 Creation of cutaneoperitoneal fistula
P1-B7890 Repair of mesentery, NOS
P1-B7892 Suture of mesentery
P1-B7894 Mesenteriopexy
Mesopexy
P1-B7895 Plication of mesentery
Mesenteriplication
P1-B7896 Epiplopexy
P1-B7897 Epiplorrhaphy

1-B7C Peritoneum, Retroperitoneum and Mesentery: Destructive Procedures

P1-B7C00 Destruction of peritoneal tissue
P1-B7C10 Destruction of intra-abdominal cysts
P1-B7C12 Destruction of intra-abdominal cysts, extensive
P1-B7C14 Destruction of intra-abdominal endometriomas
P1-B7C15 Destruction of intra-abdominal endometriomas, extensive
P1-B7C16 Destruction of intra-abdominal tumor
P1-B7C17 Destruction of intra-abdominal tumor, extensive
P1-B7C20 Destruction of retroperitoneal cysts
P1-B7C22 Destruction of retroperitoneal cysts, extensive
P1-B7C24 Destruction of retroperitoneal endometriomas
P1-B7C25 Destruction of retroperitoneal endometriomas, extensive
P1-B7C26 Destruction of retroperitoneal tumor
P1-B7C27 Destruction of retroperitoneal tumor, extensive
P1-B7C30 Lysis of adhesions of peritoneum
P1-B7C32 Lysis of adhesions of stomach
Gastrolysis
P1-B7C33 Lysis of adhesions of liver
P1-B7C34 Lysis of adhesions of intestines
Enterolysis

1-B7C Peritoneum, Retroperitoneum and Mesentery: Destructive Procedures — Continued

P1-B7C35 Lysis of adhesions of gallbladder
Lysis of adhesions of biliary tract
P1-B7C36 Lysis of adhesions of appendix
Appendicolysis
P1-B7C37 Lysis of adhesions of spleen
Splenolysis

1-B7D Peritoneum, Retroperitoneum and Mesentery: Transplantations and Transpositions

P1-B7D10 Transplantation of peritoneal tissue, NOS
P1-B7D20 Transplantation of retroperitoneal tissue, NOS
P1-B7D30 Transplantation of mesenteric tissue, NOS
P1-B7D60 Transposition of peritoneal tissue, NOS
P1-B7D70 Transposition of retroperitoneal tissue, NOS
P1-B7D80 Transposition of mesenteric tissue, NOS

1-B7E Peritoneum, Retroperitoneum and Mesentery: Manipulations

P1-B7E10 Reduction of torsion of omentum
P1-B7E20 Manual reduction of internal abdominal hernia

1-B9 OPERATIVE PROCEDURES ON THE INGUINAL REGION, PELVIS AND PERINEUM

1-B90 Inguinal Region, Pelvis and Perineum: General and Miscellaneous Operative Procedures

P1-B9070 Operation on female perineum, NOS
P1-B9080 Operation on male perineum, NOS

1-B91 Inguinal Region, Pelvis and Perineum: Incisions

P1-B9100 Incision of inguinal region, NOS
P1-B9102 Incision and exploration of inguinal region
Incision and exploration of groin
P1-B9104 Incision and evacuation of hematoma in inguinal region
Incision and evacuation of hematoma in groin region
P1-B9150 Exploration of pelvis by laparotomy
P1-B9170 Incision of perineum, NOS
Perineotomy, NOS
P1-B9172 Incision of female perineum
Schuchardt operation, nonobstetrical episiotomy
Nonobstetrical perineotomy
P1-B9174 Incision and exploration of female perineum
P1-B9176 Incision and drainage of nonobstetrical perineal abscess
P1-B9180 Incision of male perineum
P1-B9182 Incision and exploration of male perineum
P1-B9184 Incision and drainage of male perineum
P1-B9185 Incision of hematoma of male perineum
P1-B9190 Incision and drainage of iliac fossa

1-B93 Inguinal Region, Pelvis and Perineum: Excisions

P1-B9300 Excision of tissue of inguinal region, NOS
P1-B9310 Excision of lesion of inguinal region
Excision of lesion of groin region
P1-B9320 Removal of foreign body from groin region
P1-B9340 Excision of pelvic tissue, NOS
P1-B9342 Excision of lesion of pelvic wall
P1-B9344 Excision of presacral lesion, NOS
P1-B9345 Excision of presacral tumor
P1-B9350 Pelvic exenteration, NOS
P1-B9351 Pelvic exenteration, male
P1-B9352 Pelvic exenteration, female
P1-B9354 Pelvic exenteration, complete, for malignancy with removal of bladder and ureteral transplantations, NOS
P1-B9380 Biopsy of perineum, NOS
P1-B9382 Excision of lesion of male perineum
P1-B9383 Excision of lesion of female perineum
P1-B9385 Removal of foreign body from perineum, NOS
P1-B9386 Removal of foreign body from male perineum
P1-B9387 Removal of foreign body from female perineum
P1-B9388 Excision of redundant mucosa of perineum
P1-B9389 Excision of skin and subcutaneous tissue for hidradenitis of perineum

1-B95 Inguinal Region, Pelvis and Perineum: Injections and Implantations

P1-B9510 Injection into inguinal region, NOS
P1-B9520 Injection into pelvic region, NOS
P1-B9530 Injection into perineum, NOS
P1-B9560 Implantation into inguinal region, NOS
P1-B9570 Implantation into pelvic region, NOS
P1-B9580 Implantation into perineum, NOS

1-B97 Inguinal Region, Pelvis and Perineum: Endoscopy

P1-B9710 Endoscopy of inguinal region, NOS
P1-B9720 Endoscopy of pelvic region, NOS
P1-B9730 Endoscopy of perineum, NOS

1-B98 Inguinal Region, Pelvis and Perineum: Surgical Repairs, Closures and Reconstructions

P1-B9810 Repair of inguinal hernia, NOS
Inguinal herniorrhaphy, NOS
P1-B9812 Repair of inguinal hernia, under age 5
P1-B9813 Repair of inguinal hernia with hydrocelectomy, under age 5
P1-B9814 Repair of inguinal hernia, age 5 and over
P1-B9815 Repair of inguinal hernia with hydrocelectomy, age 5 and over

P1-B9820 Unilateral repair of inguinal hernia, NOS
P1-B9821 Unilateral repair of inguinal hernia, direct
P1-B9822 Unilateral repair of inguinal hernia, indirect
P1-B9824 Unilateral repair of inguinal hernia, direct and indirect
P1-B9840 Bilateral repair of inguinal hernia, NOS
P1-B9841 Bilateral repair of inguinal hernia, direct
P1-B9842 Bilateral repair of inguinal hernia, indirect
P1-B9844 Bilateral repair of inguinal hernia, direct and indirect
P1-B9846 Bilateral repair of inguinal hernia, one direct and one indirect
P1-B9850 Unilateral repair of inguinal hernia with prosthesis or graft, NOS
P1-B9851 Repair of inguinal hernia with prosthesis or graft, direct
P1-B9852 Repair of inguinal hernia with prosthesis or graft, indirect
P1-B9854 Bilateral repair of inguinal hernia with prosthesis or graft, NOS
P1-B9855 Bilateral repair inguinal hernia with prosthesis or graft, direct
P1-B9856 Bilateral repair of inguinal hernia with prosthesis or graft, indirect
P1-B9857 Bilateral repair of inguinal hernia with prosthesis or graft, direct and indirect
P1-B9860 Repair of inguinal hernia with orchiectomy
P1-B9862 Repair of inguinal hernia with orchiectomy and prosthetic replacement
P1-B9864 Repair of inguinal hernia with spermatocelectomy
P1-B9870 Repair of recurrent inguinal hernia
P1-B9872 Repair of sliding inguinal hernia
P1-B9874 Repair of incarcerated inguinal hernia
P1-B9875 Repair of strangulated inguinal hernia
P1-B9890 Gross operation, herniorrhaphy
P1-B9892 Mayo operation, herniorrhaphy
P1-B9894 Ferguson operation, herniorrhaphy
P1-B9896 Halsted operation, herniorrhaphy
P1-B9900 Femoral hernia repair
 Femoral herniorrhaphy
P1-B9901 Unilateral repair of femoral hernia
P1-B9902 Bilateral repair of femoral hernia
P1-B9906 Unilateral repair of femoral hernia with prosthesis or graft
P1-B9907 Bilateral repair of femoral hernia with prosthesis or graft
P1-B9910 Repair of femoral hernia with groin incision
P1-B9912 Repair of femoral hernia by Henry approach
P1-B9920 Repair of recurrent femoral hernia
P1-B9930 Repair of ischiatic hernia
P1-B9932 Repair of ischiorectal hernia
P1-B9942 Repair of obturator hernia
P1-B9944 Repair of pudendal hernia
P1-B9946 Repair of sciatic hernia
P1-B9948 Repair of crural hernia
P1-B9950 Repair of properitoneal hernia
P1-B9A00 Perineorrhaphy, NOS
 Suture of laceration of perineum
P1-B9A02 Suture of female perineum
P1-B9A10 Perineoplasty
 Nonobstetrical perineoplasty
P1-B9A11 Repair of female perineum
P1-B9A12 Hegar operation, perineorrhaphy
P1-B9A20 Repair of fistula of perineum
P1-B9A30 Repair of laceration of male perineum
P1-B9A40 Suture of pelvic floor
P1-B9A42 Suture of male perineum
P1-B9A82 Reconstruction of pelvic floor

1-B9C Inguinal Region, Pelvis and Perineum: Destructive Procedures

P1-B9C10 Lysis of pelvic adhesions
P1-B9C20 Lysis of adhesions of female perineum

1-B9D Inguinal Region, Pelvis and Perineum: Transplantations and Transpositions

P1-B9D10 Transplantation of tissue of inguinal region, NOS
P1-B9D20 Transplantation of tissue of pelvic region, NOS
P1-B9D30 Transplantation of tissue of perineum, NOS
P1-B9D60 Transposition of tissue of inguinal region, NOS
P1-B9D70 Transposition of tissue of pelvic region, NOS

1-B9E Inguinal Region, Pelvis and Perineum: Manipulations

P1-B9E20 Manual reduction of hernia
 Manual repair of hernia

SECTION 1-C ANESTHESIA PROCEDURES

1-C0 GENERIC ANESTHESIA PROCEDURES

P1-C0000 Anesthesia, NOS
 Anesthesia procedure, NOS
P1-C0010 General anesthesia, NOS
P1-C0020 Inhalation anesthesia, machine system, closed, rebreathing of primary agent
P1-C0030 Inhalation anesthesia, machine system, closed, no rebreathing of primary agent
P1-C0040 Inhalation anesthesia, machine system, closed, circulation of primary agent
P1-C0050 Inhalation anesthesia, machine system, semi-closed, rebreathing of primary agent
P1-C0060 Inhalation anesthesia, machine system, semi-closed, no rebreathing of primary agent
P1-C0070 Inhalation anesthesia, machine system, semi-closed, circulation of primary agent and gases
P1-C0100 Intravenous anesthesia, NOS
P1-C0200 Regional anesthesia, NOS
P1-C0205 Regional IV administration of local anesthetic agent, extremity
P1-C0210 Spinal anesthesia

1-C0 GENERIC ANESTHESIA PROCEDURES — Continued

P1-C0220 Epidural anesthesia
Peridural anesthesia
P1-C0300 Nerve block anesthesia
P1-C0310 Central block anesthesia
P1-C0320 Stellate block anesthesia
P1-C0330 Paracervical block anesthesia
P1-C0340 Paravertebral anesthesia
P1-C0350 Peripheral block anesthesia
P1-C0360 Therapeutic block anesthesia
P1-C0370 Diagnostic block anesthesia
P1-C0380 Operative block anesthesia
P1-C0400 Local anesthesia, NOS
P1-C0410 Local anesthesia, surface
Topical anesthesia
P1-C0420 Local anesthesia, surface, by refrigerant
P1-C0430 Local anesthesia, by infiltration
P1-C0500 Supplementary measure, anesthetic
P1-C0510 Supplementary agent, anesthetic
P1-C0520 Relaxant, induction and maintenance
P1-C0530 Hypotension, induction and maintenance
P1-C0540 Hypothermia, regional, induction and maintenance
P1-C0550 Hypothermia, total body, induction and maintenance
P1-C0560 Daily management of epidural or subarachnoid drug administration
P1-C0600 Anesthesia for CAT scan
P1-C0620 Anesthesia for MRI scan
P1-C0650 Anesthesia for endoscopic procedure, NOS
Anesthesia for endoscopy, NOS
P1-C0700 Anesthesia for repair of arteriovenous fistula, NOS
P1-C0720 Anesthesia for angioplasty, NOS
P1-C0800 Preoperative evaluation, anesthesia
P1-C0810 Post-operative follow-up, anesthesia
P1-C0820 Recovery room monitoring, anesthesia
P1-C0850 Resuscitation, anesthesia
P1-C0910 Anesthesia for a normal healthy patient
P1-C0912 Anesthesia for patient of extreme age, under one year and over seventy
P1-C0920 Anesthesia complicated by utilization of total body hypothermia
P1-C0926 Anesthesia complicated by utilization of controlled hypotension
P1-C0930 Anesthesia for body cast application or revision
P1-C0940 Anesthesia for a patient with severe systemic disease, life threatening
P1-C0946 Anesthesia complicated by emergency condition
P1-C0950 Anesthesia for a moribund patient requiring operation
P1-C0960 Physiological support for harvesting of organs from brain-dead patient
P1-C0980 Anesthesia for a patient with mild systemic disease
P1-C0982 Anesthesia for a patient with severe systemic disease
P1-C0A00 Acupuncture, NOS

1-C1 ANESTHESIA FOR PROCEDURES ON HEAD AND NECK

P1-C1000 Anesthesia for procedure on head and neck, NOS
P1-C1010 Anesthesia for procedure on integumentary system of head and neck
P1-C1020 Anesthesia for procedure on facial bones, NOS
P1-C1030 Anesthesia for radical surgery on facial bones, NOS
P1-C1032 Anesthesia for radical prognathism
P1-C1100 Anesthesia for intracranial procedure, NOS
P1-C1104 Anesthesia for intracranial procedure in sitting position
P1-C1120 Anesthesia for intracranial vascular procedure, NOS
P1-C1140 Anesthesia for burr holes
P1-C1142 Anesthesia for subdural taps
P1-C1144 Anesthesia for burr holes for ventriculography
P1-C1150 Anesthesia for injection procedure for pneumoencephalography
P1-C1160 Anesthesia of intracranial nerve
P1-C1180 Anesthesia for spinal fluid shunting procedure
P1-C1190 Anesthesia for electroconvulsive therapy
P1-C1200 Anesthesia for procedures on eye, NOS
P1-C1210 Anesthesia for ophthalmoscopy
P1-C1220 Anesthesia for iridectomy
P1-C1230 Anesthesia for lens surgery
P1-C1240 Anesthesia for corneal transplant
P1-C1250 Anesthesia for vitrectomy
P1-C1300 Anesthesia for procedure on external ear
P1-C1310 Anesthesia for otoscopy
P1-C1350 Anesthesia for procedure on middle and inner ear
P1-C1352 Anesthesia for tympanotomy
P1-C1400 Anesthesia for procedure on nose
P1-C1410 Anesthesia for radical surgery on nose
P1-C1440 Anesthesia for procedure on nose and accessory sinuses
P1-C1450 Anesthesia for radical surgery on accessory sinuses
P1-C1460 Anesthesia for radical surgery on nose and accessory sinuses
P1-C1500 Anesthesia for intraoral procedure, NOS
P1-C1510 Anesthesia for radical intraoral surgery
P1-C1520 Anesthesia for plastic repair of cleft lip
P1-C1540 Anesthesia for excision of retropharyngeal tumor
P1-C1600 Anesthesia for procedure on salivary glands
P1-C1800 Anesthesia for procedure on neck, NOS
P1-C1810 Anesthesia for any procedure on larynx, NOS
P1-C1820 Anesthesia for any procedure on trachea, NOS

P1-C1840 Anesthesia for any procedure on thyroid, NOS
P1-C1841 Anesthesia for needle biopsy of thyroid
P1-C1850 Anesthesia for procedure on cervical esophagus
P1-C1860 Anesthesia for procedure on major vessels of neck
P1-C1862 Anesthesia for simple ligation of major vessels of neck
P1-C1870 Anesthesia for procedures on lymphoid tissue of neck
P1-C1880 Anesthesia for vertebral arteriograms
P1-C1882 Anesthesia for carotid arteriograms
P1-C1890 Anesthesia for unlisted procedure on neck, NOS
P1-C1A00 Anesthesia for endoscopic procedure on head and neck, NOS

1-C2 ANESTHESIA FOR PROCEDURES ON THORAX, CHEST, SHOULDER AND AXILLA

P1-C2001 Anesthesia for procedure on thorax or chest, NOS
P1-C2002 Anesthesia for unlisted procedure on thorax
P1-C2003 Anesthesia for unlisted procedure on integumentary system of anterior chest
P1-C2004 Anesthesia for unlisted procedure on integumentary system of posterior chest
P1-C2020 Anesthesia for any procedure on integumentary system of shoulder and axilla
P1-C2030 Anesthesia for procedure on axilla, NOS
P1-C2100 Anesthesia for procedure on breast, NOS
P1-C2120 Anesthesia for reconstructive procedure on breast
P1-C2122 Anesthesia for augmentation mammoplasty
P1-C2124 Anesthesia for reduction mammoplasty
P1-C2130 Anesthesia for radical procedure on breast
P1-C2132 Anesthesia for modified radical procedure on breast
P1-C2134 Anesthesia for mastectomy with internal mammary node dissection
P1-C2210 Anesthesia for electrical conversion of arrhythmias
P1-C2220 Anesthesia for thoracoplasty
P1-C2230 Anesthesia for pectus excavatum
P1-C2240 Anesthesia for partial rib resection, NOS
P1-C2260 Anesthesia for procedure on clavicle and/or scapula
P1-C2262 Anesthesia for radical surgery on clavicle and/or scapula
P1-C2410 Anesthesia for shoulder disarticulation
P1-C2420 Anesthesia for interthoracoscapular, forequarter amputation
P1-C2424 Anesthesia for radical resection of shoulder
P1-C2430 Anesthesia for total shoulder replacement
P1-C2450 Anesthesia for biopsy of clavicle
P1-C2470 Anesthesia for any procedure on nerves, muscles, tendons, fascia and bursae of shoulder and axilla
P1-C2472 Anesthesia for shoulder cast procedure
P1-C2474 Anesthesia for shoulder spica procedure
P1-C2480 Anesthesia for any open procedure on humeral head and neck, sternoclavicular joint, acromioclavicular joint or shoulder joint, NOS
P1-C2490 Anesthesia for arthroscopic procedure of shoulder joint
P1-C2492 Anesthesia for any closed procedure on humeral head and neck, sternoclavicular joint, acromioclavicular joint or shoulder joint
P1-C24A0 Anesthesia for procedure on arteries of shoulder and axilla, NOS
P1-C24A4 Anesthesia for a bypass graft on arteries of shoulder and axilla
P1-C2520 Anesthesia for axillary-brachial aneurysm
P1-C2540 Anesthesia for axillary-femoral bypass graft
P1-C2590 Anesthesia for unlisted procedures on veins of shoulder and axilla
P1-C2600 Anesthesia for procedure on shoulder, NOS
P1-C2660 Anesthesia for access to central venous circulation
P1-C2700 Anesthesia for intrathoracic procedure, NOS
P1-C2710 Anesthesia for procedure on great vessels of chest with pump oxygenator
P1-C2714 Anesthesia for procedure on great vessels of chest without pump oxygenator
P1-C2730 Anesthesia for procedure on heart with pump oxygenator
P1-C2732 Anesthesia for procedure on heart without pump oxygenator
P1-C2740 Anesthesia for heart transplant
P1-C2750 Anesthesia for heart/lung transplant
P1-C2770 Anesthesia for procedure on pericardium with pump oxygenator
P1-C2772 Anesthesia for procedure on pericardium without pump oxygenator
P1-C2780 Anesthesia for cardiac catheterization including coronary arteriography and ventriculography
P1-C2790 Anesthesia for transvenous pacemaker insertion
P1-C2810 Anesthesia for procedure on thoracic esophagus
P1-C2820 Anesthesia for esophagoscopy
P1-C2900 Anesthesia for thoracotomy procedure involving lungs
P1-C2910 Anesthesia for intrathoracic repair of trauma to trachea and bronchi
P1-C2920 Anesthesia for thoracotomy procedure involving pleura
P1-C2922 Anesthesia for needle biopsy of pleura
P1-C2930 Anesthesia for pleurectomy
P1-C2932 Anesthesia for decortication of pleura
P1-C2940 Anesthesia for pulmonary resection with thoracoplasty
P1-C2950 Anesthesia for thoracotomy procedure involving diaphragm

1-C2 ANESTHESIA FOR PROCEDURES ON THORAX, CHEST, SHOULDER AND AXILLA — Continued

P1-C2970 Anesthesia for thoracotomy procedure involving mediastinum
P1-C2990 Anesthesia for thoracotomy procedure involving lungs, pleura, diaphragm and mediastinum
P1-C2A00 Anesthesia for endoscopic procedure on thorax, chest, shoulder and axilla
P1-C2A02 Anesthesia for thoracoscopy
P1-C2A04 Anesthesia for bronchoscopy
P1-C2A06 Anesthesia for mediastinoscopy
P1-C2A08 Anesthesia for pneumocentesis

1-C3 ANESTHESIA FOR PROCEDURES ON SPINE AND SPINAL CORD

P1-C3000 Anesthesia for spinal cord procedure, NOS
P1-C3020 Anesthesia for procedure on cervical spinal cord
P1-C3040 Anesthesia for procedure on thoracic spinal cord
P1-C3050 Anesthesia for procedure on lumbosacral spinal cord
P1-C3052 Anesthesia for lumbar sympathectomy
P1-C3054 Anesthesia for thoracolumbar sympathectomy
P1-C3200 Anesthesia for injection procedure for posterior fossa myelography
P1-C3220 Anesthesia for injection procedure for cervical myelography
P1-C3240 Anesthesia for injection procedure for lumbar myelography
P1-C3270 Anesthesia for injection procedure for cervical discography
P1-C3280 Anesthesia for injection procedure for lumbar discography
P1-C3290 Anesthesia for chemonucleolysis
P1-C3600 Anesthesia for procedure on spine, NOS
Anesthesia for procedure on vertebral column, NOS
P1-C3610 Anesthesia for extensive spine procedure
P1-C3620 Anesthesia for procedure on cervical spine
P1-C3630 Anesthesia for posterior cervical laminectomy in sitting position
P1-C3640 Anesthesia for procedure on thoracic spine
P1-C3660 Anesthesia for procedure in lumbar region
P1-C3670 Anesthesia for placement of Harrington rod

1-C4 ANESTHESIA FOR PROCEDURES ON THE ABDOMEN

P1-C4000 Anesthesia for procedure on abdomen, NOS
P1-C4010 Anesthesia for abdominal wound dehiscence, NOS
P1-C4020 Anesthesia for laparoscopic procedure on abdomen, NOS

1-C41-C44 Anesthesia for Procedures on The Upper Abdomen

P1-C4100 Anesthesia for upper abdominal procedure, NOS
P1-C4110 Anesthesia for procedure on upper anterior abdominal wall, NOS
P1-C4120 Anesthesia for procedure on upper posterior abdominal wall, NOS
P1-C4130 Anesthesia for laparoscopic procedure on upper abdomen
P1-C4150 Anesthesia for omphalocele
P1-C4160 Anesthesia for intraperitoneal procedure in upper abdomen, NOS
P1-C4170 Anesthesia for hernia repair in upper abdomen, NOS
P1-C4174 Anesthesia for transabdominal repair of diaphragmatic hernia
P1-C4176 Anesthesia for lumbar or ventral incisional hernia of upper abdomen
P1-C4200 Anesthesia for partial hepatectomy
P1-C4210 Anesthesia for percutaneous liver biopsy
P1-C4220 Anesthesia for liver transplant, recipient
P1-C4240 Anesthesia for pancreatectomy, total
P1-C4242 Anesthesia for pancreatectomy, partial
P1-C4300 Anesthesia for upper gastrointestinal endoscopic procedure
P1-C4400 Anesthesia for any procedure on major upper abdominal blood vessels

1-C45-C48 Anesthesia for Procedures on The Lower Abdomen

P1-C4500 Anesthesia for lower abdominal procedure, NOS
P1-C4520 Anesthesia for procedure on lower abdominal wall, NOS
P1-C4522 Anesthesia for procedure on lower anterior abdominal wall, NOS
P1-C4524 Anesthesia for procedure on lower posterior abdominal wall, NOS
P1-C4530 Anesthesia for panniculectomy
P1-C4540 Anesthesia for intraperitoneal procedure in lower abdomen, NOS
P1-C4550 Anesthesia for laparoscopic procedure on lower abdomen
P1-C4570 Anesthesia for hernia repair in lower abdomen, NOS
P1-C4572 Anesthesia for ventral or incisional hernia repair, lower abdomen
P1-C4590 Anesthesia for intestinal endoscopic procedure, NOS
P1-C4600 Anesthesia for cesarean section
P1-C4604 Anesthesia for cesarean hysterectomy
P1-C4608 Continuous epidural analgesia for labor and cesarean section
P1-C4610 Anesthesia for amniocentesis
P1-C4650 Anesthesia for radical hysterectomy

P1-C4680 Anesthesia for abdominoperineal resection
P1-C4690 Anesthesia for pelvic exenteration
P1-C4700 Anesthesia for extraperitoneal procedure in lower abdomen and urinary tract, NOS
P1-C4710 Anesthesia for lithotripsy, extracorporeal shock wave without water bath
P1-C4712 Anesthesia for lithotripsy, extracorporeal shock wave with water bath
P1-C4720 Anesthesia for renal procedure, NOS
P1-C4724 Anesthesia for renal transplant, recipient
P1-C4730 Anesthesia for cystolithotomy
P1-C4780 Anesthesia for adrenalectomy
P1-C4790 Anesthesia for total cystectomy
P1-C4800 Anesthesia for procedure on major lower abdominal vessels, NOS
P1-C4810 Anesthesia for inferior vena cava ligation
P1-C4820 Anesthesia for transvenous umbrella insertion

1-C5 ANESTHESIA FOR PROCEDURES ON PERINEUM AND PELVIS

P1-C5000 Anesthesia for procedure on perineum and pelvis, NOS
P1-C5010 Anesthesia for radical perineal procedure, nOS
P1-C5012 Anesthesia for anorectal procedure, NOS
P1-C5020 Anesthesia for procedures on perineal integumentary system
P1-C5030 Anesthesia for hysteroscopy
P1-C5040 Anesthesia for cervical cerclage
P1-C5050 Anesthesia for vaginal delivery
P1-C5054 Continuous epidural analgesia for labor and vaginal delivery
P1-C5060 Anesthesia for vulvectomy
P1-C5070 Anesthesia for colpotomy
P1-C5080 Anesthesia for procedures on seminal vesicles
P1-C5090 Anesthesia for colpectomy
P1-C5094 Anesthesia for culdoscopy
P1-C5096 Anesthesia for colporrhaphy
P1-C50B0 Anesthesia for vaginal hysterectomy
P1-C50C0 Anesthesia for procedures on labia, vagina, cervix or endometrium, NOS
P1-C5100 Anesthesia for transurethral procedure, NOS
P1-C5102 Anesthesia for transurethral resection of bladder tumor
P1-C5104 Anesthesia for transurethral resection of prostate
P1-C5110 Anesthesia for post-transurethral resection bleeding
P1-C5120 Anesthesia for procedure on male external genitalia, NOS
P1-C5150 Anesthesia for perineal prostatectomy
P1-C5160 Anesthesia for anorectal endoscopy
P1-C5180 Anesthesia for transurethral procedure with fragmentation and removal of ureteral calculus
P1-C5210 Anesthesia for complete amputation of penis
P1-C5220 Anesthesia for orchiopexy
P1-C5240 Anesthesia for insertion of penile prosthesis, perineal approach
P1-C5250 Anesthesia for radical orchiectomy, abdominal
P1-C5252 Anesthesia for radical orchiectomy, inguinal
P1-C5260 Anesthesia for radical amputation of penis with bilateral inguinal and iliac lymphadenectomy
P1-C5264 Anesthesia for radical amputation of penis with bilateral inguinal lymphadenectomy
P1-C5290 Anesthesia for biopsy of male genital system
P1-C5330 Anesthesia for procedure on undescended testis
P1-C5500 Anesthesia for procedure on pelvis, NOS
P1-C5510 Anesthesia for procedure on integumentary system of pelvis, posterior, except perineum
P1-C5540 Anesthesia for procedure on integumentary system of pelvis, anterior, except external genitalia
P1-C5600 Anesthesia for procedure on bony pelvis, NOS
P1-C5610 Anesthesia for open procedure involving symphysis pubis
P1-C5612 Anesthesia for closed procedure involving symphysis pubis
P1-C5620 Anesthesia for open procedure involving sacroiliac joint
P1-C5622 Anesthesia for closed procedure involving sacroiliac joint
P1-C5640 Anesthesia for interpelviabdominal, hindquarter amputation
P1-C5650 Anesthesia for radical procedure for tumor of pelvis, except hindquarter amputation
P1-C5710 Anesthesia for extrapelvic obturator neurectomy
P1-C5712 Anesthesia for intrapelvic obturator neurectomy
P1-C5800 Anesthesia for injection procedure for hysterosalpingography
P1-C5A00 Anesthesia for endoscopic procedure on perineum and pelvis, NOS

1-C6 ANESTHESIA FOR PROCEDURES ON LOWER EXTREMITY

P1-C6000 Anesthesia for procedure on lower extremity, NOS
  Anesthesia for procedure on lower limb, NOS
  Anesthesia for procedure on hindlimb, NOS
P1-C6010 Anesthesia for procedure on upper leg, NOS
P1-C6020 Anesthesia for unlisted procedure on integumentary system of upper leg
P1-C6110 Anesthesia for procedure involving veins of upper leg, including exploration
P1-C6120 Anesthesia for femoral artery embolectomy
P1-C6124 Anesthesia for femoral artery ligation
P1-C6130 Anesthesia for procedure involving arteries of upper leg, including bypass graft

1-C6 ANESTHESIA FOR PROCEDURES ON LOWER EXTREMITY — Continued

P1-C6140 Anesthesia for femoral arteriograms, retrograde
P1-C6200 Anesthesia for hip disarticulation
P1-C6210 Anesthesia for total hip replacement
P1-C6220 Anesthesia for total hip revision
P1-C6230 Anesthesia for closed procedure involving upper 2/3 of femur, NOS
P1-C6234 Anesthesia for open procedure involving upper 2/3 of femur, NOS
P1-C6240 Anesthesia for amputation involving upper 2/3 of femur
P1-C6244 Anesthesia for radical resection involving upper 2/3 of femur
P1-C6250 Anesthesia for unlisted procedure on nerves, muscles, tendons, fascia and bursae of upper leg
P1-C6260 Anesthesia for open procedure involving hip joint, NOS
P1-C6270 Anesthesia for unlisted closed procedure involving hip joint
P1-C6280 Anesthesia for unlisted closed procedure on lower 1/3 of femur
P1-C6286 Anesthesia for unlisted open procedure on lower 1/3 of femur
P1-C6300 Anesthesia for arthroscopic procedure of hip joint
P1-C6400 Anesthesia for procedure on knee, NOS
P1-C6410 Anesthesia for unlisted procedure on integumentary system of knee and popliteal area
P1-C6500 Anesthesia for procedure on veins of knee and popliteal area, NOS
P1-C6510 Anesthesia for procedure on arteries of knee and popliteal area, NOS
P1-C6520 Anesthesia for procedure on arteries of knee
P1-C6530 Anesthesia for arteriovenous fistula of veins of knee and popliteal area
P1-C6540 Anesthesia for popliteal excision and graft or repair for occlusion or aneurysm
P1-C6544 Anesthesia for popliteal thromboendarterectomy
P1-C6548 Anesthesia for excision and repair of popliteal aneurysm
P1-C6600 Anesthesia for open procedure on knee joint, NOS
P1-C6620 Anesthesia for total knee replacement
P1-C6630 Anesthesia for disarticulation at knee
P1-C6640 Anesthesia for open procedure on upper ends of tibia, fibula and patella, NOS
P1-C6644 Anesthesia for closed procedure on upper ends of tibia, fibula and patella, NOS
P1-C6660 Anesthesia for closed procedure on knee joint, NOS
P1-C6664 Anesthesia for arthroscopic procedure of knee joint
P1-C6680 Anesthesia for any cast procedure involving knee joint
P1-C6690 Anesthesia for procedure on nerves, muscles, tendons, fascia and bursae of knee and popliteal area, NOS
P1-C6800 Anesthesia for procedure on lower leg, NOS
P1-C6820 Anesthesia for unlisted procedure on integumentary system of lower leg, ankle and foot
P1-C6830 Anesthesia for procedure on veins of lower leg, NOS
P1-C6840 Anesthesia for procedure on arteries of lower leg with bypass graft
P1-C6850 Anesthesia for direct or catheter embolectomy on arteries of lower leg
P1-C6860 Anesthesia for direct or catheter venous thrombectomy on veins of lower leg
P1-C6880 Anesthesia for lower leg cast procedure
P1-C6900 Anesthesia for closed procedure on ankle, NOS
P1-C6910 Anesthesia for total ankle replacement
P1-C6920 Anesthesia for closed procedure on foot, NOS
P1-C6930 Anesthesia for arthroscopic procedure of ankle joint
P1-C6940 Anesthesia for procedure on nerves, muscles, tendons and fascia of lower leg, ankle and foot, NOS
P1-C6950 Anesthesia for closed procedure on lower leg, NOS
P1-C6960 Anesthesia for open procedure on bones of lower leg, ankle and foot, NOS
P1-C6964 Anesthesia for radical resection of bones of lower leg, ankle and foot
P1-C6975 Anesthesia for osteotomy or osteoplasty of tibia and/or fibula
P1-C6980 Anesthesia for gastrocnemius recession
P1-C6990 Anesthesia for repair of ruptured Achilles tendon
P1-C6A00 Anesthesia for endoscopic procedure on lower extremity, NOS

1-C7 ANESTHESIA FOR PROCEDURES ON UPPER EXTREMITY

P1-C7000 Anesthesia for procedure on upper extremity, NOS
  Anesthesia for procedure on upper limb, NOS
  Anesthesia for procedure on forelimb, NOS
P1-C7010 Anesthesia for procedure on upper arm, NOS
P1-C7020 Anesthesia for unlisted procedure on integumentary system of upper arm and elbow
P1-C7100 Anesthesia for procedure on arteries of upper arm and elbow, NOS
P1-C7104 Anesthesia for embolectomy on arteries of upper arm and elbow
P1-C7140 Anesthesia for procedure on veins of upper arm and elbow, NOS
P1-C7144 Anesthesia for phleborrhaphy on veins of upper arm and elbow

P1-C7170 Anesthesia for brachial arteriograms, retrograde
P1-C7200 Anesthesia for total elbow replacement
P1-C7220 Anesthesia for repair of malunion or nonunion of humerus
P1-C7230 Anesthesia for osteotomy of humerus
P1-C7240 Anesthesia for open procedure on humerus and elbow, NOS
P1-C7250 Anesthesia for closed procedure on humerus and elbow
P1-C7260 Anesthesia for tenodesis, rupture of long tendon of biceps
P1-C7270 Anesthesia for tenoplasty, elbow to shoulder
P1-C7280 Anesthesia for tenotomy, elbow to shoulder, open
P1-C7290 Anesthesia for procedure on nerves, muscles, tendons, fascia and bursae of upper arm and elbow
P1-C72A0 Anesthesia for arthroscopic procedure of elbow joint
P1-C72B0 Anesthesia for excision of lesion of humerus
P1-C72C0 Anesthesia for radical procedure on humerus and elbow
P1-C7500 Anesthesia for procedure on forearm, wrist or hand, NOS
P1-C7520 Anesthesia for unlisted procedure on integumentary system of forearm, wrist and hand
P1-C7540 Anesthesia for cast procedure on forearm, wrist or hand
P1-C7600 Anesthesia for vascular shunt or shunt revision
P1-C7604 Anesthesia for shunt revision, dialysis
P1-C7610 Anesthesia for procedure on veins of forearm, wrist and hand, NOS
P1-C7614 Anesthesia for phleborrhaphy on veins of forearm, wrist and hand
P1-C7630 Anesthesia for procedure on arteries of forearm, wrist and hand, NOS
P1-C7634 Anesthesia for embolectomy on arteries of forearm, wrist and hand
P1-C7700 Anesthesia for closed procedure on radius, ulna, wrist or hand bones
P1-C7720 Anesthesia for open procedure on radius, ulna, wrist or hand bones, NOS
P1-C7740 Anesthesia for total wrist replacement
P1-C7760 Anesthesia for procedure on nerves, muscles, tendons, fascia and bursae of forearm, wrist and hand
P1-C7A00 Anesthesia for endoscopic procedure on upper extremity, NOS

CHAPTER 2 — MEDICAL PROCEDURES AND SERVICES

SECTION 2-0 GENERAL MEDICAL PROCEDURES AND SERVICES INCLUDING HISTORIES AND PHYSICAL EXAMINATIONS

2-00 MEDICAL PROCEDURES: GENERAL TERMS

P2-00000 Medical procedure, NOS
P2-00010 Non-invasive medical procedure, NOS
P2-00020 Invasive medical procedure, NOS
P2-00100 General treatment, NOS
P2-00110 Preventive treatment, NOS
  Preventive service, NOS
P2-00120 Prophylactic treatment, NOS
P2-00130 Consultation, NOS
P2-00132 Limited consultation
P2-00134 Comprehensive consultation
P2-00150 Medical photography of patient, NOS
  Clinical photography, NOS
P2-00160 Cinephotography of patient, NOS

2-01 HISTORY AND PHYSICAL EXAMINATIONS

2-010 Interviews with History Taking

P2-01000 History taking, NOS
  Clinical interview, NOS
  Diagnostic interview and evaluation, NOS
P2-01010 History taking, complete
  Comprehensive interview and evaluation
P2-01020 History taking, limited
  Brief interview and evaluation
  Limited interview and evaluation
P2-01030 History taking, update
P2-01060 History taking, self-administered, questionnaire
P2-01070 History taking, self-administered, by computer terminal
P2-01090 History taking, medicolegal investigation

2-013 History and Physical Examinations

P2-01300 History and physical examination, NOS
P2-01310 History and physical examination, complete
P2-01320 History and physical examination, limited
P2-01330 History and physical examination, diagnostic
P2-01340 History and physical examination, monitoring
P2-01350 History and physical examination, follow-up
P2-01351 History and physical examination, follow-up for neoplastic disease
P2-01352 History and physical examination, follow-up examination for cardiovascular disease
P2-01353 History and physical examination, follow-up for emotional or mental disease
P2-01360 History and physical examination, administrative, NOS
P2-01361 History and physical examination, premarital
P2-01362 History and physical examination, school
P2-01363 History and physical examination, camp
P2-01364 History and physical examination, insurance
P2-01365 History and physical examination, license
P2-01366 History and physical examination, annual for health maintenance
P2-01380 History and physical examination, known or suspected contact
P2-01390 History and physical examination, known or suspected carrier
P2-013A0 History and physical examination, emergency preliminary evaluation
  Emergency examination for triage

2-014-015 Physical Examination Procedures

P2-01400 Physical examination, NOS
P2-01410 Physical examination, complete
P2-01420 Physical examination, limited
P2-01430 Specialized medical examination, NOS
P2-01431 Physical examination under local anesthesia
P2-01432 Physical examination under general anesthesia
P2-01434 Physiologic measurement, NOS
P2-01435 Anatomic measurement, NOS
P2-01436 Medical examination under sedation
P2-01440 Medical examination under hypnosis
P2-01470 Orthopedic examination under general anesthesia
P2-01480 ENT examination under general anesthesia
P2-01500 Inspection, NOS
P2-01510 Palpation, NOS
P2-01520 Digital palpation, NOS
  Digital exploration, NOS
  Digital examination, NOS
P2-01530 Bimanual palpation
  Bimanual examination
P2-01540 Mirror examination
P2-01550 Percussion, NOS
P2-01552 Immediate percussion
P2-01554 Mediate percussion
P2-01560 Auscultation, NOS
P2-01562 Immediate auscultation
P2-01564 Mediate auscultation
  Auscultation with stethoscope

2-06 GENERAL DISEASE SCREENING PROCEDURES

P2-06000 Screening procedure, NOS
P2-06010 Screening for diabetes
P2-06020 Screening for cancer
P2-06030 Screening for venereal disease
P2-06100 Multiphasic screening procedure
P2-06200 Neonatal screening, NOS
P2-06210 Infant development screening

2-07 GENERAL GENETIC INVESTIGATION PROCEDURES

P2-07000 Genetic investigation procedure, NOS
P2-07010 Family investigation, NOS
Family study, NOS

2-08 PRESCRIPTION PROCEDURES

P2-08000 Prescription, NOS
Prescription of
P2-08010 Prescription of service, NOS
P2-08020 Prescription of therapeutic agent, NOS
P2-08050 Prescription of drug, NOS
P2-08100 Prescription of prophylactic drug, NOS
P2-08110 Prescription of prophylactic antibiotic
Antibiotic coverage
P2-08120 Prescription of prophylactic anticoagulant
Anticoagulant coverage
P2-08140 Prescription of prophylactic steroid
Steroid prophylaxis
P2-08160 Prescription of prophylactic anti-malarial
Anti-malarial prophylaxis
P2-08170 Prescription of prophylactic anti-filarial
Anti-filarial prophylaxis
P2-08180 Prescription for alteration of hormonal balance by drugs
P2-08182 Prescription for alteration of hormonal balance for cancer
P2-08184 Prescription for alteration of hormonal balance for sexual aggression
P2-08300 Prescription of therapeutic regimen
Prescription of treatment plan
P2-08400 Change of prescription, NOS
P2-08500 Prescription of drug from outside authority list

2-09 VETERINARY PHYSICIANS PROCEDURES AND SERVICES

P2-09000V Veterinary clinic visit, NOS
P2-09010V Visit by veterinarian to farm
P2-09020V Visit by veterinarian to racetrack
P2-09030V Visit by veterinarian to zoo
P2-09100V Healthy animal examination, NOS
P2-09110V Breeding soundness examination
P2-09120V Selection of animals
Culling of animals
P2-09180V Animal health certification
P2-09200V Sick animal examination, NOS
P2-09212V Hip examination
P2-09214V Lameness examination
P2-09500V Animal disposition procedure, NOS
P2-09510V Euthanasia by barbiturate
P2-09512V Euthanasia by electrocution
P2-09514V Euthanasia by gunshot
P2-09600V Veterinary consultation, NOS
P2-09610V Consultation for farrier

SECTION 2-1 PHYSICIAN VISITS WITH EVALUATION AND MANAGEMENT SERVICES

2-10-11 PATIENT EVALUATION AND MANAGEMENT

P2-10000 Patient evaluation and management, NOS
History and physical examination with management of patient, NOS

2-101 Evaluation and Management — New Patients

P2-10100 Evaluation and management of new outpatient in office or other outpatient facility, NOS
History and physical examination with management of new patient, NOS
P2-10110 Problem focused history and physical with straightforward medical decision, new outpatient
Minor problem, new outpatient visit, 10 minutes
P2-10120 Expanded problem focused history and physical with straightforward medical decision, new outpatient
Minor to moderate severity problem, new outpatient visit, 20 minutes
P2-10130 Detailed history and physical with low complexity medical decision, new outpatient
Moderate severity problem, new outpatient visit, 30 minutes
P2-10140 Comprehensive history and physical with moderate complexity medical decision, new outpatient
Moderate to high severity problem, new outpatient visit, 45 minutes
P2-10150 Comprehensive history and physical with high complexity medical decision, new outpatient
High severity problem, new outpatient visit, 60 minutes

2-102 Evaluation and Management — Established Patients

P2-10200 Evaluation and management of established outpatient in office or other outpatient facility, NOS
History and physical examination with management of established patient, NOS
P2-10210 Visit by established outpatient with minimal problem
Visit by established outpatient, 5 minutes
P2-10220 Problem focused history and physical with straightforward medical decision, established outpatient
Self-limited or minor problem, established outpatient, 10 minutes
P2-10230 Expanded problem focused history and physical with low complexity medical decision, established outpatient
Low to moderate severity problem, established outpatient, 15 minutes

2-102 Evaluation and Management — Established Patients — Continued

P2-10240 Detailed history and physical with moderate complexity medical decision, established outpatient
Moderate to high severity problem, established outpatient, 25 minutes

P2-10250 Comprehensive history and physical with high complexity medical decision, established outpatient
High severity problem, established outpatient, 40 minutes

2-023 Evaluation and Management — Inpatients

P2-10300 Evaluation and management of inpatient, NOS
History and physical examination with management of inpatient, NOS

P2-10310 Initial hospital visit by physician, NOS

P2-10320 Comprehensive history and physical with straightforward or low complexity medical decision, initial inpatient visit
Low severity problem, initial inpatient visit 30 minutes

P2-10330 Comprehensive history and physical with moderate complexity medical decision, initial inpatient visit
Moderate severity problem, initial inpatient visit 50 minutes

P2-10340 Comprehensive history and physical with high complexity medical decision, initial inpatient visit
High severity problem, initial inpatient visit 70 minutes

P2-10350 Subsequent hospital visit by physician, NOS

P2-10360 Problem focused interval history and physical with straightforward or low complexity medical decision, subsequent inpatient visit
Patient stable or improving, subsequent inpatient visit 15 minutes

P2-10370 Expanded problem focused interval history and physical with moderate complexity medical decision, subsequent inpatient visit
Patient responding inadequately to therapy, subsequent inpatient visit 25 minutes

P2-10380 Detailed interval history and physical with high complexity medical decision, subsequent inpatient visit
Patient with significant complication or new problem, subsequent inpatient visit 35 minutes

P2-10390 Final inpatient visit with instructions at discharge

2-104 Medical Consultations — Office — Outpatient — Emergency Department

P2-10400 Medical consultation with outpatient, NOS

P2-10410 Office consultation with problem focused history and physical and straightforward medical decision, new or established outpatient
New or established outpatient with self-limited or minor problem, consultation visit 15 minutes

P2-10420 Office consultation with expanded problem focused history and physical and straightforward medical decision, new or established outpatient
New or established outpatient with low severity problem, consultation visit 30 minutes

P2-10430 Office consultation with detailed history and physical and low complexity medical decision, new or established outpatient
New or established outpatient with moderate severity problem, consultation visit 40 minutes

P2-10440 Office consultation with comprehensive history and physical and moderate complexity medical decision, new or established outpatient
New or established outpatient with moderate to high severity problem, consultation visit 60 minutes

P2-10450 Office consultation with comprehensive history and physical and high complexity medical decision, new or established outpatient
New or established outpatient with high severity problem, consultation visit 80 minutes

2-105 Medical Consultations — Inpatients

P2-10500 Medical consultation on inpatient, NOS

P2-10502 Medical consultation on hospital inpatient

P2-10504 Medical consultation on nursing facility inpatient

P2-10510 Inpatient consultation with problem focused history and physical and straightforward medical decision, new or established patient
New or established patient with self-limited or minor problem, 20 minute inpatient consultation visit

P2-10520 Inpatient consultation with expanded problem focused history and physical and straightforward medical decision, new or established patient
New or established patient with low severity problem, 40 minute inpatient consultation visit

P2-10530 Inpatient consultation with detailed history and physical and low complexity medical decision, new or established patient
New or established patient with moderate severity problem, 55 minute inpatient consultation visit

P2-10540 Inpatient consultation with comprehensive history and physical and moderate complexity medical decision, new or established patient
New or established patient with moderate to high severity problem, 80 minute inpatient consultation visit

P2-10550 Inpatient consultation with comprehensive history and physical and high complexity medical decision, new or established patient
New or established patient with high severity problem, 110 minute inpatient consultation visit

P2-10560 Follow-up inpatient consultation visit, NOS

P2-10570 Follow-up inpatient consultation with problem focused interval history and physical with low complexity or straightforward medical decision, established inpatient
Established inpatient stable or improving, 10 minute follow-up consultation visit

P2-10580 Follow-up inpatient consultation with expanded problem focused interval history and physical and moderate complexity medical decision, established patient
Established inpatient responding inadequately to therapy, 20 minute follow-up consultation visit

P2-10590 Follow-up inpatient consultation with detailed interval history and physical and high complexity medical decision, established patient
Established inpatient with significant complication or new problem, 30 minute follow-up consultation visit

2-106 Confirmatory Medical Consultations

P2-10600 Confirmatory medical consultation, NOS
Second or third medical opinion, NOS

P2-10610 Confirmatory consultation with problem focused history and physical and straightforward medical decision, new or established patient

P2-10620 Confirmatory consultation with expanded problem focused history and physical and straightforward medical decision, new or established patient

P2-10630 Confirmatory consultation with detailed history and physical and low complexity medical decision, new or established patient

P2-10640 Confirmatory consultation with comprehensive history and physical and moderate complexity medical decision, new or established patient

P2-10650 Confirmatory consultation with comprehensive history and physical with high complexity medical decision, new or established patient

2-107 Emergency Department Patient Visits

P2-10700 Emergency department patient visit, NOS

P2-10710 Emergency department visit with problem focused history and physical and straightforward medical decision, new or established patient

P2-10720 Emergency department visit with expanded problem focused history and physical and low complexity medical decision, new or established patient

P2-10730 Emergency department visit with expanded problem focused history and physical and low to moderate complexity medical decision, new or established patient

P2-10740 Emergency department visit with detailed history and physical and moderate complexity medical decision, new or established patient

P2-10750 Emergency department visit with comprehensive history and physical and high complexity medical decision, new or established patient

P2-10790 Physician direction of emergency medical systems

2-108 Critical Care Physician Services

P2-10800 Critical care physician services, NOS

P2-10810 Critical care diagnostic and therapeutic services, first hour

P2-10820 Critical care diagnostic and therapeutic services, each additional 30 minutes

2-109 Team Conferences and Telephone Consultations

P2-10900 Interdisciplinary medical team conference, NOS

P2-10910 Interdisciplinary medical team conference, 30 minutes

P2-10920 Interdisciplinary medical team conference, 60 minutes

P2-10950 Telephone call by physician to patient or for consultation, NOS

P2-10960 Brief telephone call by physician to patient or for consultation

P2-10970 Intermediate telephone call by physician to patient or for consultation

P2-10980 Complex or lengthy telephone call by physician to patient or for consultation

2-110 Nursing Facility Patient Evaluation and Management

P2-11000 Nursing facility patient evaluation and management, NOS
History and physical examination with evaluation and management of nursing facility patient, NOS

2-110 Nursing Facility Patient Evaluation and Management — Continued

P2-11010 Nursing facility visit with detailed interval history, comprehensive physical and straightforward or low complexity medical decision, new or established patient
Nursing facility visit to new or established patient for annual assessment, 30 minutes

P2-11020 Nursing facility visit with detailed interval history, comprehensive physical and moderate to high complexity medical decision, new or established patient
Nursing facility visit to new or established patient with major permanent change in status, 40 minutes

P2-11030 Nursing facility visit with comprehensive history and physical with high complexity medical decision, new or established patient
Nursing facility visit to new or established patient at time of initial admission, 50 minutes

P2-11050 Subsequent nursing facility visit, NOS

P2-11060 Subsequent nursing facility visit with problem focused interval history and physical and straightforward or low complexity medical decision, new or established patient
Nursing facility patient, stable or improving, subsequent visit, 15 minutes

P2-11070 Subsequent nursing facility visit with expanded problem focused history and physical and moderate complexity medical decision, new or established patient
Nursing facility patient responding inadequately to therapy, subsequent visit, 25 minutes

P2-11080 Subsequent nursing facility visit with detailed interval history and physical and moderate to high complexity medical decision, new or established patient
Nursing facility patient with significant complication or new problem, subsequent visit, 35 minutes

2-112 Domiciliary or Rest Home Patient Evaluation and Management

P2-11200 Domiciliary or rest home patient evaluation and management, NOS
History and physical examination with management of domiciliary or rest home patient, NOS

P2-11210 Domiciliary or rest home new patient evaluation with problem focused history and physical and straightforward or low complexity medical decision
Visit to domiciliary or rest home new patient presenting problems of low severity

P2-11220 Domiciliary or rest home new patient evaluation with expanded problem focused history and physical and moderate complexity medical decision
Visit to domiciliary or rest home new patient presenting problems of moderate severity

P2-11230 Domiciliary or rest home new patient evaluation with detailed history and physical and high complexity medical decision
Visit to domiciliary or rest home new patient presenting problems of high severity

P2-11250 Domiciliary or rest home established patient evaluation with problem focused interval history and physical and straightforward to low complexity medical decision
Visit to domiciliary or rest home established patient who is stable, recovering or improving

P2-11260 Domiciliary or rest home established patient evaluation with expanded problem focused interval history and physical and moderate complexity medical decision
Visit to domiciliary or rest home established patient who is responding inadequately to therapy or has minor complication

P2-11270 Domiciliary or rest home established patient evaluation with detailed interval history and physical and high complexity medical decision
Visit to domiciliary or rest home established patient who is unstable or has significant complication

2-114 Evaluation and Management of Patient at Home

P2-11400 Evaluation and management of patient at home, NOS

P2-11410 New home patient evaluation with problem focused history and physical and straightforward to low complexity medical decision
Visit to new home patient presenting problems of low severity

P2-11420 New home patient evaluation with expanded problem focused history and physical and moderate complexity medical decision
Visit to new home patient presenting problems of moderate severity

P2-11430 New home patient evaluation with detailed history and physical and high complexity medical decision
Visit to new home patient presenting problems of high severity

P2-11450 Established home patient evaluation with problem focused interval history and physical and straightforward to low complexity medical decision
Visit to established home patient who is stable, recovering or improving

P2-11460 Established home patient evaluation with expanded problem focused interval history and physical and moderate complexity medical decision
Visit to established home patient who is responding inadequately to therapy or has minor complication

P2-11470 Established home patient evaluation with detailed interval history and physical and high complexity medical decision
Visit to established home patient who is unstable or has significant complication

2-115-116 Preventive Patient Evaluation

P2-11500 Initial evaluation and management of healthy individual, NOS
Preventive evaluation of new patient, NOS
P2-11510 New well patient visit, under age one
Medical examination of well baby
Medical examination of well infant
P2-11520 New well patient visit, one through four years
P2-11530 New well patient visit, five through eleven years
P2-11540 New well patient visit, twelve through seventeen years
P2-11550 New well patient visit, eighteen through thirty-nine years
P2-11560 New well patient visit, forty through sixty-four years
P2-11570 New well patient visit, sixty-five years and over
P2-11600 Periodic reevaluation and management of healthy individual, NOS
Preventive evaluation of established patient, NOS
P2-11610 Established well patient visit, under age one
P2-11620 Established well patient visit, one through four years
P2-11630 Established well patient visit, five through eleven years
P2-11640 Established well patient visit, twelve through seventeen years
P2-11650 Established well patient visit, eighteen through thirty-nine years
P2-11660 Established well patient visit, forty through sixty-four years
P2-11670 Established well patient visit, sixty-five years and over

2-117 Preventive Medicine Counseling and Risk Factor Evaluation Services

P2-11700 Individual preventive medicine counseling, NOS
P2-11710 Individual preventive medicine counseling, 15 minutes
P2-11720 Individual preventive medicine counseling, 30 minutes
P2-11730 Individual preventive medicine counseling, 45 minutes
P2-11740 Individual preventive medicine counseling, 60 minutes
P2-11750 Group preventive medicine counseling, NOS
P2-11760 Group preventive medicine counseling, 30 minutes
P2-11770 Group preventive medicine counseling, 60 minutes
P2-11790 Physician administration and interpretation of instrument of health risk assessment
Health hazard appraisal
P2-117A0 Special preventive medicine service, explain by report

2-118 Specific Patient Counseling Sessions

P2-11800 Patient counseling, NOS
P2-11810 Family planning counseling
P2-11812 Counseling for termination of pregnancy
Counseling for abortion
P2-11816 Contraception counseling
P2-11820 Premarital counseling
P2-11822 Marital counseling
P2-11824 Sexual counseling
P2-11830 Genetic counseling
P2-11834 Maternity counseling
P2-11840 Diet counseling
P2-11850 Geriatric counseling
P2-11860 Drug addiction counseling
P2-11870 Alcoholism counseling
P2-11880 Child guidance counseling

2-11A Newborn Care Services

P2-11A00 Newborn care service, NOS
P2-11A10 History and physical of normal newborn infant with initiation of diagnosis and treatment
P2-11A20 History and physical of normal newborn infant outside hospital facility
P2-11A30 Subsequent hospital care of newborn with evaluation and management
P2-11A40 Complete infant care up to one year during regular office visit
P2-11A80 Care of high risk newborn at delivery including resuscitative measures

SECTION 2-2 MEDICAL PROCEDURES ON THE RESPIRATORY TRACT

2-20-22 GENERAL DIAGNOSTIC AND THERAPEUTIC PROCEDURES ON THE RESPIRATORY TRACT

P2-20000 Medical procedure on respiratory tract, NOS
Respiratory tract procedure, NOS
P2-20004 Nonoperative respiratory measurements, NOS
P2-20010 Pulmonary service or medical procedure, NOS
P2-20100 Medical procedure on nose, NOS
P2-20110 Direct nasal mucous membrane test
P2-20120 Nasal function study, NOS
P2-20200 Medical procedure on nasopharynx, NOS
P2-20230 Digital palpation of pharynx
P2-20232 Digital palpation of nasopharynx

2-20-22 GENERAL DIAGNOSTIC AND THERAPEUTIC PROCEDURES ON THE RESPIRATORY TRACT — Continued

P2-20250 Nose and throat examination, NOS
  Rhinolaryngologic examination
P2-20254 Laryngologic examination under general anesthesia
P2-20256 Rhinolaryngologic examination under general anesthesia
P2-20258 Follow-up examination of nose and throat
  Rhinolaryngologic follow-up evaluation
P2-20260 Binocular microscopy, otolaryngologic
P2-20300 Medical procedure on nasal sinus, NOS
P2-20310 Transillumination of nasal sinuses
P2-20400 Medical procedure on larynx, NOS
P2-20420 Laryngeal function studies
P2-20450 Complex dynamic pharyngeal and speech evaluation by cine/video recording
P2-20500 Medical procedure on trachea, NOS
P2-20550 Medical procedure on bronchus, NOS
P2-20600 Medical procedure on lung, NOS
  Pulmonary medical procedure, NOS
P2-20800 Medical procedure on pleura, NOS
P2-22000 Respiratory therapy, NOS
P2-22010 Monitoring of respiration, NOS
P2-22100 Inhalation therapy procedure, NOS
P2-22104 Inhalation bronchial challenge testing, NOS
P2-22110 Control of atmospheric pressure and composition with antigen-free air conditioning
P2-22200 Mechanical ventilation, NOS
  Assisted ventilation therapy, NOS
P2-22204 Controlled ventilation procedure and therapy, initiation and management
P2-22210 Bennett respirator therapy
P2-22212 Byrd respirator therapy
P2-22220 Fog inhalation therapy
P2-22222 Mist inhalation therapy
P2-22230 Nebulizer therapy
P2-22300 Intermittent positive pressure breathing treatment
  IPPB treatment
  Intermittent positive pressure breathing treatment without nebulized medication
P2-22310 Intermittent positive pressure breathing treatment with nebulized medication
  IPPB treatment with nebulized medication
P2-22330 Intermittent positive pressure breathing treatment for newborn infants
P2-22340 Continuous positive airway pressure ventilation treatment
  CPAP treatment
P2-22350 Continuous negative pressure ventilation treatment
  CNP treatment
P2-22360 Positive and expiratory pressure ventilation therapy, initiation and management
  PEP therapy
P2-22370 Inspiration mandatory ventilation therapy, initiation and management
  IMV therapy
P2-22390 Management of preset ventilators for assisted or controlled breathing, NOS
P2-22391 Assisted ventilation therapy, pressure or volume preset, initiation and management
P2-22392 Flow and timed ventilation procedure, initiation and management
P2-22500 Oxygen therapy, NOS
P2-22501 Intranasal oxygen therapy
P2-22700 Nonpressurized inhalation treatment for acute airway obstruction
P2-22720 Manipulation of chest wall by cupping, percussing or vibration to facilitate lung function
  Manipulation of chest wall to facilitate lung function
P2-22730 Aerosol or vapor inhalation for bronchodilation
P2-22732 Aerosol or vapor inhalation for sputum induction for diagnostic purposes
  Obtaining sputum specimen by aerosol-induced technique
  Aerosol or vapor inhalation for sputum mobilization
P2-22740 Respiratory medication administered by nebulizer
P2-22800 Breathing exercise, NOS
P2-22810 Breathing exercise, blow bottle
P2-22820 Breathing exercise, training
P2-22850 Postural drainage therapy
P2-22860 Physiotherapy of chest
P2-22900 Pulmonary resuscitation, NOS
P2-22902 Artificial respiration
P2-22904 Nonmechanical method of resuscitation
P2-22905 Respiratory assist, manual
P2-22906 Respiratory assist, mechanical
P2-22910 Resuscitation with artificial respiration
P2-22912 Mouth-to-mouth resuscitation
P2-22920 Decompression chamber therapy, NOS
  Control of atmospheric pressure and composition in decompression chamber procedure, NOS
P2-22924 Hyperbaric oxygen therapy
  Hyperbaric oxygenation
P2-22930 Helium therapy
P2-22950 Treatment by iron lung
P2-22990 Heimlich maneuver

2-25-26 PHYSIOLOGIC MEASUREMENTS OF RESPIRATORY FUNCTION

P2-25010 Measurement of respiratory function, NOS
P2-25100 Spirometry, NOS, including recording and report
  Bronchospirometry, NOS
  Spirometry including graphic record of total and timed vital capacity, expiratory flow rate and maximal voluntary ventilation
P2-25110 Spirometry for bronchospasm evaluation before and after bronchodilator, NOS

P2-25120 Spirometry for bronchospasm evaluation before and after exercise
P2-25130 Spirometry for bronchospasm with prolonged evaluation, NOS
P2-25132 Spirometry for bronchospasm with prolonged evaluation after bronchodilator
P2-25133 Spirometry for bronchospasm with prolonged evaluation after exercise
P2-25134 Spirometry for bronchospasm with prolonged evaluation after cold air
P2-25135 Spirometry for bronchospasm with prolonged evaluation after antigen exposure
P2-25136 Spirometry for bronchospasm with prolonged evaluation after methocholine
P2-25137 Spirometry for bronchospasm with prolonged evaluation after other stimulus
P2-25140 Spirometry, differential ventilation, oxygen consumption
P2-25200 Total vital capacity measurement, NOS
P2-25210 Vital capacity screening test, NOS
P2-25212 Total vital capacity with timed forced expiratory volume and peak flow rate measurement
P2-25220 Maximum breathing capacity measurement
P2-25222 Maximal voluntary ventilation measurement
P2-25230 Functional residual capacity or residual volume measurement, NOS
P2-25232 Functional residual capacity or residual volume measurement, helium method
P2-25234 Functional residual capacity or residual volume measurement, nitrogen open circuit method
P2-25250 Measurement of lung volume
Thoracic gas volume measurement
P2-25252 Collection of expired gas, quantitative
P2-25270 Multiple or single breath nitrogen washout curve
Determination of maldistribution of inspired gas by multiple breath nitrogen washout curve including alveolar nitrogen or helium equilibration time
P2-25300 Determination of resistance to airflow, NOS
Determination of airway resistance
Measurement of airway resistance, NOS
P2-25302 Determination of resistance to airflow by oscillatory method
P2-25304 Determination of resistance to airflow by plethysmographic method
P2-25310 Expiratory flow rate measurement
P2-25320 Determination of airway closing volume, single breath test
P2-25322 Amount of trapped gas, box FRC, measurement
P2-25360 CO_2 response curve measurement
Breathing response to CO_2
Ventilation response to CO_2
P2-25364 Hypoxia response curve measurement
Ventilation response to hypoxia
Breathing response to hypoxia
P2-25380 Pulmonary compliance study, NOS
Lung compliance study
P2-25390 Respiratory flow volume loop measurement
P2-25394 Respiratory quotient measurement
P2-25400 Pulmonary stress testing, NOS
P2-25402 Pulmonary stress testing, simple
P2-25404 Pulmonary stress testing, complex
P2-25600 Breath analysis, labeled hydrogen
P2-25800 Circadian respiratory pattern, continuous recording of infant
P2-25810 Pediatric pneumogram, 12 to 24 hour continuous recording
P2-26000 Non-invasive ear or pulse oximetry for oxygen saturation, NOS
P2-26020 Non-invasive ear or pulse oximetry during exercise
P2-26030 Non-invasive ear or pulse oximetry with continuous overnight monitoring
P2-26050 Oxygen uptake by expired gas analysis at rest
P2-26055 Oxygen uptake by expired gas analysis at rest and with exercise
P2-26060 Oxygen uptake by expired gas analysis including CO_2 output with percentage oxygen extracted
P2-26100 Analysis of arterial blood gases and pH
P2-26110 Analysis of arterial blood gases and pH at rest and exercise
P2-26120 Analysis of arterial blood gases and pH after O_2 administration, IPPB or exercise
P2-26150 Hemoglobin-oxygen affinity measurement
50% hemoglobin saturation with oxygen measurement
P-50 measurement
P2-26200 Carbon monoxide diffusing capacity measurement
P2-26210 Membrane diffusion capacity
P2-26220 Carbon dioxide, expired gas determination

2-28 RESPIRATORY TRACT REHABILITATION PROCEDURES

P2-28000 Pulmonary rehabilitation, NOS
P2-28100 Post-laryngectomy rehabilitation
P2-28110 Artificial voice rehabilitation
P2-28200 Nasopharyngeal rehabilitation

SECTION 2-3 MEDICAL PROCEDURES ON THE CARDIOVASCULAR SYSTEM

2-30 GENERAL MEDICAL CARDIOVASCULAR PROCEDURES INCLUDING CARDIOVERSIONS

P2-30000 Medical cardiovascular procedure, NOS
P2-30010 Medical procedure on heart, NOS
P2-30020 Cardiovascular examination and evaluation, NOS
P2-30030 Evaluation of cardiac catheterization data and report

2-30 GENERAL MEDICAL CARDIOVASCULAR PROCEDURES INCLUDING CARDIOVERSIONS — Continued

P2-30040 Cardiovascular rehabilitation procedure, NOS
P2-30042 Physician services for outpatient cardiac rehabilitation without continuous ECG monitoring
P2-30044 Physician services for outpatient cardiac rehabilitation with continuous ECG monitoring
P2-30100 Cardiac function testing, NOS
P2-30300 Cardioassist, NOS
P2-30302 External cardioassist
  Cardioassist-method of circulatory assist, external
P2-30304 Internal cardioassist
  Cardioassist-method of circulatory assist, internal
P2-30320 Cardiopulmonary resuscitation, NOS
P2-30322 Cardiac resuscitation, NOS
P2-30324 Resuscitation by cardiac cardioversion
  Resuscitation by cardiac defibrillation
P2-30330 Cardioversion, NOS
  Conversion of cardiac rhythm to sinus rhythm
  Cardiac countershock, NOS
  Conversion of cardiac rhythm, NOS
P2-30332 Elective electrical cardioversion of arrhythmia, external
  External cardioversion
P2-30336 Internal cardioversion
  Cardioversion by intracardiac catheter
P2-30338 Atrial cardioversion
P2-30600 Ballistocardiography, NOS
  Ballistocardiogram
P2-30700 Cardiac electrophysiologic stimulation and recording study, NOS
P2-30710 Intracardiac electrophysiologic procedure with ECG, NOS
P2-30720 Cardiac mapping
P2-30800V Examination of animal for heartworm
  Heartworm check

2-31 ELECTROCARDIOGRAPHIC PROCEDURES AND STRESS TESTING

P2-31000 Electrocardiographic procedure, NOS
  Electrocardiogram, NOS
  EKG
P2-31001 Electrocardiogram, rhythm
P2-31002 Electrocardiogram, single lead
P2-31003 Electrocardiogram, esophageal lead
P2-31004 Electrocardiogram, intracardiac
P2-31005 Electrocardiogram, intracardiac, His bundle recording
P2-31006 Electrocardiographic recording from artificial pacemaker
P2-31007 Continuous electrocardiogram
P2-31010 Electrocardiogram with exercise test, NOS
P2-31012 Electrocardiogram with sub-maximal exercise test
P2-31014 Electrocardiogram with maximal exercise test
P2-31020 Electrocardiogram, routine ECG with at least 12 leads, tracing only without interpretation and report
P2-31022 Electrocardiogram, routine ECG with at least 12 leads with interpretation and report
P2-31024 Electrocardiogram, routine ECG with at least 12 leads, interpretation and report only
P2-31030 Telephonic or telemetric transmission of electrocardiogram rhythm strip
P2-31032 Telephonic or telemetric transmission of electrocardiogram rhythm strip, physician review with interpretation and report only
P2-31040 Rhythm ECG, one to three leads with interpretation and report
P2-31042 Rhythm ECG, one to three leads, tracing only without interpretation and report
P2-31044 Rhythm ECG, one to three leads, interpretation and report only
P2-31100 Cardiovascular stress testing, NOS
P2-31102 Cardiovascular stress test using bicycle ergometer
P2-31103 Cardiovascular stress test using treadmill
P2-31104 Cardiovascular stress test using maximal or submaximal treadmill or bicycle exercise, continuous electrocardiographic monitoring with interpretation and report
P2-31105 Cardiovascular stress test using maximal or submaximal treadmill or bicycle exercise, tracing only without interpretation and report
P2-31106 Cardiovascular stress test using maximal or submaximal treadmill or bicycle exercise, interpretation and report only
P2-31110 Patient demand for ECG, single or multiple event recording with presymptom memory loop, transmission, physician review and interpretation
  ECG on demand by patient
P2-31120 Tracing of carotid pulse with ECG lead
P2-31130 Masters' stress test, two-step
  Testing of cardiac stress, Masters' two-step
P2-31150 Electrocardiogram with vectorcardiogram
P2-31200 Electrocardiographic monitoring, NOS
  Cardiovascular monitoring by ECG, NOS
P2-31202 Electrocardiographic monitoring for 24 hours by continuous original ECG waveform recording and storage with visual superimposition scanning includes recording, scanning analysis with report by physician
  Electrocardiographic monitoring for 24 hours by continuous original ECG waveform recording and storage with visual superimposition scanning, physician review and interpretation
P2-31210 Electrocardiographic monitoring for 24 hours by continuous original ECG waveform recording and storage without scanning utilizing a device capable of full miniaturized printout with analysis and report by physician

P2-31218 Electrocardiographic monitoring for 24 hours by continuous computerized monitoring and recording, real-time data analysis producing intermittent full-sized waveform tracings with analysis and report
P2-31323 Monitoring of cardiac output by ECG
P2-31510 Esophageal recording of atrial electrogram with or without ventricular electrogram
P2-31512 Esophageal recording of atrial electrogram with or without ventricular electrogram with pacing
P2-31600 Signal-averaged electrocardiography, NOS
SAECG, NOS

2-32 PHONOCARDIOGRAPHIC AND VECTORCARDIOGRAPHIC PROCEDURES

P2-32000 Phonocardiogram, NOS
P2-32010 Phonocardiogram with apex cardiogram
P2-32012 Phonocardiogram with artery and/or vein tracing
P2-32014 Intracardiac phonocardiogram
P2-32100 Phonocardiogram with ECG lead
P2-32101 Phonocardiogram with ECG lead with supervision during recording with interpretation and report (when equipment is supplied by the physician)
P2-32102 Phonocardiogram with ECG lead, tracing only without interpretation and report
P2-32104 Phonocardiogram with ECG lead, interpretation and report
P2-32106 Phonocardiogram with ECG lead with indirect carotid artery and/or jugular vein tracing, and/or apex cardiogram with interpretation and report
P2-32108 Phonocardiogram with ECG lead with indirect carotid artery and/or jugular vein tracing, and/or apex cardiogram, tracing only without interpretation and report
P2-32110 Phonocardiogram with ECG lead with indirect carotid artery and/or jugular vein tracing, and/or apex cardiogram, interpretation and report only
P2-32500 Vectorcardiogram, NOS
VCG, NOS
P2-32502 Vectorcardiogram with ECG
P2-32510 Vectorcardiogram with ECG, interpretation and report
P2-32512 Vectorcardiogram without ECG, interpretation and report
P2-32514 Vectorcardiogram with ECG, tracing only without interpretation and report
P2-32515 Vectorcardiogram without ECG, tracing only without interpretation and report
P2-32516 Vectorcardiogram with ECG, interpretation and report only
P2-32518 Vectorcardiogram without ECG, interpretation and report only
P2-32520 Apexcardiography
Apex cardiography
P2-32530 Apexcardiogram with ECG lead

2-34 CARDIOVASCULAR MONITORING PROCEDURES

P2-34000 Cardiovascular monitoring, NOS
Circulatory monitoring, NOS
P2-34010 Cardiac monitoring, NOS
P2-34100 Monitoring of blood pressure
P2-34102 Monitoring of pulse
P2-34110 Intra-aortic balloon counterpulsation, monitoring only
Monitoring of intra-aortic balloon counterpulsation
P2-34120 Monitoring of pacemaker
P2-34122 Monitoring of ECG at surgery
P2-34123 Electrocardiogram monitoring, 10 hour portrait
P2-34124 Monitoring of ECG, pressure, blood gases and cardiac output
P2-34126 Monitoring of ECG and pressure during major surgery
P2-34130 Systemic arterial pressure monitoring
Monitoring of systemic arterial pressure
P2-34131 Arterial pressure monitoring, invasive method
P2-34132 Arterial pressure monitoring, non-invasive method
P2-34200 Monitoring of cardiac output by oxygen consumption technique
P2-34210 Monitoring of cardiac output by indicator dilution technique
P2-34220 Monitoring of cardiac output by thermodilution indicator
P2-34230 Monitoring of cardiac output by other technique
P2-34310 Central venous pressure monitoring
P2-34320 Pulmonary artery pressure monitoring
P2-34322 Pulmonary artery wedge pressure monitoring
P2-34327 Monitoring of cardiac output by Fick method
P2-34328 Monitoring of coronary blood flow
P2-34329 Monitoring of cardiac ventricular pressure
P2-34400 Ambulatory blood pressure monitoring utilizing magnetic tape and/or computer disk for 24 hours including recording, scanning analysis, interpretation and report
P2-34402 Ambulatory blood pressure monitoring utilizing magnetic tape and/or computer disk for 24 hours with recording only
P2-34404 Ambulatory blood pressure monitoring utilizing magnetic tape and/or computer disk for 24 hours with scanning analysis and report
P2-34406 Ambulatory blood pressure monitoring utilizing magnetic tape and/or computer disk for 24 hours with physician review, interpretation and report
P2-34800 Cardiotachometry, NOS
Cardiotocogram (CTG)

2-34 CARDIOVASCULAR MONITORING PROCEDURES — Continued

P2-34810 Cardiotachometer monitoring

2-35 CARDIAC PACING PROCEDURES

P2-35000 Cardiac pacing, NOS
P2-35020 Demand pacing
P2-35030 Induction of arrhythmia by electrical pacing
P2-35100 Bundle of His recording
His bundle recording
P2-35102 Intra-atrial recording
P2-35104 Right ventricular recording
P2-35106 Left ventricular recording
P2-35200 Intra-atrial pacing
P2-35202 Intraventricular pacing
Bundle of His pacing
P2-35410 Comprehensive electrophysiologic evaluation including right atrial pacing and recording, right ventricular pacing and recording, His bundle recording and induction of arrhythmia
P2-35412 Comprehensive electrophysiologic evaluation including right atrial pacing and recording, right ventricular pacing and recording, His bundle recording and induction of arrhythmia with left atrial recording
P2-35414 Comprehensive electrophysiologic evaluation including right atrial pacing and recording, right ventricular pacing and recording, His bundle recording and induction of arrhythmia with left ventricular recording
P2-35416 Programmed stimulation and pacing after intravenous drug infusion
P2-35417 Electrophysiologic follow-up study with pacing and recording to test effectiveness of therapy
P2-35420 Intraoperative cardiac pacing and mapping
P2-35422 Intraoperative cardiac pacemaker
P2-35430 Electrophysiologic evaluation of cardioverter-defibrillator lead and/or device
P2-35440 Temporary transcutaneous pacing

2-36 CARDIOVASCULAR MEASUREMENTS

P2-36000 Cardiovascular measurement, NOS
P2-36010 Cardiometry, NOS
P2-36012 Cardiotopometry, NOS
P2-36020 Phleborheography, NOS
P2-36102 Measurement of systemic arterial pressure
Arterial pressure determination
P2-36104 Regional blood flow study
P2-36110 Determination of venous pressure
Venous pressure determination
P2-36112 Measurement of central venous pressure
P2-36120 Vascular oscillometry
P2-36130 Wedge pressure determination, NOS
P2-36132 Pulmonary artery wedge pressure determination
P2-36134 Wedge pressure determination of hepatic vein
P2-36135 Measurement of portovenous pressure
P2-36140 Vascular impedance determination, NOS
P2-36150 Circulation time, one test
P2-36152 Circulation time, two or more test materials
P2-36154 Dye dilution studies, indicator dye curves
P2-36156 Dye dilution studies, dye curves including cardiac output measurement
P2-36157 Indicator dilution studies including arterial and/or venous catheterization with cardiac output measurement as separate procedure
P2-36158 Indicator dilution flow measurement
P2-36170 Arterial cannulization with cardiac output
P2-36174 Measurement of coronary blood flow
P2-36200 Quantitative venous flow studies, NOS
P2-36202 Quantitative venous flow studies, measurement of calf venous reflux
P2-36206 Testing of internal jugular-subclavian venous reflux

2-37 NON-INVASIVE STUDIES OF THE PERIPHERAL VESSELS

P2-37000 Non-invasive study of peripheral vessel, NOS
P2-37002 Peripheral vascular disease study, NOS
P2-37100 Non-invasive studies of cerebral arteries other than carotid, ocular and ear pulse wave timing
P2-37102 Non-invasive studies of cerebral arteries other than carotid, ocular plethysmography with brachial blood pressure
P2-37110 Non-invasive studies of cerebral arteries other than carotid, vertebral arteries flow direction measurement
P2-37112 Non-invasive studies of carotid arteries, analog velocity waveform analysis
P2-37114 Non-invasive studies of carotid arteries, diastolic flow evaluation
P2-37130 Non-invasive study of veins of extremity
P2-37200 Non-invasive studies of upper extremity arteries, evocative pressure response to exercise or reactive hyperemia
P2-37210 Non-invasive studies of upper extremity arteries, flow velocity signals
P2-37300 Non-invasive studies of lower extremity arteries, evocative pressure response to exercise or reactive hyperemia
P2-37310 Non-invasive studies of lower extremity arteries, flow velocity signals

2-39 ELECTRONIC DEVICE ANALYSIS PROCEDURES

P2-39000 Check artificial pacemaker, NOS
P2-39002 Artificial pacemaker rate check
P2-39004 Check artificial pacemaker for waveform artefact
P2-39006 Check artificial pacemaker for electrode impedance
P2-39008 Check artificial pacemaker for amperage threshold

P2-39010 Check artificial pacemaker for voltage threshold
P2-39020 Check artificial pacemaker by slew rate check
P2-39100 Electronic analysis of internal pacemaker system, NOS
P2-39102 Electronic analysis of internal pacemaker system, complete
P2-39104 Electronic wave or pacemaker analysis, complete
P2-39106 Electronic wave or pacemaker analysis, remote
P2-39110 Electronic analysis of dual-chamber internal pacemaker system without reprogramming
P2-39111 Electronic analysis of dual-chamber internal pacemaker system includes rate, pulse amplitude and duration, configuration of waveform, and/or testing of sensory function of pacemaker without reprogramming
P2-39112 Electronic analysis of dual-chamber internal pacemaker system with reprogramming
P2-39114 Electronic analysis of dual-chamber internal pacemaker system by telephonic analysis
P2-39120 Electronic analysis of single-chamber internal pacemaker system without reprogramming
P2-39122 Electronic analysis of single-chamber internal pacemaker system with reprogramming
P2-39124 Electronic analysis of single-chamber internal pacemaker system by telephonic analysis
P2-39200 Assembly of pump-oxygenator for extracorporeal circulation
P2-39210 Assembly and operation of pump with oxygenator or heat exchanger with monitoring

SECTION 2-4 MEDICAL PROCEDURES RELATED TO THE SKIN AND BREAST

2-40-41 GENERAL SKIN EXAMINATION PROCEDURES AND TREATMENTS

P2-40000 Medical dermatologic procedure, NOS
    Medical skin and skin appendage procedure, NOS
P2-40010 Dermatology consultation and report, NOS
P2-40011 Dermatology consultation and report, brief
P2-40012 Dermatology consultation and report, comprehensive
P2-40020 Skin scraping for examination
P2-40021V Direct smear for ectoparasites
P2-40022 Hand microscope examination of skin, NOS
P2-40024 Skin fluorescence test by Wood's light
P2-40026 Diascopy procedure
P2-40036 Dermographia test
    Artificial urticaria test
P2-40100 Prausnitz-Kustner test
P2-40110 Mazzotti reaction test
P2-40300 Iontophoresis procedure
    Sweat collection by iontophoresis
P2-40310 Electrolysis procedure
P2-40312 Surgical galvanism
P2-40314 Medical galvanism
P2-40400 Skin snip examination, NOS
P2-40402 Skin snip examination for onchocerca
P2-40410 Curette test of skin
P2-40500 Epidermal occlusion therapy, NOS
P2-40510 Test for Nikolsky's sign
P2-40550 Preparation of skin window
P2-41000 Phototherapy, NOS
P2-41010 Actinotherapy, NOS
    Actinotherapy with ultraviolet light
    Ultraviolet light therapy
P2-41012 Local actinotherapy
P2-41014 General actinotherapy
P2-41020 Phototherapy of newborn
P2-41100 Photochemotherapy, NOS
P2-41120 Photochemotherapy with psoralens and ultraviolet A
    PUVA therapy
P2-41121 Photochemotherapy with petrolatum and ultraviolet B
P2-41122 Photochemotherapy with tar and ultraviolet B
    Goeckerman regimen
    Goeckerman treatment, photochemotherapy
P2-41126 Modified Goeckerman regimen
P2-41128 Bililite therapy with ultraviolet light
P2-41130 Photochemotherapy with tar and petrolatum

2-44 SKIN TESTS

P2-44000 Skin test, NOS
P2-44010 Allergy testing, NOS
    Percutaneous test for allergy, NOS
P2-44102 Intradermal skin test, NOS
P2-44104 Prick test, NOS
P2-44106 Scratch test, NOS
P2-44108 Patch test, NOS
P2-44109 Puncture test, NOS
P2-44120 Delayed hypersensitivity skin test
    DHST, NOS
P2-44122 Delayed hypersensitivity skin test, multitest
    Multitest skin test
P2-44130 Skin test, anergy testing
P2-44131 Delayed hypersensitivity skin test for Candida albicans
P2-44132 Delayed hypersensitivity skin test for coccidiodin
    Skin test for coccidioidomycosis
P2-44133 Delayed hypersensitivity skin test for histoplasmin
    Skin test for histoplasmosis
P2-44135 Delayed hypersensitivity skin test for phytohemagglutinin
P2-44136 Delayed hypersensitivity skin test for staphage lysate
P2-44137 Delayed hypersensitivity skin test for SK-SD
P2-44138 Delayed hypersensitivity skin test for tetanus
P2-44139 Delayed hypersensitivity skin test for diphtheria

2-44 SKIN TESTS — Continued

P2-4413A Delayed hypersensitivity skin test for mumps
  Skin test for mumps
P2-44140 Delayed hypersensitivity skin test for Trichophyton
P2-44142 Delayed hypersensitivity skin test for tuberculin PPD
  Intradermal skin test for tuberculosis
P2-44144 Skin test for tuberculosis, Tine test
P2-44148V Johnin skin test
P2-44149V Johnin intravenous test
P2-44150 Skin test for leprosy
  Lepromin skin test
P2-44152 Lepromin A skin test
  Lepromin armadillo skin test
P2-44154 Lepromin H skin test
  Lepromin human skin test
P2-44156 Fernandez reaction to lepromin
P2-44157 Mitsuda reaction to lepromin
P2-44200 Photosensitivity test, NOS
P2-44210 Ophthalmic mucous membrane test

2-45 ADMINISTRATION OF THERAPEUTIC AND PROPHYLACTIC SUBSTANCES

P2-45000 Administration of therapeutic substance, NOS
  Infusion of drug, NOS
  Injection of therapeutic substance, NOS
  Injection of medication, NOS
  Infusion of therapeutic substance, NOS
  Infusion of medication, NOS
  Injection of drug, NOS
P2-45010 Administration of anti-infective agent, NOS
  Injection of anti-infective agent, NOS
  Infusion of anti-infective agent, NOS
P2-45012 Administration of antibiotic
  Injection of antibiotic
  Infusion of antibiotic
P2-45020 Administration of hormone, NOS
  Intra-arterial infusion of hormone substance
  Hormone therapy perfusion
  Injection of hormone, NOS
  Infusion of hormone, NOS
P2-45022 Administration of steroid
  Injection of steroid
  Infusion of steroid
P2-45024 Administration of cortisone
  Injection of cortisone
  Infusion of cortisone
P2-45028 Administration of insulin
  Injection of insulin
  Infusion of insulin
P2-45040 Administration of tranquilizer
  Infusion of tranquilizer
  Injection of tranquilizer
P2-45200 Administration of immune serum
  Injection of immune serum
  Infusion of immune serum
P2-45210 Administration of Rh immune globulin
  Injection of Rh immune globulin
  Injection of gamma globulin
  Injection of Rhogam
P2-45300 Administration of antidote, NOS
  Injection of antidote, NOS
  Infusion of antidote, NOS
P2-45310 Administration of antivenin, NOS
  Injection of antivenin
  Infusion of antivenin
P2-45340 Administration of antitoxin, NOS
  Infusion of antitoxin, NOS
  Injection of antitoxin, NOS
P2-45341 Administration of tetanus antitoxin
  Infusion of tetanus antitoxin
  Injection of tetanus antitoxin
P2-45342 Administration of gas gangrene antitoxin
  Infusion of gas gangrene antitoxin
  Injection of gas gangrene antitoxin
P2-45343 Administration of botulism antitoxin
  Infusion of botulism antitoxin
  Injection of botulism antitoxin
P2-45344 Administration of diphtheria antitoxin
  Infusion of diphtheria antitoxin
  Injection of diphtheria antitoxin
P2-45345 Administration of scarlet fever antitoxin
  Infusion of scarlet fever antitoxin
  Injection of scarlet fever antitoxin
P2-45380 Administration of heavy metal antagonist, NOS
  Injection of heavy metal antagonist, NOS
  Infusion of heavy metal antagonist, NOS
P2-45400 Administration of anticoagulant, NOS
  Infusion of anticoagulant, NOS
  Injection of anticoagulant, NOS
P2-45500 Administration of electrolytes, NOS
  Infusion of electrolytes, NOS
P2-45510 Administration of saline solution
  Infusion of saline solution, NOS
  Intra-arterial infusion of saline, NOS

2-47 HUMAN VACCINATIONS

P2-47000 Vaccination, NOS
  Immunization, NOS
P2-47001 Vaccination by injection gun
P2-47002 Active immunization
P2-47004 Passive immunization
P2-47006 Booster immunization
P2-47008 Autogenous immunization
P2-47010 Cholera vaccination
  Cholera immunization
P2-47012 Typhoid vaccination
  Typhoid immunization
P2-47014 Paratyphoid fever vaccination
  Paratyphoid fever immunization
P2-47016 Typhoid-paratyphoid vaccination
  Typhoid-paratyphoid immunization

P2-47020 BCG vaccination
Tuberculosis vaccination
Tuberculosis immunization
BCG immunization
P2-47022 Plague vaccination
Plague immunization
P2-47024 Tularemia vaccination
Tularemia immunization
P2-47026 Pertussis vaccination
Whooping cough immunization
Pertussis immunization
P2-47027 Diphtheria immunization
Administration of diphtheria toxoid
P2-47028 Tetanus immunization
Administration of tetanus toxoid
P2-47030 DPT immunization
Administration of DPT toxoid
Administration of combined diphtheria pertussis tetanus toxoid
P2-47032 Poliomyelitis vaccination
Poliomyelitis immunization
P2-47034 Smallpox vaccination
Smallpox immunization
P2-47038 Rabies vaccination
Rabies immunization
Hydrophobia vaccination
P2-47040 Measles vaccination
Measles immunization
Rubeola vaccination
P2-47042 Infectious parotitis vaccination
Epidemic parotitis immunization
Mumps vaccination
Mumps immunization
P2-47046 German measles vaccination
Rubella vaccination
Rubella immunization
German measles immunization
P2-47050 Measles-mumps-rubella vaccination
MMR triple vaccination
MMR vaccination
P2-47060 Brucellosis vaccination
Undulant fever vaccination
Brucellosis immunization
P2-47062 Meningococcus vaccination
Meningococcus immunization
P2-47064 Staphylococcus vaccination
Staphylococcus immunization
P2-47066 Streptococcus vaccination
Streptococcus immunization
P2-47070 Salmonella vaccination
Salmonella immunization
P2-47080 Typhus vaccination
Typhus immunization
P2-47090 Anthrax vaccination
Anthrax immunization
P2-47100 Rocky Mountain spotted fever vaccination
P2-47120 Hemophilus influenzae immunization
P2-47400 Viral immunization, NOS
P2-47410 Vaccination for arthropod-borne virus, NOS
P2-47412 Vaccination for arthropod-borne viral encephalitis
P2-47420 Common cold vaccination
P2-47422 Influenza vaccination
Influenza immunization
P2-47424 Yellow fever vaccination
Yellow fever immunization
P2-47900 Immunization for autoimmune disease, NOS
P2-47990 Emergency immunization during epidemic
P2-47991 Elective immunization for international travel
P2-47992 Immunization in infancy

2-48 VETERINARY IMMUNIZATION PROCEDURES

P2-48000V Veterinary immunization procedure, NOS
P2-48100V Immunization for canine distemper
P2-48102V Immunization for canine distemper/hepatitis
P2-48104V Immunization for canine leptospirosis
P2-48106V Immunization for canine distemper/hepatitis/leptospirosis
P2-48108V Animal immunization for influenza
P2-48110V Immunization for rhinotracheitis/FPL/calici
P2-48112V Immunization for measles/distemper
P2-48114V Immunization for panleukopenia
P2-48116V Immunization for EIA
P2-48118V Animal immunization for rabies
Rabies animal inoculation
P2-48120V Immunization for rhinopneumonitis
P2-48122V Immunization for enterotoxemia
P2-48124V Immunization for parvovirus
P2-48126V Immunization for feline leukemia
P2-48128V Immunization for bordetella
P2-48130V Immunization for rhinotracheitis/calici
P2-48132V Immunization for rhinotracheitis
P2-48134V Immunization for encephalitis virus
P2-48135V Coronavirus vaccination

2-4A BREAST EXAMINATIONS AND PROCEDURES

P2-4A000 Examination of breast, NOS
P2-4A010 Manual examination of breast
P2-4A100 Manual extraction of milk from lactating breast
P2-4A110 Pump extraction of milk from lactating breast

SECTION 2-5 MEDICAL PROCEDURES ON THE GASTROINTESTINAL TRACT

2-50-52 GENERAL MEDICAL PROCEDURES ON THE GASTROINTESTINAL TRACT AND ORGANS

P2-50000 Digestive tract service or procedure, NOS
P2-50010 Medical procedure on gastrointestinal tract, NOS
P2-50020 Assessment of nutritional status, NOS
P2-50030V Deworming, NOS
Worming by anthelminthic

2-50-52 GENERAL MEDICAL PROCEDURES ON THE GASTROINTESTINAL TRACT AND ORGANS — Continued

P2-50060 Hyperalimentation, NOS
- PPN
- Peripheral parenteral nutrition
- TPN
- Parenteral alimentation
- Total parenteral nutrition

P2-50099 Digestive tract consultation and report, NOS
P2-50100 Medical procedure on mouth, NOS
P2-50110 Inspection of mouth
P2-50150 Medical procedure on floor of mouth, NOS
P2-50200 Medical procedure on lips, NOS
P2-50250 Medical procedure on vestibule of mouth, NOS
P2-50300 Medical procedure on tongue, NOS
P2-50400 Medical procedure on palate, NOS
P2-50450 Medical procedure on uvula, NOS
P2-50500 Medical procedure on salivary gland, NOS
P2-50600 Medical procedure on pharynx, NOS
P2-50700 Medical procedure on esophagus, NOS
P2-50760 Esophageal manometry
P2-50800 Medical procedure on stomach, NOS
P2-50850 Gastric intubation and aspiration, NOS
P2-50851 Gastric intubation and aspiration after stimulation, NOS
P2-50852 Gastric intubation, aspiration and fractional collections, one hour
P2-50854 Gastric intubation, aspiration and fractional collections, two hours
P2-50856 Gastric intubation, aspiration and fractional collections, two hours, including gastric stimulation
P2-50859 Gastric intubation, aspiration and fractional collections, three hours, including gastric stimulation
P2-50860V Rumen fluid collection and examination
P2-51000 Medical procedure on intestine, NOS
P2-51010 Medical procedure on small intestine, NOS
P2-51100 Medical procedure on duodenum, NOS
P2-51150 Digital examination of enterostomy stoma
P2-51160 Duodenal intubation and aspiration, NOS
- Duodenal intubation and aspiration, single specimen

P2-51170 Duodenal intubation and aspiration, multiple specimens with pancreatic or gallbladder stimulation
P2-51200 Medical procedure on jejunum, NOS
P2-51300 Medical procedure on ileum, NOS
P2-51360 Ileostomy management and care
P2-52000 Medical procedure on large intestine, NOS
P2-52010 Medical procedure on colon, NOS
P2-52050 Enterostomy management and care, NOS
P2-52055 Digital examination of colostomy stoma
P2-52060 Colostomy management and care
P2-52100 Medical procedure on cecum, NOS
P2-52150 Medical procedure on appendix, NOS
P2-52200 Medical procedure on sigmoid, NOS
P2-52300 Medical procedure on rectum, NOS
P2-52310 Rectal examination, NOS
- Digital palpation of rectum
- Digital examination of rectum

P2-52320 Removal of impacted feces
P2-52324 Transanal enema, NOS
P2-52330 Enema for removal of impacted feces
P2-52340 Removal of fecal impaction under anesthesia
P2-52400 Medical procedure on anus, NOS
P2-52440 Medical procedure on perirectal tissue, NOS
- Medical procedure on perianal tissue, NOS

P2-52450 Electromyography studies of anal sphincter, any technique
P2-52499 Medical procedure on rectum, rectosigmoid and perirectal tissue, NOS
P2-52610 Palpation of liver
P2-52700 Medical procedure on gallbladder, NOS
P2-52800 Medical procedure on biliary tract, NOS
P2-52820 Pressure measurement of sphincter of Oddi
P2-52830 Nonoperative removal of prosthesis of bile duct
P2-52900 Medical procedure on pancreas, NOS

2-53 GASTROINTESTINAL CONTENT ANALYSES AND MEASUREMENTS

P2-53000 Gastric analysis, NOS
P2-53010 Gastric fluid analysis, free acid measurement
P2-53012 Gastric fluid analysis, total acid measurement
P2-53013 Gastric fluid analysis, free and total acid measurement
P2-53014 Gastric fluid analysis, pH titration
- Gastric fluid analysis, pH determination

P2-53020 Gastric fluid analysis, food, forensic
P2-53030 Tubeless gastric analysis and measurement, NOS
P2-53040 Blood in gastric contents measurement
P2-53050 Guaiac test, NOS
- Screening for occult blood in feces

SECTION 2-6 MEDICAL PROCEDURES ON THE ENDOCRINE AND HEMATOPOIETIC SYSTEMS

2-60-61 MEDICAL PROCEDURES ON THE ENDOCRINE SYSTEM

P2-60000 Medical procedure on endocrine system, NOS
P2-61100 Medical procedure on adrenal gland, NOS
P2-61200 Medical procedure on pituitary gland, NOS
P2-61300 Medical procedure on pineal gland, NOS

2-66 GENERAL MEDICAL PROCEDURES ON THE HEMATOIETIC SYSTEM

P2-66000 Medical procedure on hematopoietic system, NOS

P2-66100 Medical procedure on spleen, NOS
P2-66112 Palpation of spleen
P2-66200 Medical procedure on tonsils, NOS
P2-66300 Medical procedure on adenoids, NOS
P2-66400 Medical procedure on lymphatic system, NOS
P2-66410 Medical procedure on thoracic duct, NOS
P2-66420 Perfusion of lymphatics with hyperthermia, NOS
P2-66422 Perfusion of lymphatics with hyperthermia, localized
P2-66500 Medical procedure on thymus, NOS

2-67 ONCOLOGIC PROCEDURES

P2-67000 Oncologic procedure, NOS
P2-67010 Chemotherapy, NOS
P2-67011 Parenteral chemotherapy for malignant neoplasm
P2-67012 Infusion chemotherapy for malignant neoplasm
P2-67013 Perfusion chemotherapy for malignant neoplasm
P2-67014 Intracavitary chemotherapy for malignant neoplasm
P2-67015 Oral chemotherapy for malignant neoplasm
P2-67016 Local chemotherapy for malignant neoplasm
P2-67017 Topical chemotherapy for malignant neoplasm
P2-67020 Chemotherapy for non-malignant neoplasm, NOS
P2-67021 Chemotherapy for non-neoplastic disease, NOS
P2-67030 Leukovorin rescue
P2-67040 Treatment planning for chemotherapy, NOS
P2-67042 Treatment planning for chemotherapy, primary course
P2-67044 Treatment planning for chemotherapy, secondary course
P2-67050 Chemotherapy administration, intra-arterial, push technique
P2-67051 Chemotherapy administration, intra-arterial, infusion technique
P2-67052 Chemotherapy administration, intra-arterial, infusion technique, one to 8 hours, each additional hour
P2-67053 Chemotherapy administration, intra-arterial, infusion technique, initiation of prolonged infusion, more than 8 hours, requiring the use of a portable or implantable pump
P2-67054 Chemotherapy administration, subcutaneous, with local anesthesia
P2-67055 Chemotherapy administration, subcutaneous, without local anesthesia
P2-67099 Consultation in chemotherapy

2-68 BLOOD TRANSFUSIONS

P2-68000 Transfusion, NOS
P2-68010 Transfusion of whole blood
P2-68012 Transfusion of packed red blood cells
  Transfusion of PRBC
P2-68013 Transfusion of serum
P2-68020 Transfusion of blood expander, NOS
P2-68022 Transfusion of dextran
P2-68026 Transfusion of blood component
P2-68027 Platelet transfusion
  Transfusion of thrombocytes
P2-68030 Transfusion of coagulation factors
P2-68032 Transfusion of antihemophilic factor
P2-68040 Exchange transfusion
  Transfusion replacement, total
  Exsanguination transfusion
  Exchange transfusion of blood, except newborn
P2-68050 Autotransfusion, NOS
P2-68051 Autotransfusion of whole blood
P2-68060 Intrauterine transfusion
  Fetal transfusion
P2-68100 Plasma exchange
P2-68110 Plasmapheresis
P2-68120 Leukopheresis
P2-68130 Plateletpheresis
P2-68300 Therapeutic apheresis, NOS
P2-68350 Extracorporeal photopheresis
P2-68360V Erythropoietin therapy

2-69 IMMUNOLOGIC PROCEDURES

P2-69000 In vivo immunologic procedure, NOS
P2-69010 Immunologic evaluation, NOS
  Determination of immunologic status, NOS
P2-69100 Desensitization therapy, NOS
P2-69200 Immunotherapy, NOS
P2-69300 Biological response modifier therapy, NOS
P2-69310 Cytokine therapy, NOS
P2-69320 Interleukin-2 therapy
  Il-2 therapy
P2-69350 Lymphokine activated killer cell therapy
  LAK cell therapy

SECTION 2-7 MEDICAL PROCEDURES ON THE URINARY SYSTEM

2-70 GENERAL URINARY SYSTEM PROCEDURES

P2-70000 Medical procedure on genitourinary system, NOS
P2-70010 Medical procedure on urinary system, NOS
P2-70020 Medical procedure on kidney, NOS
  Renal medical procedure, NOS
P2-70030 Medical procedure on perirenal tissue, NOS
P2-70040 Medical procedure on ureter, NOS
P2-70050 Medical procedure on bladder, NOS
P2-70060 Medical procedure on perivesical tissue, NOS
P2-70070 Medical procedure on urethra, NOS
P2-70080 Medical procedure on periurethral tissue, NOS
P2-70100 Renal function study, NOS
P2-70120 Measurement of renal clearance

2-70 GENERAL URINARY SYSTEM PROCEDURES — Continued

P2-70200 Urostomy management and care, NOS
 Stoma management and care of urinary tract, NOS
P2-70300 Calibration of urethra
P2-70310 Measurement of bulbocavernosus reflex latency time

2-71 URINARY PRESSURE AND FLOW PROCEDURES

P2-71000 Urinary pressure and flow study, NOS
P2-71010 Urinary manometry, NOS
P2-71012 Manometric studies through pyelostomy tube
P2-71014 Manometric studies through indwelling ureteral catheter
P2-71016 Manometric studies through ureterostomy
P2-71018 Manometric studies through nephrostomy tube
P2-71100 Cystometrogram, NOS
P2-71102 Simple cystometrogram
P2-71104 Complex cystometrogram
P2-71120 Voiding pressure studies of bladder, NOS
 VP studies of bladder
P2-71122 Voiding pressure studies, intra-abdominal voiding pressure
P2-71140 Urethral pressure profile study, NOS
P2-71142 Urethral sphincter function study
P2-71144 Electromyography of urethral sphincter
P2-71200 Uroflowmetry, NOS
P2-71202 Simple uroflowmetry
P2-71204 Complex uroflowmetry
P2-71210 Sound recording of external stream

2-74 URINARY BLADDER TRAINING AND REHABILITATION PROCEDURES

P2-74000 Urinary bladder training, NOS
P2-74020 Child continence training
P2-74040 Bladder retraining
P2-74100 Neurogenic bladder rehabilitation

2-77 DIALYSIS PROCEDURES

P2-77000 Hemodialysis, NOS
 Kidney dialysis, NOS
 Extracorporeal hemodialysis, NOS
 Renal dialysis, NOS
 Extracorporeal hemofiltration, NOS
 Artificial kidney dialysis, NOS
P2-77010 Initial hemodialysis
P2-77030 Stabilizing hemodialysis
P2-77040 Hemodialysis, maintenance at home
P2-77045 Hemodialysis, supervision at home
P2-77050 Hemodialysis, maintenance in hospital
P2-77060 Hemodialysis training, NOS
P2-77065 Hemodialysis training at home
P2-77080 Hemodialysis counseling
P2-77500 Peritoneal dialysis, NOS
P2-77510 Peritoneal dialysis including cannulation
P2-77520 Peritoneal dialysis excluding cannulation
P2-77530 Peritoneal dialysis counseling
P2-77540 Peritoneal dialysis training
P2-77550 Supervision of chronic ambulatory peritoneal dialysis, outpatient
P2-77590 Special dialysis procedure, explain by report

SECTION 2-8 MEDICAL PROCEDURES ON THE FEMALE GENITAL SYSTEM INCLUDING REPRODUCTION

2-80 GENERAL MEDICAL PROCEDURES AND EXAMINATIONS ON THE FEMALE GENITAL SYSTEM

P2-80000 Medical procedure on female genital system, NOS
P2-80010 Nonobstetrical medical procedure on female genital system
P2-80020 Medical procedure on labia, NOS
P2-80030 Medical procedure on vagina, NOS
P2-80040 Diagnostic procedure on uterus and supporting structures, NOS
P2-80050 Medical procedure on uterine ligament, NOS
P2-80054 Medical procedure on cervix, NOS
P2-80060 Medical procedure on ovary, NOS
P2-80070 Medical procedure on fallopian tube, NOS
P2-80080 Medical procedure on cul-de-sac, NOS
P2-80100 Gynecologic examination
P2-80110 Manual pelvic examination
P2-80112 Pelvic examination under anesthesia
 Gynecologic examination under general anesthesia
 Pelvic examination under general anesthesia
P2-80120 Gynecologic pelvimetry
P2-80200 Examination of vagina, NOS
P2-80210 Manual palpation of vagina
P2-80230 Application of medication for treatment of bacterial disease of vagina
P2-80232 Application of medication for treatment of fungoid disease of vagina
P2-80234 Application of medication for treatment of parasitic disease of vagina
P2-80300 Manual examination of uterus
 Manual exploration of uterus
P2-80310 Measurement of intrauterine pressure
P2-80320 Diaphragm fitting with instructions
P2-80322 Fitting of pessary
P2-80324 Fitting of intrauterine device
P2-80350V Acetowhitening of cervix

2-87 MEDICAL PROCEDURES AND SERVICES RELATED TO REPRODUCTION

P2-87000 Medical procedure related to reproduction, NOS

P2-87010 Pregnancy detection examination
P2-87020 Prenatal examination and care of mother
Antepartum care of mother
P2-87100 Natural childbirth instruction, class
P2-87110 Natural childbirth instruction, individual
P2-87200 Pre-admission observation, undelivered mother
P2-87250 Medical induction of labor
P2-87300 Post-partum examination and care of mother
Pregnancy follow-up examination
P2-87400 Fetal oxytocin stress test
P2-87500 Infertility study, NOS
P2-87520 Infertility therapy, NOS
P2-87522 Test tube ovum fertilization
P2-87524 Embryo transfer
P2-87600 Artificial insemination, NOS
P2-87601 Artificial insemination, homologous
P2-87602 Artificial insemination, heterologous
P2-88620 Artificial insemination with sperm washing and capacitation

SECTION 2-9 MEDICAL PROCEDURES ON THE NERVOUS SYSTEM

2-90 GENERAL NEUROLOGICAL PROCEDURES AND ASSESSMENTS

P2-90000 Medical procedure on the nervous system, NOS
P2-90010 Medical procedure on the central nervous system, NOS
P2-90020 Medical procedure on the peripheral nervous system, NOS
P2-90030 Neurological or neuromuscular medical procedure, NOS
P2-90100 Neurological examination, NOS
P2-90110 Transillumination of newborn skull
P2-90120 Stereotactic computer assisted volumetric intracranial measurement
P2-90200 Neurological mental status determination, NOS
P2-90600 Assessment and interpretation of higher cerebral function, NOS
P2-90610 Assessment and interpretation of higher cerebral function, aphasia testing
Aphasia testing and assessment
P2-90620 Assessment and interpretation of higher cerebral function, cognitive testing
Cognitive testing and assessment
P2-90630 Assessment and interpretation of higher cerebral function, developmental testing
Developmental testing and assessment

2-91 ELECTROENCEPHALOGRAPHIC PROCEDURES

P2-91000 Electroencephalographic procedure, NOS
P2-91100 Electroencephalogram, NOS
EEG, NOS
P2-91110 Portable electroencephalogram, NOS
Portable EEG, NOS
P2-91130 Electroencephalogram awake and drowsy with stimulation, NOS
P2-91134 Electroencephalogram awake and drowsy with hyperventilation and/or photic stimulation
P2-91140 Portable electroencephalogram awake and drowsy with stimulation, NOS
P2-91144 Portable electroencephalogram awake and drowsy with hyperventilation and/or photic stimulation
P2-91150 Electroencephalogram awake and asleep with stimulation, NOS
P2-91154 Electroencephalogram awake and asleep with hyperventilation and/or photic stimulation
P2-91160 Portable electroencephalogram awake and asleep with stimulation, NOS
P2-91164 Portable electroencephalogram awake and asleep with hyperventilation and/or photic stimulation
P2-91170 Electroencephalogram for monitoring at surgery
P2-91172 Electroencephalogram during nonintracranial surgery
EEG during nonintracranial surgery
P2-91174 Electroencephalogram during carotid surgery
P2-91180 Electroencephalogram with physical activation, only
P2-91190 Electroencephalogram with pharmacological activation, only
P2-91200 Sleep electroencephalogram
P2-91210 Sleep electroencephalogram, all night
P2-91220 Electroencephalogram for evaluation of cerebral death
P2-91230 Video and radio-telemetered electroencephalographic monitoring
P2-91300 Monitoring for localization of cerebral seizure focus by EEG or radiotelemetry, initial 24 hours
P2-91310 Monitoring for localization of cerebral seizure focus by EEG or radiotelemetry, each additional 24 hours
P2-91320 Monitoring for localization of cerebral seizure focus by EEG or radiotelemetry, combined electroencephalographic and video recording
P2-91330 Pharmacological activation during prolonged monitoring for localization of cerebral seizure focus
P2-91340 Wada activation test for hemispheric function including electroencephalographic EEG monitoring
Wada activation test with EEG monitoring
P2-91400 Electrocorticogram, NOS
ECoG, NOS
P2-91410 Electrocorticogram during surgery
P2-91420 Electrocorticogram with photic stimulation
P2-91500 Intracerebral electroencephalogram, NOS
Depth EEG

2-91 ELECTROENCEPHALOGRAPHIC PROCEDURES — Continued

P2-91500 (cont.) Intracerebral EEG

2-93 SENSORY AND MOTOR TESTING PROCEDURES

P2-93000 Sensory and motor testing, NOS
P2-93010 Sensory testing, NOS
P2-93020 Motor testing, NOS
P2-93100 Somatosensory testing, NOS
P2-93110 Orbicularis oculi reflex test
  Blink reflex test
P2-93120 Facial nerve function study
P2-93500 Cerebral evoked potential test, NOS
P2-93510 Evoked stimulus response testing, NOS
P2-93520 "H" reflex study by electrodiagnostic testing
P2-93530 "F" reflex study by electrodiagnostic testing
P2-93600 Nerve conduction study, NOS
P2-93610 Nerve conduction study for velocity and/or latency, NOS
P2-93630 Motor nerve conduction study for velocity and/or latency
P2-93640 Sensory nerve conduction study for velocity and/or latency
P2-93700 Neuromuscular junction testing, NOS
P2-93710 Neuromuscular junction testing by repetitive stimulation
P2-93720 Neuromuscular junction testing with paired stimuli
P2-93802 Stimulation of carotid sinus with ECG monitoring
P2-93804 Intracarotid amobarbitral test
P2-93810 Ergonovine provocation test

2-95 SLEEP DISORDER TESTS AND PROCEDURES

P2-95000 Sleep disorder function test, NOS
P2-95100 Polysomnography, NOS
  Polysomnogram, NOS
P2-95110 Polysomnograph recording, analysis and interpretation of the multiple simultaneous physiologic measurements of sleep
P2-95200 Somnocinematography
P2-95300 Sleep apnea recording, NOS
P2-95310 Sleep apnea monitoring with alarm

SECTION 2-A MEDICAL PROCEDURES ON THE EYE, EAR AND RELATED STRUCTURES

2-A0-A5 MEDICAL PROCEDURES ON THE EYE AND RELATED STRUCTURES

2-A0 GENERAL EYE EXAMINATIONS AND PROCEDURES

P2-A0000 Medical procedure on eye and related structures, NOS
P2-A0002 Ophthalmic service or procedure, NOS
P2-A0004 Medical procedure on eye, NOS
  Ophthalmologic medical procedure, NOS
  Ocular medical procedure, NOS
  Medical procedure on eyeball, NOS
P2-A0008 Medical procedure on orbit, NOS
P2-A0010 Ophthalmic examination and evaluation, NOS
  Eye examination, NOS
P2-A0012 Visual acuity testing, NOS
P2-A0014 Ophthalmic examination and evaluation, follow-up
P2-A0016V Schirmer tear test
P2-A0020 Limited eye examination
P2-A0030 Comprehensive eye examination
  Extended ophthalmologic work-up
P2-A0040 Eye examination under anesthesia, NOS
P2-A0042 Eye examination under anesthesia, limited
  Ophthalmologic examination and evaluation under general anesthesia, limited
P2-A0044 Eye examination under anesthesia, complete
  Ophthalmologic examination and evaluation under general anesthesia, complete
P2-A0050 Color vision examination, NOS
P2-A0052 Color vision examination, extended
P2-A0060 Dark adaptation study, NOS
P2-A0070 Gonioscopy with evaluation, NOS
P2-A0078 Ocular slit lamp examination
P2-A0080V Placement of collagen shield on cornea
P2-A0082V Corneal gluing
P2-A0090 Ophthalmologic counseling and instruction
P2-A0100 Ophthalmoscopy, NOS
  Ophthalmoscopic examination, NOS
  Fundoscopy, NOS
P2-A0110 Ophthalmoscopy under general anesthesia
P2-A0120 Ophthalmoscopy with medical evaluation, extended, with ophthalmodynamometry
P2-A0130 Ophthalmoscopy with medical evaluation, extended, for retinal detachment mapping
P2-A0140 Ophthalmoscopy with medical evaluation, extended, with fluorescein angiography
  Fluorescein angiography of eye
P2-A0150 Ophthalmoscopy with medical evaluation, extended, with fundus photography
P2-A0200 Visual field study, NOS

P2-A0201 Visual field examination and evaluation, limited
P2-A0202 Visual field examination and evaluation, intermediate
P2-A0203 Visual field examination and evaluation, extended
P2-A0300 Tracer study of eye, NOS
P2-A0310 P32 tracer study of eye
P2-A0510 Eikonometric examination including prescribing lenses
P2-A0800 Visual evoked potential study, NOS
  VEP study, NOS
P2-A0850 Electroretinography with medical evaluation
  Electroretinogram with medical evaluation

2-A2 OCULAR PHOTOGRAPHY AND EVALUATION

P2-A2000 External ocular photography for medical evaluation and documentation, NOS
P2-A2004 Ocular photography, close up
P2-A2010 Ocular photography for medical evaluation and documentation, goniophotography
  Goniophotography of eye
P2-A2020 Ocular photography for medical evaluation and documentation, slit lamp photography
  Slit lamp photography of eye
P2-A2030 Ocular photography for medical evaluation and documentation, stereophotography
  Stereophotography of eye
P2-A2034V Donaldson stereophotography
P2-A2040 Ocular photography of anterior segment with specular endothelial microscopy and cell count
P2-A2042 Ocular photography of anterior segment with fluorescein angiography
P2-A2050 Ocular fundus photography
P2-A2054V Kowa fundus photography

2-A3 TONOMETRY AND TONOGRAPHY PROCEDURES

P2-A3000 Tonometry-tonography with evaluation, NOS
P2-A3010 Tonography with medical evaluation, indentation tonometer method
P2-A3020 Tonography with medical evaluation, perilimbal suction method
P2-A3030 Tonography with provocative tests
P2-A3040 Tonography with water provocation
P2-A3046 Provocative test for increased intraocular pressure for glaucoma
P2-A3050 Serial tonometry-tonography with evaluation
P2-A3060 Exophthalmometry, NOS
P2-A3100 Ophthalmodynamometry, NOS
P2-A3120 Ophthalmodynamography, NOS

2-A4 OCULAR MOTILITY STUDIES AND PROCEDURES

P2-A4000 Ocular motility study, NOS
P2-A4100 Electro-oculogram examination
  Electro-oculography with medical evaluation
P2-A4120 Electromyogram examination of eye
  Oculoelectromyography with medical evaluation
P2-A4200 Nystagmus test, NOS
P2-A4202 Spontaneous nystagmus test including gaze
P2-A4204 Spontaneous nystagmus test including gaze and fixation nystagmus with recording
P2-A4210 Positional nystagmus test
P2-A4212 Positional nystagmus test with recording
P2-A4214 Positional nystagmus test with minimum of 4 positions with recording
P2-A4230 Optokinetic nystagmus test
P2-A4232 Optokinetic nystagmus test, bidirectional, with recording
P2-A4234 Optokinetic nystagmus test, bidirectional, with foveal or peripheral stimulation with recording
P2-A4250 Electronystagmogram, NOS
  Electronystagmography, NOS
  ENG examination, NOS
P2-A4252 Electronystagmography with vertical electrodes
P2-A4280 Oscillating tracking test with recording

2-A5 VISUAL CORRECTION, TRAINING AND REEDUCATION PROCEDURES

P2-A5000 Prosthetic or spectacle service, NOS
P2-A5002 Ocular prosthetic service, NOS
  Prescribing and fitting of ocular prosthesis
P2-A5004 Prescribing, fitting and supervision of ocular prosthesis
P2-A5006 Prescribing, fitting and supply of ocular prosthesis
P2-A5010 Ocular refraction procedure, NOS
P2-A5100 Fitting and dispensing of spectacles, NOS
P2-A5110 Facial measurement and fitting of spectacles, single focus
P2-A5112 Fitting of spectacles, bifocal
P2-A5113 Fitting of spectacles, monofocal
P2-A5114 Fitting of spectacles, multifocal
P2-A5120 Fitting of spectacles, low vision aid, single element
P2-A5122 Fitting of spectacles, low vision aid, telescopic or other compound lens system
P2-A5128 Dispensing of unlisted low vision aid
P2-A5130 Prescribing spectacles for aphakia, NOS
P2-A5140 Repair and refitting spectacles
P2-A5150 Supply of spectacles, NOS
P2-A5200 Prescription, fitting and dispensing of contact lens
P2-A5204 Prescribing, fitting and revision of contact lens
P2-A5206 Modification of contact lens
P2-A5210 Prescribing corneal contact lens
P2-A5220 Prescribing corneoscleral contact lens
P2-A5222 Prescribing, fitting and revision of corneoscleral contact lens

2-A5 VISUAL CORRECTION, TRAINING AND REEDUCATION PROCEDURES — Continued

P2-A5230 Prescribing contact lens for aphakia, NOS
P2-A5231 Prescribing contact lens for aphakia, unilateral
P2-A5232 Prescribing contact lens for aphakia, bilateral
P2-A5238 Replacement of contact lens
P2-A5500 Visual training and reeducation, NOS
P2-A5510 Orthoptic training, NOS
P2-A5512 Orthoptic training with continuing medical direction and evaluation
P2-A5520 Orthoptic-pleoptic training
P2-A5522 Orthoptic-pleoptic treatment
P2-A5524 Orthoptic-pleoptic evaluation with medical interpretation
P2-A5530 Pleoptic training with continuing medical direction and evaluation
P2-A5700 Visual rehabilitation, NOS
P2-A5710 Visual rehabilitation, braille reading
P2-A5720 Visual rehabilitation, eye motion defect
P2-A5730 Visual rehabilitation, visual defect

2-A7-A9 MEDICAL PROCEDURES ON THE EAR

2-A7 GENERAL MEDICAL EAR PROCEDURES AND SERVICES

P2-A7000 Medical procedure on ear, NOS
P2-A7010 Medical procedure on middle ear, NOS
P2-A7020 Medical procedure on inner ear, NOS
P2-A7030 Medical procedure on eustachian tube, NOS
P2-A7100 Medical evaluation of hearing problem, NOS
P2-A7104 Hearing examination, NOS
  Clinical test of hearing, NOS
P2-A7110 Medical evaluation of speech, language and hearing problem, NOS
P2-A7200 Consultation for hearing and/or speech problem

2-A8 AUDIOLOGIC AND AUDIOMETRIC TESTS INCLUDING VESTIBULAR FUNCTIONS

P2-A8000 Audiometric test, NOS
P2-A8004 Audiometric group testing, NOS
P2-A8010 Evoked response audiometry with EEG
  Brainstem evoked response with EEG
P2-A8020 Electrodermal audiometry
P2-A8030 Conditioning play audiometry
P2-A8040 Select picture audiometry
P2-A8100 Basic comprehensive audiometry testing
  Basic comprehensive audiometry testing pure tone, air and bone and speech, threshold and discrimination
P2-A8110 Basic pure tone audiometry, air only
P2-A8112 Basic pure tone audiometry, air and bone
P2-A8114 Basic speech audiometry, threshold only
P2-A8116 Basic speech audiometry, threshold and discrimination
P2-A8118 Speech audiometry, threshold only
P2-A8130 Speech audiometry, extended, filtered speech test
  Filtered speech test
P2-A8140 Speech audiometry, extended, staggered spondaic word test
  Staggered spondaic word test
P2-A8142 Speech audiometry, extended, Stenger test
  Stenger speech test
P2-A8146 Speech audiometry, extended, Lombard test
  Lombard speech test
P2-A8150 Speech audiometry, extended, swinging story test
  Swinging story test
P2-A8160 Speech audiometry, extended, sensorineural acuity level test
  Sensorineural acuity level test
P2-A8170 Speech audiometry, extended, synthetic sentence identification test
  Synthetic sentence identification test
P2-A8180 Speech audiometry, extended, delayed auditory feedback test
  Delayed auditory feedback test
P2-A8200 Screening test, pure tone, air only
P2-A8210 Pure tone audiometry, threshold, air only
P2-A8212 Pure tone audiometry, threshold, air and bone
P2-A8214 Pure tone audiometry, extended, Bekesy screening audiometry
  Bekesy screening audiometry
P2-A8216 Pure tone audiometry, extended, Bekesy diagnostic audiometry
  Bekesy diagnostic audiometry
P2-A8220 Pure tone audiometry, extended, loudness balance test
P2-A8222 Loudness balance test, alternate monaural
P2-A8224 Loudness balance test, alternate binaural
P2-A8240 Pure tone audiometry, extended, tone decay test
  Tone decay test
P2-A8250 Pure tone audiometry, extended, sensitivity index
  Short increment sensitivity index
  SISI index
P2-A8260 Pure tone audiometry, extended, Stenger test, pure tone
  Stenger test, pure tone
P2-A8270 Pure tone audiometry, extended, impedance testing
  Impedance testing
P2-A8300 Tympanometry testing, NOS
P2-A8500 Audiologic function test with medical evaluation, NOS
P2-A8510 Audiological evaluation
P2-A8520 Special audiometric function test, NOS
P2-A8524 Special audiologic evaluation for functional hearing loss
P2-A8530 Acoustic reflex testing
P2-A8532 Acoustic reflex decay test

P2-A8540 Central auditory function test, NOS
P2-A8550 Auditory rotation test
P2-A8554 Torsion swing test with recording
P2-A8600 Vestibular function test, NOS
P2-A8610 Vestibular function test with observation and evaluation by physician, NOS
P2-A8614 Vestibular function test with recording, NOS
P2-A8620 Caloric vestibular test, NOS
P2-A8622 Caloric vestibular test with recording
P2-A8650 Electrocochleography, NOS
P2-A8654 Use of vertical electrode in vestibular function test, NOS

2-A9 HEARING THERAPY AND AUDITORY REHABILITATION

P2-A9000 Hearing therapy, NOS
P2-A9010 Speech, language or hearing therapy with continuing medical supervision, individual
P2-A9020 Speech, language or hearing therapy with continuing medical supervision, group
P2-A9100 Evaluation for hearing aid and testing
P2-A9110 Hearing aid examination and selection, monaural
P2-A9112 Hearing aid examination and selection, binaural
P2-A9120 Electroacoustic evaluation for hearing aid, monaural
P2-A9122 Electroacoustic evaluation for hearing aid, binaural
P2-A9200 Fitting of hearing aid
P2-A9210 Hearing aid check, monaural
P2-A9212 Hearing aid check, binaural
P2-A9310 Ear protector attenuation measurements
P2-A9320 Focal application of phase control substance in middle ear
P2-A9500 Auditory rehabilitation, NOS
P2-A9600 Vestibular rehabilitation, NOS

SECTION 2-B MEDICAL PROCEDURES ON THE TOPOGRAPHIC REGIONS OF BODY

P2-B0000 Medical procedure on body region, NOS
P2-B1000 Medical procedure on thorax, NOS
  Medical procedure on chest wall, NOS
P2-B1010 Closed drainage of chest
  Closed drainage of thorax
P2-B1100 Medical procedure on mediastinum, NOS
P2-B1200 Medical procedure on diaphragm, NOS
P2-B1300 Medical procedure on abdomen, NOS
P2-B1310 Palpation of abdomen
P2-B1400 Medical procedure on peritoneum, NOS
P2-B1500 Medical procedure on retroperitoneum, NOS
P2-B1600 Medical procedure on omentum, NOS

CHAPTER 3 — LABORATORY PROCEDURES AND SERVICES

SECTION 3-0 GENERAL LABORATORY PROCEDURES AND SERVICES

3-00 GENERAL LABORATORY CONVENIENCE TERMS

P3-00010 General laboratory procedure, NOS
P3-00030 Laboratory test, NOS
P3-00040 Laboratory test order by laboratory initiative
P3-00044 Laboratory test order cancellation
P3-00050 Unsatisfactory clinical laboratory specimen identified
P3-00054 Clinical laboratory specimen rejection, NOS
P3-00060 Chain of custody procedure in laboratory specimen handling
P3-00130 Clinical laboratory specimen identification

3-02 SPECIMEN COLLECTION

P3-02000 Specimen collection, NOS
P3-02020 Venipuncture for blood test, NOS
  Phlebotomy for diagnostic test
  Venous specimen collection
P3-02040 Capillary specimen collection, NOS
P3-02041 Heel stick
P3-02042 Finger stick
  Finger puncture
  Capillary stick
P3-02043 Ear lobe stick
P3-02060 Arterial specimen collection for laboratory test
P3-02061 Radial artery puncture for laboratory test
P3-02062 Femoral artery puncture for laboratory test
P3-02063 Brachial artery puncture for laboratory test
P3-02100 Urine specimen collection, NOS
P3-02120 Urine specimen collection, 2 hours
P3-02140 Urine specimen collection, 12 hours
P3-02160 Urine specimen collection, 24 hours
  24 hour urine specimen collection
P3-02200 Urine specimen collection, clean catch
P3-02220 Urine specimen collection, catheterized
P3-02240 Urine specimen collection, closed drainage
P3-02260 Urine specimen collection, suprapubic
P3-02270 Specimen collection by drainage, NOS

3-05 SPECIMEN PROCESSING

P3-05000 Specimen processing, NOS
P3-05010 Specimen preparation, NOS
P3-05020 Specimen centrifugation
P3-05030 Specimen aliquoting
P3-05040 Specimen refrigeration
P3-05050 Specimen freezing
P3-05070 Specimen dispatch and referral, routine
P3-05074 Specimen dispatch and referral, complex

3-08 LABORATORY REPORTING

P3-08000 Laboratory reporting, NOS
P3-08010 Laboratory reporting, electronic
  Laboratory reporting, computer
P3-08020 Laboratory reporting, telephone
P3-08030 Laboratory reporting, fax
P3-08040 Laboratory reporting, verbal
P3-08060 Laboratory reporting, written report
P3-08070 Laboratory reporting, internal report
P3-08080 Laboratory reporting, cum sum

3-09 LABORATORY TEST PANELS

P3-09000 General health panel, NOS
P3-09010 Organ or system related test, NOS
  Diagnostic panel or profile, NOS
P3-09020 Arthritis panel
P3-09030 Lipid panel
P3-09100 Hepatic function panel
P3-09110 Hepatitis panel
P3-09200 Obstetric panel
P3-09300 Thyroid panel

SECTION 3-1 BLOOD COAGULATION PROCEDURES

P3-10000 Blood coagulation procedure, NOS
P3-10005 Special blood coagulation test, explain by report
P3-10010 Bleeding time, NOS
P3-10020 Bleeding time, Duke
P3-10030 Bleeding time, Ivy
P3-10040 Bleeding time, template
  Mielke template bleeding time
P3-10050 Bleeding time, quantitative
  Hemorrhagometry
P3-10070 Capillary fragility test
  Tourniquet test
  Rumpel-Leede test
P3-10100 Clot retraction, screen
P3-10120 Clot retraction, quantitative
P3-10130 Clot retraction, inhibition by drug
P3-10140 Clotting factor II assay
  Prothrombin assay
P3-10150 Clotting factor V assay
  Labile factor assay
  Proaccelerin assay
  Factor V assay
  Ac-Globulin assay
P3-10160 Clotting factor VII assay
  Factor VII assay
  Stable factor assay
  Proconvertin assay
  Autoprothrombin I assay
P3-10170 Clotting factor VIII assay, NOS
  AHF assay, NOS
  Antihemophilic factor assay, NOS
P3-10172 Factor VIII: C assay
  Factor VIII coagulation activity
P3-10180 Factor VIII C: Ag assay
  Factor VIII antigen assay

P3-10190 Factor VIII R: Ag assay
Factor VIII related antigen assay
P3-10200 Factor VIII R: WF assay
von Willebrand factor assay
Factor VIII ristocetin response
Factor VIII aggregation activity
P3-10220 Factor VIII R: R Co assay
Ristocetin cofactor assay
P3-10230 Factor VIII assay, one stage
P3-10240 Factor VIII assay, two stage
P3-10250 von Willebrand factor multimer assay
vWF multimer assay
P3-10290 Clotting factor IX assay
Autoprothrombin II assay
Christmas disease factor assay
Factor IX assay
Hemophilia B assay
Plasma thromboplastin component assay
P3-10300 Clotting factor X assay
Factor X assay
Stuart factor assay
Stuart-Prower factor assay
P3-10320 Clotting factor XI assay
Factor XI assay
Plasma thromboplastin antecedent assay
PTA assay
P3-10330 Clotting factor XII assay
Factor XII assay
Hageman factor assay
P3-10340 Clotting factor XIII assay
Factor XIII assay
Fibrinoligase assay
Laki-Lorand factor assay
Fibrin stabilizing factor assay
P3-10350 Clotting factor XIII assay, screen
P3-10360 Fitzgerald factor assay
High molecular weight kininogen assay
HMW kininogen assay
Williams-Fitzgerald Flaujeac factor assay
P3-10370 Fletcher factor assay
Prekallikrein assay
P3-10380 Antithrombin III assay, NOS
P3-10390 Antithrombin III assay, functional
P3-10400 Antithrombin III assay, immunologic
Antithrombin III assay, antigenic
P3-10410 Circulating anticoagulant assay, NOS
Clotting factor inhibitor assay, NOS
Circulating inhibitor assay, NOS
P3-10412 Fibrinogen inhibitor assay, NOS
P3-10414 Factor XIII inhibitor assay, NOS
P3-10420 Lupus anticoagulant assay, NOS
Lupus inhibitor assay, NOS
P3-10440 Tissue thromboplastin inhibitor assay
TTI assay
P3-10450 Circulating inhibitor assay, factor VIII
Factor VIII inhibitor assay
P3-10460 Circulating inhibitor assay, factor IX
Factor IX inhibitor assay
P3-10470 Circulating inhibitor assay, factor II
Factor II inhibitor assay
P3-10480 Antithrombin III, heparin cofactor assay
Heparin cofactor assay
P3-10490 Protein S assay, NOS
P3-10500 Protein S, functional assay
P3-10510 Protein S, antigenic assay
P3-10520 Protein S, free assay
P3-10530 Protein C, assay, NOS
P3-10540 Protein C, functional assay
P3-10550 Protein C, antigenic assay
P3-10560 Clotting test with substitution, NOS
Substituted clotting test, NOS
Clotting test, mixtures, NOS
P3-10570 Prothrombin time
PT
Protime
Quick one stage prothrombin time
P3-10580 Prothrombin time, substituted
P3-10590 Partial thromboplastin time, activated
APTT
PTT, activated
PTT
P3-10600 Partial thromboplastin time substituted test
APTT correction studies
Differential APTT test
PTT substitution test
P3-10610 Partial thromboplastin time inhibition test
P3-10620 Thrombin time
Fibrin time
P3-10630 Thrombin time, substituted
P3-10640 Thrombin titer
P3-10650 Coagulation time, Lee White
Lee White coagulation time
Whole blood coagulation time
P3-10660 Coagulation time, capillary
P3-10670 Coagulation time, activated
ACT
Activated clotting time
Ground glass clotting time
P3-10680 Coagulation time, HAREM test
HAREM test
Whole blood partial thromboplastin time
P3-10690 Coagulation time, Bart test
Bart test
Whole blood activated recalcification time
P3-10700 Aspirin tolerance test
ASA tolerance test
Bleeding time, aspirin tolerance test
P3-10710 Plasma recalcification time
P3-10720 Fibrinogen assay, NOS
P3-10730 Fibrinogen assay, semi-quantitative
P3-10740 Fibrinogen assay, quantitative
P3-10750 Fibrinogen assay, thrombin with plasma dilution
P3-10760 Fibrinogen assay, thrombin time dilution
P3-10770 Fibrin split products, protamine sulfate assay
Protamine sulfate test

SECTION 3-1 BLOOD COAGULATION PROCEDURES — Continued

P3-10770 (cont.) 3P test
  Triple P test
  Plasma protamine paracoagulation assay
P3-10780 Fibrin-fibrinogen split products assay, NOS
  Fibrin breakdown products assay, NOS
  Fibrin degradation products assay, NOS
  FSP assay
  FDP assay
P3-10790 Fibrin split products, agglutination assay
P3-10800 Fibrin split products, ethanol gel assay
  Ethanol gel test
P3-10810 Fibrin split products, hemagglutination inhibition microtiter assay
P3-10820 Fibrin split products, immunoelectrophoresis
P3-10830 Fibrin split products, precipitation
P3-10840 Fibrin split products, staphylococcal clumping
P3-10860 Euglobulin lysis time
P3-10870 Paracoagulation test, NOS
P3-10880 D-Dimer assay
P3-10890 Fibrinolysin assay, NOS
  Plasmin assay, NOS
P3-10900 Fibrinolysin assay, screening
  Fibrinolysis time
  Clot lysis time
  Whole blood clot lysis time
P3-10910 Plasma clot lysis time
P3-10920 Plasminogen assay, NOS
P3-10930 Plasminogen assay, antigenic
P3-10940 Alpha-2 antiplasmin assay
  Antiplasmin, functional assay
P3-10950 Plasminogen activator inhibitor assay
  PAI chromogenic assay
  PAI assay
P3-10960 Heparin assay, NOS
P3-10970 Heparin-protamine titration assay
P3-10980 Platelet function test, NOS
P3-10990 Platelet adhesiveness test, NOS
  Platelet adhesiveness, Salzman column test
  Platelet adhesiveness, glass bead
P3-11000 Platelet aggregation test, NOS
  Aggregometer test, NOS
P3-11020 Platelet aggregation with ADP test
P3-11040 Platelet aggregation with epinephrine test
P3-11060 Platelet aggregation with collagen test
P3-11080 Platelet aggregation with thrombin test
P3-11090 Platelet aggregation with drug test
P3-11100 Platelet factor 3 release test
  PF 3 release test
P3-11120 Platelet antibody assay, NOS
P3-11130 Serotonin release assay for platelet antibody
P3-11160 Prothrombin consumption time, NOS
  Serum prothrombin time
P3-11180 Prothrombin consumption time, substituted, NOS
  Serum prothrombin time, substituted
P3-11200 Dilute Russell viper venom time
  DRVVT
  Stypven time
  Reptilase time
P3-11220 Streptokinase titer
P3-11222 Streptokinase antibody measurement
P3-11230 Thromboplastin generation test, NOS
P3-11240 Thromboplastin generation test, Hicks-Pitney modification
P3-11250 Thromboplastin generation test with substitution
P3-11260 Thromboplastin generation test, Biggs-Douglas
P3-11270 Thromboelastography
P3-11280 Thromboxane B2 assay
P3-11290 Blood coagulation panel, NOS
  Blood coagulation screen, NOS
P3-11300 Blood coagulation panel, DIC
  Consumptive coagulopathy screen
  Disseminated intravascular coagulation screening panel
  DIC screen
P3-11320 Coagulation panel for thrombosis
  Thrombosis panel
  Hypercoagulable state screen

SECTION 3-2 BLOOD BANKING PROCEDURES AND SERVICES

P3-20000 Blood bank procedure, NOS
P3-20010 Special blood bank procedure, explain by report
P3-20100 Blood group typing, NOS
  Antigen typing, blood group, NOS
P3-20200 ABO typing
  Blood group typing, ABO only
P3-20220 ABO and Rho(D) typing
  Blood group typing, ABO and Rho(D)
P3-20260 Blood typing, ABO, Rho(D) and RBC antibody screening
P3-20300 Blood group typing A
P3-20310 Blood group typing A_2
P3-20330 Blood group typing B
P3-20340 Blood group typing O
P3-20400 Blood group typing Rho(D)
  Blood typing, Rho(D) only
P3-20410 Blood group typing, RH genotyping, complete
P3-20500 Blood typing, RBC antigens, other than ABO or Rho(D)
P3-20600 RBC antibody detection, NOS
  RBC agglutinin detection, NOS
P3-20620 RBC antibody detection, cold, NOS
  RBC agglutinin detection, cold, NOS
P3-20622 RBC antibody detection, cold with titration
  RBC agglutinin detection, cold with titration
P3-20660 RBC antibody detection, warm, NOS
  RBC agglutinin detection, warm, NOS
P3-20662 RBC antibody detection, warm with titration
  RBC agglutinin detection, warm with titration

P3-20710 Antibody detection, leukocyte antibody
P3-20720 Antibody detection, platelet antibody
P3-20730 RBC antibody detection with albumin
P3-20840 RBC antibody detection with saline
P3-20860 Antibody detection, RBC, saline, high protein and anti-human globulin technique
P3-20880 Antibody detection, RBC, enzyme, 1 stage technique, including anti-human globulin
P3-20900 Antibody detection, RBC, enzyme, 2 stage technique, including anti-human globulin
P3-20920 Antibody elution, RBC, NOS
  Antibody elution, RBC, any method, each elution
P3-20921 Antibody elution, ether
P3-20922 Antibody elution, heat
P3-20923 Antibody elution, alcohol
P3-21000 Pretreatment of RBC's for use in RBC antibody detection, incubation with chemical agents or drug
P3-21020 Antibody identification, RBC, NOS
  Antibody screen, RBC, each serum
P3-21040 Antibody identification, RBC, saline
P3-21042 Antibody identification, RBC, saline and AHG
P3-21044 Antibody identification, RBC, albumin
P3-21060 Hemolysin detection, NOS
P3-21062 Hemolysin detection, ABO
P3-21070 Hemolysin detection, cold, biphasic
  Donath Landsteiner test
P3-21072 Hemolysin detection, cold, quantitative
P3-21120 Antibody identification, leukocyte antibody
P3-21140 Antibody identification, platelet antibody
P3-21145 Antibody identification, RBC, albumin and AHG
P3-21160 Antibody identification, platelet associated immunoglobulin assay
P3-21200 Antibody identification, RBC antibody panel, standard technique
  Antibody identification, RBC antibody, each panel
P3-21210 Antibody identification, RBC antibody panel, cold
P3-21220 Antibody identification, RBC antibody panel, enzyme, 1 stage technique including anti-human globulin
P3-21230 Antibody identification, RBC antibody panel, enzyme, 2 stage technique including anti-human globulin
P3-21240 Pretreatment of RBC's for use in RBC antibody compatibility testing, incubation with chemical agents or drug
P3-21250 Pretreatment of RBC's for use in RBC antibody compatibility testing, incubation with enzymes
P3-21260 Pretreatment of RBC's for use in RBC antibody compatibility testing, by density gradient separation
P3-21270 Pretreatment of serum for use in RBC antibody identification, incubation with drug
P3-21280 Pretreatment of serum for use in RBC antibody identification by dilution
P3-21290 Pretreatment of serum for use in RBC antibody identification, incubation with inhibitors
P3-21292 Pretreatment of serum for use in RBC antibody identification by differential red cell absorption using patient RBC's or RBC's of known phenotype
P3-21294 Antibody absorption, RBC, cold with autoabsorption
P3-21296 Antibody absorption, RBC, differential
P3-21400 Antibody titration, anti-human globulin technique
P3-21402 Antibody titration, saline
P3-21404 Antibody titration, high protein
P3-21406 Antibody titration, enzyme
P3-22000 Direct Coombs test
  Anti-human globulin test, direct
  Anti-human globulin test, direct, broad
P3-22020 Indirect Coombs test, NOS
  Anti-human globulin test, indirect, qualitative, NOS
  Anti-human globulin test, indirect, qualitative, broad
P3-22100 Anti-human globulin test, indirect, qualitative, gamma
P3-22120 Anti-human globulin test, indirect, qualitative, non-gamma
P3-22140 Anti-human globulin test, indirect, titer, broad
P3-22160 Anti-human globulin test, indirect, titer, gamma
P3-22200 Anti-human globulin test, indirect, titer, non-gamma
P3-22220 Anti-human globulin test, enzyme technique, qualitative
P3-22240 Anti-human globulin test, enzyme technique, titer
P3-22260 Anti-human globulin test, drug sensitization and identification
P3-22300 Major crossmatch, NOS
P3-22310 Blood compatibility test, crossmatch by immediate spin technique only
P3-22320 Compatibility test, crossmatch, complete standard technique, includes typing and antibody screening of RBC
P3-22330 Blood compatibility test, crossmatch by immediate spin and anti-human globulin technique, each unit
P3-22350 Autocontrol procedure for crossmatch
P3-22380 Compatibility test, crossmatch, enzyme technique
P3-22400 Compatibility test, crossmatch, screening for compatible unit, saline and/or high protein
P3-22420 Compatibility test, crossmatch, screening for compatible unit, antiglobulin technique
P3-22440 Compatibility test, crossmatch, screening for compatible unit, enzyme technique

SECTION 3-2 BLOOD BANKING PROCEDURES AND SERVICES — Continued

P3-22460 Minor crossmatch, NOS
P3-22470 Compatibility test, crossmatch, minor, includes recipient and donor typing and antibody screening
P3-22480 Blood typing, antigen screening for compatible blood unit using reagent serum, per unit screened
P3-22500 Blood typing, antigen screening for compatible unit using patient's serum, per unit screened
P3-22510 Rhogam crossmatch
  Blood typing, anti-RH immunoglobulin testing, Rhogam type
  Compatibility test, Rho(D) immune globulin
P3-22520 Cryoprecipitate preparation
P3-22530 Cryoprecipitate thawing and pooling
P3-22540 Fresh frozen plasma preparation
P3-22550 Fresh frozen plasma thawing
P3-22560 Frozen blood preparation
P3-22562 Frozen blood preparation for freezing, each unit including processing and collection
P3-22574 Frozen blood preparation for freezing, each unit including processing and collection with thawing
P3-22576 Frozen blood preparation for freezing, each unit including processing and collection with freezing and thawing
P3-22578 Frozen blood thawing and processing
P3-22590 Blood unit collection, NOS
P3-22600 Blood unit collection for autotransfusion
  Collection, processing and storage of predeposited autologous whole blood or components
P3-22610 Blood unit collection for directed donation, donor
  Collection, processing and storage of donor directed whole blood or components
P3-22620 Collection and processing for transfusion of intraoperatively salvaged blood
P3-22670 Leukocyte poor blood preparation, NOS
P3-22680 Leukocyte poor blood preparation, nylon filter
P3-22690 Leukocyte poor blood preparation, invert-spin
P3-22700 Lymphocyte storage, NOS
P3-22710 Lymphocyte storage, liquid nitrogen
P3-22720 Lyophilized coagulation concentrate, reconstitution
P3-22730 Packed RBC preparation, NOS
P3-22740 Packed RBC preparation, sedimentation
P3-22750 Packed RBC preparation, centrifugation
P3-22760 Platelet concentrate, pooling
P3-22765 Pooling other blood products, NOS
P3-22770 Platelet rich plasma, preparation
P3-22790 Platelet concentrate, preparation
P3-22800 Reagent RBC, freeze, glycerol
P3-22810 Reagent RBC, freeze, liquid nitrogen
P3-22820 Reagent RBC, preparation A, B or O pool
P3-22830 Reagent RBC, preparation enzyme treated pool
P3-22840 Reagent RBC, preparation antibody sensitized pool
P3-22850 Reagent RBC thawing
P3-22860 Separation of blood unit into aliquots
  Splitting of blood or blood products, each
P3-22870 Washing RBC for transfusion
P3-22880 Blood unit processing, NOS
P3-22890 Blood bank inventory control
P3-22900 Blood donor rejection, clerical
P3-22910 Blood donor accounting, clerical
P3-23000 Authorization for deviation from standard blood banking procedure by physician
P3-23010 Investigation of transfusion reaction including suspicion of transmissible disease, interpretation and written report by physician
P3-23020 Difficult crossmatch and/or evaluation of irregular antibody, interpretation and written report by physician
P3-23100 Irradiation of blood products, each
P3-23200 Paternity testing, NOS
P3-23202 Paternity testing, ABO+RH factors+MN (per individual)
P3-23204 Paternity testing, ABO+RH factors+MN (per individual), each additional antigen system
P3-23300 Precipitin test for blood group, species identification
P3-23350 Saliva secretor studies, NOS

SECTION 3-3 HEMATOLOGY PROCEDURES
3-30-31 ROUTINE HEMATOLOGY PROCEDURES

P3-30000 Hematology procedure, NOS
P3-30010 Special hematology procedure, explain by report
P3-30100 Complete blood count, NOS
  CBC, NOS
P3-30110 Complete blood count with white cell differential, manual
  CBC with manual differential
P3-30120 Complete blood count with white cell differential, automated
  CBC with automated differential
P3-30130 Complete blood count without differential
  Hemogram
  CBC without differential
P3-30500 Blood cell count, NOS
P3-30510 Red blood cell count
  RBC count
P3-30520 White blood cell count
  WBC count
P3-30530 White blood cell estimate
  WBC estimate
P3-30540 Neutrophil count
P3-30542 Neutrophil band count
  Band count

P3-30550 Lymphocyte count
P3-30552 Reactive lymphocyte count
Atypical lymphocyte count
P3-30560 Monocyte count
P3-30570 Eosinophil count
P3-30571 Eosinophil count, nasal
P3-30572 Eosinophil count, stool
P3-30580 Basophil count
P3-30600 Platelet count
P3-30602 Platelet estimate
P3-30610 Cell count, body fluid, NOS
P3-30612 Cell count and differential, body fluid, NOS
P3-30620 Cell count and differential, cerebrospinal fluid
CSF cell count and differential
P3-30630 Cell count and differential, peritoneal fluid
P3-30640 Cell count and differential, pleural fluid
P3-30700 Synovial fluid analysis, NOS
P3-30710 Cell count of synovial fluid
P3-30712 Cell count of synovial fluid with differential count
P3-30720 Examination for mucin in synovial fluid
Ropes test
P3-30730 Crystal identification of synovial fluid
Crystal identification by compensated polarizing lens analysis of synovial fluid
P3-31000 Blood cell morphology, NOS
P3-31020 Peripheral blood smear interpretation
P3-31040 Red blood cell morphology
P3-31060 Red blood cell histogram evaluation
P3-31080 Red blood cell indices determination, NOS
RBC indices determination, NOS
P3-31082 Mean corpuscular hemoglobin determination
MCH determination
P3-31084 Mean corpuscular hemoglobin concentration determination
MCHC determination
P3-31086 Red cell distribution width determination
RDW determination
P3-31090 White blood cell morphology
P3-31110 White blood cell histogram evaluation
P3-31120 Buffy coat smear evaluation
P3-31200 Platelet morphology
P3-31202 Platelet mean volume determination

3-32 LABORATORY BONE MARROW PROCEDURES

P3-32000 Bone marrow laboratory procedure, NOS
P3-32010 Bone marrow smear and staining only
P3-32020 Bone marrow differential count only
P3-32030 Bone marrow staining and interpretation
P3-32032 Bone marrow interpretation of smear and cell block only
Bone marrow aspirate interpretation
P3-32040 Bone marrow biopsy interpretation only

3-33 HEMATOLOGY STAINING PROCEDURES

P3-33000 Stain, routine, blood or bone marrow
P3-33005 Special stain, blood or bone marrow, explain by report
P3-33020 Stain, iron, blood or bone marrow
Siderocyte stain
Sideroblast stain
P3-33040 Stain, peroxidase, blood or bone marrow
P3-33060 Stain, Sudan Black B, blood or bone marrow
P3-33080 Stain, PAS, blood or bone marrow
P3-33100 Stain, acid phosphatase, blood or bone marrow
P3-33120 Stain, alkaline phosphatase, blood or bone marrow
P3-33140 Stain, naphtol-AS-D-chloracetate esterase, blood or bone marrow
P3-33160 Stain, non-specific esterase, NOS, blood or bone marrow
P3-33180 Stain, alpha naphthyl acetate, blood or bone marrow
P3-33200 Stain, alpha naphthyl butyrate, blood or bone marrow
P3-33220 Stain, non-specific esterase, NaF inhibition, blood or bone marrow
P3-33240 Stain, terminal deoxynucleotidyl transferase, blood or bone marrow
TdT stain
Terminal transferase stain
P3-33260 Immunocytochemical stain, NOS

3-34 MISCELLANEOUS HEMATOLOGIC TESTS

P3-34050 Heinz body determination
P3-34052 Heinz body determination, induced
P3-34080 Hematocrit determination
P3-34100 Hemoglobin determination, NOS
P3-34120 Hemoglobin and hematocrit determination
H & H determination
P3-34160 Fetal hemoglobin determination
P3-34180 Fetal RBC determination
Kleihauer-Betke test
P3-34240 Leukocyte alkaline phosphatase score
LAP score
P3-34280 L.E. cell preparation
P3-34320 Mechanical fragility RBC
P3-34400 Osmotic fragility, NOS
P3-34402 Osmotic fragility, immediate
P3-34404 Osmotic fragility, incubated
P3-34500 Parasite detection, blood, NOS
P3-34520 Malaria smear
P3-34560 Reticulocyte count
P3-34600 Sedimentation rate, NOS
P3-34602 Sedimentation rate, Westergren
P3-34604 Sedimentation rate, Wintrobe
P3-34700 Sickle cell identification, NOS
P3-34702 Sickle cell identification, slide method
P3-34704 Sickle cell identification, solubility method
Sickling, turbidometric method
P3-34800 T cell depletion of bone marrow for transplantation, NOS

3-34 MISCELLANEOUS HEMATOLOGIC TESTS — Continued

P3-34900 WBC enzyme determination

SECTION 3-4 ANATOMIC PATHOLOGY PROCEDURES

3-40 GENERAL ANATOMIC PATHOLOGY PROCEDURES AND SERVICES

P3-40000 Anatomic pathology procedure or service, NOS
P3-40010 Special anatomic pathology procedure or service, explain by report
P3-40040 Gross organ fixation and special preparation, NOS
P3-40060 Gross organ fixation and special preparation for museum, liquid media
P3-40080 Gross organ fixation and special preparation for museum, solid plastic
P3-40120 Whole organ section preparation for special studies
P3-40140 Photography of gross organ, NOS
P3-40150 Photography, microscopic, NOS
  Photomicrography, NOS
P3-40200 Tissue autoradiography
P3-40210 Tetracycline labelling of bone
P3-40220 Stereomicroscopy
P3-40240 Cryopreservation, NOS
P3-40242 Cryopreservation for genetic studies, NOS
P3-40244 Cryopreservation technique with DMSO
P3-40246 Cryopreservation technique with glycerol
P3-40260 Nerve teasing preparation, NOS
P3-40600 Tissue processing technique, NOS
P3-40620 Tissue processing technique, routine, embed, cut and stain, per surgical specimen
P3-40640 Tissue processing technique, complex, embed, cut and stain, per surgical specimen
P3-40660 Tissue processing technique, routine, embed, cut and stain, per autopsy
P3-40680 Tissue processing technique, complex, embed, cut and stain, per autopsy
P3-40700 Tissue processing technique, cut only
P3-40720 Tissue processing technique, embed only
P3-40740 Tissue processing technique, stain only, routine
P3-40760 Tissue processing technique, stain only, special
P3-40780 Tissue processing technique, fixation only
P3-40800 Tissue decalcification technique, complete
P3-40820 Tissue frozen section technique, complete

3-41 ELECTRON MICROSCOPY AND MORPHOMETRY

P3-41000 Electron microscopic study, NOS
P3-41002 Immunoelectron microscopy study, NOS
P3-41010 Electron microscopy study, examination and report, NOS
P3-41020 Electron microscopy scanning technique, complete
P3-41022 Electron microscopy study, scanning, examination and report
P3-41024 Electron microscopy study, scanning, with X-ray analysis, examination and report
P3-41050 Electron microscopy transmission technique, complete
P3-41052 Electron microscopy study, transmission, examination and report
P3-41060 Electron microscopy technique, fixation only
P3-41070 Electron microscopy technique, blocking only
P3-41080 Electron microscopy technique, pyramid making only
P3-41190 Electron microscopy technique, cutting only
P3-41200 Electron microscopy technique, staining, thick section
P3-41210 Electron microscopy technique, staining, thin section
P3-41220 Electron microscopy technique, photography only
P3-41230 Electron microscopy technique, glass knife making
P3-41250 Electron microscopy for viral identification rapid, NOS
P3-41260 Electron microscopy for viral identification, smear, transmission
P3-41270 Electron microscopy, consultation, examination and interpretation
P3-41900 Morphometric analysis, NOS
  Morphometry, NOS
P3-41901 Morphometry, quantitative
P3-41902 Morphometric analysis, nerve
P3-41903 Morphometric analysis, tumor
P3-41904 Morphometric analysis, muscle
P3-41910 Image analysis, NOS
P3-41911 Image analysis, qualitative
P3-41912 Image analysis, quantitative
P3-41913 Image analysis, segmentation
P3-41914 Image analysis, karyometry
P3-41940 Bone histomorphometry, NOS
P3-41941 Bone histomorphometry, quantitative
P3-41942 Bone histomorphometry, aluminum stain

3-42 AUTOPSY PATHOLOGY PROCEDURES AND SERVICES

P3-42000 Autopsy examination, NOS
  Autopsy, NOS
  Necropsy, NOS
P3-42005 Special autopsy procedure, explain by report
P3-42010 Autopsy, gross examination only
P3-42040 Autopsy, gross examination with brain
P3-42060 Autopsy, gross examination with brain and spinal cord
P3-42080 Autopsy, gross examination without CNS
P3-42100 Autopsy, gross examination, infant less than 1 year
P3-42120 Autopsy, gross examination, stillborn or newborn
P3-42140 Autopsy, gross examination, macerated stillborn

P3-42160 Autopsy, gross examination, limited, NOS
P3-42180 Autopsy, gross examination, limited, single organ
P3-42200 Autopsy, gross examination, limited, regional
P3-42220 Autopsy, gross examination, limited, external exam only
P3-42240 Autopsy, gross examination, teaching, limited
P3-42260 Autopsy, gross examination, teaching, complete
P3-42280 Autopsy, gross and microscopic examination, NOS
P3-42290 Autopsy, gross and microscopic examination without CNS
P3-42300 Autopsy, gross and microscopic examination with brain
P3-42310 Autopsy, gross and microscopic examination with brain and spinal cord
P3-42320 Autopsy, gross and microscopic examination, infant less than 1 year
P3-42340 Autopsy, gross and microscopic examination, stillborn or newborn
P3-42360 Autopsy, gross and microscopic examination, stillborn or newborn without CNS
P3-42380 Autopsy, gross and microscopic examination, limited, NOS
P3-42400 Autopsy, gross and microscopic examination, single organ
P3-42420 Autopsy, gross and microscopic examination, regional
P3-42440 Forensic autopsy
P3-42442 Forensic autopsy, extensive
P3-42448 Forensic autopsy, coroner's call
P3-42500 Autopsy review, NOS
P3-42520 Autopsy review, slide only
P3-42540 Autopsy review for teaching
P3-42560 Autopsy review, consultation and report
P3-42580 Autopsy review for conference
P3-42600 Autopsy service by diener
P3-42620 Autopsy, clerical procedure
P3-42640 Autopsy, clerical with coding procedure

3-44 SURGICAL PATHOLOGY PROCEDURES AND SERVICES

P3-44000 Surgical pathology procedure, NOS
P3-44005 Special surgical pathology procedure, explain by report
P3-44010 Surgical pathology gross examination only
  Surgical pathology examination, level I
P3-44020 Surgical pathology gross and microscopic examination, identification only
  Surgical pathology examination, level II
P3-44040 Surgical pathology gross and microscopic examination, uncomplicated
  Surgical pathology examination, level III
P3-44050 Surgical pathology gross and microscopic examination, complicated without dissection
  Surgical pathology examination, level IV
P3-44070 Surgical pathology gross and microscopic examination, complicated with dissection
  Surgical pathology examination, level V
P3-44090 Surgical pathology gross and microscopic examination, complex
  Surgical pathology examination, level VI
P3-44160 Tissue immunofluorescence procedure, each antibody, direct
P3-44180 Tissue immunofluorescence procedure, each antibody, indirect
P3-44200 Immunocytochemical procedure, each antibody
P3-44202 Immunoperoxidase procedure, each antibody
P3-44204 Immunoperoxidase measurement with avidin biotin complex
P3-44300 Special stain for microorganism
P3-44320 Special stain other than microorganism
P3-44350 Histochemical stain with frozen section
P3-44400 Determinative histochemistry for chemicals
P3-44420 Determinative histochemistry for enzymes
P3-44440 Microscopic examination and diagnosis of previously processed surgical specimen
P3-44450 Surgical pathology consultation and report on referred slides prepared elsewhere
P3-44460 Pathology consultation during surgery, gross examination only
P3-44500 Pathology consultation during surgery with frozen section, single specimen
  Frozen section consultation, initial
P3-44520 Pathology consultation during surgery, each additional frozen section
  Frozen section consultation, each additional
P3-44652 Consultation and report on referred material requiring preparation of slides
P3-44700 Pathology consultation, comprehensive, records and specimen with report
P3-44800 Surgical pathology specimen, clerical procedure including coding of diagnoses

3-45 CYTOPATHOLOGY PROCEDURES AND SERVICES

P3-45000 Cytopathology procedure or service, NOS
P3-45010 Special cytopathology procedure, explain by report
P3-45020 Cytopathology, review of slides and report, genital source, by physician
P3-45060 Cytopathology, review of slides and report, nongenital source, by physician
  Cytopathology, review of slides and report, fluids, washings or brushings, by physician
  Cytopathology, review of bronchioalveolar lavage specimen
P3-45100 Cytopathology, review of slides and report, extended study, nongenital source, by physician
P3-45140 Cytopathology, screening of smear, routine, genital source, by cytotechnologist
P3-45180 Cytopathology screening of smear, routine, genital source with hormonal evaluation, by cytotechnologist

3-45 CYTOPATHOLOGY PROCEDURES AND SERVICES — Continued

P3-45220 Cytopathology screening of smear, routine, nongenital source, by cytotechnologist
P3-45260 Cytopathology procedure, preparation of smear, genital source
  PAP smear preparation
P3-45300 Cytopathology procedure, preparation of smear, nongenital source, NOS
P3-45340 Cytopathology procedure requiring centrifugation, nongenital source
  Cytopathology procedure, centrifugation of smear
  Saccomanno procedure, cytopathology
P3-45380 Cytopathology procedure, preparation, screening and interpretation, nongenital source
P3-45420 Cytopathology procedure, filtering of smear, nongenital source
P3-45460 Special cytopathology procedure, liquefaction of sputum and smear
P3-45500 Cytopathology procedure, cell block preparation
P3-45510 Cytopathology procedure, cell block and smear preparation
P3-45520 Cytopathology procedure, staining only, routine
P3-45530 Cytopathology procedure, staining only, special
P3-45600 Smear for cell identification, NOS
P3-45610 Smear for eosinophils
P3-45620 Smear for neutrophils
P3-45630 Smear for epithelial cells
P3-45640 Smear for meat fibers
P3-45650 Smear for starch granules
P3-45660 Smear for fat
P3-45840 Fine needle aspirate with immediate interpretation and report
P3-45860 Fine needle aspirate with routine interpretation and report
P3-45900 Cytopathology procedure, forensic
P3-45990 Cytopathology clerical procedure including coding

3-49 CHROMOSOME ANALYSIS, CYTOGENETIC PROCEDURES AND MOLECULAR BIOLOGY METHODS

3-490-494 Chromosome Analysis

P3-49000 Chromosome analysis, NOS
P3-49005 Special chromosome analysis, explain by report
P3-49020 Tissue culture for chromosome analysis, NOS
P3-49040 Tissue culture for chromosome analysis, lymphocytes, screening
P3-49060 Tissue culture for chromosome analysis, lymphocytes, mosaicism
P3-49080 Tissue culture for chromosome analysis, myeloid cells
P3-49100 Tissue culture for chromosome analysis, amniotic fluid
P3-49120 Tissue culture for chromosome analysis, chorionic villus
P3-49140 Tissue culture for chromosome analysis, skin
P3-49160 Tissue culture for chromosome analysis, other tissue cells
P3-49180 Tissue culture for chromosome analysis, more complex procedure with special extra counts, NOS
P3-49200 Chromosome analysis for breakage syndromes, score 25 cells, count 5 cells, 1 karyotype with banding
P3-49220 Chromosome analysis for breakage syndromes, score 100 cells, count 20 cells, 2 karyotypes with banding
P3-49240 Chromosome analysis for fragile X associated with fragile X-linked mental retardation
P3-49260 Chromosome analysis, count 5 cells, screening with banding
P3-49280 Chromosome analysis, count 5 cells, 1 karyotype with banding
P3-49300 Chromosome analysis count 15-20 cells, 2 karyotypes with banding
P3-49320 Chromosome analysis, count 45 cells for mosaicism, 2 karyotypes with banding
P3-49340 Chromosome analysis, amniotic fluid or chorionic villus, count 15 cells, 1 karyotype with banding
P3-49360 Chromosome analysis, in situ for amniotic fluid cells, count cells from 6-12 colonies, 1 karyotype with banding
P3-49380 Chromosome analysis, additional karyotypes, each study
P3-49400 Chromosome analysis, specialized banding technique, NOS
P3-49420 Chromosome analysis, specialized banding, NOR technique
P3-49440 Chromosome analysis, specialized banding, C-banding technique
P3-49460 Chromosome analysis, additional cells counted, each study
P3-49480 Chromosome analysis, additional high resolution study
P3-49490 Sex chromatin determination, Barr bodies
P3-49492 Sex chromatin determination, PMN cell drumsticks

3-495-499 Cytogenetic Procedures

P3-49500 Cytogenetic procedure, NOS
  Cytogenetic study, NOS
P3-49510 Special cytogenetic study, explain by report
P3-49520 DNA analysis, NOS
P3-49522 DNA analysis, antenatal
P3-49523 DNA analysis, antenatal, blood
P3-49524 DNA analysis, antenatal, amniotic fluid
P3-49600 Flow cytometry, NOS
P3-49605 Fluorescence activated cell sorter assay
  FACS assay, NOS

P3-49610 Flow cytometry, cell marker analysis, NOS
P3-49620 Flow cytometry, cell cycle analysis
 DNA S phase analysis
 Flow cytometry, S phase analysis
P3-49640 Flow cytometry, DNA analysis
 DNA ploidy pattern analysis
 Flow cytometry, ploidy analysis
P3-49700 DNA probe analysis, NOS
P3-49740 DNA hybridization, NOS
 Nucleic acid hybridization, NOS
P3-49760 Tissue in situ hybridization, interpretation and report
P3-49780 DNA hybridization with autoradiography
P3-49800 Carrier detection, molecular genetics, NOS
P3-49820 Alpha globulin gene analysis, NOS
P3-49821 Alpha globulin gene analysis, blood
P3-49822 Alpha globulin gene analysis, amniotic fluid
P3-49840 Breakpoint cluster region analysis, NOS
 BCR analysis, NOS
P3-49860 N MYC gene amplification
P3-49880 Immunoglobulin gene rearrangement assay, NOS
P3-49900 T cell receptor gene rearrangement, NOS
P3-49920 Cystic fibrosis carrier detection, NOS
P3-49921 Cystic fibrosis carrier detection, blood
P3-49922 Cystic fibrosis carrier detection, amniotic fluid
P3-49923 Cystic fibrosis, prenatal detection
P3-49940 Duchenne muscular dystrophy carrier detection, NOS
P3-49960 Duchenne muscular dystrophy carrier detection, blood
P3-49980 Duchenne muscular dystrophy carrier detection, amniotic fluid

3-49B-49C Molecular Biology Methods

P3-49B00 Molecular biology identification technique, NOS
P3-49B04 Restriction enzyme analysis, NOS
 REA, NOS
P3-49B05 REA of plasmid DNA, NOS
P3-49B06 REA of chromosomal DNA, NOS
P3-49B10 Ribotyping
P3-49B12 Plasmid fingerprinting, NOS
P3-49B20 Restriction fragment length polymorphism analysis
 RFLP analysis
P3-49B30 Polymerase chain reaction analysis
 PCR analysis
P3-49B40 Nucleic acid amplification, NOS
P3-49B90 Zygosity determination, NOS
P3-49C00 Transgeneic procedure, NOS
 Genetic engineering procedure, NOS
P3-49C10 Gene replacement therapy, NOS
 Gene insertion therapy, NOS

SECTION 3-5 MICROBIOLOGY PROCEDURES

3-50 GENERAL MICROBIOLOGY EXAMINATION, CULTURE AND STAINING PROCEDURES

P3-50000 Microbiology procedure, NOS
P3-50100 Microbial culture, NOS
P3-50101 Microbial culture, routine
P3-50104 Microbial culture, tissue
P3-50108 Microbial subculture, NOS
P3-50110 Microbial culture, aerobic, initial isolation
P3-50120 Microbial culture, aerobic, screen
P3-50140 Microbial culture, anaerobic, initial isolation
P3-50150 Microbial culture, anaerobic, screen
P3-50160 Microbial culture in partial CO_2, initial isolation
P3-50170 Microbial culture with overlay technique, initial isolation
P3-50180V Culture of semen, NOS
P3-50181V Culture of semen for Brucella
P3-50200 Blood culture, NOS
P3-50210 Microbial culture, slide
P3-50220 Microbial culture, complex
P3-50230 Microbial culture, room temperature
P3-50240 Mycobacteria culture, NOS
P3-50250 Mycology culture, NOS
 Fungus culture, NOS
P3-50260 Viral culture, NOS
P3-50300 Microbial smear examination, NOS
P3-50310 Microbial wet smear
P3-50312 Microbial wet smear for fungus
P3-50320 Microbial wet smear, tease preparation
P3-50330 Microbial dry smear
P3-50340 Microbial smear, phase contrast examination
P3-50350 Microbial smear, light microscopy examination
P3-50360 Microbial smear, dark field examination
P3-50370 Microbial smear, hanging drop technique
P3-50400 Microbial stain, NOS
P3-50410 Gram stain
 Bacterial stain, routine
P3-50420 Stain for viral inclusions, NOS
P3-50422 Tzanck smear
P3-50430 Stain for fungus, NOS
P3-50440 KOH stain
P3-50450 Calcoflour white stain
P3-50460 India ink stain
P3-50470 Diff-quik stain
P3-50480 Acid fast stain, NOS
P3-50482 Acid fast stain, Ziehl-Neelsen method
P3-50484 Acid fast stain, Kinyoun's cold carbolfuchsin method
P3-50486 Acid fast stain, fluorochrome method
P3-50500 Microbial ova-parasite examination, NOS
P3-50510 Microbial ova-parasite examination, fecal
P3-50512 Pinworm slide
P3-50520 Yeast identification procedure, NOS
P3-50530 Yeast identification, direct mount

3-50 GENERAL MICROBIOLOGY EXAMINATION, CULTURE AND STAINING PROCEDURES — Continued

P3-50540 Yeast identification, germ tube test
P3-50550 Yeast identification, dalmau plate test
  Yeast identification, cornmeal agar
P3-50600 Quantitative microbial culture and measurement, NOS
P3-50610 Quantitative microbial culture, pour plate method
P3-50620 Quantitative microbial culture, surface streak method
P3-50630 Quantitative microbial culture, filter paper method
P3-50640 Quantitative microbial culture, cup method
P3-50650 Quantitative microbial culture, droplet method
P3-50660 Quantitative microbial culture, pad culture method
P3-50700 In vitro hair test for molds
P3-50710 Ballistospore test for molds
P3-50720 Nutritional test for molds, NOS
P3-50730 Rice grain test for molds
P3-50740 Thermotolerance test for molds
P3-50750 Exoantigen test for molds
P3-50760 Cyclohexamide resistance test for molds
P3-50770 Mold to yeast conversion test
P3-50790 Tease mount preparation

3-51 BACTERIAL COLONY MORPHOLOGY DETERMINATIONS

P3-51000 Bacterial colony morphology, NOS
P3-51010 Bacterial colony size, NOS
P3-51020 Bacterial colony size, small
  Bacterial colony size, less than 1 mm. diameter
P3-51030 Bacterial colony size, medium
  Bacterial colony size, 1 mm. diameter
P3-51040 Bacterial colony size, large
  Bacterial colony size, greater than 1mm. diameter
P3-51050 Bacterial colony shape, NOS
P3-51060 Bacterial colony shape, circular
P3-51070 Bacterial colony shape, filamentous
P3-51080 Bacterial colony shape, irregular
P3-51090 Bacterial colony shape, punctiform
P3-51100 Bacterial colony shape, rhizoid
P3-51110 Bacterial colony shape, spindle
P3-51120 Bacterial colony elevation, NOS
P3-51130 Bacterial colony elevation, flat
P3-51140 Bacterial colony elevation, raised
P3-51150 Bacterial colony elevation, convex
P3-51160 Bacterial colony elevation, dome shaped
P3-51170 Bacterial colony elevation, umbonate
P3-51180 Bacterial colony elevation, umbilicate
P3-51190 Bacterial colony morphology, margin, NOS
P3-51200 Bacterial colony morphology, entire margin, NOS
P3-51210 Bacterial colony morphology, undulate margin, NOS
P3-51220 Bacterial colony morphology, lobate margin
P3-51230 Bacterial colony morphology, curled margin
P3-51240 Bacterial colony morphology, erose margin
P3-51250 Bacterial colony morphology, filamentous margin
P3-51260 Bacterial colony color, NOS
P3-51270 Bacterial colony surface appearance, NOS
P3-51280 Bacterial colony surface, glistening
P3-51290 Bacterial colony surface, smooth
P3-51300 Bacterial colony surface, granular
P3-51310 Bacterial colony surface, dull
P3-51320 Bacterial colony surface, rough
P3-51330 Bacterial colony surface, creamy
P3-51340 Bacterial colony density, NOS
P3-51350 Bacterial colony density, opaque
P3-51360 Bacterial colony density, transparent
P3-51370 Bacterial colony density, translucent
P3-51380 Bacterial colony consistency, NOS
P3-51390 Bacterial colony consistency, butyrous
  Bacterial colony consistency, buttery
P3-51410 Bacterial colony consistency, viscous
  Bacterial colony consistency, sticky
P3-51430 Bacterial colony consistency, friable
P3-51440 Bacterial colony consistency, brittle
P3-51450 Bacterial colony consistency, membranous
  Bacterial colony consistency, pliable
P3-51460 Bacterial colony hemolysis, NOS
P3-51470 Bacterial colony hemolysis, alpha
  Alpha hemolysis
P3-51480 Bacterial colony hemolysis, alpha prime
  Alpha prime hemolysis
P3-51490 Bacterial colony hemolysis, beta
  Beta hemolysis
P3-51510 Bacterial colony hemolysis, gamma
  Gamma hemolysis

3-52 MICROBIAL IDENTIFICATION TESTS

P3-52000 Microbial identification test, NOS
P3-52010 Microbial identification test, rapid method, NOS
P3-52020 Beta-glucuronidase test
  MUG test
P3-52030 O-nitrophenyl-beta-o-galactopyranoside test
P3-52040 Porphyrin production test
P3-52050 Tributyrin test
P3-52110 Spot indole test
P3-52120 Spot oxidase test
P3-52130 Carbohydrate fermentation test
P3-52140 Citrate utilization test
P3-52150 Decarboxylase dihydrolase test
P3-52160 Esculin hydrolysis test
P3-52170 Fluorescence identification test
P3-52180 Gelatin liquefaction test
P3-52190 Hydrogen sulfide test
P3-52200 Kligler iron test

P3-52210 Malonate test
P3-52220 Methyl red test
P3-52230 Oxidation fermentation test
P3-52240 Phenylalanine deamination test
P3-52250 Triple sugar iron test
P3-52260 Voges Proskauer test
P3-52270 Motility test
P3-52280 Urease test
P3-52290 Nitrate reduction test
P3-52300 Lipase test
P3-52310 Spore test
P3-52320 Arylsulfatase test
P3-52330 Growth on MacConkey agar without crystal violet test
P3-52340 Niacin accumulation test
P3-52350 Pyrazinamidase test
P3-52360 Sodium chloride tolerance test (6.5%)
P3-52370 Thiophene-2-carboxylic acid hydrazide test
TCH test
P3-52380 Tellurite reduction test
P3-52390 Tween 80 hydrolysis test
P3-52400 Urease test, Wayne method
P3-52410 BACTEC NAP test
P3-52420 Casein decomposition test
P3-52430 Tyrosine decomposition test
P3-52440 Xanthine decomposition agar test
P3-52450 Hypoxanthine decomposition agar test
P3-52460 Cellobiose assimilation test
P3-52470 Starch utilization test
P3-52480 Ethylene glycol opacity test
P3-52490 Lysozyme resistance test
P3-52500 Microbial growth rate test, NOS
P3-52510 Microbial growth rate, slow
P3-52520 Microbial growth rate, moderate
P3-52530 Microbial growth rate, rapid
P3-52540 Catalase test, NOS
P3-52550 Catalase test, semi-quantitative
P3-52560 Catalase test, heat-stable
P3-52570 Nitrate disk reduction test
P3-52580 Special potency disk identification test, NOS
P3-52590 Special potency disk identification, vancomycin test
P3-52600 Special potency disk identification, kanamycin test
P3-52610 Special potency disk identification, colistin test
P3-52620 Sodium polyanethol sulfonate disk test
SPS disk test
P3-52630 Bile disk test
P3-52640 Anaerobic bacterial fluorescence test
P3-52660 Clostridium difficile assay
P3-52670 Pigment production test, NOS
P3-52680 Pigment production test, nonphotochromogenic
P3-52690 Pigment production test, photochromogenic
P3-52700 Pigment production test, scotochromogenic
P3-52710 Thiacetazone test
THZ test
P3-52720 Iron uptake test
P3-52740 Utilization of inositol test
P3-52750 Utilization of mannitol test
P3-52760 Autoagglutination test
P3-52770 Coagulase test
P3-52780 Protein A test
Staphaurex method
P3-52790 Novobiocin susceptibility test
P3-52800 Trehalose-mannitol broth test
P3-52810 Rapid thermonuclease test
P3-52820 Hemolysis on sheep blood agar test
P3-52830 Bacitracin susceptibility test
P3-52840 Bile esculin test
P3-52850 Bile solubility test
P3-52860 CAMP test
P3-52870 Rapid hippurate hydrolysis test
P3-52880 Lactobacilli MRS broth test
P3-52890 Optochin susceptibility test
P3-52900 L-pyrrolidonyl-beta-naphthylamide test
PYR test

3-53 MICROBIAL IDENTIFICATION KIT METHODS

P3-53000 Microbial identification, rapid kit method, NOS
P3-53010 Microbial identification, API rapid E method
P3-53020 Microbial identification, Gonochek-II method
P3-53030 Microbial identification, identicult-Neissera method
P3-53040 Microbial identification, NET tube method
P3-53050 Microbial identification, HNID panel
P3-53060 Microbial identification, Key rapid test, NOS
P3-53070 Microbial identification, Uni yeast, TEK test
P3-53080 Microbial identification, Vitek yeast identification test
Vitek system test
P3-53090 Microbial identification, Micro-ID method
P3-53100 Microbial identification, Minitek biochemical differentiation disk method
P3-53110 Microbial identification, Minitek yeast system
P3-53120 Microbial identification, Neisseria-Kwik method
P3-53130 Microbial identification, Neisseria hemophilus identification card method
P3-53140 Microbial identification, quadFERM and method
P3-53150 Microbial identification, rapid NFT method
P3-53160 Microbial identification, rapid NH method
P3-53170 Microbial identification, rapid ANA II method
P3-53300 Microbial identification kit conventional method, NOS
P3-53310 Microbial identification kit, API 20C method
P3-53320 Microbial identification kit, API 2E method
P3-53330 Microbial identification kit, API 20A method
P3-53335 Microbial identification kit, API 20S method
P3-53340 Microbial identification kit, Enterotube II method
P3-53350 Microbial identification kit, OXI/FERM tube method

3-53 MICROBIAL IDENTIFICATION KIT METHODS — Continued

P3-53360 Microbial identification kit, N/F ferm tube method
P3-53370 Microbial identification kit, r/b ferm tube method
P3-53380 Microbial identification kit, API staph-ident method
P3-53390 Microbial identification kit, API staph-trac method
P3-53410 Microbial identification kit, rapid strep method
P3-53500 Microbial identification, automated and semiautomated methods
P3-53510 ARx advantage microbiology center system test
P3-53520 Autobac series II system test
P3-53530 Microscan system test
P3-53540 Sensititre system test
P3-53550 Sceptor system test
P3-53560 Automated microtiter identification and susceptibility test, NOS
P3-53561 Uniscept system test
P3-53562 Microbial identification and susceptibility test, NOS
P3-53580 Esteem micro media system test
P3-53590 Pasco system test

3-55 ANTIMICROBIAL SUSCEPTIBILITY TESTS

P3-55000 Antimicrobial susceptibility test, NOS
P3-55020 Disk diffusion susceptibility test
  Kirby Bauer test
P3-55060 Beta lactamase susceptibility test, NOS
P3-55080 Beta lactamase, chromogenic cephalosporin susceptibility test
P3-55100 Beta lactamase, acidimetric susceptibility test
P3-55120 Beta lactamase, iodometric susceptibility test
P3-55140 High level aminoglycoside resistance test
  HLAR test
P3-55160 HLAR agar method test
P3-55180 HLAR disk agar diffusion test
P3-55200 HLAR broth microdilution test
P3-55220 Oxacillin screen plate susceptibility test
P3-55230 Broth microdilution susceptibility test, NOS
  MIC susceptibility test, NOS
P3-55240 Broth microdilution susceptibility test for anaerobes
  MIC susceptibility test for anaerobes
P3-55300 Broth microdilution susceptibility test for Mycobacteria
P3-55340 Broth microdilution susceptibility test for Nocardia
P3-55360 Beta lactamase induction susceptibility test
P3-55380 Chloramphenicol acetyltransferase susceptibility test
P3-55400 Agar dilution MIC susceptibility test for anaerobes
P3-55420 Agar disk elution susceptibility test for Mycobacteria
P3-55440 Modified proportion agar dilution test for slow growing Mycobacteria
P3-55460 Radiometric test for slow growing Mycobacteria, NOS
P3-55500 BACTEC susceptibility test for slow growing Mycobacteria, NOS
P3-55510 BACTEC susceptibility test by direct method
P3-55520 BACTEC susceptibility test by indirect method
P3-55540 BACTEC susceptibility test by indirect method with PZA
P3-55600 Antifungal susceptibility test, NOS
P3-55604 Minimum bactericidal concentration test, NOS
  Schlicter test
P3-55608 Minimum bactericidal concentration test, macrodilution method
P3-55612 Minimum bactericidal concentration test, microdilution method
P3-55616 Time kill assay test, NOS
P3-55620 Time kill assay for synergy test
P3-55624 Serum inhibitory titer test
  SIT test
P3-55628 Synergism testing, NOS
P3-55632 Synergism testing, broth microdilution method
P3-55636 Synergism testing, broth macrodilution method
P3-55640 Synergism testing, disk dilution method

3-56 BACTERIAL TYPING PROCEDURES

P3-56000 Bacterial strain typing, NOS
P3-56004 Bacterial serotyping, NOS
P3-56008 Bacterial biotyping, NOS
P3-56010 Bacterial antibiogram analysis, NOS
P3-56014 Bacterial bacteriophage typing, NOS
  Phage typing, NOS
P3-56018 Serotyping procedure, NOS
P3-56022 Pyocin typing, NOS
P3-56026 Diene test, NOS
P3-56030 Slime test for staphylococci, NOS
P3-56034 Synergistic hemolysis test, NOS

3-58 INFECTION CONTROL PROCEDURES

P3-58000 Infection control procedure, NOS
P3-58004 Infection control culture overnight, NOS
P3-58008 Surveillance culture, NOS
P3-58012 Prospective focused infection control surveillance, NOS
P3-58016 Employee health culture, NOS
P3-58020 Environmental culture, NOS
P3-58024 Sterility testing, NOS
P3-58028 Air culture for fungus, NOS
P3-58032 Culture of biological indicator, NOS
P3-58036 Culture of dialysis fluid, NOS

P3-58040 Culture of medical device, NOS
P3-58044 Culture of environmental surface, NOS
P3-58048 Culture of blood bank product, NOS
P3-58100 Blood and body fluid laboratory precaution procedure, NOS

3-59 MISCELLANEOUS MICROBIOLOGY PROCEDURES

P3-59010 Microbiologic media preparation, NOS
P3-59020 Handling of microbiologic test report
P3-59030 Animal inoculation, NOS
P3-59032 Animal inoculation, observation only
P3-59034 Animal inoculation with autopsy, smear and culture
P3-59036 Animal inoculation for Mycobacteria
P3-59040 Endotoxin test, animal
P3-59042 Endotoxin test, chemical
P3-59058 Egg inoculation
P3-59060 Ultraviolet light examination of specimen
  Wood lamp examination of specimen
P3-59064 Concentration for ova and cysts
P3-59068 Cover slip preparation
P3-59070 Methylene blue plating test
P3-59074 Colony count on plate
P3-59078 Grinding of tissue for culture
P3-59080 Liquefaction of specimen without chemical treatment
P3-59082 Liquefaction of specimen with chemical treatment
P3-59084 Centrifugation following chemical treatment
P3-59086 Transfer of culture to holding media
P3-59088 Preparation of standardized bacterial suspension
P3-59090 Lyophilization of culture
P3-59094 Reconstitution of lyophilized culture
P3-59098 Freezing and thawing of culture
P3-59100V Dourine test
  Test for Trypanosoma equiperdum
P3-59102V Contagious equine metritis test
P3-59103V Coggins test for equine anemia
P3-59104V Knotts microfilaria test

3-5C IDENTIFICATION PROCEDURES FOR OTHER LIVING ORGANISMS

P3-5C100 Insect identification procedure, NOS
  Insect identification, NOS
P3-5C300 Plant identification procedure, NOS
  Plant identification, NOS

SECTION 3-6 IMMUNOLOGIC PROCEDURES

P3-60000 In-vitro immunologic test, NOS
P3-60010 Special in-vitro immunologic procedure, explain by report
P3-60020 Serologic test, NOS
P3-60050 Immunologic identification of antigen or antibody, NOS
P3-60054 Immunoassay for detection of antigen to infectious agent, NOS
P3-60056 Immunoassay for detection of antibody to infectious agent, NOS
P3-60058 Immunoassay for detection of antibody to infectious agent, paired sample, NOS
P3-60100 Antibody measurement, NOS
P3-60102 Agglutinin measurement, NOS
P3-60103 Warm agglutinin measurement, NOS
P3-60104 Cold agglutinin measurement, NOS
P3-60108 Qualitative non-RBC antibody measurement
P3-60109 Quantitative non-RBC antibody measurement
P3-60110 Fluorescent antibody measurement
P3-60112 Fluorescent antibody, screen
P3-60113 Fluorescent antibody, titer
P3-60115 Fluorescent antigen measurement, NOS
P3-60116 Fluorescent antigen, screen
P3-60117 Fluorescent antigen, titer
P3-60120 Agglutination assay, NOS
  Agglutination procedure, NOS
P3-60122 Passive agglutination test
P3-60130 Hemagglutination assay, NOS
P3-60132 Passive hemagglutination assay
P3-60136 Hemagglutination inhibition assay, NOS
  HAI test, NOS
P3-60140 Coated particle agglutination assay
P3-60141 Particle agglutination test for infectious agent
P3-60142 Coated particle agglutination inhibition assay
P3-60146 Latex agglutination test, NOS
P3-60147 Latex agglutination inhibition assay
P3-60200 Chemotaxis assay, NOS
P3-60220 Serum neutralization test
  SN test
P3-60240 Anti DNase test , NOS
P3-60241 Anti DNase A test
P3-60242 Anti DNase B test
P3-60243 Anti DNase C test
P3-60244 Anti DNase D test
P3-60250 Anti-A-carbohydrate test
  Anti-A-CHO test
P3-60750 Immunoprecipitin test, NOS
  Precipitin measurement, NOS
P3-60752 Immunoprecipitin test, qualitative
P3-60754 Immunoprecipitin test, quantitative
P3-61020 Antibody panel measurement, NOS
P3-61030 TORCH antibody panel measurement
P3-61040 Hypersensitivity pneumonitis panel measurement
P3-61490 Febrile agglutinins panel typhoid O & H, paratyphoid A & B, Brucella and Proteus OX-19
P3-61491 Febrile agglutinins, qualitative
P3-61492 Febrile agglutinins, quantitative
P3-61700 Rickettsial serologic study, NOS
P3-61701 Rickettsial serologic study, paired samples
P3-61711 Serologic test for Rickettsia rickettsii
P3-61712 Serologic test for Rickettsia conorii
P3-61713 Serologic test for Rickettsia typhi

SECTION 3-6 IMMUNOLOGIC PROCEDURES — Continued

P3-61714 Serologic test for Rickettsia prowazeki
P3-61715 Serologic test for Rickettsia tsutsugamushi
P3-61720 Serologic test for Rochalimaea quintana
P3-61722 Serologic test for Coxiella burnetii
P3-61723 Serologic test for Ehrlichia sennetsu
P3-61724 Serologic test for Ehrlichia chaffeensis
P3-61725 Serologic test for Ehrlichia canis
P3-61800 Fungus serologic study, NOS
P3-61801 Fungus serologic study, paired samples
P3-61810 Serologic test for Aspergillus
P3-61811 Serologic test for Blastomyces
P3-61812 Serologic test for Candida
P3-61813 Serologic test for Coccidioides
P3-61900 Parasite serologic study, NOS
P3-61901 Parasite serologic study, paired samples
P3-61A00 Viral serologic study, NOS
P3-61A01 Viral serologic study, paired samples, NOS
P3-61A10 Serologic test for cytomegalovirus
P3-61A11 Serologic test for herpes virus
P3-61A12 Serologic test for rubella
P3-61A13 Serologic test for herpes simplex
P3-61A14 Serologic test for respiratory syncytial virus
P3-61A15 Serologic test for influenza virus A
P3-61A16 Serologic test for influenza virus B
P3-61A20 Serologic test for Rotavirus, NOS
P3-62000 Anti-nuclear antibody measurement, NOS
  ANA measurement, NOS
  Deoxyribonucleic acid antibody measurement, NOS
P3-62001 Fluorescent identification of anti-nuclear antibody, NOS
P3-62002 Fluorescent identification of anti-nuclear antibody titration
P3-62004 Antibody to extractable nuclear antigen measurement, NOS
P3-62010 Antibody to double stranded DNA measurement
P3-62011 Antibody to Crithidia lucilia measurement
P3-62012 Antibody to single stranded DNA measurement
P3-62014 Antibody to single and double stranded DNA measurement
P3-62015 Quantitative anti-DNA antibody measurement
  FARR assay
P3-62016 Antibody to soluble DNA measurement
P3-62020 Antibody to histone measurement
P3-62021 Quantitative anti-histone antibody measurement
P3-62022 Antibody to SM measurement
P3-62030 Antibody to nuclear RNP measurement
P3-62034 Antibody to ribosomal RNP measurement
P3-62040 Antibody to Scl-70
P3-62044 Antibody to centromere measurement
P3-62050 Antibody to SS-A measurement
P3-62054 Antibody to SS-B measurement
P3-62060 Antibody to PM-1 measurement
P3-62062 Antibody to JO-1 measurement
P3-62064 Antibody to Mi-2 measurement
P3-62066 Antibody to Ku measurement
P3-62070 Antibody to PCNA measurement
P3-62072 Antibody to NSpI measurement
P3-62080 Antibody to nucleolus measurement
P3-62090 Antibody to nuclear matrix measurement
P3-62094 Antineuronal nuclear antibody-type I measurement
  ANNA-I measurement
P3-62100 Epstein-Barr virus serologic test, NOS
  EBV serologic test
P3-62110 Epstein-Barr nuclear antibody measurement
  EBNA antibody measurement
P3-62112 Epstein-Barr EA-R antibody measurement
P3-62114 Epstein-Barr EA-D antibody measurement
P3-62116 Epstein-Barr VCA antibody measurement
P3-62118 Epstein-Barr MA antibody measurement
P3-62130 Heterophile antibody measurement, NOS
P3-62132 Heterophile antibody screen
P3-62134 Heterophile antibody, quantitative titer
P3-62135 Heterophile antibody titer after absorption with beef cells and guinea pig kidney
P3-62140 Mono test, NOS
P3-62150 Identification of rotavirus antigen in feces
P3-62200 HIV antigen test
P3-62210 HIV-1 antibody assay, NOS
P3-62211 HIV-1 rapid latex agglutination assay
P3-62212 HIV-1 ELISA assay
P3-62216 HIV-1 passive hemagglutination assay
P3-62218 HIV-1 indirect immunofluorescence assay
P3-62220 HIV-1 antibody confirmatory test, NOS
P3-62222 HIV-1 Western blot assay
P3-62224 HIV-1 dot blot immunobinding assay
P3-62230 HIV-1 radioimmunoprecipitation assay
P3-62240 HIV-2 antigen assay
P3-62242 HIV-2 antibody assay, NOS
P3-62248 HIV-2 confirmatory assay
P3-62300 Serologic test for syphilis, NOS
  Treponema pallidum antibody measurement, NOS
P3-62302 Syphilis test, qualitative
P3-62304 Syphilis test, quantitative
P3-62308 Complement fixation test for syphilis, NOS
P3-62309 Microhemagglutination test for antibody to syphilis
P3-62310 Direct fluorescent antibody test for syphilis
  DFA-TP test
P3-62312 Fluorescent treponemal antibody absorption test
  FTA-ABS test
P3-62314 Fluorescent treponemal absorption test, double staining test
  FTA-ABS-DS test
P3-62320 Rapid plasma reagin test
  RPR test
P3-62324 VDRL test, NOS
P3-62325 VDRL, qualitative

P3-62326 VDRL, quantitative
P3-62350 Toluidine red unheated serum test
P3-62352 Unheated serum reagin test
P3-63000 Complement assay, NOS
P3-63010 Complement fixation test, NOS
P3-63012 Complement fixation titration, NOS
P3-63020 Complement assay, total
  CH_{50} assay, NOS
P3-63022 Complement hemolytic assay, NOS
P3-63030 Complement component assay, NOS
P3-63031 C_1 complement assay
P3-63032 C_1q complement assay
P3-63033 C_1r complement assay
P3-63034 C_1s complement assay
P3-63035 C_2 complement assay
P3-63036 C_3 complement assay
P3-63037 C_4 complement assay
P3-63038 C_5 complement assay
P3-63039 C_6 complement assay
P3-63040 C_7 complement assay
P3-63041 C_8 complement assay
P3-63042 C_9 complement assay
P3-63050 C_1q esterase inhibitor assay
  C_1 inhibitor assay
  C_1 inactivator assay
P3-63052 Factor B complement assay
  C_3 proactivator complement assay
  C_3 activator complement assay
P3-63053 Factor D complement assay
P3-63100 Complement typing procedure, NOS
P3-63200 Complement receptor measurement, NOS
P3-63210 CR type 1 receptor measurement
P3-63220 CR type 2 receptor measurement
P3-63230 CR type 3 receptor measurement
P3-63240 CR type 4 receptor measurement
P3-63300 DAF receptor measurement
P3-63302 MCP receptor measurement
P3-63310 C3a receptor measurement
P3-63312 C3e receptor measurement
P3-63320 Factor H receptor measurement
P3-63322 Factor B receptor measurement
P3-63330 C5a receptor measurement
P3-63340 C1q receptor measurement
P3-63430 Microcomplement consumption test
P3-63440 C1q precipitation test
P3-63442 C1q deviation test
P3-63444 C1q polyethylene glycol assay
P3-63446 C1q solid phase assay, NOS
P3-63448 Anti C3 solid phase assay, NOS
P3-63449 Anticomplement immunofluorescence test
  ACIF test
P3-63460 Conglutinin assay, NOS
P3-634A0 Immune complex assay, NOS
P3-634A2 Immune complex assay, c1q binding cell
P3-634A4 Immune complex assay, Raji cell
  Raji cell assay, NOS
P3-634B0 Plasma cell labelling index measurement
P3-63500 Immune cell phenotyping, NOS
P3-63510 Cluster of differentiation antigen detection, NOS
  CD antigen detection, NOS
P3-63550 T-cell antigen detection, NOS
  Lymphocyte T cell evaluation
P3-63560 B-cell antigen detection, NOS
  Lymphocytes, B-cell evaluation
P3-63565 Lymphocytes, T & B cell evaluation
P3-63570 Helper T-cell antigen measurement
P3-63572 Helper suppressor ratio determination
  Helper suppressor typing T-cell subsets measurement
P3-63580 Soluble CD8 T-cell antigen assay
  SCD8 T-cell assay
P3-63600 Myeloid antigen detection, NOS
P3-63620 Natural killer cell antigen detection, NOS
P3-63640 Nonlineage cell antigen detection, NOS
P3-63700 Immunoglobulin typing, NOS
P3-63710 Immunoglobulin typing, IgG
P3-63712 Immunoglobulin typing, IgM
P3-63714 Immunoglobulin typing, Inv
P3-64000 Hepatitis panel measurement
P3-64010 Hepatitis A virus measurement, NOS
P3-64012 Hepatitis A virus antibody measurement
  HAV antibody measurement
P3-64014 Hepatitis A virus antibody, IgG type
P3-64016 Hepatitis A virus antibody, IgM type
P3-64020 Hepatitis B virus measurement
P3-64021 Hepatitis B surface antigen measurement
  HBsAg measurement
P3-64022 Hepatitis B surface antibody measurement
  HBsAb measurement
P3-64030 Hepatitis B core antigen measurement
  HBcAg measurement
P3-64032 Hepatitis B core antibody measurement
  HBcAB measurement
P3-64033 Hepatitis B core antibody measurement, IgG type
P3-64034 Hepatitis B core antibody measurement, IgM type
P3-64040 Hepatitis Be antigen measurement
  HBeAg measurement
P3-64042 Hepatitis Be antibody measurement
  HBeAB measurement
P3-64050 Hepatitis C virus measurement, NOS
  HCV measurement
  Non A, non B hepatitis virus measurement, NOS
P3-64054 Hepatitis C antigen measurement
P3-64056 Hepatitis C antibody measurement
  Anti HCV measurement
  HCV antibody measurement
P3-64058 Hepatitis C virus recombinant immunoblot measurement
  HCV by RIBA measurement
P3-64070 Hepatitis D virus measurement
  HDV measurement
  Hepatitis delta agent measurement

SECTION 3-6 IMMUNOLOGIC PROCEDURES — Continued

P3-64072 Hepatitis D antigen measurement
P3-64076 Hepatitis D antibody measurement
P3-64080 Hepatitis E virus measurement
  HEV measurement
P3-64082 Hepatitis E antigen measurement
P3-64086 Hepatitis E antibody measurement
P3-65300 Radioallergosorbent test, NOS
  RAST test, NOS
  Allergen specific IgE antibody measurement
P3-65320 Radioallergosorbent test, in vitro testing for allergen-specific IGE, FAST type
  RAST test, FAST type
P3-65322 Radioallergosorbent test, in vitro testing for allergen-specific IGE, IP type
  RAST test, I type
P3-65324 Radioallergosorbent test, in vitro testing for allergen-specific IGE, MAST type
  RAST test, MAST type
P3-65326 Radioallergosorbent test, in vitro testing for allergen-specific IGE, PRIST type
  RAST test, PRIST type
P3-65350 Solid phase labelled antigen competitive binding immunoassay
  RIST assay, indirect
P3-65360 Solid phase sandwich immunometric noncompetitive immunoassay
  RIST assay, direct
P3-65362 Radioimmunosorbent test IGE, quantitative
  RIST test, quantitative
P3-65370 Liquid phase immunoprecipitation competitive binding immunoassay
P3-65380 Radioimmunoprecipitation assay
  RIP assay
P3-65400 Histamine release from basophils measurement
P3-65402 Mast cell degranulation test
  Basophil degranulation test
P3-65410 Histamine release from leukocytes measurement
P3-65420 Tryptase release from mast cell measurement
P3-65430 Direct immunobead assay
P3-65432 Indirect immunobead assay
P3-67000 Antibody to tissue specific antigen measurement, NOS
  Antibody to tissue specific organ measurement, NOS
P3-67004 Non-endocrine receptor assay, NOS
P3-67008 Striated muscle antibody, measurement
P3-67009 Smooth muscle antibody measurement
  Anti-smooth muscle antibody measurement
P3-67010 Thyroglobulin antibody measurement
  Anti-thyroglobulin antibody measurement
  Anti-thyroid antibody measurement
  Thyroid autoantibody test, NOS
P3-67011 Microsomal thyroid antibody measurement
P3-67012 Antibody to TSH receptor measurement
P3-67020 Antibody to adrenal antigen measurement
P3-67030 Antibody to mitochrondrial antigen measurement
P3-67040 Antibody to gastric parietal cell measurement
P3-67042 Intrinsic factor antibody measurement
  Intrinsic factor blocking antibody measurement
P3-67050 Antibody to islet cells of pancreas measurement
P3-67052 Insulin antibody measurement
P3-67054 Insulin factor antibody measurement
P3-67060 Antibody to epidermal antigen measurement, NOS
P3-67061 Antibody to skin antigen measurement by immunofluorescence
P3-67063 Antibody to salivary gland duct epithelium measurement
P3-67070 Antigen to cardiac tissue measurement
P3-67072 Endomysial antibody measurement
P3-67080 Antibody to spermatozoa measurement
P3-67100 Myasthenia gravis panel measurement, NOS
P3-67102 Acetylcholine receptor measurement
  Anti-Achr antibody measurement
  Acetylcholine receptor blocking antibody measurement
  Acetylcholine receptor modulating antibody measurement
P3-67120 Antineutrophil cytoplasmic antibody measurement
  ANCA measurement
  Neutrophil antibody assay, NOS
P3-67122 C-ANCA measurement
P3-67124 P-ANCA measurement
P3-67130 Leukocyte antibody measurement
P3-67150 Antiphospholipid antibody measurement
P3-67151 Anticardiolipin antibody measurement
P3-67200 Glomerular basement membrane antibody-IgG measurement
P3-67300 Tumor antigen measurement, NOS
  Immunoassay for tumor antigen, NOS
P3-67310 Tumor antibody measurement, NOS
  Anti-tumor antibody measurement, NOS
  Immunoassay for tumor antibody measurement, NOS
P3-67320 Alpha-1-Fetoprotein measurement
  AFP measurement
  Alpha Fetoprotein measurement
P3-67321 Alpha-1-Fetoprotein measurement, amniotic fluid
P3-67322 Alpha-1-Fetoprotein measurement, spinal fluid
  ASV measurement
P3-67340 Human chorionic gonadotropin measurement
  hCG measurement
  hCG, beta subunit measurement
P3-67342 Human growth hormone antibody measurement

P3-67350 Prostate specific antigen measurement
PSA measurement
P3-67352 PAP measurement
P3-67360 Antibody to CA 15-3 measurement
P3-67362 CA 15-3 measurement
P3-67370 Antibody to CA-125 measurement
P3-67372 CA 125 measurement
P3-67380 Breast tumor mucin measurement, NOS
P3-67382 CA 19-9 measurement
P3-67400 Antibody to cell surface receptor measurement
P3-67420 Estrogen receptor assay (ERA) measurement
P3-67422 Progesterone receptor assay measurement
P3-67424 Estrogen-progesterone receptor assay measurement
P3-68000 Lymphocyte blast cell transformation assay, NOS
Lymphocyte transformation assay, NOS
P3-68002 Lymphocyte transformation, spontaneous blastogenesis
P3-68004 Lymphocyte transformation, antigen induced
P3-68010 Mixed lymphocyte culture assay, NOS
Allogeneic mixed lymphocyte assay, NOS
MLC assay, NOS
P3-68020 Lymphocyte transformation with mitogen culture, NOS
P3-68030 Lymphocyte transformation, phytomitogen
P3-68031 Lymphocyte transformation, PHA
Phytohemagglutination assay
PHA assay
P3-68032 Concanavalin A assay
Con A assay
P3-68034 Pokeweed mitogen assay
P3-68050 Phorbol myristate acetate-ionomycin stimulation assay
P3-68070 Migration inhibitory factor test, NOS
MIF test, NOS
P3-68072 Leukocyte migration factor assay
P3-68073 Leukocyte migration inhibitor factor assay
P3-68074 Granulocyte migration factor assay
P3-68075 Granulocyte migration inhibitor factor assay
P3-68076 Lymphocyte migration factor assay
P3-68077 Lymphocyte migration inhibitor factor assay
P3-68078 Macrophage migration factor assay
P3-68079 Macrophage migration inhibitor factor assay
P3-68080 Phagocytosis assay, NOS
P3-68100 Cytokine assay, NOS
P3-68102 Lymphokine assay, NOS
P3-68106 Protein kinase C activity assay
P3-68107 Intracellular free calcium assay
P3-68108 Mononuclear cell function assay, NOS
P3-68109 TNF, Beta assay
P3-68110 IL-1 Alpha assay
P3-68112 IL-1 Beta assay
P3-68114 IL-2 assay
P3-68116 IL-3 assay
P3-68118 IL-4 assay
P3-68120 IL-5 assay
P3-68122 IL-6 assay
P3-68124 Il-7 assay
P3-68126 IL-8 assay
P3-68130 Interferon assay, NOS
IFN assay
P3-68132 Interferon alpha assay, NOS
P3-68134 Interferon beta assay, NOS
P3-68136 Interferon gamma assay, NOS
P3-68140 Tumor necrosis factor assay, NOS
Peripheral blood mononuclear cell assay, NOS
PBMC assay, NOS
MNC function assay, NOS
TNF assay, NOS
P3-68141 Mononuclear cell direct cytotoxicity assay
MTT reduction assay
P3-68142 Mononuclear cell growth inhibitor assay
P3-68143 Mononuclear cell hydrogen peroxide generation assay
P3-68144 Mononuclear cell neopterin production assay
P3-68146 Neutrophil staphylocidal assay
P3-68150 Tumor growth factor assay, NOS
P3-68151 Nitro Blue tetrazolium assay
NBT assay
P3-68152 TGF-Alpha assay
P3-68154 TGF-Beta assay
P3-68156 Cr^{51} release assay, NOS
P3-68190 Anticytokine antibody assay, NOS
P3-68200 Colony forming unit assay, NOS
Hematopoietic growth factor assay, NOS
CFU assay, NOS
P3-68210 Colony forming unit-granulocyte assay
CFU-G assay
P3-68220 Colony forming unit-macrophage assay
CFU-M assay
P3-68230 Colony forming unit-granulocyte/macrophage assay
CFU-GM assay
P3-68240 Colony forming unit-granulocyte-monocyte-erythroid-megakaryocyte assay
CFU-GEMM assay
P3-68250 Colony forming unit-mixed
CFU-mixed
P3-68260 Burst forming unit-erythroid assay
BFU-E assay
P3-68300 Antigen proliferation assay, NOS
P3-68310 Proliferative T lymphocyte assay
PTL assay
P3-68314 T cell antigen receptor assay, NOS
TCR assay, NOS
P3-68320 Primed lymphocyte test
PLT
P3-68330 Cell mediated lympholysis assay
CML assay
P3-68350 Antigen capture assay
P3-68352 Antigen capture EIA test
P3-68360 Antibody capture EIA test

SECTION 3-6 IMMUNOLOGIC PROCEDURES — Continued

P3-68500 Cytotoxicity assay, NOS
P3-68502 Complement mediated cytotoxicity assay
  Complement mediated cytotoxicity assay, dye exclusion assay
P3-68504 Antibody dependent cellular cytotoxicity assay
  ADCC assay
P3-68510 Cytotoxicity assay for endothelial/monocyte antigen
P3-68514 Cytotoxicity assay for epithelial/endothelial antigen
P3-68520 Cytotoxicity assay for autoantibody to HLA antigens, NOS
P3-68522 HLA class I serotyping
P3-68524 HLA class II serotyping
P3-68530 HLA-A serotyping, NOS
  Tissue typing for HLA, NOS
  Histocompatibility testing for HLA antigens, NOS
P3-68540 HLA-B serotyping, NOS
P3-68550 HLA-C serotyping, NOS
P3-68560 HLA-DR serotyping, NOS
P3-68570 HLA-DQ serotyping, NOS
P3-68590 Cytotoxicity assay for autoantibody, NOS
P3-68600 Histocompatibility crossmatch, NOS
  Histocompatibility crossmatch testing, NOS
P3-68610 Micro cytotoxicity crossmatch, NOS
P3-68612 Micro cytotoxicity crossmatch, NIH type
P3-68614 Micro cytotoxicity crossmatch, Amos wash type
P3-68616 Micro cytotoxicity crossmatch, anti human globulin type
P3-68618 Micro cytotoxicity crossmatch, long incubation type
P3-68619 Micro cytotoxicity crossmatch, B cell type
P3-68620 Lymphocytotoxicity assay, visual crossmatch with titration
P3-68622 Lymphocytotoxicity assay, visual crossmatch without titration
P3-68630 Flow cytometric crossmatch, NOS
P3-68632 Flow cytometric crossmatch, single color
P3-68634 Flow cytometric crossmatch, two colors
P3-68640 Serum screening for cytotoxic percent reactive antibody, standard method
  Serum screening for cytotoxic PRA, standard method
P3-68642 Serum screening for cytotoxic percent reactive antibody, quick method
  Serum screening for cytotoxic PRA, quick method
P3-68700 Non-sensitized spontaneous sheep erythrocyte binding, E-rosette
P3-68702 Detection of erythrocyte IgG antibody complex binding
  Ea rosette test
P3-68704 Detection of erythrocyte antibody complement complex binding
  Eac rosette test
P3-68710 Detection of aggregated IGG binding
P3-68712 Fc receptor test
  Fc receptor assay
P3-69010 ASO test
  Antistreptolysin O test
P3-69011 Antistreptolysin O screen
P3-69012 Antistreptolysin O titer
P3-69060 C-reactive protein measurement
P3-69080 Anti-streptokinase assay
P3-69100 Immunoassay for chemical constituent
P3-69200 Rheumatoid factor measurement, NOS
P3-69201 Rheumatoid factor, qualitative
P3-69202 Rheumatoid factor, quantitative
P3-69210 Colloidal gold test
P3-69240 Reticulin antibody measurement
P3-69280 Transfer factor test
P3-69290 Toxoplasmosis dye test
P3-69300 Autogenous vaccine preparation
P3-69310 Cardiolipin antigen preparation
P3-69330 Preparation of sensitized rbc for complement fixation
P3-6A050 Cell hybridization
P3-6A052 Cell fusion
P3-6A100 Tissue culture antitoxin assay, NOS
  Toxin or antitoxin assay in tissue culture
P3-6A101 Clostridium difficile toxin assay
  Clostridium difficile cytotoxicity assay in feces
P3-6A110 Virus identification by inoculation of embryonated eggs or small animal includes observation
P3-6A112 Virus identification by inoculation of embryonated eggs or small animal includes observation and dissection
P3-6A130 Virus identification by tissue culture inoculation and observation
P3-6A138 Virus identification in tissue culture with additional studies
P3-6A150 Mouse toxin neutralization test
P3-6A200 Viral neutralization test
P3-6A220 Human papillomavirus DNA detection
  HPV DNA detection
P3-6A222 Human papillomavirus typing
  HPV typing

SECTION 3-7 CHEMISTRY PROCEDURES

3-70 CHEMISTRY METHODS

P3-70000 Chemical procedure, NOS
  Chemical measurement, NOS
  Chemical test, NOS
P3-70010 Chemical method, NOS
  Chemical technique, NOS
  Chemical methodology, NOS
P3-70020 Special chemical test, explain by report
P3-70030 Chemical test, qualitative
P3-70050 Chemical test, semi-quantitative
P3-70070 Chemical test, quantitative

P3-70080 Chemical test, qualitative and quantitative
P3-70082 Test kit method, NOS
P3-70090 Spectrophotometric measurement, NOS
P3-70110 Spectrophotometric measurement, qualitative
P3-70130 Spectrophotometric measurement, quantitative
P3-70132 UV-VIS spectrophotometric measurement
P3-70200 Enzyme immunoassay, NOS
  EIA, NOS
  Immunoenzymatic assay, NOS
P3-70210 Enzyme-linked immunosorbant assay
  ELISA assay
P3-70211 Enzyme-linked immunoassay, competitive
P3-70212 Enzyme-linked immunoassay, noncompetitive
P3-70213 ELISA by avidin biotin peroxidase complex method
P3-70214 ELISA by peroxidase-antiperoxidase method
P3-70230 Enzyme-multiplied immunoassay technique
  EMIT assay
P3-70242 Capillary electrophoresis, NOS
P3-70270 Radioimmunoassay, NOS
  RIA
P3-70271 Solid phase radioimmunoassay
  SPRIA
P3-70272 Radioreceptor assay, NOS
  Immunoradiometric assay
  RRA, NOS
  IRMA
P3-70274 Radioimmunofocus assay
P3-70275 Solid phase fluoroimmunoassay
P3-70276 Autoradiographic cell labelling index measurement
P3-70290 Fluorescent immunoassay, NOS
  Immunofluorescence assay, NOS
  IMF assay
P3-70292 Fluorescence polarization immunoassay, NOS
P3-70293 Immunofluorescence cell labelling index measurement
P3-70294 Fluorescence polarization immunoassay, heterogenous
P3-70295 Fluorescence polarization immunoassay, homogeneous
P3-70296 Time resolved fluorescence immunoassay
P3-70300 Chemiluminescence assay
P3-70302 Immunochemiluminescent assay, NOS
P3-70310 Receptor binding site activity
P3-70315 Competitive protein binding assay, NOS
P3-70320 Immunodiffusion measurement, NOS
  ID measurement
P3-70321 Immunodiffusion, qualitative
P3-70322 Immunodiffusion, qualitative by Ouchterlony technique
P3-70324 Immunodiffusion, quantitative
P3-70326 Radial immunodiffusion measurement
  RID measurement
P3-70340 Electrophoresis measurement, NOS
  Zone electrophoresis measurement, NOS
P3-70341 Protein electrophoresis, NOS
P3-70342 Serum protein electrophoresis
P3-70343 Urine protein electrophoresis
P3-70344 CSF protein electrophoresis
P3-70345 Body fluid protein electrophoresis
P3-70350 Immunoelectrophoresis, NOS
  IEP
P3-70351 Serum immunoelectrophoresis
P3-70352 Immunofixation electrophoresis
  IFE
P3-70354 Counterimmunoelectrophoresis measurement
  CIE measurement
P3-70355 Crossed immunoelectrophoresis measurement
P3-70356 Countercurrent electrophoresis measurement
  CEP measurement
P3-70358 Isoelectric focusing measurement
  Electrofocusing measurement
P3-70359 Isotachyphoresis measurement, NOS
P3-70370 Plasma emission spectroscopy inductively coupled measurement, NOS
  Inductively coupled plasma emission spectroscopy
  ICPES measurement
P3-70380 Nuclear magnetic resonance measurement, NOS
P3-70384 Electron spin resonance measurement, NOS
P3-70392 Free radical assay technique measurement
  FRAT measurement
P3-703A0 Pharmacokinetic study, NOS
P3-70400 Atomic absorption measurement, NOS
P3-70401 Atomic absorption, flame type
P3-70402 Atomic absorption, Delves cup type
P3-70403 Atomic absorption, furnace type
P3-70404 Atomic absorption, flameless type
  Atomic absorption, cold vapor type
P3-70410 Mass spectrometry measurement, NOS
  Mass spectroscopy measurement, NOS
P3-70411 Mass spectrometry, electron impact type
P3-70412 Mass spectrometry, chemical ionization type
P3-70413 Mass spectrometry, field ionization type
P3-70414 Mass spectrometry, field desorption type
P3-70415 Mass spectrometry, plasma desorption type
P3-70420 Atomic emission measurement, NOS
P3-70440 Ion selective electrode measurement, NOS
  Specific ion electrode measurement
P3-70442 Anodic stripping voltammetry measurement
P3-70460 Chromatography measurement, NOS
P3-70470 Gas chromatography measurement, NOS
P3-70480 Gas liquid chromatography measurement, NOS
P3-70481 Gas liquid chromatography, flame ionization type
P3-70482 Gas liquid chromatography, electron capture type
P3-70483 Gas liquid chromatography, flame photometric type
P3-70484 Gas liquid chromatography, microwave plasma type

3-70 CHEMISTRY METHODS — Continued

P3-70485 Gas liquid chromatography, alkali flame ionization type
Gas liquid chromatography, thermionic type
P3-70486 Gas liquid chromatography, microcoulometric type
P3-70487 Gas liquid chromatography, Coulson conductivity type
P3-70488 Gas liquid chromatography, Hall conductivity type
P3-70489 Gas liquid chromatography, mass analyzer type
P3-70490 Liquid chromatography measurement, NOS
P3-70500 High performance liquid chromatography measurement, NOS
HPLC measurement, NOS
P3-70501 High performance liquid chromatography, refractive index type
P3-70502 High performance liquid chromatography, UV type
P3-70503 High performance liquid chromatography, fluorescence type
P3-70504 High performance liquid chromatography, mass analyzer type
P3-70505 High performance liquid chromatography, electrochemical type
P3-70506 High performance liquid chromatography, ion exchange type
P3-70510 Paper chromatography measurement
P3-70520 Thin layer chromatography measurement
P3-70530 Affinity chromatography measurement
P3-70531 Boronate affinity chromatography measurement
P3-70540 Immunoblot assay, NOS
P3-70550 Western blot assay
P3-70560 Southern blot assay
P3-70572 Northern blot assay
P3-70580 Tolerance test, NOS
P3-70590 Tolerance test, oral
P3-70600 Tolerance test, intravenous
P3-70610 Stimulation test
P3-70620 Activation test
P3-70630 Suppression test
P3-70640 Inhibition test
P3-70650 Provocative test
P3-70660 Rate measurement, NOS
P3-70670 Resorption rate measurement, NOS
P3-70680 Resorption rate measurement, renal tubule
P3-70690 Resorption rate measurement, gastrointestinal
P3-70700 Clearance rate measurement, NOS
P3-70710 Clearance rate measurement, renal
P3-70712 Creatinine clearance study
P3-70720 Clearance ratio measurement
P3-70730 Filtration rate measurement
P3-70740 Refractometer measurement, NOS
P3-70750 DNA hybridization assay, NOS
P3-70760 Turbidity test, NOS
Nephelometric measurement, NOS
Light scatter measurement, NOS
P3-70764 Turbidity test, quantitative
P3-70766 Turbidity test, qualitative
P3-70768 Flocculation test
P3-70770 Viscosity measurement
P3-70780 Centrifugation, NOS
P3-70782 Ultracentrifugation, NOS
P3-70786 Sucrose density gradient centrifugation technique
P3-70790 Polarographic measurement
P3-70800 Differential solubility measurement
P3-70810 Specific gravity measurement, NOS
P3-70820 Osmolality measurement
P3-70822 Osmolarity measurement
P3-70840 Laboratory calculation, NOS
P3-70842 Laboratory ratio determination, NOS
P3-70860 Uptake measurement
P3-70862 Excretion measurement
P3-70880 Electron probe scan, NOS
P3-70881 Electron probe scan, heavy metal
P3-70900 Chemical test for occult blood, NOS
Guaiac test
P3-70910 Spot test, NOS
P3-70920 Membrane stability test
Bubble stability test
P3-70930 Calculus analysis, NOS
P3-70931 Calculus analysis, qualitative
P3-70932 Calculus analysis, quantitative
P3-70933 Calculus analysis, quantitative, infrared spectroscopy
P3-70934 Calculus analysis, quantitative, X-ray diffraction
P3-70935 Common duct stone analysis
P3-70936 Gallstone analysis
P3-70937 Kidney stone analysis
P3-70938 Bladder stone analysis
P3-70940 Crystal identification, chemical, NOS
P3-70944 Crystal identification, polarization microscopy
P3-70950 Cytochemical test, NOS
P3-70960 Bioassay, NOS
P3-70961 Bioassay, qualitative
P3-70962 Bioassay, quantitative

3-71-74 SPECIFIC SUBSTANCE CHEMISTRY TESTS

P3-71080 Acetylcholinesterase measurement, NOS
P3-71081 Acetylcholinesterase measurement, amniotic fluid
AChE-AF measurement
P3-71082 Acetylcholinesterase, red blood cell measurement
Red cell cholinesterase measurement
Acetylcholinesterase, RBC measurement
Cholinesterase, erythrocytic measurement
P3-71086 True cholinesterase measurement
P3-71090 Acid mucopolysaccharides measurement

P3-71160 Acid phosphatase measurement
Prostatic acid phosphatase measurement
P3-71200 Adrenocorticotropic hormone measurement
Corticotropin measurement
ACTH measurement
P3-71220 Alanine aminotransferase measurement
GPT measurement
Glutamic pyruvate transaminase measurement
SGPT measurement
ALT measurement
P3-71240 Albumin/Globulin ratio
A/G ratio
P3-71260 Albumin measurement
P3-71280 Aldolase measurement
P3-71300 Aldosterone measurement
P3-71301 Aldosterone measurement, serum
P3-71302 Aldosterone measurement, standing, normal salt diet
P3-71303 Aldosterone measurement, recumbent, normal salt diet
P3-71306 Aldosterone measurement, urine
P3-71307 Aldosterone measurement, normal salt diet, urine
P3-71308 Aldosterone measurement low salt diet, urine
P3-71309 Aldosterone measurement, high salt diet, urine
P3-71310 Androstenedione measurement
P3-71320 Antidiuretic hormone measurement
Arginine vasopressin measurement
P3-71350 Alkaline phosphatase measurement
P3-71351 Alkaline phosphatase isoenzymes measurement
P3-71352 Placental alkaline phosphatase measurement
PLAP measurement
P3-71353 Intestinal alkaline phosphatase measurement
IAP measurement
P3-71354 Germ cell alkaline phosphatase measurement
GCAP measurement
P3-71359 Alkaline phosphatase, heat stable measurement
Thermostable alkaline phosphatase measurement
P3-71370 Alpha-1-antitrypsin measurement
P3-71380 Alpha-1-antitrypsin clearance, feces and serum
P3-71390 Alpha-1-antitrypsin phenotyping
Alpha-1-Protease inhibitor
P3-71440 Alpha-fucosidase measurement
P3-71441 Alpha-fucosidase measurement, fibroblasts
P3-71442 Alpha-fucosidase measurement, leukocytes
P3-71460 Alpha-galactosidase measurement
P3-71461 Alpha-galactosidase measurement, leukocytes
P3-71462 Alpha-galactosidase measurement, fibroblasts
P3-71520 Alpha-1-iduronidase measurement
P3-71521 Alpha-1-iduronidase measurement, leukocytes
P3-71522 Alpha-1-iduronidase measurement, fibroblasts
P3-71540 Alpha-mannosidase measurement
P3-71541 Alpha-mannosidase measurement, leukocytes
P3-71542 Alpha-mannosidase measurement, fibroblasts
P3-71560 Alpha-n-acetylglucosaminidase measurement
P3-71561 Alpha-n-acetylglucosaminidase measurement, fibroblasts
P3-71580 Alpha-subunit of pituitary glycoprotein hormone measurement
Alpha-PGH measurement
P3-71590 Paraaminohippurate measurement
Aminohippurate, para measurement
P3-71620 Amino acids measurement, NOS
P3-71622 Amino acids measurement, quantitative, urine
P3-71630 Amino acid screen
Metabolic screen for amino acids
P3-71700 Inborn errors of metabolism screen
P3-71760 Aminolevulinic acid dehydratase measurement
ALA-D measurement
P3-71780 Ammonia measurement
NH3 measurement
P3-71800 Amniotic fluid analysis for erythroblastosis fetalis
Liley test
Amniotic fluid analysis for hemolytic disease of the newborn
Amniotic fluid spectral analysis
P3-71820 Amniotic fluid lecithin/sphingomyelin ratio
Phospholipid profile, amniotic fluid
Fetal lung maturity profile
L/S ratio, amniotic fluid
P3-71840 Amniotic fluid pulmonary surfactant test
Pulmonary surfactant test
Shake test
P3-71860 Amylase measurement, NOS
P3-71861 Amylase measurement, pleural fluid
P3-71862 Amylase measurement, serum
P3-71863 Amylase measurement, urine
P3-71865 Amylase measurement, peritoneal fluid
P3-71900 Angiotensin converting enzyme measurement
ACE measurement
Angiotensin-I-converting enzyme measurement
P3-71920 Anion gap measurement
Ion gap measurement
P3-71924 Arachidonate measurement
P3-71930 Arginine tolerance test
P3-71940 Arylsulfatase A measurement, NOS
P3-71941 Arylsulfatase A measurement, urine
P3-71942 Arylsulfatase A measurement, leukocytes
P3-71943 Arylsulfatase A measurement, fibroblasts
P3-71950 Arylsulfatase B measurement, NOS
P3-71951 Arylsulfatase B measurement, fibroblasts
P3-71980 Ascorbic acid measurement
Vitamin C measurement
P3-72000 Aspartate aminotransferase measurement
AST measurement
Glutamic oxaloacetic transaminase measurement

3-71-74 SPECIFIC SUBSTANCE CHEMISTRY TESTS — Continued

P3-72000 (cont.) GOT measurement
SGOT measurement
P3-72010 Atrial natriuretic factor (ANF) measurement
P3-72040 Beta-galactosidase measurement, NOS
P3-72041 Beta-galactosidase measurement, fibroblasts
P3-72042 Beta-galactosidase measurement, leukocytes
P3-72060 Beta-glucosidase measurement, NOS
P3-72061 Beta-glucosidase measurement, fibroblasts
P3-72062 Beta-glucosidase measurement, leukocytes
P3-72080 Beta-glucuronidase measurement, NOS
P3-72081 Beta-glucuronidase measurement, fibroblasts
P3-72082 Beta-glucuronidase measurement, spinal fluid
P3-72120 Beta-2-microglobulin measurement
P3-72130 Bicarbonate loading test
P3-72132 Bicarbonate excretion measurement
P3-72140 Bilirubin, total measurement
Bilirubin measurement, amniotic fluid
Bilirubin measurement, urine
P3-72144 Total bile acids measurement
P3-72145 Cholylglycine measurement
P3-72150 Bilirubin, direct measurement
Bilirubin, conjugated measurement
P3-72160 Bilirubin, neonatal measurement
Total bilirubin, neonatal measurement
Microbilirubin measurement
Baby bilirubin measurement
P3-72170 Blood gases, arterial measurement
ABGs measurement
Gases, arterial measurement
P3-72171 Blood gases, venous measurement
P3-72172 Blood gases, capillary measurement
P3-72173V Bromsulphalein clearance
P3-72180 BUN/Creatinine ratio
P3-72200 Biotinidase measurement
P3-72220 Calcitonin measurement
Thyrocalcitonin measurement
P3-72230 Calcium measurement, NOS
P3-72231 Calcium measurement, urine
P3-72232 Calcium, serum, ionized measurement
Ionized calcium measurement
P3-72236 Calcium excretion, 2-hour collection, fasting, urine
P3-72240 Carbohydrate measurement, NOS
P3-72250 Carbon dioxide content measurement
CO_2 content measurement
P3-72252 Carbon dioxide measurement, partial pressure
PaCO2 measurement
P3-72260 Carboxyhemoglobin measurement
COHb measurement
Carbon monoxide measurement
P3-72270 Carcinoembryonic antigen measurement
CEA measurement
P3-72280 Cardiac enzymes/isoenzymes measurement, NOS
CK and/or LD isoenzymes measurement, NOS
P3-72300 Carotene measurement
P3-72310 Carnitine measurement, NOS
P3-72311 Carnitine measurement, serum
P3-72312 Carnitine measurement, tissue
P3-72320 Catecholamines, fractionation measurement, plasma
Pressor amines measurement, plasma
P3-72322 Catecholamines, fractionation measurement, urine
Free catecholamine fractionation measurement, urine
P3-72330 Cerebrospinal fluid immunoglobulin G
CSF gamma G
CSF IgG
Cerebrospinal fluid IgG
P3-72332 Cerebrospinal fluid oligoclonal bands
P3-72340 Cerebrospinal fluid protein
CSF protein
Protein, CSF
Protein, spinal fluid
P3-72341 Pandy test
P3-72350 Cerebrospinal fluid protein electrophoresis
Spinal fluid protein electrophoresis
CSF electrophoresis
P3-72360 Cerebrospinal fluid IgG ratio and IgG index
CSF IgG/CSF albumin ratio
P3-72364 Cerebrospinal fluid IgG synthesis rate
P3-72370 Myelin basic protein measurement, spinal fluid
MBP assay, spinal fluid
CSF myelin basic protein measurement
P3-72400 Ceruloplasmin measurement
P3-72410 Cholesterol measurement
P3-72412 Cholesteryl esters measurement
Cholesterol esters measurement
P3-72420 Chloride measurement, NOS
P3-72421 Chloride measurement, urine
P3-72430 Chorionic gonadotropin, beta-subunit measurement
Chorionic gonadotropin, beta-subunit measurement, spinal fluid
P3-72440 Chromium measurement, urine
P3-72450 Citrate measurement
P3-72452 Citrate excretion measurement, urine
P3-72460 Clomiphene test
Clomid test
P3-72470 Copper measurement, NOS
P3-72471 Copper measurement, urine
P3-72472 Copper measurement, liver tissue
P3-72473 Copper measurement, serum
P3-72500 Coproporphyrin measurement, NOS
P3-72510 Coproporphyrin I measurement
P3-72520 Coproporphyrin III measurement
P3-72530 Coproporphyrin isomers, series I & III, urine
P3-72540 Coproporphyrinogen oxidase measurement erythrocytes
P3-72550 Cortisol measurement, NOS
Hydrocortisone measurement

P3-72550 (cont.) Compound F measurement
P3-72552 Cortisol measurement, free, urine
P3-72553 11-deoxycortisol measurement
P3-72560 Cosyntropin test
  Cortisol response to cosyntropin test
  Rapid ACTH test
P3-72570 Creatine measurement, amniotic fluid
P3-72580 Creatine kinase measurement
  Creatine phosphokinase measurement
  CK measurement
  CPK measurement
P3-72590 Creatine kinase isoenzymes measurement
  CPK isoenzymes measurement
  CK isoenzymes measurement
  Creatine kinase isoforms measurement
P3-72600 Creatinine measurement, NOS
P3-72601 Creatinine measurement, serum
P3-72603 Creatinine measurement, 12 hour urine
P3-72604 Creatinine measurement, 24 hour urine
P3-72620 Cyclic adenosine monophosphate measurement
  Cyclic AMP measurement, urine
  Cyclic AMP measurement
  cAMP measurement
  Cyclic adenosine monophosphate measurement, urine
  cAMP measurement, urine
P3-72625 Cystic fibrosis sweat test
  Chloride measurement, sweat
P3-72630 Cystine measurement, qualitative
P3-72632 Cystine measurement, quantitative
P3-72640 Dehydroepiandosterone sulfate measurement
  DHEA-S measurement
P3-72650 Delta aminolevulinic acid measurement, urine
  ALA measurement, urine
  Aminolevulinic acid measurement, urine
  Delta-ALA measurement, urine
P3-72660 Delta base, blood
  Actual base excess
  Base excess
P3-72670 Deoxycorticosteroids measurement
P3-72680 Dibucaine number
  Cholinesterase inhibition by dibucaine measurement
  Pseudocholinesterase inhibition measurement
P3-72700 2,3-diphosphoglycerate measurement, erythrocytes
P3-72705 Dopamine measurement, NOS
P3-72706 Dopamine measurement, blood
P3-72707 Dopamine measurement, urine
P3-72710 Electrolytes measurement, NOS
P3-72711 Electrolytes measurement, urine
P3-72712 Electrolytes measurement, serum
P3-72713 Electrolytes measurement, plasma
P3-72714V BSP clearance
P3-72715 Congo red test
P3-72720 Epinephrine measurement, NOS
P3-72722 Epinephrine measurement, supine
P3-72724 Epinephrine measurement, standing
P3-72730 Erythropoietin measurement
  EPO assay
P3-72740 Estradiol measurement
P3-72750 Estriol measurement, NOS
P3-72751 Estriol measurement, serum
P3-72752 Estriol measurement, urine
P3-72760 Estrogen measurement, NOS
P3-72761 Estrogen measurement, urine
  Total urine estrogens
P3-72762 Etiocholanalone measurement
P3-72770 Fatty acid profile measurement, NOS
P3-72780 Fecal analysis, NOS
  Feces analysis, NOS
  Stool analysis, NOS
P3-72781 Fecal fat screening
P3-72782 Stool fat, quantitative measurement
P3-72783 Fecal fat measurement, 24-hour collection
P3-72784 Fecal fat measurement, 72-hour collection
P3-72785 Fecal fat differential, quantitative
P3-72786 Fecal trypsin, qualitative 24-hour specimen
P3-72787 Fecal trypsin, quantitative
P3-72789 Trypsin, duodenal fluid
P3-72790 Ferritin measurement
P3-72800 Folic acid measurement, serum
  Serum folate measurement
P3-72802 Folic acid measurement, RBC
  RBC folate measurement
P3-72810 Follicle stimulating hormone measurement
  FSH measurement
P3-72820 Free fatty acids measurement
P3-72830 Free thyroxine index
  FT4 index
  FTI
  FT4I
P3-72840 Fructosamine measurement
  Glycated protein measurement
P3-72850 Galactokinase measurement
P3-72860 Galactose-1-phosphate measurement
P3-72870 Galactose-1-phosphate uridyltransferase measurement
P3-72880 Galactose screening test for galactosemia
  Beutler test
  Paigen test
P3-72890 Galactose measurement, NOS
P3-72891 Galactose measurement, urine
P3-72900 Galactosylceramide beta-galactosidase measurement, NOS
P3-72901 Galactosylceramide beta-galactosidase measurement, fibroblasts
P3-72902 Galactosylceramide beta-galactosidase measurement, leukocytes
P3-72910 Gamma glutamyl transferase measurement
  Gamma glutamyl transpeptidase measurement
  GTP measurement

3-71-74 SPECIFIC SUBSTANCE CHEMISTRY TESTS — Continued

P3-72910 (cont.) GGT measurement
GGTP measurement
P3-72920 Gastrin measurement
P3-72922 Gibberelic acid measurement
P3-72930 Glucagon measurement
P3-72940 Glucose measurement, NOS
P3-72941 Glucose measurement, CSF
P3-72942 Glucose measurement, serum
P3-72943 Glucose measurement, plasma
P3-72944 Glucose measurement, urine
P3-72945 Glucose measurement, blood
P3-72946 Glucose measurement, fasting
P3-72947 Glucose measurement, random
P3-72948 Glucose measurement, 2 hour post prandial
P3-72949 Glucose measurement by monitoring device
Glucose monitoring at home
P3-72950 Glucose tolerance test, NOS
P3-72952 Glucose tolerance test, 2 hours
P3-72954 Glucose tolerance test, 3 hours
P3-72956 Glucose tolerance test, 5 hours
P3-72960 Glucose phosphate isomerase measurement
P3-72970 Glutathione measurement
P3-72980 Glucohemoglobin measurement, NOS
Glycosylated hemoglobin measurement
Glycated hemoglobin measurement
P3-72982 Hemoglobin A1c measurement
P3-72990 Growth hormone measurement
Somatotropin measurement
P3-73000 Haptoglobin measurement, electrophoresis
P3-73002 Haptoglobin measurement, chemical
P3-73010 Bicarbonate measurement
HCO_3- measurement
P3-73020 Hemoquant feces
P3-73030 Hemosiderin, quantitative measurement
P3-73040 Hexosaminidase A and total hexosaminidase measurement, NOS
P3-73041 Hexosaminidase A and total hexosaminidase measurement, amniotic fluid cells
P3-73042 Hexosaminidase A and total hexosaminidase measurement, serum
P3-73043 Hexosaminidase A and total hexosaminidase measurement, leukocytes
P3-73044 Hexosaminidase A and total hexosaminidase measurement, serum and leukocytes
P3-73045 Hexosaminidase A and total hexosaminidase measurement, fibroblasts
P3-73050 High density lipoprotein measurement
P3-73052 High density lipoprotein cholesterol measurement
HDL measurement
P3-73060 Histamine measurement
P3-73064 Homovanillic acid measurement
HVA measurement
P3-73070 Homogentisic acid measurement
P3-73080 Hydroxycorticosteroids measurement, urine
Porter-Silber chromogens measurement, urine
17-OHCS measurement
P3-73090 5-Hydroxyindoleacetic acid measurement, quantitative, urine
5-HIAA quantitative, urine
P3-73100 17 Hydroxyprogesterone measurement, NOS
P3-73101 17 Hydroxyprogesterone measurement, amniotic fluid
P3-73102 17 Hydroxyprogesterone measurement, serum
P3-73110 Hydroxyproline measurement, NOS
P3-73111 Hydroxyproline measurement, urine, total
P3-73114 Hydroxyproline measurement, free, urine
P3-73140 Immunoglobulin measurement, NOS
P3-73142 Secretory immunoglobulin A measurement
P3-73143 Immunoglobulin A measurement
P3-73144 Immunoglobulin M measurement
P3-73145 Immunoglobulin D measurement
P3-73146 Immunoglobulin E measurement
P3-73150 Immunoglobulin G measurement
P3-73151 Immunoglobulin G subclass measurement, NOS
P3-73152 Immunoglobulin G subclass, G1 measurement
P3-73153 Immunoglobulin G subclass, G2 measurement
P3-73154 Immunoglobulin G subclass, G3 measurement
P3-73155 Immunoglobulin G subclass, G4 measurement
P3-73170 Cryoglobulin measurement, NOS
P3-73171 Cryoglobulin measurement, type I
P3-73172 Cryoglobulin measurement, type II
P3-73173 Cryoglobulin measurement, type III
P3-73180 Anti-IgA assay
IgG anti-IgA assay
P3-73300 Insulin measurement
P3-73302 Immunoreactive insulin measurement
P3-73304 Insulin C-peptide measurement
Proinsulin C-peptide measurement
Connecting peptide insulin measurement
C-peptide measurement
P3-73320 Iodine, urine free measurement
P3-73330 Iron measurement, NOS
P3-73331 Iron measurement, liver tissue
P3-73332 Iron measurement, urine
P3-73340 Transferrin measurement
Total iron binding capacity measurement
P3-73341 Unsaturated iron binding capacity measurement
Iron, percent saturation, calculated
P3-73350 D-lactate measurement, NOS
P3-73351 D-lactate measurement, urine
P3-73360 Ketone bodies measurement, qualitative
Beta-hydroxybutyrate measurement
Acetoacetate measurement
Acetone measurement
Nitroprusside reaction, blood
P3-73361 Ketone bodies measurement, quantitative
P3-73370 17-Ketogenic steroids measurement
17-Ketosteroids measurement, total, urine
17-KS measurement
17-KGS measurement

P3-73372 17-Ketosteroids measurement, fractionation, urine
17-KS measurement, fractionation
P3-73380 Lactate dehydrogenase measurement
LD measurement
Lactic acid dehydrogenase measurement
LDH measurement
P3-73382 Lactate dehydrogenase isoenzymes measurement
LDH isoenzymes measurement
Lactic acid dehydrogenase isoenzymes measurement
LD isoenzymes measurement
P3-73390 Lactic acid measurement
P3-73400 Lactose tolerance test
P3-73410 Low density lipoprotein measurement, NOS
P3-73414 Low density lipoprotein cholesterol measurement
LDL cholesterol measurement
P3-73430 Leucine aminopeptidase measurement
Arylamidase measurement
LAP measurement
P3-73435 Linoleate measurement
P3-73440 Lipase measurement
P3-73450 Lipoprotein electrophoresis
Lipoprotein phenotyping
P3-73460 Lysozyme measurement, urine
Muramidase measurement
P3-73470 Luteinizing hormone measurement
Interstitial cell stimulating hormone measurement
LH measurement
ICSH measurement
P3-73480 Magnesium measurement, NOS
P3-73481 Magnesium measurement, serum
P3-73482 Magnesium measurement, urine
P3-73490 Manganese measurement, NOS
P3-73491 Manganese measurement, serum
P3-73492 Manganese measurement, urine
P3-73500 Metanephrines measurement, total
Metanephrines measurement, urine
P3-73510 Methemoglobin reductase measurement
P3-73512 Methemoglobin measurement, qualitative
P3-73514 Methemoglobin measurement, quantitative
P3-73520 Metyrapone test
P3-73530 N-methylimidazoleacetic acid measurement, urine
MIAA measurement, urine
P3-73540 MHPG measurement, urine
3-Methoxy-4-hydroxyphenylglycol measurement, urine
P3-73550 Microalbuminuria measurement, NOS
P3-73552 Microalbuminuria measurement, 10-hour collection, urine
P3-73554 Microalbuminuria measurement, 24-hour collection, urine
P3-73570 N-acetylglucosaminidase A & B measurement
P3-73580 Myoglobin measurement, NOS
P3-73581 Myoglobin measurement, urine
P3-73585 Neopterin measurement, NOS
P3-73590 Neuron-specific enolase measurement
S-NSE measurement
NSE measurement
P3-73595 Norepinephrine measurement
P3-73596 Norepinephrine measurement, standing
P3-73597 Norepinephrine measurement, supine
P3-73600 5' Nucleotidase measurement
P3-73610 Orotic acid measurement
P3-73620 Osmolality measurement, calculated
P3-73622 Osmolality measurement, serum
P3-73624 Osmolality measurement, urine
P3-73630 Oxalate measurement
Calcium oxalate measurement, urine
P3-73640 Oxygen saturation measurement, arterial
Hemoglobin saturation measurement
P3-73642 Oxygen measurement, partial pressure, arterial
PaO_2 measurement
P3-73650 P-50 blood gas measurement
PO_2 measurement
PO_2 at half saturation measurement
P3-73660 Palmitate measurement
P3-73670 Pancreatic polypeptide measurement
Human pancreatic polypeptide measurement
P3-73680 Parathyroid hormone measurement
Parathormone measurement
PTH measurement
Immunoreactive PTH measurement
P3-73681 Parathyroid related protein measurement
P3-73682 Parathyroid hormone measurement, C-terminal
PTH-C measurement
P3-73684 Parathyroid hormone measurement, functional N-terminal
P3-73686 Parathyroid hormone (PTH) immunochemiluminescent measurement
P3-73690 Carbon dioxide measurement
PCO_2, blood
P3-73700 pH measurement, NOS
P3-73702 pH measurement, arterial
P3-73704 pH measurement, venous
P3-73706 pH measurement, body fluid
P3-73720 Phenolphthalein measurement, urine
PSP test, urine
P3-73721 Phenolphthalein measurement, feces
P3-73730 Phosphatidylinositol measurement
P3-73740 Phosphatidylglycerol measurement, NOS
P3-73741 Phosphatidylglycerol measurement, semi-quantitative, amniotic fluid
P3-73750 Phenylalanine measurement
Guthrie test
Phenylalanine screening test, blood
P3-73752 Phenylketonuria test
PKU test
Hyperphenylalaninemia screen

3-71-74 SPECIFIC SUBSTANCE CHEMISTRY TESTS — Continued

P3-73752 (cont.) Phenylketone measurement, urine
P3-73760 Phosphofructokinase measurement, erythrocytes
P3-73770 Phospholipid measurement
P3-73780 Phosphorus measurement, NOS
  Phosphate, inorganic measurement
P3-73781 Phosphorus measurement, urine
P3-73785 Phytanate measurement
P3-73787 Pituitary gonadotropin measurement, NOS
P3-73790 Placental lactogen measurement
  Human chorionic somatomammotropin measurement
  Human placental lactogen measurement
  Chorionic somatomammotropin measurement
P3-73800 Porphobilinogen measurement, qualitative, urine
  Watson-Schwartz test
P3-73810 Porphyrin measurement, fractionation, erythrocytes
P3-73811 Porphyrin measurement, 24-hours, feces
P3-73812 Porphyrin measurement, total, erythrocytes
P3-73813 Porphyrin measurement, total, plasma
P3-73814 Porphyrin, quantitative measurement, urine
P3-73815 Porphyrin, feces, quantitative
P3-73816 Fecal urobilin, quantitative
P3-73817 Fecal urobilinogen, quantitative
P3-73818 Fecal stercobilin, qualitative
P3-73820 Uroporphyrin measurement
P3-73850 Potassium measurement, NOS
P3-73851 Potassium measurement, urine
P3-73860 Prealbumin measurement
P3-73870 Pregnanetriol measurement
P3-73872 Pregnanediol measurement
P3-73880 Progesterone measurement
P3-73890 Prolactin measurement
P3-73900 Prostacyclin measurement
  6-Keto-PG-F-1 measurement
P3-73920 Protein measurement, NOS
P3-73921 Protein measurement, urine
P3-73922 Protein measurement, urine, quantitative 24 hour
P3-73924 Oligoclonal protein measurement
P3-73930 Protoporphyrin measurement
  Protoporphyrins fractionation, erythrocytes
  Protoporphyrin, free erythrocyte
  RBC protoporphyrin measurement
P3-73940 Pseudocholinesterase measurement
  Cholinesterase measurement
P3-73950 Pyruvate kinase measurement, NOS
P3-73951 Pyruvate kinase measurement, erythrocytes
P3-73960 Renin measurement
P3-73961 Renin, normal salt intake measurement, recumbent, 6 hours
P3-73962 Renin, normal salt intake measurement, upright, 4 hours
P3-73963 Renin, low salt intake measurement, recumbent, 6 hours
P3-73964 Renin, low salt intake measurement, upright, 4 hours
P3-73965 Renin, low salt intake measurement, upright, 4 hours with diuretic
P3-73970 Retinoids measurement
P3-73990 Serotonin measurement
  5-Hydroxytryptamine measurement
P3-74010 Sex hormone binding globulin measurement
  SHBG measurement
P3-74020 Sodium measurement
  Sodium measurement, urine
P3-74040 Somatomedin-C measurement
  Insulin-like growth factor-1 measurement
P3-74050 Sphingomyelinase measurement, NOS
P3-74051 Sphingomyelinase measurement, fibroblasts
P3-74060 T3 reverse measurement
  Tri-iodothyronine reverse measurement
P3-74070 T3 uptake measurement
  Tri-iodothyronine resin uptake measurement
  T3U measurement
P3-74080 T4 free measurement
  FT4 measurement
  Free thyroxine measurement
  Unbound T4 measurement
  Free T4 measurement
P3-74090 T4 newborn screen
  Thyroid screen for newborn
  T4 neonatal screen
P3-74100 Testosterone measurement, total
P3-74102 Testosterone measurement, unbound
P3-74110 Thyroglobulin measurement
P3-74120 Thyroid stimulating hormone measurement
  TSH measurement
  Thyrotropin measurement
  Thyrotropin stimulating hormone measurement
P3-74130 Thyroxine measurement
  T4 measurement
  Tetraiodothyronine measurement
P3-74132 Thyroid hormone binding index measurement
  T4/TBG ratio
P3-74140 Thyroxine binding globulin measurement
  T4-binding globulin measurement
  TBG measurement
P3-74150 Tyrosine measurement
P3-74160 Siderophilin measurement
P3-74170 Triglycerides measurement
  Triacylglycerols measurement
P3-74180 Tri-iodothyronine measurement, total
  T3, total measurement
P3-74190 Urea nitrogen measurement
  Blood urea nitrogen measurement
  BUN measurement
P3-74200 Uric acid measurement, NOS
  Urate measurement, NOS

P3-74201 Uric acid measurement, urine
P3-74210 Urobilinogen measurement, NOS
P3-74211 Urobilinogen measurement, urine
P3-74212 Urobilinogen measurement, 48-hour, feces
P3-74220 Uroporphyrinogendecarboxylase measurement, erythrocytes
P3-74230 Uroporphyrinogen-I-synthase measurement
P3-74231 Uroporphyrinogen-I-synthase measurement, erythrocyte
Erythrocyte PBG-deaminase measurement
P3-74240 Vanillylmandelic acid measurement
VMA measurement
3-Methoxy-4-hydroxymandelic acid measurement
P3-74250 Vasoactive intestinal polypeptide measurement
VIP measurement
P3-74260 Very long chain fatty acids measurement
P3-74270 Vitamin A measurement
P3-74280 Vitamin B6 measurement
Pyridoxal phosphate measurement
Pyridoxine measurement
P3-74290 Vitamin B12 measurement
Cyanocobalamin, true measurement
Antipernicious anemia factor measurement
P3-74292 Vitamin B12 binding capacity measurement
P3-74300 Vitamin D measurement, NOS
Cholecalciferol measurement, NOS
Vitamin D3 measurement, NOS
P3-74301 Vitamin D, 1,25-dihydroxy measurement
P3-74302 Vitamin D, 25-hydroxy measurement
P3-74320 Vitamin E measurement
Alpha tocopherol measurement
Tocopherol measurement
P3-74330 Zinc measurement, NOS
P3-74331 Zinc measurement, urine
P3-74340 D-xylose, blood
P3-74341 D-xylose, urine

3-77 GENERAL DRUG MONITORING PROCEDURES AND TOXICOLOGY SCREENS

P3-77020 Pharmacometric study, NOS
P3-77040 Therapeutic drug monitoring assay, NOS
P3-77080 Therapeutic drug monitoring, quantitative
P3-77090 Therapeutic drug monitoring, qualitative
P3-77140 Antibiotic measurement, NOS
Antimicrobial measurement, NOS
P3-77142 Serum antimicrobial level, bioassay method
P3-77144 Serum antimicrobial level, immunoassay method
P3-77146 Serum antimicrobial level, radioimmunoassay method
P3-77180 Drug of abuse screen, NOS
Narcotics screen, NOS
P3-77181 Drug of abuse, qualitative screen
P3-77182 Drug of abuse, quantitative screen, includes amphetamines, barbiturates, benzodiazepines, cannabinoids, cocaine, methadone, methaqualone, opiates, phencyclidines and propoxyphene
P3-77183 Drug of abuse screen on urine
P3-77184 Drug of abuse screen on gastric fluid
P3-77185 Drug of abuse screen on bile
P3-77220 Drug screen for alkaloids, NOS
P3-77260 Heavy metal screen, NOS
P3-77261 Heavy metal screen, qualitative
P3-77262 Heavy metal screen, quantitative, includes antimony, arsenic, bismuth, boron, cadmium, cobalt, lead, mercury, selenium, tellurium, thallium and zinc
P3-77263 Heavy metal screen on blood
P3-77264 Heavy metal screen on urine
P3-77265 Heavy metal screen on gastric fluid
P3-77266 Heavy metal screen on bile
P3-77300 Organic acid screen, NOS
P3-77340 Organic acid screen, qualitative
P3-77380 Organic acid screen, quantitative
P3-77420 Volatile substance screen, includes acetone, ethanol, isopropanol, methanol, acetic anhydride, carbon tetrachloride, dichloroethane, dichloromethane and diethylether
P3-77460 Neuroleptic drug screen, NOS
P3-77500 Pesticides screen
P3-77540 Chlorinated hydrocarbon screen
P3-77620 Essential elements screen
P3-77660 Toxicology screen, general, NOS
P3-77700 Toxicology screen, sedatives, NOS

3-78 SPECIFIC DRUG AND TOXICOLOGY TESTS

P3-78000 Toxicology substance measurement, NOS
P3-78004 Therapeutic compound measurement, NOS
P3-78010 Acetominophen measurement, NOS
P3-78011 Acetaminophen measurement, urine
P3-78015 Acetozolamide measurement
P3-78018 Acetaldehyde measurement
P3-78020 Acetylsalicylic acid measurement, quantitative
P3-78025 Acetylsalicylic acid measurement, qualitative
P3-78030 Alcohol measurement, NOS
Ethanol measurement, NOS
P3-78031 Alcohol measurement, urine
P3-78032 Alcohol measurement, breath
P3-78035 Alcohol, isopropyl measurement
P3-78037 Alcohol, methyl measurement
Methanol measurement
P3-78045 Alkaloids measurement, tissue screening
Alkaloids measurement, tissue quantitative
P3-78046 Alkaloids measurement, urine screening
Alkaloids measurement, urine quantitative
P3-78050 Aluminum measurement, NOS
P3-78051 Aluminum measurement, blood
P3-78052 Aluminum measurement, tissue
P3-78053 Aluminum measurement, urine
P3-78055 Amikacin measurement
P3-78065 Amitriptyline measurement
P3-78070 Amphetamine measurement
P3-78075 Amphotericin measurement
Fungizone measurement

3-78 SPECIFIC DRUG AND TOXICOLOGY TESTS — Continued

P3-78080 Amoxapine measurement
P3-78085 Aniline measurement
P3-78090 Antimony measurement, NOS
P3-78091 Antimony measurement, urine
P3-78100 Azidothymidine measurement
Azt measurement
P3-78104 Arsenic measurement, NOS
P3-78105 Arsenic measurement, blood
P3-78106 Arsenic measurement, urine
P3-78107 Arsenic measurement, hair
P3-78108 Arsenic measurement, gastric
P3-78109 Arsenic measurement, nails
P3-78110 Barbiturates measurement, qualitative
P3-78115 Barbiturates measurement, quantitative
P3-78120 Barbiturates measurement, quantitative and qualitative
P3-78125 Barium measurement
P3-78130 Benzodiazepine measurement, NOS
P3-78135 Beryllium measurement
P3-78138 Beta lactamase measurement
P3-78140 Bismuth measurement
P3-78145 Boric acid measurement, NOS
Boron measurement
P3-78146 Boric acid measurement, blood
P3-78147 Boric acid measurement, urine
P3-78150 Bromides measurement, NOS
P3-78151 Bromides measurement, blood
P3-78152 Bromides measurement, urine
P3-78155 Butabarbital measurement
P3-78160 Butalbital measurement
P3-78165 Cadmium measurement, NOS
P3-78166 Cadmium measurement, urine
P3-78170 Caffeine measurement
P3-78175 Cannabinoids measurement, NOS
Hashish measurement
Marijuana measurement
Tetracannibinol measurement
P3-78180 Carbamazepine measurement
Tegretol measurement
P3-78185 Chloral hydrate measurement, NOS
P3-78186 Chloral hydrate measurement, blood
P3-78187 Chloral hydrate measurement, urine
P3-78190 Chloramphenicol measurement
Chloromycetin measurement
P3-78195 Chlorazepate dipotassium measurement
P3-78200 Chlordiazepoxide measurement, NOS
Librium measurement, NOS
P3-78201 Chlordiazepoxide measurement, blood
P3-78202 Chlordiazepoxide measurement, urine
P3-78203 Chlorpromazine measurement
P3-78205 Chromium measurement
P3-78210 Clonazepam measurement
Cobalt measurement
P3-78215 Cocaine measurement
P3-78220 Cotinine measurement
P3-78225 Cyanide measurement, NOS
P3-78226 Cyanide measurement, blood
P3-78227 Cyanide measurement, tissue
P3-78230 Cyclosporine measurement
P3-78235 Diazepam measurement
Valium measurement
Nordiazepam measurement
P3-78240 Desipramine measurement
P3-78245 Digitoxin measurement
Digitalis measurement
P3-78250 Digoxin measurement
P3-78260 Dihydrocodeinone measurement
P3-78265 Dihydromorphinone measurement
P3-78270 Disopyramide measurement
P3-78275 Dimethadione measurement
P3-78280 Doxepin measurement
P3-78285 Encainide measurement
P3-78290 Ethchlorvynol measurement, NOS
Placidyl measurement, NOS
P3-78291 Ethchlorvynol measurement, blood
P3-78292 Ethchlorvynol measurement, urine
P3-78295 Ethosuximide measurement
P3-78300 Ethylene glycol measurement
Antifreeze measurement
P3-78305 Flecainide measurement
P3-78310 Flucytosine measurement
5-Fluorocytosine measurement
P3-78315 Prozac measurement
P3-78320 Fluoride measurement
P3-78325 Fluphenazine measurement
P3-78330 Flurazepam measurement
Dalmane measurement
P3-78335 Gadolinium measurement
P3-78340 Gallium measurement
P3-78345 Gentamicin measurement
P3-78350 Germanium measurement
P3-78355 Glutethimide measurement
Doriden measurement
P3-78360 Gold measurement
P3-78365 Haloperidol measurement
Haldol measurement
P3-78370 Isonicotinic acid hydrazide measurement
INH measurement
P3-78375 Kanamycin measurement
P3-78380 Lead screening, NOS
P3-78381 Lead screening, blood
P3-78382 Lead screening, urine
P3-78385 Lead measurement, quantitative, NOS
P3-78386 Lead measurement, quantitative, blood
P3-78387 Lead measurement, quantitative, urine
P3-78390 Lidocaine measurement
Xylocaine measurement
P3-78395 Lithium measurement
P3-78400 Lysergic acid diethylamide measurement
LSD measurement
P3-78405 Maprotiline measurement
P3-78410 Meperidine measurement
P3-78415 Mephenytoin measurement
Mesantoin measurement

P3-78420 Mephobarbital measurement
P3-78425 Meprobamate measurement, NOS
Equanil measurement, NOS
P3-78426 Meprobamate measurement, urine
P3-78430 Mercury measurement, NOS
P3-78431 Mercury measurement, blood
P3-78432 Mercury measurement, urine
P3-78433 Mercury measurement, hair
P3-78434 Mercury measurement, nails
P3-78435 Methadone measurement
P3-78440 Methamphetamine measurement
P3-78445 Methapyrilene measurement
Lude measurement
P3-78450 Methotrexate measurement
P3-78455 Methsuximide measurement
P3-78460 Methyprylon measurement
P3-78465 Mexilitene measurement
P3-78470 Molybdenum measurement
P3-78475 Monoethylglycinexylidide measurement
P3-78480 Morphine measurement screening
P3-78485 Morphine measurement, quantitative
P3-78490 Methaqualone
P3-78495 Nalorphine measurement
P3-78500 Nickel measurement
P3-78502 Nicotine measurement
P3-78505 Nortryptyline measurement
P3-78510 Opiates, NOS
P3-78515 Opiates, qualitative
P3-78520 Opiates, quantitative
P3-78525 Ouabain measurement
P3-78530 Oxazepam measurement
P3-78535 Oxybutyric acid measurement
P3-78540 Oxycodinone measurement
P3-78545 Oxytocinase measurement
P3-78550 Paraldehyde measurement
P3-78555 Penicillin measurement
P3-78557 Penicillinase measurement
P3-78560 Pentazocine measurement
P3-78565 Pentobarbital measurement
Phenobarbital measurement
P3-78570 Phencyclidine measurement
PCP measurement
Angel dust measurement
P3-78575 Phenol measurement, NOS
P3-78576 Phenol measurement, blood
P3-78577 Phenol measurement, urine
P3-78580 Phenothiazine measurement, NOS
Thorazine measurement
Compazine measurement
P3-78585 Phenothiazine measurement, qualitative
P3-78590 Phenothiazine measurement, quantitative
P3-78595 Phenylbutazone measurement
P3-78600 Phenylpropanolamine measurement
P3-78605 Phenytoin measurement
Diphenylhydantoin measurement
Dilantin measurement
P3-78610 Platinum measurement
P3-78615 Primidone measurement
Mysoline measurement
P3-78620 Procainamide measurement
Pronestyl measurement
P3-78625 Propoxyphene measurement
Darvon measurement
Darvocet measurement
P3-78630 Propranolol measurement
P3-78635 Protriptyline measurement
P3-78640 Quinine measurement
P3-78645 Quinidine measurement
P3-78650 Salicylate measurement
Acetylsalicylic acid measurement
Aspirin measurement
P3-78655 Secobarbital measurement
P3-78660 Selenium measurement, NOS
P3-78661 Selenium measurement, blood
P3-78662 Selenium measurement, urine
P3-78663 Selenium measurement, tissue
P3-78670 Silica measurement, NOS
P3-78671 Silica measurement, blood
P3-78672 Silica measurement, tissue
P3-78673 Silica measurement, urine
P3-78675 Silver measurement
P3-78680 Strychnine measurement
P3-78690 Sulfonamide measurement
P3-78692 Sulfadizine measurement
P3-78694 Sulfapyridine measurement
P3-78696 Sulfisoxazole measurement
P3-78700 Tetracaine measurement
P3-78705 Thallium measurement, blood
P3-78706 Thallium measurement, urine
P3-78710 Theophylline measurement, NOS
Aminophyline measurement, NOS
P3-78711 Theophylline measurement, blood
P3-78712 Theophylline measurement, saliva
P3-78715 Thiocyanate measurement, blood
P3-78720 Thioridazine measurement
P3-78725 Tin measurement
P3-78730 Titanium measurement
P3-78735 Tocainide measurement
P3-78737 Tobramycin measurement
P3-78740 Trazodone measurement
P3-78741 Tricyclic antidepressant measurement, NOS
P3-78745 Trifluoperazine measurement
P3-78750 Trimethadione measurement
P3-78755 Valproic acid measurement
P3-78760 Vancomycin measurement
P3-78765 Verapamil measurement
P3-78770 Warfarin measurement
Dicumarol measurement
P3-78780V Toxicology testing for insecticide, NOS
P3-78781V Toxicology testing for Cl-HC insecticide
P3-78782V Toxicology testing for organophosphate insecticide
P3-78783V Toxicology testing for ANTU

SECTION 3-9 URINE AND SEMEN ANALYSIS

P3-90000 Urinalysis, NOS
Urinalysis procedure, NOS

SECTION 3-9 URINE AND SEMEN ANALYSIS — Continued

P3-90010 Urinalysis, routine and microscopic
Urinalysis, reagent strip with microscopy
Urinalysis, complete
P3-90012 Urinalysis, reagent strip without microscopy
Urinalysis, dipstick method
Urinalysis, qualitative, chemical
Rapid urine screening test, NOS
P3-90030 Urinalysis, microscopic only, NOS
P3-90032 Urinalysis, sediment examination, centrifuged
P3-90034 Urinalysis, sediment examination, uncentrifuged
P3-90100 Urinalysis, glucose, qualitative
P3-90140 Urinalysis, bacteriuria screen
Urine nitrite test
Urinalysis, WBC esterase method
P3-90150 Rapid urine screening test, enzyme tube test, NOS
P3-90160 Urinalysis, protein, qualitative
P3-90170 Rapid urine screening test, bioluminescence, NOS
P3-90180 Urinalysis, blood, qualitative
Chemical test for occult blood, urine
P3-90200 Urinalysis, acetone or ketone bodies measurement
P3-90220 Urinalysis, acetoacetic acid-diacetic acid measurement
P3-90240 Urinalysis, specific gravity measurement
P3-90260 Tritratable acidity, urine measurement
P3-90280 Calcium, urine, qualitative
Sulkowitch test
P3-90300 Bile pigment measurement, urine
P3-90310 Ferric chloride test, urine
P3-90320 Hemosiderin measurement, urine
P3-90340 Indican measurement, urine
P3-90350 Melanin measurement, urine, qualitative
P3-90370 Protein, urine, Bence-Jones
P3-90380 Urobilin, urine, qualitative
P3-90390 Fat stain, urine
P3-90400 Crystal identification, urine
P3-90410 Water load test
P3-90420 Urine concentration test
P3-90430 Urine dilution test
P3-90990 Urinalysis, automated, NOS
P3-91000 Semen analysis, NOS
P3-91002 Semen analysis, post vasectomy
P3-91010 Complete semen analysis
Complete semen analysis with volume, count, motility and differential
P3-91020 Semen analysis, presence only
P3-91030 Semen analysis, presence and motility of sperm
P3-91035 Semen analysis, motility and count
P3-91100 Seminal fluid detection, NOS
P3-91110 Seminal fluid detection by acid phosphatase method
P3-91200 Sperm evaluation by hamster penetration test
P3-91210 Sperm evaluation by cervical mucus penetration test
Huhner test
P3-91230 Fructose measurement, semen

SECTION 3-A FOOD ANALYSIS PROCEDURES

P3-A0000 Food analysis, NOS
Feed analysis, NOS
P3-A0010V Water analysis, NOS
P3-A0100V Proximate feed analysis
P3-A0101V Feed analysis for salt
P3-A0102V Feed analysis for non-protein nitrogen
P3-A0103V Feed analysis for moisture
P3-A0104V Feed analysis for total sugars
P3-A0105V Feed analysis for moisture-protein-fiber
P3-A0106V Feed analysis for protein-fat-CHO-calories
P3-A0108V Feed analysis for fat
P3-A0109V Feed analysis for acid insoluble ash
Feed analysis for ash
P3-A010AV Feed analysis for fiber
P3-A0110V Feed analysis for pepsin digestibility
P3-A0112V Feed analysis for protein
P3-A0114V Feed analysis for fat-fiber-protein
P3-A0120V Premix analysis
P3-A0122V Feed antibiotic assay
P3-A0130V Meat inspection for toxicology
P3-A0131V Feed analysis for mycotoxin
P3-A0132V Meat inspection for bacterial culture

CHAPTER 5 — RADIOLOGY, RADIOTHERAPY, NUCLEAR MEDICINE AND ULTRASOUND PROCEDURES

SECTION 5-0 GENERAL RADIOLOGY PROCEDURES, TECHNIQUES AND SERVICES

5-00 GENERAL DIAGNOSTIC RADIOGRAPHIC PROCEDURES

P5-00005 Special radiologic procedure or service, explain by report
  Special diagnostic radiologic procedure, explain by report
P5-00010 Diagnostic radiologic examination, NOS
  Diagnostic radiography, NOS
  X-ray, NOS
P5-00012 Diagnostic radiography, right
P5-00014 Diagnostic radiography, left
P5-00016 Diagnostic radiography, bilateral
P5-00018 Diagnostic radiography, lateral
P5-00020 Diagnostic radiography, anteroposterior (AP)
P5-00022 Diagnostic radiography, posteroanterior (PA)
P5-00024 Diagnostic radiography, oblique, standard
P5-00026 Diagnostic radiography, oblique, special
P5-00030 Diagnostic radiography, stereo
P5-00032 Diagnostic radiography, stereotactic localization
P5-00040 Diagnostic radiography, combined PA and lateral
P5-00042 Diagnostic radiography, combined AP and lateral
P5-00044 Diagnostic radiography, lateral decubitus studies
P5-00046 Diagnostic radiography, supine and erect studies
P5-00048 Diagnostic radiography, flexion and/or extension studies
P5-00050 Diagnostic radiography, minifilm
P5-00060 Diagnostic radiography during operative procedure
P5-00062 Diagnostic radiography for foreign body detection and localization
P5-00070 Diagnostic radiography with measurements
P5-00080 Diagnostic radiography, survey, NOS
P5-00090 Diagnostic radiography, special views
P5-00100 Diagnostic radiography with contrast media, NOS
  Diagnostic radiologic examination with contrast media, NOS
P5-00101 Subtraction in conjunction with contrast studies
P5-00102 Diagnostic radiography with contrast media, unilateral
P5-00104 Diagnostic radiography with contrast media, bilateral
P5-00106 Diagnostic radiography with oral contrast
  Diagnostic radiography with contrast media by ingestion
P5-00110 Roentgenography, negative contrast, NOS
P5-00112 Diagnostic radiography with gas-air, negative contrast
P5-00114 Diagnostic radiography with contrast media by injection, negative contrast, NOS
P5-00120 Diagnostic radiography with contrast media by injection, unilateral
P5-00121 Diagnostic radiography with contrast media by injection, bilateral
P5-00122 Diagnostic radiography with contrast media by injection, positive contrast, NOS
P5-00124 Diagnostic radiography with contrast media by injection, positive contrast, unilateral
P5-00126 Diagnostic radiography with contrast media by injection, positive contrast, bilateral
P5-00130 Diagnostic radiography with contrast media by injection, positive contrast, operative
P5-00132 Diagnostic radiography with contrast media by injection, positive contrast, post-operative
P5-00134 Diagnostic radiography double contrast, NOS
  Diagnostic radiography with contrast media by injection, positive and negative contrast, NOS
P5-00136 Diagnostic radiography with contrast media by injection, positive and negative contrast, unilateral
P5-00138 Diagnostic radiography with contrast media by injection, positive and negative contrast, bilateral
P5-00140 Diagnostic radiography, serial films, NOS
  Serialography, NOS
P5-00142 Serialography, single plane
P5-00144 Serialography, multi-plane
P5-00150 Diagnostic tomography, NOS
  Diagnostic laminographic examination, NOS
  Diagnostic tomographic examination, NOS
P5-00152 Polytomography, NOS
P5-00160 Cineradiography, NOS
P5-00162 Cineradiography to complement routine examination
P5-00170 Xeroradiography, NOS
  Xerography, NOS
P5-00210 Diagnostic video sound tape
P5-00220 Diagnostic radiography of fistula or sinus tract, positive contrast
  Fistulogram
P5-00221 Radiologic examination of fistula or sinus tract with radiological supervision and interpretation
P5-00300 Skeletal X-ray, NOS
P5-00312 Radiologic examination, osseous survey, complete
  Skeletal series, NOS
  Radiography for bone survey

5-00 GENERAL DIAGNOSTIC RADIOGRAPHIC PROCEDURES — Continued

P5-00312 (cont.) Complete skeletal series

P5-00314 Radiologic examination, osseous survey, limited
Diagnostic radiography, osseous survey, limited

P5-00316 Radiologic examination osseous survey, infant

P5-00320 Radiography for bone age studies
Bone age studies by X-ray

P5-00340 Radiography for bone length studies
Orthoroentgenogram

P5-00380 Arthrography, NOS
Arthrogram, NOS

P5-00382 Joint survey, single view of one or more joints

P5-00400 Injection of contrast media for radiography, NOS
Radiological injection procedure, NOS

P5-00410 Injection of contrast media for radiography by direct puncture

P5-00420 Injection of contrast media for radiography by catheter, NOS

P5-00422 Injection of contrast media for radiography by catheter, non-selective

P5-00424 Injection of contrast media for radiography by catheter, selective

P5-00426 Injection of contrast media for radiography by catheter, supraselective

P5-00428 Injection of contrast media for radiography by catheter, retrograde

P5-00500 Diagnostic radiography of soft tissues, NOS

P5-00600 Diagnostic radiography with special study, NOS
Diagnostic radiologic examination with special study, NOS

P5-00610 Radiologic examination, complex motion body section, other than with urography, unilateral
Hypercycloidal radiologic examination, unilateral

P5-00612 Radiologic examination, complex motion body section, other than with urography, bilateral
Hypercycloidal radiologic examination, bilateral

P5-00900 Radiologic supervision and interpretation of procedure, NOS

P5-00910 Consultation and report by radiologist

P5-00920 Consultation on X-ray examination made elsewhere, written report

P5-00990 Diagnostic imaging, NOS

5-05 THERMOGRAPHY

P5-05000 Thermography, NOS
Thermogram, NOS

P5-05020 Peripheral thermogram

P5-05060 Osteoarticular thermography

P5-05070 Bone thermography

P5-05080 Muscle thermography

5-06 FLUOROSCOPY

P5-06000 Fluoroscopy, NOS

P5-06010 Diagnostic radiologic examination with fluoroscopy
Fluoroscopic monitoring with radiography

P5-06040 Fluoroscopic localization for needle biopsy

P5-06042 Fluoroscopic localization for fine needle aspiration

P5-06060 Fluoroscopy, serial films

P5-06070 Fluoroscopy during operation

P5-06072 Fluoroscopy, post-operative

P5-06080 Fluoroscopy for foreign body localization

P5-06084 Fluoroscopy to assist endoscopic maneuver

P5-06086 Fluoroscopic guidance for percutaneous drainage of abscess or specimen collection, radiological supervision and interpretation

P5-06090 Fluoroscopy, up to one hour physician time

P5-06092 Fluoroscopy of more than one hour, assisting a non-radiologic physician

5-08 COMPUTERIZED TOMOGRAPHY

P5-08000 Computerized axial tomography, NOS
Computerized transaxial tomography without IV contrast
Computerized tomography without IV contrast
CT scan without IV contrast
CAT scan, NOS
Computerized transaxial tomography, NOS

P5-08010 Computerized tomography with IV contrast

P5-08020 Computerized tomography without IV contrast followed by IV contrast and more sections

P5-08040 Computerized tomography, additional views

P5-08050 Computerized tomography, limited studies

P5-08060 Computerized tomography, follow-up
Computerized tomography, limited or localized follow-up study

P5-08070 Computerized tomography, bone density study

P5-08100 Computerized tomography, sagittal

P5-08101 Computerized tomography, coronal

P5-08102 Computerized tomography, oblique

P5-08104 Computerized tomography, multi-plane

P5-08106 Computerized tomography, 3 dimensional reconstruction

P5-08110 Computerized tomography for guidance-localization, NOS

P5-08112 Computerized tomography guidance for stereotactic localization

P5-08120 Computerized tomography guidance for percutaneous drainage of abscess or specimen collection, radiological supervision and interpretation

P5-08130 CT guidance for needle biopsy
Computerized tomography guidance for needle biopsy, radiological supervision and interpretation

P5-08140 CT guidance for cyst aspiration
Computerized tomography guidance for cyst aspiration, radiological supervision and interpretation
P5-08150 CT guidance for treatment planning, teletherapy
Computerized tomography guidance for placement of radiation therapy fields

5-09 MAGNETIC RESONANCE IMAGING

P5-09000 Magnetic resonance imaging, NOS
MRI, NOS
P5-09001 Magnetic resonance imaging without contrast
P5-09002 Magnetic resonance imaging with contrast
P5-09004 Magnetic resonance imaging without IV contrast followed by contrast and more sections
P5-09010 Magnetic resonance imaging of musculoskeletal structures
P5-09012 Magnetic resonance imaging for bone marrow blood supply

5-0A POSITRON EMISSION TOMOGRAPHY

P5-0A000 Positron emission tomography, NOS
PET scan, NOS

SECTIONS 5-1-9 TOPOGRAPHY SPECIFIC RADIOLOGIC PROCEDURES

SECTION 5-1 RADIOLOGIC PROCEDURES ON THE FACE, HEAD AND NECK

P5-10000 Radiography of face, head and neck, NOS
P5-10002 Soft tissue X-ray of face, head and neck, NOS
P5-10010 Radiography of head, NOS
P5-10012 Diagnostic radiography, stereotactic localization in head
P5-10020 Diagnostic radiography of skull
P5-10021 Radiologic examination of skull, less than four views without stereo
P5-10022 Radiologic examination of skull, less than four views with stereo
P5-10031 Radiologic examination of skull, complete, minimum of four views without stereo
P5-10032 Radiologic examination of skull, complete, minimum of four views with stereo
P5-10040 Radiologic examination of sella turcica
Diagnostic radiography of sella turcica
P5-10042 Clivogram
P5-10090 Magnetic resonance imaging of face
P5-10092 Magnetic resonance imaging of orbit, face and neck
P5-10099 X-ray of skull
P5-10100 Computerized axial tomography of brain, NOS
Computerized axial tomography of head
CAT scan of head
Computerized tomography of head
P5-10102 Computerized axial tomography of head or brain without contrast
P5-10104 Computerized axial tomography of head or brain with contrast
Computerized tomography of head with contrast
P5-10106 Computerized axial tomography of head or brain without contrast followed by contrast and further sections
Computerized tomography of head without contrast followed by IV contrast and more sections
P5-10110 Computerized axial tomography of posterior fossa without contrast
P5-10112 Computerized axial tomography of posterior fossa with contrast
P5-10114 Computerized axial tomography of posterior fossa without contrast followed by contrast and further sections
P5-10130 Magnetic resonance imaging of brain and brain stem, NOS
P5-10131 Magnetic resonance imaging of brain including brain stem without contrast
P5-10132 Magnetic resonance imaging of brain including brain stem with contrast
P5-10134 Magnetic resonance imaging of brain including brain stem without contrast followed by contrast and further sections
P5-10160 Myelogram of posterior fossa
P5-10170 Cisternography
Pneumocisternogram
P5-10190 Cerebral thermography
Cephalic thermogram
P5-10200 Contrast radiography of brain, NOS
Cephalogram
P5-10210 Pneumoencephalography
Pneumoencephalogram
P5-10220 Cerebral ventriculography
P5-10224 Cerebral ventriculography, air contrast
Cerebral pneumoventriculogram
P5-10226 Cerebral ventriculography, positive contrast
P5-10300 Diagnostic radiography of facial bones
Radiography of facial bones, NOS
X-ray of facial bones
P5-10302 Radiologic examination of facial bones, less than three views
P5-10304 Radiologic examination of facial bones, complete, three or more views
P5-10306 Radiography of supraorbital area
P5-10310 Radiography of maxilla
P5-10312 Radiography of zygomaticomaxillary complex
P5-10314 Computerized axial tomography of maxillofacial area without contrast
P5-10316 Computerized axial tomography of maxillofacial area with contrast
P5-10318 Computerized axial tomography of maxillofacial area without contrast followed by contrast and further sections

SECTION 5-1 RADIOLOGIC PROCEDURES ON THE FACE, HEAD AND NECK — Continued

P5-10320 Radiography of mandible
P5-10322 Radiologic examination of mandible, partial, less than four views
P5-10324 Radiologic examination of mandible, complete, four or more views
P5-10326 Radiography of symphysis menti
P5-10330 Diagnostic radiography of temporomandibular joint, NOS
P5-10332 Radiologic examination of temporomandibular joint, open and closed mouth, unilateral
P5-10334 Radiologic examination of temporomandibular joint, open and closed mouth, bilateral
P5-10336 Arthrogram of temporomandibular joint
  Temporomandibular contrast arthrogram
P5-10338 Magnetic resonance imaging of temporomandibular joint
P5-10340 Diagnostic radiography of mastoids
P5-10342 Radiologic examination of mastoids, less than three views per side
P5-10344 Radiologic examination of mastoids, complete, three or more views per side
P5-10350 Diagnostic radiography of nasal bones
  Radiography of nose
P5-10352 Radiologic examination of nasal bones, complete, three or more views
P5-10354 Radiography of nasal sinuses, NOS
  Diagnostic radiography of paranasal sinuses
P5-10355 Radiologic examination of paranasal sinuses, less than three views
P5-10356 Radiologic examination of paranasal sinuses, complete, minimum of three views
P5-10358 Contrast radiography of nasal sinuses
  Contrast radiography of paranasal sinuses
P5-10360 Radiologic examination of internal auditory meatus, complete
P5-10365 Computerized axial tomography of outer, middle or inner ear without contrast
P5-10366 Computerized axial tomography of outer, middle or inner ear with contrast
P5-10367 Computerized axial tomography of outer, middle or inner ear without contrast followed by contrast and further sections
P5-10371 Radiography of uvula
P5-10374 Radiography of salivary gland
  Sialography
  Sialogram
P5-10375 Diagnostic radiography of salivary gland for calculus
  Radiologic examination of salivary gland for calculus
P5-10380 Radiography of nasolacrimal duct
P5-10382 Contrast radiography of nasolacrimal ducts
P5-10383 Dacryocystography
  Dacryocystogram
P5-10384 Contrast dacryocystogram
P5-10400 Diagnostic radiography of orbits, NOS
  Radiography of orbit, NOS
P5-10410 Radiologic examination of orbits, complete, four views or more
P5-10420 Diagnostic radiography of optic foramina
  Radiologic examination of optic foramina
P5-10430 Diagnostic radiography of eye for detection and localization of foreign body
P5-10450 Contrast radiography of orbit, NOS
P5-10452 Air contrast orbitography
  Pneumogram of orbit
P5-10458 Ocular thermography
  Eye thermography
P5-10480 Computerized axial tomography of orbit and sella without contrast
P5-10482 Computerized axial tomography of orbit and sella with contrast
P5-10484 Computerized axial tomography of orbit and sella without contrast followed by contrast and further sections
P5-10490 Magnetic resonance imaging of orbit
P5-10600 Radiologic examination of neck
  Diagnostic radiography of neck
P5-10602 Computerized axial tomography of soft tissue of neck without contrast
P5-10603 Computerized axial tomography of soft tissue of neck with contrast
P5-10604 Computerized axial tomography of soft tissue of neck without contrast followed by contrast and further sections
P5-10608 Radiography of thyroid region
P5-10610 Magnetic resonance imaging of neck
P5-10620 Diagnostic radiography of larynx
  Radiography of larynx
P5-10624 Diagnostic radiography of pharynx
P5-10626 Pharyngogram
P5-10628 Cineradiography of pharynx
P5-10630 Laryngogram, NOS
P5-10632 Positive contrast laryngography
P5-10640 Radiologic examination of pharynx or larynx including fluoroscopy and magnification
  Diagnostic radiologic examination with fluoroscopy of larynx
  Diagnostic radiologic examination of pharynx with fluoroscopy
P5-10644 Complex dynamic pharyngeal and speech evaluation by cineradiography or video recording
P5-10650 Radiography of tonsils and adenoids
P5-10652 Radiography of adenoids
P5-10660 Radiography of nasopharynx
P5-10662 Contrast radiography of nasopharynx
  Nasopharyngogram
P5-11000 Radiography of teeth, NOS
  Dental radiography
  Dental X-ray
P5-11002 Radiologic examination of teeth, single view
P5-11004 Radiologic examination of teeth, partial examination, less than full mouth

P5-11006 Radiologic examination of teeth, complete, full mouth
 Diagnostic radiography of full mouth
 Full-mouth X-ray of teeth
P5-11010 Orthodontic cephalogram
 Orthodontic cephalometry
 Dental cephalogram
P5-11020 Orthopantogram
P5-11030 Radiography of root canal
P5-11040 Panorex examination of mandible

SECTION 5-2 RADIOLOGIC PROCEDURES ON THE CHEST AND ABDOMEN

P5-20000 Radiography of chest, NOS
 Radiologic examination of chest, NOS
P5-20010 Routine chest X-ray
P5-20020 Diagnostic radiography of chest, lateral
P5-20030 Diagnostic radiography of chest, stereo
P5-20032 Radiologic examination of chest, stereo, frontal
P5-20040 Diagnostic radiography of chest, PA
P5-20050 Diagnostic radiography of chest, minifilm
P5-20060 Diagnostic radiography of chest, oblique, standard
P5-20070 Radiologic examination of chest, single view, frontal
P5-20080 Radiologic examination of chest, two views, frontal and lateral
P5-20100 Diagnostic radiography of chest, combined PA and lateral
P5-20110 Radiologic examination of chest, two views, frontal and lateral with apical lordotic procedure
P5-20120 Radiologic examination of chest, two views, frontal and lateral with oblique projections
P5-20130 Radiologic examination of chest, two views, frontal and lateral with fluoroscopy
P5-20140 Radiologic examination of chest, complete, minimum of four views
P5-20150 Radiologic examination of chest, complete, minimum of four views with fluoroscopy
P5-20160 Radiologic examination of chest, special views, NOS
P5-20170 Radiologic examination of chest, special views, lateral decubitus
P5-20180 Radiologic examination of chest, special views, Bucky studies
P5-20200 Fluoroscopy of chest
P5-20202 Diagnostic radiologic examination with fluoroscopy of chest
P5-20210 Fluoroscopic localization for needle biopsy in chest
 Fluoroscopic localization for needle biopsy of intrathoracic lesion including follow-up films
P5-20240 Fluoroscopic localization for transbronchial biopsy
P5-20242 Fluoroscopic localization for transbronchial biopsy and brushing
P5-20400 Endotracheal bronchography, NOS
 Endotracheal bronchogram, NOS
P5-20410 Positive contrast bronchography, unilateral
 Unilateral bronchography
P5-20420 Positive contrast bronchography, bilateral
 Bilateral bronchography
P5-20450 Transcricoid bronchography
 Transcricoid bronchogram
P5-20458 Contrast bronchogram, NOS
P5-20460 Tracheography, NOS
P5-20500 Mediastinal pneumogram
 Pneumomediastinography
P5-20600 Radiography of ribs, NOS
P5-20610 Radiologic examination of ribs, unilateral, two views
P5-20620 Radiologic examination of ribs, unilateral including posteroanterior chest, three or more views
P5-20640 Diagnostic radiography of ribs, bilateral
P5-20642 Radiologic examination of ribs, bilateral, three views
P5-20644 Radiologic examination of ribs, bilateral including posteroanterior chest, four or more views
P5-20660 Radiologic examination of ribs, sternum and clavicle
 X-ray of ribs, sternum and clavicle
P5-20670 Radiography of sternum
P5-20672 Radiologic examination of sternum, two or more views
P5-20674 Radiologic examination of sternoclavicular joints, three or more views
P5-20700 Computerized axial tomography of thorax without contrast
 Computerized tomography of thorax
 Computerized axial tomography of thorax
P5-20702 Computerized axial tomography of thorax with contrast
P5-20704 Computerized axial tomography of thorax without contrast followed by contrast and further sections
P5-20800 Magnetic resonance imaging of chest
P5-20810 Magnetic resonance imaging of chest and myocardium
P5-20820 Magnetic resonance imaging of mediastinum
P5-20900 Radiography of chest wall, NOS
 X-ray of chest wall, NOS
P5-20904 Soft tissue X-ray of chest wall
P5-20910 Fistulogram of chest wall
 Sinogram of chest wall
P5-27000 Radiologic examination of abdomen, NOS
 X-ray of abdomen, NOS
 Radiologic procedure on abdomen, NOS
P5-27010 Radiologic examination of abdomen, single anteroposterior view
 Abdominal flat plate

SECTION 5-2 RADIOLOGIC PROCEDURES ON THE CHEST AND ABDOMEN — Continued

P5-27010 (cont.) Diagnostic radiography of abdomen, AP

P5-27020 Diagnostic radiography of abdomen, oblique standard

P5-27030 Radiologic examination of abdomen, anteroposterior, oblique and cone views

P5-27040 Diagnostic radiography of abdomen, decubitus and erect
  Radiologic examination of abdomen, complete including decubitus and erect views

P5-27050 Radiologic examination of abdomen, complete acute abdomen series

P5-27100 Computerized axial tomography of abdomen without contrast
  Computerized tomography of abdomen
  Computerized axial tomography of abdomen
  CAT scan of abdomen

P5-27102 Computerized tomography of abdomen with contrast

P5-27104 Computerized axial tomography of abdomen without contrast followed by contrast and further sections

P5-27200 Fistulogram of abdominal wall
  Sinogram of abdominal wall

P5-27210 Retroperitoneal fistulogram
  Sinogram of retroperitoneum

P5-27220 Soft tissue X-ray of abdominal wall

P5-27300 Gas contrast radiography of pelvis
  Pelvic pneumography

P5-27330 Radiography of retroperitoneum, NOS
  Retroperitoneal X-ray, NOS

P5-27332 Pneumography of retroperitoneum
  Pneumoperitoneum, air contrast

SECTION 5-3 RADIOLOGIC PROCEDURES ON THE CARDIOVASCULAR SYSTEM

P5-30000 Radiography of heart, NOS
  Diagnostic radiography of heart, NOS

P5-30004 Cardiac tomography

P5-30010 Angiocardiography, negative contrast
  Angiocardiography with carbon dioxide negative contrast
  Negative contrast cardiac roentgenography

P5-30012 Angiocardiography, positive contrast
  Cardiac radiography, positive contrast

P5-30030 Angiocardiography, NOS
  Angiography of heart, NOS

P5-30032 Angiocardiography by serialography, single plane

P5-30034 Angiocardiography by serialography, multi-plane

P5-30040 Cineradiography of cardiovascular system
  Cineangiocardiography

P5-30050 Angiocardiography of right heart
  Ventriculography of right ventricle
  Selective cardiac catheterization of right heart for ventriculography
  Selective right atrial injection for angiography
  Selective right ventricular injection for angiography
  Injection procedure during cardiac catheterization for selective right ventricular or right atrial angiography

P5-30060 Angiocardiography of left heart
  Ventriculography of left ventricle
  Selective cardiac catheterization of left heart for ventriculography
  Selective left atrial injection for angiography
  Selective left ventricular injection for angiography
  Injection procedure during cardiac catheterization for selective left ventricular or left atrial angiography
  Combined left heart catheterization and left ventricular angiography

P5-30070 Angiocardiography of combined right and left heart for ventriculography
  Cardiac catheterization of right and left heart for ventriculography
  Ventriculography of right and left heart
  Combined right and left heart angiocardiography

P5-30080 Selective angiocardiography, NOS

P5-30100 Coronary angiography, NOS
  Angiography of coronary arteries, NOS
  Coronary arteriography, NOS

P5-30104 Coronary arteriography using a single catheter

P5-30105 Coronary arteriography using two catheters

P5-30108 Coronary angiography using root injection

P5-30109 Injection procedure during cardiac catheterization for selective coronary angiography
  Selective coronary artery injection for arteriography

P5-30120 Coronary angiography, unilateral
  Coronary angiography, unilateral selective injection includes angiogram and recording

P5-30130 Angiography of coronary arteries, bilateral
  Coronary angiography, bilateral selective injection includes angiogram and recording

P5-30180 Angiography of coronary bypass, unilateral selective injection

P5-30182 Angiography of coronary bypass, multiple selective injections

P5-30200 Cardiac fluoroscopy, NOS

P5-30210 Fluoroscopic monitoring and radiography for cardiac pacemaker insertion

P5-30300 Magnetic resonance imaging of myocardium, NOS

P5-30400 Angiocardiography by cineradiography
P5-31010 Combined left heart catheterization, selective coronary angiography, one or more coronary arteries, and selective left ventricular angiography
P5-31012 Combined left heart catheterization, selective coronary angiography, one or more coronary arteries, selective left ventriculography, with aortic root aortography
P5-31014 Combined right and left heart catheterization, selective coronary angiography, one or more coronary arteries, and selective left ventricular angiography
P5-31016 Combined right and left heart catheterization, selective coronary angiography, one or more coronary arteries, and selective left ventricular angiography with selective visualization of bypass graft
P5-31018 Selective opacification of aortocoronary bypass grafts, one or more coronary arteries
P5-31020 Combined left heart catheterization, selective coronary angiography, one or more coronary arteries, selective left ventricular cineangiography and visualization of bypass grafts
P5-31022 Combined left heart catheterization, selective coronary angiography, one or more coronary arteries, selective left ventricular cineangiography and visualization of bypass grafts with aortic root
P5-31500 Percutaneous transluminal balloon angioplasty, NOS
  Dotter operation for transluminal angioplasty
P5-31510 Infusion of intra-arterial thrombolytic agent with percutaneous transluminal coronary angioplasty
P5-31512 Infusion of intra-arterial thrombolytic agent with percutaneous transluminal coronary angioplasty, single vessel
P5-31514 Infusion of intra-arterial thrombolytic agent with percutaneous transluminal coronary angioplasty, multiple vessels
P5-31520 Percutaneous transluminal coronary angioplasty
P5-31522 Percutaneous transluminal coronary angioplasty, single vessel
P5-31523 Single vessel percutaneous transluminal coronary angioplasty without mention of thrombolytic agent
P5-31524 Single vessel percutaneous transluminal coronary angioplasty with thrombolytic agent infusion
P5-31525 Percutaneous transluminal coronary angioplasty, multiple vessels
  Balloon angioplasty of coronary artery, multiple vessels
P5-31530 Percutaneous transluminal iliac artery balloon angioplasty
P5-31532 Percutaneous transluminal renal artery balloon angioplasty
P5-31536 Percutaneous transluminal femoropopliteal artery balloon angioplasty
P5-32000 Non-coronary arterial angiography, NOS
  Selective angiography
P5-32006 Angiography of arteriovenous shunt
P5-32008 Blood vessel thermography
P5-32009 Arteriography of unlisted site
P5-32090 Arteriography of head and neck
P5-32092 Angiography of neck
P5-32100 Arteriography of cerebral arteries, NOS
  Angiography of intracranial vessels
P5-32102 Angiography of carotid artery, unilateral
P5-32104 Angiography of carotid arteries, bilateral
P5-32106 Angiography of cervical carotid artery, unilateral
P5-32108 Angiography of cervical carotid arteries, bilateral
P5-32109 Angiography of cervicocerebral arteries
P5-32110 Angiography of internal carotid artery, unilateral
P5-32112 Angiography of internal carotid arteries, bilateral
P5-32114 Angiography of external carotid artery, unilateral
P5-32115 Angiography of external carotid arteries, bilateral
P5-32118 Angiography of cervical vertebral artery, unilateral
  Angiography of vertebral artery, unilateral
P5-32119 Angiography of cervical vertebral arteries, bilateral
  Angiography of posterior cerebral circulation
  Angiography of vertebral arteries, bilateral
P5-3211A Angiography of cervical vertebral and intracranial arteries
P5-32120 Angiography of intrathoracic vessels, NOS
  Intrathoracic arteriography, NOS
P5-32124 Angiography of internal mammary artery
P5-32126 Arteriography of pulmonary arteries
  Pulmonary angiography
  Pulmonary arteriography
P5-32127 Angiography of pulmonary artery, unilateral
P5-32128 Angiography of pulmonary arteries, bilateral
P5-32129 Angiography of pulmonary arteries by non-selective catheter or venous injection
P5-3212A Injection procedure during cardiac catheterization for pulmonary angiography
P5-32130 Aortography, NOS
P5-32131 Thoracic aortography with serialography
P5-32132 Thoracic aortography without serialography
P5-32133 Thoracic aortography, positive contrast
P5-32134 Injection procedure during cardiac catheterization for aortography
  Selective aortic root injection for aortography

SECTION 5-3 RADIOLOGIC PROCEDURES ON THE CARDIOVASCULAR SYSTEM — Continued

P5-32135 Intra-abdominal arteriography, NOS
  Intra-abdominal angiography, NOS
P5-32136 Abdominal aortography, positive contrast
P5-32137 Translumbar aortogram
P5-32138 Abdominal aortography, translumbar with serialography
P5-32139 Abdominal aortography with bilateral iliofemoral arteries with serialography
P5-32142 Visceral angiography, selective or supraselective
P5-32144 Celiac angiography
P5-32146 Arteriography of superior mesenteric artery
P5-32149 Arteriography of unlisted intra-abdominal arteries
P5-32150 Splenogram
P5-32152 Splenoportography, positive contrast
P5-32160 Renal arteriography, NOS
  Renal angiography, NOS
P5-32161 Angiography of renal artery, unilateral
P5-32162 Angiography of renal arteries, bilateral
P5-32170 Angiography of pelvic arteries, selective or supraselective
P5-32190 Angiography of adrenal artery, unilateral
P5-32192 Angiography of adrenal arteries, bilateral
P5-32200 Spinal angiography, selective, NOS
P5-32300 Angiography of arteries of extremity, NOS
P5-32302 Angiography of arteries of extremity, unilateral
P5-32306 Angiography of arteries of extremities, bilateral
P5-32308 Angiography of arteries of extremity with serialography
P5-32350 Angiography of upper extremity arteries, NOS
P5-32351 Angiography of upper extremity arteries, unilateral
P5-32352 Angiography of upper extremity arteries, bilateral
P5-32353 Angiography of upper extremity arteries with serialography
P5-32354 Retrograde angiography of brachial artery
P5-32356 Angiography of brachial artery
P5-32400 Arteriography of lower extremity arteries, NOS
  Angiography of lower extremity arteries, NOS
P5-32404 Angiography of lower extremity arteries, unilateral
P5-32406 Angiography of lower extremity arteries, bilateral
P5-32408 Angiography of lower extremity arteries with serialography
P5-32410 Femoral arteriography
  Femoral angiography
P5-36000 Phlebography, NOS
P5-36004 Impedance phlebography
P5-36010 Phlebography of veins of head and neck
P5-36014 Phlebography of head
P5-36016 Venography of superior sagittal sinus
P5-36017 Epidural venography
P5-36020 Orbital venography
P5-36030 Phlebography of neck, NOS
P5-36032 Venography of jugular vein
  Sinus or jugular venography
P5-36050 Intrathoracic phlebography, NOS
P5-36052 Pulmonary phlebography
P5-36054 Azygography
  Venography of azygos vein
P5-36100 Intra-abdominal phlebography
P5-36110 Hepatic venography with hemodynamic evaluation
P5-36112 Hepatic venography without hemodynamic evaluation
P5-36116 Percutaneous transhepatic portography with hemodynamic evaluation
P5-36118 Percutaneous transhepatic portography without hemodynamic evaluation
P5-36130 Venography of vena cava, NOS
  Phlebography of vena cava, NOS
P5-36132 Venography of inferior vena cava with serialography
P5-36134 Venography of superior vena cava with serialography
P5-36140 Venography of renal vein, unilateral
P5-36142 Venography of renal vein, bilateral
P5-36150 Phlebography of portal system
P5-36160 Venography of adrenal, NOS
P5-36162 Venography of adrenal, unilateral
P5-36164 Venography of adrenal, bilateral
P5-36170 Splenoportogram by splenic arteriography
  Splenoportography
P5-36176 Hepatic venography
  Hepatic phlebography
P5-36180 Deep vein thermography
P5-36310 Venography of upper extremity, NOS
P5-36312 Venography of upper extremity, unilateral
P5-36314 Venography of upper extremities, bilateral, radiological supervision and interpretation
P5-36400 Venography of lower extremity, NOS
P5-36402 Venography of lower extremity, unilateral
P5-36404 Venography of lower extremity, bilateral
P5-36410 Femoral phlebography
P5-36420 Intraosseous venography
P5-36600 Lymphangiogram, NOS
  Lymphangiography, NOS
P5-36604 Lymph gland thermography
P5-36610 Cervical lymphangiogram
P5-36620 Intrathoracic lymphangiogram
P5-36630 Abdominal lymphangiogram, NOS
P5-36632 Abdominal lymphangiography, unilateral
P5-36634 Abdominal lymphangiography, bilateral
P5-36650 Pelvic lymphangiogram, NOS
P5-36652 Pelvic lymphangiography, unilateral
P5-36654 Pelvic lymphangiography, bilateral
P5-36660 Pelvic and abdominal lymphangiography, unilateral

P5-36662 Pelvic and abdominal lymphangiography, bilateral
P5-36680 Lymphangiogram of upper extremity, NOS
P5-36682 Lymphangiography of upper extremity, unilateral
P5-36684 Lymphangiography of upper extremities, bilateral
P5-36690 Lymphangiography of lower extremity, NOS
Lymphangiogram of lower extremity, NOS
P5-36692 Lymphangiography of lower extremity, unilateral
P5-36694 Lymphangiography of lower extremities, bilateral
P5-39000 Transcatheter therapy, NOS
Transcatheter therapeutic procedure, NOS
P5-39010 Transcatheter therapy for embolization, NOS
P5-39012 Transcatheter therapy for embolization with angiography
P5-39020 Transcatheter therapy by infusion, NOS
P5-39022 Transcatheter therapy by infusion with angiography
P5-39034 Angiogram through existing catheter for follow-up study for transcatheter therapy
P5-39040 Transcatheter biopsy with radiologic supervision and interpretation
P5-39044 Radiologic guidance for percutaneous specimen collection
P5-39050 Percutaneous retrieval of intravascular foreign body, NOS
P5-39052 Percutaneous retrieval of fractured venous or arterial catheter
P5-39060 Radiologic guidance for percutaneous drainage of abscess
P5-39064 Replacement of percutaneous drainage catheter with contrast monitoring
P5-39090 Transcatheter therapy with bougienage, NOS
P5-39100 Percutaneous transluminal angioplasty, NOS
P5-39110 Percutaneous transluminal angioplasty of peripheral artery
P5-39114 Percutaneous transluminal angioplasty of multiple arteries
P5-39120 Percutaneous transluminal angioplasty of renal artery
P5-39130 Percutaneous transluminal angioplasty of visceral artery
P5-39134 Percutaneous transluminal angioplasty of multiple visceral arteries
P5-39160 Percutaneous transluminal angioplasty of vein, NOS
P5-39190 Percutaneous insertion of inferior vena cava filter

SECTION 5-4 RADIOLOGIC PROCEDURES FOR OBSTETRICS AND GYNECOLOGY

P5-40010 Mammography, NOS
Radiographic examination of breast, NOS
Mammogram, NOS
P5-40012 Unilateral mammography
P5-40014 Bilateral mammography
P5-40018 Screening mammography
P5-40020 Radiologic localization of breast nodule, single lesion
P5-40022 Radiologic localization of breast nodule, multiple lesions
P5-40030 Specimen mammography
Specimen radiography of breast
P5-40040 Breast thermography
P5-40050 Xeromammography
Xerography of breast
P5-40060 Mammary ductogram, NOS
P5-40061 Mammary ductogram of single duct
Mammary galactogram of single duct
P5-40064 Mammary ductogram of multiple ducts
Mammary galactogram of multiple ducts
P5-41000 Radiography of female genital organs, NOS
X-ray of female genital organs, NOS
P5-41010 Radiography of uterus, NOS
P5-41012 Radiography of gravid uterus
X-ray of gravid uterus
P5-41020 Hysterogram, NOS
P5-41022 Percutaneous hysterogram
P5-41040 Diagnostic radiography of uterus for fetal age, fetal position and/or placental localization
P5-41044 Placentography
Arteriography of placenta
Angiography of placenta
Placentogram
Placental imaging
P5-41045 Amniography
P5-41046 Molegraphy
P5-41050 Pelvimetry
P5-41051 Pelvimetry without placental localization
P5-41052 Pelvimetry with placental localization
P5-41070 Fetography
Diagnostic radiography of fetus with intrauterine contrast visualization
P5-41074 Obstetric cephalometry
P5-41100 Pneumogynecography, NOS
P5-41110 Hysterosalpingography, NOS
Hysterosalpingography with positive contrast
P5-41112 Hysterosalpingography with gas contrast
P5-41120 Salpingography, NOS
Radiography of fallopian tubes
P5-41130 Vaginogram
P5-41134 Perineogram

SECTION 5-5 RADIOLOGIC PROCEDURES ON THE GASTROINTESTINAL TRACT

P5-50000 Radiography of digestive tract, NOS
P5-50030 Radiologic examination from nose to rectum for foreign body, single film, child
P5-50100 Radiography of intestine, NOS

SECTION 5-5 RADIOLOGIC PROCEDURES ON THE GASTROINTESTINAL TRACT — Continued

P5-50110 Radiologic examination of upper gastrointestinal tract without KUB
  Upper GI series
P5-50112 Radiologic examination of upper gastrointestinal tract with KUB
P5-50114 Upper gastrointestinal tract examination with air contrast without KUB
P5-50116 Upper gastrointestinal tract examination with air contrast with KUB
P5-50120 Diagnostic radiography of upper gastrointestinal tract with serial films
P5-50122 Radiologic examination of upper gastrointestinal tract and small bowel with serial films
P5-50124 Upper gastrointestinal tract examination with air contrast with small bowel follow through
P5-50140 Radiography of esophagus, NOS
  Radiologic examination of esophagus, NOS
P5-50141 Barium swallow
  Contrast radiography of esophagus
P5-50142 Diagnostic radiography of cervical esophagus
P5-50144 Radiologic examination of pharynx and cervical esophagus
P5-50146 Swallowing function of pharynx and esophagus with cineradiography and video recording
  Cineradiography of esophagus
P5-50147 Gastroesophageal reflux study
P5-50148 Fluoroscopy for removal of foreign body from esophagus with balloon catheter
P5-50152 Gastric emptying study
P5-50156 Oral contrast duodenography
P5-50158 Hypotonic duodenography
P5-50170 Small bowel series
  Radiography of digestive tract, small bowel series
  Diagnostic radiography of small bowel, serial films
  Radiologic examination of small bowel, serial films
P5-50180 Barium enema, NOS
  Lower GI series
  Radiologic examination of colon with barium
P5-50182 Air contrast barium enema
  Radiologic examination of colon by air contrast
P5-50184 Radiologic examination of colon by air contrast with specific high density barium with glucagon
P5-50186 Therapeutic barium enema for reduction of intussusception
P5-50200 Oral contrast cholecystography
  Cholecystogram
P5-50204 Oral contrast cholecystography, multiple examinations
P5-50210 Cholangiogram, NOS
  Contrast radiography of bile ducts, NOS
  Cholangiography
P5-50212 Oral contrast cholangiography
P5-50214 Intravenous cholangiogram
P5-50216 Intraoperative cholangiogram
  Cholangiography during surgery
P5-50218 Postoperative cholangiography
P5-50219 Percutaneous transhepatic cholangiogram
  Percutaneous transhepatic cholangiography
P5-5021A Intraoperative transhepatic cholangiogram
P5-5021E Endoscopic retrograde cholangiopancreatography
P5-50220 Cholecystocholangiogram
P5-50250 Fluoroscopic monitoring and guidance for endoscopic catheterization of the biliary ductal system
P5-50252 Fluoroscopic monitoring and guidance for endoscopic catheterization of the pancreatic ductal system
P5-50254 Fluoroscopic monitoring and radiography for combined endoscopic catheterization of the biliary and pancreatic ductal systems
P5-50256 Fluoroscopic monitoring and radiography for percutaneous biliary duct stone removal
P5-50260 Pancreatogram, NOS
P5-50262 Pancreatography during surgery
P5-50266 Postoperative pancreatography
P5-50288 Radiologic guidance for percutaneous transhepatic biliary drainage
  Radiologic guidance for percutaneous insertion of catheter or stent for biliary drainage
P5-50300 Introduction of long gastrointestinal tube with multiple fluoroscopies and films
P5-50310 Radiologic guidance for percutaneous placement of gastrostomy tube
P5-50320 Radiologic guidance for intraluminal dilation of strictures and/or obstructions of gastrointestinal tract
P5-50340 Radiologic guidance for percutaneous placement of enteroclysis tube

SECTION 5-6 RADIOLOGIC PROCEDURES ON THE GENITOURINARY SYSTEM

P5-60000 Radiography of urinary system, NOS
P5-60002 Radiography of kidney-ureter-bladder
  KUB X-ray
P5-60003 Nephrotomogram, NOS
  Nephrotomography, NOS
  Tomography of kidney, NOS
P5-60004 Unilateral nephrotomography
P5-60005 Bilateral nephrotomography
P5-60010 Intravenous pyelogram, NOS
  Intravenous urography, NOS
  Intravenous urography without KUB
  Intravenous pyelogram without KUB

P5-60020 Intravenous pyelogram with KUB
  Intravenous urography with KUB
P5-60022 Intravenous pyelogram with special hypertensive contrast concentration and clearance studies
P5-60030 Infusion urography by drip or bolus technique, NOS
  Infusion pyelogram, NOS
P5-60032 Infusion urography by drip or bolus technique with nephrotomography
P5-60040 Retrograde pyelogram, NOS
  Retrograde urography without KUB
  Retrograde ureteropyelography
  Retrograde urography
P5-60041 Retrograde urography with KUB
P5-60042 Unilateral retrograde pyelography
P5-60044 Bilateral retrograde pyelography
P5-60050 Antegrade urography
  Nephrostogram
  Antegrade pyelogram
  Loopogram
P5-60060 Radiologic examination of renal cyst, translumbar approach
P5-60064 Radiologic guidance for percutaneous catheterization into renal pelvis for drainage or injection
P5-60066 Radiologic guidance for percutaneous catheterization of ureter through renal pelvis for drainage or injection
P5-60068 Radiologic guidance for dilation of nephrostomy
P5-60080 Computerized axial tomography of kidney
  CAT scan of kidney
P5-60090 Magnetic resonance imaging of prostate
P5-60092 Magnetic resonance imaging of urinary bladder
P5-60094 Magnetic resonance imaging of pelvis, prostate and bladder
P5-60100 Cystography, NOS
  Contrast radiography of bladder, NOS
P5-60104 Cystography with three or more views
P5-60110 Retrograde cystourethrogram
  Retrograde urethrocystography
P5-60116 Voiding urethrocystography
P5-60118 Radiologic guidance for dilation of urethra
P5-60119 Radiologic guidance for dilation of ureters
P5-60120 Radiologic guidance for ileal conduitogram
  Ileoloopogram
P5-60200 Radiography of male genital organs, NOS
P5-60210 Epididymography
  Epididymogram
P5-60220 Vasography
  Vasogram
P5-60230 Vesiculography
  Vesiculogram of seminal vesicles
  Seminal vesiculogram
P5-60234 X-ray of epididymis and vas deferens
P5-60240 Radiography of prostate, NOS
P5-60250 Radiography of penis
P5-60252 Corpora cavernosography

SECTION 5-7 RADIOLOGIC PROCEDURES ON THE SPINE AND PELVIS

P5-70010 Radiography of spine, NOS
  X-ray of spine, NOS
P5-70020 Radiologic examination of complete spine, anteroposterior and lateral
  Diagnostic radiography of spine, combined AP and lateral
P5-70024 Radiologic examination of spine, single view, NOS
P5-70030 Radiologic examination of spine, scoliosis study with supine and erect studies
P5-70040 Diagnostic radiography of spine with flexion and extension studies
P5-70050 Diagnostic radiography of spine, survey study
P5-70100 Radiography of cervical spine, NOS
  X-ray of cervical spine, NOS
P5-70102 Radiologic examination of cervical spine, single view
P5-70104 Radiologic examination of cervical spine, anteroposterior and lateral
  Diagnostic radiography of cervical spine, combined AP and lateral
P5-70106 Radiologic examination of cervical spine, four or more views
P5-70110 Radiologic examination of cervical spine, complete with oblique flexion and extension studies
P5-70180 Computerized axial tomography of cervical spine without contrast
P5-70182 Computerized axial tomography of cervical spine with contrast
P5-70184 Computerized axial tomography of cervical spine without contrast followed by contrast and further sections
P5-70190 Magnetic resonance imaging of cervical spine without contrast
P5-70192 Magnetic resonance imaging of cervical spine with contrast
P5-70194 Magnetic resonance imaging of cervical spine without contrast followed by contrast
P5-70200 Radiography of thoracic spine, NOS
  X-ray of thoracic spine, NOS
P5-70204 Radiologic examination of thoracic spine, single view
P5-70206 Radiologic examination of thoracic spine, anteroposterior and lateral
P5-70220 Radiologic examination of thoracic spine, anteroposterior and lateral with swimmer's view of the cervicothoracic junction
P5-70230 Radiologic examination of thoracic spine, complete with obliques, four or more views
P5-70250 Radiologic examination of thoracolumbar spine, standing

SECTION 5-7 RADIOLOGIC PROCEDURES ON THE SPINE AND PELVIS — Continued

P5-70254 Radiologic examination of thoracolumbar spine, anteroposterior and lateral
 Diagnostic radiography of thoracolumbar spine, combined AP and lateral
P5-70260 Diagnostic radiography of thoracolumbar spine, supine and erect for scoliosis
P5-70280 Computerized axial tomography of thoracic spine without contrast
P5-70282 Computerized axial tomography of thoracic spine with contrast
P5-70284 Computerized axial tomography of thoracic spine without contrast followed by contrast and further sections
P5-70290 Magnetic resonance imaging of thoracic spine without contrast
P5-70292 Magnetic resonance imaging of thoracic spine with contrast
P5-70294 Magnetic resonance imaging of thoracic spine without contrast followed by contrast
P5-70300 Diagnostic radiography of lumbar spine
P5-70304 Radiologic examination of lumbar spine, single view
P5-70310 Diagnostic radiography of lumbar spine, combined AP and lateral
P5-70380 Computerized axial tomography of lumbar spine without contrast
P5-70382 Computerized axial tomography of lumbar spine with contrast
P5-70384 Computerized axial tomography of lumbar spine without contrast followed by contrast and further sections
P5-70390 Magnetic resonance imaging of lumbar spine without contrast
P5-70392 Magnetic resonance imaging of lumbar spine with contrast
P5-70394 Magnetic resonance imaging of lumbar spine without contrast followed by contrast
P5-70400 X-ray of lumbosacral spine, NOS
 Radiography of lumbosacral spine, NOS
P5-70410 Radiologic examination of lumbosacral spine, anteroposterior and lateral
 Diagnostic radiography of lumbosacral spine, combined AP and lateral
P5-70420 Radiologic examination of lumbosacral spine, complete, with oblique views
P5-70424 Radiologic examination of lumbosacral spine, complete, with bending views
P5-70428 Radiologic examination of lumbosacral spine with bending views only, four or more views
P5-70500 Diagnostic radiography of sacrum, NOS
P5-70510 Diagnostic radiography of sacral spine, combined AP and lateral
P5-70520 Diagnostic radiography of sacroiliac joints
P5-70522 Radiologic examination of sacroiliac joints, more than three views
 Radiologic examination of sacroiliac joints, three or more views
P5-70530 Radiography of sacrococcygeal spine
 Diagnostic radiography of sacrum and coccyx
P5-70532 Radiologic examination of sacrum and coccyx, two or more views
P5-70534 Diagnostic radiography of sacrococcygeal joint
P5-70536 Diagnostic radiography of coccyx
P5-70600 Radiography of pelvic bones
P5-70602 Diagnostic radiography of pelvis, stereo views
P5-70604 Radiologic examination of pelvis, anteroposterior only
 Diagnostic radiography of pelvis, AP
P5-70610 Radiologic examination of pelvis, three or more views
P5-70620 Skeletal X-ray of pelvis and hip
P5-70660 Radiography of pelvic soft tissue
P5-70680 Computerized axial tomography of pelvis without contrast
P5-70682 Computerized axial tomography of pelvis with contrast
P5-70684 Computerized axial tomography of pelvis without contrast followed by contrast and further sections
P5-70690 Magnetic resonance imaging of pelvis
P5-70700 Myelogram, NOS
 Myelography, NOS
 Epidurography, NOS
P5-70710 Myelography of entire spinal canal
P5-70720 Cervical myelography
P5-70730 Thoracic myelography
P5-70740 Lumbosacral myelography
P5-70800 Discogram, NOS
 Diskogram, NOS
P5-70810 Cervical discography
P5-70820 Thoracic discography
P5-70830 Lumbar discography

SECTION 5-8 RADIOLOGIC PROCEDURES ON THE UPPER EXTREMITY AND SHOULDER

P5-80010 Radiography of upper limb, NOS
P5-80012V Arthrogram of forelimb
P5-80020 Skeletal X-ray of shoulder and upper limb
P5-80030 Skeletal X-ray of upper limb, NOS
P5-80032 Radiography of humerus, NOS
P5-80034 Radiologic examination of humerus, two or more views
P5-80036 Radiologic examination of upper extremity of infant, two or more views
P5-80040 Soft tissue X-ray of shoulder and upper limb
P5-80044 Radiography of upper limb soft tissue, NOS
P5-80046 Radiography of soft tissue of upper arm
P5-80070 Radiography of shoulder, NOS
P5-80072 Radiologic examination of shoulder, one view
P5-80074 Radiologic examination of shoulder, two or more views
P5-80075 Arthrography of shoulder
P5-80078 Radiography of soft tissue of shoulder

P5-80080 Radiologic examination of clavicle, complete
Radiography of clavicle, complete
P5-80084 Radiologic examination of acromioclavicular joints, bilateral without weighted distraction
P5-80086 Radiologic examination of acromioclavicular joints, bilateral with weighted distraction
P5-80090 Diagnostic radiography of scapula, NOS
Radiologic examination of scapula, NOS
P5-80100 Radiography of elbow, NOS
P5-80102 Radiologic examination of elbow, anteroposterior and lateral views
Diagnostic radiography of elbow, combined AP and lateral
P5-80104 Radiologic examination of elbow, complete, three or more views
P5-80106 Radiography of soft tissue of elbow
P5-80110 Arthrography of elbow
P5-80118 Arthrography of wrist
P5-80120 Radiography of forearm
P5-80122 Radiologic examination of forearm, anteroposterior and lateral views
Diagnostic radiography of forearm, combined AP and lateral
P5-80124 Skeletal X-ray of elbow and forearm
P5-80126 Radiography of soft tissue of forearm
P5-80130 Radiography of wrist, NOS
P5-80132 Radiologic examination of wrist, anteroposterior and lateral views
Diagnostic radiography of wrist, combined AP and lateral
P5-80134 Radiologic examination of wrist, complete, three or more views
P5-80136 Skeletal X-ray of wrist and hand
P5-80140 Radiography of hand, NOS
P5-80141V Arthrogram of fetlock of forelimb
P5-80142 Radiologic examination of hand, two views
P5-80144 Radiologic examination of hand, three or more views
P5-80146 Radiography of soft tissue of hand
P5-80147 Diagnostic radiography of finger, NOS
P5-80148 Radiologic examination of fingers, two or more views
P5-80149 Diagnostic radiography of all fingers
P5-80300 Computerized axial tomography of upper extremity without contrast
P5-80302 Computerized axial tomography of upper extremity with contrast
P5-80304 Computerized axial tomography of upper extremity without contrast followed by contrast and further sections
P5-80320 Magnetic resonance imaging of upper extremity, except joint
P5-80324 Magnetic resonance imaging of joint of upper extremity

SECTION 5-9 RADIOLOGIC PROCEDURES ON THE LOWER EXTREMITY AND HIP

P5-90000 Radiologic procedure on lower extremity and pelvis, NOS
P5-90020 Skeletal X-ray of lower limb, NOS
P5-90022V Arthrogram of hindlimb
P5-90040 Soft tissue X-ray of lower limb
P5-90100 Radiography of hip, NOS
Arthrogram of coxofemoral joint
P5-90102 Radiologic examination of pelvis and hips of infant or child, two or more views
P5-90103 Radiologic examination of hip, unilateral, one view
P5-90104 Radiologic examination of hip, complete, two or more views
P5-90106 Diagnostic radiography of hip, bilateral
P5-90108 Radiologic examination of hips, bilateral, two or more views of each hip, including anteroposterior view of pelvis
P5-90110 Radiologic examination of hip during operative procedure
P5-90114 Radiography of soft tissue of hip
P5-90122 Radiologic examination of lower extremity of infant, two or more views
P5-90130 Radiologic examination of femur, anteroposterior and lateral views
Radiography of thigh
Diagnostic radiography of femur, combined AP and lateral
P5-90134 Radiography of soft tissue of thigh
P5-90140 Radiologic examination of knee, NOS
Arthrogram of stifle joint
P5-90142 Radiologic examination of knee, anteroposterior and lateral views
Diagnostic radiography of knee, AP and lateral
P5-90144 Radiologic examination of knee, anteroposterior and lateral with obliques, three or more views
P5-90146 Radiologic examination of knee, standing anteroposterior
P5-90148 Radiography of soft tissue of knee
P5-90160 Radiologic examination of tibia and fibula, anteroposterior and lateral views
P5-90162 Diagnostic radiography of tibia, combined AP and lateral
P5-90164 Diagnostic radiography of fibula, combined AP and lateral
P5-90170 Radiography of ankle, NOS
P5-90171V Arthrogram of tarsal joint
P5-90172 Radiologic examination of ankle, anteroposterior and lateral views
Diagnostic radiography of ankle, combined AP and lateral
P5-90174 Radiologic examination of ankle, three or more views
P5-90176 Radiography of soft tissue of ankle

SECTION 5-9 RADIOLOGIC PROCEDURES ON THE LOWER EXTREMITY AND HIP — Continued

P5-90178 Skeletal X-ray of ankle and foot
P5-90200 Radiography of foot, NOS
P5-90201V Arthrogram of fetlock of hindlimb
P5-90202 Radiologic examination of foot, anteroposterior and lateral views
  Diagnostic radiography of foot, combined AP and lateral
P5-90204 Radiologic examination of foot, complete, three or more views
P5-90206 Diagnostic radiography of calcaneus
P5-90208 Radiologic examination of calcaneus, two or more views
P5-90220 Diagnostic radiography of toes, NOS
P5-90222 Radiologic examination of toes, two or more views
P5-90300 Computerized axial tomography of lower extremity without contrast
P5-90302 Computerized axial tomography of lower extremity with contrast
P5-90304 Computerized axial tomography of lower extremity without contrast followed by contrast and further sections
P5-90320 Magnetic resonance imaging of lower extremity
P5-90322 Magnetic resonance imaging of lower extremity, except joint
P5-90324 Magnetic resonance imaging of joint of lower extremity
P5-90400 Arthrography of hip with positive contrast
P5-90410 Arthrography of knee with positive contrast
P5-90420 Arthrography of ankle with positive contrast

SECTION 5-B ULTRASOUND PROCEDURES
5-B0 GENERAL ULTRASOUND PROCEDURES

P5-B0000 Ultrasonography, NOS
  Diagnostic ultrasonography, NOS
  Echography, NOS
P5-B0002 Intraoperative echography
P5-B0004 Ultrasound study follow-up
P5-B0006 Ultrasound for foreign body localization
P5-B0008 Ultrasonography of total body
P5-B0009 Ultrasonography of multiple sites
P5-B0010 Echography, A-mode
P5-B0012 Echography, A-mode with amplitude quantitation
P5-B0016 Echography, B-scan, NOS
P5-B0017 Echography, B-scan, complete
P5-B0018 Echography, B-scan, limited
P5-B0020 Echography, contact B-scan
P5-B0024 Echography, immersion B-scan
P5-B0030 Echography, scan C-mode
P5-B0040 Echography, M-mode, NOS
P5-B0042 Echography, M-mode, complete
P5-B0046 Echography, M-mode, limited
P5-B0050 Real time scan, NOS
P5-B0060 Special echography procedure, NOS
P5-B0090 Therapeutic ultrasound, NOS
  Ultrasound therapy, NOS
P5-B0100 Ultrasound peripheral imaging, NOS
P5-B0102 Ultrasound peripheral imaging, B-scan
P5-B0104 Ultrasound peripheral imaging, real time scan
P5-B0110 Diagnostic Doppler ultrasonography, NOS
P5-B0111 Ultrasound peripheral vascular flow study, NOS
  Doppler peripheral vascular flow study
  Echography of peripheral vascular system
  Ultrasonography of peripheral vascular system
  Diagnostic ultrasound of peripheral vascular system
P5-B0112 Doppler color flow velocity mapping
P5-B0113 Ultrasound peripheral vascular flow study, arterial only
P5-B0114 Ultrasound peripheral vascular flow study, venous only
P5-B0115 Ultrasonography for deep vein thrombosis
P5-B0116 Ultrasound peripheral vascular flow study, arterial and venous
P5-B0500 Plethysmometry, NOS
P5-B0510 Plethysmography, NOS
  Plethysmogram, NOS
P5-B0512 Total body plethysmography
P5-B0514 Regional plethysmography
P5-B0520 Photoplethysmography, NOS
P5-B0530 Quantitative photoplethysmography, NOS
P5-B0532 Quantitative photoplethysmography, hollow organ
P5-B0540 Quantitative photoplethysmography, vascular, NOS
P5-B0542 Quantitative photoplethysmography, venous
P5-B0544 Quantitative photoplethysmography, arterial
P5-B0700 Ultrasonic guidance procedure, NOS
P5-B0702 Ultrasonic guidance for needle biopsy
P5-B0710 Ultrasonic guidance for aspiration of cyst
P5-B0714 Ultrasound guidance for percutaneous drainage of abscess or specimen collection
P5-B0770 Echography, scan B-mode for placement of radiation fields
P5-B0772 Ultrasonic guidance for placement of radiation therapy fields, other than B-scan
P5-B0774 Echography for placement of radiation therapy fields, B-scan
P5-B0799 Ultrasonic guidance for unlisted procedure
P5-B0990 Special ultrasonic display or imaging technique, NOS

5-B3 ULTRASOUND PROCEDURES ON THE CARDIOVASCULAR SYSTEM

P5-B3000 Echocardiography, NOS
  Ultrasonography of heart, NOS
  Diagnostic ultrasound of heart

P5-B3000 (cont.) Echocardiographic procedure, NOS

P5-B3010 Doppler flow mapping of heart

P5-B3020 Echocardiography, real-time with image documentation with M-mode recording, complete

P5-B3021 Echocardiography, real-time with image documentation without M-mode recording, complete

P5-B3022 Echocardiography, real-time with image documentation with M-mode, limited

P5-B3024 Echocardiography, real time with image documentation without M-mode, limited

P5-B3025 Echocardiography, real time with image documentation with M-mode, follow-up

P5-B3028 Echocardiography, real-time with image documentation, without M-mode, follow-up

P5-B3030 Echocardiography, real-time with image documentation, with M-mode recording, during rest and cardiovascular stress test

P5-B3032 Echocardiography, real-time with image documentation, without M-mode recording, during rest and cardiovascular stress test

P5-B3034 Echocardiography, real time with image documentation with M-mode recording, transesophageal

P5-B3036 Echocardiography, real time with image documentation without M-mode recording, transesophageal

P5-B3040 Doppler echocardiography, pulsed wave and/or continuous wave with spectral display, limited study

P5-B3041 Doppler echocardiography, pulsed wave and/or continuous wave with spectral display, follow-up

P5-B3042 Doppler echocardiography, pulsed wave and/or continuous wave with spectral display, complete

P5-B3100 Echocardiography for determining posterior left ventricular wall thickness

P5-B3102 Echocardiography for determining interventricular septal thickness

P5-B3104 Echocardiography for detecting cardiac output

P5-B3105 Echocardiography for determining prosthetic valve motion

P5-B3106 Echocardiography for determining mitral valve motion

P5-B3108 Echocardiography for determining mitral, aortic and tricuspid valve motion

P5-B3109 Echocardiography for determining mitral and tricuspid valve motion

P5-B3110 Echocardiography for determining pericardial effusion

P5-B3120 Echocardiography for determining size of ventricular chambers

P5-B3121 Echocardiography for determining ventricular contraction

P5-B3150 Ultrasonography of aortic arch

P5-B3160 Doppler flow mapping of aortic arch

P5-B3200 Three dimensional ultrasound imaging of heart, NOS
 Three dimensional echocardiography, NOS

P5-B3210 Four dimensional ultrasound imaging of heart, NOS
 Four dimensional echocardiography, NOS

P5-B3500 Imaging of cerebral arteries, NOS

P5-B3502 Non-invasive studies of cerebral arteries other than carotid by periorbital flow direction with arterial compression

P5-B3600 Imaging of carotid arteries, NOS
 Carotid imaging

P5-B3606 Imaging of carotid arteries by Doppler flow scan with spectrum analysis

P5-B3608 Imaging of carotid arteries by duplex scan with spectrum analysis

P5-B3610 Imaging of carotid arteries with resolution B-scan with pulsed Doppler flow evaluation, Doppler flow or duplex scan with spectrum analysis

P5-B3612 Imaging of carotid arteries with high resolution B-scan without pulsed Doppler flow evaluation, Doppler flow or duplex scan with spectrum analysis

P5-B3634 Doppler study of intracranial arteries, complete

P5-B3700 Doppler study of intracranial arteries, limited

P5-B3702 Non-invasive physiologic studies of bilateral extracranial arteries by ocular plethysmography

P5-B3704 Non-invasive physiologic studies of bilateral extracranial arteries by Doppler ultrasound technique

P5-B3800 Imaging of arteries of extremities, NOS

P5-B3810 Imaging of arteries of upper extremity, NOS

P5-B3820 Continuous wave Doppler analog wave form analysis of upper extremity arteries

P5-B3822 Photoplethysmographic or pulse volume digit wave form analysis of upper extremity arteries

P5-B3824 Imaging of arteries of lower extremities, NOS

P5-B3830 Continuous wave Doppler analog wave form analysis of lower extremity arteries

P5-B3832 Photoplethysmographic or pulse volume digit wave form analysis of lower extremity arteries

P5-B3850 Ultrasonic guidance for endomyocardial biopsy

P5-B3854 Ultrasonic guidance for pericardiocentesis

5-B5 ULTRASOUND PROCEDURES ON THE GASTROINTESTINAL SYSTEM

P5-B5000 Ultrasonography of digestive system, NOS
 Ultrasonography of intestine, NOS

P5-B5200 Ultrasonography of biliary tract, NOS

5-B6 ULTRASOUND PROCEDURES ON THE ENDOCRINE SYSTEM

P5-B6110 Echography of thyroid, A-mode
P5-B6112 Echography of thyroid, B-scan

5-B7 ULTRASOUND PROCEDURES ON THE URINARY AND MALE GENITAL SYSTEMS

P5-B7000 Ultrasonography of urinary system, NOS
P5-B7100 Echography of kidney, NOS
P5-B7110 Echography of transplanted kidney, B-scan and/or real time with image documentation with duplex Doppler studies
P5-B7112 Echography of transplanted kidney, B-scan and/or real time with image documentation without duplex Doppler studies
P5-B7120 Ultrasonic fragmentation of urinary stones
P5-B7130 Ultrasonic guidance for renal pelvis aspiration
P5-B7300 Echography of scrotum and contents
P5-B7320 Echography of prostate, transrectal approach

5-B8 ULTRASOUND PROCEDURES ON THE FEMALE GENITAL SYSTEM AND PREGNANCY RELATED STRUCTURES

P5-B8000 Echogynography, NOS
P5-B8010 Ultrasonography of uterus, NOS
P5-B8012 Transvaginal echography
P5-B8020 Diagnostic ultrasound of gravid uterus, NOS
  Ultrasonography of gravid uterus, NOS
P5-B8022 Echography of pregnant uterus, B-scan and/or real time with image documentation, limited
P5-B8024 Echography of pregnant uterus, B-scan and/or real time with image documentation, complete
  Echography, scan B-mode for pregnancy, complete series
P5-B8028 Echography of pregnant uterus, B-scan and/or real time with image documentation, complete, multiple gestation
P5-B8100 Echography, scan B-mode for placental localization
  Echoplacentogram
P5-B8200 Ultrasound cephalometrics
  Echocephalometry
P5-B8210 Fetal biophysical profile
P5-B8220 Fetal echocardiography, real time with image documentation (2D) without M-mode recording
P5-B8222 Fetal echocardiography, real time with image documentation (2D) with M-mode recording
P5-B8224 Ultrasonography for antepartum monitoring of fetus
  Intrapartum monitoring of fetus with pulsed Doppler ultrasound
P5-B8226 Echography, scan B-mode for fetal age determination
P5-B8228 Echography, scan B-mode for fetal growth rate
P5-B8300 Ultrasonic guidance for aspiration of ova
P5-B8310 Ultrasonic guidance for amniocentesis
P5-B8500 Ultrasonography of breast
  Ultrasonic examination of breast
P5-B8502 Echography of breast, A-mode
P5-B8504 Echography of breast, B-scan
P5-B8506 Echography of breast, B-scan and real time with image documentation

5-B9 ULTRASOUND PROCEDURES ON THE NERVOUS SYSTEM AND SPECIAL SENSE ORGANS

P5-B9000 Echoencephalography, NOS
P5-B9010 Echoencephalography, A-mode
P5-B9020 Echoencephalography, B-scan and real time with image documentation including A-mode encephalography
P5-B9120 Ultrasonography for midline shift of brain
P5-B9130 Ultrasound of inner ear
P5-B9150 Ultrasound study of eye, NOS
P5-B9152 Ophthalmic echography, A-mode
P5-B9154 Ophthalmic echography with amplitude quantitation, A-mode
P5-B9156 Ophthalmic echography, B-scan, limited
P5-B9158 Ophthalmic echography, contact B-scan
P5-B9159 Ophthalmic echography, immersion B-scan
P5-B9160 Ophthalmic biometry by ultrasound echography, A-mode
P5-B9162 Ophthalmic biometry by ultrasound echography, A-mode with intraocular lens power calculation
P5-B9170 Ophthalmic ultrasonic foreign body localization
P5-B9500 Echography of spinal canal and contents

5-BB ULTRASOUND PROCEDURES ON TOPOGRAPHIC REGIONS

P5-BB000 Ultrasonography of head and neck, NOS
  Diagnostic ultrasound of head and neck, NOS
P5-BB010 Echography, soft tissues of head and neck, B-scan and/or real time with image documentation
P5-BB020 Doppler flow mapping of head and neck
P5-BB100 Ultrasonography of thorax, NOS
P5-BB102 Echography of chest, A-mode
P5-BB104 Echography of chest, B-scan
P5-BB105 Echography of chest, B-scan with image documentation
P5-BB106 Echography of chest, real time with image documentation
P5-BB108 Echography of chest, B-scan and real time with image documentation
P5-BB120 Doppler flow mapping of thorax
P5-BB130 Ultrasonic guidance for thoracentesis
P5-BB150 Ultrasonography of lung

P5-BB200 Ultrasonography of abdomen, NOS
P5-BB204 Echography of abdomen, B-scan, limited
P5-BB206 Echography of abdomen, B-scan, complete
P5-BB208 Echography of abdomen, B-scan and real time with image documentation, limited
P5-BB209 Echography of abdomen, B-scan and real time with image documentation, complete
P5-BB300 Ultrasonography of retroperitoneum, NOS
P5-BB302 Retroperitoneal echography, B-scan, limited
P5-BB304 Retroperitoneal echography, B-scan, complete
P5-BB306 Retroperitoneal echography, B-scan and real time with image documentation, limited
P5-BB308 Retroperitoneal echography, B-scan and real time with image documentation, complete
P5-BB320 Diagnostic ultrasound of abdomen and retroperitoneum, NOS
P5-BB400 Pelvic echography, NOS
P5-BB402 Pelvic echography, B-scan, limited
P5-BB404 Pelvic echography, B-scan, complete
P5-BB410 Diagnostic Doppler ultrasonography of pelvic area
P5-BB420 Pelvic echography, nonobstetric, B-scan and/or real time with image documentation, complete
P5-BB422 Echography, pelvic, nonobstetric, B-scan and/or real time with image documentation, limited or follow-up
P5-BB500 Echography of extremity, non-vascular, B-scan and/or real time with image documentation
P5-BB510V Ultrasound examination of forelimb
P5-BB512V Ultrasound examination of hindlimb
P5-BB514V Ultrasound examination of joint, NOS

SECTION 5-C RADIATION AND RADIONUCLIDE THERAPEUTIC PROCEDURES

5-C0 RADIATION ONCOLOGY AND RADIOTHERAPY

P5-C0000 Radiation therapy procedure or service, NOS
P5-C0005 Special radiation therapy procedure or service, explain by report
P5-C0010 General radiation therapy consultation and report
P5-C0012 Consultation in teletherapy, NOS
P5-C0014 Consultation in computer dosimetry and isodose chart, teletherapy
P5-C0020 Radiation physics consultation, NOS
P5-C0022 Radiation physics consultation, special
P5-C0024 Radiation physics consultation with therapeutic radiologist
P5-C0026 Unlisted procedure, medical radiation physics, dosimetry and treatment devices
P5-C0050 Total body irradiation
P5-C0052 Hemibody irradiation
P5-C0054 Vaginal cone irradiation
P5-C0056 Oral radiation
P5-C0100 Radiation therapy treatment planning service, NOS
P5-C0101 Treatment planning for teletherapy, NOS
P5-C0102 Therapeutic radiation treatment planning, simple
P5-C0104 Therapeutic radiation treatment planning, intermediate
P5-C0106 Therapeutic radiation treatment planning, complex
P5-C0108 Radiation therapy treatment planning, patient contour and localization of internal structures
P5-C0109 Radiation therapy treatment planning, setting of each treatment port
P5-C0120 Radiation therapy simulator aided field setting, NOS
P5-C0122 Radiation therapy simulator aided field setting, simple
P5-C0124 Radiation therapy simulator aided field setting, intermediate
P5-C0126 Radiation therapy simulator aided field setting, complex
P5-C0130 Radiation therapy, central axis depth dose computation, NOS
P5-C0132 Basic radiation dosimetry calculation, central axis depth dose, TDF, NSD, GAP calculation, off axis factor, tissue inhomogeneity factors
P5-C0134 Radiation therapy, tissue and geometric inhomogeneity correction
P5-C0136 Special dosimetry, NOS
P5-C0137 Special dosimetry, microdosimetry
P5-C0138 Special dosimetry, TLD
P5-C0140 Isodose computation for teletherapy, NOS
P5-C0142 Radiation therapy isodose plan, simple
Teletherapy isodose plan, simple
P5-C0144 Radiation therapy isodose plan, intermediate
Teletherapy isodose plan, intermediate
P5-C0145 Radiation therapy isodose plan, complex
Teletherapy isodose plan, complex
P5-C0160 Radiation therapy isodose plan, arc field
P5-C0161 Radiation therapy isodose plan, wedge fields
P5-C0162 Radiation therapy isodose plan, rotation field
P5-C0163 Radiation therapy isodose plan, moving strip field
P5-C0164 Radiation therapy isodose plan, isocentric
P5-C0190 Special teletherapy port plan, particles, hemibody or total body
P5-C0192 Radiation therapy treatment planning, interpretation of special testing ordered by radiation therapist
P5-C0194 Therapeutic radiology port film interpretation and verification
P5-C0198 Unlisted procedure, therapeutic radiology clinical treatment planning
P5-C0200 Design and construction of treatment devices, simple
P5-C0202 Design and construction of treatment devices, intermediate
P5-C0204 Design and construction of treatment devices, complex
P5-C0210 Preparation of radiation therapy aid, NOS

5-C0 RADIATION ONCOLOGY AND RADIOTHERAPY — Continued

P5-C0212 Wedge filter design and fabrication
P5-C0214 Bolus design and fabrication
P5-C0216 Field block design and fabrication
P5-C0218 Compensating filter design and fabrication
P5-C0220 Provision of moulds or casts for immobilization
P5-C0222 Provision of stents or bite blocks
P5-C0224 Provision of external compensating shield
P5-C0300 Radiation therapy, NOS
 Radiotherapy, NOS
P5-C0310 Teleradiotherapy procedure, NOS
 Teletherapy procedure, NOS
P5-C0320 Superficial teletherapy procedure, Grenz type
 Therapy radiation contact, 150 KVP or less
 Teletherapy, Grenz type
 Superficial radiation therapy, 150 KVP or less
 Radiation therapy low voltage, 150 KVP or less
 Superficial radiation
P5-C0330 Deep radiation therapy, 200-300 KVP
 Orthovoltage radiation therapy
 Orthovoltage radiation
 High voltage radiation therapy, 200-300 KVP
P5-C0340 Teleradiotherapy of 1 to 25 MEV protons
P5-C0350 Betatron teleradiotherapy
P5-C0360 Megavoltage radiation therapy
 Supervoltage radiation therapy
P5-C0362 Teleradiotherapy by linear accelerator
P5-C0370 Teleradiotherapy using electrons
 Teleradiotherapy beta particles
P5-C0380 Teleradiotherapy particulate radiation, NOS
P5-C0382 Teleradiotherapy neutrons
P5-C0384 Teleradiotherapy protons
P5-C0386 Cobalt-60 therapy
P5-C0389 Teleradiotherapy of unlisted particulate radiation
P5-C0390 Stereotactic focused gamma radiosurgery of cerebrum
P5-C0391 Stereotactic focused proton beam on cerebrum
P5-C0400 Radiation treatment delivery, superficial or ortho voltage
P5-C0402 Radiation treatment delivery of single treatment area, up to 5 MEV
P5-C0404 Radiation treatment delivery of single treatment area, 6-10 MEV
P5-C0406 Radiation treatment delivery of single treatment area, 11-19 MEV
P5-C0408 Radiation treatment delivery of single treatment area, 20 MEV or greater
P5-C0410 Radiation treatment delivery of two separate treatment areas, up to 5 MEV
P5-C0412 Radiation treatment delivery of two separate treatment areas, 6-10 MEV
P5-C0414 Radiation treatment delivery of two separate treatment areas, 11-19 MEV
P5-C0416 Radiation treatment delivery of two separate treatment areas, 20 MEV or greater
P5-C0420 Radiation treatment delivery of three or more separate treatment areas, up to 5 MEV
P5-C0422 Radiation treatment delivery of three or more separate treatment areas, 6-10 MEV
P5-C0424 Radiation treatment delivery of three or more separate treatment areas, 11-19 MEV
P5-C0426 Radiation treatment delivery of three or more separate treatment areas, 20 MEV or greater
P5-C0500 Radiation therapy treatment management, NOS
P5-C0504 Radiation therapy management for course of one or two fractions
P5-C0510 Weekly megavoltage treatment management, simple
 Radiation therapy treatment management, simple
P5-C0512 Weekly megavoltage treatment management, intermediate
 Radiation therapy treatment management, intermediate
P5-C0514 Weekly megavoltage treatment management, complex
 Radiation therapy treatment management, complex
P5-C0600 Brachytherapy procedure, NOS
 Contact radiation therapy procedure, NOS
P5-C0602 Surface brachytherapy, NOS
 Surface application of radioelement
 Surface radioactive source application
P5-C0610 Intracavitary brachytherapy
P5-C0612 Intracavitary radioelement application, simple
P5-C0614 Intracavitary radioelement application, intermediate
P5-C0616 Intracavitary radioelement application, complex
P5-C0618 Intracavitary radium application
P5-C0619 Uterine implantation of radium
P5-C0620 Interstitial brachytherapy
P5-C0622 Interstitial radioelement application, simple
P5-C0624 Interstitial radioelement application, intermediate
P5-C0626 Interstitial radioelement application, complex
P5-C0628 Interstitial radium application
P5-C0650 Remote afterloading high intensity brachytherapy, 1-4 source positions
P5-C0652 Remote afterloading high intensity brachytherapy, 5-8 source positions
P5-C0654 Remote afterloading high intensity brachytherapy, 9-12 source positions
P5-C0656 Remote afterloading high intensity brachytherapy, over 12 source positions
P5-C0670 Treatment planning for brachytherapy, NOS
P5-C0671 Isodose computation for brachytherapy, NOS
P5-C0672 Brachytherapy isodose calculation, simple

P5-C0674 Brachytherapy isodose calculation, intermediate
P5-C0676 Brachytherapy isodose calculation, complex
P5-C0690 Consultation in brachytherapy, NOS
P5-C0692 Consultation in computer dosimetry and isodose chart for brachytherapy
P5-C0699 Unlisted procedure in clinical brachytherapy
P5-C0700 Hyperthermia treatment, NOS
P5-C0702 Hyperthermia treatment of cancer
P5-C0710 Hyperthermia, externally generated, superficial with depth of 4 cm or less
P5-C0712 Hyperthermia, externally generated, deep with depths greater than 4 cm
P5-C0720 Hyperthermia generated by interstitial probes, 5 or fewer interstitial applicators
P5-C0722 Hyperthermia generated by interstitial probes, more than 5 interstitial applicators
P5-C0730 Hyperthermia generated by intracavitary probes
P5-C0800 Preparation of radioactive source
P5-C0802 Disposal of radioactive source
P5-C0810 Supervision, handling and loading of radioelement

5-C1 THERAPEUTIC RADIONUCLIDE PROCEDURES

P5-C1100 Radionuclide therapy, NOS
  Radioisotope teleradiotherapy, NOS
P5-C1105 Gamma ray therapy
P5-C1110 Teleradiotherapy with iodine-125
P5-C1112 Teleradiotherapy with radioactive cesium
P5-C1114 Therapy with cobalt-60
  Teleradiotherapy with cobalt-60
P5-C1116 Radium therapy
P5-C1150 Intracavitary radionuclide therapy
  Intracavitary instillation of radioisotope
  Intracavitary radioactive colloid therapy
P5-C1160 Interstitial radionuclide therapy
  Interstitial radioactive colloid therapy
P5-C1164 Intra-articular radionuclide therapy
P5-C1170 Intravascular radionuclide therapy
  Intravenous injection of radioisotope
P5-C1172 Intravascular radionuclide therapy, particulate
P5-C1300 Radionuclide therapy for glandular suppression, NOS
P5-C1302 Radionuclide therapy for gland ablation, NOS
P5-C1310 Radionuclide therapy for hyperthyroidism, NOS
P5-C1312 Radionuclide therapy for hyperthyroidism, initial
P5-C1316 Radionuclide therapy for thyroid suppression
P5-C1320 Radionuclide ablation of thyroid gland, NOS
P5-C1322 Radionuclide ablation of gland for thyroid carcinoma
P5-C1324 Radionuclide therapy for metastases of thyroid carcinoma
P5-C1330 Radionuclide therapy for polycythemia vera
P5-C1340 Radionuclide therapy for chronic leukemia
P5-C1400 Radionuclide therapy, nonthyroid, nonhematologic
P5-C1500 Insertion of radioactive isotope
  Implantation of radioactive isotope
P5-C1502 Infusion or instillation of radioelement solution
  Injection or instillation of radioisotope

SECTION 5-D NUCLEAR MEDICINE DIAGNOSTIC PROCEDURES

5-D0 GENERAL NUCLEAR MEDICINE DIAGNOSTIC PROCEDURES

P5-D0000 Nuclear medicine procedure, NOS
  Radionuclide procedure, NOS
  Diagnostic radionuclide study, NOS
P5-D0005 Special radioisotope function studies, explain by report
P5-D0010 Radionuclide scanning, NOS
P5-D0012 Radionuclide scanning for hot spot
P5-D0014 Radionuclide scanning for cold spot
P5-D0017 Radionuclide special dynamic function study, NOS
P5-D0018 Serial scanning, NOS
P5-D0019 Radioisotope scan of unlisted site
P5-D0020 Radionuclide dynamic function study, NOS
  Dynamic scanning study, NOS
P5-D0024 Radionuclide uptake study, NOS
P5-D0026 Radionuclide tissue clearance study
P5-D0027 Radionuclide lacrimal flow study
P5-D0028 Radionuclide dynamic function study with multiple probes, NOS
P5-D0030 Radionuclide volume dilution study, NOS
P5-D0032 Radionuclide volume dilution of body spaces
P5-D0036 Radionuclide localization of abscess of limited area
P5-D0038 Radionuclide localization of abscess of whole body
P5-D0040 Radionuclide localization of tumor, NOS
P5-D0042 Radionuclide localization of tumor, limited area
P5-D0044 Radionuclide localization of tumor, multiple areas
P5-D0046 Radionuclide localization of tumor, whole body
P5-D0050 Scanning or imaging with vascular flow, NOS
  Radionuclide vascular imaging
  Scanning or imaging, perfusion study, NOS
P5-D0052 Scanning or imaging, perfusion study, particulate
P5-D0054 Scanning or imaging, perfusion study, gaseous
P5-D0080 Generation of automated data by nuclear physician, simple, less than 30 minutes
P5-D0082 Generation of automated data by nuclear physician, complex, more than 30 minutes
P5-D0086 Special radionuclide imaging technique, NOS

5-D0 GENERAL NUCLEAR MEDICINE DIAGNOSTIC PROCEDURES — Continued

P5-D0088 Multi-plane radionuclide tomography, NOS
P5-D0090 Provision of diagnostic radioisotope
  Provision of diagnostic radionuclide
P5-D0092 Provision of therapeutic radionuclide

5-D1-D9 SPECIFIC DIAGNOSTIC NUCLEAR MEDICINE PROCEDURES

5-D1 NUCLEAR MEDICINE DIAGNOSTIC PROCEDURES ON THE MUSCULOSKELETAL SYSTEM

P5-D1000 Radioisotope study of musculoskeletal system, NOS
P5-D1005 Special musculoskeletal diagnostic nuclear medicine procedure, explain by report
P5-D1010 Radioisotope scan of bone, NOS
  Bone scan, NOS
  Bone imaging, NOS
P5-D1020 Total body scan
  Whole body bone imaging
  Radioisotope scan of total body
P5-D1022 Bone imaging of limited area
P5-D1024 Bone imaging of multiple areas
P5-D1030 Bone imaging, vascular flow study
P5-D1040 Bone imaging, three phase technique
P5-D1050 Bone imaging, tomographic
P5-D1100 Bone density study, single photon absorptiometry
  Bone mineral content study, single photon absorptiometry
P5-D1110 Bone density study, dual photon absorptiometry
  Bone mineral content study, dual photon absorptiometry
P5-D1150 Transmission bone density study, NOS
  Transmission bone imaging, NOS
P5-D1160 Radiocalcium absorption study
P5-D1170 Joint imaging

5-D2 NUCLEAR MEDICINE DIAGNOSTIC PROCEDURES ON THE RESPIRATORY SYSTEM

P5-D2000 Radioisotope study of respiratory system, NOS
P5-D2005 Special respiratory diagnostic nuclear medicine procedure, explain by report
P5-D2010 Pulmonary scan, NOS
  Transmission imaging of lung, NOS
  Radioisotope scan of lung, NOS
P5-D2100 Pulmonary perfusion study, NOS
P5-D2102 Pulmonary perfusion imaging, particulate
P5-D2104 Pulmonary perfusion imaging, particulate with ventilation, single breath
P5-D2106 Pulmonary perfusion imaging, particulate with ventilation, rebreathing and washout with or without single breath
P5-D2110 Pulmonary perfusion imaging, gaseous
P5-D2112 Pulmonary perfusion imaging, gaseous, with ventilation, rebreathing and washout
P5-D2200 Pulmonary ventilation study, NOS
P5-D2201 Pulmonary ventilation study, gaseous
P5-D2202 Pulmonary ventilation study, total
P5-D2204 Pulmonary inhalation study
P5-D2210 Pulmonary ventilation study, gaseous, single breath only
P5-D2212 Pulmonary ventilation study, gaseous, rebreathing and washout only
P5-D2300 Pulmonary ventilation imaging, gaseous, single breath, single projection
P5-D2310 Pulmonary ventilation imaging, gaseous, with rebreathing and washout with or without single breath, single projection
P5-D2320 Pulmonary ventilation imaging, gaseous, with rebreathing and washout with or without single breath, multiple projections
P5-D2400 Pulmonary ventilation study, aerosol
P5-D2410 Pulmonary ventilation imaging, aerosol, single projection
P5-D2420 Pulmonary ventilation imaging, aerosol, multiple projections
P5-D2500 Pulmonary ventilation perfusion study, NOS
  Pulmonary ventilation-perfusion study by radionuclide gas, NOS
  Pulmonary quantitative differential function study
P5-D2512 Pulmonary ventilation-perfusion study by radioactive oxygen
P5-D2514 Pulmonary ventilation-perfusion study by radioactive carbon
P5-D2516 Pulmonary ventilation-perfusion study by radioactive nitrogen
P5-D2518 Pulmonary ventilation-perfusion study by radioactive krypton
P5-D2519 Pulmonary ventilation-perfusion study by radioactive xenon
  Pulmonary xenon flow study

5-D3 NUCLEAR MEDICINE DIAGNOSTIC PROCEDURES ON THE CARDIOVASCULAR SYSTEM

P5-D3000 Radioisotope study of cardiovascular system, NOS
P5-D3005 Special cardiovascular diagnostic nuclear medicine procedure, explain by report
P5-D3010 Radioisotope scan of cardiovascular system
P5-D3014 Xenon flow scan of cardiovascular system
P5-D3030 Myocardial imaging
  Transmission imaging of heart
P5-D3100 Cardiac flow imaging, NOS
P5-D3102 Cardiac blood pool imaging, first pass technique, wall motion study with ejection fraction, single study at rest
P5-D3104 Cardiac blood pool imaging, first pass technique, multiple studies, resting and with stress

P5-D3106 Cardiac blood pool imaging, gated equilibrium, wall motion study plus ejection fraction, single study at rest

P5-D3108 Cardiac blood pool imaging, gated equilibrium, wall motion study plus ejection fraction, multiple studies, resting and with stress

P5-D3200 Radioisotope scan for myocardial infarction

P5-D3210 Myocardial imaging for infarct, planar technique

P5-D3220 Myocardial imaging for infarct with ejection fraction, first pass technique

P5-D3230 Myocardial imaging for infarct, tomographic SPECT, qualitative or quantitative

P5-D3300 Radionuclide cardiac ventriculography

P5-D3302 Cardiovascular flow study imaging
  Cardiac flow study imaging

P5-D3304 Cardiac blood pool imaging

P5-D3310 Myocardial perfusion imaging, resting or stress, quantitative or qualitative, single study

P5-D3320 Myocardial perfusion imaging, resting or stress, redistribution or rest injection, qualitative or quantitative, multiple studies

P5-D3330 Myocardial perfusion imaging, tomographic, resting or stress, quantitative or qualitative, single study

P5-D3332 Myocardial perfusion imaging, tomographic, resting or stress, redistribution or rest injection, qualitative or quantitative, multiple studies

P5-D3336 Myocardial perfusion study with wall motion, qualitative or quantitative

P5-D3340 Determination of ventricular ejection fraction with probe technique

P5-D3342 Radionuclide study of cardiac output
  Radioisotope scan of cardiac output
  Myocardial perfusion study with ejection fraction

P5-D3370 Determination of central cardiovascular hemodynamics with or without exercise, single or multiple sites

P5-D3400 Radionuclide study of coronary blood flow

P5-D3600 Radionuclide venous thrombosis study, NOS

P5-D3602 Venous thrombosis study with radioactive fibrinogen

P5-D3604 Venous thrombosis imaging, unilateral
  Radionuclide venogram, unilateral

P5-D3606 Venous thrombosis imaging, bilateral
  Radionuclide venogram, bilateral

P5-D3700 Cardiac shunt detection

5-D5 NUCLEAR MEDICINE DIAGNOSTIC PROCEDURES ON THE GASTROINTESTINAL SYSTEM

P5-D5000 Radioisotope study of gastrointestinal system, NOS

P5-D5005 Special gastrointestinal diagnostic nuclear medicine procedure, explain by report

P5-D5010 Radioisotope scan of gastrointestinal system, NOS

P5-D5011 Radioisotope scan of intestine
  Radioisotope scan of bowel
  Bowel imaging, NOS

P5-D5012 Bowel imaging for Meckel's diverticulum

P5-D5014 Bowel imaging for volvulus

P5-D5016 Bowel imaging for ectopic gastric mucosa

P5-D5017 Gastric mucosa imaging

P5-D5018 Large bowel imaging

P5-D5020 Isotope study for gastrointestinal blood loss
  Gastrointestinal blood loss study

P5-D5022 Acute gastrointestinal blood loss imaging

P5-D5024 Gastrointestinal aspirate for localization of blood loss

P5-D5026 Gastrointestinal blood loss study by stool counting

P5-D5030 Gastrointestinal protein loss study

P5-D5040 Gastrointestinal isotope fat absorption study

P5-D5042 Radioiodinated triolein study

P5-D5044 Radioiodinated oleic acid study

P5-D5050 Radioisotope function study of liver
  Liver scan
  Liver imaging
  Radionuclide hepatic function study

P5-D5051 Liver imaging, static only

P5-D5052 Liver function study with serial images

P5-D5054 Liver imaging with vascular flow

P5-D5056 Radionuclide biliary patency study

P5-D5057 Hepatobiliary ductal system imaging including gallbladder

P5-D5058 Radioiodinated rose bengal study of liver

P5-D5062 Liver and spleen imaging

P5-D5064 Liver and spleen imaging, static only

P5-D5065 Liver and spleen imaging with vascular flow

P5-D5068 Radioisotope scan of pancreas

P5-D5070 Esophageal motility study

P5-D5080 Salivary gland imaging

P5-D5082 Salivary gland imaging with serial views

P5-D5084 Salivary gland function study

P5-D5090 Schilling test, NOS
  Schilling test without intrinsic factor
  Vitamin B_{12} absorption study without intrinsic factor

P5-D5092 Schilling test with intrinsic factor
  Vitamin B_{12} absorption study with intrinsic factor

P5-D5094 Vitamin B_{12} absorption studies combined, with and without intrinsic factor
  Vitamin B_{12} absorption study, combined

5-D6 NUCLEAR MEDICINE DIAGNOSTIC PROCEDURES ON THE ENDOCRINE AND HEMATOPOIETIC SYSTEMS

5-D60-D61 Nuclear Medicine Diagnostic Procedures on The Endocrine System

P5-D6000 Radioisotope study of endocrine system, NOS
  Endocrine diagnostic nuclear medicine procedure, NOS
P5-D6010 Radioiodine uptake study
P5-D6100 Thyroid imaging, NOS
  Thyroid scan and radioisotope function studies, NOS
  Thyroid scan, NOS
P5-D6102 Thyroid uptake, single determination
  Thyroid imaging with uptake, single determination
P5-D6104 Thyroid uptake, multiple determinations
  Thyroid imaging with uptake, multiple determinations
P5-D6106 Thyroid uptake with thyroid stimulation
  Radioiodine uptake study with thyroid stimulation
P5-D6108 Thyroid uptake with thyroid suppression
P5-D6109 Thyroid uptake with discharge
  Radioactive study with thyroid washout
P5-D6120 Thyroid imaging with vascular flow
P5-D6130 Thyroid imaging for metastatic carcinoma, limited area
P5-D6132 Neck imaging for metastatic carcinoma of thyroid
P5-D6133 Chest imaging for metastatic carcinoma of thyroid
P5-D6134 Thyroid imaging for metastatic carcinoma, multiple areas
P5-D6136 Thyroid imaging for metastatic carcinoma, whole body
P5-D6138 Thyroid imaging for metastatic carcinoma, with additional studies
P5-D6140 Parathyroid imaging, NOS
  Parathyroid scan, NOS
  Radioisotope scan of parathyroid
P5-D6150 Adrenal imaging, NOS
  Adrenal radioisotope scan, NOS
P5-D6152 Imaging of adrenal cortex
P5-D6160 Radioisotope scan of pituitary

5-D65-D66 Nuclear Medicine Diagnostic Procedures on The Hematopoietic System

P5-D6500 Radioisotope study of hematopoietic system, NOS
P5-D6510 Special hematopoietic, reticuloendothelial or lymphatic diagnostic nuclear medicine procedure, explain by report
P5-D6600 Radioisotope scan of hematopoietic system, NOS
P5-D6610 Bone marrow imaging
  Radioisotope scan of bone marrow
P5-D6612 Bone marrow imaging, limited area
P5-D6614 Bone marrow imaging, multiple areas
P5-D6616 Bone marrow imaging, whole body
P5-D6620 Isotope study of blood volume
P5-D6622 Whole blood volume determination, including separate measurement of plasma volume and red cell volume
P5-D6630 Isotope study for plasma volume
P5-D6632 Plasma volume by radionuclide volume dilution technique, single sample
P5-D6633 Plasma volume by radionuclide volume dilution technique, multiple samples
P5-D6640 Red cell volume determination, single sample
  Isotope study for red cell mass determination
P5-D6642 Red cell volume determination, multiple samples
P5-D6650 Red cell survival study, NOS
  Isotope study for red blood cell survival
P5-D6652 Isotope study for red blood cell survival with sequestration, NOS
  Isotope study for red blood cell sequestration
P5-D6654 Red cell survival study with hepatic sequestration
  Isotope study for red blood cell hepatic sequestration
P5-D6655 Red cell survival study with splenic sequestration
  Isotope study for red blood cell splenic sequestration
P5-D6656 Red cell survival study for splenic and hepatic sequestration
  Red cell splenic and hepatic sequestration study
P5-D6660 Iron kinetics study, NOS
P5-D6661 Plasma radioiron turnover rate
  Plasma radioiron clearance
  Plasma radioiron disappearance rate
P5-D6662 Iron chelation study, NOS
  Total body iron with chelatable radioiron study
P5-D6664 Red cell iron utilization study
  Radioiron red cell utilization
P5-D6666 Radioiron oral absorption study
  Radioiron absorption study
P5-D6668 Radioiron body distribution study
P5-D6670 Platelet survival study, NOS
P5-D6674 White blood cell localization, limited area scanning
P5-D6675 White blood cell localization, whole body
P5-D6680 Spleen imaging, NOS
  Radioisotope scan of spleen
P5-D6682 Spleen imaging with vascular flow
P5-D6690 Radioisotope scan of lymphatic system
  Lymphatics imaging

P5-D6690 (cont.) Lymphatics and lymph gland imaging
Scan of lymphatic system
Radionuclide lymphangiogram
P5-D66A0 Dynamic function study, blood clearance
P5-D66A2 Radioiodine plasma clearance study
P5-D66A4 Radionuclide study, circulation time
P5-D66A6 Radionuclide study, protein kinetics

5-D7 NUCLEAR MEDICINE DIAGNOSTIC PROCEDURES ON THE GENITOURINARY SYSTEM

P5-D7000 Radioisotope study of genitourinary system, NOS
P5-D7005 Special genitourinary diagnostic nuclear medicine procedure, explain by report
P5-D7010 Kidney imaging, NOS
Isotopic renogram, NOS
P5-D7012 Kidney imaging with function study
Renal scan
Kidney radioisotope scan
Renal scan and radioisotope function study
Renal radioisotope scan
P5-D7020 Radioiodohippurate sodium renogram, serial imaging
P5-D7022 Radioiodohippurate sodium renogram, multiple probes
P5-D7030 Kidney imaging with dynamic function study
P5-D7032 Renal function study with serial imaging
P5-D7040 Kidney function study only
Kidney vascular flow study only
P5-D7042 Kidney function study only with pharmacologic intervention
P5-D7060 Kidney imaging, SPECT technique
P5-D7062 Kidney imaging, static only
P5-D7070 Kidney imaging with vascular flow
P5-D7072 Kidney imaging with vascular flow and function study
P5-D7100 Isotope study for glomerular filtration rate
P5-D7110 Isotope study for renal plasma flow
P5-D7120 Isotope study for renal clearance
P5-D7130 Isotope study for urinary recovery
P5-D7200 Kidney transplant evaluation
P5-D7300 Urinary bladder residual urine study
Isotope study for residual urine
P5-D7310 Ureteral reflux study
Isotope study for ureteral reflux
P5-D7400 Testicular imaging
P5-D7410 Testicular imaging with vascular flow

5-D9 NUCLEAR MEDICINE DIAGNOSTIC PROCEDURES ON THE NERVOUS SYSTEM

P5-D9000 Radioisotope study of central nervous system, NOS
P5-D9005 Special nervous system diagnostic nuclear medicine procedure, explain by report
P5-D9010 Radioisotope scan of head, NOS
P5-D9020 Brain imaging, NOS
Radioisotope scan of brain, NOS
Positrocephalogram, NOS
Cerebral scan, NOS
P5-D9100 Brain imaging, limited study, static
P5-D9104 Brain imaging, complete study, static
P5-D9110 Brain imaging with vascular flow, NOS
P5-D9112 Brain imaging, limited study with vascular flow
P5-D9114 Brain imaging, complete study with vascular flow
P5-D9120 Brain imaging, complete study, tomographic technique
P5-D9200 Cerebral blood flow radionuclide study, NOS
P5-D9300 Cerebrospinal fluid flow imaging, NOS
P5-D9310 Cerebrospinal fluid flow imaging, cisternography
P5-D9320 Cerebrospinal fluid flow imaging, ventriculography
P5-D9330 Cerebrospinal fluid flow imaging, shunt evaluation
P5-D9332 Peritoneal venous shunt patency test for Leveen shunt
Peritoneal venous shunt patency test
Leveen shunt patency test
P5-D9334 Denver shunt patency test
P5-D9340 Cerebrospinal fluid flow imaging for CSF leakage detection and localization
Cerebrospinal fluid leakage study
P5-D9350 Cerebrospinal fluid flow imaging, tomographic
P5-D9500 Radionuclide identification of eye tumor
P5-D9600 Radionuclide dacryocystography

5-DB MISCELLANEOUS NUCLEAR MEDICINE DIAGNOSTIC PROCEDURES

P5-DB100 Placental scan
Localization of placenta by RISA injection
Placentography with radioisotope
P5-DB110 Radioisotope scan of uterus

CHAPTER 7 — PHYSICAL MEDICINE AND PHYSIOTHERAPY PROCEDURES AND SERVICES

SECTION 7-0 GENERAL PHYSICAL MEDICINE PROCEDURES

P7-00000 Physical medicine procedure, NOS
  Physiatric procedure, NOS
P7-00020 Physical medicine service, NOS
  Physiatric service, NOS
P7-00060 Physical therapy procedure, NOS
  Physiotherapy procedure, NOS
P7-00070 Diagnostic physical therapy procedure, NOS
P7-00100 Physical medicine, initial examination, evaluation and treatment program planning, NOS
  Physiatric initial examination, evaluation and treatment planning, NOS
P7-00120 Physical medicine, initial examination, review and planning of physiotherapy program or procedure
P7-00140 Physical medicine evaluation of functional activities, initial 30 minutes
P7-00180 Physical medicine consultation and report
P7-00200 Counseling by physiotherapist, NOS
P7-00400 Physical medicine service to one body area, NOS
P7-00410 Physical medicine service to two body areas, NOS
P7-00420 Physical medicine service to three or more body areas, NOS
P7-00500 Therapeutic mechanical traction
P7-00504 Physical medicine treatment to one area by mechanical traction
P7-00510 Intermittent mechanical traction
P7-00520 Therapeutic manual traction
P7-00524 Physical medicine manual traction, initial 30 minutes
P7-00530 Intermittent manual traction
P7-00550 Manual and mechanical traction
P7-00600 Therapeutic electrical stimulation
P7-00602 Therapeutic electrical stimulation for bone healing
P7-00604 Physical medicine treatment to one area with electrical stimulation
P7-00610 Physical medicine treatment with electrical manual stimulation
P7-00620 Therapeutic application of vasopneumatic device
  Physical medicine treatment to one area with vasopneumatic device
P7-01050 Massage physiotherapy
  Physical medicine massage, initial 30 minutes
P7-01060 Effleurage
P7-01070 Bandaging therapy
P7-01090 Combined physical therapy without mention of the components
P7-01100 Body measurement
P7-01110 Measurement of girth
P7-01120 Measurement of skin fold thickness
P7-01130 Measurement of skull circumference

SECTION 7-1 PHYSICAL MANIPULATIONS
7-10 PHYSIATRIC MANIPULATIONS

P7-10000 Physiatric manipulation, NOS
  Forcible correction of musculoskeletal deformity, NOS
P7-10010 Passive manipulation
P7-10020 Active manipulation
P7-10100 Lysis of adhesions of muscle by stretching or manipulation
  Physiatric manipulation of muscle structures
  Myotasis
  Physiatric stretching of muscle
P7-10160 Lysis of adhesions of tendon by stretching or manipulation
  Physiatric stretching of tendon
P7-10210 Lysis of adhesions of bursa by stretching or manipulation
P7-10240 Physiatric stretching of fascia
P7-10250 Measurement of limb length
P7-10280 Forced extension of limb
P7-10320 Arthrolysis by stretching or manipulation
  Physiatric manipulation of joint adhesions
  Brisement forcé
  Lysis of adhesions of cartilage of joint by stretching or manipulation
  Physiatric manual rupture of joint adhesions
P7-10324 Physiatric mobilization of joint, NOS
  Physiatric remobilization of joint, NOS
P7-10360 Physiatric hyperextension of joint
P7-10400 Physiatric manipulation of back
  Physiatric mobilization of spine
P7-10410 Physiatric manipulation of nuchal region
  Physiatric cervical manipulation
P7-10420 Physiatric manipulation of thoracic region
  Physiatric thoracic manipulation
P7-10430 Physiatric manipulation of lumbosacral region
  Physiatric lumbosacral manipulation
P7-10440 Physiatric manipulation of sacroiliac region
  Physiatric sacroiliac manipulation
P7-10500 Physiatric manipulation of hand
  Lysis of adhesions of hand by stretching or manipulation
P7-10520 Physiatric manipulation of wrist

7-11 OSTEOPATHIC MANIPULATIONS

P7-11000 Osteopathic manipulation, NOS
Osteopathic manipulative therapy, NOS
P7-11010 Osteopathic manipulation for general mobilization, general articulation
P7-11020 Osteopathic manipulation, high-velocity, low-amplitude forces, thrusting
P7-11030 Osteopathic manipulation, low-velocity, high-amplitude forces, springing
P7-11040 Osteopathic manipulation, isotonic, isometric forces
P7-11050 Osteopathic manipulation, indirect forces
P7-11080 Osteopathic manipulation to move tissue fluids

7-12 CHIROPRACTIC MANIPULATIONS

P7-12000 Chiropractic manipulation, NOS
P7-12100 Chiropractic consultation
P7-12102 Chiropractic consultation with history
P7-12104 Chiropractic examination
P7-12106 Chiropractic consultation, history and examination
P7-12110 Chiropractic visit, NOS
P7-12120 Chiropractic interpretation of X-rays
P7-12200 Chiropractic application of ice
P7-12210 Chiropractic application of heat
P7-12220 Chiropractic ultrasound
P7-12230 Chiropractic diathermy
P7-12240 Chiropractic vibration therapy
P7-12300 Chiropractic adjustment of single cervical spine subluxation
P7-12304 Chiropractic adjustment of multiple cervical spine subluxations
P7-12310 Chiropractic adjustment of single thoracic spine subluxation
P7-12314 Chiropractic adjustment of multiple thoracic spine subluxations
P7-12320 Chiropractic adjustment of single lumbar spine subluxation
P7-12324 Chiropractic adjustment of multiple lumbar spine subluxations
P7-12330 Chiropractic adjustment of coccyx subluxation
P7-12334 Chiropractic adjustment of sacral subluxation
P7-12340 Chiropractic adjustment of temporomandibular joint subluxation
P7-12344 Chiropractic adjustment of shoulder subluxation
P7-12350 Chiropractic adjustment of knee subluxation
P7-12360 Chiropractic adjustment of hip subluxation
P7-12400 Chiropractic patient education and instruction

SECTION 7-2 PHYSIOTHERAPY TRAINING

P7-20000 Physiotherapy training, NOS
P7-20010 Physical medicine neuromuscular reeducation, NOS
P7-20100 Training of joint movements, NOS
P7-20110 Gait training procedure, NOS
Gait training
P7-20120 Ambulation and gait training
Ambulation training
P7-20130 Gait evaluation
P7-20140 Gait reeducation
P7-20200 Transfer training, NOS
P7-20210 Standing transfer training
P7-20220 Bathtub transfer training
P7-20230 Sliding transfer training
P7-20240 Swinging transfer training
P7-20250 Car transfer training
P7-20400 Activities of daily living therapy, NOS
Housing activities training
Home making activities training
Domestic tasks therapy
P7-20404 Training in activities of daily living, NOS
P7-20600 Body function training activity, NOS
P7-20610 Functional independence training
P7-20620 Post-cardiac rehabilitation training
Cardiac retraining
P7-20720 Child care training

SECTION 7-3 THERAPEUTIC EXERCISES

P7-30000 Therapeutic exercise, NOS
P7-30100 Musculoskeletal exercise, active, NOS
P7-30110 Musculoskeletal exercise, passive, NOS
P7-30120 Individual exercises, NOS
P7-30130 General calisthenic exercise regimen
P7-30140 Remedial exercise
P7-30150 Assisting exercise
P7-30160 Coordination exercise
P7-30170 Resistive exercise
P7-30180 Breathing exercise
P7-30200 Range of motion exercise
P7-30210 Muscular strength development exercise
P7-30220 Relaxation exercise
P7-30230 Isometric exercise
P7-30240 Isotonic exercise
P7-30300 Mobilizing exercises
Mobilization physiotherapy
P7-30310 Immobilization physiotherapy
P7-30400 Kinetic activities for coordination, NOS
Kinetic activities to increase coordination, NOS
P7-30410 Kinetic activities for range of motion
Kinetic activities to increase range of motion
P7-30420 Kinetic activities for strengthening
Kinetic activities to increase strength
P7-30450 Muscular endurance development exercise

SECTION 7-4 PHYSIOTHERAPY CLASS ACTIVITIES

P7-40000 Physiotherapy class activities, NOS
P7-40100 Class in calisthenics

SECTION 7-4 PHYSIOTHERAPY CLASS ACTIVITIES — Continued

P7-40120 Class in general exercises
  Class in physical fitness and conditioning
P7-40200 Orthopedic class in walking reeducation, musculoskeletal
P7-40210 Instruction in use of crutch
  Training in crutch walking
P7-40230 Class in walking reeducation, nervous system
P7-40240 Class in walking reeducation, amputee
P7-40280 Instruction in use of walker
P7-40290 Instruction in use of cane
P7-40400 Use of tilt table
P7-40410 Use of sling suspension
P7-40430 Use of pulley apparatus
P7-40450 Use of ergometer bicycle
P7-40460 Use of treadmill

SECTION 7-5 HYDROTHERAPY AND DIATHERMY PROCEDURES

P7-50000 Hydrotherapy, NOS
  Therapeutic bath, NOS
P7-50010 Hydrotherapy in Hubbard tank
P7-50030 Pool therapy or Hubbard tank with therapeutic exercises
  Hydrotherapy with assisted exercise in pool
P7-50040 Hot water bath hydrotherapy
P7-50050 Cold water bath hydrotherapy
P7-50060 Contrast water bath hydrotherapy
P7-50080 Shower hydrotherapy
  Douche hydrotherapy
P7-50100 Hydrotherapy with hot packs or compresses
  Thermotherapy with hot packs
  Therapy with hot packs
P7-50140 Hydrotherapy with cold packs or compresses
P7-50150 Physical medicine treatment to one area with hot or cold packs
P7-50160 Therapeutic paraffin bath
  Physical medicine treatment to one area with paraffin bath
P7-50200 Hydrotherapy with whirlpool bath
  Physical medicine treatment to one area with whirlpool bath
  Whirlpool treatment
P7-50600 Diathermy, NOS
  Physical medicine diathermy treatment to one area
P7-50610 Short wave diathermy
P7-50612 Ultrashort wave diathermy
P7-50620 Microwave diathermy
  Physical medicine microwave treatment to one area
P7-50630 Physical medicine ultrasound treatment
P7-50640 Physical medicine ultraviolet treatment to one area
P7-50650 Physical medicine infrared treatment to one area
  Infrared therapy
P7-50660 Physical medicine iontophoresis
P7-50800 Heat therapy, NOS
  Hyperthermia therapy, NOS
  Therapeutic heat application
  Therapeutic application of conductive heat
P7-50820 Moxibustion
P7-50840 Cryotherapy, NOS
  Therapeutic application of cold

SECTION 7-6 MUSCLE FUNCTION STUDIES

P7-60000 Muscle function study, NOS
P7-60050 Neuromuscular procedure, NOS
P7-60100 Electromyography, NOS
P7-60110 Electromyography, limited study of specific muscles
P7-60120 Electromyography, single fiber, any technique
P7-60130 Electromyography, one extremity and related paraspinal areas
P7-60140 Electromyography, two extremities and related paraspinal areas
P7-60150 Electromyography, three extremities and related paraspinal areas
P7-60160 Electromyography, four extremities and related paraspinal areas
P7-60400 Electromyography, cranial nerve supplied muscles, unilateral
P7-60410 Electromyography, cranial nerve supplied muscles, bilateral
P7-60500 Edrophonium chloride test for myasthenia gravis
  Tensilon test for myasthenia gravis
P7-60510 Edrophonium chloride test with electromyographic recording
  Tensilon test with electromyographic recording
P7-60520 Ischemic forearm exercise test
P7-60530 Ischemic limb exercise with EMG and lactic acid determination
P7-60540 Measurement of interstitial fluid pressure, NOS
P7-60542 Measurement of interstitial fluid pressure in muscle compartment
P7-60600 Manual testing of muscle function, NOS
P7-60610 Manual muscle-testing of extremity or trunk
P7-60620 Manual muscle-testing of total body including hands
  Manual muscle-testing with total evaluation of body
P7-60624 Manual muscle-testing of total body excluding hands
P7-60630 Manual muscle-testing of hand
  Grip strength testing
P7-60800 Electrical muscle-testing, NOS
P7-60810 Muscle-testing electrodiagnosis with chronaximetry
P7-60820 Muscle-testing with strength duration curve, each nerve

P7-60830 Extremity testing for strength, dexterity or stamina
P7-60840 Muscle-testing with torque curves during isometric and isokinetic exercise
P7-60900 Range of motion testing, NOS
P7-60910 Range of motion measurements and report for each extremity
P7-60920 Range of motion measurements and report for hand
P7-60950 Muscle-testing by bicycle dynamometer
Bicycle dynamometer

SECTION 7-7 ORTHOTIC AND PROSTHETIC PROCEDURES

7-70 ORTHOTIC PROCEDURES

P7-70000 Orthotic procedure, NOS
P7-70010 Physical medicine evaluation and review for orthotic program
Orthotic check-out
Orthotic evaluation
P7-70020 Physical medicine initial examination for orthotic program
Office visit, orthotic check-out
P7-70100 Orthotics training of upper extremities, NOS
P7-70200 Orthotic evaluation for brace fitting
P7-70220 Orthotic device construction and fitting
P7-70230 Fitting of orthotic device
P7-70240 Orthotic splinting
P7-70250 Orthotic bracing
P7-70300 Orthotic check-out readjustment

7-71 PROSTHETIC PROCEDURES

P7-71000 Prosthetic procedure, NOS
P7-71010 Physical medicine evaluation and review for prosthetic program
Prosthetic evaluation
Prosthetic check-out
Office visit, prosthetic check-out
P7-71020 Physical medicine initial examination for prosthetic program
P7-71100 Prosthetic evaluation for artificial limb fitting
P7-71110 Prosthetic construction and fitting
P7-71120 Prosthetic readjustment
Adjustment of prosthesis
P7-71200 Training in use of prosthetic device, NOS
Instruction in use of prosthesis
Prosthetic training

SECTION 7-8 SPEECH PATHOLOGY PROCEDURES

P7-80000 Speech pathology procedure, NOS
P7-80020 Medical evaluation for speech, language and/or hearing problems
P7-80030 Speech, language or hearing therapy with individual medical supervision
P7-80040 Speech, language or hearing therapy with group medical supervision
P7-80200 Speech therapy, NOS
P7-80210 Dysphasia training
P7-80220 Speech defect training
P7-80300 Language therapy, NOS
P7-80310 Dyslexia training
P7-80320 Voice training
P7-80330 Esophageal speech training
P7-80340 Sign language training
P7-80350 Training for lip reading

SECTION 7-9 OTHER PHYSICAL REHABILITATION THERAPY PROCEDURES

P7-90000 Rehabilitation therapy, NOS
Rehabilitation, NOS
P7-90002 Physical medicine initial examination and planning for rehabilitation program
P7-90010 Post-amputation rehabilitation
P7-90020 Neurological rehabilitation, NOS
P7-90022 Stroke rehabilitation
P7-90024 Stroke-hemiplegia rehabilitation
P7-90026 Cerebral palsy rehabilitation
P7-90028 Paraplegia-paraparesis rehabilitation
P7-90030 Spinal cord injury rehabilitation
P7-90032 Flail extremity rehabilitation
P7-90034 Head injury rehabilitation
P7-90036 Congenital spinal cord disease rehabilitation
P7-90037 Progressive central nervous system disease rehabilitation
P7-90038 Peripheral nervous system disease rehabilitation
P7-90040 Back disease and deformity rehabilitation
P7-90042 Joint disease rehabilitation
P7-90044 Post-fracture rehabilitation
P7-90046 Musculoskeletal injury rehabilitation
P7-90100 Diversional therapy
P7-90110 Recreational therapy
P7-90130 Organized games therapy
P7-90140 Dance therapy
P7-90200 Educational therapy
P7-90240 Education of bed-bound child
P7-90250 Special schooling for handicapped person
P7-90300 Occupational therapy
P7-90400 Vocational rehabilitation
P7-90404 Vocational schooling
P7-90410 Vocational assessment
P7-90420 Vocational training
P7-90430 Vocational retraining
P7-90450 Sheltered employment
P7-90500 Blind rehabilitation therapy, NOS
P7-90510 Training in Braille or Moon
P7-90520 Activities of daily living training for the blind
P7-90550 Training in use of lead dog for the blind

CHAPTER 8 — DENTAL PROCEDURES AND SERVICES

SECTION 8-0 GENERAL DENTAL PROCEDURES AND SERVICES

P8-00100 Dental-oral procedure or service, NOS
P8-00110 Dental consultation and report, NOS
P8-00120 Diagnostic dental procedure, NOS
P8-00200 Initial oral examination
P8-00210 Periodic oral examination
P8-00220 Emergency oral examination
P8-00250 Oral hygiene instruction
P8-00260 Nutritional counseling for control of dental disease
P8-00300 Dental examination for personal identification, NOS
P8-00310 Direct dental examination for personal identification
P8-00320 Radiographic dental examination for personal identification
P8-00340 Forensic bite mark comparison technique
P8-00400 Caries susceptibility test
P8-00420 Pulp vitality test
P8-00490 Diagnostic model construction
P8-00500 Diagnostic dental cast
P8-00510 Diagnostic dental photographs

SECTION 8-1 TOOTH EXTRACTIONS AND IMPLANTATIONS

8-10 TOOTH EXTRACTIONS

P8-10000 Tooth extraction, NOS
  Exodontia procedure, NOS
P8-10040 Tooth extraction, single
P8-10042 Tooth extraction, each additional tooth
P8-10080 Extraction of deciduous tooth
P8-10120 Extraction of permanent tooth
P8-10160 Extraction of wisdom tooth
P8-10200 Tooth extraction, multiple
P8-10240 Tooth extraction, complete upper
  Extraction of all maxillary teeth
P8-10280 Tooth extraction, complete lower
  Extraction of all mandibular teeth
P8-10320 Tooth extraction, complete mouth
P8-10440 Tooth extraction, root removal of exposed roots
P8-10480 Surgical removal of erupted tooth requiring elevation of mucoperiosteal flap and removal of bone and/or section of tooth
P8-10520 Removal of impacted tooth, soft tissue
P8-10560 Removal of impacted tooth, partially bony
P8-10600 Removal of impacted tooth, completely bony
P8-10640 Removal of impacted tooth, completely bony, with unusual surgical complications
P8-10680 Surgical removal of residual tooth roots

8-16 TOOTH IMPLANTATIONS

P8-16000 Tooth implantation, NOS
  Tooth transplantation, NOS
P8-16040 Dental endosseous implant
P8-16080 Dental subperiosteal implant
P8-16120 Dental transosseous implant
P8-16160 Dental implant connecting bar
P8-16200 Dental implant maintenance procedure
P8-16240 Repair of dental implant
P8-16280 Removal of dental implant
P8-16320 Tooth reimplantation and/or stabilization of accidentally evulsed or displaced tooth and/or alveolus

SECTION 8-3 PREVENTIVE DENTAL SERVICES AND PROCEDURES

P8-30000 Preventive dental service, NOS
P8-30030 Preventive dental procedure, NOS
P8-30040 Dental prophylaxis, adult
P8-30080 Dental prophylaxis, children
P8-30100V Dental debridement, NOS
P8-30120 Dental scaling and polishing
  Scale teeth
P8-30124V Filing of floating teeth
  Float teeth
P8-30160 Dental fluoride treatment
P8-30200 Topical application of fluoride including prophylaxis, child
P8-30240 Topical application of fluoride excluding prophylaxis, child
P8-30280 Topical application of fluoride including prophylaxis, adult
P8-30320 Topical application of fluoride excluding prophylaxis, adult
P8-30400 Space maintainer, NOS
P8-30440 Fixed space maintainer, unilateral
P8-30480 Fixed space maintainer, bilateral
P8-30520 Removable space maintainer, unilateral
P8-30560 Removable space maintainer, bilateral
P8-30600 Recementation of space maintainer
P8-30640 Space maintainer, fixed band type
P8-30680 Space maintainer fixed, stainless steel crown type
P8-30720 Space maintainer, fixed, cast type
P8-30760 Removable space maintainer, acrylic
P8-30780 Space maintainer, additional clasps and/or activating wires

SECTION 8-4 ORTHODONTIC PROCEDURES

P8-40000 Orthodontic service, NOS
P8-40010 Orthodontic procedure, NOS
P8-40020 Orthodontic dental consultation and report
P8-40100 Removable appliance therapy, NOS
P8-40110 Removable appliance therapy for tooth guidance
P8-40120 Removable appliance therapy to control harmful habit

P8-40160 Removable appliance therapy for interceptive orthodontic treatment
P8-40200 Fixed appliance therapy, NOS
P8-40210 Fixed appliance therapy for tooth guidance
P8-40220 Fixed appliance therapy for control of harmful habit
P8-40260 Fixed appliance therapy for interceptive orthodontic treatment
P8-40310 Comprehensive orthodontic treatment, transitional dentition, for class I malocclusion
P8-40320 Comprehensive orthodontic treatment, transitional dentition, for class II malocclusion
P8-40330 Comprehensive orthodontic treatment, transitional dentition, for class III malocclusion
P8-40350 Comprehensive orthodontic treatment, permanent dentition, for class I malocclusion
P8-40360 Comprehensive orthodontic treatment, permanent dentition, for class II malocclusion
P8-40370 Comprehensive orthodontic treatment, permanent dentition, for class III malocclusion
P8-40400 Dental application of desensitizing medicament
P8-40420 Dental behavior management, NOS
P8-40450 Occlusal guard therapy
P8-40460 Fabrication of athletic mouth guards
P8-40470 Occlusion analysis, mounted case
P8-40480 Occlusal adjustment, limited
P8-40490 Occlusal adjustment, complete
P8-40500 Posttreatment stabilization, orthodontic device

SECTION 8-5 RESTORATIVE DENTAL PROCEDURES

P8-50000 Dental restorative procedure, NOS
P8-50040 Amalgam restoration, one surface, primary
P8-50080 Amalgam restoration, two surfaces, primary
P8-50120 Amalgam restoration, three surfaces, primary
P8-50160 Amalgam restoration, four or more surfaces, primary
P8-50200 Amalgam restoration, one surface, permanent
P8-50220 Amalgam restoration, two surfaces, permanent
P8-50230 Amalgam restoration, three surfaces, permanent
P8-50240 Amalgam restoration, four or more surfaces, permanent
P8-50250 Reinforced pin amalgam, Markley type procedure
P8-50400 Restoration, silicate, NOS
P8-50410 Silicate cement, per restoration
P8-50440 Restoration, resin, NOS
P8-50480 Restoration, resin, one surface, anterior
P8-50520 Restoration, resin, two surfaces, anterior
P8-50560 Restoration, resin, three surfaces, anterior
P8-50600 Restorations resin, four or more surfaces or involving anterior incisal angle
P8-50640 Restoration, composite resin crown, anterior, primary
P8-50680 Restoration, resin, one surface, posterior, primary
P8-50720 Restoration, resin, two surfaces, posterior, primary
P8-50760 Restoration, resin, three or more surfaces, posterior, primary
P8-50800 Restoration, resin, one surface, posterior, permanent
P8-50840 Restoration, resin, two surfaces, posterior, permanent
P8-50850 Restoration, resin, three or more surfaces, posterior, permanent
P8-50900 Restoration, gold foil, NOS
P8-50920 Restoration, gold foil, one surface
P8-50960 Restoration, gold foil, two surfaces
P8-50980 Restoration, gold foil, three surfaces
P8-51000 Restoration, inlay, NOS
P8-51100 Restoration, inlay, metallic, NOS
P8-51110 Restoration, inlay, metallic, one surface
P8-51120 Restoration, inlay, metallic, two surfaces
P8-51130 Restoration, inlay, metallic, three surfaces
P8-51140 Restoration, inlay, metallic, per tooth, in addition to inlay
P8-51200 Restoration, inlay, porcelain/ceramic, NOS
P8-51210 Restoration, inlay, porcelain/ceramic, one surface
P8-51220 Restoration, inlay, porcelain/ceramic, two surfaces
P8-51230 Restoration, inlay, porcelain/ceramic, three surfaces
P8-51250 Restoration, inlay, porcelain/ceramic, per tooth, in addition to inlay
P8-51300 Restoration, inlay, composite/resin, NOS
P8-51310 Restoration, inlay, composite/resin, one surface, laboratory processed
P8-51320 Restoration, inlay, composite/resin, two surfaces, laboratory processed
P8-51330 Restoration, inlay, composite/resin, three surfaces, laboratory processed
P8-51350 Restoration, inlay, composite/resin, per tooth, in addition to inlay, laboratory processed
P8-51400 Restoration, crown, single
P8-51410 Restoration, crown, resin, laboratory
P8-51420 Restoration, crown, resin with high noble metal
P8-51430 Restoration, crown, resin with predominantly base metal
P8-51440 Restoration, crown, resin with noble metal
P8-51450 Restoration, crown, porcelain/ceramic substrate
P8-51460 Restoration, crown, porcelain fused to high noble metal
P8-51470 Restoration, crown, porcelain fused to predominantly base metal
P8-51480 Restoration, crown, porcelain fused to noble metal

SECTION 8-5 RESTORATIVE DENTAL PROCEDURES — Continued

P8-51500 Restoration, crown, full cast, high noble metal
P8-51510 Restoration, crown, full cast, predominantly base metal
P8-51520 Restoration, crown, full cast, noble metal
P8-51530 Restoration, crown, 3/4 cast, metallic
P8-52020 Recement inlay
P8-52030 Recement crown
P8-52050 Sedative filling
P8-52100 Prefabricated stainless steel crown, primary tooth
P8-52110 Prefabricated stainless steel crown, permanent tooth
P8-52120 Prefabricated resin crown
P8-52130 Prefabricated stainless steel crown with resin window
P8-52200 Labial veneer, laminate, chairside
P8-52210 Labial veneer, resin laminate, laboratory
P8-52220 Labial veneer, porcelain laminate, laboratory
P8-52300 Pin retention, per tooth, in addition to restoration
P8-52310 Dental core buildup, including any pins
P8-52320 Cast post and core in addition to crown
P8-52330 Temporary crown for fractured tooth
P8-52340 Prefabricated post and core in addition to crown
P8-52350 Crown repair, NOS
P8-52490 Unlisted restorative service

SECTION 8-6 ENDODONTIC PROCEDURES

P8-60000 Endodontic procedure, NOS
P8-60010 Emergency endodontic procedure
P8-60020 Endodontic dental consultation and report
P8-60100 Pulp capping, NOS
P8-60110 Pulp cap, direct, excluding final restoration
P8-60120 Pulp cap, indirect, excluding final restoration
P8-60200 Recalcification, CaOH, temporary restoration, per tooth
P8-60210 Pulpotomy, therapeutic, excluding final restoration
P8-60220 Therapeutic apical closure
P8-60230 Vital pulpotomy
P8-60300 Root canal therapy, comprehensive, NOS
P8-60310 Root canal therapy, anterior, excluding final restoration
P8-60320 Root canal therapy, bicuspid, excluding final restoration
P8-60330 Root canal therapy, molar, excluding final restoration
P8-60340 Root canal therapy, retreatment, anterior, by report
P8-60350 Root canal therapy retreatment, bicuspid, by report
P8-60360 Root canal therapy, retreatment of molar, by report
P8-60370 Apexification/recalcification, initial visit
P8-60380 Apexification/recalcification, interim visit
P8-60390 Apexification/recalcification, final visit
P8-60500 Apicoectomy/periradicular surgery, anterior
P8-60510 Apicoectomy/periradicular surgery, bicuspid
P8-60520 Apicoectomy/periradicular surgery, molar
P8-60530 Apicoectomy/periradicular surgery, each additional root
P8-60600 Retrograde filling per root
P8-60610 Root amputation, per root
P8-60620 Endodontic endosseous implant
P8-60630 Intentional replantation with splinting
P8-60640 Surgical procedure for isolation of tooth with rubber dam
P8-60650 Hemisection of tooth
P8-60660 Canal preparation and fitting of preformed dowel or post
P8-60670 Bleaching of discolored tooth

SECTION 8-7 PERIODONTIC PROCEDURES

P8-70000 Periodontic procedure, NOS
P8-70010 Periodontic dental consultation and report
P8-70040 Dental surgical procedure, NOS
  Dental operation, NOS
P8-70100 Gingivectomy or gingivoplasty, per quadrant
P8-70110 Gingivectomy or gingivoplasty, per tooth
P8-70130 Gingival flap procedure, including root planing, per quadrant
P8-70140 Crown lengthening, hard and soft tissue
P8-70150 Mucogingival surgery, per quadrant
P8-70160 Drainage of abscess of dentoalveolar structures
P8-70170 Drainage of cyst of dentoalveolar structures
P8-70180 Drainage of hematoma of dentoalveolar structures
P8-70200 Dentoalveolar bone osseous surgery, including flap entry and closure, per quadrant
P8-70210 Dentoalveolar bone replacement graft, single site, including flap entry and closure
P8-70220 Dentoalveolar bone replacement graft, multiple sites, including flap entry and closure
P8-70230 Surgical exposure of impacted or unerupted tooth to aid eruption
P8-70260 Removal of embedded foreign body from dentoalveolar bone
P8-70270 Removal of embedded foreign body from dentoalveolar soft tissues
P8-70300 Guided dentoalveolar tissue regeneration, including surgery and re-entry
P8-70310 Pedicle soft dentoalveolar tissue graft procedure
P8-70320 Surgical exposure of impacted or unerupted tooth for orthodontic reason
P8-70360 Free soft dentoalveolar tissue graft procedure, including donor site
P8-70400 Operculectomy
  Excision of pericoronal tissues

P8-70410 Excision of fibrous tuberosities of dentoalveolar structures
P8-70420 Excision of osseous tuberosities of dentoalveolar structures
P8-70430 Excision of lesion of dentoalveolar structures without repair
P8-70440 Excision of lesion of dentoalveolar structures with simple repair
P8-70450 Excision of lesion of dentoalveolar structures with complex repair
P8-70460 Excision of hyperplastic alveolar mucosa, each quadrant
P8-70470 Excision of hyperplastic alveolar mucosa, each sextant
P8-70480 Alveolectomy, including curettage of osteitis
P8-70482 Subgingival curettage, NOS
P8-70484 Gingival curettage, surgical, per quadrant
P8-70490 Alveolectomy, including sequestrectomy
P8-70500 Periodontic adjunctive service, NOS
P8-70510 Training in personal periodontal care, plaque control
P8-70520 Provisional splinting, intracoronal
P8-70530 Provisional splinting, extracoronal
P8-70540 Periodontal scaling and root planing, entire mouth
P8-70550 Periodontal scaling and root planing, per quadrant
P8-70560 Tooth movement for periodontal purposes
P8-70570 Preventive periodontal procedure, periodontal prophylaxis
P8-70580 Unscheduled dressing change, by other than treating dentist
P8-70800 Case patterns section, NOS
P8-70810 Type I, gingivitis, shallow pocket therapy
P8-70820 Type II, early periodontitis, moderate pocket therapy
P8-70830 Type III, moderate periodontitis, moderate to deep pocket therapy
P8-70840 Type IV, advanced periodontitis, deep pocket therapy
P8-70880 Destruction of lesion of dentoalveolar structures

SECTION 8-8 PROSTHODONTIC PROCEDURES AND SERVICES

8-80 REMOVABLE PROSTHODONTIC PROCEDURES

P8-80000 Prosthodontic procedure, NOS
P8-80010 Prosthodontic dental consultation and report
P8-80020 Removable prosthodontic procedure, NOS
P8-80100 Complete denture, including adjustments, NOS
P8-80110 Complete upper denture
P8-80120 Complete lower denture
P8-80130 Immediate upper denture
P8-80140 Immediate lower denture
P8-80150 Interim complete upper denture
P8-80160 Interim complete lower denture
P8-80170 Interim partial upper denture
P8-80180 Interim partial lower denture
P8-80200 Partial denture, including adjustments, NOS
P8-80210 Upper partial denture, resin base, including any conventional clasps, rests and teeth
P8-80220 Lower partial denture, resin base, including any conventional clasps, rests and teeth
P8-80230 Upper partial denture, cast metal base without resin saddles, including any conventional clasps, rests and teeth
P8-80240 Lower partial denture, cast metal base with resin saddles, including any conventional clasps, rests and teeth
P8-80250 Removable unilateral partial denture, one piece cast metal, including clasps and pontics
P8-80300 Adjust complete denture, upper
P8-80310 Adjust complete denture, lower
P8-80320 Adjust partial denture, upper
P8-80330 Adjust partial denture, lower
P8-80380 Adjustments to denture by other than dentist providing appliances
P8-80500 Repair to denture, NOS
P8-80510 Repair of broken complete denture base
P8-80520 Replace missing or broken teeth, complete denture, each tooth
P8-80530 Repair of resin saddle or base, partial denture
P8-80540 Repair of cast framework, partial denture
P8-80550 Repair or replace broken clasp, partial denture
P8-80560 Replace broken teeth, per tooth, partial denture
P8-80570 Add tooth to existing partial denture
P8-80580 Add clasp to existing partial denture
P8-80600 Rebase of complete upper denture
P8-80610 Rebase of complete lower denture
P8-80620 Rebase of upper partial denture
P8-80630 Rebase of lower partial denture
P8-80700 Reline complete upper denture, chairside
P8-80710 Reline complete lower denture, chairside
P8-80720 Reline upper partial denture, chairside
P8-80730 Reline lower partial denture, chairside
P8-80740 Reline complete upper denture, laboratory
P8-80750 Reline complete lower denture, laboratory
P8-80760 Reline upper partial denture, laboratory
P8-80770 Reline lower partial denture, laboratory
P8-80840 Tissue conditioning, upper, per denture unit
P8-80850 Tissue conditioning, lower, per denture unit
P8-80860 Complete overdenture
P8-80870 Partial overdenture
P8-80880 Precision attachment denture

8-85 FIXED PROSTHODONTIC PROCEDURES

P8-85000 Fixed prosthodontic procedure, NOS
P8-85100 Bridge pontic, NOS
P8-85110 Pontic cast, high noble metal
P8-85120 Pontic cast, predominantly base metal

8-85 FIXED PROSTHODONTIC PROCEDURES — Continued

P8-85130 Pontic cast, noble metal
P8-85140 Pontic, porcelain fused to high noble metal
P8-85150 Pontic, porcelain fused to predominantly base metal
P8-85160 Pontic, porcelain fused to noble metal
P8-85170 Pontic, resin with high noble metal
P8-85180 Pontic, resin with predominantly base metal
P8-85190 Pontic, resin with noble metal
P8-85310 Retainers inlay, metallic, two surfaces
P8-85320 Retainers inlay, metallic, three or more surfaces
P8-85330 Retainers inlay, metallic, per tooth, in addition to inlay
P8-85340 Retainers, cast metal for acid etched fixed prosthesis
P8-85410 Crown, resin with high noble metal
P8-85420 Crown, resin with predominantly base metal
P8-85430 Crown, resin with noble metal
P8-85440 Crown, porcelain fused to high noble metal
P8-85450 Crown, porcelain fused to predominantly base metal
P8-85460 Crown, porcelain fused to noble metal
P8-85470 Crown, 3/4 cast high noble metal
P8-85500 Crown, full cast high noble metal
P8-85510 Crown, full cast predominantly base metal
P8-85520 Crown, full cast noble metal
P8-85600 Recement bridge
P8-85610 Stress breaker
P8-85620 Precision attachment
P8-85630 Cast post and core in addition to bridge retainer
P8-85640 Cast post as part of bridge retainer
P8-85650 Prefabricated post and core in addition to bridge retainer
P8-85660 Core build up for retainer, including any pins
P8-85670 Metal coping
P8-85680 Bridge repair by report

CHAPTER 9 — PSYCHOLOGIC AND PSYCHIATRIC PROCEDURES AND SERVICES

SECTION 9-0 PSYCHOLOGIC EVALUATION AND TEST PROCEDURES

P9-00000 Psychologic evaluation or test procedure, NOS
P9-00010 Psychological testing by physician with written report, per hour
P9-00100 Intelligence test, NOS
P9-00300 Intelligence test/WB1
P9-00400 Intelligence test/WB2
P9-00500 Intelligence test/WAIS
  Wechsler adult intelligence scale
P9-00600 Intelligence test/WISC
  Wechsler intelligence scale for children
P9-00700 Intelligence test/S-B
  Stanford-Binet test
P9-01000 Psychologic test, NOS
P9-01100 Psychologic test, organic battery
P9-01200 Psychologic test, Wechsler memory scale
P9-01300 Psychologic test, Bender visual-motor gestalt test
P9-01400 Psychologic test, Benton visual retention test
P9-02100 Purdue pegboard test
P9-02200 Figure drawing test
  Draw a man test
P9-02300 Rorschach test
P9-02400 Thematic apperception test
P9-02500 Vineland social maturity test
P9-02600 Merrill Palmer preschool performance
P9-02700 Catell infant intelligence scale
P9-02800 Grace Arthur point scale
P9-02900 Eisenson test for aphasia
P9-03100 Porteus mazes
P9-03200 Child apperception test
P9-03300 Minnesota multiphasic personality inventory
  MMPI test
P9-03400 Psychologic cognitive testing and assessment
P9-03410 Incomplete sentence test
P9-03500 Word association test
P9-04000 Automated psychologic testing, NOS
P9-06000 Clinical psychologic mental status determination
P9-07000 Character analysis, NOS
  Character type determination
P9-07020 Personality assessment
P9-07400 Graphology analysis
  Hand writing analysis
P9-09900 Unlisted psychologic test, explain by report

SECTION 9-1 PSYCHIATRIC PROCEDURES, SERVICES AND PSYCHOANALYSIS

9-10-15 GENERAL PSYCHIATRIC PROCEDURES, INTERVIEWS AND CONSULTATIONS

P9-10000 Psychiatry procedure or service, NOS
P9-10010 Psychiatric interview and evaluation, NOS
P9-10012 Psychiatric diagnostic interview, examination, history, mental status and disposition
P9-10020 Psychiatric evaluation of records, psychiatric reports or psychometric tests for medical diagnostic purposes
P9-10030 Environmental intervention on a psychiatric patient's behalf with agencies
P9-10040 Environmental intervention on a psychiatric patient's behalf with employers
P9-10050 Environmental intervention on a psychiatric patient's behalf with institutions
P9-10060 Interpretation of results of psychiatric examinations and data
P9-10080 Preparation of nonlegal report of patient's psychiatric status, history, treatment and progress
P9-10100 Interactive medical psychiatric diagnostic interview, NOS
P9-10110 Initial psychiatric interview with data recording by aide or social worker
P9-10130 Initial psychiatric interview with mental status and evaluation
P9-10200 Mental status determination, NOS
P9-10210 Clinical psychiatric mental status determination
  Assessment of mental status by psychiatrist
P9-10230 Medico-legal mental status determination
P9-10300 Psychiatric interview, continuation or follow-up
P9-10400 Regular psychiatric visit, routine, established patient
P9-10420 Reevaluation of established psychiatric patient
P9-10430 Psychiatric telephone consultation or therapy with patient
P9-10440 Comprehensive report of psychiatric patient for third party
P9-10500 Psychiatric interview of family of patient
P9-10510 Psychiatric interpretation to family or parents of patient
P9-12000 Psychiatric commitment procedure, NOS
P9-12200 Psychiatric pre-commitment interview and report
P9-12500 Psychiatric commitment to psychiatric institution
  Commitment to psychiatric institution

9-10-15 GENERAL PSYCHIATRIC PROCEDURES, INTERVIEWS AND CONSULTATIONS — Continued

P9-13000 Psychiatric evaluation of patient for testimentary capacity with report
  Assessment of fitness to testify
P9-13400 Psychiatric evaluation of patient for criminal responsibility with report
P9-13600 Evaluation of psychiatric state of patient
P9-13700 Legal testimony of psychiatric state of patient
P9-13900 Supervision of psychiatric therapist or aide
P9-14000 Daily full psychiatric care of inpatient
P9-14200 Psychiatric day care by day
P9-14400 Psychiatric follow-up
P9-14450 Psychiatric rehabilitation
P9-14990 Unlisted psychiatric service, NOS

9-16-18 PSYCHOANALYSIS

P9-16500 Psychoanalysis, NOS
P9-16600 Structural analysis
P9-16700 Transactional analysis
P9-16800 Game analysis
P9-16900 Script analysis
P9-17000 Psychoanalysis in depth
P9-17100 Psychoanalysis of transference
P9-17200 Psychoanalysis of ego
  Ego analysis
P9-18000 Hypnotherapy
  Hypnosis
  Hypnotism
  Mesmerism
P9-18100 Hypnodrama
P9-18110 Psychiatric catharsis method

SECTIONS 9-2-3 PSYCHIATRIC THERAPEUTIC PROCEDURES
9-20-23 GENERAL AND INDIVIDUAL PSYCHOTHERAPY PROCEDURES

P9-20000 Psychiatric therapeutic procedure, NOS
P9-20100 Psychotherapy, NOS
P9-20500 Gestalt therapy
P9-20600 Logotherapy
P9-21000 Individual psychotherapy, NOS
  Dyadic therapy
P9-21010 Individual medical psychotherapy with medical diagnostic evaluation and drug management when indicated with insight oriented, behavior modifying or supportive psychotherapy, time unspecified
P9-21175 Interactive individual medical psychotherapy
P9-21200 Conjoint psychotherapy, NOS
  Triadic therapy
P9-21400 Aversive psychotherapy
P9-22000 Behavioral therapy
  Behavior conditioning therapy
  Behavior modification
  Behavior modification psychotherapy
P9-22400 Operant conditioning
P9-22600 Transcendental meditation therapy
P9-22620 Desensitization therapy
  Psychologic desensitization
P9-22622 Psychologic desensitization, flooding
P9-22624 Psychologic desensitization, implosion
P9-22640 Extinction therapy
P9-22660 Relaxation training therapy
P9-22680 Token economy therapy
P9-23000 Confrontation therapy
  Confrontation technique
P9-23500 Existential therapy
P9-23600 Suppressive psychotherapy
P9-23700 Supportive verbal psychotherapy
P9-23800 Relationship psychotherapy
P9-23900 Expressive psychotherapy
  Exploratory verbal psychotherapy

9-24 CRISIS INTERVENTION

P9-24000 Crisis intervention, NOS
P9-24200 Crisis intervention with medication
P9-24400 Crisis intervention with follow-up
P9-24600 Crisis intervention by group therapy

9-25 ENVIRONMENTAL INTERVENTION

P9-25000 Environmental intervention, NOS
  Milieu therapy
P9-25200 Institutional environmental intervention
P9-25400 Employment environmental intervention
P9-25600 Interpersonal intervention

9-26-28 GROUP PSYCHOTHERAPY PROCEDURES

P9-26000 Group psychotherapy, NOS
P9-26020 Group medical psychotherapy with continuing medical diagnostic evaluation and drug management when indicated
P9-26100 Interactive group medical psychotherapy
P9-26300 Group analytical psychotherapy
P9-26500 Activity group therapy
P9-26600 Body contact-exploration therapy
  Body contact-exploration maneuver
P9-26700 Group marathon therapy
  Accelerated interaction
P9-26800 Client-centered psychotherapy
  Supportive therapy
P9-27000 Group primal therapy
P9-27100 Brief group psychotherapy
P9-27200 Group reassurance
P9-28000 Combined therapy, NOS
  Group co-therapy
  Cooperative therapy
  Dual leadership therapy
  Multiple therapy
  Three cornered therapy
P9-28400 Encounter group therapy
  Sensitivity training

9-29 FAMILY PSYCHOTHERAPY PROCEDURES

P9-29000 Family therapy, NOS
P9-29100 Family therapy without patient present
P9-29110 Family medical psychotherapy, conjoint with continuing medical diagnostic evaluation and drug management when indicated
P9-29120 Extended family therapy
  Multiple family group therapy
P9-29130 Multiple-family group medical psychotherapy with continuing medical diagnostic evaluation and drug management when indicated
P9-29300 Social network therapy

9-30 SEXUAL PSYCHOTHERAPY PROCEDURES

P9-30000 Sexual psychotherapy, NOS
P9-30100 Sexual psychotherapy, male therapist — female patient
P9-30200 Sexual psychotherapy, female therapist — male patient
P9-30300 Sexual psychotherapy, male therapist — male patient
P9-30400 Sexual psychotherapy, female therapist — female patient
P9-30450 Sexual psychotherapy, group, NOS
P9-30500 Sexual psychotherapy, group, all male
P9-30600 Sexual psychotherapy, group, all female
P9-30700 Sexual psychotherapy, group, male and female

9-33-34 SOCIAL PSYCHOTHERAPY PROCEDURES

P9-33500 Social psychotherapy, NOS
P9-33600 Occupational social therapy, NOS
P9-33710 Art therapy
P9-33720 Manual arts therapy
P9-33850 Music therapy
P9-34100 Psychodrama
P9-34110 Play psychotherapy
P9-34400 Recreational therapy, NOS
P9-34410 Diversional therapy, NOS
P9-34420 Play therapy
P9-34430 Competitive games psychotherapy
P9-34500 Educational therapy, NOS

9-35-36 PSYCHIATRIC DRUG THERAPY PROCEDURES

P9-35000 Psychiatric somatotherapy, NOS
P9-35100 Psychiatric drug therapy, NOS
  Neuroleptic therapy, NOS
  Psychiatric pharmacologic management
P9-35200 Initial drug therapy for mental disorder
P9-35300 Maintenance drug therapy for mental disorder
P9-35500 Narcotherapy
  Narcoanalysis
  Narcosynthesis
P9-35510 Amobarbital interview
P9-36000 Electroconvulsive therapy, NOS
  ECT therapy
  Electroshock therapy, NOS
  EST therapy
P9-36100 Subconvulsive electroshock therapy
P9-36110 Electroconvulsive therapy, multiple seizures per day
P9-36150 Chemical shock therapy, NOS
P9-36180 Electronarcosis
P9-36200 Insulin shock therapy
  Insulin coma therapy
P9-36400 Lithium therapy
P9-36500 Carbon dioxide therapy
P9-36600 Flurothyl therapy

9-37 DRUG DETOXIFICATION THERAPY PROCEDURES

P9-37000 Detoxification therapy, NOS
  Detoxication therapy, NOS
P9-37010 Detoxication therapy for alcoholism
  Alcohol detoxification
P9-37020 Alcohol rehabilitation
P9-37030 Alcohol rehabilitation and detoxification
P9-37100 Drug detoxification
P9-37110 Drug rehabilitation
P9-37120 Drug rehabilitation and detoxification
P9-37200 Combined alcohol and drug detoxification
P9-37210 Combined alcohol and drug rehabilitation
P9-37220 Combined alcohol and drug rehabilitation and detoxification

SECTION 9-4 BIOFEEDBACK PROCEDURES

P9-40000 Biofeedback procedure, NOS
P9-40500 Biofeedback, autogenic training
P9-40600 Biofeedback, autogenic treatment
P9-41000 Biofeedback, strain gage
P9-41200 Biofeedback, thermal
P9-41400 Biofeedback, respiratory air volume
P9-41600 Biofeedback, electrocardiogram
  Biofeedback, ECG
P9-41610 Biofeedback training in conduction disorder, arrythmia
P9-41800 Biofeedback, pulse wave velocity
P9-41850 Biofeedback, regulation of blood pressure
P9-41860 Biofeedback training in regulation of blood pressure for essential hypertension
P9-41900 Biofeedback, electro-oculogram
P9-41910 Biofeedback training by electro-oculogram application in blepharospasm
P9-42000 Biofeedback, gastric secretion pH
P9-42200 Biofeedback, three channel rectal balloon
P9-42400 Biofeedback, intestinal borborygmi
P9-42600 Biofeedback, galvanic skin response
P9-42610 Biofeedback training in regulation of skin temperature or peripheral blood flow
P9-43000 Electromyographic biofeedback, NOS

SECTION 9-4 BIOFEEDBACK PROCEDURES — Continued

P9-43010 Electromyographic biofeedback, single unit implanted electrodes

P9-43012 Electromyographic biofeedback, surface electrodes

P9-43020 Biofeedback training by electromyogram application in tension headache

P9-44000 Electroencephalographic biofeedback, NOS
  EEG biofeedback, NOS

P9-44020 Biofeedback training by electroencephalogram application in anxiety

P9-44100 Electroencephalographic biofeedback, alpha wave
  EEG biofeedback, alpha wave

P9-44200 Electroencephalographic biofeedback, theta wave
  EEG biofeedback, theta wave

P9-44300 Electroencephalographic biofeedback, central cortical wave 13-15 hz
  EEG biofeedback, central cortical wave, 13-15 hz

P9-44400 Electroencephalographic biofeedback, central synchrony
  EEG biofeedback, central synchrony

P9-44999 Unlisted biofeedback training

CHAPTER A — NURSING PROCEDURES

SECTION A-0 GENERAL CARE NURSING PROCEDURES

PA-00000N Nursing procedure, NOS
PA-00100N Nursing ward administrative procedure, NOS
PA-00110N Nursing consultation and report, NOS
PA-00120N Nursing evaluation of patient and report, NOS
PA-00130N Nursing care quality assurance procedure, NOS
  Nursing care QA, NOS
PA-00140N Nursing care planning session
PA-00145N Participation in ward rounds
PA-00150N Nursing care management session
PA-00160N Charting patient information
PA-00170N Nursing report session
PA-00180N Nursing conference
PA-00190N Assisting physician with procedure, NOS
PA-00200N Nursing history taking, NOS
PA-00210N Nursing physical examination, NOS
PA-00300N General nursing care, NOS
PA-00310N General day care of adult
PA-00320N General afternoon and evening care of adult
PA-00330N General night care of adult
PA-00340N General day care of child
PA-00350N General afternoon and evening care of child
PA-00360N General night care of child
PA-00380N Weighing patient
PA-00390N Measuring height of patient
PA-00400N Moving a patient, NOS
PA-00402N Moving a patient in bed
  Turning patient in bed
PA-00403N Moving a patient to a stretcher
PA-00404N Sitting a patient up in a chair
PA-00410N Placing a patient on a bedpan
PA-00412N Give bedpan, remove and clean
PA-00414N Give urinal, remove and clean
PA-00420N Ambulating patient
PA-00440N Bathing patient, NOS
  Giving patient a bath, NOS
PA-00442N Bathing patient in bed
PA-00443N Bathing patient with alcohol sponge
PA-00444N Bathing patient in sitz bath
PA-00445N Bathing patient with tepid sponge
PA-00446N Bathing patient in starch bath
PA-00447N Bathing patient in tub
PA-00448N Bathing patient in incubator
PA-00449N Bathing patient in isolette
PA-0044AN Bathing patient in shower
PA-00460N Making patient bed, NOS
PA-00461N Making open bed
PA-00462N Making occupied bed
PA-00463N Making unoccupied bed
PA-00464N Making Foster bed
PA-00465N Making anesthesia bed
PA-00466N Making circolectric bed
PA-00467N Making orthopedic bed
PA-00500N Taking patient vital signs, NOS
  Vital signs, NOS
  Observing patient vital signs, NOS
PA-00510N Pulse taking, NOS
PA-00511N Radial pulse taking
PA-00512N Apical pulse taking
PA-00513N Pedal pulse taking
PA-00530N Temperature taking, NOS
PA-00532N Oral temperature taking
PA-00534N Rectal temperature taking
PA-00540N Blood pressure taking, NOS
PA-00542N Taking arterial blood pressure
PA-00544N Taking central venous pressure
PA-00550N Respirations counting and evaluation
PA-00570N Taking neurologic vital signs, NOS
PA-00572N Pupillary reaction to light
PA-00600N Feeding patient, NOS
PA-00602N Routine feeding of patient
PA-00605N Food intake encouragement
PA-00606N Fluid intake encouragement
PA-00607N Mealtime assistance
PA-00609N Fluid restriction
PA-00610N Intravenous feeding of patient
PA-00620N Tube feeding of patient
  Tube feeding
  Gavage
PA-00622N Tube feeding by Barron pump
PA-00624N Tube feeding by syringe method
PA-00628N Tube feeding by drip method
PA-00630N Forced feeding of patient
PA-00640N Hyperalimentation procedure
PA-00700N Measuring intake
PA-00710N Measuring intake and output
  Ingesta et excreta
  I and O measurement
PA-00720N Measuring output
PA-00800N Giving patient an enema, NOS
  Enema, NOS
PA-00802N Disposable enema
PA-00804N Funnel enema
PA-00806N Irrigating can enema
PA-00900N Care of hair, NOS
PA-00902N Combing of hair
PA-00910N Routine shampoo of hair
PA-00912N Shampoo of hair on stretcher
PA-00914N Shampoo of hair in bed
PA-00920N Pediculosis treatment of hair
PA-00950N Clipping nails of patient
PA-00A00N Care of patient's personal effects, NOS
PA-00A10N Care of patient clothing (record)
PA-00A20N Care of patient valuables

A-10 NURSING PRECAUTIONARY AND SECURITY PROCEDURES — Continued

SECTION A-1 NURSING PRECAUTIONARY AND SPECIAL PROCEDURES

A-10 NURSING PRECAUTIONARY AND SECURITY PROCEDURES

PA-10000N Precautionary nursing procedure, NOS
PA-10004N Verification routine
PA-10010N Isolation procedure
  Isolation technique
PA-10012N Quarantine
  Isolation after contact with infectious disease
PA-10020N General gown technique
PA-10022N Nursery gown technique
PA-10024N Reverse isolation technique
PA-10030N Bleeding precautions
PA-10032N Subarachnoid hemorrhage precautions
PA-10034N Application of tourniquet
PA-10040N Seizure precautions
PA-10050N Suicide precautions
PA-10060N Blood and fluids precautions
PA-10100N Nursing patient security measure, NOS
PA-10110N Placing cribguard
PA-10112N Placing bedrails
PA-10120N Holding patient
PA-10130N Placing restraint
PA-10132N Restraint maintenance
PA-10134N Restraint removal
PA-10140N Search for dangerous objects
PA-10150N Secluding patient
PA-10152N Protection of individual from surroundings
PA-10154N Protection of surroundings from individual
PA-10160N Reorienting patient
PA-10170N Baby-sitting patient
  Keeping patient company

A-11 SPECIAL NURSING PROCEDURES

A-110-113 Special Ward Care Nursing Procedures

PA-11000N Specific or special nursing care, NOS
PA-11010N Special back care
PA-11020N Dressing change under anesthesia, other than burn
PA-11030N Special care of neurological patient, with neurological vital signs
PA-11040N Special care of gastrointestinal tube patient
PA-11050N Special care of patient with seizures
PA-11060N Special care of patient with contagious disease
PA-11070N Special care of immunosuppressed patient
PA-11080N Special care of patient in operating room
PA-11200N Special care of mouth
  Oral hygiene procedure
PA-11202N Special care of dentures
PA-11210N Special care of wound
PA-11220N Special care of eye
PA-11230N Special nursing care of burned patient
PA-11240N Special nursing care of unconscious patient
PA-11250N Special nursing care in intensive care unit
PA-11260N Passive exercises of patient
PA-11290N Special postmortem body preparation
PA-11300N Application of electric heating pad
PA-11304N Application of hot water bottle
PA-11310N Application of ice, NOS
PA-11312N Application of ice collar, cap or bag
PA-11320N Application of support hose
PA-11330N Application of Fazio bag
PA-11340N Application of eye pad
PA-11350N Application of surgically clean compresses
PA-11354N Application of pressure binder
PA-11360N Soak, NOS
PA-11362N Warm soak of an extremity

A-114 Nursing Procedures Related to Obstetrics and Gynecology

PA-11400N Delivery by midwife
PA-11410N Delivery by nurse
PA-11420N Amniotomy by nurse
  Puncture of membranes by nurse
PA-11430N Special care of patient in delivery room
PA-11434N Special postpartum nursing care
PA-11440N Perineal care in obstetrics
PA-11442N Nursing care of episiotomy wound
PA-11444N Nursing care of obstetrical laceration
PA-11450N Vaginal irrigation
  Vaginal douche
PA-11460N Removal of intrauterine device
PA-11470N Care of nursing breast
PA-11472N Application of manual or electric breast pump
  Breast pumping
PA-11474N Application of breast binder
PA-11480N Application of heat lamp to perineum

A-117 Nursing Care of Newborn

PA-11700N General care of newborn
  Routine care of newborn
PA-11704N Bottle feeding of patient
PA-11708N Suction of newborn
PA-11710N Special care of baby in nursery, NOS
PA-11714N Special care of premature baby
  Premature baby care
PA-11720N Nursing care of circumcision
PA-11730N Foot printing of newborn infant

A-118 Preoperative Nursing Procedures

PA-11800N Preoperative preparation of skin, NOS
PA-11802N Preoperative shaving of skin
PA-11804N Preoperative disinfection of skin

A-12 NURSING PROCEDURES RELATED TO TUBES AND DRAINS

PA-12010N Respiratory care and adjustment, NOS
PA-12012N Deep breathing, clapping and postural drainage
PA-12020N Operation of Ambu resuscitator
PA-12024N Operation of Puritan heated aerosol nebulizer
PA-12100N Suction of patient, NOS
PA-12110N Closed chest suction
PA-12120N Maintenance of thoracic drain
PA-12122N Clamping of thoracic drain
PA-12124N Measuring output from thoracic drain
PA-12126N Maintenance of newborn thoracic drain
PA-12128N Measuring output from newborn thoracic drain
PA-12130N Suction and cleaning of tracheostomy tube
PA-12132N Changing tracheostomy tube
PA-12136N Application of tracheostomy mask using jet humidifier
PA-12140N Suction and cleaning of endotracheal tube
PA-12200N Insertion of nasogastric tube
PA-12202N Nasogastric tube maintenance
PA-12203N Nasogastric tube irrigation
PA-12204N Nasogastric tube aspiration
PA-12206N Nasogastric tube removal
PA-12212N Nasoenteric tube maintenance
PA-12214N Nasoenteric tube aspiration
PA-12216N Nasoenteric tube irrigation
PA-12218N Nasoenteric tube removal
PA-12220N T-tube maintenance
PA-12222N T-tube clamping
PA-12230N Penrose maintenance
PA-12234N Jackson Pratt maintenance
PA-12240N Hemovac pump use, care and adjustment
PA-12250N Peritoneal dialysis catheter maintenance
PA-12252N Empty and measure peritoneal dialysis fluid
PA-12254N Removal of peritoneal dialysis catheter
PA-12260N Care of venous dissection
PA-12270N Subcutaneous clysis of patient for fluid administration

A-13 NURSING PROCEDURES RELATED TO THE MUSCULOSKELETAL SYSTEM

PA-13100N Application of back brace
PA-13102N Removal of back brace
PA-13110N Application of clavicular bandage
PA-13112N Removal of clavicular bandage
PA-13120N Application of elastic bandage
PA-13122N Maintenance of elastic bandage
PA-13124N Removal of elastic bandage
PA-13130N Application of cervical collar
PA-13132N Maintenance of cervical collar
PA-13134N Removal of cervical collar
PA-13140N Application of knee immobilizer
PA-13142N Maintenance of knee immobilizer
PA-13144N Removal of knee immobilizer
PA-13150N Elevation of arm
PA-13160N Elevation of leg
PA-13170N Aspiration of joint
PA-13180N Pin/tong site care
PA-13190N Bivalving of cast
PA-13192N Removal of cast
PA-13200N Application of sling
PA-13202N Sling maintenance
PA-13204N Sling removal
PA-13210N Application of splint
PA-13212N Splint maintenance
PA-13214N Splint removal
PA-13220N Removal of staples
PA-13230N Application of traction
PA-13232N Traction maintenance
PA-13234N Traction removal

SECTION A-2 SPECIMEN COLLECTION AND WARD LABORATORY PROCEDURES

PA-20000N Collection of specimen by nursing, NOS
PA-20010N Collection of urine and strain for calculus
PA-20020N Collection of pinworm specimen
PA-20030N Collection of sweat test
PA-20034N Collection of sweat test, pediatric overnight
PA-20040N Collection of string test
PA-20050N Collection of sputum, NOS
PA-20052N Collection of sputum, Lukens tube
PA-20100N Collection of routine urine specimen for laboratory
PA-20102N Collection of 24-hour urine specimen for laboratory
PA-20110N Collection of blood specimen for laboratory
PA-20130N Collection of specimen for culture by laboratory
PA-20200N Ward laboratory procedure, screening, NOS
PA-20210N Ward urine dip stick testing, NOS
PA-20212N Ward urine dip stick testing for sugar
PA-20214N Ward urine dip stick testing for acetone
PA-20220N Ward glucometer test
PA-20230N Ward guaiac test
PA-20240N Ward specific gravity test

SECTION A-3 ADMINISTRATION OF MEDICATION

PA-30000N Administration of medication, NOS
PA-30010N Routine administration of medication
PA-30020N Special administration of medication
PA-30030N Emergency administration of medication
PA-30040N Administration of therapeutic medication
PA-30050N Administration of prophylactic medication
PA-30080N Administration of dermatologic formulation, NOS
PA-33090N Administration of skin test by nurse, NOS

SECTION A-5 MONITORING PROCEDURES BY NURSING STAFF

PA-50000N Monitoring procedure by nursing staff, NOS

SECTION A-5 MONITORING PROCEDURES BY NURSING STAFF — Continued

PA-50010N Routine patient monitoring by nurse
PA-50020N Monitoring of cardiac output/cardiac index
PA-50022N Cardiac monitor surveillance
PA-50024N Cardiac monitor removal
PA-50030N Hemodynamic measurements
PA-50040N Internal fetal monitoring during labor
PA-50042N Internal fetal monitor maintenance
PA-50044N Internal fetal monitor removal
PA-50050N Intraaortic balloon pump maintenance
PA-50052N Intraaortic balloon pump weaning
PA-50054N Intraaortic balloon pump removal
PA-50060N Intracranial/cerebral perfusion pressure monitoring
PA-50062N Intracranial pressure monitor maintenance
PA-50064N Intracranial pressure monitor removal
PA-50070N Apnea monitor surveillance
PA-50072N Apnea monitor removal
PA-50080N External fetal monitor surveillance
PA-50082N External fetal monitor surveillance during multiple pregnancy
PA-50084N External fetal monitor removal
PA-50090N Pulmonary artery pressure monitoring
PA-50094N Pulmonary artery wedge pressure monitoring
PA-50100N Rhythm strip monitoring
PA-50110N IV/irrigation monitoring
PA-50120N Uterine contraction monitor maintenance
PA-50124N Uterine contraction monitor removal

SECTION A-6 NURSING EDUCATIONAL SERVICES

A-60 PATIENT EDUCATION BY NURSING PERSONNEL

PA-60000N Patient education, NOS
Teaching session by nurse with patient, NOS
PA-60002N Treatment or procedure explanation with education, NOS
PA-60004N Disease process or condition education
PA-60010N Allergy education
PA-60020N Amputation education
PA-60030N Body alignment education
PA-60040N CPR education
PA-60050N Alternative communication technique education
PA-60060N Tonsils and adenoids postoperative education
T and A education
PA-60100N Cardiac catheterization education
PA-60110N Diet education
PA-60120N Child security measures education
PA-60130N Basic nutrition education
PA-60140N Diabetic patient education
PA-60150N Decubitus ulcer prevention education
PA-60160N Intestinal function reeducation education
PA-60170N Respiratory technique education
PA-60180N Blood pressure education
PA-60190N Growth and development education
PA-60200N Halo traction education
PA-60210N Home apnea monitor education
PA-60220N Home oxygen therapy education
PA-60230N Home safety education
PA-60240N Hygiene education
PA-60250N Hypertension education
PA-60260N Infant care education
PA-60270N Contraceptive use education
PA-60272N Condom use education
PA-60276N Diaphragm use education
PA-60280N Infection prevention education
PA-60300N Medication education
PA-60310N Myocardial infarction education
PA-60320N Myringotomy with tubes discharge education
PA-60330N Pain control techniques education
PA-60360N Preoperative education
PA-60370N Wound treatment education
PA-60380N Specimen collection education
PA-60400N Walker reinforcement education
PA-60410N Obstetrical perineal care education
PA-60500N Individual natural childbirth education
PA-60510N Natural childbirth class education
PA-60520N Labor and delivery educational tour
PA-60540N Postpartum education
PA-60550N Prenatal care education
PA-60570N Breast self-examination technique education
PA-60580N Breast feeding education
Teaching mother breast feeding technique

A-62 PSYCHOSOCIAL NURSING PROCEDURES

PA-62000N Psychosocial nursing procedure, NOS
PA-62010N Nurse and patient conference
PA-62020N Role clarification by nurse
PA-62100N Bonding encouragement by nurse
PA-62110N Comfort measures by nurse
PA-62120N Communication of alternative technique by nurse
PA-62130N Decision making encouragement by nurse
PA-62140N Emotional support by nurse
PA-62150N Grieving support by nurse
PA-62160N Social interaction encouragement by nurse

A-63 HOME CARE AND SOCIAL SERVICES

PA-63000N Home care of patient, NOS
PA-63010N Home care by visiting nurse
PA-63100N Social service at home, NOS
PA-63110N Social service interview of patient
PA-63120N Social service interview of family
PA-63130N Social service interview of other agency
PA-63140N Social service interview of planning
PA-63150N Social service referral of home patient

SECTION A-9 SPECIFIC VETERINARY NURSING AND GROOMING PROCEDURES

PA-90100V Dressing and fixation procedure, NOS

PA-90101V Removal of dressing of skin of feet
PA-90102V Removal of dressing from claw
PA-90104V Apply dressing with fixation of hoof
PA-90105V Removal of dressing of hoof
PA-90106V Removal of dressing of foredigit
PA-90108V Removal of dressing of coccygeal vertebra
PA-90109V Removal of dressing of tail
PA-90110V Removal of dressing of hindfoot
PA-90112V Apply dressing with fixation of claw
PA-90120V Removal of dressing of forelimb
PA-90122V Removal of dressing of hindlimb
PA-90124V Removal of dressing of skin of forelimb
PA-90126V Apply dressing with fixation of skin of forelimb
PA-90130V Removal of dressing of stifle ligament
PA-90132V Apply dressing with fixation of hindlimb
PA-90134V Apply dressing with fixation of foredigit
PA-90136V Apply dressing with fixation of forelimb
PA-90140V Clip and clean wound site
PA-90150V Bandaging of animal, NOS
PA-90152V Bandaging of large animal
PA-90154V Bandaging of small animal
PA-90158V Robert Jones bandaging
PA-90200V Grooming of animal, NOS
PA-90210V Trimming of nail
Nail trim
PA-90220V Trimming of hoof
Hoof trim
PA-90230V Cutting of animal hair
PA-90232V Shearing
PA-90240V Clipping of feathers
Cutting of feathers
PA-90242V Removal of feathers
PA-90250V Clipping of beak
PA-90300V Washing of animal, NOS
PA-90302V Animal ear washing
PA-90310V Delousing of animal, NOS
Parasite dip, NOS
PA-90320V Flushing of gluteal pouch
PA-90324V Bull sheath washing
PA-90326V Cleaning of animal penis
PA-90340V Induction of vomiting in animal
PA-90500V Boarding of animal, NOS
PA-90510V Boarding and feeding of animal
PA-90520V Withholding feed from animal
PA-90522V Withholding feed and water from animal

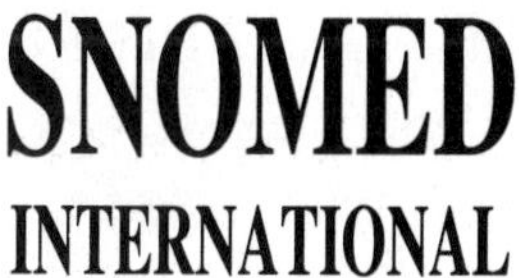

Source documents and references

AHFS Drug Information. Bethesda, MD: American Society of Hospital Pharmacists; 1990

Baillière's Comprehensive Veterinary Dictionary. London, England: Baillière, Tindall; 1988

Bates B, *A Guide to Physical Examination and History Taking,* 5th ed. Philadelphia, PA: JB Lippincott; 1991

Beaver PC and Jung RC, *Animal Agents and Vectors of Human Disease,* 5th ed. Philadelphia, PA: Lea and Febiger; 1985

Braunwald E, Isselbacher KJ, Petersdorg RG, Wilson JD, Martin JB, and Fauci AS, *Harrison's Principles of Internal Medicine,* 11th ed. New York, NY: McGraw-Hill; 1987

Churchill's Illustrated Medical Dictionary, New York, NY: Churchill Livingstone; 1989

Cotran RS, Kumar V, and Robbins SL. *Robbins Pathologic Basis of Disease,* 4th ed. Philadelphia, PA: WB Saunders; 1989

Diagnostic and Statistical Manual of Mental Disorders, 3rd ed, revised. Washington, DC: American Psychiatric Association; 1987

Dorland's Illustrated Medical Dictionary, 27th ed. Philadelphia, PA: WB Saunders Co: 1988

Dyce KM, Sack WO, and Wensing CJ. *Textbook of Veterinary Anatomy.* Philadelphia, PA: WB Saunders; 1987

Garcia LS and Bruckner DA, *Diagnostic Medical Parasitology.* New York, NY: Elsevier; 1988

Goldsmith R and Heyneman D. *Tropical Medicine and Parasitology.* San Mateo, CA: Appleton and Lange; 1989

Gordon M. *Nursing Diagnosis – Process and Application,* 2nd ed. New York, NY: McGraw-Hill; 1987

Guyton AC. *Textbook of Medical Physiology,* 8th ed. Philadelphia, PA: WB Saunders; 1991

Index for Radiological Diagnoses, 3rd ed, revised. Reston, VA: American College of Radiology; 1985

International Classification of Diseases for Oncology (ICD–O), 2nd ed. Geneva, Switzerland: WHO; 1990

International Classification of Diseases, 9th ed, revised–1975. Geneva, Switzerland: WHO; 1979

International Classification of Diseases, Clinical Modification, 9th ed, revised. Publication DHHS (PHS) 89-1260. Washington, DC; US Government Printing Offfice; 1979

International Nomenclature of Diseases, Vol II, Parts 1 to 4, Infectious Diseases. Geneva, Switzerland: CIOMS and WHO; 1982-87

International Nomenclature of Diseases, Vol III, Diseases of the Lower Respiratory Tract. Geneva, Switzerland: CIOMS and WHO; 1979

International Nomenclature of Diseases, Vol V, Cardiac and Vascular Diseases. Geneva, Switzerland: CIOMS and WHO; 1989

International Nomenclature of Diseases, Vol VI, Metabolic, Nutritional, and Endocrine Disorders. Geneva, Switzerland: CIOMS and WHO; 1991

International Standard Classification of Occupations, Rev ed. Geneva, Switzerland: International Labour Office; 1968

International Union of Biochemists, *Enzyme Nomenclature*, Orlando, FL: Academic Press; 1984

Isenberg HD, ed. *Clinical Microbiology Procedures Handbook.* Washington, DC: American Society for Microbiology; 1992

Jacobs DS, Kasten BL Jr., DeMott WR, and Wolfson WL. *Laboratory Test Handbook*, 2nd ed. Baltimore, MD: Williams and Wilkins; 1990

Jones KL. *Smith's Recognizable Patterns of Human Malformation*, 4th ed. Philadelphia, PA: WB Saunders; 1989

Kansky B. *Review of Medical Embryology.* New York, NY: Macmillan: 1982

Lewis WH and Elvin-Lewis MP. *Medical Botany.* New York, NY: John Wiley and Sons; 1977

Magalini SI and Scrascia E, *Dictionary of Medical Syndromes*, 2nd ed. Philadelphia, PA: JB Lippincott:; 1981

McLay ALC and Toner P. *Subcellular Taxonomy – An Ultrastructural Classification System with Diagnostic Applications.* Washington, DC: Hemisphere Publishing; 1985

Netter FH, *Atlas of Human Anatomy.* West Caldwell, NJ: Ciba-Geigy; 1989

Noble ER, Noble GA, Schad GA, and Macinnes AJ. *Parasitology – Biology of Animal Parasites*, 6th ed. Philadelphia: Lea and Febiger; 1989

Nomina Anatomica, 6th ed. London, England: Churchill Livingstone; 1989

Nomina Embryologica, 3rd ed. London, England: Churchill Livingstone; 1989

Nomina Histologica, 3rd ed. London, England: Churchill Livingstone; 1989

Physicians' Current Procedural Terminology (CPT). Chicago: American Medical Associaiton; 1992

Rippon JW. *Medical Mycology*, 3rd ed. Phildelphia, PA: WB Saunders; 1988

Rose NR, DeMacario EW, Fahey JL, Friedman H, Penn GM. *Manual of Clinical Laboratory Immunology.* Washington, DC: American Soceity for Microbiology; 1992

Schwartz MH. *Textbook of Physical Diagnosis.* Philadelphia, PA: WB Saunders; 1989

Stedman's Medical Dictionary, 25th ed. Baltimore, MD: Williams & Wilkins; 1990

The Merck Index – An Encyclopedia of Chemicals, Drugs, and Biologicals, 11th ed. Rahway, NJ: Merck & Co; 1989

Universal Medical Device Nomenclature System. Plymouth Meeting, PA: ECRI; 1990

Warwick R and Williams PL, *Gray's Anatomy*, 35th ed. London, England: Longman Group; 1973

Williams WJ, Beutler E, Erslev AJ, and Lichtman MA, *Hematology.* New York, NY: McGraw-Hill; 1992